The Language
of Medicine

DAVI-ELLEN CHABNER, BA, MAT

The Language
of Medicine

11TH EDITION

ELSEVIER

ELSEVIER

3251 Riverport Lane
St. Louis, Missouri 63043

Notices

Knowledge and best practice in this field are constantly changing. As new research and experience broaden our understanding, changes in research methods, professional practices, or medical treatment may become necessary.

Practitioners and researchers must always rely on their own experience and knowledge in evaluating and using any information, methods, compounds, or experiments described herein. In using such information or methods they should be mindful of their own safety and the safety of others, including parties for whom they have a professional responsibility.

With respect to any drug or pharmaceutical products identified, readers are advised to check the most current information provided (i) on procedures featured or (ii) by the manufacturer of each product to be administered, to verify the recommended dose or formula, the method and duration of administration, and contraindications. It is the responsibility of practitioners, relying on their own experience and knowledge of their patients, to make diagnoses, to determine dosages and the best treatment for each individual patient, and to take all appropriate safety precautions.

To the fullest extent of the law, neither the Publisher nor the authors, contributors, or editors, assume any liability for any injury and/or damage to persons or property as a matter of products liability, negligence or otherwise, or from any use or operation of any methods, products, instructions, or ideas contained in the material herein.

Library of Congress Cataloging-in-Publication Data

Names: Chabner, Davi-Ellen, author.
Title: The language of medicine / Davi-Ellen Chabner.
Description: 11th edition. | St. Louis, Missouri : Elsevier, [2017] | Includes bibliographical references and index.
Identifiers: LCCN 2015050598 | ISBN 9780323370813 (pbk.)
Subjects: | MESH: Terminology as Topic | Problems and Exercises
Classification: LCC R123 | NLM W 15 | DDC 610.1/4–dc23 LC record available at http://lccn.loc.gov/2015050598

International Standard Book Number: 978-0-323-37081-3

Senior Content Strategist: Linda Woodard
Content Development Manager: Luke Held
Senior Content Development Specialist: Diane Chatman
Publishing Services Manager: Julie Eddy
Book Production Specialist: Celeste Clingan
Design Direction: Brian Salisbury

Printed in the United States of America

Last digit is the print number:
9 8 7 6 5 4 3 2 1

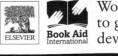

Working together
to grow libraries in
developing countries

www.elsevier.com • www.bookaid.org

For Catherine ("Kay") F. Scott

With enduring gratitude for your

vision, inspiration, and encouragement

from the very beginning.

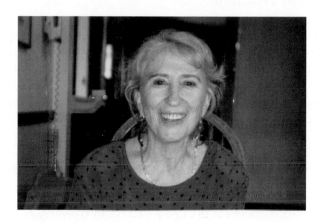

AND

To Gus, Ben, Bebe, Solomon, Amari, and Louisa

You make it all worthwhile.

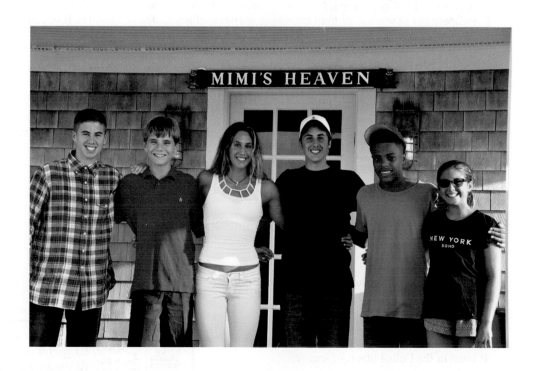

Preface

WELCOME TO THE 11TH EDITION OF THE LANGUAGE OF MEDICINE

The continuing focus of this new edition is its cutting-edge relevance to real-life medical practice. Drawing on the newest technology, state-of-the-art medical procedures, and treatments, *The Language of Medicine* brings medical terminology to life. The newly-drawn dynamic images and up-to-date photography plus compelling patient stories further illustrate medical terminology in action.

I am honored that this text continues to be the book instructors return to, year after year, because their students tell them that it works! As a student, you will find that *The Language of Medicine* speaks to you no matter what your background or level of education. It is written in simple, non-technical language that creates an exceptionally accessible pathway to learning. Since it is a workbook-text combination, you engage and interact on practically every page through writing and reviewing terms, labeling diagrams, and answering questions. Terminology is explained so that you understand medical terms in their proper context, which is the structure and function of the human body in health and disease.

Throughout the process of writing this text over its 11 editions, I have listened to hundreds of students and instructors and incorporated their insightful suggestions.

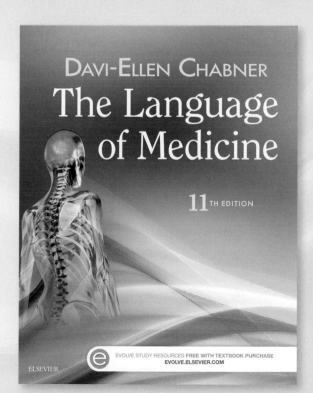

Expert medical reviewers have once again helped me to ensure that the terminology included reflects cutting edge clinical practice. New information and illustrations throughout are the result of recommendations from all those who have so generously provided feedback. My continuing goal in writing *The Language of Medicine* is to help you not only learn medical terminology but also to enjoy learning! You will find that medical terminology comes alive and stays with you when you use my interactive, logical, and easy-to-follow method. Undeniably, the study of this language requires commitment and hard work, but the benefits are great. Knowledge of medical terminology will give you a strong start in your career.

NEW TO THE 11TH EDITION

While the essential elements of *The Language of Medicine* remain in place, the new 11th edition is even more relevant to real-life medical situations.

The 11th edition includes helpful hints to point out important facts and make things clear. There are also new, first-hand stories of medical conditions and procedures. These personal accounts make medical terminology more understandable.

IN PERSON: HODGKIN LYMPHOMA

When I began noticing persistent back pain and fatigue in 2006, my doctor and I didn't take the symptoms seriously until 2007, when I noticed I was losing weight and short of breath. I saw a lung specialist, who took a chest x-ray and discovered a mass the size of a grapefruit in my mediastinum. Immediately, my stress level went sky high, and being 25 in New York City on my own (my family was in California and my mother was going through metastatic breast cancer treatment), I felt afraid and alone.

I was scheduled for a PET-CT scan and visited a friend who was a radiation oncologist. She was alarmed by my symptoms and appearance and through her father, a medical oncologist, immediat[e] contact with a cancer specialist. The results from the bronchoscopy with a biopsy, and a bone marrow biopsy c[...] I had Stage 2B Hodgkin lymphoma with "bulky disease" mass] in my mediastinum. This diagnosis was really scar[...] watching my mother go through her difficult battle with [...] made me realize that if I emulated her positive attitude, i[...] life easier for my entire family.

The treatment was six cycles of chemotherapy. After tw[...] I shaved my head. A Powerport was installed in my upp[...] more quickly and with less pain. Because I was so young, [...] menopause, to preserve my fertility.

Three months into my treatment a PET-CT showed [...] that I would need radiation to my chest after the che[...] chemotherapy, I was having a difficult time coping with [...] Nevertheless, I rallied and traveled to Boston for 4 week[...] felt lucky to be receiving this cutting-edge treatment, del[...] the country.

My radiation treatment ended in 2008, and a follow-[...] treatment. I remember when the doctor told me that the [...] outside and cried on a bench for an hour. More recently, I'[...] I'm relieved when the scan is clear, but I am also afraid [...] developing a secondary cancer as a result of the extensive [...] in 2013, I've been getting regular mammograms, and be[...] I'm taking thyroid hormone to treat hypothyroidism.

I know that my Hodgkin lymphoma experience will alwa[...] attitude, which has enabled and empowered me to start [...] about the future.

Lenore Estrada is the CEO and Co-Founder of Three [...] to bring awareness to the economic, social [...] communities. She is also the President of the Boa[...]

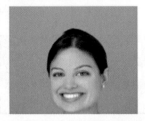

IN PERSON: PROPHYLACTIC MASTECTOMY

This first-person narrative describes a woman who elected to undergo prophylactic mastectomy.

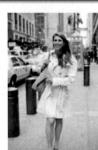

Whenever May rolls around I think about my surgery and the decision I made many years ago to have prophylactic mastectomies. I grew up in a family of strong women. They were determined to work, play sports, and raise their families, except they all had breast cancer. It was a bump in the road for each one of them and, at age 36, I had 4 children, a wonderful career and a husband and abnormal mammograms. I had friends, holidays, and biopsies, and being a physician (radiation oncologist) and the daughter of a medical oncologist, I was worried about my own health.

When my mother tested negative for the BRCA gene, it did not relieve my anxiety. It just intensified it. What was causing the breast cancer in my family? Genetic counselors explained that only about 15% of breast cancer can be attributed to the BRCA genes; the rest are caused by other "faulty genes" or just changes in the breast cells.

I heard about a new procedure that physicians were pioneering—direct-to-implant breast reconstruction after mastectomy. One step and one surgery would drop my risk from 40% to close to 2% or 3%. I could preserve my anatomy and get rid of those breast cells that might kill me someday. It had a lot to do with my family and career. I did not want to have breast cancer.

So I decided, after much research and discussion, to have prophylactic mastectomies with reconstruction. On a Tuesday in the first week of May 2006, I had my surgery. My mother was there when I woke up from anesthesia, and I have never seen her so relieved. My husband took care of the kids, closed the car doors for me, and took over mowing the lawn for a while. I didn't discus my surgery, especially not with the freedom that Angelina Jolie did in 2013. In 2006, no one had heard of my surgery; they couldn't even pronounce the name of it. But I was convinced that it meant I might very well "dodge a bullet."

Nine years later, I smile when I see morning television shows talk about the "Angelina Effect"—implants and breast reconstruction, nipples, and risk reduction, all in the same story. It's wonderful that women can talk about their "faulty parts" without feeling shame. It's a great example for our daughters as well.

In March of 2015, Angelina wrote another op-ed discussing her oophorectomy and salpingectomy surgery (removal of both ovaries and both fallopian tubes). Women with BRCA genes have an increased risk not only for breast cancer but also for ovarian cancer. And this was the disease that took Angelina's mother's life. Ovarian cancer, unlike breast cancer, is often diagnosed at a very late stage. A majority of breast cancers are diagnosed at stage 1 or 2 or even at a "pre-cancer" DCIS [ductal carcinoma in situ] stage. Ovarian cancer, on the other hand, often is diagnosed after the cancer has already spread. Angelina also discussed another "taboo" subject: Removing ovaries and the fallopian tubes in a premenopausal woman (Angelina was 39 years old at the time of her surgery) sends her into early menopause. Hot flashes, skin changes, dryness (you know where) are hard topics to discuss in public. She put it out there, front and center, to destigmatize the subject for all women.

✳ **HINT:** Don't confuse *pleural* with *plural*, which means more than one!

New ✳ **HINTS** make things clear and point out important facts.

✳ *HINT: You may be familiar with a **TIA (transient ischemic attack)**, which is a "**mini-stroke**" that occurs when blood is held back from tissue in the brain.*

✳ **HINT:** The extra n in -thyronine (pronounced THĪ-rō-nēn) avoids the combination of two vowels (o and i).

New clinical photographs and drawings dynamically illustrate medical terminology, conditions, and treatments.

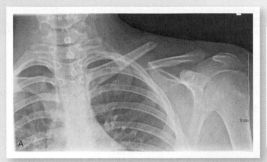

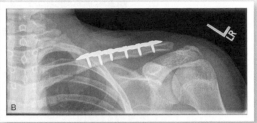

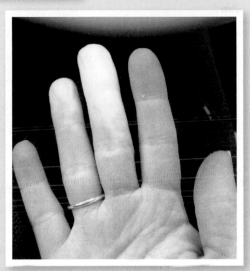

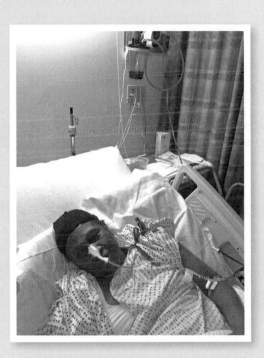

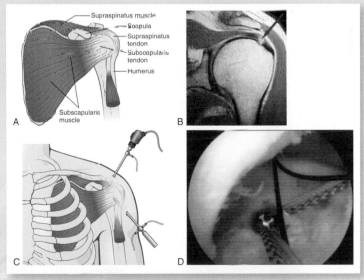

Supraspinatus muscle
Scapula
Supraspinatus tendon
Subscapularis tendon
Humerus
Subscapularis muscle

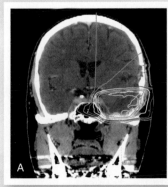

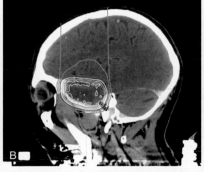

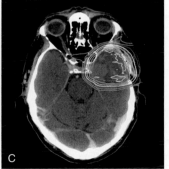

HOW TO USE THE BOOK

The Language of Medicine makes learning easy. The book guides and coaches you step by step through the learning experience. Don't get overwhelmed! Approach learning systematically, step by step. I've helped you study each chapter by organizing the information in small pieces. Icons are provided to help you navigate the sections of the text.

VOCABULARY

The following list reviews many of the terms introduced in this chapter. Short definitions and additional information reinforce your understanding of the terms. All of the terms are included in the *Pronunciation of Terms* section later in the chapter.

absorption	Passage of materials through the walls of the small intestine into the bloodstream.
amino acids	Small building blocks of proteins (like links in a chain), released when proteins are digested.
amylase	Enzyme (-ase) secreted by the pancreas and salivary glands to digest starch (amyl/o).
anus	Terminal end or opening of the digestive tract to the outside of the body.
appendix	Blind pouch hanging from the cecum (in the right lower quadrant [RLQ]). It literally means hanging (pend/o) onto (ap-, which is a form of ad-).
bile	Digestive juice made in the live[...] up (emulsifies) large fat globul[...] *bilis*, meaning gall or anger), p[...] composed of bile pigments (col[...] salts.

 After basic material in the chapter is introduced, the key terms you need to learn are presented in Vocabulary lists. These lists help you study and stay focused.

 You cannot get lost using *The Language of Medicine*. You learn and engage in small incremental steps. The book imparts the most important concepts, allowing you to concentrate on what is essential.

TERMINOLOGY

Write the meanings of the medical terms in the spaces provided.

COMBINING FORMS

COMBINING FORM	MEANING	TERMINOLOGY	MEANING
adenoid/o	adenoids	adenoidectomy ___	
		adenoid hypertrophy ___	
alveol/o	alveolus, air sac	alveolar ___	
bronch/o bronchi/o	bronchial tube, bronchus	bronchospasm ___ *This tightening of the bronchus is a chief characteristic of asthma and bronchitis.*	
		bronchiectasis ___ *Caused by weakening of the bronchial wall from infection.*	
		bronchodilator ___ *This drug causes dilation, or enlargement, of the opening of a bronchus to improve ventilation to the lungs. An example is albuterol, delivered via an inhaler.*	
		bronchopleural ___ *A **bronchopleural fistula** is an abnormal connection between the bronchial tube and the pleural cavity (space). Occurring as a result of lung disease or surgical complication, this can cause an air leak into the pleural space.*	
bronchiol/o	bronchiole, small bronchus	bronchiolitis ___ *This is an acute viral infection occurring in infants younger than 18 months of age.*	
capn/o	carbon dioxide	hypercapnia ___	

 Anabolic Steroids

These drugs are similar to androgens (male hormones) in their effects on the body. They build up protein within cells.

 Metabolism and the Thyroid Gland

The thyroid gland secretes thyroid hormone (thyroxine, or T4), which stimulates metabolism in cells. Increased levels of hormone speed up metabolism (increased energy and weight loss) and decreased levels of hormone slow down metabolism (sluggishness and weight gain).

Epinephrine and Adrenaline

These are the SAME hormone! Two different names for the same substance secreted by the adrenal glands (above the kidneys).

 Throughout the text, Spotlights enhance the relevance of medical terms.

PRACTICAL APPLICATIONS

CASE STUDY: A PATIENT'S ACCOUNT OF ULNAR NERVE NEUROPATHY

I am definitely not one of those ambidextrous people. I am a true righty, so the "experiment" of making me a lefty out of necessity didn't go so well. Over the past decade, I had slowly lost sensation in my right pinky, and a fair amount of function, in my right hand. You might think that I should have taken care of treating it when it initially presented itself with an electric shock down my arm from hitting my "funny

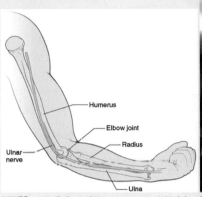

FIGURE 10-25   Pathway of ulnar nerve running behind the   FIGUR
elbow joint (median epicondyle of the humerus) and toward   surgery
the hand.

During an exam by an orthopedic elbow specialist, testi
right hand muscles. My grip strength was also affected an
than my right.

Surgery was scheduled immediately with hopes of halting
sensation in my pinky. My surgeon performed an Eaton proc
its vulnerable path to a position over the medial epicondyle
placed sutures to hold the ulnar nerve in its new place un
He created a little "curtain" with the fascia to keep the nerv
the nerve to take a "short cut" on the way to my hand w
keeping it away from the bony prominence of the elbow.

When I awoke from the anesthesia, I could immediatel
hand. I had tingling in my previously numb fingers and soc
my palm. These findings demonstrated the return of the aut

Medical terminology is connected to real life with case reports and case studies throughout the text and on the companion Evolve website.

PRACTICAL APPLICATIONS

CASE STUDY: TARGETED THERAPY FOR LUNG CANCER

In 2008, Sarah Broom was a 35-year-old literature instructor and poet living in New Zealand. Married with two young sons, she was pregnant with her third child when she noticed shortness of breath accompanied by a persistent cough. An x-ray of her lungs during her 7th month of pregnancy showed a large mass in

one lung. After a cesarean section (her daughter was born safely), she had a biopsy and other tests, which revealed advanced lung cancer. Sarah was a nonsmoker.

The doctors in New Zealand told her that her care would be palliative and that she had only a few months to live.

Sarah was desperate to explore every option, and through a personal connection, she sent her biopsy slides to the MGH Cancer Center in Boston. The slides were analyzed using cutting edge technology, and her tumor was found to have a mutation called EML4-ALK, which occurs in only 5% of lung cancers. The doctors at MGH knew of a new drug called crizotinib that was being evaluated to treat lung cancers with this specific mutation. Finding a specific mutation in a tumor and targeting that mutation with particular drug is a cutting edge approach to cancer treatment.

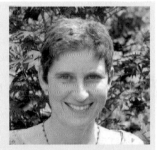

Sarah was given the new drug—and her tumors shrunk! She was in remission for over 2 years. In 2010, the tumors returned, and Sarah traveled back to Boston for further drug treatment, which was not successful. She developed brain metastases.

Her doctors in Boston knew of one more targeted therapy drug called ceritinib that was still in clinical trials and therefore would not be available for patients. However, through coordinated and persistent efforts, the pharmaceutical company allowed her advance, compassionate access to the drug, and it worked for 2 years! Because it was seen that this drug was effective against lung cancer in patients with relapsed

Study sections organize information and help you learn.

STUDY SECTION 5

Practice spelling each term, and know its meaning.

anterior (ventral)	Front surface of the body.
deep	Away from the surface.
distal	Far from the point of attachment to the trunk or far from the beginning of a structure.
frontal (coronal) plane	Vertical plane dividing the body or structure into anterior and posterior portions.
inferior (caudal)	Below another structure; pertaining to the tail or lower portion of the body.
lateral	Pertaining to the side.
medial	Pertaining to the middle or near the medial plane of the body.
posterior (dorsal)	Back surface of the body.
prone	Lying on the belly (face down, palms down).
proximal	Near the point of attachment to the trunk or near the beginning of a structure.
sagittal (lateral) plane	Lengthwise, vertical plane dividing the body or structure into right and left sides. From the Latin *sagitta*, meaning arrow. As an arrow is shot from a bow it enters the body in the sagittal plane, dividing right from left. The **midsagittal** plane divides the body into right and left halves.
superficial	On the surface.
superior (cephalic)	Above another structure; pertaining to the head.
supine	Lying on the back (face up, palms up).
transverse (axial) plane	Horizontal (cross-sectional) plane dividing the body into upper and lower portions.

As you study with *The Language of Medicine,* you are engaged in each step of the learning process. On nearly every page, you are actively involved in labeling diagrams, dividing words into component parts, writing meanings to terms, testing, reviewing, and evaluating your learning.

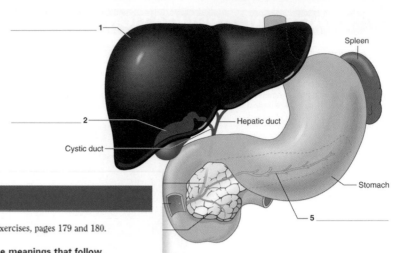

EXERCISES

Remember to check your answers carefully with the Answers to Exercises, pages 179 and 180.

A **Match the listed digestive system structures with the meanings that follow.**

anus	esophagus	liver
cecum	gallbladder	pancreas
colon	ileum	pharynx
duodenum	jejunum	sigmoid colon

1. consists of ascending, transverse, descending, and sigmoid sections _____
2. small sac under the liver; stores bile _____
3. first part of the large intestine _____
4. end of the digestive tract opening to the outside of
5. second part of the small intestine _____
6. tube connecting the throat to the stomach _____
7. third part of the small intestine _____
8. large organ in the RUQ; secretes bile, stores sugar,
9. throat _____
10. lowest part of the colon _____
11. first part of the small intestine _____
12. organ under the stomach; produces insulin and dig

Abbreviations are listed and explained in each body system chapter.

ABBREVIATIONS

AC	acromioclavicular (joint)	**NSAID**	nonsteroidal anti-inflammatory drug—often prescribed to treat musculoskeletal disorders
ACL	anterior cruciate ligament of the knee		
		OA	osteoarthritis
ANA	antinuclear antibody—indicator of systemic lupus erythematosus	**ORIF**	open reduction (of fracture)/internal fixation
BKA	below-knee amputation		
BMD	bone mineral density	**ortho**	orthopedics (*or* orthopaedics)
C1 to C7	cervical vertebrae	**OT**	occupational therapy—helps patients with impaired musculoskeletal function perform activities of daily
Ca	calcium		

 A Review Sheet at the end of each chapter helps you organize and test yourself on what you have learned!

REVIEW SHEET

This Review Sheet and the others that follow each chapter are complete lists of the word elements contained in the chapter. They are designed to pull together the terminology and to reinforce your learning by giving you the opportunity to write the meanings of each word part in the spaces provided and to **test yourself.** Check your answers with the information in the chapter or in the Glossary (Medical Word Parts—English), at the end of the book. It's a good idea to tab the Glossary so that you can easily locate it.

Combining Forms

COMBINING FORM	MEANING	COMBINING FORM	MEANING
aden/o	_____	hem/o, hemat/o	_____
arthr/o	_____	hepat/o	_____
bi/o	_____	iatr/o	_____
carcin/o	_____	leuk/o	_____
cardi/o	_____	log/o	_____
cephal/o	_____	nephr/o	_____
cerebr/o	_____	neur/o	_____
cis/o	_____	onc/o	_____
crin/o	_____	ophthalm/o	_____
cyst/o	_____	oste/o	_____
cyt/o	_____	path/o	_____
derm/o, dermat/o	_____	ped/o	_____
electr/o	_____	psych/o	_____
encephal/o	_____	radi/o	_____
enter/o	_____	ren/o	_____

PRONUNCIATION OF TERMS

To test your understanding of the terminology in this chapter, write the meaning of each term in the space provided. In addition, you may wish to cover the terms and write them by looking at your definitions. Make sure your spelling is correct. The CAPITAL letters indicate the accented syllable. The page number after each term indicates where it is defined or used in the book, so you can easily check your responses. You will find complete definitions for all of these terms and their audio pronunciations on the Evolve website.

Pronunciation Guide
ā as in āpe   ă as in ăpple
ē as in ēven   ĕ as in ĕvery
ī as in īce   ĭ as in ĭnterest
ō as in ōpen   ŏ as in pŏt
ū as in ūnit   ŭ as in ŭnder

TERM	PRONUNCIATION	MEANING
abdomen (47)	ĂB-dō-mĕn	_____
abdominal cavity (47)	ăb-DŎM-ĭ-năl KĂ-vĭ-tē	_____
adipose (41)	ĂD-ĭ-pōs	_____
anabolism (37)	ă-NĂB-ō-lĭzm	_____
anterior (52)	an-TĒ-rē-ŏr	_____
cartilage (41)	KĂR-tĭ-lĭj	_____
catabolism (37)	kă-TĂB-ō-lĭzm	_____
caudal (52)	KĂW-dăl	_____
cell membrane (37)	sĕl MĔM-brăn	_____
cephalic (52)	SĔF-ă-lĭk	_____
cervical (51)	SĔR-vĭ-kăl	_____
chondroma (56)	kŏn-DRŌ-mă	_____
chondrosarcoma (56)	kŏn-drŏ-sar-KŌ-mă	_____
chromosome (37)	KRŌ-mō-sōm	_____

The Pronunciation of Terms section shows you how to pronounce each new term in the chapter and gives you the chance to practice writing its meaning. You can also hear these terms pronounced on the companion Evolve website. The answers to the Pronunciation of Terms section are found on the Evolve website as well.

ALSO AVAILABLE

evolve **STUDENT EVOLVE RESOURCES** (COMPLIMENTARY ACCESS INCLUDED WITH PURCHASE OF THIS TEXT)

All student resources are now available online on the Evolve website. The student website accompanying this new edition is packed with activities, games, additional information, and video clips to expand your understanding and test your knowledge. Chapter by chapter you will find quizzes, case studies, examples of medical records, and a wealth of images to illustrate terminology. Additionally, on the website, you can hear the terms corresponding to the Pronunciation of Terms section in each chapter (more than 3,000 terms in all). Access your resources at: http://evolve.elsevier.com/Chabner/language.

New to the Student Evolve Website for the 11th Edition

- Updated interface enabling convenient online access to your resources.

- The Mobile Dictionary has been updated for this edition. Access this complimentary resource from the Evolve site on your desktop or mobile device and have easy access to definitions of all terms found in the text. This resource helps you study each chapter and also will be a reference for you in the workplace. Each definition has been crafted carefully to explain terms using plain, nontechnical language.

- The Quick Quiz feature has also been revised, enabling students to get a snapshot assessment of their knowledge of a chapter's content.

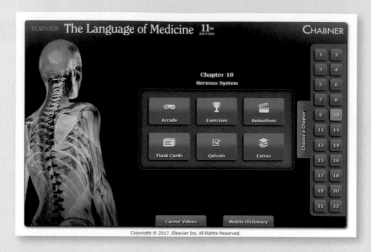

iTerms Study Companion (for sale separately)

- The iTerms audio study guide provides pronunciation and enables you to hear each term pronounced with its definition, in a portable format. This audio companion is available for download. Also included are short review quizzes and coaching tips to help you make the most of your study.

- The iTerms Study Companion, Mobile Dictionary, Quick Quizzes, and updated Flash Cards have been optimized for use on mobile devices, providing convenient access for on-the-go studying.

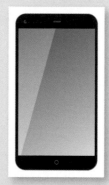

MEDICAL LANGUAGE INSTANT TRANSLATOR (for sale separately)

The *Medical Language Instant Translator* is a uniquely useful resource for all allied health professionals and students of medical terminology. It is a pocket-sized medical terminology reference with convenient information at your fingertips!

- NEW updates to correlate with the revision of *The Language of Medicine*

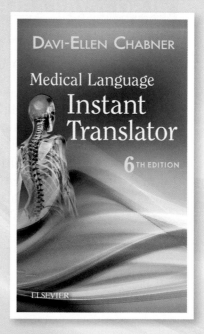

INSTRUCTOR'S RESOURCE MANUAL

The Language of Medicine Instructor's Resource Manual (includes instructor's manual, ExamView test bank, PowerPoints, and an image collection) is available with even more new quizzes, teaching suggestions, crossword puzzles, medical reports, and reference material. The image collection contains all figures and photos from the 11th edition. The instructor materials plus a test bank can be accessed online at http://evolve.elsevier.com/Chabner/language.

The fundamental features you have come to trust in learning and teaching medical terminology remain strong in this new edition. These are:

- Simple, nontechnical explanations of medical terms.
- Workbook format with ample space to write answers.
- Explanations of clinical procedures, laboratory tests, and abbreviations related to each body system.
- Pronunciation of Terms sections with phonetic spellings and spaces to write meanings of terms.
- Practical Applications sections with case reports, operative and diagnostic tests, and laboratory and x-ray reports.
- Exercises that test your understanding of terminology as you work through the text step by step (answers are included).
- Review Sheets that pull together terminology to help you study.
- Comprehensive glossaries and appendices for reference in class and on the job.

Each student and teacher who selects *The Language of Medicine* becomes my partner in the exciting adventure of learning medical terms. Continuity is crucial. Continue to communicate with me through email (daviellenchabner@gmail.com) with your suggestions and comments so that future printings and editions may benefit. A website connected to *The Language of Medicine* and dedicated to helping students and teachers is located at http://evolve.elsevier.com/Chabner/language. I hope you will tell me about additional resources you would like to see on that website so that we can make it an even more useful part of the learning process. You should know that I still experience the thrill and joy of teaching new students. I love being in a classroom and feel privileged to continue to write this text. I hope that my enthusiasm and passion for the medical language are transmitted to you through these pages.

Work hard, but have fun with
The Language of Medicine!

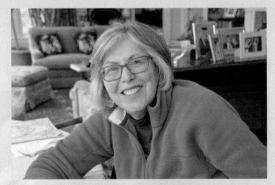

DAVI-ELLEN CHABNER

Acknowledgments

Maureen Pfeifer has been my extraordinary and indispensable editorial partner for the last 18 years. Her phenomenal expertise in all facets of communication, coordination, production, editing, updating, and management is amazing. She has the unique ability to "make things happen" and "make things right." Both personally and professionally, I am grateful for her unique insight and capabilities. She is intelligent, calm, and upbeat in the face of any issue affecting *The Language of Medicine* and its ancillaries. Most of all, I rely on her loyalty and her confidence that we are creating an eminently useful and valuable textbook and resource for both students and instructors. Thank you, Maureen, for everything you do for me, especially when you take things "off my plate."

Bruce A. Chabner, MD, and Elizabeth Chabner Thompson, MD, MPH, continue to be amazing resources to me for expert and up-to-date medical advice. Their contributions were essential in reviewing and editing all chapters and glossaries. My devoted friend, Dan Longo, MD, never turned me down for valuable medical advice and editing of chapters. He was also a wonderful resource for helping identify expert reviewers.

For many editions of this and my other books, Elizabeth Galbraith has copyedited and proofread the manuscript with her characteristic expert attention to grammatical detail and medical accuracy. Thanks to her, students will read and study the text with greater ease.

Jim Perkins, Assistant Professor of Medical Illustration, Rochester Institute of Technology, has been associated with *The Language of Medicine* since its 6th edition. He has worked with me to create drawings that are not only attractive but also essential in making the terminology more understandable. I have come to rely on his unique talent for clarity, accuracy, and detail.

I am indebted to the many medical reviewers listed on pages xv-xvi who offered essential advice and comments on specific chapters. Their insights and expertise make this 11th edition reflect what is current, accurate, and cutting edge in medicine today.

The classroom instructors listed on pages xvi-xvii extensively and carefully reviewed the text, and I have listened to their comments, which are integrated into this new edition. Many other instructors contacted me personally through email with helpful suggestions. Special thank you to Robert Boyd, Martha J. Payne, Heather LaJoie, and Dorothy Price.

I am always pleased to hear from students who comment on the book and ask important questions. I try to answer each as quickly and accurately as possible. Thanks to Jennifer Trup, Michelle Sabri, Hannah Hickerson, Winnie Mei, Anna Spiro, Elizabeth Ramirez, Jared Rodriquez, Al-Yasha Andersen, and Sam Brondfield.

The In Person stories throughout the text are first-hand personal accounts of individuals dealing with illness and medical procedures. The writers of these stories are extraordinarily generous to share their insights and reactions so that we all benefit. A very special thank you to: Stan Ber, Nancy J. Brandwein, Mary Braun, Bruce A. Chabner, Lenore Estrada, Sidra DeKoven Ezrahi, Elizabeth F. Fideler, Tanzie Johnson, Kevin Mahoney,

Frank McGinnis, Brenda Melson, John Melson, Laura Claridge Oppenheimer, Carolyn Peter, Bob Rowe, Ruthellen Sheldon, Elizabeth Chabner Thompson, and Cathy Ward.

The superb staff at Elsevier Health Sciences continues to be vital to the success of *The Language of Medicine*. Luke Held, Content Development Manager, was always responsive, available, and effective in managing the many details of the project. Diane Chatman, Senior Content Development Specialist, coordinated countless facets of this edition. I appreciate Linda Woodard, Senior Content Strategist, and Jeanne Olson, Director of PSE & Professional Reference, for their expert management and their steadfast support of my books.

I am grateful to Michelle Harness, Director, Book Production, Gayle May, Book Production Manager, and Julie Eddy, Publishing Services Manager, for their superb production efforts. Celeste Clingan, Book Production Specialist, tirelessly and effectively handled the day-to-day aspects of the production process. Thank you, Celeste! Brian Salisbury created the design for this edition. I appreciate his expertise and responsiveness.

I continue to be impressed by the talents of the entire marketing team, especially Bianca Janosevic, Senior Vice President, Trade/Digital Channels, Julie Burchett, Director of Product Solutions Marketing, and Traci Cahill, Associate Marketing Manager, Nursing and Health Professions Marketing. They do a phenomenal job keeping *The Language of Medicine* in-step with the needs of instructors and students.

Thanks to Joe Gramlich, Multimedia Producer and Jeanne Crook, Team Manager, Multimedia, for their work on the electronic products associated with this new edition.

A very special note of gratitude to the extraordinary and devoted sales team at Elsevier Health Sciences, which is beyond compare! Led by Jerry Pianto, Senior Vice President of Sales, and Linda Morris, Director of Sales Operations, Nursing and Health Professions, they work tirelessly to bring my books and learning system to the marketplace. You are the best!

My family and friends continue to be my greatest comfort and support. The kids, Brandon, Marla, Noonie, and Dave, are always "in my corner." The grandkids, Bebe, Solomon, Ben, Gus, Louisa, and Amari make me feel "on top of the world." Juliana DoCarmo, by managing so many day-to-day responsibilities, allows me the luxury of being able to work and concentrate. Bruce, my husband of 52 years, has always encouraged my passion for teaching and writing, and given me the space and time to enjoy it. His calm and reassurance trumps any doubt or angst. Lastly, our canine kids, Greta and Owen, remain the love of our lives, providing countless hours of relaxation.

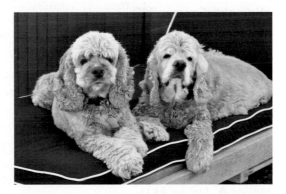

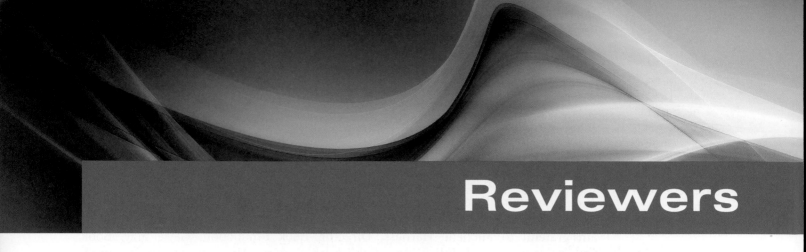

Reviewers

The following persons reviewed the text and/or the ancillaries:

MEDICAL REVIEWERS

Elizabeth Chabner Thompson, MD, MPH
CEO/Founder of BFFL Co
Scarsdale, New York

Bruce A. Chabner, MD
Director of Clinical Research
Massachusetts General Hospital Cancer Center
Professor of Medicine
Harvard Medical School
Boston, Massachusetts

Michael J. Curtin, MD
Medical Director, St. Luke's Sports Medicine
Orthopedic Surgery and Sports Medicine
St. Luke's Clinic
Boise, Idaho

Michael F. Greene, MD
Professor of Obstetrics, Gynecology, and
    Reproductive Biology
Harvard Medical School
Vincent Department of Obstetrics and Gynecology
Massachusetts General Hospital
Boston, Massachusetts

Thomas K. Fehring, MD
Co-Director Orthocarolina Hip and Knee Center
Charlotte, North Carolina

Morris A. Fisher, M.D.
Attending Neurologist
Edward Hines Jr. Veterans Hospital
Hines, Illinois
Professor of Neurology Loyola University
Chicago Stritch School of Medicine
Maywood, Illinois

Lipika Goyal, MD, MPhil
Instructor, Internal Medicine
Harvard Medical School
Boston, Massachusetts

Carlos A. Jamis-Dow, M.D.
Associate Professor of Radiology
Penn State
Milton S. Hershey Medical Center
Hershey, Pennsylvania

Jay Loeffler, MD
Chief of Radiation Oncology
Massachusetts General Hospital Cancer Center
Herman and Joan Suit Professor
Harvard Medical School
Boston, Massachusetts

Dan L. Longo, MD
Deputy Editor
New England Journal of Medicine
Professor of Medicine
Harvard Medical School
Boston, Massachusetts

Ann Sacher, MD
Scarsdale, New York

Henry E. Schniewind, MD
Boston, Massachusetts

Noëlle S. Sherber, MD, FAAD
Dermatologist
Co-Founder, Sherber+Rad
Washington, DC

Leigh H. Simmons, MD
Assistant Professor of Medicine
Harvard Medical School
Division of General Internal Medicine
Massachusetts General Hospital
Boston, Massachusetts

Daniel I. Simon, MD
President, University Hospitals Case Medical Center
President, Harrington Heart & Vascular Institute
Chief, Division of Cardiovascular Medicine
University Hospitals Health System
Herman K. Hellerstein Chair of Cardiovascular
    Research and Professor of Medicine
Case Western Reserve University School of Medicine
Cleveland, OH

Norman M. Simon, MD
Evanston Northwestern Healthcare
Professor of Medicine
Northwestern University
Feinberg School of Medicine
Chicago, Illinois

Jill Smith, MD
Chief of Ophthalmology
Newton-Wellesley Hospital
Newton, Massachusetts

Marcy L. Schwartz, MD
Department of Pediatric Cardiology
The Cleveland Clinic Foundation
Cleveland, Ohio

INSTRUCTOR REVIEWERS

Teresa S. Boyer, MSN, APN-BC, PMHNP
Associate Professor of Nursing
Motlow College
Lynchburg, Tennessee

Cheryl Christopher, RHIA
Adjunct
Borough of Manhattan Community College
New York, New York

**Mary Jane Durksen, Medical Office Administrator
    Diploma**
Lead Virtual Instructor/Courseware Developer
AOLC
Ontario, Canada

Shelba Durston, MSN, RN, CCRN, SAFE
Professor of Nursing
San Joaquin Delta College
Stockton, California

Erin J. Fitzgerald, RN, BSN, MBA
Norwalk Community College
Norwalk, Connecticut

Rosalie Griffith, RN, MSN, MA.Ed
Nursing Success Coordinator
Chesapeake College
Wye Mills, Maryland

Shawn McGowan
Manager, Healthcare Division
AOLC
Ontario, Canada

Angela J. Moore, RN, MSN Ed.
Assistant Director of Nurses
Career Care Institute
Lancaster, California

José L. Mosqueda
Healthcare Lead Instructor
Erie Neighborhood House
Chicago, Illinois

Mary Prorok, RN, MSN
Instructor
South Hills School of Business & Technology
Altoona, Pennsylvania

Danielle Robel, MBA
Professor, Health Sciences
AAMA, Milwaukee Area Technical College
Milwaukee Wisconsin

Deb Stockberger MSN, RN
Health Division Instructor
North Iowa Area Community College
Mason City, Iowa

Donna J. Wilde, MPA, RHIA
Professor, Health Informatics and Information
    Management
Shoreline Community College
Seattle, Washington

Charles K. Williston BA, MS, CPC
Instructor
Traviss Career Center
Lakeland, Florida

**Lynda Wilson, Masters in the Art of Teaching,
    EMT-Paramedic**
Professor of Medical Terminology
Valencia College
Orlando, Florida

Mindy Wray, MA, CMA (AAMA), RMA
Program Director, Medical Assisting
ECPI University
Greensboro, North Carolina

Carole Zeglin, MSEd, BSMT, RMA
Associate Professor/Director Medical Laboratory
    Technology, Medical Assisting, and Phlebotomy/
    Specimen Processing Programs
Westmoreland County Community College
Youngwood, Pennsylvania

Contents

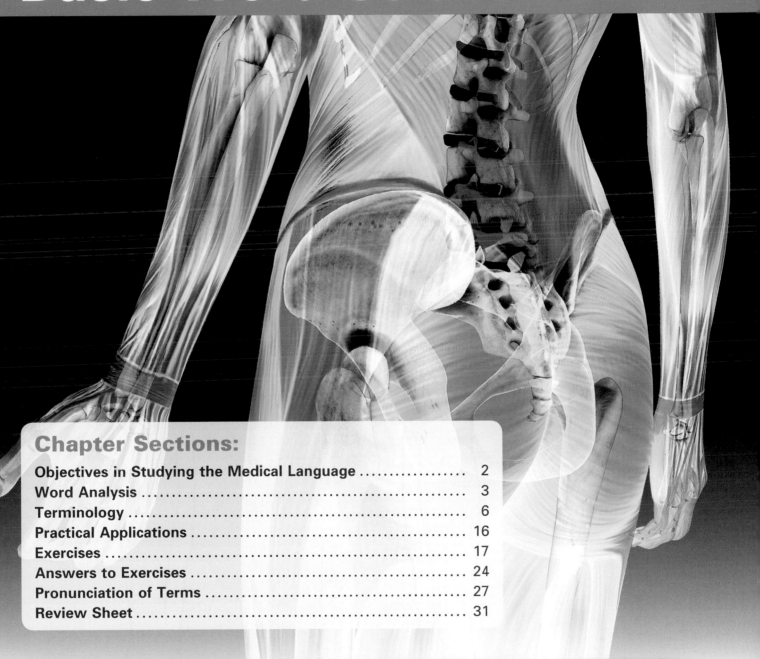

Basic Word Structure

Chapter Sections:

CHAPTER GOALS

- Identify basic objectives to guide your study of the medical language.
- Divide medical words into their component parts.
- Learn the meanings of basic combining forms, suffixes, and prefixes of the medical language.
- Use these combining forms, suffixes, and prefixes to build medical words.

OBJECTIVES IN STUDYING THE MEDICAL LANGUAGE

There are three objectives to keep in mind as you study medical terminology:

- **Analyze words by dividing them into component parts.**

  Your goal is to learn the *tools* of word analysis that will make understanding complex terminology easier. Do not simply memorize terms; think about dividing terms into their component parts—the building blocks of terminology. This book shows how to separate both complicated and simple terms into understandable word elements. Medical terms are much like jigsaw puzzles in that they are constructed of small pieces that make each word unique, with one major difference: The pieces can be shuffled up and used in lots of combinations to make other words as well. As you become familiar with word parts and learn what each means, you will be able to recognize those word parts in totally new combinations in other terms.

- **Relate the medical terms to the structure and function of the human body.**

  Memorization of terms, although essential to retention of the language, should not become the primary objective of your study. A major focus of this book is to *explain* terms in the context of how the body works in health and disease. Medical terms explained in their proper context also will be easier to remember. Thus, the term **hepatitis,** meaning inflammation (**-itis**) of the liver (**hepat**), is better understood when you know where the liver is and how it functions. No previous knowledge of biology, anatomy, or physiology is needed for this study. Explanations in this book are straightforward and basic.

- **Be aware of spelling and pronunciation problems.**

  Some medical terms are pronounced alike but are spelled differently, which accounts for their different meanings. For example, **ilium** and **ileum** have identical pronunciations, but the first term, **ilium,** means a part of the hip bone, whereas the second term, **ileum,** refers to a part of the small intestine (Figure 1-1). Even when terms are spelled correctly,

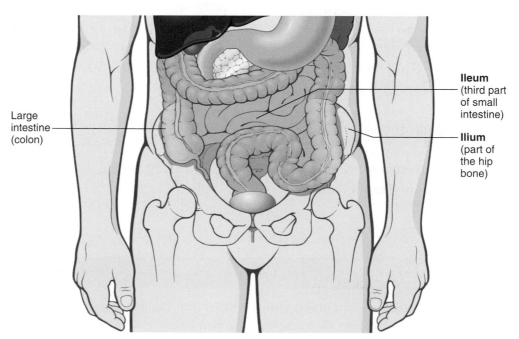

Large intestine (colon)

Ileum (third part of small intestine)

Ilium (part of the hip bone)

FIGURE 1-1   The terms **ileum** and **ilium** can be confusing because they are pronounced alike and refer to body parts located in the same general region of the body. ✱ **HINT:** The **ileum**, with an "**e**," is part of the digestive tract, which has to do with **e**ating.

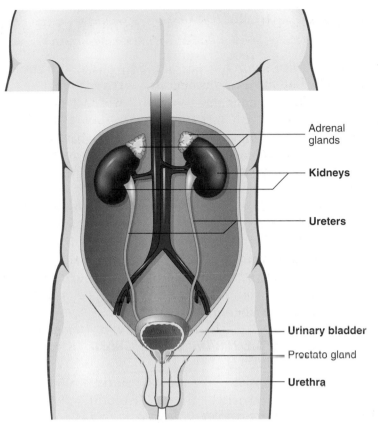

Adrenal
glands

Kidneys

Ureters

Urinary bladder

Prostate gland

Urethra

FIGURE 1-2   Male urinary tract. The terms **urethra** and **ureter** can be confusing because they are both tubes of the urinary system, but spellings and pronunciations are different. Notice their locations: **two ureters** between the kidneys and urinary bladder and **one urethra** between the urinary bladder and the outside of the body. ✳ **HINT:** Ureter has two "e's" and urethra has just one "e."

they can be misunderstood because of incorrect pronunciation. For example, the **urethra** (ū-RĒ-thrăh) is the tube leading from the urinary bladder to the outside of the body, whereas a **ureter** (ŪR-ĕ-tĕr) is one of two tubes each leading from a single kidney and inserting into the urinary bladder. Figure 1-2 illustrates the different anatomy of the urethra and the ureters.

WORD ANALYSIS

Studying medical terminology is very similar to learning a new language. At first, the words seem strange and complicated, although they may stand for commonly known disorders and terms. For example, **cephalgia** means "headache," and an **ophthalmologist** is an "eye doctor."

Your first job in learning the language of medicine is to understand how to divide words into their component parts. Logically, most terms, whether complex or simple, can be broken down into basic parts and then understood. For example, consider the following term, which is divided into three parts:

HEMAT/O/LOGY

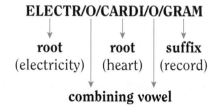

root | suffix
(blood) | (process of study)

combining vowel

The **root** is the *foundation of the word*. All medical terms have one or more roots. For example, the root **hemat** means **blood.**

The **suffix** is the *word ending*. All medical terms have a suffix. The suffix **-logy** means **process of study.**

The **combining vowel**—usually **o**, as in this term—*links the root to the suffix or the root to another root.* A combining vowel has no meaning of its own; it joins one word part to another.

It is useful to read the meaning of medical terms *starting from the suffix and then going back to the beginning of the term.* Thus, the term **hematology** means **process of study of blood.**

Here is another familiar medical term:

ELECTR/O/CARDI/O/GRAM

root | root | suffix
(electricity) | (heart) | (record)

combining vowel

Electrocardiogram, reading from the suffix back to the beginning of the term, means **record of the electricity in the heart.**

Notice that there are two combining vowels—both **o**—in this term. The first o links the two roots **electr** and **cardi**; the second o links the root **cardi** and the suffix **-gram.**

Try another term:

GASTR/ITIS

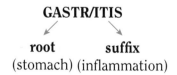

root   suffix
(stomach)   (inflammation)

Gastritis, reading from the end of the term (suffix) to the beginning, means **inflammation of the stomach.**

Notice that the combining vowel, o, is missing in this term. This is because the suffix, **-itis,** begins with a vowel. The combining vowel is dropped before a suffix that begins with a vowel. It is retained, however, between two roots, even if the second root begins with a vowel.

Consider the following term:

GASTR/O/ENTER/O/LOGY

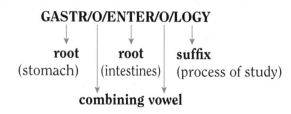

root | root | suffix
(stomach) | (intestines) | (process of study)

combining vowel

The entire term means **process of study of the stomach and intestines.**

Notice that the combining vowel is retained between **gastr** and **enter,** even though the second root, **enter,** begins with a vowel. When a term contains two or more roots related to parts of the body, anatomic position often determines which root goes before the other. For example, the stomach receives food first, before the small intestine—so the word is formed as **gastroenterology,** not "enterogastrology."

In summary, remember **three general rules:**
1. **READ** the meaning of medical terms from the suffix back to the beginning of the term and across.
2. **DROP** the combining vowel (usually o) before a suffix beginning with a vowel: **gastritis,** *not* "gastroitis."
3. **KEEP** the combining vowel between two roots: **gastroenterology,** *not* "gastrenterology."

In addition to the root, suffix, and combining vowel, two other word parts are commonly found in medical terms. These are the combining form and the **prefix.** The combining form is simply the root plus the combining vowel. For example, you already are familiar with the following combining forms and their meanings:

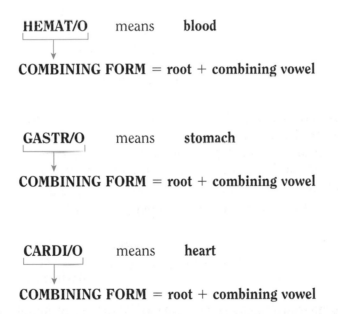

HEMAT/O   means   **blood**

COMBINING FORM = root + combining vowel

GASTR/O   means   **stomach**

COMBINING FORM = root + combining vowel

CARDI/O   means   **heart**

COMBINING FORM = root + combining vowel

Combining forms are used with many different suffixes. Remembering the meaning of a combining form will help you understand unfamiliar medical terms.

The **prefix** is a small part attached to the *beginning* of a term. Not all medical terms contain prefixes, but the prefix can have an important influence on the meaning. Consider the following examples:

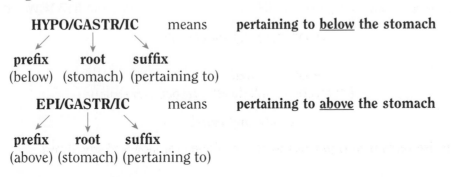

HYPO/GASTR/IC   means   **pertaining to <u>below</u> the stomach**

prefix   root   suffix
(below) (stomach) (pertaining to)

EPI/GASTR/IC   means   **pertaining to <u>above</u> the stomach**

prefix   root   suffix
(above) (stomach) (pertaining to)

In summary, the **important elements of medical terms** are the following:
1. **ROOT:** foundation of the term
2. **SUFFIX:** word ending
3. **PREFIX:** word beginning
4. **COMBINING VOWEL:** vowel (usually o) that links the root to the suffix or the root to another root
5. **COMBINING FORM:** combination of the root and the combining vowel

TERMINOLOGY

In previous examples you have been introduced to the combining forms **gastr/o** (stomach), **hemat/o** (blood), and **cardi/o** (heart). This section of the chapter presents a list of additional combining forms, suffixes, and prefixes, with examples of medical words using those word parts. Similar lists are included for each chapter in the book. Write the *meaning* of the medical term in the space provided. Then check the correct pronunciation for each term with the Pronunciation of Terms list on pages 27 to 30. The Evolve website for *The Language of Medicine* contains definitions and audio pronunciations for each term. **Use it!**

Most medical terms are derived from Greek and Latin roots. Greek, Roman, and Arabic physicians had developed medically useful concepts and associated vocabularies long before the 21st century. Greek and Latin origins for medical terms are presented for your interest on the Evolve website.

CHAPTER STUDY GUIDE

1. **Use slashes to divide each term** into component parts (*aden/oma*), and **write its meaning** (*tumor of a gland*) in the space provided. Although most medical terms are divided easily into component parts and understood, others defy simple explanation. Information in *italics* under a medical term helps you define and understand the term. You can check meanings on the Evolve site.
2. **Complete the Exercises,** pages 17 to 23, and **check your answers** on pages 24 to 26.
3. **Write meanings for terms on the Pronunciation of Terms list,** pages 27 to 30. Definitions are on the Evolve site.
4. **Complete the Review Sheet,** pages 31 and 32. Check your answers with the Glossary, page 959. Then, **test yourself** by writing Review Sheet terms and meanings on a separate sheet of paper.
5. **Make your own flash cards.** Using the Review Sheet as a guide, create flash cards that can be transported wherever you study!
6. **Create your own book tabs** to have easy access to key concepts and frequently used sections—for example, the **Glossary of Word Parts,** beginning on page 961.
7. **Review terms** using the audio pronunciations found on the Evolve website.

Notice that you are actively engaging in the learning process by writing terms and their meanings and testing yourself repeatedly. Here is your study mantra: **READ, WRITE, RECITE,** and **REVIEW.** I guarantee success if you follow these simple steps. This is a proven method—it really works!

COMBINING FORMS

Write the *meaning* of each medical term in the space provided.

Remember: You will find every term phonetically pronounced starting on page 27, and you can hear the pronunciations on the Evolve website.

COMBINING FORM	MEANING	TERMINOLOGY	MEANING
aden/o	gland	adenoma *tumor of a gland*	
		The suffix -oma means tumor or mass.	
		adenitis	
		The suffix -itis means inflammation.	
arthr/o	joint	arthritis	
bi/o	life	biology	
		The suffix -logy is composed of the root log (study) and the final suffix -y (process or condition).	
		biopsy	
		The suffix -opsy means process of viewing. Living tissue is removed from the body and viewed under a microscope.	
carcin/o	cancerous, cancer	carcinoma	
		A carcinoma is a cancerous tumor. Carcinomas grow from the epithelial (surface or skin) cells that cover the outside of the body and line organs, cavities, and tubes within the body (Figure 1-3).	
cardi/o	heart	cardiology	
cephal/o	head	cephalic	
		(sĕ-FĂL-ĭk) The suffix -ic means pertaining to. A cephalic presentation describes a "head first" position for the delivery of an infant.	

1

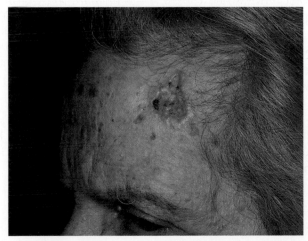

FIGURE 1-3 Carcinoma of the skin. This is a **basal cell carcinoma,** the most common form of skin cancer. It usually occurs on sun-damaged skin.

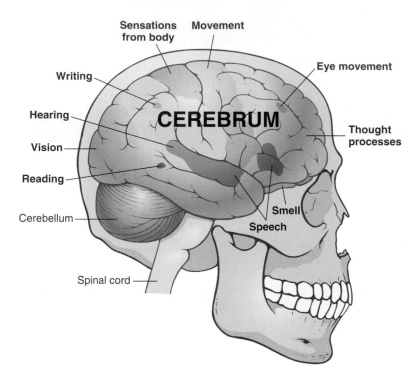

FIGURE 1-4 **Cerebrum** and the functions it controls. A **cerebrovascular accident** (**CVA**), or **stroke,** occurs when blood vessels (vascul/o means blood vessel) are damaged in the cerebrum and blood is prevented from reaching functional areas of the brain. Cells, deprived of oxygen and nutrients, are damaged, causing loss of movement or speech and other signs and symptoms of a CVA.

COMBINING FORM	MEANING	TERMINOLOGY	MEANING
cerebr/o	cerebrum (largest part of the brain)	cerebral _____ *The suffix -al means pertaining to. Figure 1-4 shows the cerebrum and its many functional areas.*	
cis/o	to cut	incision _____ *The prefix in- means into, and the suffix -ion means process.*	
		excision _____ *The prefix ex- means out.*	
crin/o	to secrete (to form and give off)	endocrine glands _____ *The prefix endo- means within; **endocrine glands** (e.g., thyroid, pituitary, and adrenal glands) secrete hormones directly within (into) the bloodstream. Other glands, called **exocrine glands,** release their secretions (e.g., saliva, sweat, tears, milk) through tubes (ducts) to the outside of the body.*	
cyst/o	urinary bladder; a sac or a cyst (sac containing fluid)	cystoscopy _____ *(sĭs-TŎS-kō-pē) The suffix -scopy is a **complex suffix** that includes the root scop, meaning visual examination, and the final suffix -y, meaning process.*	

 Complex Suffixes

Many suffixes, like **-scopy**, contain an embedded root word. Other examples are **-opsy** (ops is a root) and **-logy** (log is a root).

COMBINING FORM	MEANING	TERMINOLOGY	MEANING
cyt/o	cell	cytology _____ *See Figure 1-5 for examples of blood cells.*	
derm/o **dermat/o**	skin	dermatitis _____ hypodermic _____ *The prefix hypo- means under or below.*	
electr/o	electricity	electrocardiogram _____ *The suffix -gram means record. Abbreviated ECG (or sometimes EKG).*	
encephal/o	brain	electroencephalogram _____ *Abbreviated EEG.*	
enter/o	intestines (usually the small intestine)	enteritis _____ *The small intestine is narrower but much longer than the large intestine (colon). See Figure 1-1 on page 2, which shows the small and large intestines.*	
erythr/o	red	erythrocyte _____ *The suffix -cyte means cell. Erythrocytes carry oxygen in the blood.*	
gastr/o	stomach	gastrectomy _____ *The suffix -ectomy means excision or removal. All or, more commonly, part of the stomach is removed.* gastrotomy _____ *The suffix -tomy is another complex suffix, which contains the root tom, meaning to cut, and the final suffix -y, meaning process of.*	

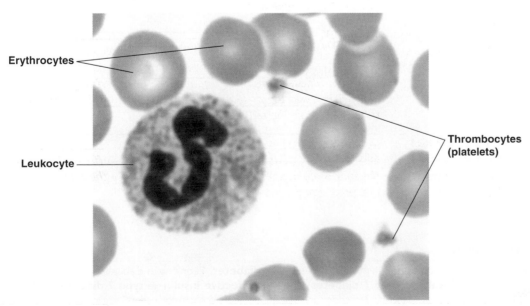

FIGURE 1-5 Blood cells. Notice red blood cells (erythrocytes), a white blood cell (leukocyte), and clotting cells (thrombocytes or platelets).

COMBINING FORM	MEANING	TERMINOLOGY	MEANING
glyc/o	sugar	hyperglycemia ◨ _____ *The prefix hyper- means excessive, above, or more than normal. The suffix -emia means blood condition.*	
gnos/o	knowledge	diagnosis _____ *The prefix dia- means complete. The suffix -sis means state or condition of. A diagnosis is made after sufficient information has been obtained about the patient's condition. Literally, it is a "state of complete knowledge."*	
		prognosis _____ *The prefix pro- means before. Literally "knowledge before," a prognosis is a prediction about the outcome of an illness, but it is always given after the diagnosis has been determined.*	
gynec/o	woman, female	gynecology _____	
hemat/o **hem/o**	blood	hematology _____	
		hematoma _____ *In this term, -oma means a mass or collection of blood, rather than a growth of cells (tumor). A hematoma forms when blood escapes from blood vessels and collects as a clot in a cavity or organ or under the skin. See Figure 1-6.*	
		hemoglobin _____ *The suffix -globin means protein. Hemoglobin carries oxygen in red blood cells.*	
hepat/o	liver	hepatitis _____	
iatr/o	treatment, physician	iatrogenic _____ *The suffix -genic means pertaining to producing, produced by, or produced in. Iatrogenic conditions are adverse effects that result from treatment or intervention by a physician.*	
leuk/o	white	leukocyte _____ *This blood cell helps the body fight disease.*	
log/o	study of	dermatology _____	
nephr/o	kidney	nephritis _____	
		nephrology _____	
neur/o	nerve	neurology _____	

Hyperglycemia and Diabetes

Hyperglycemia (high blood sugar) most frequently is associated with **diabetes.** People with diabetes have high blood sugar levels because they **lack insulin** (in **type 1 diabetes**) or have **ineffective insulin** (in **type 2 diabetes**). Insulin is the hormone normally released by the pancreas (an endocrine gland near the stomach) to "escort" sugar from the bloodstream into cells. Sugar (glucose) is then broken down in cells to release energy. When insulin is not present, sugar cannot enter cells and builds up in the bloodstream (hyperglycemia).

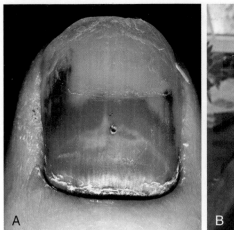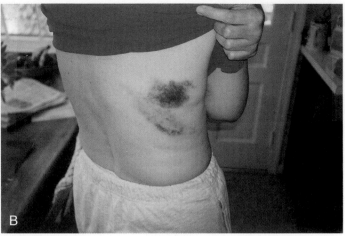

FIGURE 1-6 **A,** Notice the **hematoma** under the nail. **B, Hematoma** from broken ribs.

1

COMBINING FORM	MEANING	TERMINOLOGY	MEANING
onc/o	tumor (cancerous)	oncology _____	
		oncologist _____ *The suffix -ist means one who specializes in a field of medicine (or other profession).*	
ophthalm/o	eye	ophthalmoscope _____ *(ŏf-THĂL-mō-skōp) The suffix -scope means an instrument for visual examination.* ✱ **HINT**: *Pronunciation helps! The first syllable is "ŏf" and here the "f" sound is spelled "ph."*	
oste/o	bone	osteitis _____	
		osteoarthritis _____ *This condition of aging is actually a degeneration of bones and joints often accompanied by inflammation.*	
path/o	disease	pathology _____	
		pathologist _____ *A pathologist examines biopsy samples microscopically and examines dead bodies to determine the cause of death.*	
ped/o	child	pediatric _____ *Notice that ped/o is also in the term orthopedist. Orthopedists once were doctors who straightened (orth/o means straight) children's bones and corrected deformities. Nowadays, orthopedists specialize in disorders of bones and muscles in people of all ages.*	

COMBINING FORM	MEANING	TERMINOLOGY	MEANING
psych/o	mind	psychology _____	
		psychiatrist _____	
radi/o	x-rays	radiology _____ *Low-energy x-rays are used for diagnostic imaging.*	
ren/o	kidney	renal _____ *Ren/o (Latin) and nephr/o (Greek) both mean kidney. Ren/o is used with -al (Latin) to describe the kidney, whereas nephr/o is used with other suffixes such as -osis, -itis, and -ectomy (Greek) to describe abnormal conditions and operative procedures.*	
rhin/o	nose	rhinitis _____	
sarc/o	flesh	sarcoma _____ *This is a **cancerous (malignant) tumor.** A **sarcoma** (Figure 1-7) grows from cells of "fleshy" connective tissue such as muscle, bone, and fat, whereas a **carcinoma** (another type of **cancerous tumor**) grows from epithelial cells that line the outside of the body or the inside of organs in the body.*	
sect/o	to cut	resection _____ *The prefix re- means back. A resection is a cutting back in the sense of cutting out or removal (excision). A gastric resection is a gastrectomy, or excision of the stomach.*	
thromb/o	clot, clotting	thrombocyte _____ *Also known as platelets, these cells help clot blood. A **thrombus** is the actual clot that forms, and **thrombosis** (-osis means condition) is the condition of clot formation.*	
ur/o	urinary tract, urine	urologist _____	

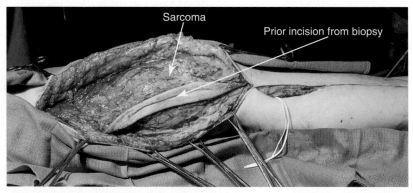

FIGURE 1-7   Sarcoma of muscle in the thigh. *(Courtesy Dr. Sam Yoon, Sloan Kettering Hospital, New York City.)*

Urologist and Nephrologist

A **urologist** is a **surgeon** who operates on the urinary tract and the organs of the male reproductive system.
A **nephrologist** is an **internal medicine specialist** (nonsurgical) who diagnoses and treats disorders of kidneys.
Both urologists and nephrologists are medical doctors.

SUFFIXES

SUFFIX	MEANING	TERMINOLOGY	MEANING
-ac	pertaining to	cardi<u>ac</u> _____	
-al	pertaining to	neur<u>al</u> _____	
-algia	pain	arthr<u>algia</u> _____	
		neur<u>algia</u> _____	
-cyte	cell	erythro<u>cyte</u> _____	
-ectomy	excision, removal	nephr<u>ectomy</u> _____	
-emia	blood condition	leuk<u>emia</u> _____ *Literally, this term means "a blood condition of white (blood cells)." Actually, it is a condition of blood in which cancerous white blood cells proliferate (increase in number).*	
-genic	pertaining to producing, produced by, or produced in	carcino<u>genic</u> _____ *Cigarette smoke is carcinogenic.* patho<u>genic</u> _____ *Many viruses and bacteria are pathogenic organisms.* iatro<u>genic</u> _____ *In this term, -genic means produced by.*	
-globin	protein	hemo<u>globin</u> _____	
-gram	record	electroencephalo<u>gram</u> _____	
-ic, -ical	pertaining to	gastr<u>ic</u> _____ neurolog<u>ic</u> _____ *Log/o means study of.*	
-ion	process	excis<u>ion</u> _____	
-ist	specialist	ophthalmolog<u>ist</u> _____	
-itis	inflammation	cyst<u>itis</u> _____	
-logy	process of study	endocrino<u>logy</u> _____	
-oma	tumor, mass, swelling	hepat<u>oma</u> _____ *A hepatoma **(hepatocellular carcinoma)** is a malignant tumor of the liver.*	
-opsy	process of viewing	bi<u>opsy</u> _____ *Biopsy specimens are obtained and viewed under a microscope.*	

Ophthalmologist, Optometrist, Optician

An **ophthalmologist** is a **physician** who specializes in diagnosing and treating (surgically and medically) disorders of the eye. An **optometrist** is a **health care professional** who examines (metr/o = to measure) eyes and prescribes corrective lenses and may treat eye diseases. An **optician** grinds lenses and fits glasses but does *not* examine eyes, prescribe corrective lenses, or treat eye diseases.

SUFFIX	MEANING	TERMINOLOGY	MEANING
-osis	condition, usually abnormal (slight increase in numbers when used with blood cells)	nephr<u>osis</u> _____ leukocyt<u>osis</u> _____ *This condition, a slight increase in normal white blood cells, occurs as white blood cells multiply to fight an infection. Don't confuse **leukocytosis** with **leukemia,** which is a cancerous (malignant) condition marked by high levels of abnormal, immature white blood cells.*	
-pathy	disease condition	entero<u>pathy</u> _____ (ĕn-tĕ-RŎP-ă-thē) adeno<u>pathy</u> _____ (ă-dĕ-NŎP-ă-thē)	
-scope	instrument to visually examine	endo<u>scope</u> _____ *Endo- means within. A cystoscope is a type of endoscope. A periscope is a nonmedical term meaning an instrument to visually examine an area around (peri-) an obstacle.*	
-scopy	process of visually examining	endo<u>scopy</u> _____ (ĕn-DŎS-kō-pē) *Endoscopy is performed with an endoscope. A common endoscopic procedure is a **colonoscopy** (colon/o = colon or large intestine).*	
-sis	state of; condition	progno<u>sis</u> _____	
-tomy	process of cutting, incision	osteo<u>tomy</u> _____ (ŏs-tē-ŎT-tō-mē)	
-y	process, condition	gastroenterolog<u>y</u> _____	

PREFIXES

PREFIX	MEANING	TERMINOLOGY	MEANING
a-, an-	no, not, without	<u>an</u>emia _____ *Anemia is a decreased number of erythrocytes or an abnormality of the hemoglobin (a chemical) within the red blood cells. This results in decreased delivery of oxygen to cells of the body. Anemic patients look so pale that early physicians thought they were literally "without blood."*	
aut-, auto-	self, own	<u>aut</u>opsy _____ *This term literally means "process of viewing by oneself." Hence, an autopsy is the examination of a dead body with one's own eyes to determine the cause of death and nature of disease.*	

Other Suffixes Meaning Process or Condition

Examples are **-ia** as in **-algia** (condition of pain) and **-ism** as in hyperthyroid**ism** (condition of high thyroid hormone).

PREFIX	MEANING	TERMINOLOGY	MEANING
dia-	complete, through	diagnosis _____ *The plural of diagnosis is diagnoses.*	
endo-	within	endocrinologist _____	
epi-	above, upon	epigastric _____	
		epidermis _____ *This outermost layer of skin lies above the middle layer of skin, known as the dermis.*	
ex-, exo-	out, outside of, outward	excision _____	
		exocrine glands _____	
hyper-	excessive, above, more than normal	hyperthyroidism _____ *The suffix -ism means process or condition.*	
hypo-	deficient, below, under, less than normal	hypogastric _____ *When hypo- is used with a part of the body, it means below.*	
		hypoglycemia _____ *In this term, hypo- means deficient.*	
in-	into, in	incision _____	
peri-	surrounding, around	pericardium _____ *The suffix -um means a structure. The pericardium is the membrane that surrounds the heart.*	
pro-	before, forward	prostate gland _____ *This exocrine gland "stands" (-state) before or in front of the male urinary bladder (see Figure 1-2). It produces semen, which contains fluid and sperm cells.*	
re-	back, backward, again	resection _____ *This is an operation in which tissue is "cut back" or removed. The Latin resectio means a trimming or pruning.*	
retro-	behind	retrocardiac _____	
sub-	below, under	subhepatic _____	
trans-	across, through	transhepatic _____	

Plurals

Terms ending in **-is** (diagnosis, prognosis) form their plural by dropping the **-is** and adding **-es.** See Appendix I, page 981, for other rules on formation of plurals.

Understanding Hyperthyroidism

In **hyperthyroidism,** a **hyperactive thyroid gland** (an endocrine gland in the neck) secretes a greater than normal amount of **thyroxine** (thyroid hormone, or **T₄**). Because thyroxine causes cells to burn fuel and release energy, signs and symptoms of hyperthyroidism are **increased energy level** and **nervousness, tachycardia** (increased heart rate), **weight loss,** and **exophthalmos** (bulging eyeballs).

PRACTICAL APPLICATIONS

This section provides an opportunity for you to use your skill in understanding medical terms in this chapters and to increase your knowledge of new terms. Be sure to check your answers with the Answers to Practical Applications on page 26. You should find helpful explanations there.

SPECIALISTS

Match the **abnormal condition** in Column I with the **physician (specialist)** who treats it in Column II. Write the letter of the correct specialist in the space provided.

COLUMN I: Abnormal Conditions

1. heart attack _____

2. ovarian cysts _____

3. bipolar (manic-depressive) disorder _____

4. breast adenocarcinoma _____

5. iron deficiency anemia _____

6. retinopathy _____

7. cerebrovascular accident (stroke) _____

8. renal failure _____

9. inflammatory bowel disease _____

10. prostatic adenocarcinoma _____

COLUMN II: Physicians (Specialists)

A. gastroenterologist
B. hematologist
C. nephrologist
D. cardiologist
E. oncologist
F. gynecologist
G. urologist
H. ophthalmologist
I. neurologist
J. psychiatrist

1

EXERCISES

The exercises that follow are designed to help you learn the terms presented in the chapter. **Writing terms over and over again is a good way to study this new language.** You will find the answers to these exercises starting on page 24. This makes it easy to **check your work.** As you check each answer, you not only will reinforce your understanding of a term but often will gain additional information from the answer.

Each exercise is designed not as a test, but rather as an opportunity for you to learn the material.

A **Complete the following sentences.**

1. Word beginnings are called _____.

2. Word endings are called _____.

3. The foundation of a word is known as the _____.

4. A letter linking a suffix and a root, or linking two roots, in a term is the

   _____.

5. The combination of a root and a combining vowel is known as the _____.

B **Give the meanings of the following combining forms.**

1. cardi/o _____   7. carcin/o _____

2. aden/o _____   8. cyst/o _____

3. bi/o _____   9. cyt/o _____

4. cerebr/o _____   10. derm/o or dermat/o _____

5. cephal/o _____   11. encephal/o _____

6. arthr/o _____   12. electr/o _____

C **Give the meanings of the following suffixes.**

1. -oma _____   5. -scopy _____

2. -al _____   6. -ic _____

3. -itis _____   7. -gram _____

4. -logy _____   8. -opsy _____

1

D Using slashes, divide the following terms into parts, and give the meaning of the entire term.

1. cerebral _____

2. biopsy _____

3. adenitis _____

4. cephalic _____

5. carcinoma _____

6. cystoscopy _____

7. electrocardiogram _____

8. cardiology _____

9. electroencephalogram _____

10. dermatitis _____

11. arthroscopy _____

12. cytology _____

E Give the meanings of the following combining forms.

1. erythr/o _____

2. enter/o _____

3. gastr/o _____

4. gnos/o _____

5. hemat/o _____

6. cis/o _____

7. nephr/o _____

8. leuk/o _____

9. iatr/o _____

10. hepat/o _____

11. neur/o _____

12. gynec/o _____

F Complete the medical term, based on its meaning as provided.

1. white blood cell: _____cyte

2. inflammation of the stomach: gastr_____

3. pertaining to being produced by treatment: _____genic

4. study of kidneys: _____logy

5. red blood cell: _____cyte

6. mass of blood: _____oma

7. process of viewing living tissue (using a microscope): bi_____

8. pain of nerves: neur_____

9. process of visual examination of the eye: _____scopy

10. inflammation of the small intestine: _____itis

G Select from the combining forms below to match the numbered English terms. Write the correct combining form in the space provided.

onc/o   path/o   ren/o   sect/o
ophthalm/o   psych/o   rhin/o   thromb/o
oste/o   radi/o   sarc/o   ur/o

English Terms

1. kidney _____   7. mind _____

2. disease _____   8. urinary tract _____

3. eye _____   9. bone _____

4. to cut _____   10. x-rays _____

5. nose _____   11. clotting _____

6. flesh _____   12. tumor _____

H <u>Underline</u> the suffix in each term, and then give the meaning of the term.

1. ophthalmoscopy _____

2. ophthalmoscope _____

3. oncology _____

4. osteitis _____

5. psychosis _____

6. thrombocyte _____

7. renal _____

8. nephrectomy _____

9. osteotomy _____

10. resection _____

11. carcinogenic _____

12. sarcoma _____

I Match the suffix in Column I with its meaning in Column II. Write the correct meaning in the space provided.

COLUMN I
Suffix

COLUMN II
Meaning

1. -algia _____

2. -ion _____

3. -emia _____

4. -gram _____

5. -scope _____

6. -osis _____

7. -ectomy _____

8. -genic _____

9. -pathy _____

10. -tomy _____

11. -itis _____

12. -cyte _____

13. -globin _____

condition, usually abnormal
blood condition
cell
disease condition
process of cutting, incision
inflammation
instrument to visually examine
pain
pertaining to producing, produced by, or produced in
process
protein
record
excision, removal (resection)

J Select from the listed terms to complete the sentences that follow.

arthralgia
carcinogenic
cystitis
endocrine
exocrine

hematoma
hepatoma (hepatocellular
    carcinoma)
encephalopathy

iatrogenic
leukemia
leukocytosis
neuralgia

1. When Paul smoked cigarettes, he inhaled a _____ substance with each puff.

2. Sally's sore throat, fever, and chills made her doctor order a white blood cell count. The results, indicating infection, showed a slight increase in normal cells, a condition called

_____.

3. Mr. Smith's liver enlarged, giving him abdominal pain. His radiologic tests and biopsy revealed a

malignant tumor, or _____.

4. Mrs. Rose complained of pain in her hip joints, knees, and shoulders each morning. She was

told that she had painful joints, or _____.

5. Dr. Black was trained to treat disorders of the pancreas, thyroid gland, adrenal glands, and

pituitary gland. Thus, he was an expert in the _____ glands.

6. Ms. Walsh told her doctor she had pain when urinating. After tests, the doctor's diagnosis was

inflammation of the urinary bladder, or _____.

7. Elizabeth's overhead tennis shot hit David in the thigh, producing a large _____. His skin looked bruised and the affected area was tender.

8. Mr. Bell's white blood cell count is 10 times higher than normal. Examination of his blood

   shows cancerous white blood cells. His diagnosis is _____.

9. Mr. Kay was resuscitated (revived from potential or apparent death) in the emergency department after experiencing a heart attack. Unfortunately, he suffered a broken rib as a result of the

   physician's chest compressions. This is an example of a/an _____ fracture.

10. After playing one season for a professional football team, Bill Smith decided to retire because he worried about the dangers of concussions and head trauma—a condition called CTE, or chronic

    traumatic _____.

K **Give the meanings of the following prefixes.**

1. dia- _____

8. endo- _____

2. pro- _____

9. retro- _____

3. aut-, auto- _____

10. trans- _____

4. a-, an- _____

11. peri- _____

5. hyper- _____

12. ex-, exo- _____

6. hypo- _____

13. sub- _____

7. epi- _____

14. re- _____

L **Underline the prefix in the following terms, and then give the meaning of the entire term.**

1. diagnosis _____

2. prognosis _____

3. subhepatic _____

4. pericardium _____

5. hyperglycemia _____

6. hypodermic _____

7. epigastric _____

8. resection _____

9. hypoglycemia _____

10. anemia _____

1

M **Complete the following terms (describing areas of medicine), based on their meanings as given.**

1. study of the urinary tract: _____ logy

2. study of women and women's diseases: _____ logy

3. study of blood: _____ logy

4. study of tumors: _____ logy

5. study of the kidneys: _____ logy

6. study of nerves: _____ logy

7. treatment of children: _____ iatrics

8. study of x-rays in diagnostic imaging: _____ logy

9. study of the eyes: _____ logy

10. study of the stomach and intestines: _____ logy

11. study of glands that secrete hormones: _____ logy

12. treatment of the mind: _____ iatry

13. study of disease: _____ logy

14. study of the heart: _____ logy

N **Give the meaning of the underlined word part, and then define the term.**

1. <u>cerebro</u>vascular accident _____

2. <u>encephal</u>itis _____

3. <u>cysto</u>scope _____

4. <u>trans</u>hepatic _____

5. <u>iatro</u>genic _____

6. <u>hypo</u>gastric _____

7. <u>endo</u>crine glands _____

8. nephr<u>ectomy</u> _____

9. <u>exo</u>crine glands _____

10. neur<u>algia</u> _____

O **Select from the terms listed below to complete the sentences that follow.**

anemia	oncogenic	psychiatrist
biopsy	oncologist	psychologist
diagnosis	osteoarthritis	thrombocyte
leukemia	pathogenic	thrombosis
nephrologist	prognosis	urologist
neuropathy		

1. Pamela Crick is 72 years old and suffers from a degenerative joint disease that is caused by the wearing away of tissue around her joints. This disease, which literally means "inflammation of bones and joints," is _____.

2. The _____ sample was removed during surgery and sent to a pathologist to be examined under a microscope for a proper diagnosis.

3. A/An _____ performed surgery to remove Mr. Simon's cancerous kidney.

4. Ms. Rose has suffered from diabetes with hyperglycemia for many years. This condition can lead to long-term complications, such as the disease of nerves called diabetic _____.

5. A virus or a bacterium produces disease and is therefore a/an _____ organism.

6. Jordan has a disease caused by abnormal hemoglobin in his erythrocytes. The erythrocytes change shape, collapsing to form sickle-shaped cells that can become clots and stop the flow of blood. His condition is called sickle cell _____.

7. Dr. Max Shelby is a physician who treats carcinomas and sarcomas. He is a/an _____.

8. Bill had difficulty stopping the bleeding from a cut on his face while shaving. He knew his medication caused him to have decreased platelets, or a low _____ count, and that probably was the reason his blood was not clotting very well.

9. Dr. Susan Parker told Paul that his condition would improve with treatment in a few weeks. She said his _____ is excellent and he can expect total recovery.

10. After fleeing the World Trade Center on September 11, 2001, Mrs. Jones had many problems with her job, her husband, and her family relationships. She went to see a _____, who prescribed drugs to treat her depression.

P Circle the correct term to complete each sentence.

1. Ms. Brody had a cough and fever. Her doctor instructed her to go to the (**pathology, radiology, hematology**) department for a chest x-ray examination.

2. After she gave birth to her fourth child, Ms. Thompson had problems holding her urine (a condition known as urinary incontinence). She made an appointment with a (**gastroenterologist, pathologist, urologist**) to evaluate her condition.

3. Dr. Monroe told a new mother she had lost much blood during delivery of her child. She had (**anemia, leukocytosis, adenitis**) and needed a blood transfusion immediately.

4. Mr. Preston was having chest pain during his morning walks. He made an appointment to discuss his new symptom with a (**nephrologist, neurologist, cardiologist**).

5. After my skiing accident, Dr. Curtin suggested (**cystoscopy, biopsy, arthroscopy**) to visually examine my swollen, painful knee.

ANSWERS TO EXERCISES

A

1. prefixes
2. suffixes
3. root
4. combining vowel
5. combining form

B

1. heart
2. gland
3. life
4. cerebrum, largest part of the brain
5. head
6. joint
7. cancer, cancerous
8. urinary bladder
9. cell
10. skin
11. brain
12. electricity

C

1. tumor, mass, swelling
2. pertaining to
3. inflammation
4. process of study
5. process of visual examination
6. pertaining to
7. record (image)
8. process of viewing

D

1. cerebr/al—pertaining to the cerebrum, or largest part of the brain
2. bi/opsy—process of viewing life (removal of living tissue and viewing it under a microscope)
3. aden/itis—inflammation of a gland
4. cephal/ic—pertaining to the head
5. carcin/oma—tumor that is cancerous (cancerous tumor)
6. cyst/o/scopy—process of visually examining the urinary bladder
7. electr/o/cardi/o/gram—record of the electricity in the heart
8. cardi/o/logy—process of study of the heart
9. electr/o/encephal/o/gram—record of the electricity in the brain
10. dermat/itis—inflammation of the skin
11. arthr/o/scopy—process of visual examination of a joint
12. cyt/o/logy—process of study of cells

E

1. red
2. intestines (usually small intestine)
3. stomach
4. knowledge
5. blood
6. to cut
7. kidney
8. white
9. treatment, physician
10. liver
11. nerve
12. woman, female

F

1. leukocyte
2. gastritis
3. iatrogenic
4. nephrology
5. erythrocyte
6. hematoma
7. biopsy
8. neuralgia
9. ophthalmoscopy
10. enteritis

G

1. ren/o
2. path/o
3. ophthalm/o
4. sect/o
5. rhin/o
6. sarc/o
7. psych/o
8. ur/o
9. oste/o
10. radi/o
11. thromb/o
12. onc/o

H

1. ophthalmo<u>scopy</u>—process of visual examination of the eye
2. ophthalmo<u>scope</u>—instrument to visually examine the eye
3. onco<u>logy</u>—study of tumors
4. oste<u>itis</u>—inflammation of bone
5. psych<u>osis</u>—abnormal condition of the mind
6. thrombo<u>cyte</u>—clotting cell (platelet)
7. <u>renal</u>—pertaining to the kidney
8. neph<u>rectomy</u>—removal (excision or resection) of the kidney
9. osteo<u>tomy</u>—incision of (process of cutting into) a bone
10. resec<u>tion</u>—process of cutting back (in the sense of "cutting out" or removal)
11. carcino<u>genic</u>—pertaining to producing cancer
12. sarc<u>oma</u>—tumor of flesh (cancerous tumor of flesh tissue, such as bone, fat, and muscle)

1

I

1. pain
2. process
3. blood condition
4. record (image)
5. instrument to visually examine
6. condition, usually abnormal
7. excision, removal (resection)
8. pertaining to producing, produced by, or produced in
9. disease condition
10. process of cutting, incision
11. inflammation
12. cell
13. protein

J

1. carcinogenic
2. leukocytosis
3. hepatoma (hepatocellular carcinoma)
4. arthralgia
5. endocrine
6. cystitis
7. hematoma
8. leukemia
9. iatrogenic
10. encephalopathy

K

1. complete, through
2. before
3. self, own
4. no, not, without
5. excessive, above, more than normal
6. deficient, below, less than normal
7. above, upon
8. within
9. behind
10. across, through
11. surrounding
12. out
13. below, under
14. back

L

1. diagnosis   complete knowledge; a decision about the nature of the patient's condition after the appropriate tests are done
2. prognosis—before knowledge; a prediction about the outcome of treatment, given after the diagnosis
3. subhepatic—pertaining to below the liver. A combining vowel is not needed between the prefix and the root.
4. pericardium—the membrane surrounding the heart
5. hyperglycemia—condition of excessive sugar in the blood
6. hypodermic—pertaining to under the skin
7. epigastric—pertaining to above the stomach
8. resection—process of cutting back (in the sense of cutting out)
9. hypoglycemia—condition of deficient (low) sugar in the blood
10. anemia—condition of low numbers of erythrocytes (red blood cells) or deficient hemoglobin in these cells. Notice that the root in this term is *em*, which is shortened from *hem*, meaning blood.

M

1. urology
2. gynecology
3. hematology
4. oncology
5. nephrology
6. neurology
7. pediatrics (combining vowel o has been dropped between *ped* and *iatr*)
8. radiology
9. ophthalmology
10. gastroenterology
11. endocrinology
12. psychiatry
13. pathology
14. cardiology

N

1. cerebrum (largest part of the brain). A cerebrovascular accident, or stroke, is damage to the blood vessels of the cerebrum, leading to death of brain cells.
2. brain. Encephalitis is inflammation of the brain.
3. urinary bladder. A cystoscope is an instrument used to visually examine the urinary bladder. The cystoscope is inserted into the urethra and urinary bladder.
4. across, through. Transhepatic means pertaining to across or through the liver.
5. treatment. Iatrogenic means pertaining to an adverse side effect produced by treatment.
6. under, below, deficient. Hypogastric means pertaining to below the stomach.
7. within. Endocrine glands secrete hormones within the body. Examples of these are the
pituitary, thyroid, and adrenal glands.
8. excision or resection. Nephrectomy is the removal of a kidney.
9. outside. Exocrine glands secrete chemicals to the outside of the body. Examples are the sweat, lacrimal or tear-producing, prostate, and salivary glands.
10. pain. Neuralgia is nerve pain.

1

O

1. osteoarthritis
2. biopsy
3. urologist (a nephrologist is a medical doctor who treats kidney disorders but does not operate on patients)

4. neuropathy
5. pathogenic
6. anemia
7. oncologist
8. thrombocyte
9. prognosis

10. psychiatrist (a psychologist can treat mentally ill patients but is not a medical doctor and cannot prescribe medications)

P

1. radiology
2. urologist
3. anemia

4. cardiologist
5. arthroscopy

Answers to Practical Applications

1. **D** A **cardiologist** is an internal medicine specialist who takes additional (fellowship) training in the diagnosis and treatment of heart disease.

2. **F** A **gynecologist** specializes in surgery and internal medicine to diagnose and treat disorders of the female reproductive system. Ovarian cysts are sacs of fluid that form on and in the ovaries (female organs that produce eggs and hormones).

3. **J** A **psychiatrist** is a specialist in diagnosing and treating mental illness. In bipolar disorder (manic-depressive illness), the mood switches periodically from excessive mania (excitability) to deep depression (sadness, despair, and discouragement).

4. **E** An **oncologist** is an internal medicine specialist who takes fellowship training in the diagnosis and medical (drug) treatment of cancer.

5. **B** A **hematologist** is an internal medicine specialist who takes fellowship training in the diagnosis and treatment of blood disorders such as anemia and clotting diseases.

6. **H** An **ophthalmologist** trains in both surgery and internal medicine in order to diagnose and treat disorders of the eye. The retina is a sensitive layer of light receptor cells in the back of the eye. Retinopathy can occur as a secondary complication of chronic diabetes (from hyperglycemia).

7. **I** A **neurologist** is an internal medicine specialist who takes fellowship training in the diagnosis and treatment of disorders of nervous tissue (brain, spinal cord, and nerves). A **CVA** causes damage to areas of the brain, resulting in loss of function.

8. **C** A **nephrologist** is an internal medicine specialist who takes fellowship training in the

diagnosis and medical treatment of kidney disease. A nephrologist does not perform surgery on the urinary tract, but treats kidney disease with drugs.

9. **A** A **gastroenterologist** is an internal medicine specialist who takes fellowship training in the diagnosis and treatment of disorders of the gastrointestinal tract. Examples of inflammatory bowel disease are ulcerative colitis (inflammation of the large intestine) and Crohn disease (inflammation of the last part of the small intestine).

10. **G** A **urologist** is a surgeon who operates on organs of the urinary tract and the male reproductive system (such as the prostate gland). Urologists also prescribe drugs for some conditions.

PRONUNCIATION OF TERMS

The markings ‾ and ˇ above the vowels—a, e, i, o, and u—indicate the proper sounds of the vowels in a term. When ‾ is above a vowel, its sound is long—that is, exactly like its name. The ˇ marking indicates a short vowel sound. The CAPITAL letters indicate the accented syllable.

To test your understanding of the terminology in this chapter, write the meaning of each term in the space provided. In addition, you may wish to cover the terms and write them by looking at your definitions. Make sure your spelling is correct. The page number after each term indicates where it is defined or used in the book, so you can easily check your responses. You will find complete definitions for all of these terms and their audio pronunciations on the Evolve website.

Pronunciation Guide

ā as in āpe	ă as in ăpple
ē as in ēven	ĕ as in ĕvery
ī as in īce	ĭ as in ĭnterest
ō as in ōpen	ŏ as in pŏt
ū as in ūnit	ŭ as in ŭnder

TERM	PRONUNCIATION	MEANING
adenitis (7)	ăd-ĕ-NĪ-tĭs	
adenoma (7)	ăd-ĕ-NŌ-mă	
adenopathy (14)	ăd-ĕ-NŎP-ă-thē	
anemia (14)	ă-NĒ-mē-ă	
arthralgia (13)	ăr-THRĂL-jă	
arthritis (7)	ăr-THRĪ-tĭs	
autopsy (14)	ĂW-tŏp-sē	
biology (7)	bī-ŎL-ō-jē	
biopsy (7)	BĪ-ŏp-sē	
carcinogenic (13)	kăr-sĭ-nō-JĔN-ĭk	
carcinoma (7)	kăr-sĭ-NŌ-mă	
cardiac (13)	KĂR-dē-ăk	
cardiology (7)	kăr-dē-ŎL-ō-jē	
cephalic (7)	sĕ-FĂL-ĭk	
cerebral (8)	sĕ-RĒ-brăl *or* SĔR-ĕ-brăl	
cystitis (13)	sĭs-TĪ-tĭs	
cystoscopy (8)	sĭs-TŎS-kō-pē	
cytology (9)	sī-TŎL-ō-jē	
dermatitis (9)	dĕr-mă-TĪ-tĭs	

1

TERM	PRONUNCIATION	MEANING
dermatology (10)	dĕr-mă-TŎL-ō-jē	_____
diagnosis (15)	dī-ăg-NŌ-sĭs	_____
electrocardiogram (9)	ē-lĕk-trō-KĂR-dē-ō-grăm	_____
electroencephalogram (9)	ē-lĕk-trō-ĕn-SĔF-ă-lō-grăm	_____
endocrine glands (8)	ĔN-dō-krĭn glăndz	_____
endocrinologist (15)	ĕn-dō-krĭ-NŎL-ō-jĭst	_____
endocrinology (13)	ĕn-dō-krĭ-NŎL-ō-jē	_____
endoscope (14)	ĔN-dō-skōp	_____
endoscopy (14)	ĕn-DŎS-kō-pē	_____
enteritis (9)	ĕn-tĕ-RĪ-tĭs	_____
enteropathy (14)	ĕn-tĕ-RŎP-ă-thē	_____
epidermis (15)	ĕp-ĭ-DĔR-mĭs	_____
epigastric (15)	ĕp-ĭ-GĂS-trĭk	_____
erythrocyte (9)	ĕ-RĬTH-rō-sīt	_____
excision (8)	ĕk-SĬ-zhŭn	_____
exocrine glands (15)	ĔK-sō-krĭn glăndz	_____
gastrectomy (9)	găs-TRĔK-tō-mē	_____
gastric (13)	GĂS-trĭk	_____
gastroenterology (14)	găs-trō-ĕn-tĕr-ŎL-ō-jē	_____
gastrotomy (9)	găs-TRŎT-ō-mē	_____
gynecologist (26)	gī-nĕ-KŎL-ō-jĭst	_____
gynecology (10)	gī-nĕ-KŎL-ō-jē	_____
hematology (10)	hē-mă-TŎL-ō-jē	_____
hematoma (10)	hē-mă-TŌ-mă	_____
hemoglobin (10)	HĒ-mō-glō-bĭn	_____
hepatitis (10)	hĕp-ă-TĪ-tĭs	_____
hepatoma (13)	hĕp-ă-TŌ-mă	_____
hyperglycemia (10)	hī-pĕr-glī-SĒ-mē-ă	_____
hyperthyroidism (15)	hī-pĕr-THĪ-rŏyd-ĭsm	_____
hypodermic (9)	hī-pō-DĔR-mĭk	_____

1

TERM	PRONUNCIATION	MEANING
hypogastric (15)	hī-pō-GĂS-trĭk	_____
hypoglycemia (15)	hī-pō-glī-SĒ-mē-ă	_____
iatrogenic (10)	ī-ăt-rō-JĔN-ĭk	_____
incision (8)	ĭn-SĬ-zhŭn	_____
leukemia (13)	loo-KĒ-mē-ă	_____
leukocyte (10)	LOO-kō-sīt	_____
leukocytosis (14)	loo-kō-sī-TŌ-sĭs	_____
nephrectomy (13)	nĕ-FRĔK-tō-mē	_____
nephritis (10)	nĕ-FRĪ-tĭs	_____
nephrology (10)	nĕ-FRŎL-ō-jē	_____
nephrosis (14)	nĕ-FRŌ-sĭs	_____
neural (13)	NŪ-răl	_____
neuralgia (13)	nū-RĂL-jă	_____
neurologic (13)	nū-rō-LŎJ-ĭk	_____
neurology (10)	nū-RŎL-ō-jē	_____
oncologist (11)	ŏn-KŎL-ō-jĭst	_____
oncology (11)	ŏn-KŎL-ō-jē	_____
ophthalmologist (13)	ŏf-thăl-MŎL-ō-jĭst	_____
ophthalmoscope (11)	ŏf-THĂL-mō-skōp	_____
osteitis (11)	ŏs-tē-Ī-tĭs	_____
osteoarthritis (11)	ŏs-tē-ō-ăr-THRĪ-tĭs	_____
osteotomy (14)	ŏs-tē-ŎT-ō-mē	_____
pathogenic (13)	păth-ō-JĔN-ĭk	_____
pathologist (11)	pă-THŎL-ō-jĭst	_____
pathology (11)	pă-THŎL-ō-jē	_____
pediatric (11)	pē-dē-ĂT-rĭk	_____
pericardium (15)	pĕr-ĭ-KĂR-dē-ŭm	_____
prognosis (10)	prŏg-NŌ-sĭs	_____
prostate gland (15)	PRŎS-tāt glănd	_____
psychiatrist (12)	sī-KĪ-ă-trĭst	_____

TERM	PRONUNCIATION	MEANING
psychology (12)	sī-KŎL-ō-jē	_____
radiology (12)	rā-dē-ŎL-ō-jē	_____
renal (12)	RĒ-năl	_____
resection (12)	rē-SĔK-shŭn	_____
retrocardiac (15)	rĕ-trō-KĂR-dē-ăc	_____
rhinitis (12)	rī-NĪ-tĭs	_____
sarcoma (12)	săr-KŌ-mă	_____
subhepatic (15)	sŭb-hĕ-PĂT-ĭk	_____
thrombocyte (12)	THRŎM-bō-sīt	_____
transhepatic (15)	trănz-hĕ-PĂT-ĭk	_____
urologist (12)	ū-RŎL-ō-jĭst	_____

1

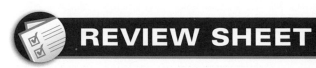

REVIEW SHEET

This Review Sheet and the others that follow each chapter are complete lists of the word elements contained in the chapter. They are designed to pull together the terminology and to reinforce your learning by giving you the opportunity to write the meanings of each word part in the spaces provided and to **test yourself.** Check your answers with the information in the chapter or in the *Glossary (Medical Word Parts—English),* at the end of the book. It's a good idea to tab the Glossary so that you can easily locate it.

Combining Forms

COMBINING FORM	MEANING	COMBINING FORM	MEANING
aden/o		hem/o, hemat/o	
arthr/o		hepat/o	
bi/o		iatr/o	
carcin/o		leuk/o	
cardi/o		log/o	
cephal/o		nephr/o	
cerebr/o		neur/o	
cis/o		onc/o	
crin/o		ophthalm/o	
cyst/o		oste/o	
cyt/o		path/o	
derm/o, dermat/o		ped/o	
electr/o		psych/o	
encephal/o		radi/o	
enter/o		ren/o	
erythr/o		rhin/o	
gastr/o		sarc/o	
glyc/o		sect/o	
gnos/o		thromb/o	
gynec/o		ur/o	

1

Suffixes

SUFFIX	MEANING	SUFFIX	MEANING
-ac ◤	_____	-itis	_____
-al	_____	-logy	_____
-algia	_____	-oma	_____
-cyte	_____	-opsy	_____
-ectomy	_____	-osis	_____
-emia	_____	-pathy	_____
-genic	_____	-scope	_____
-globin	_____	-scopy	_____
-gram	_____	-sis	_____
-ic, -ical	_____	-tomy	_____
-ion	_____	-y	_____
-ist	_____		

Prefixes

PREFIX	MEANING	PREFIX	MEANING
a-, an-	_____	in-	_____
aut-, auto-	_____	peri-	_____
dia-	_____	pro-	_____
endo-	_____	re-	_____
epi-	_____	retro-	_____
ex-, exo-	_____	sub-	_____
hyper-	_____	trans-	_____
hypo-	_____		

Suffixes Meaning Pertaining To

There are many suffixes that mean "pertaining to." In this chapter, you have learned -ac, -al, -ic, and -ical. For a more comprehensive list, see the **Glossary (English to Medical Word Parts)**, page 959.

evolve   *Please visit the Evolve website for additional exercises, games, and images related to this chapter.*

Terms Pertaining to the Body as a Whole

CHAPTER GOALS

- Define terms that apply to the structural organization of the body.
- Identify the body cavities and recognize the organs contained within those cavities.
- Locate and identify the anatomic and clinical divisions of the abdomen.
- Locate and name the anatomic divisions of the back.
- Become acquainted with terms that describe positions, directions, and planes of the body.
- Identify the meanings for new word elements and use them to understand medical terms.

STRUCTURAL ORGANIZATION OF THE BODY

This chapter provides you with an orientation to the body as a whole—cells, tissues, organs, and systems—along with terminology describing positions and directions within the body. We begin with the smallest living unit, the **cell**, and build to an understanding of complex body systems. In order to know how organs function in both health and disease, it is important to appreciate the workings of their individual cellular units.

CELLS

The cell is the fundamental unit of all living things (animal or plant). Cells are everywhere in the human body—every tissue, every organ is made up of these individual units.

Similarity in Cells

All cells are similar in that they contain a gelatinous substance composed of water, protein, sugar, acids, fats, and various minerals. Several parts of a cell, described next, are pictured in Figure 2-1 as they might look when photographed with an electron microscope. Label the structures on Figure 2-1. Throughout the book, numbers or letters in brackets indicate that the boldface term preceding it is to be used in labeling.

The **cell membrane** [1] not only surrounds and protects the cell but also regulates what passes into and out of the cell.

The **nucleus** [2] controls the operations of the cell. It directs cell division and determines the structure and function of the cell.

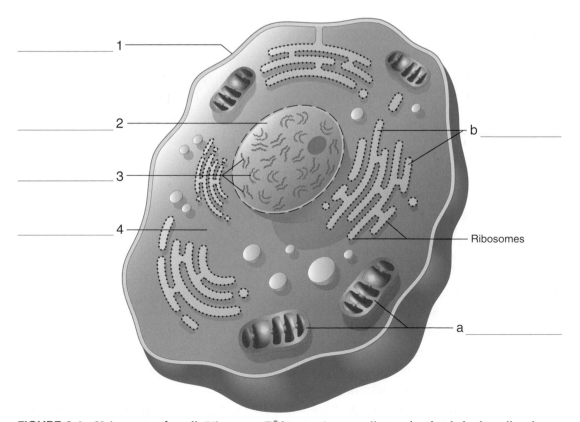

FIGURE 2-1   Major parts of a cell. Ribosomes (RĪ-bō-sōmz) are small granules that help the cell make proteins.

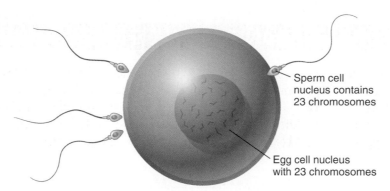

FIGURE 2-2 **Egg and sperm cells,** each containing 23 chromosomes.

Chromosomes [3] are rod-like structures within the nucleus. All human body cells—except for the sex cells, the egg and the sperm (short for spermatozoon)—contain 23 pairs of chromosomes. Each sperm and each egg cell have only 23 unpaired chromosomes. After an egg and a sperm cell unite to form the embryo, each cell of the embryo then has 46 chromosomes (23 pairs) (Figure 2-2).

Chromosomes contain regions called **genes.** There are several thousand genes, in an orderly sequence, on every chromosome. Each gene contains a chemical called **DNA** (deoxyribonucleic acid). DNA regulates the activities of the cell according to its sequence (arrangement into genes) on each chromosome. The DNA sequence resembles a series of recipes in code. This code, when passed out of the nucleus to the rest of the cell, directs the activities of the cell, such as cell division and synthesis of proteins.

A **karyotype** is a photograph of an individual's chromosomes, arranged by size, shape, and number (Figure 2-3). Karyotyping can determine whether chromosomes are normal.

2

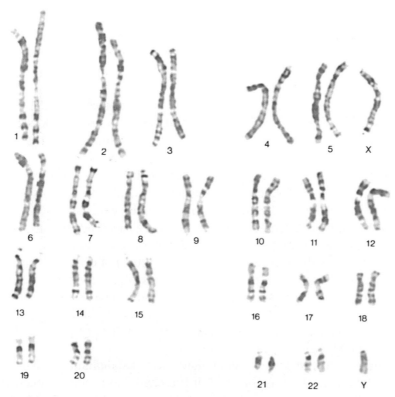

FIGURE 2-3 **Karyotype of a normal male.** Twenty-three pairs of chromosomes are shown. The 23rd pair is the XY pair present in normal males. In normal females, the 23rd pair is XX. For this karyotype, the chromosomes were treated with chemicals so that bands of light and dark areas are seen.

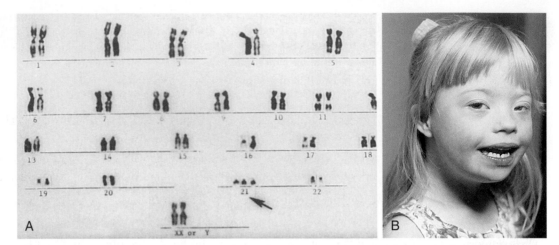

FIGURE 2-4 **A, Karyotype of a Down syndrome female** patient showing trisomy 21. There is an extra copy of chromosome 21, in addition to the usual pair, for a total of three (tri-). **B,** Photograph of a child with the typical facial appearance in Down syndrome. Features include a small, somewhat flat nose and upward slant of the eyes. Other characteristics of patients with Down syndrome are mental deficiency and heart defects.

For example, an obstetrician may recommend amniocentesis (puncture of the sac around the fetus for removal of fluid and cells) for a pregnant woman so that the karyotype of the baby can be examined.

If a baby is born with a chromosomal abnormality, serious problems can result. In Down syndrome, the karyotype shows 47 chromosomes instead of the normal number, 46 (Figure 2-4). The extra chromosome 21 results in the development of a child with Down syndrome (also called trisomy 21 syndrome). Its incidence is about 1 in every 750 live births, but as the mother's age increases, the presence of the chromosomal abnormality increases.

Continue labeling Figure 2-1.

The **cytoplasm** [4] (cyt/o = cell, -plasm = formation) includes all of the material outside the nucleus and enclosed by the cell membrane. It carries on the work of the cell (e.g., in a muscle cell, it does the contracting; in a nerve cell, it transmits impulses). The cytoplasm contains specialized apparatus to supply the chemical needs of the cell.

Mitochondria [a] are small sausage-shaped bodies that provide the principal source of energy for the cell. They use nutrients and oxygen to release energy that is stored in food. During the chemical process called **catabolism,** complex foods such as sugar and fat are broken down into simpler substances and energy is released by the mitochondria. Thus, catabolism provides the energy for cells to do the work of the body.

The **endoplasmic reticulum** [b] is a network (reticulum) of canals within the cell. These canals are cellular tunnel systems that manufacture proteins for the cell. Attached to the endoplasmic reticulum are **ribosomes,** which build long chains of proteins. **Anabolism,** occurring on the endoplasmic reticulum, is the process of building large proteins from small protein pieces called amino acids. Examples of important proteins for cell growth are hormones and enzymes.

Together, these two processes—**anabolism** and **catabolism**—make up the cell's **metabolism.** Metabolism, then, is the total of the chemical processes occurring in a cell. If a person has a "fast metabolism," foods such as sugar and fat are used up very quickly, and energy is released. If a person has a "slow metabolism," foods are burned slowly, and fat accumulates in cells.

STUDY SECTION 1

Practice spelling each term, and know its meaning.

anabolism	Process of building up large proteins from small protein pieces called amino acids. Ana- means up, bol means to cast, and -ism is a process.
catabolism	Process whereby complex nutrients are broken down to simpler substances and energy is released. Cata- means down, bol means to cast, and -ism is a process.
cell membrane	Structure surrounding and protecting the cell. It determines what enters and leaves the cell.
chromosomes	Rod-shaped structures in the nucleus that contain regions of DNA called genes. There are 46 chromosomes (23 pairs) in every cell except for the egg and sperm cells, which contain only 23 individual, unpaired chromosomes.
cytoplasm	All of the material that is outside the nucleus and yet contained within the cell membrane.
DNA	Chemical found within each chromosome. Arranged like a sequence of recipes in code, it directs the activities of the cell.
endoplasmic reticulum	Network of canals within the cytoplasm of the cell. Here, large proteins are made from smaller protein pieces.
genes	Regions of DNA within each chromosome.
karyotype	Picture of chromosomes in the nucleus of a cell. The chromosomes are arranged in numerical order to determine their number and structure.
metabolism	Total of the chemical processes in a cell. It includes catabolism and anabolism. Meta- means change, bol means to cast, and -ism means a process.
mitochondria	Structures in the cytoplasm that provide the principal source of energy (miniature "power plants") for the cell. **Catabolism** is the process that occurs in mitochondria. (From the Greek *mitos* meaning thread and *chondrion* meaning granule.) ⊛ **HINT:** Think of "mighty" mitochondria!
nucleus	Control center of the cell. It contains chromosomes and directs the activities of the cell.

Anabolic Steroids

These drugs are similar to **androgens** (male hormones) in their effects on the body. They build up protein within cells.

Metabolism and the Thyroid Gland

The thyroid gland secretes thyroid hormone (thyroxine, or T_4), which stimulates metabolism in cells. Increased levels of hormone speed up metabolism (increased energy and weight loss) and decreased levels of hormone slow down metabolism (sluggishness and weight gain).

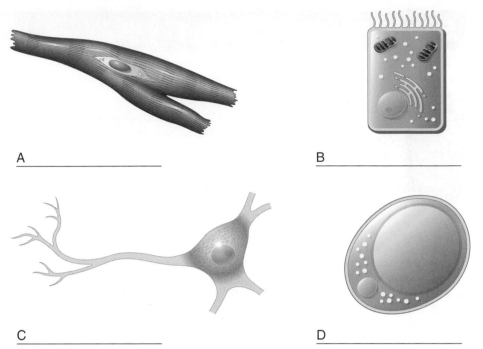

A _____   B _____

C _____   D _____

FIGURE 2-5   **Types of cells. A, muscle cell; B, epithelial cell; C, nerve cell; and D, fat cell.**

Differences in Cells

While we have just seen how cells contain similar structures, as they develop in the embryo, cells change to form many different types. Cells are different, or specialized, throughout the body to carry out their individual functions. For example, a **muscle cell** is long and slender and contains fibers that aid in contracting and relaxing; an **epithelial cell** (a lining and skin cell) may be square and flat to provide protection; a **nerve cell** may be long and have various fibrous extensions that aid in its job of carrying impulses; a **fat cell** contains large, empty spaces for fat storage. These are only a few of the many types of cells in the body. Figure 2-5 illustrates the different sizes and shapes of muscle, epithelial, nerve, and fat cells.

TISSUES

A tissue is a group of similar cells working together to do a specific job. A **histologist** (hist/o = tissue) is a scientist who specializes in the study of tissues. Several different types of tissue are recognized. Tissues of the same type may be located in various regions of the body. Figure 2-6 illustrates four types of tissues.

Epithelial Tissue

Epithelial tissue, located all over the body, forms the linings of internal organs, and the outer surface of the skin covering the body. It also lines exocrine and endocrine glands and is responsible for the secretions that the glands produce. The term **epithelial** originally referred to the tissue on (epi-) the breast nipple (thel/o). Now it describes all tissue that covers the outside of the body and lines the inner surface of internal organs.

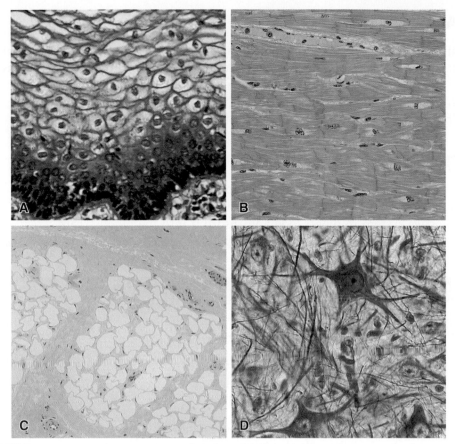

FIGURE 2-6   Types of tissues. A, Epithelial. B, Muscle. C, Connective tissue (Fat). D, Nerve.

Muscle Tissue

Voluntary muscle is found in arms and legs and parts of the body where movement is under conscious control. Involuntary muscle, found in the heart and digestive system, as well as other organs, allows movement that is not under conscious control. Cardiac muscle is a specialized type of muscle found only in the heart. Contractions of this muscle type can be seen as a beating heart in an ultrasound scan of a 6-week-old fetus.

Connective Tissue

Examples are **adipose** (fat) tissue, **cartilage** (elastic, fibrous tissue attached to bones), bone, and blood.

Nerve Tissue

Nerve tissue conducts impulses all over the body.

ORGANS

Different types of tissue combine to form an organ. For example, an organ such as the stomach is composed of muscle tissue, nerve tissue, and glandular epithelial tissue. The medical term for internal organs is **viscera** (singular: **viscus**). Examples of abdominal viscera (organs located in the abdomen) are the liver, stomach, intestines, pancreas, spleen, and gallbladder.

SYSTEMS

Systems are groups of organs working together to perform complex functions. For example, the mouth, esophagus, stomach, and small and large intestines are organs that do the work of the digestive system to digest food and absorb it into the bloodstream.

The body systems with their individual organs are listed next. Learn to spell and identify the organs in **boldface.**

SYSTEM	ORGANS
Digestive	Mouth, **pharynx** (throat), esophagus, stomach, intestines (small and large), liver, gallbladder, pancreas
Urinary or excretory	Kidneys, **ureters** (tubes from the kidneys to the urinary bladder), urinary bladder, **urethra** (tube from the bladder to the outside of the body)
Respiratory	Nose, pharynx, **larynx** (voice box), **trachea** (windpipe), bronchial tubes, lungs (where the exchange of gases takes place)
Reproductive	*Female*: Ovaries, fallopian tubes, **uterus** (womb), vagina, mammary glands *Male*: Testes and associated tubes, urethra, penis, prostate gland
Endocrine	**Thyroid gland** (in the neck), **pituitary gland** (at the base of the brain), sex glands (ovaries and testes), adrenal glands, pancreas (islets of Langerhans), parathyroid glands
Nervous	Brain, spinal cord, nerves, and collections of nerves
Circulatory	Heart, blood vessels (arteries, veins, and capillaries), lymphatic vessels and nodes, spleen, thymus gland
Musculoskeletal	Muscles, bones, and joints
Skin and sense organs	Skin, hair, nails, sweat glands, and sebaceous (oil) glands; eye, ear, nose, and tongue

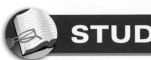

STUDY SECTION 2

Practice spelling each term, and know its meaning.

adipose tissue	Collection of fat cells.
cartilage	Flexible connective tissue often attached to bones at joints. Cartilage forms part of the external ear and the nose. Rings of cartilage surround the trachea.
epithelial cells	Skin cells that cover the outside of the body line the internal surfaces of organs.
histologist	Specialist in the study of tissues.
larynx (LĂR-ĭnks)	Voice box; located at the upper part of the trachea. ✱ **HINT**: Think of the word *laryngitis,* which means inflammation of the voice box, and may result in losing your voice!
pharynx (FĂR-ĭnks)	Throat. The pharynx serves as the common passageway for food (from the mouth going to the esophagus) and air (from the nose to the trachea). ✱ **HINT**: Note that "y" comes before "n" in both pha**ryn**x and la**ryn**x.
pituitary gland	Endocrine gland at the base of the brain.
thyroid gland	Endocrine gland that surrounds the trachea in the neck.
trachea	Windpipe (tube leading from the throat to the bronchial tubes).
ureter	One of two tubes, each leading from a single kidney to the urinary bladder. ✱ **HINT**: *Spelling clue*: Ureter has two **e**'s, and there are two ureters.
urethra	Tube from the urinary bladder to the outside of the body. ✱ **HINT**: *Spelling clue*: Urethra has one **e**, and there is only one urethra.
uterus	Womb; the organ that holds the embryo/fetus as it develops.
viscera	Internal organs.

2

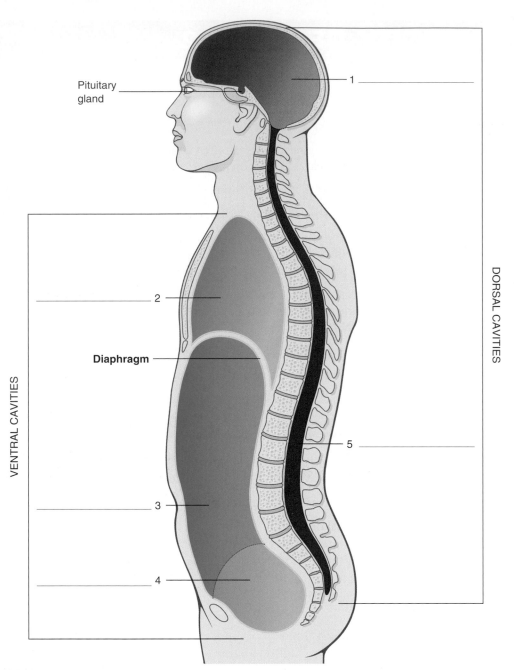

FIGURE 2-7   **Body cavities. Ventral** (anterior) cavities are in the front of the body (*blue*). **Dorsal** (posterior) cavities are in the back (*red*).

BODY CAVITIES

A body cavity is a space within the body that contains internal organs (viscera). Label Figure 2-7 as you learn the names of the body cavities. Some of the important organs contained within those cavities are listed as well.

CAVITY	ORGANS
Cranial [1]	Brain, pituitary gland.
Thoracic [2]	Lungs, heart, esophagus, trachea, bronchial tubes, thymus gland, aorta (large artery).

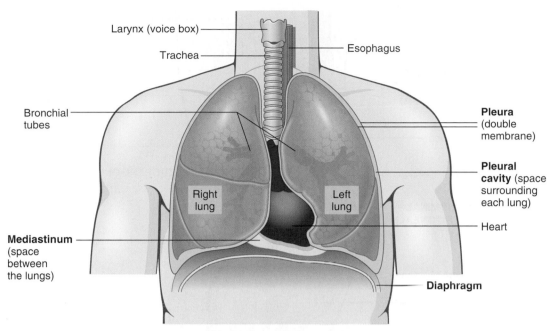

FIGURE 2-8   Thoracic Cavity.

CAVITY	ORGANS

The thoracic cavity is divided into two smaller cavities (Figure 2-8):
- a. **Pleural cavity**—space surrounding each lung. The **pleura** is a double membrane that surrounds the lungs and protects them. If the **pleura** is inflamed (as in pleuritis or pleurisy), the pleural cavity may fill with fluid.
- b. **Mediastinum**—centrally located space outside of and between the lungs. It contains the heart, aorta, trachea, esophagus, thymus gland, bronchial tubes, and many lymph nodes.

Continue labeling Figure 2-7.

Abdominal [3]   The **peritoneum** is the double-folded membrane surrounding the abdominal cavity (Figure 2-9). It attaches the abdominal organs to the abdominal muscles and surrounds each organ to hold it in place. The kidneys are two bean-shaped organs situated behind (retroperitoneal area) the abdominal cavity on either side of the backbone (see Figures 2-9 and 2-11). Also contains the stomach, small and large intestines, spleen, pancreas, liver, and gallbladder. The **diaphragm** (a muscular wall) divides the abdominal and thoracic cavities (see Figure 2-7).

Pelvic [4]   Portions of the small and large intestines, rectum, urinary bladder, urethra, and ureters; uterus and vagina in the female.

Spinal [5]   Nerves of the spinal cord.

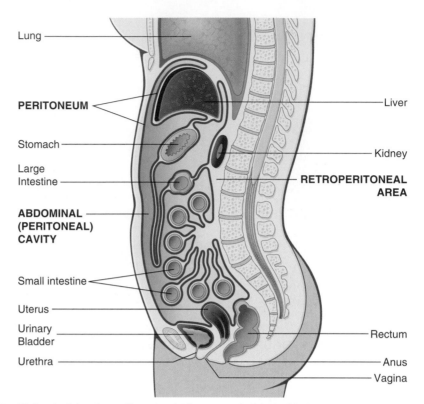

Lung

PERITONEUM

Stomach

Large Intestine

ABDOMINAL (PERITONEAL) CAVITY

Small intestine

Uterus

Urinary Bladder

Urethra

Liver

Kidney

RETROPERITONEAL AREA

Rectum

Anus

Vagina

FIGURE 2-9 **Abdominal (peritoneal) cavity** (*side view* and in *light blue*). Notice the **peritoneum,** which is a membrane surrounding the organs in the abdominal cavity. The **retroperitoneal area** is behind the peritoneum.

The cranial and spinal cavities are the dorsal (dors/o = back) body cavity because of their location on the back or posterior portion of the body. The thoracic, abdominal, and pelvic cavities are ventral (ventr/o = belly) body cavities because they are on the front (anterior) portion of the body (see Figure 2-7).

While the thoracic and abdominal cavities are separated by a muscular wall called the **diaphragm,** the abdominal and pelvic cavities are not separated and are referred to together as the **abdominopelvic cavity.** Figures 2-10 and 2-11 show the abdominal and thoracic viscera from anterior (ventral) and posterior (dorsal) views.

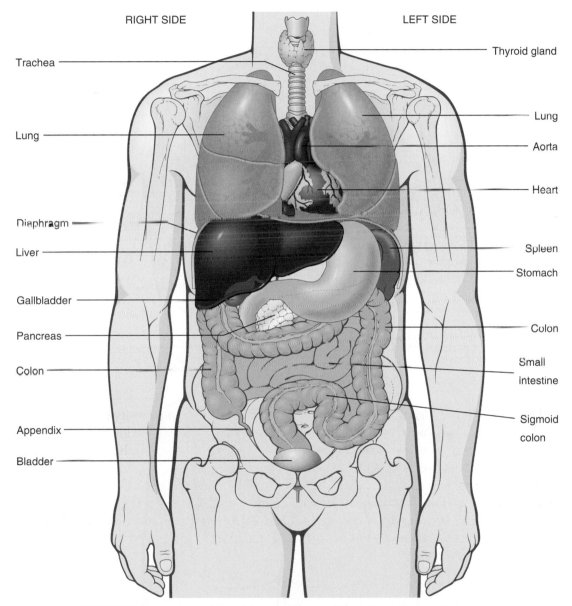

RIGHT SIDE

LEFT SIDE

Trachea

Lung

Diaphragm

Liver

Gallbladder

Pancreas

Colon

Appendix

Bladder

Thyroid gland

Lung

Aorta

Heart

Spleen

Stomach

Colon

Small intestine

Sigmoid colon

FIGURE 2-10   Organs of the abdominopelvic and thoracic cavities, anterior view.

2

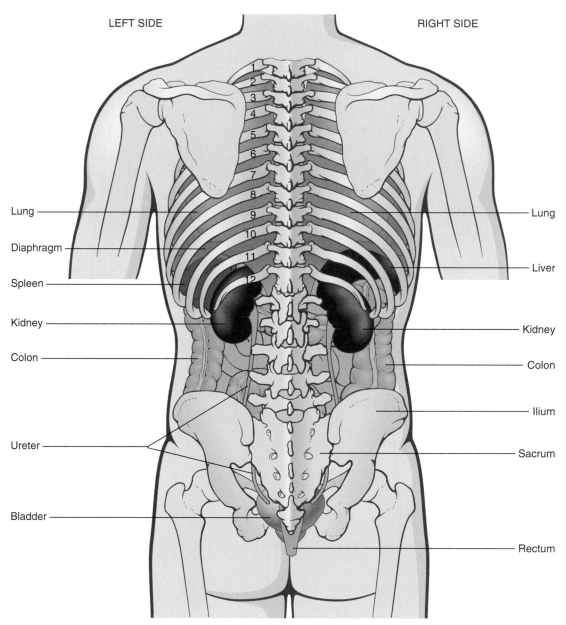

LEFT SIDE

RIGHT SIDE

Lung

Diaphragm

Spleen

Kidney

Colon

Ureter

Bladder

Lung

Liver

Kidney

Colon

Ilium

Sacrum

Rectum

FIGURE 2-11 Organs of the abdominopelvic and thoracic cavities, posterior view.

STUDY SECTION 3

Practice spelling each term, and know its meaning.

abdominal cavity	Space below the chest containing organs such as the liver, stomach, gallbladder, and intestines; also called the **abdomen** or **peritoneal cavity.**
cranial cavity	Space in the head containing the brain and surrounded by the skull. **Cranial** means **pertaining to the skull.**
diaphragm	Muscle separating the abdominal and thoracic cavities. The diaphragm moves up and down and aids in breathing.
dorsal (posterior)	Pertaining to the back.
mediastinum	Centrally located space outside of and between the lungs.
pelvic cavity	Space below the abdomen containing portions of the intestines, rectum, urinary bladder, and reproductive organs. **Pelvic** means **pertaining to the pelvis,** composed of the hip bones surrounding the pelvic cavity.
peritoneum	Double-folded membrane surrounding the abdominal cavity. The peritoneum attaches abdominal viscera to muscles and functions as a protective membrane (containing blood vessels and nerves) around the organs.
pleura	Double-folded membrane surrounding each lung. Pleural means pertaining to the pleura. ✱ **HINT:** Don't confuse *pleural* with *plural,* which means more than one!
pleural cavity	Space between the pleural layers.
spinal cavity	Space within the spinal column (backbones) containing the spinal cord. Also called the **spinal canal.**
thoracic cavity	Space in the chest containing the heart, lungs, bronchial tubes, trachea, esophagus, and other organs.
ventral (anterior)	Pertaining to the front.

2

Peritoneum and Other Membranes

Many vital organs are covered and protected by membranes. The **peritoneum** surrounds abdominal viscera (liver, small and large intestines, stomach), the **pleura** covers the lungs, the **periosteum** protects bones, and the **meninges** are membranes surrounding the brain and spinal cord.

You can visualize the way organs are surrounded by a double membrane by imagining your fist pushing deep into a soft balloon. The balloon is then in two layers folded over your fist, just the way the pleura surrounds the lungs and the peritoneum surrounds the abdominal organs. Double wrapping around organs provides protection and cushioning, as well as a site for attachment to muscles. In the event of inflammation or disease of organs or membranes, fluid may collect in the space between the membranes surrounding the organs. This collection of fluid in the pleural cavity is called a **pleural effusion.** A collection of fluid in the peritoneal cavity is called **ascites.**

ABDOMINOPELVIC REGIONS AND QUADRANTS

REGIONS

Doctors divide the abdominopelvic area into nine regions. Label these regions in Figure 2-12.

Right hypochondriac region [1]: right upper region below (hypo-) the cartilage (chondr/o) of the ribs that extend over the abdomen

Left hypochondriac region [2]: left upper region below the rib cartilage

Epigastric region [3]: region above the stomach

Right lumbar region [4]: right middle region near the waist

Left lumbar region [5]: left middle region near the waist

Umbilical region [6]: region of the navel or umbilicus

Right inguinal region [7]: right lower region near the groin (inguin/o = groin), which is the area where the legs join the trunk of the body. This region also is known as the **right iliac region** because it lies near the ilium (the upper portion of the hip bone).

Left inguinal region [8]: left lower region near the groin. Also called the **left iliac region.**

Hypogastric region [9]: middle lower region below the umbilical region.

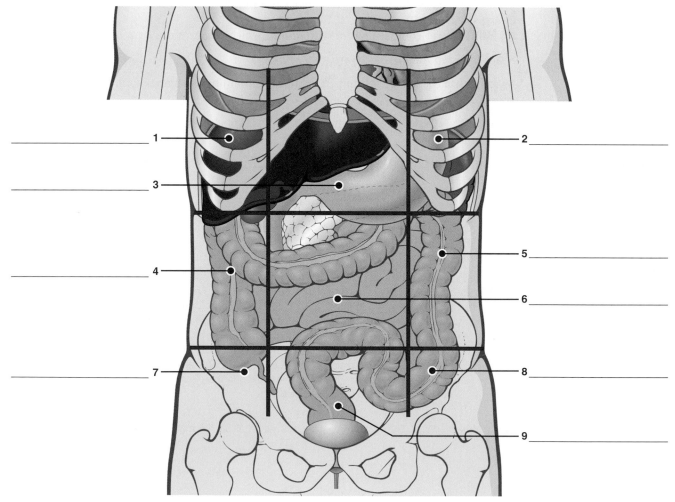

FIGURE 2-12 Abdominopelvic regions. These regions can be used clinically to locate internal organs.

QUADRANTS

The abdominopelvic area can be divided into four quadrants by two imaginary lines—one horizontal and one vertical—that cross at the midsection of the body. Figure 2-13 shows the four abdominopelvic quadrants; add the proper abbreviation on the line under each label on the diagram.

Right upper quadrant (RUQ)—contains the liver (right lobe), gallbladder, part of the pancreas, parts of the small and large intestines

Left upper quadrant (LUQ)—contains the liver (left lobe), stomach, spleen, part of the pancreas, parts of the small and large intestines

Right lower quadrant (RLQ)—contains parts of the small and large intestines, right ovary, right fallopian tube, appendix, right ureter

Left lower quadrant (LLQ)—contains parts of the small and large intestines, left ovary, left fallopian tube, left ureter

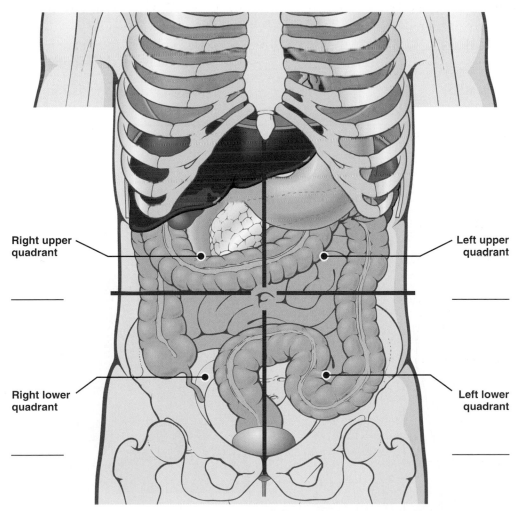

Right upper quadrant

Left upper quadrant

Right lower quadrant

Left lower quadrant

FIGURE 2-13   Abdominopelvic quadrants. Write the abbreviation for each quadrant on the line provided.

DIVISIONS OF THE BACK (SPINAL COLUMN)

The spinal column is composed of a series of bones that extend from the neck to the tailbone. Each bone is a **vertebra** (plural: **vertebrae**).

Label the divisions of the back on Figure 2-14A as you study the following:

DIVISION OF THE BACK	ABBREVIATION	LOCATION
Cervical [1]	C	Neck region. There are seven cervical vertebrae (C1 to C7).
Thoracic [2]	T	Chest region. There are 12 thoracic vertebrae (T1 to T12). Each bone is joined to a rib.
Lumbar [3]	L	Loin (waist) or flank region (between the ribs and the hipbone). There are five lumbar vertebrae (L1 to L5).
Sacral [4]	S	Five bones (S1 to S5) are fused to form one bone, the **sacrum**.
Coccygeal [5]		The **coccyx** (tailbone) is a small bone composed of four fused pieces.

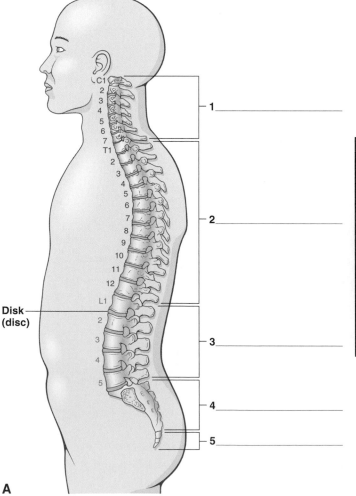

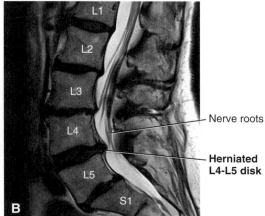

FIGURE 2-14 **A, Anatomic divisions of the back (spinal column).** A **disk (disc)** is a small pad of cartilage between each backbone. **B, MRI (magnetic resonance image)** of a **herniated disk** at the L4-L5 level of the spinal column.

Do not confuse the **spinal column** (backbones or vertebrae) with the **spinal cord** (nerves surrounded by the column). The **spinal column** is **bone tissue**, whereas the **spinal cord** is **nervous tissue**.

The spaces between the vertebrae (intervertebral spaces) are identified according to the two vertebrae between which they occur—for example, the L5–S1 space is between the fifth lumbar vertebra and the first sacral vertebra; T2–3 is between the second and third thoracic vertebrae. Within the space and between vertebrae is a small pad called a **disk,** or **disc.** The disk, composed of water and cartilage, is a shock absorber. Occasionally, a disk may move out of place (herniate) and put pressure on a nerve (see Figure 2-14B). This **"slipped disk"** can cause pain in an area of the body affected by the nerve.

 STUDY SECTION 4

Practice spelling each term, and know its meaning.

ABDOMINOPELVIC REGIONS

hypochondriac	Right and left upper regions beneath the ribs.
epigastric	Middle upper region above the stomach.
lumbar	Right and left middle regions near the waist.
umbilical	Central region near the navel.
inguinal	Right and left lower regions near the groin. Also called iliac regions.
hypogastric	Middle lower region below the umbilical region.

ABDOMINOPELVIC QUADRANTS

RUQ	Right upper quadrant.
LUQ	Left upper quadrant.
RLQ	Right lower quadrant.
LLQ	Left lower quadrant.

DIVISIONS OF THE BACK

cervical	Neck region (C1 to C7).
thoracic	Chest region (T1 to T12).
lumbar	Loin (waist) region (L1 to L5).
sacral	Region of the sacrum (S1 to S5).
coccygeal	Region of the coccyx (tailbone).

RELATED TERMS

vertebra	Single backbone.
vertebrae	Backbones.
spinal column	Bone tissue surrounding the spinal cavity.
spinal cord	Nervous tissue within the spinal cavity.
disk (disc)	Pad of cartilage between vertebrae.

2

2

POSITIONAL AND DIRECTIONAL TERMS

Label Figure 2-15 to identify the following positional and directional terms.

LOCATION	RELATIONSHIP
Anterior (ventral) [1]	**Front side of the body.** *Example*: The forehead is on the anterior side of the body.
Posterior (dorsal) [2]	**Back side of the body.** *Example*: The back of the head is posterior (dorsal) to the face.
Deep [3]	**Away from the surface.** *Example*: The stab wound penetrated deep into the abdomen.
Superficial [4]	**On the surface.** *Example*: Superficial veins can be viewed through the skin.
Proximal [5]	**Near the point of attachment to the trunk or near the beginning of a structure.** *Example*: The proximal end of the thigh bone (femur) joins with the hip socket.
Distal [6]	**Far from the point of attachment to the trunk or far from the beginning of a structure.** *Example*: At its distal end, the femur joins with the knee.
Inferior [7]	**Below another structure.** *Example*: The feet are at the inferior part of the body. They are inferior to the knees. The term **caudal** (pertaining to the tail, or to the lower portion of the body) also means away from the head or below another structure.
Superior [8]	**Above another structure.** *Example*: The head lies **superior** to the neck. **Cephalic** (pertaining to the head) also means above another structure.
Medial [9]	**Pertaining to the middle, or nearer the medial plane of the body.** *Example*: When in the anatomic position (palms of the hands facing outward), the fifth (little) finger is medial.
Lateral [10]	**Pertaining to the side.** *Example*: When in the anatomic position (palms of the hands facing outward), the thumb is lateral.
Supine [11]	**Lying on the back.** *Example*: The patient lies **supine** during an examination of the abdomen and, in females, during a pelvic (gynecologic) exam. See Figure 2-19 on page 65.
Prone [12]	**Lying on the belly.** *Example*: The backbones are examined with the patient in a **prone** position. A patient lies **on** his/her stomach in the pr**on**e position.

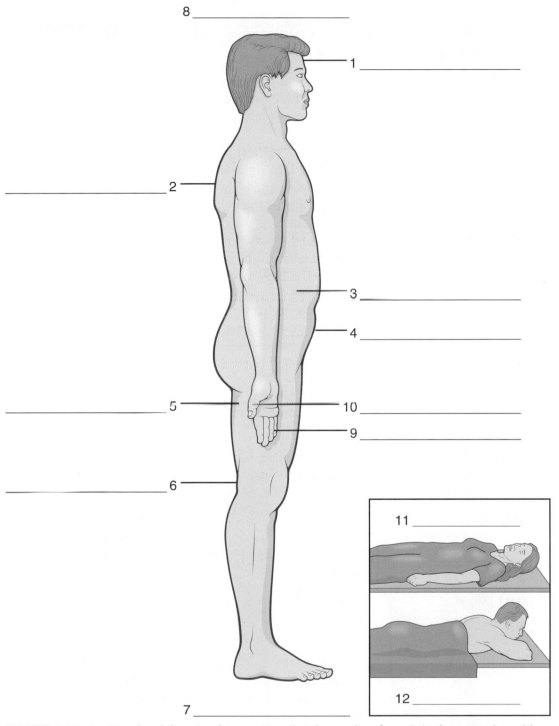

FIGURE 2-15   Positional and directional terms. Note that the standing figure is in the **anatomic position**, with the palms of the hands facing outward and the fifth (little) finger in a medial position (closer to the center of the body). The thumb is lateral.

PLANES OF THE BODY

A **plane** is an **imaginary** flat surface. Label Figure 2-16 to identify the following planes of the body:

PLANE	LOCATION
Frontal (coronal) plane [1]	**Vertical plane dividing the body or structure into anterior and posterior portions.** A common chest x-ray view is a PA (posteroanterior—viewed from back to front) view, which is in the frontal (coronal) plane. See Figure 2-16.
Sagittal (lateral) plane [2]	**Lengthwise vertical plane dividing the body or structure into right and left sides.** The **midsagittal** plane divides the body into right and left halves. A lateral (side-to-side) chest x-ray film is taken in the sagittal plane.
Transverse (axial) plane [3]	**Horizontal (cross-sectional) plane running across the body parallel to the ground.** This cross-sectional plane divides the body or structure into upper and lower portions. A CT (computed tomography) scan is one of a series of x-ray pictures taken in the transverse (axial or cross-sectional) plane.

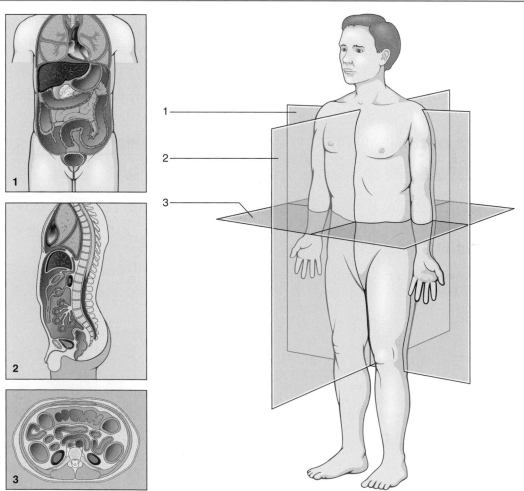

FIGURE 2-16 Planes of the body. The figure is in the **anatomic position.** Note the views of the body represented by each plane.

STUDY SECTION 5

Practice spelling each term, and know its meaning.

anterior (ventral)	Front surface of the body.
deep	Away from the surface.
distal	Far from the point of attachment to the trunk or far from the beginning of a structure.
frontal (coronal) plane	Vertical plane dividing the body or structure into anterior and posterior portions.
inferior (caudal)	Below another structure; pertaining to the tail or lower portion of the body.
lateral	Pertaining to the side.
medial	Pertaining to the middle or near the medial plane of the body.
posterior (dorsal)	Back surface of the body.
prone	Lying on the belly (face down, palms down).
proximal	Near the point of attachment to the trunk or near the beginning of a structure.
sagittal (lateral) plane	Lengthwise, vertical plane dividing the body or structure into right and left sides. From the Latin *sagitta*, meaning arrow. As an arrow is shot from a bow it enters the body in the sagittal plane, dividing right from left. The **midsagittal** plane divides the body into right and left halves.
superficial	On the surface.
superior (cephalic)	Above another structure; pertaining to the head.
supine	Lying on the back (face up, palms up).
transverse (axial) plane	Horizontal (cross-sectional) plane dividing the body into upper and lower portions.

2

TERMINOLOGY

Divide each term into its component parts, and write its meaning in the space provided.

COMBINING FORMS

COMBINING FORM	MEANING	TERMINOLOGY	MEANING
abdomin/o	abdomen	abdominal _____ *The abdomen is the region below the chest containing internal organs (such as the liver, intestines, stomach, and gallbladder).*	
adip/o	fat	adipose _____ *The suffix -ose means pertaining to or full of. Another combining form meaning fat is lip/o. Lipids are fats.*	
anter/o	front	anterior _____ *The suffix -ior means pertaining to.*	

COMBINING FORM	MEANING	TERMINOLOGY	MEANING
cervic/o	neck (of the body or of the uterus)	cervical *The **cervix** is the neck of the uterus. See Figure 2-17.*	
chondr/o	cartilage (type of connective tissue)	chondroma _____ *This is a benign tumor.* chondrosarcoma _____ *This is a malignant tumor. The root sarc indicates that the malignant tumor arises from a type of flesh or connective tissue.*	
chrom/o	color	chromosomes _____ *These nuclear structures absorb the color of dyes used to stain the cell. The suffix -somes means bodies. Literally, this term means "bodies of color," because this is how they appeared to researchers who first saw them under the microscope.*	
coccyg/o	coccyx (tailbone)	coccygeal _____	
crani/o	skull	craniotomy _____	
cyt/o	cell	cytoplasm _____ *The suffix -plasm means formation.*	
dist/o	far, distant	distal _____	
dors/o	back portion of the body	dorsal _____	
hist/o	tissue	histology _____	
ili/o	ilium (upper part of the pelvic bone)	iliac _____ *See Figure 2-18 for a picture of the ilium.*	
inguin/o	groin	inguinal _____	
kary/o	nucleus	karyotype _____ *The suffix -type means classification or picture.*	

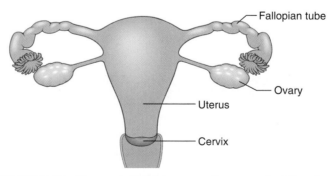

FIGURE 2-17 The cervix is the lower portion or neck of the uterus.

 Cervical

The term **cervical** can have two different meanings depending on where it is used. In a gynecologic report, cervical means the lower portion or neck of the uterus **(cervix).** In a spinal radiologic report about cervical vertebrae, cervical refers to the neck of the body.

In a gynecologic report cervical mean cervix, the neck.

In a spinal radiologic report, cervical refers to the neck of the body.

COMBINING FORM	MEANING	TERMINOLOGY	MEANING
later/o	side	lateral _____	
lumb/o	lower back (side and back between the ribs and the pelvis)	lumbosacral _____	
medi/o	middle	medial _____	
nucle/o	nucleus	nucleic _____	
pelv/i	pelvis	pelvic _____	
		The pelvis includes all the bones that surround the pelvic cavity (Figure 2-18).	
poster/o	back, behind	posterior _____	
proxim/o	nearest	proximal _____	
sacr/o	sacrum	sacral _____	
sarc/o	flesh	sarcoma _____	
spin/o	spine, backbone	spinal _____	

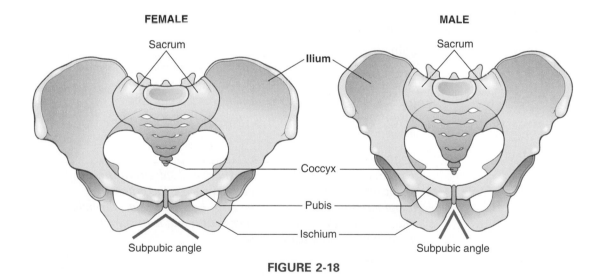

FEMALE   MALE

Sacrum   Ilium   Sacrum

Coccyx

Pubis

Ischium

Subpubic angle   Subpubic angle

FIGURE 2-18

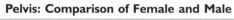

Pelvis: Comparison of Female and Male

The female pelvis is wider and more massive than the male pelvis. The female pelvic opening is a larger, rounded, oval shape, whereas the male pelvic opening is deep, narrow, and funnel- or heart-shaped. Thus, the female pelvis can accommodate the fetus during pregnancy and its downward passage through the pelvic cavity in childbirth.

COMBINING FORM	MEANING	TERMINOLOGY	MEANING
thel/o, theli/o	nipple	epithelial cell _____ *This cell, originally identified in the skin of the nipples, lies on body surfaces, externally (outside the body) and internally (lining cavities and organs).*	
thorac/o	chest	thoracic _____	
		thoracotomy _____	
trache/o	trachea, windpipe	tracheal _____	
umbilic/o	navel, umbilicus	umbilical _____	
ventr/o	belly side of the body	ventral _____	
vertebr/o	vertebra(e), backbone(s)	vertebral _____	
viscer/o	internal organs	visceral _____	

PREFIXES

PREFIX	MEANING	TERMINOLOGY	MEANING
ana-	up	anabolism _____ *In this cellular process, proteins are built **up** from simpler substances (amino acids).*	
cata-	down	catabolism _____ *Complex nutrients are broken **down** into simpler substances and energy is released.*	
epi-	above	epinephrine _____ *The suffix -ine means a substance. Epinephrine is a hormone secreted by the adrenal glands, located above (epi-) the kidneys (nephr/o). It is used as a treatment (as with an EpiPen®) for severe allergic reactions. It opens airways and increases heart rate in medical emergencies.*	
hypo-	below	hypochondriac region _____ *The Greeks thought that organs (liver and spleen) in the hypochondriac region of the abdomen were the origin of imaginary illnesses—hence the term hypochondriac, a person with unusual anxiety about his or her health and with symptoms not attributable to any disease process.*	
inter-	between	intervertebral _____ *A disk (disc) is an intervertebral structure.*	
intra-	within	intravenous _____ *The abbreviation for intravenous is **IV**.*	
meta-	change	metabolism _____ *Literally, to cast (bol/o) a change (meta-), meaning the chemical changes (processes) that occur in a cell.*	

Epinephrine and Adrenaline

These are the SAME hormone! Two different names for the same substance secreted by the adrenal glands (above the kidneys).

SUFFIXES

The following are some new suffixes introduced in this chapter. See the **Glossary (Medical Word Parts—English)** at the end of the book for additional suffixes meaning "pertaining to."

SUFFIX	MEANING	SUFFIX	MEANING
-eal	pertaining to	-ose	pertaining to, full of
-iac	pertaining to	-plasm	formation
-ior	pertaining to	-somes	bodies
-ism	process, condition	-type	picture, classification

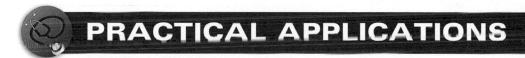

PRACTICAL APPLICATIONS

Be sure to check your answers with the Answers to Practical Applications on page 67.

SURGICAL PROCEDURES

Match the surgical procedure in Column I with an indication for performing it in Column II. *Note:* You are not looking for the exact meaning of each surgical procedure, but rather why it would be performed.

COLUMN I

Procedures

1. Craniotomy _____

2. Thoracotomy _____

3. Diskectomy _____

4. Mediastinoscopy _____

5. Tracheotomy _____

6. Laryngectomy _____

7. Arthroscopy _____

8. Peritoneoscopy _____

COLUMN II

Indications

A. Emergency effort to remove foreign material from the windpipe
B. Inspection and repair of torn cartilage in the knee
C. Removal of a diseased or injured portion of the brain
D. Inspection of lymph nodes* in the region between the lungs
E. Removal of a squamous cell[†] carcinoma in the voice box
F. Open heart surgery, or removal of lung tissue
G. Inspection of abdominal organs and removal of diseased tissue
H. Relief of symptoms from a bulging intervertebral disk

*Lymph nodes are collections of tissue containing white blood cells called lymphocytes.
[†]A squamous cell is a type of epithelial cell.

X-RAY VIEWS

Circle the correct answers in the following sentences related to each x-ray view of the chest.

FIGURE A

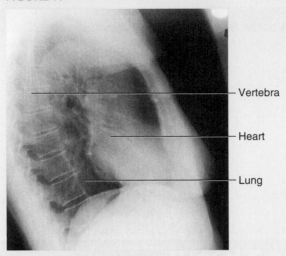

Vertebra

Heart

Lung

1. This is a/an (**coronal, sagittal, axial**) view. The heart lies (**anterior, posterior, dorsal**) to the vertebrae.

FIGURE B

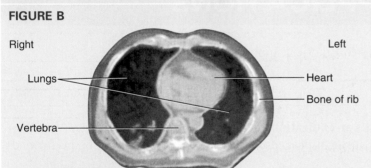

Right

Left

Lungs

Heart

Bone of rib

Vertebra

2. This is a/an (**coronal, sagittal, axial**) view. It is a/an (**CT, traditional x-ray**) image.

FIGURE C

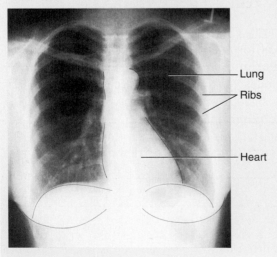

Lung

Ribs

Heart

3. This is a/an (**coronal, sagittal, axial**) view. It is a/an (**lateral, transverse, anterior/posterior**) image.

2

? EXERCISES

Remember to check your answers carefully with the Answers to Exercises, page 66.

A **The listed terms are parts of a cell. Match each term with its correct meaning.**

cell membrane   DNA   mitochondria
chromosomes   endoplasmic reticulum   nucleus
cytoplasm   genes

1. material of the cell located outside the nucleus and yet enclosed by the cell membrane

   _____

2. regions of DNA within each chromosome _____

3. small sausage-shaped structures that are the principal source of energy for the cell

   _____

4. network of canals within the cytoplasm; the site of protein synthesis _____

5. structure that surrounds and protects the cell _____

6. control center of the cell, containing chromosomes _____

7. chemical found within each chromosome _____

8. rod-shaped structures in the nucleus that contain regions called genes _____

B **Use medical terms or numbers to complete the following sentences.**

1. A picture of chromosomes in the nucleus of a cell is a/an _____.

2. The number of chromosomes in a normal male's muscle cell is _____.

3. The number of chromosomes in a female's egg cell is _____.

4. The process of building up proteins in a cell is _____.

5. Complex nutrients are broken down to similar substances and energy is released

   _____.

6. The total of the chemical processes in a cell is _____.

7. A scientist who studies tissues is a/an _____.

8. The medical term for internal organs is _____.

2

C Match the listed body parts or tissues with their correct descriptions that follow.

adipose tissue	pharynx	trachea
cartilage	pituitary gland	ureter
epithelial tissue	pleura	urethra
larynx	thyroid gland	uterus

1. voice box _____

2. membrane surrounding the lungs _____

3. throat _____

4. tube from the kidney to the urinary bladder _____

5. collection of fat cells _____

6. endocrine organ located at the base of the brain _____

7. windpipe _____

8. flexible connective tissue attached to bones at joints _____

9. skin cells that cover the outside of the body and line internal organs _____

10. endocrine gland surrounding the windpipe in the neck _____

11. womb _____

12. tube leading from the urinary bladder to the outside of the body _____

D Name the five cavities of the body.

1. cavity surrounded by the skull _____

2. cavity in the chest surrounded by the ribs _____

3. cavity below the chest containing the stomach, liver, and gallbladder _____

4. cavity surrounded by the hip bones _____

5. cavity surrounded by the bones of the back _____

E Select from the following to define the terms listed on the next page.
space surrounding each lung
space between the lungs
muscle separating the abdominal and thoracic cavities
membrane surrounding the abdominal organs
area below the umbilicus (as well as below the stomach)
area above the stomach
area of the navel
areas near the groin
nervous tissue within the spinal cavity
bony tissue surrounding the spinal cavity
pad of cartilage between two adjoining vertebrae

1. hypogastric region _____

2. mediastinum _____

3. spinal cord _____

4. diaphragm _____

5. intervertebral disk _____

6. pleural cavity _____

7. spinal column _____

8. inguinal regions _____

9. peritoneum _____

10. umbilical region _____

11. epigastric region _____

F Name the five divisions of the back.

1. region of the neck _____

2. region of the chest _____

3. region of the waist _____

4. region of the sacrum _____

5. region of the tailbone _____

G Give the meanings of the following abbreviations.

1. LLQ _____

2. L5–S1 _____

3. RUQ _____

4. C3–C4 _____

5. RLQ _____

H Give the opposites of the following terms.

1. deep _____   4. medial _____

2. proximal _____   5. dorsal _____

3. supine _____   6. superior _____

2

I **Select from the following medical terms to complete the sentences below.**

distal   midsagittal   transverse (axial)
frontal (coronal)   proximal   vertebra
inferior (caudal)   superior (cephalic)   vertebrae
lateral

1. The kidney lies to side of or _____ of the spinal cord.

2. The _____ end of the thigh bone (femur) joins with the kneecap (patella).

3. The _____ plane divides the body into an anterior and a posterior portion.

4. Each backbone is a/an _____.

5. Several backbones are _____.

6. The diaphragm lies _____ to the organs in the thoracic cavity.

7. The _____ plane divides the body into right and left halves.

8. The _____ end of the upper arm bone (humerus) is at the shoulder.

9. The _____ plane divides the body into upper and lower portions.

10. The pharynx is located _____ to the esophagus.

J **Use slashes to divide the following terms into component parts, and give meanings for each.**

1. craniotomy _____

2. cervical _____

3. chondroma _____

4. chondrosarcoma _____

5. nucleic _____

6. epinephrine _____

7. intravenous _____

K **Give the medical term for the following definitions. Pay attention to spelling!**

1. space below the chest containing the liver, stomach, gallbladder, and intestines

   _____

2. flexible connective tissue attached to bones at joints _____

3. rod-shaped structures in the cell nucleus, containing regions of DNA _____

4. muscle separating the abdominal and thoracic cavities _____

5. voice box _____

6. vertical plane dividing the body into right and left sides _____

7. pertaining to the neck _____

8. tumor (benign) of cartilage _____

9. control center of the cell; directs the activities of the cell _____

10. pertaining to the windpipe _____

L **Complete each term based on the meaning provided.**

1. pertaining to internal organs: _____ al

2. tumor of flesh tissue (malignant): _____ oma

3. pertaining to the chest: _____ ic

4. picture of the chromosomes in the cell nucleus: _____ type

5. sausage-shaped cellular structures in which catabolism takes place: mito

   _____

6. space between the lungs: media _____

7. endocrine gland at the base of the brain: _____ ary gland

8. pertaining to skin (surface) cells: epi _____

9. pertaining to far from the beginning of a structure: _____ al

10. on the surface of the body: super _____

M **Circle the correct term to complete each sentence.**

1. Dr. Curnen said the (**inguinal, superior, superficial**) wound barely scratched the surface.

2. Because the liver and spleen are on opposite sides of the body, the liver is in the (**RUQ, LUQ, LLQ**) of the abdominopelvic cavity and the spleen is in the (**RUQ, LUQ, RLQ**).

3. When a gynecologist performs a pelvic examination, the patient lies on her back in the (**ventral, dorsal, medial**) lithotomy position (Figure 2-19).

4. Sally complained of pain in the area surrounding her navel. The doctor described the pain as (**periumbilical, epigastric, hypogastric**).

5. After sampling the fluid surrounding her 16-week-old fetus and reviewing the chromosomal picture, the doctor explained to Mrs. Jones that the fetus had trisomy 21. The diagnosis was made by analysis of an abnormal (**urine sample, x-ray film, karyotype**).

6. The (**spinal, sagittal, abdominal**) cavity contains digestive organs.

7. The emergency department physician suspected appendicitis when Brandon was admitted with sharp (**LLQ, RLQ, RUQ**) pain.

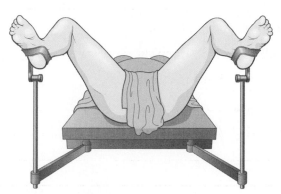

FIGURE 2-19   Dorsal lithotomy position. Lithotomy means incision to remove a stone (lith/o = stone). This supine position is used for pelvic (gynecologic) examinations and for removal of stones from the urinary tract.

8. Susan had hiccups after rapidly eating spicy Indian food. Her physician explained that the hiccups were involuntary contractions or spasms of the (**umbilicus, diaphragm, mediastinum**) resulting in uncontrolled breathing in of air.

9. Everyone in the society pages was noticeably slimmer this year. Could the popularity of liposuction surgery to remove unwanted (**cartilage, epithelial tissue, adipose tissue**) have something to do with this phenomenon?

10. Maria's coughing and sneezing were a result of an allergy to animal dander that affected her (**respiratory, cardiovascular, urinary**) system.

11. While ice skating, Natalie fell and landed on her buttocks. She had persistent (**cervical, thoracic, coccygeal**) pain for a few weeks but no broken bones on x-ray examination.

ANSWERS TO EXERCISES

A

1. cytoplasm
2. genes
3. mitochondria
4. endoplasmic reticulum
5. cell membrane
6. nucleus
7. DNA
8. chromosomes

B

1. karyotype
2. 46 (23 pairs)
3. 23
4. anabolism
5. catabolism
6. metabolism
7. histologist
8. viscera

C

1. larynx
2. pleura
3. pharynx
4. ureter
5. adipose tissue
6. pituitary gland
7. trachea
8. cartilage
9. epithelial tissue
10. thyroid gland
11. uterus
12. urethra

D

1. cranial
2. thoracic
3. abdominal
4. pelvic
5. spinal

E

1. area below the umbilicus
2. space between the lungs
3. nervous tissue within the spinal cavity
4. muscle separating the abdominal and thoracic cavities
5. pad of cartilage between two adjoining vertebrae
6. space surrounding each lung
7. bony tissue surrounding the spinal cavity
8. areas near the groin
9. membrane surrounding the abdominal organs
10. area of the navel
11. area above the stomach

F

1. cervical
2. thoracic
3. lumbar
4. sacral
5. coccygeal

2

G

1. left lower quadrant (of the abdominopelvic cavity)
2. between the fifth lumbar vertebra and the first sacral vertebra (a
3. right upper quadrant (of the abdominopelvic cavity)
4. between the third and fourth cervical vertebrae
5. right lower quadrant (of the abdominopelvic cavity)

common place for a herniated disk)

H

1. superficial
2. distal
3. prone
4. lateral
5. ventral (anterior)
6. inferior (caudal)

I

1. lateral
2. distal
3. frontal (coronal)
4. vertebra
5. vertebrae
6. inferior (caudal)
7. midsagittal
8. proximal
9. transverse (cross-sectional)
10. superior (cephalic)

J

1. crani/o/tomy—incision of the skull
2. cervic/al—pertaining to the neck (of the body or the cervix of the uterus)
3. chondr/oma—tumor of cartilage (benign or noncancerous tumor)
4. chondr/o/sarc/oma—flesh tumor of cartilage (cancerous, malignant tumor)
5. nucle/ic—pertaining to the nucleus
6. epi/nephr/ine—substance (hormone) secreted by the adrenal glands (epi- = above; nephr- = kidney)
7. intra/ven/ous—pertaining to within a vein

K

1. abdomen or abdominal cavity
2. cartilage
3. chromosomes
4. diaphragm
5. larynx
6. sagittal—note spelling with two t's
7. cervical
8. chondroma
9. nucleus
10. tracheal

L

1. visceral
2. sarcoma
3. thoracic
4. karyotype
5. mitochondria—*memory tip*: **cat**abolism and **mit**ochondria, **cat** and **m**ouse!
6. mediastinum
7. pituitary gland
8. epithelial
9. distal
10. superficial

M

1. superficial
2. RUQ; LUQ
3. dorsal; often called the dorsolithotomy position
4. periumbilical
5. karyotype
6. abdominal
7. RLQ
8. diaphragm
9. adipose tissue
10. respiratory
11. coccygeal

Answers to Practical Applications

Surgical Procedures

1. **C** A trephine is a type of circular saw used for craniotomy.
2. **F**
3. **H** Endoscopic diskectomy is performed through a small incision on the back, lateral to the spine. All or a portion of the disk is removed.
4. **D** A small incision is made above the breastbone and an endoscope is inserted to inspect the lymph nodes around the trachea.
5. **A**
6. **E**
7. **B**
8. **G** A small incision is made near the navel, and a laparoscope is inserted. The procedure, also called laparoscopy (lapar/o means abdomen) or minimally invasive surgery, is used to examine organs and perform less complex surgical operations, such as removal of the gallbladder or appendix or tying off of the fallopian tubes.

X-ray Views

1. sagittal, anterior
2. axial, CT
3. coronal, anterior/posterior

2

PRONUNCIATION OF TERMS

To test your understanding of the terminology in this chapter, write the meaning of each term in the space provided. In addition, you may wish to cover the terms and write them by looking at your definitions. Make sure your spelling is correct. The CAPITAL letters indicate the accented syllable. The page number after each term indicates where it is defined or used in the book, so you can easily check your responses. You will find complete definitions for all of these terms and their audio pronunciations on the Evolve website.

Pronunciation Guide

ā as in āpe	ă as in ăpple
ē as in ēven	ĕ as in ĕvery
ī as in īce	ĭ as in ĭnterest
ō as in ōpen	ŏ as in pŏt
ū as in ūnit	ŭ as in ŭnder

TERM	PRONUNCIATION	MEANING
abdomen (47)	ĂB-dō-mĕn	_____
abdominal cavity (47)	ăb-DŎM-ĭ-năl KĂ-vĭ-tē	_____
adipose (41)	ĂD-ĭ-pōs	_____
anabolism (37)	ă-NĂB-ō-lĭzm	_____
anterior (52)	an-TĒ-rē-ŏr	_____
cartilage (41)	KĂR-tĭ-lĭj	_____
catabolism (37)	kă-TĂB-ō-lĭzm	_____
caudal (52)	KĂW-dăl	_____
cell membrane (37)	sĕl MĔM-brān	_____
cephalic (52)	SĔF-ă-lĭk	_____
cervical (51)	SĔR-vĭ-kăl	_____
chondroma (56)	kŏn-DRŌ-mă	_____
chondrosarcoma (56)	kŏn-drō-săr-KŌ-mă	_____
chromosome (37)	KRŌ-mō-sōm	_____
coccygeal (50)	kŏk-sĭ-JĒ-ăl	_____
coccyx (50)	KŎK-sĭks	_____
cranial cavity (47)	KRĀ-nē-ăl KĂ-vĭ-tē	_____
craniotomy (56)	krā-nē-ŎT-ō-mē	_____
cytoplasm (37)	SĪ-tō-plăzm	_____
deep (52)	dēp	_____
diaphragm (47)	DĪ-ă-frăm	_____
disk (disc) (51)	dĭsk	_____

TERM	PRONUNCIATION	MEANING
distal (52)	DĬS-tăl	
dorsal (47)	DŎR-săl	
endoplasmic reticulum (37)	ĕn-dō-PLĂZ-mĭk rē-TĬK-ū-lŭm	
epigastric region (51)	ĕp-ĭ-GĂS-trĭk RĒ-jŭn	
epinephrine (58)	ĕp-ĭ-NĔ-frĭn	
epithelial cells (41)	ĕp-ĭ-THĒ-lē-ăl sĕlz	
frontal plane (52)	FRŬN-tăl plān	
genes (37)	jēnz	
histology (56)	hĭs-TŎL-ō-jē	
hypochondriac region (51)	hī-pō-KŎN-drē-ăk RĒ-jŭn	
hypogastric region (51)	hĭ-po-GĂS-trĭk RĒ-jŭn	
iliac (56)	ĬL-ē-ăk	
inferior (52)	in-FĒR-ē-ŭr	
inguinal region (51)	ĬNG-gwĭ-năl RĒ-jŭn	
intervertebral (58)	ĭn-tĕr-VĔR-tĕ-brăl	
intravenous (58)	ĭn-tră-VĒ-nŭs	
karyotype (37)	KĂR-ē-ō-tīp	
larynx (41)	LĂR-ĭnks	
lateral (52)	LĂT-ĕr-al	
lumbar region (51)	LŬM-băr RĒ-jŭn	
lumbosacral (57)	lŭm-bō-SĀ-krăl	
medial (52)	MĒ-dē-ăl	
mediastinum (47)	mē-dē-ă-STĪ-nŭm	
metabolism (37)	mĕ-TĂB-ō-lĭzm	
mitochondria (37)	mī-tō-KŎN-drē-ă	
nucleic (57)	nū-KLĒ-ĭk	
nucleus (37)	NŪ-klē-ŭs	
pelvic cavity (47)	PĔL-vĭk KĂ-vĭ-tē	
peritoneum (47)	pĕ-rĭ-tō-NĒ-uŭm	
pharynx (41)	FĂR-ĭnks	
pituitary gland (41)	pĭ-TOO-ĭ-tăr-ē glănd	

2

TERM	PRONUNCIATION	MEANING
pleura (47)	PLOO-ră	
pleural cavity (47)	PLOOR-ăl KĂ-vĭ-tē	
posterior (52)	pŏs-TĒR-ē-ŏr	
prone (52)	prōn	
proximal (52)	PRŎKS-ĭ-măl	
sacral (51)	SĀ-krăl	
sacrum (50)	SĀ-krŭm	
sagittal plane (54)	SĂJ-ĭ-tăl plān	
sarcoma (57)	săr-KŌ-mă	
spinal cavity (47)	SPĪ-năl KĂ-vĭ-tē	
spinal column (51)	SPĪ-năl KŎL-ŭm	
spinal cord (51)	SPĪ-năl kŏrd	
superficial (52)	soo-pĕr-FĬSH-ăl	
superior (52)	soo-PĒR-ē-ŭr	
supine (52)	SOO-pīn	
thoracic cavity (47)	thō-RĂS-ĭk KĂ-vĭ-tē	
thoracotomy (58)	thō-ră-KŎT-ō-mē	
thyroid gland (41)	THĪ-royd glănd	
trachea (41)	TRĀ-kē-ă	
tracheal (58)	TRĀ-kē-ăl	
transverse plane (52)	trănz-VĔRS plān	
umbilical region (51)	ŭm-BĬL-ĭ-kăl RĒ-jŭn	
ureter (41)	Ū-rĕ-tĕr *or* ū-RĒ-tĕr	
urethra (41)	ū-RĒ-thră	
uterus (41)	Ū-tĕ-rŭs	
ventral (47)	VĔN-trăl	
vertebra (51)	VĔR-tĕ-bră	
vertebrae (51)	VĔR-tĕ-brā	
vertebral (58)	VĔR-tĕ-brăl *or* vĕr-TĒ-brăl	
viscera (41)	VĬS-ĕr-ă	
visceral (58)	VĬS-ĕr-ăl	

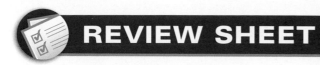

REVIEW SHEET

Write the meaning of each combining form, prefix, or suffix in the space provided, and test yourself. Check your answers with the information in the chapter or in the **Glossary (Medical Word Parts—English),** at the end of the book.

Combining Forms

COMBINING FORM	MEANING	COMBINING FORM	MEANING
abdomin/o		lumb/o	
adip/o		medi/o	
anter/o		nucle/o	
cervic/o		pelv/i	
chondr/o		poster/o	
chrom/o		proxim/o	
coccyg/o		sacr/o	
crani/o		sarc/o	
cyt/o		spin/o	
dist/o		thel/o, theli/o	
dors/o		thorac/o	
hist/o		trache/o	
ili/o		umbilic/o	
inguin/o		ventr/o	
kary/o		vertebr/o	
later/o		viscer/o	

Prefixes

PREFIX	MEANING	PREFIX	MEANING
ana-		hypo-	
cata-		inter-	
epi-		meta-	

2

Suffixes

SUFFIX	MEANING	SUFFIX	MEANING
-al	_____	-oma	_____
-eal	_____	-ose	_____
-ectomy	_____	-plasm	_____
-iac	_____	-somes	_____
-ior	_____	-tomy	_____
-ism	_____	-type	_____

Label the regions and quadrants (use abbreviations) of the abdominopelvic cavity. Check your answers in the chapter, pages 48 and 49.

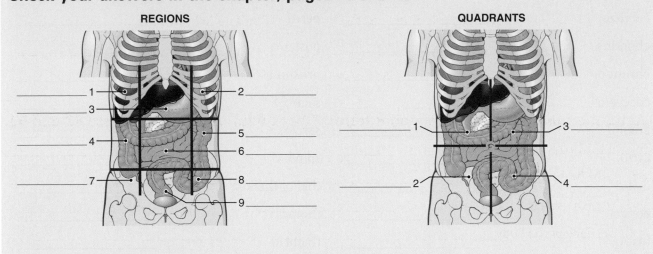

REGIONS

QUADRANTS

1 _____
3 _____
_____ 4
_____ 7
5 _____
6 _____
8 _____
9 _____

1 _____
2 _____
3 _____
4 _____

Name the divisions of the spinal column. Check your answers on page 50.

neck region (C1 to C7) _____

chest region (T1 to T12) _____

lower back (loin) region (L1 to L5) _____

region of the sacrum (S1 to S5) _____

tailbone region _____

2

Name the planes of the head as pictured below. Check your answers on page 54.

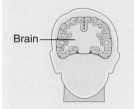

Brain

vertical plane that divides the body into anterior and posterior portions

_____

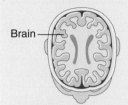

Brain

horizontal plane that divides the body into upper and lower portions

_____

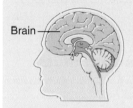

Brain

vertical plane that divides the body into right and left portions

_____

Name the positional and directional terms. Check your answers on pages 52 and 53.

front of the body _____

back of the body _____

away from the surface of the body _____

on the surface of the body _____

far from the point of attachment to the trunk or far from the beginning of a structure

_____

near the point of attachment to the trunk or near the beginning of a structure

_____

below another structure _____

above another structure _____

pertaining to the side _____

pertaining to the middle _____

lying on the belly _____

lying on the back _____

2

Give the meanings of the following terms that pertain to the cell. Check your answers with Study Section 1, page 37.

chromosomes _____

mitochondria _____

nucleus _____

DNA _____

endoplasmic reticulum _____

cell membrane _____

catabolism _____

anabolism _____

metabolism _____

Give the term that suits the meaning provided. Check your answers with Study Section 2, page 41.

membrane surrounding the lungs _____

membrane surrounding the abdominal viscera _____

muscular wall separating the thoracic and abdominal cavities _____

space between the lungs, containing the heart, windpipe, aorta _____

a backbone _____

a pad of cartilage between each backbone and the next _____

2

evolve *Please refer to the Evolve website for additional exercises, games, and images related to this chapter.*

Suffixes

CHAPTER GOALS

- Define new suffixes and review those presented in previous chapters.
- Gain practice in word analysis by using these suffixes with combining forms to build and understand terms.
- Identify the functions of the different types of blood cells in the body.

INTRODUCTION

In this chapter you will encounter many of the most common suffixes in the medical language. As you work through the entire book, these suffixes will appear often. An additional group of suffixes is presented in Chapter 6.

Additional combining forms are presented in this chapter to use in making words with suffixes. Your mastery of this material and your analysis of the words in the section on Suffixes and Terminology will increase your medical language vocabulary.

COMBINING FORMS

Use the following list of combining forms as you write the meanings of terms starting on page 78.

COMBINING FORM	MEANING	COMBINING FORM	MEANING
abdomin/o	abdomen	carcin/o	cancer
acr/o	extremities, top, extreme point	cardi/o	heart
		chem/o	drug, chemical
acu/o	sharp, severe, sudden	chondr/o	cartilage
aden/o	gland		
adip/o	fat	chron/o	time
amni/o	amnion (sac surrounding the embryo in the uterus)	col/o	colon (large intestine)
		cyst/o	urinary bladder
angi/o	vessel	encephal/o	brain
arteri/o	artery	erythr/o	red
arthr/o	joint	hem/o	blood
axill/o	armpit		
bi/o	life	hepat/o	liver
blephar/o	eyelid	hydr/o	water, fluid
		inguin/o	groin
bronch/o	bronchial tubes (two tubes, one right and one left, that branch from the trachea to enter the lungs)	isch/o	to hold back
		lapar/o	abdomen, abdominal wall

Encephal/o, Cerebr/o, Cephal/o, Crani/o, and Psych/o

Don't confuse the meanings of these combining forms!

Encephal/o = brain
Cerebr/o = cerebrum (largest part of the brain)
Cephal/o = head
Crani/o = skull
Psych/o = mind

COMBINING FORM	MEANING	COMBINING FORM	MEANING
laryng/o	larynx	path/o	disease
leuk/o	white	peritone/o	peritoneum
lymph/o	lymph *Lymph, a clear fluid that bathes tissue spaces, is contained in special lymph vessels and nodes throughout the body.*	phag/o	to eat, swallow
		phleb/o	vein
		plas/o	formation, development
		pleur/o	pleura (membrane surrounding lungs and adjacent to chest wall)
mamm/o	breast		
mast/o	breast	pneumon/o	lungs
morph/o	shape, form	pulmon/o	lungs
muc/o	mucus	radi/o	x-rays
my/o	muscle	rect/o	rectum
myel/o	spinal cord, bone marrow *Context of usage indicates the meaning intended.*	ren/o	kidney
		rhin/o	nose
necr/o	death (of cells or whole body)	sarc/o	flesh
		splen/o	spleen
nephr/o	kidney	staphyl/o	clusters
neur/o	nerve	strept/o	twisted chains
neutr/o	neutrophil (a white blood cell)	thorac/o	chest
		thromb/o	clot
nucle/o	nucleus	tonsill/o	tonsils
ophthalm/o	eye	trache/o	trachea (windpipe)
oste/o	bone	ven/o	vein
ot/o	ear		

Larynx and Other Parts of the Body Ending in x

coccy**x** = tailbone
laryn**x** = voice box
pharyn**x** = throat
phalan**x** = finger or toe

To make combining forms for parts of the body that end in x, **substitute g for x:**

coccy**g**/o
laryn**g**/o
pharyn**g**/o
phalan**g**/o

SUFFIXES AND TERMINOLOGY

NOUN SUFFIXES

The following list includes common noun suffixes. After the meaning of each suffix, terminology illustrates the use of the suffix in various words. Recall the basic rule for building a medical term: Use a combining vowel, such as o, to connect the root to the suffix. However, drop the combining vowel if the suffix begins with a vowel—for example, **gastr/itis,** *not* "gastr/o/itis."

Beginning on page 86, more detail is given about specific terms. This section, called **A Closer Look,** will give you a fuller understanding of the terminology.

SUFFIX	MEANING	TERMINOLOGY	MEANING
-algia	pain	arthr<u>algia</u> _____	
		ot<u>algia</u> _____	
		neur<u>algia</u> _____	
		my<u>algia</u> _____	
-cele	hernia (see **A Closer Look: Hernia,** page 86)	recto<u>cele</u> _____	
		cysto<u>cele</u> _____	
-centesis	surgical puncture to remove fluid	thora<u>centesis</u> _____ *Notice that this term is shortened from* thoracocentesis.	
		amnio<u>centesis</u> _____ *The amnion is the sac (membrane) surrounding the embryo (fetus after the 8th week) in the uterus. Fluid accumulates within the amnion and may be withdrawn for analysis between the 12th and 18th weeks of pregnancy. See Figure 3-1.*	
		abdomino<u>centesis</u> _____ *This procedure is more commonly known as abdominal* **paracentesis** *(para- means beside or near). A tube is placed through an incision in the abdomen and fluid is removed from the peritoneal cavity (beside the abdominal organs).*	
-coccus (*singular*) **-cocci** (*plural*)	berry-shaped bacterium (*plural:* bacteria)	strepto<u>coccus</u> _____ *See **A Closer Look: Streptococcus,** page 87.*	
		staphylo<u>cocci</u> _____ (stăf-ĭ-lō-KŎK-sī) *Microbiologists often refer to bacteria in clusters as "staph."*	

3

Formation of Plurals

Words ending in **-us** commonly form their plural by dropping **-us** and adding **-i**. Other examples of **-us** plural formation follow:

    nucle**us** → nucle**i**
    bronch**us** → bronch**i**
    thromb**us** → thromb**i**

See Appendix I at the end of the book for additional information about plural formation.

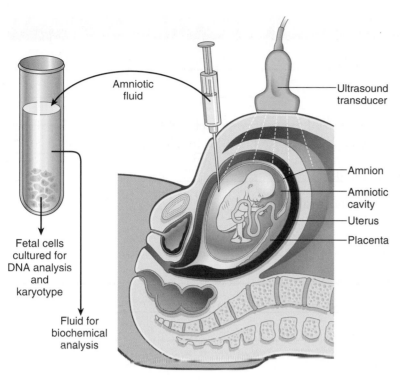

Amniotic
fluid

Ultrasound
transducer

Amnion

Amniotic
cavity

Uterus

Placenta

Fetal cells
cultured for
DNA analysis
and
karyotype

Fluid for
biochemical
analysis

FIGURE 3-1   Amniocentesis. Under ultrasound guidance (imaging based on high-frequency sound waves), the physician inserts a needle through the uterine wall and amnion, into the amniotic cavity. Amniotic fluid, containing fetal cells, is withdrawn and grown (cultured) for microscopic analysis. A karyotype is made to study chromosomes. Fluid is examined for chemicals that indicate fetal defects.

3

SUFFIX	MEANING	TERMINOLOGY	MEANING
-cyte	cell	erythro<u>cyte</u> _____ See **A Closer Look: Blood Cells,** *page 88.*	
		leuko<u>cyte</u> _____	
		thrombo<u>cyte</u> _____	
-dynia	pain	pleuro<u>dynia</u> _____ *Pain in the chest wall muscles that is aggravated by breathing.*	
-ectomy	excision, removal, resection	laryng<u>ectomy</u> _____	
		mast<u>ectomy</u> _____	
-emia	blood condition	an<u>emia</u> ◤ _____	
		isch<u>emia</u> _____ *Literally, to hold back (isch/o) blood (-emia) from a part of the body or tissue. Because of a decrease in blood supply (blood clot in a vessel or narrowing and closing off of a vessel), tissue becomes* ***ischemic*** *and can even die if it is deprived of oxygen long enough.* ✷ ***HINT:*** *You may be familiar with a* ***TIA (transient ischemic attack),*** *which is a "**mini-stroke**" that occurs when blood is held back from tissue in the brain.*	

◤ Anemia

While anemia literally means "no blood," it is actually a condition marked by **reduction** in the number of erythrocytes or in the amount of hemoglobin in blood. Examples of types of anemias are:
- **iron deficiency anemia** (iron is needed to make hemoglobin)
- **sickle cell anemia** (erythrocytes assume an abnormal sickle shape and clog blood vessels)
- **aplastic anemia** (erythrocytes, leukocytes, and thrombocytes are not formed in bone marrow)

SUFFIX	MEANING	TERMINOLOGY	MEANING
-genesis	condition of producing, forming	carcino<u>genesis</u> _____	
		patho<u>genesis</u> _____	
		angio<u>genesis</u> _____	
-gram	record	electroencephalo<u>gram</u> _____	
		mammo<u>gram</u> _____	
-graph	instrument for recording	electroencephalo<u>graph</u> _____	
-graphy	process of recording	electroencephalo<u>graphy</u> _____	
		angio<u>graphy</u> _____	
-itis	inflammation	bronch<u>itis</u> _____	
		myel<u>itis</u> _____ _Myel/o means spinal cord in this term._	
		tonsill<u>itis</u> _____ _Tonsils (notice the spelling with one letter, whereas the combining form has a double letter) are lymphatic tissue in the back of the throat. See Figure 3-2._	
		thrombophleb<u>itis</u> _____ _Also called phlebitis._	
-logy	study of	ophthalmo<u>logy</u> _____	
		morpho<u>logy</u> _____	
-lysis	breakdown, destruction, separation	hemo<u>lysis</u> _____ _Breakdown of red blood cells with release of hemoglobin._	
-malacia	softening	osteo<u>malacia</u> _____	
		chondro<u>malacia</u> _____	

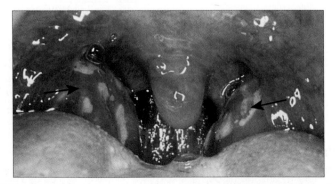

FIGURE 3-2   Tonsillitis. This shows streptococcal tonsillitis with intense erythema (redness) of the tonsils (see arrows) and a creamy-yellow exudate (pus containing leukocytes and bacteria). Normally, tonsils contain lymphocytes that fight bacteria. When they become infected and inflamed, **tonsillectomy** may be necessary.

SUFFIX	MEANING	TERMINOLOGY	MEANING
-megaly	enlargement	acromegaly _____ *See **A Closer Look: Acromegaly,** page 89.*	
		splenomegaly _____	
-oma	tumor, mass, collection of fluid	myoma _____ *A benign tumor.*	
		myosarcoma _____ *A malignant tumor. Muscle is a type of flesh (sarc/o) tissue.*	
		multiple myeloma _____ *Myel/o means bone marrow in this term. This malignant tumor occurs in bone marrow tissue throughout the body.*	
		hematoma _____	
-opsy	to view	biopsy _____	
		necropsy _____ *This is an autopsy or postmortem examination.*	
-osis	condition, usually abnormal	necrosis _____	
		hydronephrosis _____	
		leukocytosis _____	
-pathy	disease condition	cardiomyopathy _____ *Primary disease of the heart muscle in the absence of a known underlying etiology (cause).*	
-penia	deficiency	erythropenia _____	
		neutropenia _____ *In this term, neutr/o indicates neutrophil (a type of white blood cell).*	
		thrombocytopenia _____	
-phobia	fear	acrophobia _____ *Fear of heights. Acr/o means extremities, in the sense of extreme or far points.* ✳ **HINT:** *Think of **acrobats** who perform high-wire acts.*	
		agoraphobia _____ *Agora means marketplace. This is an anxiety disorder marked by fear of being outside of home alone; being in open or enclosed places or using public transportation.*	

3

 Splenomegaly

The spleen is an organ in left upper quadrant (LUQ) of the abdomen (below the diaphragm and to the side of the stomach). Composed of lymph tissue and blood vessels, it disposes of dying red blood cells and contains white blood cells to fight disease. **Splenomegaly** occurs with development of high blood pressure in hepatic veins and hemolytic blood diseases (anemias involving excessive destruction or lysis of red blood cells). If the spleen is removed (splenectomy), other organs carry out its functions.

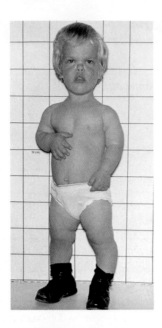

FIGURE 3-3   Achondroplasia. A boy with achondroplasia. His abnormalities include short stature with normal length of the trunk, short limbs and fingers, bowed legs, prominent forehead, and depressed nasal bridge. *(Courtesy A.E. Chudley, MD, Section of Genetics and Metabolism, Department of Pediatrics and Child Health, Children's Hospital, Winnipeg, Manitoba, Canada.)*

SUFFIX	MEANING	TERMINOLOGY	MEANING
-plasia	development, formation, growth	achondro<u>plasia</u> _____ *This is an inherited disorder or can be the result of a mutation (change) in a specific gene. Bones of the arms and legs do not grow to normal size because of a defect in cartilage and bone formation. Dwarfism results, marked by short limbs, but normal-sized head and trunk and normal intelligence. See Figure 3-3.*	
-plasty	surgical repair	angio<u>plasty</u> _____ *An interventional cardiologist opens a narrowed blood vessel (artery) using a balloon that is inflated after insertion into the vessel. Stents, or slotted tubes, are then put in place to keep the artery open.*	
-ptosis	drooping, falling, prolapse	blepharo<u>ptosis</u> _____ *Physicians use **ptosis** (TŌ-sĭs) alone to indicate drooping of the upper eyelids or the breasts. See Figure 3-4.*	
-rrhea	flow, discharge	rhino<u>rrhea</u> _____	

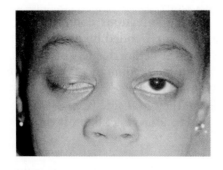

FIGURE 3-4   Ptosis of the upper eyelid (blepharoptosis). This condition may be congenital (appear at birth), can occur with aging, or may be associated with stroke (cerebrovascular accident), cranial nerve damage, and other neurologic disorders. The eyelid droops because of muscle weakness.

 Common Surgical Repair Procedures

Popular procedures include:
  abdominoplasty—abdomen
  blepharoplasty—eyelid
  mammoplasty—breast
  rhinoplasty—nose

SUFFIX	MEANING	TERMINOLOGY	MEANING
-sclerosis	hardening	arterio<u>sclerosis</u> _____	
		In **atherosclerosis** *(a form of arteriosclerosis), deposits of fat (ather/o means fatty material) collect in an artery.*	
-scope	instrument for visual examination	laparo<u>scope</u> _____	
-scopy	process of visual examination (with an endoscope)	laparo<u>scopy</u> _____	
		*See **A Closer Look: Laparoscopy,** page 90.*	
-stasis	controlling, stopping	meta<u>stasis</u> _____	
		Meta- means beyond. A metastasis is the spread of a malignant tumor beyond its original site to a secondary organ or location.	
		hemo<u>stasis</u> _____	
		*Blood flow is stopped naturally by clotting or artificially by compression or suturing of a wound. A **hemostat** is a surgical clamp used in operating rooms to stop blood flow. See Figure 3-5.*	
-stomy	opening to form a mouth (stoma)	colo<u>stomy</u> _____	
		tracheo<u>stomy</u> _____	
-therapy	treatment	hydro<u>therapy</u> _____	
		chemo<u>therapy</u> _____	
		radio<u>therapy</u> _____	
		High-energy radiation is used to treat, not diagnose, illness.	
-tomy	incision, cutting into	laparo<u>tomy</u> _____	
		Also referred to as a "lap," this procedure is creation of a large incision into the peritoneal cavity, often performed on an exploratory basis.	
		phlebo<u>tomy</u> _____	
		tracheo<u>tomy</u> _____	
		*See **A Closer Look: Tracheotomy,** page 91.*	
-trophy	development, nourishment	hyper<u>trophy</u> _____	
		(hī-PĔR-trō-fē) *Cells increase in size, not number. Muscles of weight lifters often hypertrophy.*	
		a<u>trophy</u> _____	
		Cells decrease in size. Muscles atrophy when immobilized in a cast and not in use.	

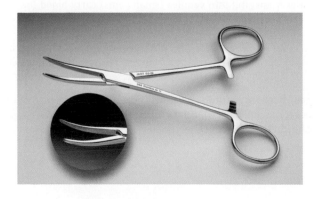

FIGURE 3-5 Hemostat.

The following are shorter noun suffixes that usually are attached to roots in words.

SUFFIX	MEANING	TERMINOLOGY	MEANING
-er	one who	radiograph<u>er</u> _____ *A technologist who assists in the making of diagnostic x-ray pictures.*	
-ia	condition	leukem<u>ia</u> _____	
		pneumon<u>ia</u> _____	
-ist	specialist	nephrolog<u>ist</u> _____	
-ole	little, small	arter<u>iole</u> _____ *See Figure 3-6.*	
-ule	little, small	ven<u>ule</u> _____ *See Figure 3-6.*	
-um, -ium	structure, tissue	pericard<u>ium</u> _____ *This membrane surrounds the heart.*	
-us	structure, substance	muc<u>us</u> _____	
		esophag<u>us</u> _____ *Eso- means within or inward.*	
-y	condition, process	nephropath<u>y</u> _____	

3

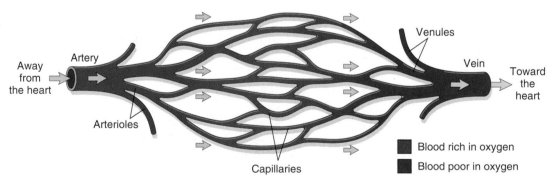

FIGURE 3-6   Relationship of blood vessels. An **artery** carries blood rich in oxygen from the heart to the organs of the body. In the organs, the artery narrows to form **arterioles** (small arteries) that branch into capillaries (the smallest blood vessels). Through the thin walls of capillaries, oxygen leaves the blood and enters cells. Thus, the capillaries branching into **venules** (small veins) carry blood low in oxygen. Venules lead to a vein that brings oxygen-poor blood back to the heart.

Leukemia and Lymphoma

Leukemia is a malignancy of white blood cells, such as **granulocytes,** that derive from bone marrow **(myeloid)** tissue. An example of a type of leukemia is acute myelogenous leukemia (AML). **Lymphoma,** however, is a malignancy of white blood cells **(lymphocytes)** that derive from **lymphoid** tissue such as lymph nodes. Examples of lymphomas are Hodgkin disease and non-Hodgkin lymphoma.

ADJECTIVE SUFFIXES

The following are adjective suffixes. No simple rule will explain which suffix meaning "pertaining to" is used with a specific combining form. Concentrate on identifying the suffix in each term; then write the meaning of the term.

SUFFIX	MEANING	TERMINOLOGY	MEANING
-ac, -iac	pertaining to	cardiac _____	
-al	pertaining to	peritoneal _____	
		inguinal _____	
		pleural _____	
-ar	pertaining to	tonsillar _____	
-ary	pertaining to	pulmonary _____	
		axillary _____	
-eal	pertaining to	laryngeal _____	
-genic	pertaining to producing, produced by or in	carcinogenic _____	
		osteogenic _____	
		An osteogenic sarcoma is a malignant tumor produced in bone.	
-ic, -ical	pertaining to	chronic _____	
		Acute *is the opposite of chronic. It describes a disease that is of rapid onset and has severe symptoms and brief duration.*	
		pathologic _____	
-oid	resembling, derived from	adenoids _____	
		See ***A Closer Look: Adenoids***, *page 91.*	
		mucoid _____	
-ose	pertaining to, full of	adipose _____	
-ous	pertaining to	mucous membrane _____	
		Mucous *(an adjective)* ***membranes*** *produce the sticky secretion called* ***mucus*** *(a noun).*	
-tic	pertaining to	necrotic _____	

Axillary Lymph Nodes and Breast Cancer

Axillary lymph nodes are particularly important in breast cancer. Breast cancer cells often spread to lymph nodes under the arm (armpit). When this occurs, the tumor found in the axillary lymph nodes is a breast cancer metastasis.

A CLOSER LOOK

HERNIA

A **hernia** is protrusion of an organ or the muscular wall of an organ through the cavity that normally contains it. A **hiatal hernia** occurs when the stomach protrudes upward into the mediastinum through the esophageal opening in the diaphragm, and an **inguinal hernia** occurs when part of the intestine protrudes downward into the groin region and commonly into the scrotal sac in the male. A **cystocele** occurs when part of the urinary bladder herniates through the vaginal wall as a result of weakness of the pelvic muscles (Figure 3-7). A **rectocele** is the protrusion of a portion of the rectum toward the vagina (Figure 3-7). An **omphalocele** (omphal/o = umbilicus, navel) is a herniation of the intestines through a weakness in the abdominal wall around the navel occurring in infants at birth. See Figure 3-8.

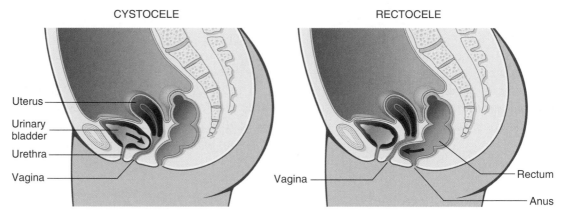

FIGURE 3-7   Hernias: cystocele and rectocele. *Arrows* point to the areas of herniation. In a cystocele, a portion of the urinary bladder herniates posteriorly toward the vagina. In a rectocele, a portion of the rectum herniates anteriorly toward the vagina.

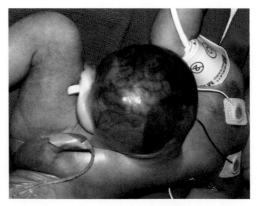

FIGURE 3-8   Omphalocele. This baby was born with large omphalocele containing intra-abdominal viscera. His parents were advised to wait and have surgery performed when his abdominal muscles had grown large enough to close over the hernia. Surgery was performed at 7.5 months to permanently repair the hernia.

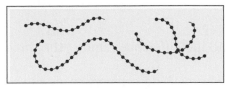
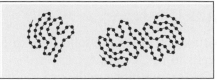
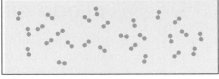

| Streptococci | Staphylococci | Diplococci |

FIGURE 3-9   **Types of coccal bacteria.** Notice the berry or rounded shape of each bacterium. Streptococci and staphylococci are **gram-positive bacteria**, meaning that they retain the light purple color of the stain used in Gram's method (named for Hans C.J. Gram, Danish physician, 1853-1938.) **Gram-negative bacteria (such as diplococci) have the pink color of the counterstain (safranin) used in Gram's method**.

STREPTOCOCCUS

Streptococcus, a berry-shaped bacterium, grows in twisted chains. One group of **streptococci** causes such conditions as "strep throat," tonsillitis, rheumatic fever, and certain kidney ailments, whereas another group causes infections in teeth, within the sinuses (cavities) of the nose and face, and in the valves of the heart.

Staphylococci, other berry-shaped bacteria, grow in small clusters like grapes. Staphylococcal lesions may be external (skin abscesses, boils, styes) or internal (abscesses in bone and kidney). An **abscess** is a collection of pus, white blood cells, and protein that is present at the site of infection. **MRSA** (methicillin-resistant *Staphylococcus aureus*) is a serious staphylococcal condition that is difficult to treat with antibiotics.

Examples of **diplococci** (berry-shaped bacteria organized in pairs; dipl/o = two) are **pneumococci** (pneum/o = lungs) and **gonococci** (gon/o = seed). Pneumococci cause bacterial pneumonia, and gonococci invade the reproductive organs, causing gonorrhea (a sexually transmitted infection). Figure 3-9 illustrates the different growth patterns of streptococci, staphylococci, and diplococci.

3

BLOOD CELLS

Refer to Figure 3-10 as you read the following, to note the differences among the three different types of cells in the blood.

ERYTHROCYTES, or **red blood cells**, are the first type. These cells are made in the bone marrow (soft tissue in the center of certain bones). They carry oxygen from the lungs through the blood to all body cells. Body cells use oxygen to burn food and release energy (catabolism). **Hemoglobin** (globin = protein), an important protein in erythrocytes, carries the oxygen through the bloodstream.

LEUKOCYTES, or **white blood cells**, are the second type. There are five different kinds of leukocytes: three granulocytes, or polymorphonuclear cells, and two mononuclear cells.

- **Granulocytes** contain dark-staining granules in their cytoplasm and have a multilobed nucleus. They are formed in the bone marrow. There are three types:
  1. **Eosinophils** (granules stain red [eosin/o = rosy] with acidic stain) are increased in number in allergic conditions such as asthma. About 3% of leukocytes are eosinophils.
  2. **Basophils** (granules stain blue with basic [bas/o = basic] stain). The function of basophils is not clear, but the number of these cells increases in the healing phase of inflammation. Less than 1% of leukocytes are basophils.
  3. **Neutrophils** (granules stain a pale purple with neutral stain) are the most important disease-fighting cells and the most numerous. About 50% to 60% of all leukocytes are neutrophils. They are **phagocytes** (phag/o = eating, swallowing)—engulfing and digesting bacteria like circulating "pac-men." Neutrophils are referred to as "polys" or **polymorphonuclear leukocytes** (poly = many, morph/o = shape) because of their multilobed nucleus.
- **Mononuclear cells** have one large nucleus (mononuclear) and only a few granules in their cytoplasm. They are produced in bone marrow as well as in lymph nodes and spleen. There are two types of mononuclear leukocytes (see Figure 3-10):
  4. **Lymphocytes** (lymph cells) fight disease by producing antibodies, thereby destroying foreign cells. They also may attach directly to foreign cells and destroy them. Two types of lymphocytes are T cells and B cells. About 32% of white blood cells are lymphocytes. In AIDS (acquired immunodeficiency syndrome), patients have a serious depletion of T lymphocytes (T cells).
  5. **Monocytes** (containing one [mon/o = one] very large nucleus) engulf and destroy cellular debris after neutrophils have attacked foreign cells. Monocytes leave the bloodstream and enter tissues (such as lung and liver) to become **macrophages,** which are large phagocytes. Monocytes make up about 4% of all leukocytes.

See Table 3-1 to review the five types of leukocytes. Each type fights infection in a specific manner. This is similar to the five branches of the armed forces (Navy, Army, Air Force, Marines, and Coast Guard), each of which is equipped with specialized skills and procedures.

THROMBOCYTES or **PLATELETS** (**clotting cells**) are the third type of blood cell. These are actually tiny fragments of cells formed in the bone marrow and are necessary for blood clotting.

| TABLE 3-1 | FIVE TYPES OF LEUKOCYTES (WHITE BLOOD CELLS) |

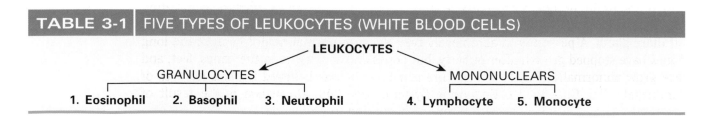

ERYTHROCYTES
(no nucleus;
contain hemoglobin)

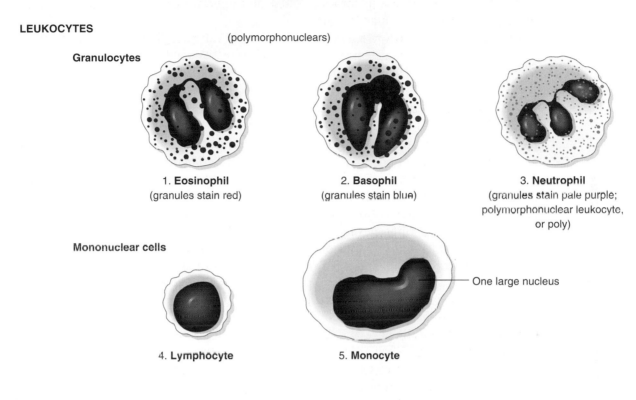

(side view)

LEUKOCYTES

(polymorphonuclears)

Granulocytes

1. **Eosinophil**
(granules stain red)

2. **Basophil**
(granules stain blue)

3. **Neutrophil**
(granules stain pale purple;
polymorphonuclear leukocyte,
or poly)

Mononuclear cells

One large nucleus

4. **Lymphocyte**

5. **Monocyte**

**THROMBOCYTES
(PLATELETS)**

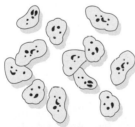

FIGURE 3-10   Types of blood cells. ✳ **HINT:** Here's an easy way to remember the names of the five leukocytes:
Never (neutrophil)
Let (lymphocyte)
Monkeys (monocyte)
Eat (eosinophil)
Bananas (basophil)

ACROMEGALY

Acromegaly is an endocrine disorder. It occurs when the **pituitary gland,** attached to the base of the brain, produces an excessive amount of growth hormone *after* the completion of puberty. The excess growth hormone most often results from a benign tumor of the pituitary gland. A person with acromegaly typically is of normal height because the long bones have stopped growth after puberty, but bones and soft tissue in the hands, feet, and face grow abnormally (Figure 3-11). Abraham Lincoln was believed to have features of acromegaly. See Chapter 18, Endocrine System, page 749. **Gigantism** is the result of overproduction of pituitary growth hormone beginning in childhood.

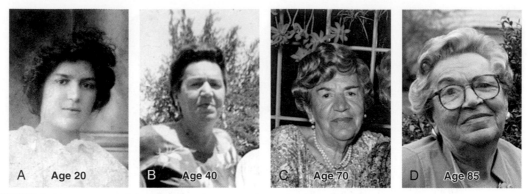

FIGURE 3-11   Acromegaly. Notice the changes in facial features (shape of face and protruding nose, jaw, and brow) of my grandmother, Bessie Brandwein.

LAPAROSCOPY

Laparoscopy (a form of **minimally invasive surgery**) is visual examination of the abdominal cavity using a laparoscope. A surgeon inserts the laparoscope, a lighted telescopic instrument, through an incision in the abdomen near the navel. Then, gas (carbon dioxide) is infused into the peritoneal cavity, to separate and prevent injury to abdominal structures during surgery. Surgeons use laparoscopy to examine abdominal viscera for evidence of disease (performing biopsies) or for procedures such as removal of the appendix, gallbladder, adrenal gland, spleen, or ovary, colon resection, and repair of hernias. In tubal ligation, the laparoscope contains an instrument to clip and collapse the fallopian tubes, which prevents sperm cells from reaching eggs that leave the ovary (Figure 3-12).

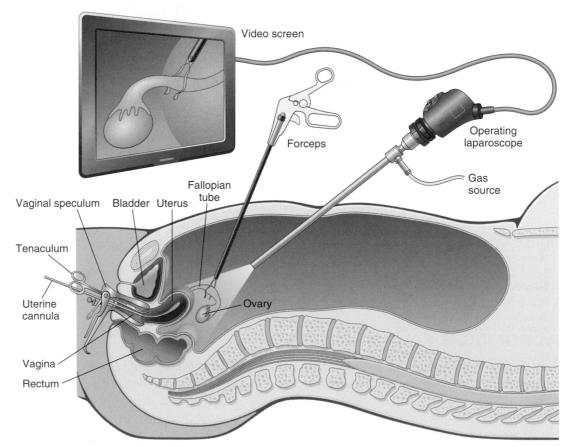

FIGURE 3-12   Laparoscopy for tubal ligation (interruption of the continuity of the fallopian tubes) as a means of preventing future pregnancy. The **tenaculum** grasps the cervix. The **vaginal speculum** keeps the vaginal cavity open. The **uterine cannula** is a tube placed into the uterus to manipulate the uterus during the procedure. **Forceps**, placed through the laparoscope, grasp or move tissue.

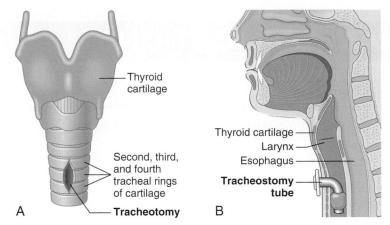

FIGURE 3-13 A, Tracheotomy. B, Tracheostomy.

TRACHEOTOMY

A **tracheotomy** is an incision into the trachea typically done to open it below a blockage. Tracheotomy may be performed to remove a foreign body or to obtain a biopsy specimen (Figure 3-13A).

A **tracheostomy** is an opening into the trachea through which an indwelling tube is inserted. The tube is required to allow air to flow into the lungs or to help remove secretions (mucus) from the bronchial tubes. When a temporary tracheostomy is performed, extreme care is used to insert the tracheostomy tube below the larynx so that the vocal cords are not damaged (Figure 3-13B).

ADENOIDS

The **adenoids** are small masses of lymphatic tissue in the part of the pharynx (throat) near the nose and nasal passages. The literal meaning, "resembling glands," is appropriate because they are neither endocrine nor exocrine glands. Enlargement of adenoids may cause blockage of the airway from the nose to the pharynx, and adenoidectomy may be advised. The **tonsils** also are lymphatic tissue, and their location as well as that of the adenoids is indicated in Figure 3-14.

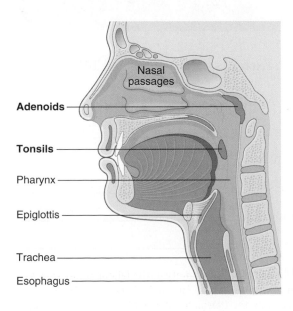

FIGURE 3-14 **Adenoids and tonsils.** The adenoids and tonsils are lymphatic tissue in the pharynx (throat).

PRACTICAL APPLICATIONS

PROCEDURES AND THEIR DEFINITIONS

Choose the correct diagnostic or treatment procedure for each of the numbered definitions. Answers are on page 101.

amniocentesis	colostomy	mastectomy	thoracentesis
angiography	laparoscopy	paracentesis	tonsillectomy
angioplasty	laparotomy	(abdominocentesis)	

1. removal of abdominal fluid (ascites) from the peritoneal space _____

2. large abdominal incision to remove an ovarian adenocarcinoma _____

3. removal of the breast _____

4. a method used to determine the karyotype of a fetus _____

5. surgical procedure to remove pharyngeal lymphatic tissue _____

6. surgical procedure to open clogged coronary arteries _____

7. method of removing fluid from the chest (pleural effusion) _____

8. procedure to drain waste from the body after bowel resection _____

9. x-ray procedure used to examine blood vessels before surgery _____

10. minimally invasive surgery within the abdomen _____

EXERCISES

Remember to check your answers carefully with the Answers to Exercises on pages 100 and 101.

A **Give the meanings for the following suffixes.**

1. -cele _____

2. -emia _____

3. -coccus _____

4. -gram _____

5. -cyte _____

6. -algia _____

7. -ectomy _____

8. -centesis _____

9. -genesis _____

10. -graph _____

11. -itis _____

12. -graphy _____

B **Using the listed combining forms and your knowledge of suffixes, build medical terms for the definitions that follow.**

amni/o	cyst/o	myel/o
angi/o	isch/o	rhin/o
arthr/o	laryng/o	staphyl/o
bronch/o	mast/o	strept/o
carcin/o	my/o	thorac/o

1. hernia of the urinary bladder _____

2. pain of muscle _____

3. process of producing cancer _____

4. inflammation of the spinal cord _____

5. berry-shaped bacteria in twisted chains _____

6. surgical puncture to remove fluid from the chest _____

7. removal of the breast _____

8. inflammation of the tubes leading from the windpipe to the lungs _____

9. to hold back blood from cells _____

10. process of recording (x-ray) blood vessels _____

11. visual examination of joints _____

12. berry-shaped bacteria in clusters _____

13. resection of the voice box _____

14. surgical procedure to remove fluid from the sac around a fetus _____

15. discharge from the nose _____

C **Match the listed terms, which describe blood cells, with the meanings that follow.**

basophil	lymphocyte	neutrophil
eosinophil	monocyte	thrombocyte
erythrocyte		

1. granulocytic white blood cell (granules stain purple) that destroys foreign cells by engulfing and digesting them; also called a polymorphonuclear leukocyte _____

2. mononuclear white blood cell that destroys foreign cells by making antibodies

_____

3. clotting cell; also called a platelet _____

4. leukocyte with reddish staining granules and numbers elevated in allergic reactions

_____

5. red blood cell _____

6. mononuclear white blood cell that engulfs and digests cellular debris; contains one large nucleus

_____

7. granulocytic white blood cell that increases during the healing phase of inflammation

_____

D Give the meanings of the following suffixes.

1. -logy _____

2. -lysis _____

3. -pathy _____

4. -penia _____

5. -malacia _____

6. -osis _____

7. -phobia _____

8. -megaly _____

9. -oma _____

10. -opsy _____

11. -plasia _____

12. -plasty _____

13. -sclerosis _____

14. -stasis _____

E Using the combining forms below and your knowledge of suffixes, build medical terms for the following definitions.

acr/o   chondr/o   myel/o
arteri/o   hem/o   phleb/o
bi/o   hydr/o   rhin/o
blephar/o   morph/o   sarc/o
cardi/o   my/o   splen/o

1. enlargement of the spleen _____

2. study of the shape (of cells) _____

3. softening of cartilage _____

4. abnormal condition of water (fluid) in the kidney _____

5. disease condition of heart muscle _____

6. hardening of arteries _____

7. tumor (benign) of muscle _____

8. flesh tumor (malignant) of muscle _____

9. surgical repair of the nose _____

10. tumor of bone marrow _____

11. fear of heights _____

12. view of living tissue under a microscope _____

13. stoppage of the flow of blood (by mechanical or natural means) _____

14. inflammation of the eyelid _____

15. incision of a vein _____

3

F Give the plural formations of the following terms:

1. bacterium _____

2. metastasis _____

3. vertebra _____

4. streptococcus _____

5. nucleus _____

6. prognosis _____

G Match the following terms with their meanings.

achondroplasia   colostomy   laparoscopy
acromegaly   hydrotherapy   metastasis
atrophy   hypertrophy   necrosis
chemotherapy   laparoscope   osteomalacia

1. treatment using drugs _____

2. condition of death (of cells) _____

3. softening of bone _____

4. opening of the large intestine to the outside of the body _____

5. no development; shrinkage of cells _____

6. beyond control; spread of a cancerous tumor to another organ _____

7. instrument to visually examine the abdomen _____

8. enlargement of extremities; an endocrine disorder that causes excess growth hormone to be produced by the pituitary gland after puberty _____

9. condition of improper formation of cartilage in the embryo that leads to short bones and dwarfism _____

10. process of viewing the peritoneal (abdominal) cavity _____

11. treatment using water _____

12. excessive development of cells (increase in size of individual cells) _____

H Give the meanings of the following suffixes.

1. -ia _____

2. -trophy _____

3. -stasis _____

4. -stomy _____

5. -tomy _____

6. -ole _____

7. -um _____

8. -ule _____

9. -y _____

10. -oid _____

11. -genic _____

12. -ptosis _____

I Using the lists of combining forms and suffixes below, build medical terms for the following definitions.

COMBINING FORMS

arteri/o	pleur/o
lapar/o	pneumon/o
mamm/o	radi/o
nephr/o	ven/o

SUFFIXES

-dynia	-ole	-therapy
-ectomy	-pathy	-tomy
-gram	-plasty	-ule
-ia	-scopy	

1. incision of the abdomen _____

2. process of visual examination of the abdomen _____

3. a small artery _____

4. condition of the lungs _____

5. treatment using x-rays _____

6. record (x-ray film) of the breast _____

7. pain of the chest wall and the membranes surrounding the lungs _____

8. a small vein _____

9. disease condition of the kidney _____

10. surgical repair of the breast _____

J Underline the suffix in the following terms, and give the meaning of the entire term.

1. laryngeal _____

2. inguinal _____

3. chronic _____

4. pulmonary _____

5. adipose _____

6. peritoneal _____

7. axillary _____

8. necrotic _____

9. mucoid _____

10. mucous _____

11. agoraphobia _____

12. esophagus _____

K **Select from the listed terms relating to blood and blood vessels to complete the sentences that follow.**

anemia	hemolysis	leukocytosis
angioplasty	hemostasis	multiple myeloma
arterioles	ischemia	thrombocytopenia
hematoma	leukemia	venules

1. Billy was diagnosed with excessively high numbers of cancerous white blood cells, or

   _____. His doctor prescribed chemotherapy and expected an excellent prognosis.

2. Mr. Clark's angiogram showed that he had serious atherosclerosis of one of the arteries

   supplying blood to his heart. His doctor recommended that _____ would be helpful to open up his clogged artery by threading a catheter (tube) through his artery and opening a balloon at the end of the catheter to widen the artery.

3. Mrs. Jackson's blood count showed a reduced number of red blood cells, indicating

   _____. Her erythrocytes were being destroyed by _____.

4. Doctors refused to operate on Joe because of his low platelet count, a condition called

   _____.

5. Blockage of an artery leading to Mr. Stein's brain led to the holding back of blood flow to nerve

   tissue in his brain. This condition, called _____, could lead to necrosis of tissue and a cerebrovascular accident.

6. Small arteries, or _____, were broken under Ms. Bein's scalp when she was struck on the head with a rock. She soon developed a mass of blood, a/an

   _____, under the skin in that region of her head.

7. Sarah Jones had a staphylococcal infection, causing elevation of her white blood cell count,

   known as _____. She was treated with antibiotics, and her blood count returned to normal.

8. Within the body, the bone marrow (soft tissue within bones) is the "factory" for making blood

   cells. Mr. Scott developed _____, a malignant condition of the bone marrow cells in his hip, upper arm, and thigh bones.

9. During operations, surgeons use clamps to close off blood vessels and prevent blood loss. In this

   way, they maintain _____ and avoid blood transfusions.

10. Small vessels that carry blood toward the heart from capillaries and tissues are

    _____.

3

L Complete the medical term for the following definitions.

DEFINITION   MEDICAL TERM

1. membrane surrounding the heart   peri _____

2. hardening of arteries   arterio _____

3. enlargement of the liver   hepato _____

4. new opening of the windpipe to the outside of the body   tracheo _____

5. inflammation of the tonsils   _____ itis

6. surgical puncture to remove fluid from the abdomen   abdomino _____

7. muscle pain   my _____

8. pertaining to the membranes surrounding the lungs   _____ al

9. study of the eye   _____ logy

10. berry-shaped (spheroidal) bacteria in clusters   _____ cocci

11. beyond control (spread of a cancerous tumor)   meta _____

12. pertaining to the voice box   _____ eal

M Select from the meanings in Column II to match the suffixes in Column I. Write each meaning in the space provided.

COLUMN I   COLUMN II

Suffixes: Conditions   *Meanings*

1. -algia or -dynia _____   blood condition
                                                                            controlling; stopping
2. -cele _____   deficiency
                                                                            destruction; breakdown
3. -megaly _____   development; nourishment
                                                                            falling; drooping; prolapse
4. -oma _____   enlargement
                                                                            fear
5. -penia _____   formation
                                                                            hardening
6. -phobia _____   hernia
                                                                            inflammation
7. -plasia _____   pain
                                                                            softening
8. -emia _____   tumor; mass

9. -itis _____

10. -trophy _____

11. -stasis _____

12. -sclerosis _____

13. -lysis _____

14. -ptosis _____

15. -malacia _____

3

N **Select from the meanings in Column II to match the suffixes in Column I. Write each meaning in the space provided.**

COLUMN I

Suffixes: Procedures

1. -centesis _____
2. -opsy _____
3. -ectomy _____
4. -tomy _____
5. -stomy _____
6. -therapy _____
7. -plasty _____
8. -scopy _____
9. -scope _____
10. -graphy _____
11. -gram _____
12. -graph _____

COLUMN II

Meanings

excision
incision
instrument to record
instrument to visually examine
new opening
process of recording
process of visual examination
record
surgical puncture to remove fluid
surgical repair
to view
treatment

O **Circle the correct term to complete the following sentences.**

1. Ms. Daley, who has nine children, visited her general practitioner because she was experiencing problems with urination. After examining her, the doctor found that her bladder was protruding into her vagina and told her she had a (**rectocele, cystocele, hiatal hernia**).

2. Susan coughed constantly for a week. Her physician told her that her chest x-ray examination showed evidence of pneumonia. Her sputum (material coughed up from the bronchial tubes) was found to contain (**ischemic, pleuritic, pneumococcal**) bacteria.

3. Mr. Manion went to see his family doctor because he couldn't keep his left upper eyelid from sagging. His doctor told him that he had a neurologic problem called Horner syndrome, characterized by (**necrosis, hydronephrosis, ptosis**) of his eyelid.

4. Jill broke her left arm in a fall while mountain biking. After 6 weeks in a cast to treat the fracture, her left arm was noticeably smaller and weaker than her right arm—the muscles had (**atrophied, hypertrophied, metastasized**). Her physician recommended physical therapy to strengthen the affected arm.

5. Ms. Brody was diagnosed with breast cancer. The first phase of her treatment included a (**nephrectomy, mastectomy, pulmonary resection**) to remove her breast and the tumor. After the surgery, her doctors recommended (**chemotherapy, radiotherapy, hydrotherapy**) using drugs such as doxorubicin (Adriamycin) and paclitaxel (Taxol).

6. At age 29, Kevin's facial features became coarser and his hands and tongue enlarged. After a head CT (computed tomography) scan, doctors diagnosed the cause of these changes as (**hyperglycemia, hyperthyroidism, acromegaly**), a slowly progressive endocrine condition involving the pituitary gland.

7. Each winter during "cold and flu season," Daisy developed (**chondromalacia, bronchitis, cardiomyopathy**). Her doctor prescribed antibiotics and respiratory therapy to help her recover.

8. After undergoing (**arthroscopy, laparotomy, radiotherapy**) on his knee, Alan noticed swelling and inflammation near the small incisions. Dr. Nicholas assured him that this was a common side effect of the procedure that would resolve spontaneously.

9. Under the microscope, Dr. Vance could see grape-like clusters of bacteria called (**eosinophils, streptococci, staphylococci**). She made the diagnosis of (**staphylococcemia, eosinophilia, streptococcemia**), and the patient was started on antibiotic therapy.

10. David enjoyed weight lifting, but he recently noticed a bulge in his right groin region. He visited his doctor, who made the diagnosis of (**hiatal hernia, rectocele, inguinal hernia**) and recommended surgical repair.

ANSWERS TO EXERCISES

A

1. hernia
2. blood condition
3. berry-shaped bacterium
4. record
5. cell
6. pain
7. removal, excision, resection
8. surgical puncture to remove fluid
9. process of producing, forming
10. instrument to record
11. inflammation
12. process of recording

B

1. cystocele
2. myalgia ("myodynia" is not used)
3. carcinogenesis
4. myelitis
5. streptococci (*bacteria* is a plural term)
6. thoracentesis or thoracocentesis
7. mastectomy
8. bronchitis
9. ischemia
10. angiography
11. arthroscopy
12. staphylococci
13. laryngectomy
14. amniocentesis
15. rhinorrhea

C

1. neutrophil
2. lymphocyte
3. thrombocyte
4. eosinophil
5. erythrocyte
6. monocyte
7. basophil

D

1. process of study
2. breakdown, separation, destruction
3. process of disease
4. deficiency, less than normal
5. softening
6. condition, abnormal condition
7. fear of
8. enlargement
9. tumor, mass
10. process of viewing
11. condition of formation, growth
12. surgical repair
13. hardening, to harden
14. to stop, control

E

1. splenomegaly
2. morphology
3. chondromalacia
4. hydronephrosis
5. cardiomyopathy
6. arteriosclerosis
7. myoma
8. myosarcoma
9. rhinoplasty
10. myeloma (called multiple myeloma)
11. acrophobia
12. biopsy
13. hemostasis
14. blepharitis
15. phlebotomy

F

1. bacteria
2. metastases
3. vertebrae
4. streptococci
5. nuclei
6. prognoses

G

1. chemotherapy
2. necrosis
3. osteomalacia
4. colostomy
5. atrophy
6. metastasis
7. laparoscope
8. acromegaly
9. achondroplasia
10. laparoscopy
11. hydrotherapy
12. hypertrophy

H

1. condition
2. development, nourishment
3. to stop, control
4. new opening
5. incision, cut into
6. small, little
7. structure
8. small, little
9. condition, process
10. resembling
11. pertaining to producing, produced by or in
12. falling, drooping, prolapse

I

1. laparotomy
2. laparoscopy
3. arteriole
4. pneumonia (this condition is actually *pneumonitis*)
5. radiotherapy
6. mammogram
7. pleurodynia
8. venule
9. nephropathy
10. mammoplasty

J

1. laryngeal—pertaining to the voice box
2. inguinal—pertaining to the groin
3. chronic—pertaining to time (over a long period of time); the opposite of chronic is acute
4. pulmonary—pertaining to the lung
5. adipose—pertaining to (or full of) fat
6. peritoneal—pertaining to the peritoneum (membrane around the abdominal organs)
7. axillary—pertaining to the armpit, under arm
8. necrotic—pertaining to death
9. mucoid—resembling mucus
10. mucous—pertaining to mucus
11. agoraphobia—fear of open spaces and being away from home alone (agora means marketplace)
12. esophagus—tube leading from the throat to the stomach

K

1. leukemia
2. angioplasty
3. anemia; hemolysis
4. thrombocytopenia
5. ischemia
6. arterioles; hematoma
7. leukocytosis
8. multiple myeloma
9. hemostasis
10. venules

L

1. pericardium
2. arteriosclerosis
3. hepatomegaly
4. tracheostomy
5. tonsillitis
6. abdominocentesis (this procedure also is known as paracentesis)
7. myalgia
8. pleural
9. ophthalmology
10. staphylococci
11. metastasis
12. laryngeal

M

1. pain
2. hernia
3. enlargement
4. tumor; mass
5. deficiency
6. fear
7. formation
8. blood condition
9. inflammation
10. development; nourishment
11. controlling; stopping
12. hardening
13. destruction; breakdown
14. falling; drooping; prolapse
15. softening

N

1. surgical puncture to remove fluid
2. to view
3. excision
4. incision
5. new opening
6. treatment
7. surgical repair
8. process of visual examination
9. instrument to visually examine
10. process of recording
11. record
12. instrument to record

O

1. cystocele
2. pneumococcal
3. ptosis
4. atrophied
5. mastectomy; chemotherapy
6. acromegaly
7. bronchitis
8. arthroscopy
9. staphylococci; staphylococcemia
10. inguinal hernia

Answers to Practical Applications

1. paracentesis (abdominocentesis)
2. laparotomy
3. mastectomy
4. amniocentesis
5. tonsillectomy
6. angioplasty
7. thoracentesis
8. colostomy
9. angiography
10. laparoscopy

3

PRONUNCIATION OF TERMS

To test your understanding of the terminology in this chapter, write the meaning of each term in the space provided. In addition, you may wish to cover the terms and write them by looking at your definitions. Make sure your spelling is correct. The CAPITAL letters indicate the accented syllable. The page number after each term indicates where it is defined or used in the text, so you can check your responses. You will find complete definitions for all of these terms and their audio pronunciations on the Evolve site.

Pronunciation Guide

ā as in āpe   ă as in ăpple
ē as in ēven   ĕ as in ĕvery
ī as in īce   ĭ as in ĭnterest
ō as in ōpen   ŏ as in pŏt
ū as in ūnit   ŭ as in ŭnder

TERM	PRONUNCIATION	MEANING
abdominocentesis (78)	ăb-dŏm-ĭ-nō-sĕn-TĒ-sĭs	_____
achondroplasia (82)	ā-kŏn-drō-PLĀ-zē-ă	_____
acromegaly (81)	ăk-rō-MĔG-ă-lē	_____
acrophobia (81)	ăk-rō-FŌ-bē-ă	_____
acute (85)	ă-KŪT	_____
adenoids (85)	ĂD-ĕ-noydz	_____
adipose (85)	Ă-dĭ-pōs	_____
agoraphobia (81)	ă-gŏr-ă-FŌ-bē-ă	_____
amniocentesis (78)	ăm-nē-ō-sĕn-TĒ-sĭs	_____
anemia (79)	ă-NĒ-mē-ă	_____
angiogenesis (80)	ăn-jē-ō-JĔN-ĕ-sĭs	_____
angiography (80)	ăn-jē-ŎG-ră-fē	_____
angioplasty (82)	ăn-jē-ō-PLĂS-tē	_____
arteriole (84)	ăr-TĒR-ē-ōl	_____
arteriosclerosis (83)	ăr-tē-rē-ō-sklĕ-RŌ-sĭs	_____
arthralgia (78)	ăr-THRĂL-jă	_____
atrophy (83)	ĂT-rō-fē	_____
axillary (85)	ĂK-sĭ-lār-ē	_____
basophil (87)	BĀ-sō-fĭl	_____
biopsy (81)	BĪ-ŏp-sē	_____
blepharoptosis (82)	blĕf-ă-rŏp-TŌ-sĭs	_____
bronchitis (80)	brŏng-KĪ-tĭs	_____

TERM	PRONUNCIATION	MEANING
carcinogenesis (80)	kăr-sĭ-nō-JĔN-ĕ-sĭs	
carcinogenic (85)	kăr-sĭ-nō-JĔN-ik	
cardiac (85)	KĂR-dē-ăk	
cardiomyopathy (81)	kăr-dē-ō-mī-ŎP-ă-thē	
chemotherapy (83)	kē-mō-THĔR-ĕ-pē	
chondromalacia (80)	kŏn-drō-mă-LĀ-shă	
chronic (85)	KRŎN-ĭk	
colostomy (83)	kō-LŎS-tō-mē	
cystocele (78)	SĬS-tō-sēl	
electroencephalogram (80)	ē-lĕk-trō-ĕn-SĔF-ă-lō-grăm	
electroencephalograph (80)	ē-lĕk-trō-ĕn-SĔF-ă-lō-grăf	
electroencephalography (80)	ē-lĕk-trō-ĕn-sĕf-ă-LŎG-ră fē	
eosinophil (87)	ē-ō-SĬN-ō-fĭl	
erythrocyte (79)	ĕ-RĬTH-rō-sīt	
erythropenia (81)	ĕ-rĭth-rō-PĒ-nē-ă	
esophagus (84)	ĕ-SŎF-ă-gus	
hematoma (81)	hē-mă-TŌ-mă	
hemolysis (80)	hē-MŎL-ĭ-sĭs	
hemostasis (83)	hē-mō-STĀ-sĭs	
hydronephrosis (81)	hī-drō-nĕ-FRŌ-sĭs	
hydrotherapy (83)	hī-drō-THĔR-ă-pē	
hypertrophy (83)	hī-PĔR-trō-fē	
inguinal (85)	ĬNG-wĭ-năl	
ischemia (79)	ĭs-KĒ-mē-ă	
laparoscope (83)	LĂP-ă-rō-skōp	
laparoscopy (83)	lă-pă-RŎS-kō-pē	
laparotomy (83)	lăp-ă-RŎT-ō-mē	
laryngeal (85)	lă-RĬN-jē-ăl or lăr-ĭn-JĒ-ăl	
laryngectomy (79)	lăr-ĭn-JĔK-tō-mē	
leukemia (84)	lū-KĒ-mē-ă	
leukocyte (79)	LOO-kō-sīt	

TERM	PRONUNCIATION	MEANING
leukocytosis (81)	loo-kō-sī-TŌ-sĭs	_____
lymphocyte (87)	LĬM-fō-sīt	_____
mammogram (80)	MĂM-mō-grăm	_____
mastectomy (79)	măs-TĔK-tō-mē	_____
metastasis (83)	mĕ-TĂS-tă-sĭs	_____
monocyte (87)	MŎN-ō-sīt	_____
morphology (80)	mŏr-FŎL-ō-jē	_____
mucoid (85)	MŪ-koyd	_____
mucous membrane (85)	MŪ-kŭs MĔM-brān	_____
mucus (84)	MŪ-kŭs	_____
myalgia (78)	mī-ĂL-jă	_____
myelitis (80)	MĪ-ĕ-LĪ-tĭs	_____
myeloma (81)	mī-ĕ-LŌ-mă	_____
myoma (81)	mī-Ō-mă	_____
myosarcoma (81)	mī-ō-săr-KŌ-mă	_____
necropsy (81)	NĔ-krŏp-sē	_____
necrosis (81)	nĕ-KRŌ-sĭs	_____
necrotic (85)	nĕ-KRŎT-ĭk	_____
nephrologist (84)	nĕ-FRŎL-ō-jĭst	_____
nephropathy (84)	nĕ-FRŎP-ă-thē	_____
neuralgia (78)	nū-RĂL-jă	_____
neutropenia (81)	nū-trō-PĒ-nē-ă	_____
neutrophil (87)	NOO-trō-fĭl	_____
ophthalmology (80)	ŏf-thăl-MŎL-ō-jē	_____
osteogenic (85)	ŏs-tē-ō-JĔN-ĭk	_____
osteomalacia (80)	ŏs-tē-ō-mă-LĀ-shă	_____
otalgia (78)	ō-TĂL-jă	_____
paracentesis (78)	pă-ră-cĕn-TĒ-sĭs	_____
pathogenesis (80)	păth-ŏ-JĔN-ĕ-sĭs	_____
pathologic (85)	păth-ō-LŎJ-ĭk	_____
pericardium (84)	pĕr-ē-KĂR-dē-ŭm	_____

3

TERM	PRONUNCIATION	MEANING
peritoneal (85)	pĕr-ĭ-tō-NĒ-ăl	_____
phlebotomy (83)	flĕ-BŎT-ō-mē	_____
platelet (87)	PLĀT-lĕt	_____
pleural (85)	PLŬR-ăl	_____
pleurodynia (79)	plūr-ō-DĬN-ē-ă	_____
pneumonia (84)	noo-MŌN-yă	_____
polymorphonuclear leukocyte (87)	pŏl-ē-mŏr-fō-NŪ-klē-ăr LU-kō-sīt	_____
ptosis (82)	TŌ-sĭs	_____
pulmonary (85)	PŪL-mō-nā-rē	_____
radiographer (84)	rā-dē-ŎG-ră-fĕr	_____
radiotherapy (83)	rā-dē-ō-THĔR-ă-pe	_____
rectocele (78)	RĔK-tō-sēl	_____
rhinorrhea (82)	rī-nō-RĒ-ă	_____
splenomegaly (81)	splē-nō-MĔG-ă-lē	_____
staphylococci (78)	stăf-ĭ-lō-KŎK-sī	_____
streptococcus (78)	strĕp-tō-KŎK-ŭs	_____
thoracentesis (78)	thō-ră-sĕn-TĒ-sĭs	_____
thrombocyte (79)	THRŌM-bō-sīt	_____
thrombocytopenia (81)	thrŏm-bō-sī-tō-PĒ-nē-ă	_____
thrombophlebitis (80)	thrŏm-bō-flĕ-BĪ-tĭs	_____
tonsillar (85)	TŎN-sĭ-lăr	_____
tonsillitis (80)	tŏn-sĭ-LĪ-tĭs	_____
tracheostomy (83)	trā-kē-ŎS-tō-mē	_____
tracheotomy (83)	trā-kē-ŎT-ō-mē	_____
venule (84)	VĔN-ūl	_____

3

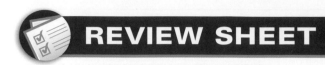

REVIEW SHEET

Write the meanings of each word part in the space provided and test yourself. Check your answers with the information in the chapter or in the **Glossary (Medical Word Parts—English),** at the end of this book.

Noun Suffixes

SUFFIX	MEANING	SUFFIX	MEANING
-algia		-opsy	
-cele		-osis	
-centesis		-pathy	
-coccus (-cocci)		-penia	
-cyte		-phobia	
-dynia		-plasia	
-ectomy		-plasty	
-emia		-ptosis	
-er		-rrhea	
-genesis		-sclerosis	
-gram		-scope	
-graph		-scopy	
-graphy		-stasis	
-ia		-stomy	
-ist		-therapy	
-itis		-tomy	
-logy		-trophy	
-lysis		-ule	
-malacia		-um, -ium	
-megaly		-us	
-ole		-y	
-oma			

3

Adjective Suffixes

SUFFIX	MEANING	SUFFIX	MEANING
-ac, -iac	_____	-ic, -ical	_____
-al	_____	-oid	_____
-ar	_____	-ose	_____
-ary	_____	-ous	_____
-eal	_____	-tic	_____
-genic	_____		

Combining Forms

COMBINING FORM	MEANING	COMBINING FORM	MEANING
abdomin/o	_____	erythr/o	_____
acr/o	_____	hem/o	_____
acu/o	_____	hepat/o	_____
aden/o	_____	hydr/o	_____
adip/o	_____	inguin/o	_____
amni/o	_____	isch/o	_____
angi/o	_____	lapar/o	_____
arteri/o	_____	laryng/o	_____
arthr/o	_____	leuk/o	_____
axill/o	_____	lymph/o	_____
bi/o	_____	mamm/o	_____
blephar/o	_____	mast/o	_____
bronch/o	_____	morph/o	_____
carcin/o	_____	muc/o	_____
cardi/o	_____	my/o	_____
chem/o	_____	myel/o	_____
chondr/o	_____	necr/o	_____
chron/o	_____	nephr/o	_____
col/o	_____	neur/o	_____
cyst/o	_____	neutr/o	_____
encephal/o	_____	nucle/o	_____

3

COMBINING FORM	MEANING	COMBINING FORM	MEANING
ophthalm/o	_____	rect/o	_____
oste/o	_____	ren/o	_____
ot/o	_____	rhin/o	_____
path/o	_____	sarc/o	_____
peritone/o	_____	splen/o	_____
phag/o	_____	staphyl/o	_____
phleb/o	_____	strept/o	_____
plas/o	_____	thorac/o	_____
pleur/o	_____	thromb/o	_____
pneumon/o	_____	tonsill/o	_____
pulmon/o	_____	trache/o	_____
radi/o	_____	ven/o	_____

Give the medical term for the following blood cells.

red blood cell _____

clotting cell _____

white blood cell _____

Name five different types of white blood cells (the first letter is given).

e _____

b _____

n _____

l _____

m _____

Prefixes

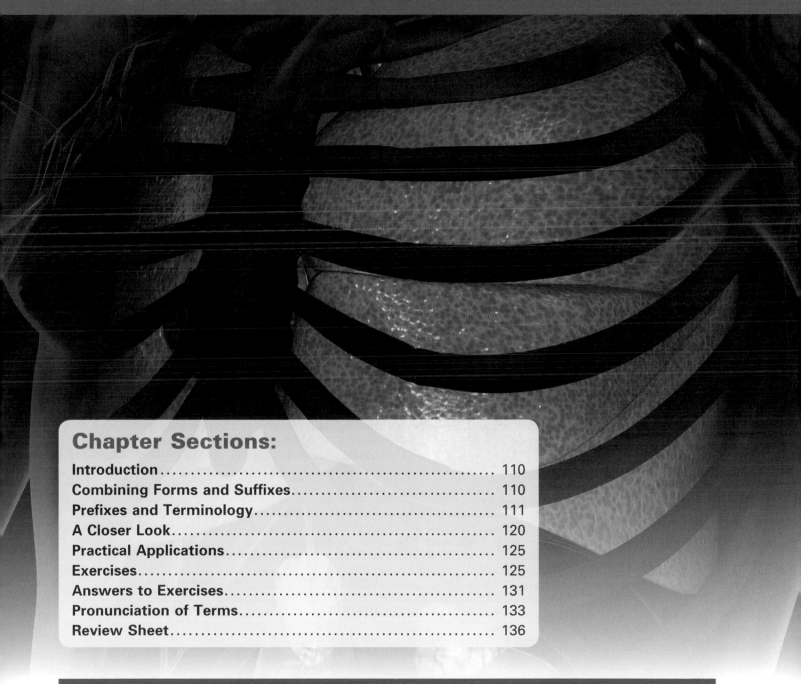

CHAPTER GOALS

- Define basic prefixes used in the medical language.
- Analyze medical terms that combine prefixes and other word elements.
- Learn about the Rh condition as an example of an antigen-antibody reaction.

INTRODUCTION

This chapter on prefixes, like the preceding chapter on suffixes, gives you practice in word analysis and provides a foundation for the study of the terminology of body systems that follows.

The list of combining forms, suffixes, and meanings helps you analyze terminology in the rest of the chapter. To support a broader understanding, *A Closer Look,* beginning on page 120, contains more detailed explanations of new terms.

COMBINING FORMS AND SUFFIXES

COMBINING FORMS

COMBINING FORM	MEANING	COMBINING FORM	MEANING
carp/o	wrist bones	pub/o	pubis (pubic bone); anterior portion of the pelvic or hipbone
cis/o	to cut		
cost/o	rib		
cutane/o	skin	seps/o	infection
dactyl/o	fingers, toes	somn/o	sleep
duct/o	to lead, carry	son/o	sound
flex/o	to bend	the/o	to put, place
gloss/o	tongue	thel/o, theli/o	nipple
glyc/o	sugar	thyr/o	thyroid gland; shield (the shape of the thyroid gland resembled [-oid] a shield to those who named it)
immun/o	protection		
morph/o	shape, form		
mort/o	death		
nat/i	birth	top/o	place, position, location
norm/o	rule, order	tox/o	poison
ox/o	oxygen	trache/o	windpipe, trachea
		urethr/o	urethra

4

SUFFIXES

These suffixes are used in this chapter in combination with prefixes. Some are complex suffixes that contain roots. For example, the suffix -pnea contains a root pne, meaning breathing, and a final suffix **-a,** meaning condition.

SUFFIX	MEANING	SUFFIX	MEANING
-blast	embryonic, immature	**-partum**	birth, labor
-crine	to secrete	**-phoria**	to bear, carry; feeling (mental state)
-drome	to run	**-physis**	to grow
-fusion	coming together; to pour	**-plasia**	development, formation, growth
-gen	substance that produces	**-plasm**	structure or formation
-lapse	to slide, fall, sag	**-pnea**	breathing
-lysis	breakdown, destruction, separation	**-ptosis**	falling, drooping, prolapse
-meter	to measure	**-rrhea**	flow, discharge
-mission	to send	**-stasis**	stopping, controlling
-or	one who	**-trophy**	development, nourishment
-oxia	oxygen		

4

PREFIXES AND TERMINOLOGY

Write the meaning of the medical term in the space provided. Remember: the Evolve website provides the definition and audio pronunciation for each term.

PREFIX	MEANING	TERMINOLOGY	MEANING
a-, an-	no, not, without	<u>a</u>pnea _____	
		<u>an</u>oxia _____	
ab-	away from	<u>ab</u>normal _____	
		<u>ab</u>ductor _____	

*A muscle that draws a limb **away** from the body.*

⊛ *HINT: Notice that in **ab**ductor, the **b** faces away from the **a**.*

PREFIX	MEANING	TERMINOLOGY	MEANING
ad-	toward	adductor _____ *A muscle that draws a limb* **toward** *the body.* ✳ **HINT:** *Notice that in* **ad***ductor, the* **d** *faces toward the* **a**. adrenal glands _____ *These glands actually lie on top of each kidney. See Figure 4-1.*	
ana-	up, apart	anabolism _____ analysis _____ *Urinalysis (urin/o + [an]/alysis) is a laboratory examination of urine that aids in the diagnosis of many medical conditions. In this term, -lysis means separation.*	
ante-	before, forward	ante cibum _____ *The word cibum means meals. The notation a.c., seen on prescription orders, means before meals. You can guess that p.c. means after (post) meals.* anteflexion _____ antepartum _____	

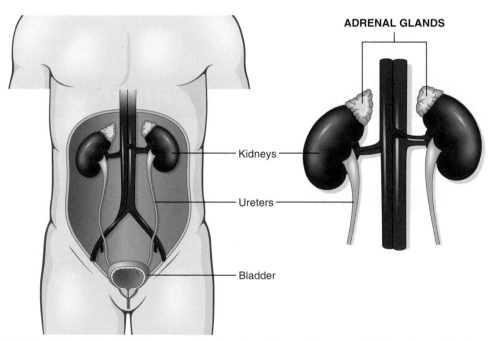

FIGURE 4-1 Adrenal glands. These are endocrine glands located above each kidney. One of the hormones they secrete is adrenaline (epinephrine). It causes bronchial tubes to widen, the heart to beat more rapidly and blood pressure to rise.

PREFIX	MEANING	TERMINOLOGY	MEANING
anti-	against	antibiotic _____ *Antibiotics destroy or inhibit the growth of microorganisms such as bacteria. Penicillin was the first antibiotic discovered in immature plants called molds, and was in widespread use by the 1940s. In early 2015, a new antibiotic called teixobactin was discovered. It has shown activity against antibiotic-resistant bacterial infections.* antibody _____ *Protein produced against an antigen (foreign body).* antigen _____ *In this term, anti- is short for antibody. An antigen (bacterium or virus) is a substance that produces (-gen) an antibody.* **See A Closer Look: Antigens and Antibodies,** *page 120.* antisepsis _____ *An antiseptic (-sis changes to -tic to form an adjective) substance fights infection.* antitoxin _____ *This is an antibody, often from an animal (such as a horse), that acts against a toxin. An example is tetanus antitoxin given against tetanus, an acute bacterial infection of the nervous system.*	
auto-	self, own	autoimmune disease _____	
bi-	two	bifurcation _____ *Normal splitting into two branches, such as bifurcation of the trachea to form the bronchi. The root furc means branching or forking.* bilateral _____	
brady-	slow	bradycardia _____ *Usually, a pulse of less than 60; a slow heart rate. Tachycardia (tachy- means fast) is a pulse of more than 100 beats per minute.*	
cata-	down	catabolism _____	
con-	with, together	congenital anomaly **See A Closer Look: Congenital Anomaly,** *page 122.* connective _____ *The root nect means to tie or bind. Connective tissue supports and binds other body tissue and parts. Bone, cartilage, and fibrous tissue are connective tissues.*	

Anti- and Ante-

Be careful not to confuse these prefixes. Pay close attention to their different pronunciations. **Anti-** is pronounced ăn-tǐ, and **ante-** is pronounced ăn-tē.

Autoimmune Disease

In an **autoimmune disease,** the body makes antibodies against its own good cells and tissues, causing inflammation and injury. Examples of autoimmune disorders are **rheumatoid arthritis,** affecting joints; **celiac disease,** affecting the intestinal tract; and **Graves disease,** affecting the thyroid gland.

PREFIX	MEANING	TERMINOLOGY	MEANING
contra-	against, opposite	<u>contra</u>indication _____ *Contra- means against in this term.* <u>contra</u>lateral _____ *Contra- means opposite in this term. A stroke affecting the right side of the brain may cause* **contralateral** *paralysis affecting the left arm and leg. The opposite of contralateral is* **ipsilateral.** *(ipsi- means same).*	
de-	down, lack of	<u>de</u>hydration _____	
dia-	through, complete	<u>dia</u>meter _____ <u>dia</u>rrhea _____ <u>dia</u>lysis _____ *Literal meaning is complete (dia-) separation (-lysis). In* **hemodialysis,** *waste materials are separated from the blood via a machine (artificial kidney) when the kidneys no longer function. See Figure 7-15, page 234, for an illustration of hemodialysis.*	
dys-	bad, painful, difficult, abnormal	<u>dys</u>pnea _____ *Often caused by respiratory or cardiac conditions, strenuous exercise, or anxiety.* <u>dys</u>entery _____ <u>dys</u>plasia _____	
ec-	out, outside	<u>ec</u>topic pregnancy _____ *Ectopic means pertaining to out of place and modifies the noun "pregnancy." See Figure 4-2.*	

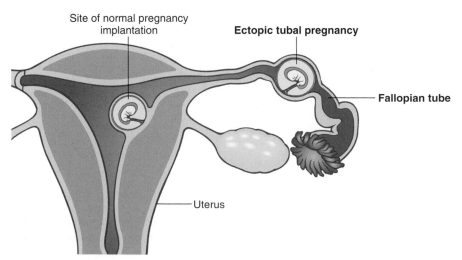

FIGURE 4-2   Ectopic pregnancy. Normal pregnancy implantation is in the upper portion of the uterus. Ectopic pregnancy occurs most commonly in a **fallopian tube** (i.e., tubal pregnancy). In this condition, the fetus is not viable. Surgery often is necessary to remove the ectopic tissue. Tubal surgery may damage a fallopian tube, and scar tissue can cause future pregnancy problems.

PREFIX	MEANING	TERMINOLOGY	MEANING
endo-	in, within	endocardium _____	
		endoscope _____	
		endotracheal _____ *An endotracheal tube, placed through the mouth into the trachea, is used for giving oxygen and in general anesthesia procedures.*	
epi-	upon, on, above	epithelium _____	
eu-	good, normal	euphoria _____ *Feeling of well-being.*	
		euthyroid _____ *Normal thyroid function.*	
ex-	out, outside	exophthalmos _____ *Protrusion of the eyeball associated with enlargement and overactivity of the thyroid gland; also called proptosis (pro- = forward, -ptosis =prolapse).*	
hemi-	half	hemiglossectomy _____	
hyper-	excessive, above	hyperglycemia _____ *This is a sign of diabetes mellitus. Lack of insulin (type 1 diabetes) or ineffective insulin (type 2 diabetes) causes high levels of sugar in the blood.*	
		hyperplasia _____ *Increase in cell numbers. Hyperplasia is a characteristic of tumor growth.*	
		hypertrophy _____ *Increase in size of individual cells. Muscle, cardiac, and renal cells exhibit hypertrophy when workload is increased.*	
hypo-	deficient, under	hypodermic injection _____	
		hypoglycemia _____	
in-	not	insomniac _____	
in-	into, within	incision _____	

4

Signs and Symptoms

A **sign** is **an objective finding that is perceived by an examiner,** such as fever, rash, or abnormal blood cell counts. A **symptom** (from Greek, *symptoma,* meaning that which happens) is **a subjective change in condition as perceived by the patient.** Examples of symptoms are loss of appetite, abdominal pain, and fatigue (tiredness). Both signs and symptoms are useful clues in the diagnosis of a disease, such as diabetes mellitus.

PREFIX	MEANING	TERMINOLOGY	MEANING
infra-	beneath, under	infracostal _____	
inter-	between	intercostal _____ *Intercostal muscles lie between adjacent ribs.*	
intra-	in, within, into	intravenous _____	
macro-	large	macrocephaly _____ *This is a congenital anomaly.*	
mal-	bad	malaise _____ (măl-ĀZ) *This is a French word meaning discomfort. It is a symptom of illness often marking the onset of a disease.*	
		malignant _____ *From the Latin ignis, meaning fire.* **Benign** (ben- = good) *is noncancerous, whereas* **malignant** *means cancerous.*	
meta-	beyond, change	metacarpal bones _____ *The five hand bones lie beyond the wrist bones but before the finger bones (phalanges).*	
		metamorphosis _____ *Meta- means change in this term. The change in development from the larval (caterpillar) stage to the adult (butterfly) is a form of metamorphosis. Embryonic (immature)* **stem cells** *spontaneously change (undergo metamorphosis) to form different types of mature cells.*	
		metastasis _____ *Meta- = beyond and -stasis = controlling, stopping. A metastasis is a malignant tumor that has spread to a secondary location.*	
micro-	small	microscope _____	
neo-	new	neonatal _____ *The neonatal period is the interval from birth to 28 days.*	
		neoplasm _____ *A neoplasm may be benign or malignant.*	
pan-	all	pancytopenia _____ *Deficiency of erythrocytes, leukocytes, and thrombocytes.*	

Intra-, Inter-, Infra-

Be careful not to confuse these prefixes: **intra-** means in, within, into; **inter-** means between; **infra-** means beneath, under.

PREFIX	MEANING	TERMINOLOGY	MEANING
para-	abnormal, beside, near	paralysis _____	
		Abnormal disruption of the connection between nerve and muscle. Originally from the Greek paralusis, meaning separation or loosening on one side, describing the loss of movement on one side of the body (occurring in stroke patients).	
		parathyroid glands _____	
		Para- means beside. The four parathyroid glands are located behind the thyroid gland. They secrete a hormone that regulates the calcium levels in blood and tissues.	
per-	through	percutaneous _____	
peri-	surrounding	pericardium _____	
poly-	many, much	polymorphonuclear _____	
		polyneuritis _____	
post-	after, behind	postmortem _____	
		postpartum _____	
pre-	before, in front of	precancerous _____	
		prenatal _____	
pro-	before, forward	prodrome _____	
		***Prodromal** signs and symptoms (rash, fever) appear before the actual illness (such as chickenpox) and signal its onset. Altered mood, fatigue, flashes of light, or stiff muscles may accompany the prodromal migraine aura that occurs before the actual headache.*	
		prolapse _____	
		The suffix -lapse means to slide, sag, or fall. See Figure 4-3.	

FIRST-DEGREE PROLAPSE   **SECOND-DEGREE PROLAPSE**

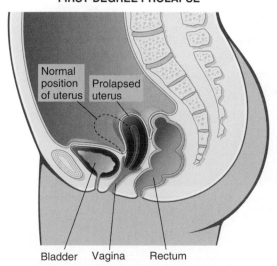
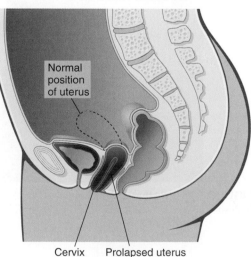

FIGURE 4-3   Prolapse of the uterus. In **first-degree prolapse,** the uterus descends into the vaginal canal. In **second-degree prolapse,** the body of the uterus is still within the vagina, but the cervix protrudes from the vaginal orifice (opening). In **third-degree prolapse** (*not pictured*), the entire uterus projects outside the orifice. As treatment, the uterus may be held in position by a plastic pessary (oval supporting object) that is inserted into the vagina. Some affected women may require hysterectomy (removal of the uterus).

PREFIX	MEANING	TERMINOLOGY	MEANING
pros-	before, forward	prosthesis _____ *An artificial limb is a prosthesis. Figure 4-4 shows Amy Palmiero-Winters running with a prosthetic leg.*	
re-	back, again	relapse _____ *A disease or its signs and symptoms return after an apparent recovery.*	
		remission _____ *Signs and symptoms lessen and the patient feels better. Remission may be spontaneous or the result of treatment. In some cases, a permanent remission means the disease is cured.*	
		recombinant DNA _____ *Genetic engineering uses recombinant DNA techniques.* See ***A Closer Look: Recombinant DNA***, page 122.	
retro-	behind, backward	retroperitoneal _____	
		retroflexion _____ *An abnormal position of an organ, such as the uterus, bent or tilted backward.*	
sub-	under	subcutaneous _____	

4

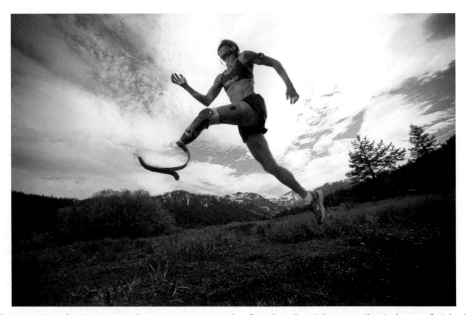

FIGURE 4-4   Prosthesis. Amy Palmeiro-Winters is the first female with a prosthetic leg to finish the Badwater 135, a 135-mile race from Badwater in Death Valley to Mount Whitney, California.

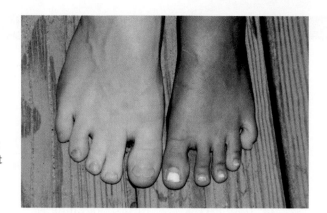

FIGURE 4-5 **Syndactyly.** The foot on the left (*pale*) shows syndactyly (webbed toes). The foot on the right (*darker*) shows normal toes. Syndactyly is a hereditary, congenital anomaly of fingers or toes.

PREFIX	MEANING	TERMINOLOGY	MEANING
supra-	above, upper	suprapubic _____ *The pubis is one of a pair of pubic bones that forms the anterior part of the pelvic (hip) bone. Pubic bones are pictured in Figure 4-6.*	
syn-, sym-	together, with	syndactyly _____ *See Figure 4-5.*	
		synthesis _____ *In protein synthesis, complex proteins are built up from simpler amino acids.*	
		syndrome _____ *See A Closer Look: Syndromes, page 123.*	
		symbiosis _____ *Before the letters b, m, and p, syn- becomes sym-.* ✱ **HINT:** *The term symptom is an important example. Be careful about spelling! Don't forget the p in symptom.*	
		symmetry _____ *Equality of parts on opposite sides of the body. What is asymmetry?*	
		symphysis _____ *A symphysis is a joint in which the bony surfaces are firmly united by a layer of fibrocartilage. See Figure 4-6.*	

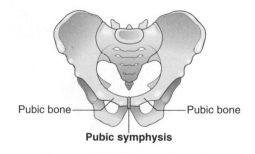

Pubic bone — — Pubic bone

Pubic symphysis

FIGURE 4-6 **Pubic symphysis.** This is the area in which the pubic bones of the pelvis have grown together. Another example of a symphysis is the solid connection between the two halves of the mandible (lower jawbone), which unite before birth.

Symbiosis

Symbiosis occurs when two organisms live together in close association, either for mutual benefit or not. Examples are:
- bacteria in the intestines and the cells lining the intestines benefit each other.
- parasites (tapeworms and fleas) live off another organism and are harmful to the host.

In psychiatry, symbiosis is a relationship between two people who are emotionally dependent on each other.

PREFIX	MEANING	TERMINOLOGY	MEANING
tachy-	fast	tachypnea _____ *(tă-KĬP-nē-ă)*	
trans-	across, through	transfusion _____ *Transfer of blood or blood parts from one person to another.*	
		transurethral _____ See ***A Closer Look: Transurethral Resection of the Prostate Gland,*** page 124.	
ultra-	beyond, excess	ultrasonography _____ See ***A Closer Look: Ultrasonography,*** page 124.	
uni-	one	unilateral _____	

A CLOSER LOOK

ANTIGENS AND ANTIBODIES; THE Rh CONDITION

An **antigen,** usually a foreign substance (such as a poison, virus, or bacterium), stimulates the production of **antibodies.** Antibodies are protein substances made by white blood cells in response to the presence of foreign antigens. For example, the flu virus (antigen) enters the body, causing the production of antibodies in the bloodstream. These antibodies then bind to and mark for destruction the antigens (viruses) that produced them. The reaction between an antigen and an antibody is an **immune response** (immun/o means protection). See Figure 4-7. When you receive a **vaccine,** you actually are receiving dead or weakened antigens that stimulate white blood cells (lymphocytes) to make antibodies. These antibodies remain in your blood to protect against those specific antigens when encountered in the future.

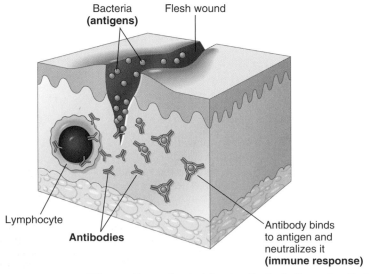

FIGURE 4-7 Immune response. When antigens (bacteria) enter the body through a flesh wound, antibodies are produced to destroy the antigens.

Another example of an antigen-antibody reaction is the **Rh condition.** A person who is Rh-positive (Rh⁺) has a protein coating (antigen) on his or her red blood cells (RBCs). This specific antigen factor is something that the person is born with and is normal. People who are Rh-negative (Rh⁻) have normal RBCs as well, but their red cells lack the Rh factor antigen.

If an Rh⁻ woman and an Rh⁺ man conceive an embryo, the embryo may be Rh⁻ or Rh⁺. A dangerous condition arises only when the embryo is Rh⁺ (because this is different from the Rh⁻ mother). During delivery of the first Rh⁺ baby, some of the baby's blood cells containing Rh⁺ antigens can escape into the mother's bloodstream. This sensitizes the mother so that she produces a low level of antibodies to the Rh⁺ antigen. Because this occurs at delivery, the first baby is generally not affected and is normal at birth. Sensitization can also occur after a miscarriage, abortion, or blood transfusions (with Rh⁺ blood).

Difficulties arise with the second Rh⁺ pregnancy. If this embryo also is Rh⁺, during pregnancy the mother's acquired antibodies (from the first pregnancy) enter the embryo's bloodstream. These antibodies attack and destroy the embryo's Rh⁺ RBCs. The embryo attempts to compensate for this loss by making many new but immature RBCs called erythroblasts (-blast = immature). The affected infant is born with **hemolytic disease of the newborn (HDN)** or **erythroblastosis fetalis.** HDN can occur in the first pregnancy if a mother has had an Rh⁺ blood transfusion.

One of the clinical signs of HDN is **jaundice** (yellow skin pigmentation). Jaundice results from excessive destruction of RBCs. When RBCs break down (hemolysis), the hemoglobin within the cells produces **bilirubin** (a chemical pigment). High levels of bilirubin in the bloodstream (hyperbilirubinemia) cause jaundice. To prevent bilirubin from affecting the brain cells of the infant, newborns are treated with exposure to bright lights (phototherapy). The light decomposes the bilirubin, which is then excreted from the infant's body.

Physicians administer Rh immunoglobulin to an Rh⁻ woman within 72 hours after each Rh⁺ delivery, abortion, or miscarriage. The globulin binds to Rh⁺ cells that escape into the mother's circulation and prevents formation of Rh⁺ antibodies. This protects future babies from developing HDN. Figure 4-8 reviews the Rh antigen-antibody reaction.

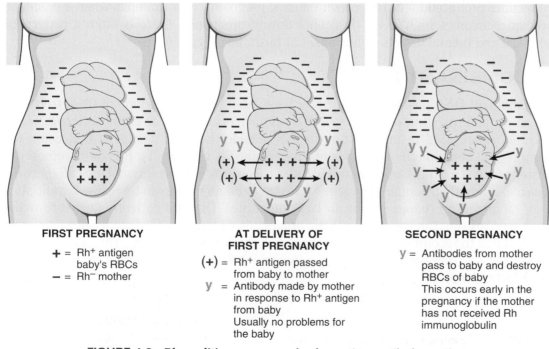

FIRST PREGNANCY

+ = Rh⁺ antigen
    baby's RBCs
− = Rh⁻ mother

AT DELIVERY OF FIRST PREGNANCY

(+) = Rh⁺ antigen passed
    from baby to mother
y = Antibody made by mother
    in response to Rh⁺ antigen
    from baby
    Usually no problems for
    the baby

SECOND PREGNANCY

y = Antibodies from mother
    pass to baby and destroy
    RBCs of baby
    This occurs early in the
    pregnancy if the mother
    has not received Rh
    immunoglobulin

FIGURE 4-8 **Rh condition** as an example of an antigen-antibody reaction.

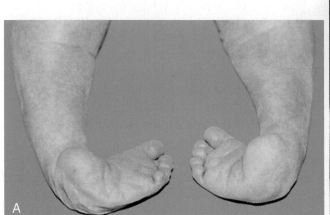
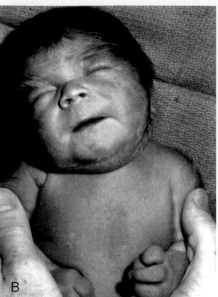

FIGURE 4-9 **Congenital anomalies. A, Clubfoot** is a hereditary congenital anomaly. The "clubbing" may affect one or both feet. **B, Fetal alcohol syndrome (FAS)** is a congenital anomaly caused by environmental factors during pregnancy. Notice the facial features of FAS: skin folds in corners of eyes, long, smooth groove between the nose and upper lip, thin upper lip, and flat nasal bridge.

CONGENITAL ANOMALY

An anomaly is an irregularity in a structure or organ. Examples of **congenital anomalies** (those that an infant is born with) include webbed fingers or toes (syndactyly), heart defects, and clubbed feet. See Figure 4-9A. Some congenital anomalies are hereditary (passed to the infant through chromosomes from the father or mother, or both), whereas others are produced by factors present during pregnancy. For example, when a pregnant woman consumes high levels of alcohol during pregnancy, there is often a pattern of physical and mental defects in her infant at birth. See Figure 4-9B.

RECOMBINANT DNA

Recombinant DNA technology is the process of taking a gene (a region of DNA) from one organism and inserting it into the DNA of another organism. For example, recombinant techniques are used to manufacture insulin outside the body. The gene that codes for insulin (i.e., contains the recipe for making insulin) is cut out of a human chromosome (using special enzymes) and transferred into a bacterium, such as *Escherichia coli* (*E. coli*). The bacterium then contains the gene for making human insulin and, because it multiplies very rapidly, can produce insulin in large quantities. Diabetic patients, unable to make their own insulin, can use this synthetic product (see Figure 4-10). Another term you may hear related to recombinant DNA is **polymerase chain reaction** (**PCR**). This is a method of producing multiple copies of a single gene, which is an important tool in recombinant DNA technology.

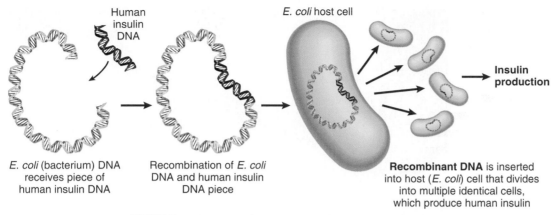

Human insulin DNA

E. coli host cell

Insulin production

E. coli (bacterium) DNA receives piece of human insulin DNA

Recombination of *E. coli* DNA and human insulin DNA piece

Recombinant DNA is inserted into host (*E. coli*) cell that divides into multiple identical cells, which produce human insulin

FIGURE 4-10   Recombinant DNA and insulin production.

SYNDROMES

A **syndrome** (from the Greek *dromos*, meaning a course for running) is a group of signs or symptoms that appear together to produce a typical clinical picture of a disease or inherited abnormality. For example, **Reye syndrome** is characterized by vomiting, swelling of the brain, increased intracranial pressure, hypoglycemia, and dysfunction of the liver. It may occur in children after a viral infection that has been treated with aspirin.

Marfan syndrome is an inherited connective tissue disorder marked by a tall, thin body type with long, "spidery" fingers and toes (arachnodactyly), elongated head, and heart, blood vessel, and ophthalmic abnormalities (see Figure 4-11).

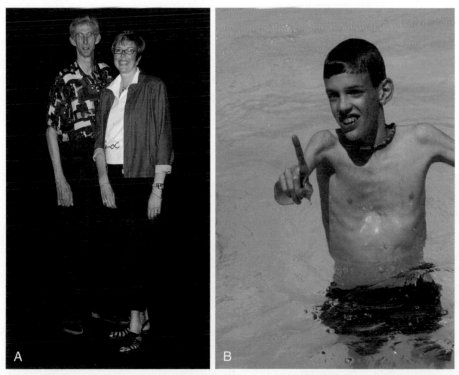

FIGURE 4-11   Marfan syndrome. A and **B** show people with Marfan's. Note the unusually tall body type and long, spidery fingers. The Olympic swimmer Michael Phelps (not pictured) has Marfan syndrome. His height is 6″4′ and his arm span is 6″7′.

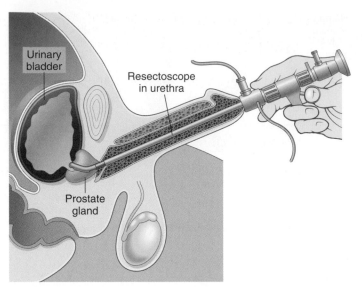

FIGURE 4-12   Transurethral resection of the prostate (TURP). The resectoscope contains a light, valves for controlling irrigated fluid, and an electrical loop that cuts tissue and seals blood vessels.

TRANSURETHRAL RESECTION OF THE PROSTATE GLAND

In **transurethral resection of the prostate gland** (**TURP**), a portion of the prostate gland is removed with an instrument (resectoscope) passed through (**trans-**) the urethra. The procedure is indicated when prostatic tissue increases (hyperplasia) and interferes with urination. Figure 4-12 shows a TURP procedure.

ULTRASONOGRAPHY

Ultrasonography is a diagnostic technique using ultrasound waves (inaudible sound waves) to produce an image of an organ or tissue. A machine records ultrasonic echoes as they pass through different types of tissue. **Echocardiograms** are ultrasound images of the heart. Figure 4-13 shows a fetal ultrasound image **(sonogram).**

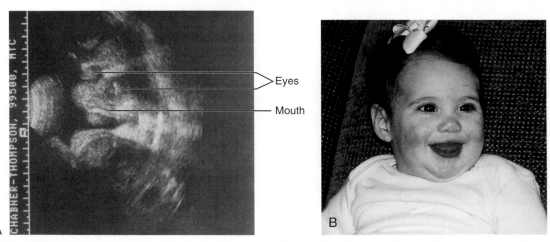

FIGURE 4-13   Ultrasonography. A, Notice the facial features of this beautiful 30-week-old fetus, in a (very) early "baby picture" of my granddaughter, Beatrix Bess Thompson! **B,** Bebe, smiling, at 3 months of age. *(Courtesy Dr. Elizabeth Chabner Thompson.)*

PRACTICAL APPLICATIONS

Check your answers with the Answers to Practical Applications on page 132. You should find helpful explanations there.

MATCHING: INDICATIONS AND PROCEDURES

Choose the correct procedure or treatment for each of the numbered indications.

INDICATIONS

1. Diagnose hepatopathy _____

2. Treat renal failure _____

3. Obtain prenatal images _____

4. Determine the postmortem status of organs _____

5. Treat carcinoma of the tongue _____

6. Treat benign prostatic hyperplasia _____

7. Diagnose disease in the stomach _____

8. Establish an airway during surgery _____

9. Treat pancytopenia _____

10. Treat staphylococcemia _____

PROCEDURES

a. antibiotics
b. autopsy
c. dialysis
d. endotracheal intubation
e. gastric endoscopy
f. hemiglossectomy
g. percutaneous liver biopsy
h. transfusion of blood cells
i. transurethral resection
j. ultrasonography

? EXERCISES

Remember to check your answers carefully with the Answers to Exercises, pages 131 and 132.

A Give the meanings of the following prefixes.

1. ante- _____

2. ab- _____

3. ana- _____

4. anti- _____

5. a-, an- _____

6. ad- _____

7. auto- _____

8. cata- _____

9. brady- _____

10. contra- _____

11. bi- _____

12. con- _____

B **Match the listed terms with the meanings that follow.**

adductor   anteflexion   bilateral
adrenal   antepartum   bradycardia
analysis   antisepsis   congenital anomaly
anoxia   apnea   contralateral

1. bending forward _____

2. muscle that carries the limb toward the body _____

3. before birth _____

4. slow heartbeat _____

5. gland located near (above) each kidney _____

6. absence of breathing _____

7. pertaining to the opposite side _____

8. against infection _____

9. to separate _____

10. pertaining to two (both) sides _____

11. condition of no oxygen in tissues _____

12. irregularity present at birth _____

C **Select from the listed terms to match the descriptions that follow.**

anabolism   antigen   catabolism
antibiotic   antitoxin   congenital anomaly
antibody   autoimmune disease   contraindication

1. chemical substance, such as erythromycin (-mycin = mold), made from molds and used against

   bacterial life _____

2. process of burning food (breaking it down) and releasing the energy stored in the food

   _____

3. reason that a doctor would advise against taking a specific medication

   _____

4. disorder in which the body's own leukocytes make antibodies that damage its own good tissue

   _____

5. a foreign agent (virus or bacterium) that causes production of antibodies

   _____

6. an antibody that acts against poisons that enter the body _____

7. process of building up proteins in cells by putting together small pieces of proteins called amino

   acids _____

8. protein made by lymphocytes in response to the presence in the blood of a specific antigen

   _____

4

D Give the meanings of the following prefixes.

1. ec- _____

2. dys- _____

3. de- _____

4. dia- _____

5. hemi- _____

6. hypo- _____

7. epi- _____

8. hyper- _____

9. endo- _____

10. eu- _____

11. in- _____

12. inter- _____

13. intra- _____

14. infra- _____

15. macro- _____

E Complete the following terms, based on their meanings as given.

1. normal thyroid function: _____ thyroid

2. painful breathing: _____ _____ pnea

3. pregnancy that is out of place (outside the uterus): _____ topic

4. instrument to visually examine within the body: endo _____

5. removal of half of the tongue: _____ glossectomy

6. good (exaggerated) feeling (of well-being): _____ phoria

7. pertaining to within the windpipe: endo _____

8. blood condition of less than normal sugar: _____ glycemia

9. condition (congenital anomaly) of large head: _____ cephaly

10. pertaining to between the ribs: _____ costal

11. pertaining to within a vein: intra _____

12. condition of bad (abnormal) formation (of cells): dys _____

13. condition of excessive formation (numbers of cells): _____ plasia

14. structure (membrane) that forms the inner lining of the heart: endo _____

15. pertaining to below the ribs: infra _____

16. blood condition of excessive amount of sugar: hyper _____

4

F **Match the listed terms with the meanings that follow.**

dehydration	incision	metamorphosis
dialysis	insomnia	metastasis
diarrhea	malaise	microscope
exophthalmos (proptosis)	malignant	pancytopenia

1. vague feeling of bodily discomfort _____

2. inability to sleep _____

3. lack of water _____

4. spread of a cancerous tumor to a secondary organ or tissue

_____

5. instrument used to view small objects _____

6. to cut into an organ or tissue _____

7. outward bulging of the eyeballs _____

8. condition of change in shape or form _____

9. watery discharge of wastes from the colon _____

10. deficiency of all (blood) cells _____

11. separation of wastes from the blood by using a machine that does the job of the kidney

_____

12. harmful, cancerous _____

G **Give the meanings of the following prefixes.**

1. mal- _____   11. sub- _____

2. pan- _____   12. supra- _____

3. per- _____   13. re- _____

4. meta- _____   14. retro- _____

5. para- _____   15. tachy- _____

6. peri- _____   16. syn- _____

7. poly- _____   17. uni- _____

8. post- _____   18. trans- _____

9. pro- _____   19. neo- _____

10. pre- _____   20. epi- _____

H <u>Underline</u> **the prefix in the following terms, and give the meaning of the entire term.**

1. pericardium _____

2. percutaneous _____

3. retroperitoneal _____

4. suprapubic _____

5. polyneuritis _____

6. retroflexion _____

7. transurethral _____

8. subcutaneous _____

9. tachypnea _____

10. unilateral _____

11. prosthesis _____

12. bilateral _____

13. symptom _____

14. syndrome _____

I **Match the listed terms with the meanings that follow.**

adrenal   prodrome   remission
neoplasm   prolapse   syndactyly
paralysis   recombinant DNA   syndrome
parathyroid   relapse   ultrasonography

1. return of a disease or its symptoms _____

2. loss of movement in muscles _____

3. congenital anomaly in which fingers or toes are webbed (formed together)

   _____

4. four endocrine glands that are located near (behind) another endocrine gland in the neck

   _____

5. glands that are located above the kidneys _____

6. symptoms that come before the actual illness _____

7. technique of transferring genetic material from one organism into another

   _____

8. sliding, sagging downward or forward _____

9. new growth or tumor _____

10. process of using sound waves to create an image of organs and structures in the body

    _____

11. group of signs and symptoms that occur together and indicate a particular disorder

    _____

12. symptoms lessen and a patient feels better _____

4

J Complete the following terms, based on their meanings as given.

1. pertaining to new birth: neo _____

2. after death: post _____

3. spread of a cancerous tumor: meta _____

4. branching into two: bi _____

5. increase in development (size of cells): hyper _____

6. pertaining to a chemical that works against bacterial life: _____ biotic

7. hand bones (beyond the wrist): _____ carpals

8. protein produced by leukocytes to fight foreign organisms: anti _____

9. group of symptoms that occur together: _____ drome

10. surface or skin tissue of the body: _____ thelium

K Circle the correct bold term to complete the following sentences.

1. Dr. Tate felt that Mrs. Snow's condition of thrombocytopenia was a clear (**analysis, contraindication, synthesis**) to performing elective surgery.

2. Medical science was revolutionized by the introduction of (**antigens, antibiotics, antibodies**) in the 1940s. Now some infections can be treated with only one dose.

3. Robert's 82-year-old grandfather complained of (**malaise, dialysis, insomnia**) despite taking the sleeping medication that his doctor prescribed.

4. During her pregnancy, Ms. Payne described pressure on her (**pituitary gland, parathyroid gland, pubic symphysis**), making it difficult for her to find a comfortable position, even when seated.

5. Many times, people with diabetes accidentally take too much insulin. This results in lowering their blood sugar so much that they may be admitted to the emergency department with (**hyperplasia, hypoglycemia, hyperglycemia**).

6. Before his migraine headaches began, John noticed changes in his eyesight, such as bright spots, zigzag lines, and double vision. His physician told him that these were (**symbiotic, exophthalmic, prodromal**) symptoms.

7. After hiking in the Grand Canyon without an adequate water supply, Julie experienced (**hyperglycemia, dehydration, hypothyroidism**).

8. At 65 years of age, Paul Smith often felt fullness in his urinary bladder but had difficulty urinating. He visited his (**cardiologist, nephrologist, urologist**), who examined his prostate gland and diagnosed (**hyperplasia, atrophy, ischemia**). The doctor advised (**intracostal, transurethral, peritoneal**) resection of Paul's prostate.

9. After running the Boston Marathon, Elizabeth felt nauseated and dizzy. She realized that she was experiencing (**malaise, euphoria, hypoglycemia**) and drank a sports drink containing sugar, which made her feel better.

10. While she was taking an antibiotic that reacted with sunlight, Ruth's physician advised her that sunbathing was (**unilateral, contraindicated, contralateral**) and might cause a serious sunburn.

11. Puerperal (pertaining to childbirth) fever was an iatrogenic infection; it was carried from one woman to another by the doctor before the days of (**antigens, antibodies, antisepsis**).

12. Dysplastic nevi (abnormal pigmented lesions or moles) on a patient's skin may be a (**precancerous, metastatic, unilateral**) sign of malignant skin cancer called melanoma.

13. Nerve cells of the brain may (**relapse, hypertrophy, atrophy**) in old age because of ischemia caused by restricted blood flow.

14. Changes in cell growth resulting in cells that differ in size, shape, and appearance are the result of chronic inflammation and irritation. When the condition occurs in the uterine cervix, it is known as cervical (**prolapse, paralysis, dysplasia**).

4

ANSWERS TO EXERCISES

A

1. before, forward
2. away from
3. up, apart
4. against
5. no, not, without
6. toward
7. self, own
8. down
9. slow
10. against, opposite
11. two
12. together, with

B

1. anteflexion
2. adductor
3. antepartum
4. bradycardia
5. adrenal
6. apnea
7. contralateral
8. antisepsis
9. analysis
10. bilateral
11. anoxia
12. congenital anomaly

C

1. antibiotic
2. catabolism
3. contraindication
4. autoimmune disease
5. antigen
6. antitoxin
7. anabolism
8. antibody

D

1. out, outside
2. bad, painful, difficult
3. down, lack of
4. through, complete
5. half
6. deficient, under
7. upon, on, above
8. excessive, above, beyond
9. in, within
10. good, well
11. in, not
12. between
13. within
14. below, inferior
15. large

E

1. euthyroid
2. dyspnea
3. ectopic
4. endoscope
5. hemiglossectomy
6. euphoria
7. endotracheal
8. hypoglycemia
9. macrocephaly
10. intercostal
11. intravenous
12. dysplasia
13. hyperplasia
14. endocardium
15. infracostal
16. hyperglycemia

F

1. malaise
2. insomnia
3. dehydration
4. metastasis
5. microscope
6. incision
7. exophthalmos (proptosis)
8. metamorphosis
9. diarrhea
10. pancytopenia
11. dialysis
12. malignant

G

1. bad
2. all
3. through
4. change, beyond
5. near, beside, abnormal
6. surrounding
7. many, much
8. after, behind
9. before, forward
10. before, in front of
11. under
12. above
13. back, again
14. behind, backward
15. fast
16. together, with
17. one
18. across, through
19. new
20. above, upon, on

H

1. pericardium—membrane surrounding the heart
2. percutaneous—pertaining to through the skin
3. retroperitoneal—pertaining to behind the peritoneum
4. suprapubic—above the pubic bone
5. polyneuritis—inflammation of many nerves
6. retroflexion—bending backward
7. transurethral—pertaining to through the urethra
8. subcutaneous—pertaining to below the skin
9. tachypnea—rapid, fast breathing
10. unilateral—pertaining to one side
11. prosthesis—artificial limb or part of the body (literally, to put or place forward)
12. bilateral—both sides
13. symptom—subjective change of condition as observed by a patient
14. syndrome—group of objective findings that characterize an abnormal condition

4

I

1. relapse
2. paralysis
3. syndactyly
4. parathyroid

5. adrenal
6. prodrome
7. recombinant DNA
8. prolapse

9. neoplasm
10. ultrasonography
11. syndrome
12. remission

J

1. neonatal
2. postmortem
3. metastasis
4. bifurcation

5. hypertrophy
6. antibiotic
7. metacarpals
8. antibody

9. syndrome
10. epithelium

K

1. contraindication
2. antibiotics
3. insomnia
4. pubic symphysis
5. hypoglycemia

6. prodromal
7. dehydration
8. urologist; hyperplasia; transurethral
9. hypoglycemia

10. contraindicated
11. antisepsis
12. precancerous
13. atrophy
14. dysplasia

Answers to Practical Applications

1. **G—percutaneous liver biopsy** Diseases such as hepatitis or hepatoma are diagnosed by performing a liver biopsy.
2. **C—dialysis** Patients experiencing loss of kidney function need dialysis to remove waste materials from the blood.
3. **J—ultrasonography** Ultrasonography is especially useful to detect fetal structures because no x-rays are used.
4. **B—autopsy** A veterinarian performs postmortem examination of animals, which is called necropsy.

5. **F—hemiglossectomy** Malignancies of the oral (mouth) cavity often are treated with surgery to remove the cancerous growth.
6. **I—transurethral resection** A TURP is a transurethral resection of the prostate gland.
7. **F—gastric endoscopy** Placement of an endoscope through the mouth and esophagus and into the stomach is used to diagnose gastric (stomach) disease.
8. **D—endotracheal intubation** This is necessary during surgery in which general anesthesia is used.

9. **H—transfusion of blood cells** Transfusion of leukocytes, erythrocytes, and platelets will increase numbers of these cells in the bloodstream.
10. **A—antibiotics** Examples are penicillin, erythromycin, and amoxicillin.

4

PRONUNCIATION OF TERMS

To test your understanding of the terminology in this chapter, write the meaning of each term in the space provided. In addition, you may wish to cover the terms and write them by looking at your definitions. Make sure your spelling is correct. The CAPITAL letters indicate the accented syllable. The page number after each term indicates where it is defined or used in the book, so you can easily check your responses. You will find complete definitions for all of these terms and their audio pronunciations on the Evolve website.

Pronunciation Guide

ā as in āpe	ă as in ăpple
ē as in ēven	ĕ as in ĕvery
ī as in īce	ĭ as in ĭnterest
ō as in ōpen	ŏ as in pŏt
ū as in ūnit	ŭ as in ŭnder

TERM	PRONUNCIATION	MEANING
abductor (111)	ăb-DŬK-tŏr	
abnormal (111)	ăb-NŌR-măl	
adductor (112)	ă-DŬK-tŏr	
adrenal glands (112)	ă-DRĒ-năl glăndz	
anabolism (112)	ă-NĂ-bō-lĭzm	
analysis (112)	ă-NĂL-ĭ-sĭs	
anoxia (111)	ă-NŎK-sē-ă	
ante cibum (112)	ĂN-tē SĒ-bŭm	
anteflexion (112)	ăn-tē-FLĔK-shŭn	
antepartum (112)	ăn-tē-PĂR-tŭm	
antibiotic (113)	ăn-tĭ-bī-ŎT-ĭk	
antibody (113)	ĂN-tĭ-bŏd-ē	
antigen (113)	ĂN-tĭ-jĕn	
antisepsis (113)	ăn-tĭ-SĔP-sĭs	
antitoxin (113)	ăn-tĭ-TŎK-sĭn	
apnea (111)	ĂP-nē-ă *or* ăp-NĒ-ă	
autoimmune disease (113)	aw-tō-ĭ-MŪN dĭ-ZĒZ	
benign (116)	bē-NĪN	
bifurcation (113)	bī-fŭr-KĀ-shŭn	
bilateral (113)	bī-LĂT-ĕr-ăl	
bradycardia (113)	brăd-ē-KĂR-dē-ă	
catabolism (113)	kă-TĂB-ō-lĭzm	
congenital anomaly (113)	kŏn-JĔN-ĭ-tăl ă-NŎM-ă-lē	
connective tissue (113)	kŏn-NĔK-tĭv TĬ-shū	
contraindication (114)	kŏn-tră-ĭn-dĭ-KĀ-shŭn	

4

TERM	PRONUNCIATION	MEANING
contralateral (114)	kŏn-tră-LĂT-ĕr-ăl	_____
dehydration (114)	dē-hī-DRĀ-shŭn	_____
dialysis (114)	dī-ĂL-ĭ-sĭs	_____
diameter (114)	dī-ĂM-ĭ-tĕr	_____
diarrhea (114)	dī-ă-RĒ-ă	_____
dysentery (114)	DĬS-ĕn-tĕ-rē	_____
dysplasia (114)	dĭs-PLĀ-zē-ă	_____
dyspnea (114)	DĬSP-nē-ă _or_ dĭsp-NĒ-ă	_____
ectopic pregnancy (114)	ĕk-TŎP-ĭk PRĔG-năn-sē	_____
endocardium (115)	ĕn-dō-KĂR-dē-ŭm	_____
endoscope (115)	ĔN-dō-skōp	_____
endotracheal (115)	ĕn-dō-TRĀ-kē-ăl	_____
epithelium (115)	ĕp-ĭ-THĒ-lē-ŭm	_____
euphoria (115)	ū-FŎR-ē-ă	_____
euthyroid (115)	ū-THĪ-royd	_____
exophthalmos (115)	ĕk-sŏf-THĂL-mŏs	_____
hemiglossectomy (115)	hĕm-ē-glŏs-SĔK-tō-mē	_____
hyperglycemia (115)	hī-pĕr-glī-SĒ-mē-ă	_____
hyperplasia (115)	hī-pĕr-PLĀ-zē-ă	_____
hypertrophy (115)	hī-PĔR-trō-fē	_____
hypodermic injection (115)	hī-pō-DĔR-mĭk ĭn-JĔK-shŭn	_____
hypoglycemia (115)	hī-pō-glī-SĒ-mē-ă	_____
incision (115)	ĭn-SĬZ-Ŏn	_____
infracostal (116)	ĭn-fră-KŎS-tăl	_____
insomniac (115)	ĭn-SŎM-nē-ăk	_____
intercostal (116)	ĭn-tĕr-KŎS-tăl	_____
intravenous (116)	ĭn-tră-VĒ-nŭs	_____
macrocephaly (116)	măk-rō-SĔF-ă-lē	_____
malaise (116)	măl-ĀZ	_____
malignant (116)	mă-LĬG-nănt	_____
metacarpal bones (116)	mĕ-tă-KĂR-păl bōnz	_____
metamorphosis (116)	mĕt-ă-MŎR-fŏ-sĭs	_____
metastasis (116)	mĕ-TĂS-tă-sĭs	_____
microscope (116)	MĪ-krō-skōp	_____
neonatal (116)	nē-ō-NĀ-tăl	_____

4

TERM	PRONUNCIATION	MEANING
neoplasm (116)	NĒ-ō-plăzm	
pancytopenia (116)	păn-sī-tō-PĒ-ne-ă	
paralysis (117)	pă-RĂL-ĭ-sĭs	
parathyroid glands (117)	păr-ă-THĪ-royd glănz	
percutaneous (117)	pĕr-kū-TĀ-nē-ŭs	
pericardium (117)	pĕ-rē-KĂR-dē-ŭm	
polymorphonuclear (117)	pŏl-ĕ-mŏr-fō-NŪ-klē-ăr	
polyneuritis (117)	pŏl-ē-nū-RĪ-tĭs	
postmortem (117)	pōst-MŎR-tĕm	
postpartum (117)	pōst-PĂR-tŭm	
precancerous (117)	prē-KĂN-sĕr-ŭs	
prenatal (117)	prē-NĀ-tăl	
prodrome (117)	PRŌ-drōm	
prolapse (117)	PRŌ-lăps	
prosthesis (118)	prŏs-THĒ-sĭs	
recombinant DNA (118)	rē-KŎM-bĭ nănt DNA	
relapse (118)	RĒ-lăps	
remission (118)	rē-MĬ-shŭn	
retroflexion (116)	rĕt-rō-FLĔK-shŭn	
retroperitoneal (118)	rĕt-rō-pĕr-ĭ-tō-NĒ-ăl	
subcutaneous (118)	sŭb-kū-TĀ-nē-ŭs	
suprapubic (118)	sū-pră-PŪ-bĭk	
symbiosis (119)	sĭm-bē-Ō-sĭs	
symmetry (119)	SĬM-mĕ-trē	
symphysis (119)	SĬM-fĭ-sĭs	
symptom (119)	SĬMP-tŭm	
syndactyly (119)	sĭn-DĂK-tĭ-lē	
syndrome (119)	SĬN-drōm	
synthesis (119)	SĬN-thĕ-sĭs	
tachypnea (120)	tă-KĬP-nē-ă *or* tăk-ĭp-NĒ-ă	
transfusion (120)	trăns-FŪ-zhŭn	
transurethral (120)	trăns-ū-RĒ-thrăl	
ultrasonography (120)	ŭl-tră-sŏ-NŎG-ră-fē	
unilateral (120)	ū-nĭ-LĂT-ĕr-ăl	

4

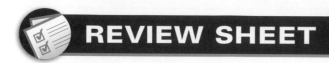

REVIEW SHEET

Write the meanings of each word part in the space provided, and test yourself. Check your answers with the information in the chapter or in the *Glossary (Medical Word Parts—English)* at the end of the book.

4

Prefixes

PREFIX	MEANING	PREFIX	MEANING
a-, an-	_____	inter-	_____
ab-	_____	intra-	_____
ad-	_____	macro-	_____
ana-	_____	mal-	_____
ante-	_____	meta-	_____
anti-	_____	micro-	_____
auto-	_____	neo-	_____
bi-	_____	pan-	_____
brady-	_____	para-	_____
cata-	_____	per-	_____
con-	_____	peri-	_____
contra-	_____	poly-	_____
de-	_____	post-	_____
dia-	_____	pre-	_____
dys-	_____	pro-	_____
ec-	_____	pros-	_____
en-, endo-	_____	re-	_____
epi-	_____	retro-	_____
eu-	_____	sub-	_____
ex-	_____	supra-	_____
hemi-	_____	syn-, sym-	_____
hyper-	_____	tachy-	_____
hypo-	_____	trans-	_____
in-	_____	ultra-	_____
infra-	_____	uni-	_____

Prefixes with Similar Meanings

PREFIX	MEANING	PREFIX	MEANING
a-, an-, in-	_____	ec-, ecto-, ex-	_____
ante-, pre-, pro-	_____	endo-, in-, intra-	_____
anti-, contra-	_____	epi-, hyper-, supra-	_____
con-, syn-, sym-	_____	hypo-, infra-, sub-	_____
de-, cata-	_____	re-, retro-, post-	_____
dia-, per-, trans-	_____	ultra-, meta-	_____
dys-, mal-	_____		

Combining Forms

COMBINING FORM	MEANING	COMBINING FORM	MEANING
carp/o	_____	ophthalm/o	_____
cost/o	_____	ox/o	_____
cutane/o	_____	pub/o	_____
dactyl/o	_____	ren/o	_____
duct/o	_____	seps/o	_____
flex/o	_____	somn/o	_____
gloss/o	_____	son/o	_____
glyc/o	_____	the/o	_____
immun/o	_____	thyr/o	_____
later/o	_____	top/o	_____
morph/o	_____	tox/o	_____
mort/o	_____	trache/o	_____
nat/i	_____	urethr/o	_____
necr/o	_____	ven/o	_____
norm/o	_____		

4

Suffixes

SUFFIX	MEANING	SUFFIX	MEANING
-blast	_____	-partum	_____
-crine	_____	-phoria	_____
-drome	_____	-physis	_____
-fusion	_____	-plasia	_____
-gen	_____	-plasm	_____
-lapse	_____	-pnea	_____
-lysis	_____	-ptosis	_____
-meter	_____	-rrhea	_____
-mission	_____	-stasis	_____
-or	_____	-trophy	_____

evolve   *Please visit the Evolve website for additional exercises, games, and images related to this chapter.*

4

Digestive System

Chapter Sections:

CHAPTER GOALS

- Name the organs of the digestive system and describe their locations and functions.
- Define combining forms for organs and know the meaning of related terminology.
- Describe signs, symptoms, and disease conditions affecting the digestive system.

INTRODUCTION

The digestive system is divided between Chapters 5 and 6. Chapter 5 covers the anatomy, physiology, pathology, and basic terminology of the system. Chapter 6 introduces additional terminology and review of digestive system terms, plus laboratory tests, clinical procedures, and abbreviations. My reason for not combining the chapters is that I did not want to overwhelm you with an extraordinarily long chapter so early in your study. In my own teaching, I find that my students are grateful for this separation, and especially for the breather and review of terminology in Chapter 6.

My choice to begin with the digestive system is based on a perception that this body system (resembling a long conveyor belt with the mouth at the entrance and anus at the exit) is one of the more straightforward and easiest to understand. Keep in mind, however, that the book is organized so that you may begin study of the body systems with any chapter to create the order that best reflects your interests.

The digestive or **gastrointestinal tract** begins with the mouth, where food enters, and ends with the anus, where solid waste material leaves the body. The four functions of the system are **ingestion, digestion, absorption,** and **elimination.**

First, complex food material taken into the mouth is **ingested.** Second, it is **digested,** or broken down, mechanically and chemically, as it travels through the gastrointestinal tract. Digestive **enzymes** speed up chemical reactions and aid the breakdown (digestion) of complex nutrients. Complex proteins are digested to simpler **amino acids;** complicated sugars are reduced to simple sugars, such as **glucose;** and large fat or lipid molecules are broken down to simpler substances such as **fatty acids** and **triglycerides** (three parts fatty acids and one part glycerol). Digestion occurs in the mouth, stomach, and small intestine.

Third, through **absorption,** nutrients from digested food pass through the lining cells or epithelium of the small intestine and into the bloodstream. Nutrients then travel to all cells of the body. Cells then break down nutrients in the presence of oxygen to release energy. Cells also use amino acid nutrients to build up large protein molecules needed for growth and development. In addition, fat molecules are absorbed into lymphatic vessels from the intestine.

The fourth function of the digestive system is **elimination** of the solid waste materials that cannot be absorbed into the bloodstream. The large intestine concentrates these solid wastes, called **feces,** and the wastes finally pass out of the body through the anus.

ANATOMY AND PHYSIOLOGY

ORAL CAVITY

The gastrointestinal tract begins with the **oral cavity.** Oral means pertaining to the mouth (or/o). Label Figure 5-1 as you learn the major parts of the oral cavity.

The **cheeks** [1] form the walls of the oval-shaped oral cavity, and the **lips** [2] surround the opening to the cavity.

The **hard palate** [3] forms the anterior portion of the roof of the mouth, and the muscular **soft palate** [4] lies posterior to it. **Rugae** are irregular ridges in the mucous membrane covering the anterior portion of the hard palate. The **uvula** [5], a small soft tissue projection, hangs from the soft palate. It aids production of sounds and speech.

The **tongue** [6] extends across the floor of the oral cavity, and muscles attach it to the lower jawbone. It moves food around during **mastication** (chewing) and **deglutition** (swallowing). **Papillae,** small raised areas on the tongue, contain taste buds that are sensitive to the chemical nature of foods and allow discrimination of different tastes as food moves across the tongue.

COMBINING FORMS
1. bucc/o
2. cheil/o, labi/o
3. palat/o
4. palat/o
5. uvul/o
6. gloss/o, lingu/o
7. tonsill/o
8. gingiv/o
9. dent/i, odont/o

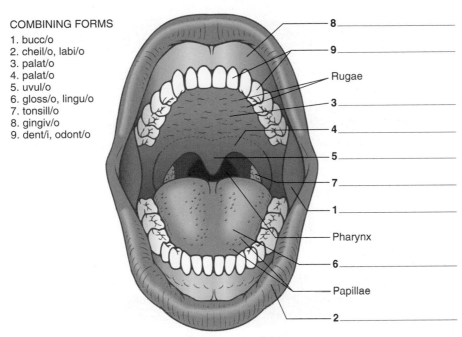

8 _____
9 _____
Rugae
3 _____
4 _____
5 _____
7 _____
1 _____
Pharynx
6 _____
Papillae
2 _____

FIGURE 5-1 Oral cavity.

The **tonsils** [7], masses of lymphatic tissue located in depressions of the mucous membranes, lie on both sides of the oropharynx (part of the throat near the mouth). They are filters to protect the body from the invasion of microorganisms and produce lymphocytes, disease-fighting white blood cells.

The **gums** [8] are the fleshy tissue surrounding the sockets of the **teeth** [9]. Figure 5-2 shows a dental arch with 16 permanent teeth (there are 32 permanent teeth in the entire oral cavity). The names of the teeth are labeled in Figure 5-2.

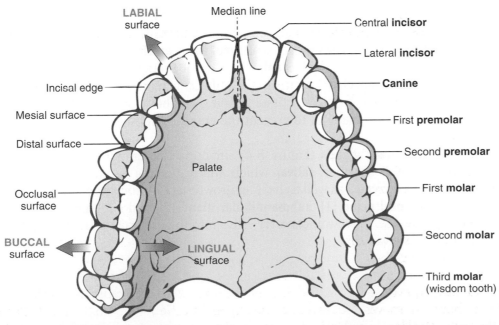

LABIAL surface
Median line
Central **incisor**
Lateral **incisor**
Canine
Incisal edge
Mesial surface
Distal surface
First **premolar**
Second **premolar**
Palate
First **molar**
Occlusal surface
Second **molar**
BUCCAL surface
LINGUAL surface
Third **molar** (wisdom tooth)

FIGURE 5-2 Upper permanent teeth within the dental arch. The **buccal** surface faces the cheek, whereas the **lingual** surface faces the tongue. The **labial** surface faces the lips. Dentists refer to the labial and buccal surfaces as the **facial** (faci/o = face) surface.

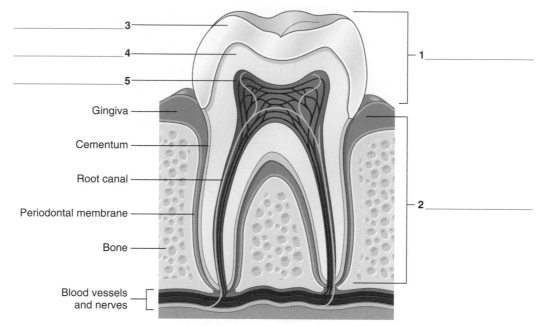

Gingiva

Cementum

Root canal

Periodontal membrane

Bone

Blood vessels
and nerves

FIGURE 5-3   Anatomy of a tooth.

Figure 5-3 shows the inner anatomy of a tooth. Label it as you read the following description:

A tooth consists of a **crown** [1], which shows above the gum line, and a **root** [2], which lies within the bony tooth socket. The outermost layer of the crown, the **enamel** [3], protects the tooth. It is the hardest tissue in the human body. **Dentin** [4], the main substance of the tooth, lies beneath the enamel and extends throughout the crown. Dentin's color ranges from creamy white to yellow, and it affects the color of teeth because enamel is translucent. The **cementum** covers, protects, and supports the dentin in the root. A **periodontal membrane** surrounds the cementum and holds the tooth in place in the tooth socket.

The **pulp** [5] lies underneath the dentin. This soft and delicate tissue fills the center of the tooth. Blood vessels, nerve endings, connective tissue, and lymphatic vessels are within the pulp canal (also called the **root canal**). Root canal therapy often is necessary when disease or abscess (pus collection) occurs in the pulp canal. A dentist opens the tooth from above and cleans the canal of infected tissue, nerves, and blood vessels. The canal is then disinfected and filled with material to prevent the entrance of microorganisms that could cause decay.

Three pairs of **salivary glands** (Figure 5-4) surround and empty into the oral cavity. These exocrine glands produce **saliva,** which lubricates the mouth. Saliva contains important digestive **enzymes** as well as healing growth factors such as cytokines. Saliva is released from a **parotid gland** [1], **submandibular gland** [2], and **sublingual gland** [3] on both sides of the mouth. Narrow ducts carry saliva into the oral cavity. The glands produce about 1.5 liters of saliva daily.

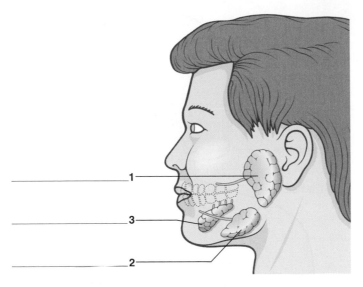

FIGURE 5-4   Salivary glands.

PHARYNX

Refer to Figure 5-5. The **pharynx** or **throat** is a muscular tube, about 5 inches long, lined with a mucous membrane. It serves as a passageway both for air traveling from the nose (nasal cavity) to the windpipe (trachea) and for food traveling from the oral cavity to the **esophagus.** When swallowing (**deglutition**) occurs, a cartilaginous flap of tissue, the epiglottis, covers the trachea so that food cannot enter and become lodged there. See Figure 5-5A and B.

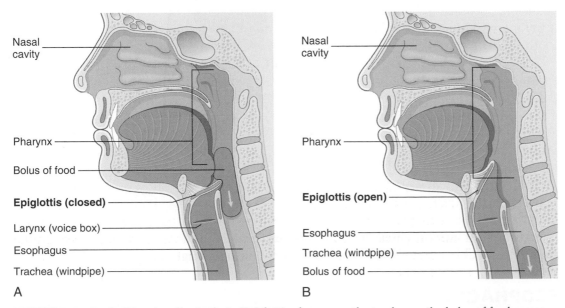

FIGURE 5-5   Deglutition (swallowing). A, Epiglottis closes over the trachea as the bolus of food passes down the pharynx toward the esophagus. **B, Epiglottis opens** as the bolus moves down the esophagus.

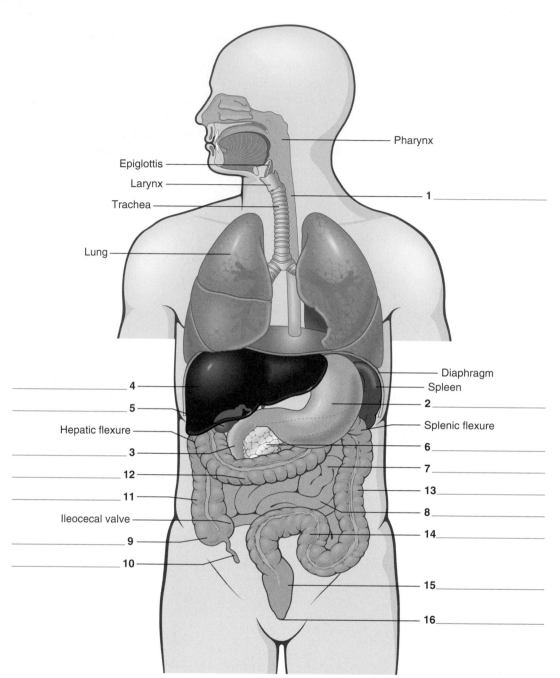

FIGURE 5-6   The gastrointestinal tract.

Figure 5-6 shows the passageway for food as it travels from the esophagus through the gastrointestinal tract. Label it as you read the following paragraphs.

ESOPHAGUS

The **esophagus** [1] is a 9- to 10-inch muscular tube extending from the pharynx to the stomach. **Peristalsis** is the involuntary, progressive, rhythmic contraction of muscles in the wall of the esophagus (and other gastrointestinal organs) propelling a **bolus** (mass of food) down toward the stomach. The process is like squeezing a marble through a rubber tube.

STOMACH

Food passes from the esophagus into the **stomach** [2]. The stomach (Figure 5-7) has three main parts: **fundus** (upper portion), **body** (middle section), and **antrum** (lower portion). Rings of muscle called **sphincters** control the openings into and leading out of the stomach. They prevent food from regurgitating (flowing backward from the normal direction). The **lower esophageal sphincter** (**LES**) relaxes and contracts to move food from the esophagus into the stomach. The **pyloric sphincter** allows food to leave the stomach and enter the small intestine when it is ready. Folds in the mucous membrane **(mucosa)** lining the stomach are called **rugae.** The rugae increase surface area for digestion and contain glands that produce the enzyme **pepsin** to begin digestion of proteins. **Hydrochloric acid** also is secreted to digest protein and kill any bacteria remaining in food.

The stomach prepares food for the small intestine, where further digestion and absorption into the bloodstream take place. Food leaves the stomach in 1 to 4 hours or longer, depending on the amount and type of food eaten.

SMALL INTESTINE (SMALL BOWEL)

(Continue labeling Figure 5-6 on page 144.)

The **small intestine (small bowel)** extends for 20 feet from the pyloric sphincter to the first part of the large intestine. It has three parts. The first section, the **duodenum** [3], is only 1 foot long. It receives food from the stomach as well as **bile** from the **liver** [4] and **gallbladder** [5] and pancreatic juice from the **pancreas** [6]. Enzymes and bile help digest food before it passes into the second part of the small intestine, the **jejunum** [7], about 8 feet long. The jejunum connects with the third section, the **ileum** [8], about 11 feet long. The ileum attaches to the first part of the large intestine.

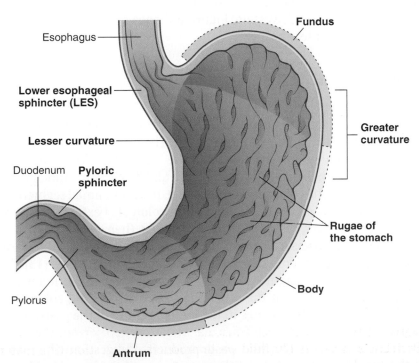

FIGURE 5-7   Parts of the stomach. The **fundus** and **body** (often referred to collectively as the fundus) are a reservoir for ingested food and an area for action by acid and pepsin (gastric enzyme). The **antrum** is a muscular grinding chamber that breaks up food and feeds it gradually into the duodenum.

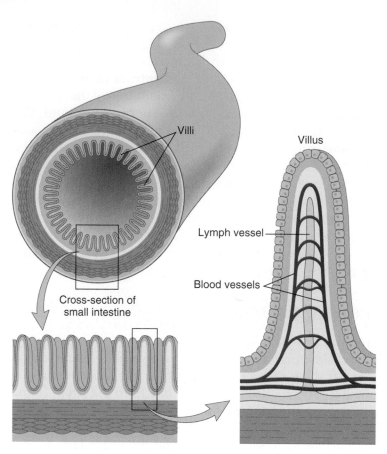

Villi

Villus

Lymph vessel

Blood vessels

Cross-section of
small intestine

**FIGURE 5-8 Villi in the
lining of the small intestine.**
Villi increase the surface area
for absorption of nutrients.

Millions of tiny, microscopic projections called **villi** line the walls of the small intestine. The tiny capillaries (microscopic blood vessels) in the villi absorb the digested nutrients into the bloodstream and lymph vessels. Figure 5-8 shows several different views of villi in the lining of the small intestine.

LARGE INTESTINE (LARGE BOWEL)

(Continue labeling Figure 5-6 on page 144.)

The large intestine extends from the end of the ileum to the anus. It has three main components: the cecum, the colon, and the rectum. The **cecum** [9] is a pouch on the right side that connects to the ileum at the ileocecal valve (sphincter). The **appendix** [10] hangs from the cecum. The appendix has no clear function and can become inflamed and infected when clogged or blocked. The **colon**, about 5 feet long, has four named segments: ascending, descending, transverse, and sigmoid. The **ascending colon** [11] extends from the cecum to the undersurface of the liver, where it turns to the left (hepatic flexure) to become the **transverse colon** [12]. The transverse colon passes horizontally to the left toward the spleen and then turns downward (splenic flexure) into the **descending colon** [13]. The **sigmoid colon** [14], shaped like an S (sigmoid means resembling the Greek letter sigma, which curves like the letter S), begins at the distal end of the descending colon and leads into the **rectum** [15]. The rectum terminates in the lower opening of the gastrointestinal tract, the **anus** [16].

The large intestine receives the fluid waste products of digestion (the material unable to pass into the bloodstream) and stores these wastes until they can be released from the body. Because the large intestine absorbs most of the water within the waste material, the body can expel solid **feces** (stools). **Defecation** is the expulsion or passage of feces from the body through the anus. Diarrhea, or passage of watery stools, results from reduced water absorption into the bloodstream through the walls of the large intestine.

LIVER, GALLBLADDER, AND PANCREAS

Three important additional organs of the digestive system—the liver, gallbladder, and pancreas—play crucial roles in the proper digestion and absorption of nutrients. Label Figure 5-9 as you study the following:

The **liver** [1], located in the right upper quadrant (RUQ) of the abdomen, manufactures a thick, orange-black, sometimes greenish, fluid called **bile.** Bile contains cholesterol (a fatty substance), bile acids, and several bile pigments. One of these pigments, **bilirubin,** is produced from the breakdown of hemoglobin during normal red blood cell destruction. Bilirubin travels via the bloodstream to the liver, where it is conjugated or converted into a water-soluble form. Conjugated bilirubin is then added to bile and enters the intestine (duodenum). Bacteria in the colon degrade bilirubin into a variety of pigments that give feces a brownish color. Bilirubin and bile leave the body in feces.

If the bile duct is blocked or the liver damaged and unable to excrete bilirubin into bile, the bilirubin remains in the bloodstream, causing **jaundice (hyperbilirubinemia)**—yellow discoloration of the skin, whites of the eyes, and mucous membranes. Figure 5-10 reviews the path of bilirubin from red blood cell destruction (hemolysis) to elimination with bile in the feces.

(Continue labeling Figure 5-9.)

The liver continuously releases bile, which then travels through the **hepatic duct** to the **cystic duct.** The cystic duct leads to the **gallbladder** [2], a pear-shaped sac under the liver, which stores and concentrates the bile for later use. After meals, in response to the presence of food in the stomach and duodenum, the gallbladder contracts, forcing the bile out the cystic duct into the **common bile duct** [3]. Meanwhile, the **pancreas** [4] secretes pancreatic juices (enzymes) that are released into the **pancreatic duct** [5], which joins with the common bile duct just as it enters the **duodenum** [6]. The duodenum thus receives a mixture of bile and pancreatic juices.

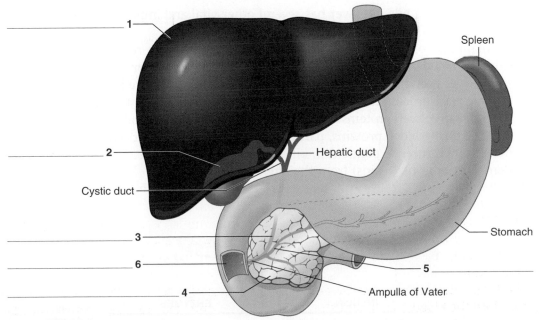

FIGURE 5-9   Liver, gallbladder, and pancreas. The **ampulla of Vater** is at the junction of the pancreatic duct and common bile duct entering the duodenum.

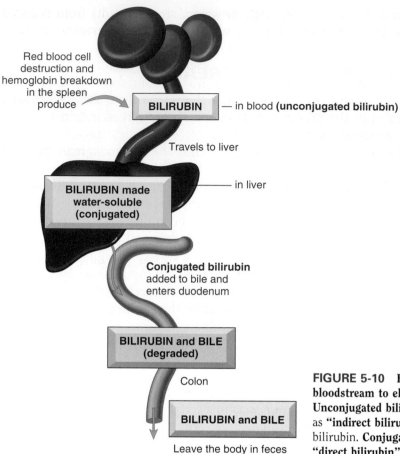

Red blood cell destruction and hemoglobin breakdown in the spleen produce

BILIRUBIN — in blood (unconjugated bilirubin)

Travels to liver

BILIRUBIN made water-soluble (conjugated) — in liver

Conjugated bilirubin added to bile and enters duodenum

BILIRUBIN and BILE (degraded)

Colon

BILIRUBIN and BILE

Leave the body in feces

FIGURE 5-10 **Bilirubin pathway from bloodstream to elimination in feces.** **Unconjugated bilirubin** (measured in lab tests as **"indirect bilirubin"**) is prehepatic, free bilirubin. **Conjugated bilirubin** (measured as **"direct bilirubin"**) is posthepatic bilirubin.

Bile has a detergent-like effect on fats in the duodenum. In the process of **emulsification,** bile breaks apart large fat globules, creating more surface area so that enzymes from the pancreas can digest the fats. Without bile, most of the fat taken into the body remains undigested.

Besides producing bile, the liver has several other vital and important functions:

- Maintaining normal blood **glucose** (sugar) levels. The liver removes excess glucose from the bloodstream and stores it as **glycogen** (starch) in liver cells. When the blood sugar level becomes dangerously low, the liver converts stored glycogen back into glucose via a process called **glycogenolysis.** In addition, when the body needs sugar, the liver can convert proteins and fats into glucose, by a process called **gluconeogenesis.**
- Manufacturing blood proteins, particularly those necessary for blood clotting
- Releasing bilirubin, a pigment in bile
- Removing poisons (toxins) from the blood

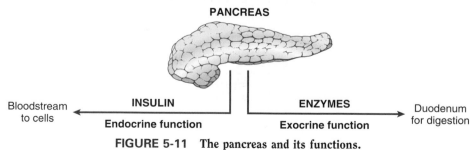

PANCREAS

Bloodstream to cells

INSULIN
Endocrine function

ENZYMES
Exocrine function

Duodenum for digestion

FIGURE 5-11   **The pancreas and its functions.**

The **portal vein** brings blood to the liver from the intestines. Nutrients from digested foods pass into the portal vein directly after being absorbed into the capillaries of the small intestine, thus giving the liver the first chance to use the nutrients.

The **pancreas** (Figure 5-11) is both an **exocrine** and an **endocrine** organ. As an exocrine gland, it produces enzymes to digest starch, such as **amylase** (amyl/o = starch, -ase = enzyme), to digest fat, such as **lipase** (lip/o = fat), and to digest proteins, such as **protease** (prote/o = protein). These pass into the duodenum through the pancreatic duct.

As an endocrine gland (secreting into the bloodstream), the pancreas secretes **insulin.** This hormone, needed to help release sugar from the blood, acts as a carrier to bring glucose into cells of the body to be used for energy.

Figure 5-12 is a flow chart that traces the pathway of food through the gastrointestinal tract.

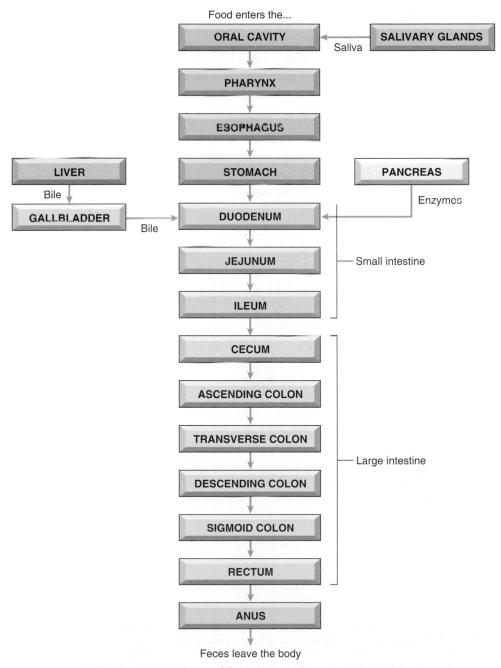

FIGURE 5-12 Pathway of food through the gastrointestinal tract.

VOCABULARY

The following list reviews many of the terms introduced in this chapter. Short definitions and additional information reinforce your understanding of the terms. All of the terms are included in the Pronunciation of Terms section later in the chapter.

absorption	Passage of materials through the walls of the small intestine into the bloodstream.
amino acids	Small building blocks of proteins (like links in a chain), released when proteins are digested.
amylase	Enzyme (-ase) secreted by the pancreas and salivary glands to digest starch (amyl/o).
anus	Terminal end or opening of the digestive tract to the outside of the body.
appendix	Blind pouch hanging from the cecum (in the right lower quadrant [RLQ]). It literally means hanging (pend/o) onto (ap-, which is a form of ad-).
bile	Digestive juice made in the liver and stored in the gallbladder. It breaks up (emulsifies) large fat globules. Bile originally was called gall (Latin *bilis*, meaning gall or anger), probably because it has a bitter taste. It is composed of bile pigments (colored materials), cholesterol, and bile salts.
bilirubin	Pigment released by the liver in bile.
bowel	Intestine.
canine teeth	Pointed, dog-like teeth (canine means pertaining to dog) next to the incisors. Also called cuspids or eyeteeth.
cecum	First part of the large intestine.
colon	Portion of the large intestine consisting of the ascending, transverse, descending, and sigmoid segments.
common bile duct	Carries bile from the liver and gallbladder to the duodenum. Also called the choledochus.
defecation	Elimination of feces from the digestive tract through the anus.
deglutition	Swallowing.
dentin	Primary material found in teeth. It is covered by the enamel in the crown and a protective layer of cementum in the root.
digestion	Breakdown of complex foods to simpler forms.
duodenum	First part of the small intestine. Duo = 2, den = 10; the duodenum measures 12 inches long.
elimination	Act of removal of materials from the body; in the digestive system, the removal of indigestible materials as feces.
emulsification	Physical process of breaking up large fat globules into smaller globules, thereby increasing the surface area that enzymes can use to digest the fat.

5

enamel	Hard, outermost layer of a tooth.
enzyme	Chemical that speeds up a reaction between substances. Digestive enzymes break down complex foods to simpler substances. Enzymes are given names that end in -ase.
esophagus	Tube connecting the throat to the stomach. Eso- means inward; phag/o means swallowing.
fatty acids	Substances produced when fats are digested. Fatty acids are a category of lipids.
feces	Solid wastes; stool.
gallbladder	Small sac under the liver; stores bile. ✳ **HINT:** gallbladder is one word!
glucose	Simple sugar.
glycogen	Starch; glucose is stored in the form of glycogen in liver cells.
hydrochloric acid	Substance produced in the stomach; necessary for digestion of food.
ileum	Third part of the small intestine; from the Greek *eilos,* meaning twisted. When the abdomen was viewed at autopsy, the intestine appeared twisted, and the ileum often was an area of obstruction.
incisor	Any one of four front teeth in the dental arch.
insulin	Hormone produced by the endocrine cells of the pancreas. It transports sugar from the blood into cells and stimulates glycogen formation by the liver.
jejunum	Second part of the small intestine. The Latin *jejunus* means empty; this part of the intestine was always empty when a body was examined after death.
lipase	Pancreatic enzyme necessary to digest fats.
liver	Large organ located in the RUQ of the abdomen. The liver secretes bile; stores sugar, iron, and vitamins; produces blood proteins; destroys worn-out red blood cells; and filters out toxins. The normal adult liver weighs about 2½ to 3 pounds.
lower esophageal sphincter (LES)	Ring of muscles between the esophagus and the stomach. Also called **cardiac sphincter.**
mastication	Chewing.
molar teeth	Sixth, seventh, and eighth teeth from the middle on either side of the dental arch. **Premolar teeth** are the fourth and fifth teeth, before the molars.
palate	Roof of the mouth. The hard palate lies anterior to the soft palate and is supported by the upper jawbone (maxilla). The soft palate is the posterior fleshy part between the mouth and the throat.
pancreas	Organ behind the stomach; produces insulin (for transport of sugar into cells) and enzymes (for digestion of foods).
papillae (*singular*: papilla)	Small projections on the tongue. A papilla is a nipple-like elevation.
parotid gland	Salivary gland within the cheek, just anterior to the ear. Note the literal meaning of parotid (par- = near; ot/o = ear).

5

peristalsis	Rhythmic contractions of the tubular organs. In the gastrointestinal tract, peristalsis moves the contents through at different rates: stomach, 0.5 to 2 hours; small intestine, 2 to 6 hours; and colon, 6 to 72 hours. Peri- means surrounding; -stalsis is constriction.
pharynx	Throat, the common passageway for food from the mouth and for air from the nose.
portal vein	Large vein bringing blood to the liver from the intestines.
protease	Enzyme that digests protein.
pulp	Soft tissue within a tooth, containing nerves and blood vessels.
pyloric sphincter	Ring of muscle at the end of the stomach, near the duodenum. From the Greek *pyloros*, meaning gatekeeper. It is normally closed, but opens when a wave of peristalsis passes over it.
pylorus	Distal region of the stomach, opening to the duodenum.
rectum	Last section of the large intestine, connecting the end of the colon and the anus.
rugae	Ridges on the hard palate and the wall of the stomach.
saliva	Digestive juice produced by salivary glands. Saliva contains the enzyme amylase, which begins the digestion of starch to sugar.
salivary glands	Parotid, sublingual, and submandibular glands.
sigmoid colon	Fourth and last, S-shaped segment of the colon, just before the rectum; empties into the rectum.
sphincter	Circular ring of muscle that constricts a passage or closes a natural opening.
stomach	Muscular organ that receives food from the esophagus. The stomach's parts are the fundus (proximal section), body (middle section), and antrum (distal section).

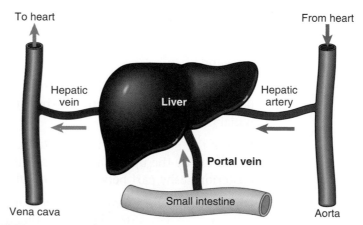

FIGURE 5-13 **Portal vein** and its relationship to the liver and small intestine.

Portal Vein

Notice the relationship of the **portal vein** (also called **hepatic portal vein**) between the intestines and the liver (Figure 5-13). This vein is not a true vein because it doesn't conduct blood directly to the heart as do other veins. In liver disease, blood backs up into the portal vein, causing **portal hypertension** (high blood pressure) and **esophageal varices**. See page 162.

triglycerides	Fat molecules composed of three parts fatty acids and one part glycerol. Triglycerides (fats) are a subgroup of **lipids.** Another type of lipid is cholesterol.
uvula	Soft tissue hanging from the middle of the soft palate. The Latin *uva* means bunch of grapes.
villi (*singular*: villus)	Microscopic projections in the wall of the small intestine that absorb nutrients into the bloodstream.

TERMINOLOGY

Write the meaning of the medical term in the space provided. Check the Pronunciation of Terms on pages 181 to 186 for any unfamiliar words.

PARTS OF THE BODY

COMBINING FORM	MEANING	TERMINOLOGY	MEANING
an/o	anus	perianal _____	
append/o	appendix	appendectomy _____	
appendic/o		appendicitis _____ *See Figure 5-14.*	
bucc/o	cheek	buccal mucosa _____ *A mucosa is a **mucous membrane** lining cavities or canals that open to the outside of the body.*	
cec/o	cecum	cecal _____	
celi/o	belly, abdomen	celiac _____ *Abdomin/o and lapar/o also mean abdomen. With combining forms that have the same basic meaning, no rule exists for the proper usage of one or the other. You will learn to recognize each in its proper context.*	

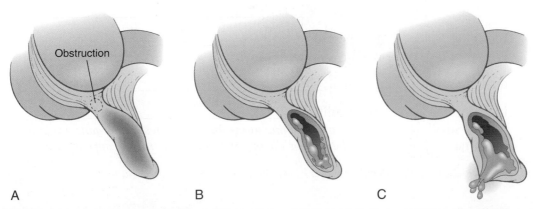

A   B   C

FIGURE 5-14   Stages of appendicitis. A, Obstruction and bacterial infection cause red, swollen, and inflamed appendix. **B,** Pus and bacteria invade the wall of the appendix. **C,** Pus perforates (ruptures through) the wall of the appendix into the abdomen, leading to peritonitis (inflammation of the peritoneum).

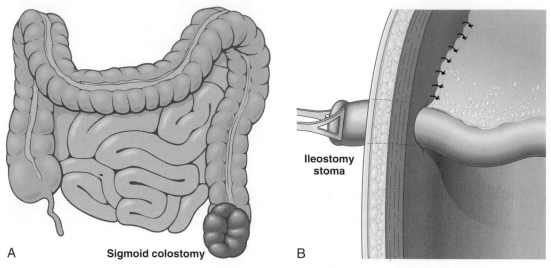

A   Sigmoid colostomy   B

FIGURE 5-15 **Different types of stomas. A, Sigmoid colostomy** after resection of the rectum and part of the sigmoid colon. The stoma is at the end of the colon and attached to the abdominal wall. **B, Ileostomy** after resection of the entire colon. The ileum is drawn through the abdominal wall to form an **ileostomy stoma.**

COMBINING FORM	MEANING	TERMINOLOGY	MEANING
cheil/o	lip	cheilosis _____ *Labi/o also means lip.*	
cholecyst/o ◼	gallbladder	cholecystectomy _____ *Chol/e = gall, bile.*	
choledoch/o	common bile duct	choledochotomy _____	
col/o	colon	colostomy _____ *The suffix -stomy, when used with a combining form for an organ, means an opening to the outside of the body. A **stoma** is an opening between an organ and the surface of the body (Figure 5-15).*	
colon/o	colon	colonic _____	
		colonoscopy _____	
dent/i	tooth	dentibuccal _____ *Odont/o also means tooth.*	
duoden/o	duodenum	duodenal _____	
enter/o	intestines, usually small intestine	enterocolitis _____ *When two combining forms for gastrointestinal organs are in a term, the one for the organ closer to the mouth appears first.*	

Cholecyst/o and Cyst/o

Don't confuse **cholecyst/o (gallbladder)** with **cyst/o**, which is the **urinary bladder.**

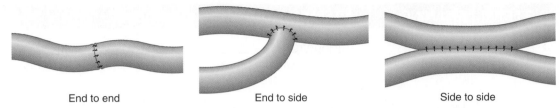

| End to end | End to side | Side to side |

FIGURE 5-16 Three types of anastomoses. These are examples of an enteroenterostomy. The suffix -stomy, when used with two or more combining forms (enter/o and enter/o), indicates the surgical creation of a new opening between those parts of the body.

COMBINING FORM	MEANING	TERMINOLOGY	MEANING
		entero<u>enter</u>ostomy _____ *New opening between two previously unconnected parts of the small intestine. This is an **anastomosis,** which is any surgical connection between two parts, such us vessels, ducts, or bowel segments (ana = up, stom = opening, -sis = state of) (Figure 5-16).*	
		mes<u>enter</u>y _____ *Part of the double fold of peritoneum that stretches around the organs in the abdomen, the mesentery holds the organs in place. Literally, it lies in the middle (mes-) of the intestines, a membrane attaching the intestines to the muscle wall at the back of the abdomen (Figure 5-17).*	
		par<u>enter</u>al _____ *Par (from para-) means apart from in this term. An intravenous line brings **parenteral nutrition** directly into the bloodstream, bypassing the intestinal tract (**enteral** nutrition). Parenteral injections may be subcutaneous or intramuscular as well.*	

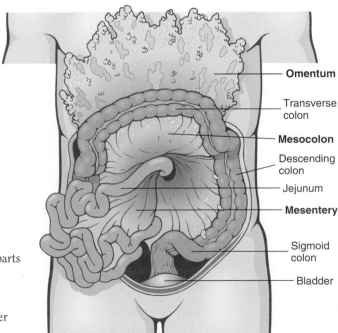

- Omentum
- Transverse colon
- **Mesocolon**
- Descending colon
- Jejunum
- **Mesentery**
- Sigmoid colon
- Bladder

FIGURE 5-17 Mesentery. The **omentum** and **mesocolon** are parts of the mesentery. The omentum (raised in this figure) actually hangs down like an apron over the intestines. The mesentery contains blood and lymph vessels. The lymph nodes in the mesentery are important indicators in the spread of colon cancer (staging of colon cancer).

5

COMBINING FORM	MEANING	TERMINOLOGY	MEANING
esophag/o	esophagus	esophageal _____ Note: *Changing the suffix from -al to -eal softens the final g (ĕ-sŏf-ă-JĒ-ăl).*	
faci/o	face	facial _____	
gastr/o	stomach	gastrostomy _____	
gingiv/o	gums	gingivitis _____	
gloss/o	tongue	hypoglossal _____ *Lingu/o also means tongue.*	
hepat/o	liver	hepatoma _____ *Also called **hepatocellular carcinoma.*** hepatomegaly _____	
ile/o	ileum	ileocecal sphincter _____ *Also called the ileocecal valve.* ileitis _____ ileostomy _____ *See Figure 5-15B, page 154.*	
jejun/o	jejunum	choledochojejunostomy _____ *An anastomosis.* gastrojejunostomy _____ *This is part of a **gastric bypass** procedure. See Figure 6-7, page 197.*	
labi/o	lip	labial _____	
lapar/o	abdomen	laparoscopy _____ *A form of **minimally invasive surgery (MIS).** Examples are laparoscopic cholecystectomy (Figure 5-28, page 168) and laparoscopic appendectomy.*	
lingu/o	tongue	sublingual _____	
mandibul/o	lower jaw, mandible	submandibular _____	
odont/o	tooth	orthodontist _____ *Orth/o means straight.* periodontist _____ endodontist _____ *Performs root canal therapy.*	

Ileum and Ilium

Don't confuse the **ileum,** which is the third part of the small intestine, with the **ilium,** uppermost and largest part of the pelvis (hip bone).

COMBINING FORM	MEANING	TERMINOLOGY	MEANING
or/o	mouth	oral _____ *Stomat/o also means mouth.*	
palat/o	palate	palatoplasty _____ *Procedure to repair cleft palate and cleft lip; repair of a cleft palate.*	
pancreat/o	pancreas	pancreatitis _____	
peritone/o	peritoneum	peritonitis _____ *The e of the root has been dropped in this term.*	
pharyng/o	throat	pharyngeal _____	
		palatopharyngoplasty _____ *Used to treat cases of snoring or sleep apnea caused by obstructions in the throat or nose.*	
proct/o	anus and rectum	proctologist _____	
pylor/o	pyloric sphincter	pyloroplasty _____	
rect/o	rectum	rectocele _____	
sialaden/o	salivary gland	sialadenitis _____	
sigmoid/o	sigmoid colon	sigmoidoscopy _____	
stomat/o	mouth	stomatitis _____	
uvul/o	uvula	uvulectomy _____	

SUBSTANCES

COMBINING FORM	MEANING	TERMINOLOGY	MEANING
amyl/o	starch	amylase _____ *The suffix -ase means enzyme.*	
bil/i	gall, bile	biliary _____ *The **biliary tract** includes the organs (liver and gallbladder) and ducts (hepatic, cystic, and common bile ducts) that secrete, store, and empty bile into the duodenum.*	
bilirubin/o	bilirubin (bile pigment)	hyperbilirubinemia _____	
chol/e ◼	gall, bile	cholelithiasis _____ *Lith/o means stone or calculus; -iasis means abnormal condition.*	

Chol/e and Col/o

Don't confuse **chol/e,** which means gall or bile, with **col/o,** which indicates the colon! The context of the term will help you determine the correct spelling.

COMBINING FORM	MEANING	TERMINOLOGY	MEANING
chlorhydr/o	hydrochloric acid	a<u>chlorhydr</u>ia *Absence of gastric juice is associated with gastric carcinoma.*	
gluc/o	sugar	<u>gluc</u>oneogenesis *Liver cells make new sugar from fats and proteins.*	
glyc/o	sugar	hyper<u>glyc</u>emia	
glycogen/o	glycogen, animal starch	<u>glycogen</u>olysis *Liver cells change glycogen back to glucose when blood sugar levels drop.*	
lip/o	fat, lipid	<u>lip</u>oma	
lith/o	stone	<u>lith</u>ogenesis	
prote/o	protein	<u>prote</u>ase	
py/o	pus	<u>py</u>orrhea *Periodontitis; an advanced stage of periodontal disease (gingivitis).*	
sial/o	saliva, salivary	<u>sial</u>olith	
steat/o	fat	<u>steat</u>orrhea *Improperly digested (malabsorbed) fats will appear in the feces.*	

SUFFIXES

SUFFIX	MEANING	TERMINOLOGY	MEANING
-ase	enzyme	lip<u>ase</u> *Enzymes speed up chemical reactions. Lipase aids in the digestion of fats. In all types of liver disease, liver enzyme levels may be elevated, indicating damage to liver cells. Signs and symptoms include malaise, anorexia, hepatomegaly, jaundice, and abdominal pain.*	
-chezia	defecation, elimination of wastes	hemato<u>chezia</u> *(hē-mă-tō-KĒ-zē-ă) Bright red blood is found in the feces.*	
-iasis	abnormal condition	choledocholith<u>iasis</u>	
-prandial	meal	post<u>prandial</u> ***Post cibum (p.c.),** seen on written prescriptions, also means after meals.*	

Pyorrhea and Pyuria

Pyorrhea is discharge (-rrhea) of pus from gums, and **pyuria** is presence of pus in urine (sign of a urinary tract infection).

PATHOLOGY OF THE DIGESTIVE SYSTEM

This section presents medical terms that describe **signs and symptoms** (clinical indications of illness) and pathologic conditions of the gastrointestinal tract. Sentences following each definition describe the **etiology** (eti/o = cause) of the illness and treatment. When the etiology (cause) is not understood, the condition is **idiopathic** (idi/o = unknown). You can find a list of drugs prescribed to treat gastrointestinal signs and symptoms and conditions in Chapter 21, Pharmacology.

SIGNS AND SYMPTOMS

anorexia

Lack of appetite.

Anorexia (-orexia = appetite) often is a sign of malignancy or liver disease. **Anorexia nervosa** is loss of appetite associated with emotional problems such as anger, anxiety, and irrational fear of weight gain. It is an eating disorder and is discussed along with a similar eating disorder, bulimia nervosa, in Chapter 22.

ascites

Abnormal accumulation of fluid in the abdomen.

This condition occurs when fluid passes from the bloodstream and collects in the peritoneal cavity. It can be a sign of neoplasm or inflammatory disorders in the abdomen, venous hypertension (high blood pressure) caused by liver disease (cirrhosis), or heart failure (Figure 5-18). Treatment for ascites includes administration of diuretic drugs and paracentesis to remove abdominal fluid.

borborygmi
(*singular:* borborygmus)

Rumbling or gurgling noises produced by the movement of gas, fluid, or both in the gastrointestinal tract.

Signs of hyperactive intestinal peristalsis, **borborygmi (bowel sounds)** often are present in cases of gastroenteritis and diarrhea.

constipation

Difficulty in passing stools (feces).

When peristalsis is slow, stools are dry and hard. A diet with plentiful fruits, vegetables, and water is helpful. **Laxatives** and **cathartics** are medications to promote movement of stools.

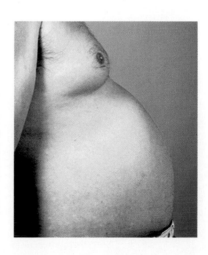

FIGURE 5-18 Ascites in a male patient. The photograph was taken after **paracentesis** (puncture to remove fluid from the abdomen) was performed. Notice the gynecomastia (condition of female-type breasts) in this patient due to an excess of estrogen, which can accompany cirrhosis, especially in persons with alcoholism.

Signs and Symptoms

A **sign** is an **objective** finding—such as an increase in body temperature, a rash, or a sound heard on listening to the chest—indicating the presence of disease as **perceived by an examiner.** By contrast, a **symptom** is a **subjective** sensation or change in health—such as itching, pain, fatigue, or nausea—as **experienced by the patient.** Clearly, the same feature may be noticed by both doctor and patient, which makes it at once both a sign and a symptom!

5

diarrhea	**Frequent passage of loose, watery stools.** Abrupt onset of diarrhea immediately after eating suggests acute infection or toxin in the gastrointestinal tract. Untreated, severe diarrhea may lead to dehydration. Antidiarrheal drugs are helpful.
dysphagia	**Difficulty in swallowing.** This sensation feels like a "lump in the throat" when a swallowed bolus fails to progress, either because of a physical obstruction (obstructive dysphagia) or because of a motor disorder in which esophageal peristalsis is not coordinated (motor dysphagia).
eructation	**Gas expelled from the stomach through the mouth.** Eructation produces a characteristic sound and also is called **belching.**
flatus	**Gas expelled through the anus.** Flatulence is the presence of excessive gas in the stomach and the intestines. One sign of a bowel obstruction is the inability to pass flatus.
hematochezia	**Passage of fresh, bright red blood from the rectum.** The cause of hematochezia is usually hemorrhoids, but can also be colitis, ulcers, polyps, or cancer.
jaundice (icterus)	**Yellow-orange coloration of the skin and whites of the eyes caused by high levels of bilirubin in the blood (hyperbilirubinemia).** See Figure 5-19. Jaundice can occur when (1) excessive destruction of erythrocytes, as in **hemolysis,** causes excess bilirubin in the blood; (2) malfunction of liver cells (hepatocytes) due to **liver disease** prevents the liver from excreting bilirubin with bile; or (3) **obstruction of bile flow,** such as from choledocholithiasis or tumor, prevents bilirubin in bile from being excreted into the duodenum.

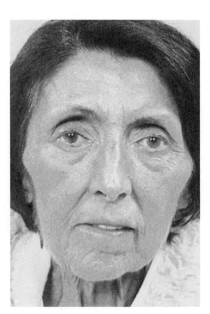

FIGURE 5-19 Jaundice due to liver disease.

melena	**Black, tarry stools; feces containing digested blood.**
	This clinical sign usually reflects a condition in which blood has had time to be digested (acted on by intestinal juices) and results from bleeding in the upper gastrointestinal tract (duodenal ulcer). A positive result on **stool guaiac testing** (see page 193) indicates blood in the stool.
nausea	**Unpleasant sensation in the stomach with a tendency to vomit.**
	Common causes are motion sickness, early pregnancy, and viral gastroenteritis. Nausea and vomiting may be symptomatic of a perforation (hole in the wall) of an abdominal organ; obstruction of a bile duct, stomach, or intestine; or exposure to poisons.
steatorrhea	**Fat in the feces.**
	Steatorrhea is production of frothy, foul-smelling fecal matter that often floats in the toilet. Improper digestion or absorption of fat causes fat to remain in the intestine. This may occur with disease of the pancreas (pancreatitis) when pancreatic enzymes are not excreted. It also is a sign of intestinal disease that involves malabsorption of fat.

PATHOLOGIC CONDITIONS

ORAL CAVITY AND TEETH

aphthous stomatitis	**Inflammation of the mouth with small, painful ulcers.**
	The ulcers associated with this condition are commonly called **canker** (KĂNK-ĕr) **sores**; the cause is unknown (Figure 5-20B).
dental caries	**Tooth decay.**
	Dental plaque results from the accumulation of foods, proteins from saliva, and necrotic debris on the tooth enamel. Bacteria grow in the plaque and cause production of acid that dissolves the tooth enamel, resulting in a cavity (area of decay) (Figure 5-20C). If the bacterial infection reaches the pulp of the tooth, root canal therapy may be necessary.

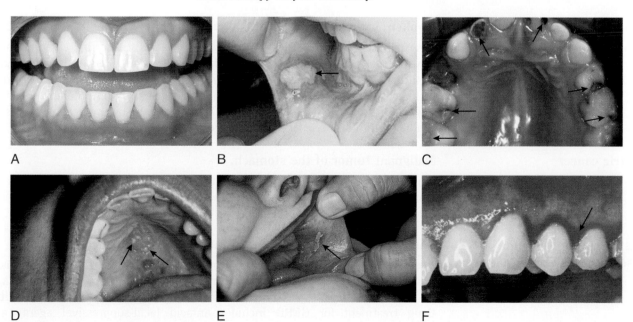

A   B   C

D   E   F

FIGURE 5-20   Normal teeth and gums and pathologic conditions. **A**, Normal teeth and gums. **B**, Aphthous stomatitis. **C**, Dental caries. **D**, Herpetic stomatitis. **E**, Oral leukoplakia. **F**, Gingivitis.

herpetic stomatitis	**Inflammation of the mouth caused by infection with the herpesvirus.**

Painful fluid-filled blisters on the lips, palate, gums, and tongue, commonly called **fever blisters** or **cold sores** (Figure 5-20D). It is caused by herpes simplex virus type 1 (HSV1). Herpes genitalis (due to HSV2) involves the reproductive organs. Both conditions are highly contagious.

oral leukoplakia	**White plaques or patches on the mucosa of the mouth.**

This precancerous lesion (Figure 5-20E) can result from chronic tobacco use (pipe smoking or chewing tobacco). Malignant potential is assessed by microscopic study of biopsied tissue.

periodontal disease	**Inflammation and degeneration of gums, teeth, and surrounding bone.**

Gingivitis (Figure 5-20F) occurs as a result of accumulation of **dental plaque** and **dental calculus** or **tartar** (a yellow-brown calcified deposit on teeth). In **gingivectomy**, the periodontist uses a metal instrument to scrape away plaque and tartar from teeth; any pockets of pus (pyorrhea) are then drained and removed to allow new tissue to form. Localized infections are treated with systemic antibiotics.

UPPER GASTROINTESTINAL TRACT

achalasia	**Failure of the lower esophagus sphincter (LES) muscle to relax.**

Achalasia (-chalasia = relaxation) results from the loss of peristalsis so that food cannot pass easily through the esophagus. Both failure of the LES to relax and the loss of peristalsis cause dilatation (widening) of the esophagus above the constriction. Physicians recommend a bland diet low in bulk and mechanical stretching of the LES to relieve symptoms.

esophageal cancer	**Malignant tumor of the esophagus.**

The most common symptom of esophageal cancer is difficulty swallowing (dysphagia). Smoking and chronic alcohol use are major risk factors. Long-term irritation of the esophagus caused by gastric reflux is a premalignant condition called **Barrett esophagus.** Surgery, radiation therapy, and chemotherapy are treatment options.

esophageal varices	**Swollen, varicose veins at the lower end of the esophagus** (Figure 5-21**).**

Liver disease (such as cirrhosis and chronic hepatitis) causes increased pressure in veins near and around the liver (**portal hypertension**). This leads to enlarged, tortuous esophageal veins with danger of hemorrhage (bleeding). Treatment may include banding (tying off the swollen esophageal veins) or sclerotherapy (injecting veins with a solution that closes them). Drug therapy to lower portal hypertension can be used to decrease the risk of variceal bleeding.

gastric cancer	**Malignant tumor of the stomach.**

Smoking, alcohol use, and chronic gastritis associated with bacterial infection are major risk factors for gastric carcinoma. Gastric endoscopy and biopsy diagnose the condition. Cure depends on early detection and surgical removal.

gastroesophageal reflux disease (GERD)	**Solids and fluids return to the mouth from the stomach.**

Heartburn is a burning sensation caused by regurgitation of hydrochloric acid from the stomach to the esophagus. Chronic exposure of esophageal mucosa to gastric acid and pepsin (an enzyme that digests protein) leads to **reflux esophagitis.** Drug treatment for GERD includes antacid (acid-suppressive) agents and medication to increase the tone of the LES.

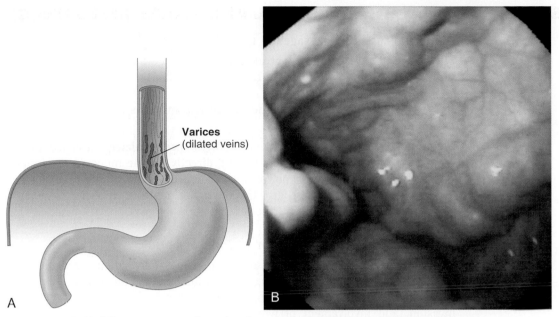

FIGURE 5-21   A, Esophageal varices. B, Endoscopic view of esophageal varices.

hernia	**Protrusion of an organ or part through the tissues and muscles normally containing it.**

A **hiatal hernia** occurs when the upper part of the stomach protrudes upward through the diaphragm (Figure 5-22A). This condition can lead to GERD. An **inguinal hernia** occurs when a small loop of bowel protrudes through a weak lower abdominal wall tissue (fascia) surrounding muscles (Figure 5-22B). Surgical repair of inguinal hernias is known as herniorrhaphy (-rrhaphy means suture).

peptic ulcer	**Open sore in the lining of the stomach or duodenum.**

A bacterium, *Helicobacter pylori* (*H. pylori*), is responsible for many cases of peptic ulcer disease. The combination of bacteria, hyperacidity, and gastric juice damages epithelial linings. Drug treatment includes antibiotics, antacids, and agents to protect the lining of the stomach and intestine.

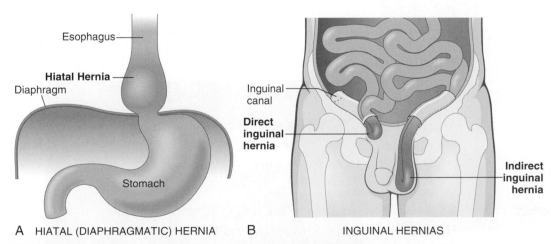

A   HIATAL (DIAPHRAGMATIC) HERNIA   B   INGUINAL HERNIAS

FIGURE 5-22   Hernias. A, Hiatal hernia. B, Inguinal hernias. A direct inguinal hernia occurs through the abdominal wall in an area of muscular weakness. An **indirect inguinal hernia** occurs through the inguinal canal (passageway in the lower abdomen), where the herniated tissue/bowel descends into the scrotal sac.

LOWER GASTROINTESTINAL TRACT (SMALL AND LARGE INTESTINES)

anal fistula

Abnormal tube-like passageway near the anus.

The fistula often results from a break or **fissure** in the wall of the anus or rectum, or from an **abscess** (infected area) there (Figure 5-23A).

colonic polyps

Polyps (benign growths) protrude from the mucous membrane of the colon.

Figure 5-23A illustrates two types of polyps: **pedunculated** (attached to the membrane by a stalk) and **sessile** (sitting directly on the mucous membrane). Figure 5-23B shows multiple polyps of the colon. Many polyps are premalignant (adenomatous polyps); these growths often are removed (polypectomy) as a preventative measure and for further examination (biopsy).

colorectal cancer

Adenocarcinoma of the colon or rectum, or both.

Colorectal cancer (Figure 5-24) can arise from polyps in the colon or rectal region. Diagnosis is determined by detecting blood in stool and by colonoscopy. Prognosis depends on the stage (extent of spread) of the tumor, including size, depth of invasion, and involvement of lymph nodes. Surgical treatment may require excision of a major section of colon with rejoining of the cut ends (anastomosis). Chemotherapy and radiotherapy are administered as needed.

Crohn disease ("Crohn's")

Chronic inflammation of the intestinal tract.

Crohn's can occur anywhere from mouth to anus but most commonly in the ileum (ileitis) and colon. Signs and symptoms include diarrhea, severe abdominal pain, fever, anorexia, weakness, and weight loss. Both Crohn disease and ulcerative colitis are forms of **inflammatory bowel disease (IBD).** Treatment is with drugs that control inflammation and other symptoms or by surgical removal of diseased portions of the intestine, with anastomosis of remaining parts. Read the ***In Person: Living with Crohn's*** story on page 170.

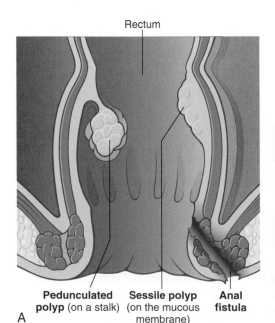

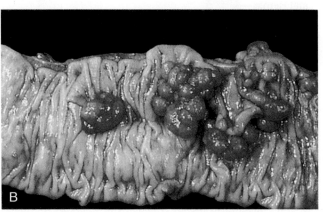

Rectum

Pedunculated polyp (on a stalk)   **Sessile polyp** (on the mucous membrane)   **Anal fistula**

A

B

FIGURE 5-23   Anal fistula and colonic polyps. A, Anal fistula and two types of polyps. **B,** Multiple polyps of the colon.

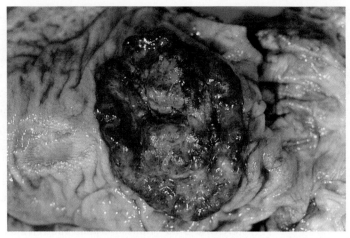

FIGURE 5-24   Adenocarcinoma of the colon. This tumor has "heaped-up" edges and an ulcerated central portion.

diverticulosis

Abnormal outpouchings (diverticula) in the intestinal wall of the colon. See Figure 5-25A.

Diverticulitis is a complication of diverticulosis. When fecal matter becomes trapped in diverticula, diverticulitis can occur. Pain and rectal bleeding are symptoms. Figure 5-25B and C shows diverticulitis in a section through the sigmoid colon. Initial treatment for an attack of diverticulitis includes a liquid diet and oral antibiotics. In severe cases, the patient may need hospitalization, intravenous antibiotics, and surgery to remove the affected area of the colon with anastomosis of the cut ends.

dysentery

Painful inflammation of the intestines commonly caused by bacterial infection.

Often occurring in the colon, dysentery results from ingestion of food or water containing bacteria (salmonellae or shigellae), amebae (one-celled organisms), or viruses. Symptoms are bloody stools, abdominal pain, and sometimes fever.

hemorrhoids

Swollen, twisted, varicose veins in the rectal region.

Varicose veins can be internal (within the rectum) or external (outside the anal sphincter). Pregnancy and chronic constipation, which put pressure on anal veins, often cause hemorrhoids.

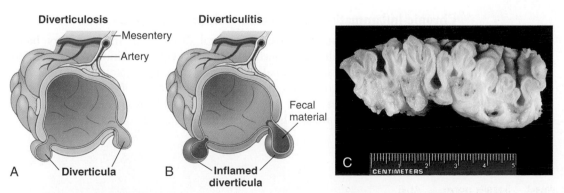

FIGURE 5-25   A, Diverticula (resulting in **diverticulosis**) form when the mucous membrane lining of the colon bulges through the weakened muscular wall. **B** and **C, Diverticulitis** can result when fecal material lodges in diverticula. Avoidance of foods with seeds and nuts decreases the risk of this condition.

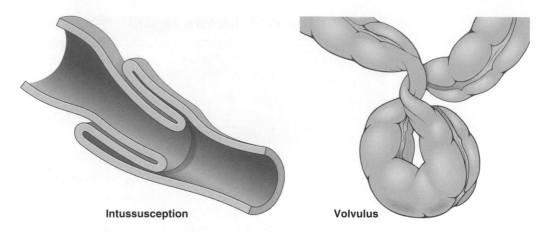

Intussusception   Volvulus

FIGURE 5-26   Intussusception and volvulus.

ileus	**Loss of peristalsis with resulting obstruction of the intestines.**

Surgery, trauma, or bacterial injury to the peritoneum can lead to a **paralytic ileus** (acute, transient loss of peristalsis).

inflammatory bowel disease (IBD)	**Inflammation of the colon and small intestine.** See **Crohn disease** and **ulcerative colitis.**

intussusception	**Telescoping of the intestines.**

In this condition, one segment of the bowel collapses into the opening of another segment (Figure 5-26). It often occurs in children and at the ileocecal region. Intestinal obstruction with pain and vomiting can occur. A barium enema can diagnose and may successfully reduce the intussusception. Otherwise, surgery to remove the affected segment of bowel (followed by anastomosis) may be necessary.

irritable bowel syndrome (IBS)	**Group of GI symptoms (abdominal pain, bloating, diarrhea, constipation), but without defined abnormalities in the intestines.**

IBS may be associated with stress or occur after infection. Treatment includes a diet high in bran and fiber and laxatives plus antidiarrheals to establish regular bowel movements. Other names for IBS are **irritable colon** and **spastic colon.** IBS is a type of **functional gastrointestinal disorder (FGID).** These are disorders of how the gastrointestinal tract functions, but without structural or biochemical abnormalities.

ulcerative colitis	**Chronic inflammation of the colon with presence of ulcers.**

This idiopathic, chronic, recurrent diarrheal disease (an **inflammatory bowel disease**) manifests with rectal bleeding and pain. Often beginning in the colon, the inflammation spreads proximally, involving the entire colon. Drug treatment and careful attention to diet are recommended. Resection of diseased bowel with ileostomy may be necessary. In some cases it is cured by total colectomy. Patients with ulcerative colitis are at a higher risk for developing colon cancer.

Irritable Bowel Syndrome (IBS) and Inflammatory Bowel Disease (IBD)

While **IBS** is a condition with no structural abnormalities of the intestines, **IBD** (**Crohn's** and **ulcerative colitis**) involves structural abnormalities.

volvulus	**Twisting of the intestine on itself.**

Volvulus causes intestinal obstruction. Severe pain, nausea and vomiting, and absence of bowel sounds are clinical features. Surgical correction is necessary to prevent necrosis of the affected segment of the bowel (see Figure 5-26).

LIVER, GALLBLADDER, AND PANCREAS

cholelithiasis	**Gallstones in the gallbladder.**

Calculi (stones) prevent bile from leaving the gallbladder and bile ducts (Figure 5-27). Many patients remain asymptomatic and do not require treatment; symptoms related to gallbladder stones are either **biliary colic** (pain from blocked ducts) or **cholecystitis** (inflammation and infection of the gallbladder), both of which require treatment. Currently, **laparoscopic** or **minimally invasive surgery (laparoscopic cholecystectomy)** can be performed to remove the gallbladder and stones (Figure 5-28A and B).

5

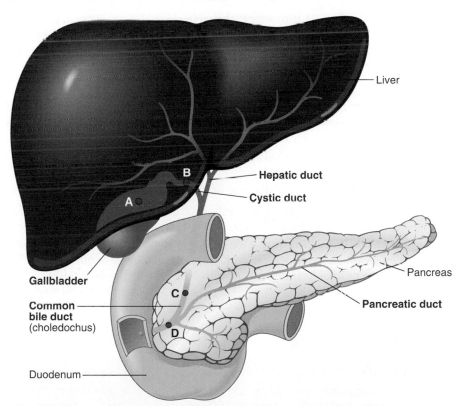

FIGURE 5-27 Gallstone positions in the gallbladder and bile ducts. A, Stone in the gallbladder causing mild or no symptoms. **B,** Stone obstructing the cystic duct, causing pain. **C,** Stone obstructing the common bile duct, causing pain and jaundice. **D,** Stone at the lower end of the common bile duct and pancreatic duct, causing pain, jaundice, and pancreatitis.

What's "in" Gallstones?

Gallstones are composed of cholesterol, bilirubin (pigment in bile), and calcium salts. They can vary in size and shape—ranging from as small as a grain of sand to as large as a golf ball!

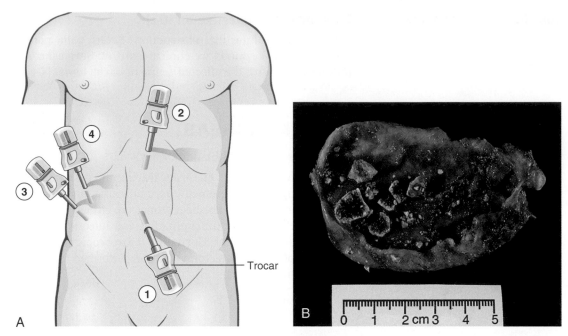

FIGURE 5-28 **A, Trocars in place for laparoscopic cholecystectomy.** Trocars are used to puncture and enter the abdomen. These devices are metal sleeves consisting of a hollow metal tube (cannula) into which fits an obturator (a solid, removable metal instrument with a sharp, three-cornered tip) used to puncture the wall. *Circled numbers* show common positions for trocar insertion: **1** is an umbilical 10/11-mm trocar (the largest trocar diameter is 15). **2** is a 10/11-mm trocar at the midline. **3** and **4** are 5-mm trocars placed in the right upper quadrant of the abdomen. **B, Gallstones.** Mechanical manipulation during laparoscopic cholecystectomy has caused fragmentation of several cholesterol gallstones, revealing interiors that are pigmented because of entrapped bile pigments. The gallbladder mucosa is reddened and irregular as a result.

5

cirrhosis

Chronic degenerative disease of the liver.

Cirrhosis is commonly the result of chronic alcoholism, viral hepatitis, iron overload, or other causes. Lobes of the liver become scarred with fibrous tissue, hepatic cells degenerate, and the liver is infiltrated with fat. Cirrh/o means yellow-orange, which describes the liver's color caused by fat accumulation. Figure 5-29 shows a normal liver and a liver with alcoholic cirrhosis.

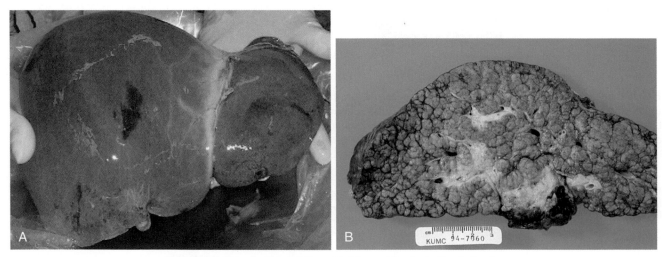

FIGURE 5-29 **A,** Normal liver. **B,** Liver with alcoholic cirrhosis.

hepatocellular carcinoma (HCC)	**Liver cancer.** Cancer that starts in the liver is primary liver cancer (as opposed to secondary liver cancer, which starts in another organ and metastasizes to the liver). HCC is commonly associated with hepatitis B and C virus infections and cirrhosis due to chronic alcohol use. **Nonalcoholic steatohepatitis (NASH)** is fatty infiltration of the liver, which may progress to cirrhosis and HCC. Surgery and chemotherapy are therapeutic options. Hepatocellular carcinomas produce **alpha-fetoprotein (AFP)**, a tumor marker that is elevated in the blood in patients with this cancer. AFP is used as a screen for HCC in patients with cirrhosis. Liver cancers that begin in the bile ducts are called **cholangiocarcinomas**. Bile duct cancers also can arise from the gallbladder.
pancreatic cancer	**Malignant tumor of the pancreas.** It often occurs in the head of the pancreas (closer to the duodenum), where it can block ducts. Although the cause is unknown, pancreatic cancer is more common in smokers and people with diabetes and chronic pancreatitis. Symptoms and signs are abdominal or back pain, fatigue, jaundice, anorexia, diarrhea, and weight loss. The standard surgical treatment is a **pancreatoduodenectomy (Whipple procedure)**.
pancreatitis	**Inflammation of the pancreas.** Digestive enzymes attack pancreatic tissue and damage the gland. Other etiologic factors include chronic alcoholism, drug toxicity, gallstone obstruction of the common bile duct, and viral infections. Treatment includes medications to relieve epigastric pain, intravenous fluids, bowel rest, and subtotal pancreatectomy if necessary.
viral hepatitis	**Inflammation of the liver caused by a virus.** **Hepatitis A** is viral hepatitis caused by the hepatitis A virus (**HAV**). It is a disorder spread by contaminated food or water and characterized by slow onset of symptoms. **Hepatitis B** is caused by the hepatitis B virus (**HBV**) and is transmitted by sexual contact, blood transfusions, or the use of contaminated needles or may be acquired by maternal to fetal transmission. Severe infection can cause destruction of liver cells, cirrhosis, or death. A vaccine that provides immunity is available and recommended for persons at risk for exposure. **Hepatitis C** is caused by the hepatitis C virus (**HCV**) and is transmitted by blood transfusions or needle inoculation (such as among intravenous drug users sharing needles). The acute illness may progress to chronic hepatitis and hepatocellular carcinoma. Two new drugs, simeprevir (Olysio) and sofosbuvir (Sovaldi), are effective for treating HCV infection. In all types, liver enzyme levels may be elevated, indicating damage to liver cells. Signs and symptoms include malaise, anorexia, hepatomegaly, jaundice, and abdominal pain.

Whipple Procedure for Pancreatic Cancer

This surgery consists of:
- removal of the distal half of the stomach (antrectomy)
- removal of gallbladder and common bile duct (cholecystectomy and choledochectomy)
- removal of part of the pancreas and duodenum (pancreatoduodenectomy)
- reconstruction consists of pancreatojejunostomy, hepaticojejunostomy, and gastrojejunostomy

Steve Jobs, cofounder of Apple Inc., and Luciano Pavarotti, opera singer, had this surgery.

IN PERSON: LIVING WITH CROHN'S

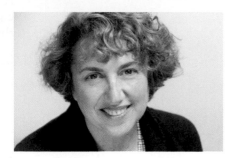

When a friend told me she was sick with the flu yesterday, I was jealous. To someone with a chronic illness, like me, having something acute always seems luxurious. Lie in bed, read glossy magazines, take over-the-counter meds, sleep it off, and in a matter of days you're okay. I have Crohn disease, a chronic inflammation of the small intestine, which is characterized by flare-ups and remission. During flare-ups, I've experienced fever, diarrhea, vomiting, pain, and intestinal obstruction. Even in remission I am never "okay."

Right now I have been in remission two years after a third surgery to remove yet another portion of my small bowel. This time internal bleeding, a rather rare symptom of Crohn's, necessitated the surgery. I was enduring weekly iron infusions, which turned into bimonthly blood transfusions, as my hemoglobin plummeted to 6 (12 is normal). It was no way to live. After the surgery, the bleeding stopped, but I had bouts of urgent, watery diarrhea for a year. That was no way to live either, and unfortunately, as wonderful as my doctor is, I've found that few gastroenterologists want to address aftereffects of small bowel surgery. After visiting several doctors and by trial and error, I finally got these symptoms under control with codeine, Lomotil, and Metamucil, but I will never be able to absorb vitamin B_{12}, so I must inject it monthly for the rest of my life. In addition to taking medicine to cope with having less and less small bowel, I take medicine in the hopes of preventing the next flare-up. Every few weeks, I inject myself with a biologic medicine, Humira, but I must eventually be weaned off this drug because it has possible long-term side effects, the scariest of which is lymphoma. At 52 and with two school-age children, however, I have learned to think of valuing my present quality of life the most, over possible unknown dangers lurking in the future.

I do often think about the past. What would my life be like if our family doctor hadn't told my parents that my constant episodes of diarrhea—which occurred since I was a child—were caused by "nerves?" By the time I was 21, my weight had dropped below 100 pounds, and I was twisted in pain after every meal. My dad arranged for me to visit his own doctor, who gave me a small bowel series that showed I had Crohn's and that a portion of my small intestine was "as narrow as a pencil." By then it was too late for even prednisone (then the drug of choice despite side effects ranging from puffy face to psychosis) to open up the inflamed passage, and I had my first surgery just months after I was diagnosed. Thinking of those times—as well as all the other flare-up times—makes me flinch. While you can never relive pain, you can remember what it felt like. In my case, it was as if a large metal bike lock chain was being forced through my tender gut.

Before that first surgery, I was just out of college and longing to make my mark on the world, but I spent most of my evenings curled up in my small bedroom, listening to the soothing strains of "Make Believe Ballroom Hour" on the radio. Or, because vomiting and diarrhea usually accompanied the pain, I lay with my back pressed against the cold tiles of the bathroom floor. Later on, as a mom with two young children, I would lie on the couch watching life swirl around me, feeling guilty that I could not take part.

There was a silver lining to those flare-ups, and that is the tender affection of those around me: husband, family, and friends. When you have Crohn's, no one knows you have it until things get unbearable. It's not the kind of illness you discuss, but when you have pain and fever, you can kind of approximate those times of being felled by the flu. Yet you know that it will take more than a dose of Nyquil or a night's sleep to get "better." You know you'll face another course of medications—often untried ones—or that you will likely end up in the hospital undergoing yet another surgery.

Nancy J. Brandwein is a writer, editor, and food columnist.

? EXERCISES

Remember to check your answers carefully with the Answers to Exercises, pages 179 and 180.

A **Match the following digestive system structures with their meanings below.**

anus	esophagus	liver
cecum	gallbladder	pancreas
colon	ileum	pharynx
duodenum	jejunum	sigmoid colon

1. consists of ascending, transverse, descending, and sigmoid sections _____

2. small sac under the liver; stores bile _____

3. first part of the large intestine _____

4. end of the digestive tract opening to the outside of the body _____

5. second part of the small intestine _____

6. tube connecting the throat to the stomach _____

7. third part of the small intestine _____

8. large organ in the RUQ; secretes bile, stores sugar, produces blood proteins _____

9. throat _____

10. lowest part of the colon _____

11. first part of the small intestine _____

12. organ under the stomach; produces insulin and digestive enzymes _____

5

B Label the following flow chart of the pathway of food through the gastrointestinal tract. The terms you will need are listed below:

anus
ascending colon
cecum
descending colon
duodenum
esophagus

gallbladder
ileum
jejunum
liver
pancreas
pharynx

rectum
salivary glands
sigmoid colon
stomach
transverse colon

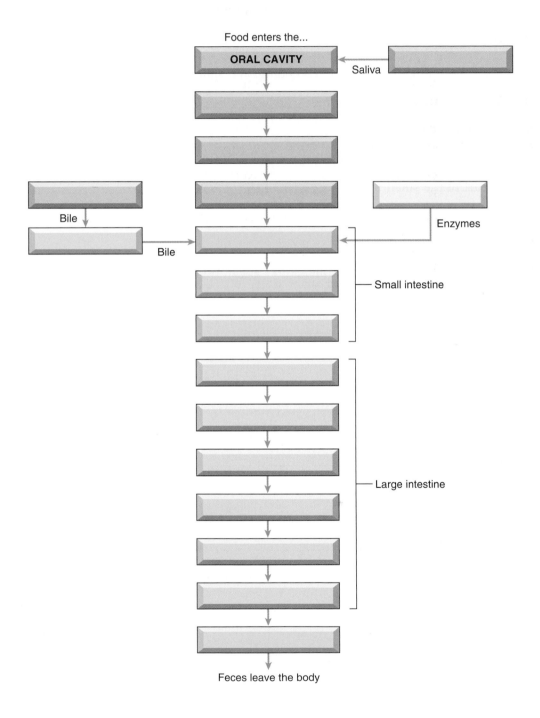

Food enters the...

ORAL CAVITY

Saliva

Bile

Bile

Enzymes

Small intestine

Large intestine

Feces leave the body

5

C Circle the bold term that fits the given definition. You should be able to define the other terms as well!

1. microscopic projections in the walls of the small intestine:
   papillae   villi   rugae

2. salivary gland near the ear:
   submandibular   sublingual   parotid

3. ring of muscle at the end of the stomach:
   pyloric sphincter   uvula   lower esophageal sphincter

4. soft, inner section of a tooth:
   dentin   enamel   pulp

5. chemical that speeds up reactions and helps digest foods:
   triglyceride   amino acid   enzyme

6. pigment released with bile:
   glycogen   bilirubin   melena

7. hormone produced by endocrine cells of the pancreas:
   insulin   amylase   lipase

8. rhythm-like contraction of the muscles in the walls of the gastrointestinal tract:
   deglutition   mastication   peristalsis

9. breakdown of large fat globules:
   absorption   emulsification   anabolism

10. pointed, dog-like tooth medial to premolars:
    incisor   canine   molar

D Complete the following.

1. Labi/o and cheil/o mean _____

2. Gloss/o and lingu/o mean _____

3. Or/o and stomat/o mean _____

4. Dent/i and odont/o mean _____

5. Lapar/o and celi/o mean _____

6. Gluc/o and glyc/o mean _____

7. Lip/o, steat/o, and adip/o mean _____

8. The suffixes -iasis and -osis mean _____

9. Chol/e and bil/i mean _____

10. Resection and -ectomy mean _____

E **Build medical terms based on the given definitions.**

1. removal of a salivary gland _____

2. pertaining to the throat _____

3. hernia of the rectum _____

4. enlargement of the liver _____

5. surgical repair of the roof of the mouth _____

6. after meals _____

7. visual examination of the anal and rectal region _____

8. study of the cause (of disease) _____

9. incision of the common bile duct _____

10. pertaining to teeth and cheek _____

11. disease condition of the small intestine _____

12. new opening between the common bile duct and the jejunum _____

13. pertaining to surrounding the anus _____

14. new opening from the colon to the outside of the body _____

15. under the lower jaw _____

16. pertaining to the face _____

F **Match the following doctors or dentists with their specialties.**

colorectal surgeon	nephrologist	periodontist
endodontist	oral surgeon	proctologist
gastroenterologist	orthodontist	urologist

1. treats disorders of the anus and rectum _____

2. operates on the organs of the urinary tract _____

3. straightens teeth _____

4. performs root canal therapy _____

5. operates on the mouth and teeth _____

6. treats kidney disorders _____

7. diagnoses and treats gastrointestinal disorders _____

8. treats gum disease _____

9. operates on the intestinal tract _____

G Build medical terms to describe the following inflammations.

1. inflammation of the appendix _____

2. inflammation of the large intestine _____

3. inflammation of the passageway from the throat to the stomach _____

4. inflammation of the membrane surrounding the abdomen _____

5. inflammation of the gallbladder _____

6. inflammation of the third part of the small intestine _____

7. inflammation of the pancreas _____

8. inflammation of the gums _____

9. inflammation of the liver _____

10. inflammation of the mouth _____

11. inflammation of the salivary gland _____

12. inflammation of the small and large intestines _____

H Match the listed terms with the meanings that follow.

anastomosis	gluconeogenesis	mesentery
biliary	glycogenolysis	mucosa
defecation	hyperbilirubinemia	parenteral
cheilitis	hyperglycemia	portal vein

1. high level of blood sugar _____

2. inflammation of the lip _____

3. pertaining to administration of medicines and fluid other than by mouth _____

4. mucous membrane _____

5. expulsion of feces from the body through the anus _____

6. breakdown (conversion) of starch to sugar _____

7. fan-like membrane that connects the small intestine to the abdominal wall _____

8. large vessel that takes blood to the liver from the intestines _____

9. new surgical connection between structures or organs _____

10. pertaining to bile ducts _____

11. process of forming new sugar from proteins and fats _____

12. high levels of a bile pigment in the bloodstream _____

5

I Give the names of the following gastrointestinal signs or symptoms based on their descriptions.

1. passage of bright red blood from the rectum _____

2. lack of appetite _____

3. fat in the feces _____

4. black, tarry stools; feces containing digested blood _____

5. abnormal accumulation of fluid in the abdomen _____

6. rumbling noises produced by gas in the gastrointestinal tract _____

7. gas expelled through the anus _____

8. an unpleasant sensation in the stomach and a tendency to vomit _____

9. loose, watery stools _____

10. difficulty in passing stools (feces) _____

11. difficulty in swallowing _____

12. gas expelled from the stomach through the mouth _____

J Write short answers for the following questions.

1. What is jaundice? _____

2. List three ways in which a patient can become jaundiced:

   a. _____

   b. _____

   c. _____

3. What does it mean when a disease is described as *idiopathic*? _____

K Select from the list of pathologic conditions to make a diagnosis.

achalasia	colorectal cancer	herpetic stomatitis
anal fistula	Crohn disease (Crohn's)	oral leukoplakia
aphthous stomatitis	dental caries	pancreatic cancer
colonic polyps	esophageal cancer	periodontal disease

1. Mr. Jones, a smoker and heavy drinker, complained of dysphagia in recent months. A longstanding condition of Barrett esophagus resulted in his malignant condition.

   Diagnosis: _____.

2. An abnormal tube-like passageway near his anus caused Mr. Rosen's proctalgia. His doctor

   performed surgery to close off the abnormality. Diagnosis: _____.

3. Carol's dentist informed her that the enamel of three teeth was damaged by bacteria-producing

   acid. Diagnosis: _____.

4. Paola's symptoms of chronic diarrhea, abdominal cramps, and fever led her doctor to suspect that she suffered from an inflammatory bowel disease affecting the distal portion of her ileum. The doctor prescribed steroid drugs to heal her condition.

   Diagnosis: _____.

5. Mr. Hart learned that his colonoscopy showed the presence of small benign growths protruding

   from the mucous membrane of his large intestine. Diagnosis: _____.

6. During a routine dental checkup, Dr. Friedman discovered white plaques on Mr. Longo's buccal mucosa. He advised Mr. Longo, who was a chronic smoker and heavy drinker, to have these

   precancerous lesions removed. Diagnosis: _____.

7. Every time Carl had a stressful time at work, he developed a fever blister (cold sore) on his lip, resulting from reactivation of a previous viral infection. His doctor told him that there was no treatment 100% effective in preventing the reappearance of these lesions.

   Diagnosis: _____.

8. Mr. Green had a biopsy of a neoplastic lesion in his descending colon. The pathology report indicated a malignancy. A partial colectomy was necessary.

   Diagnosis: _____.

9. Small ulcers (canker sores) appeared on Diane's gums. They were painful and annoying.

   Diagnosis: _____.

10. Sharon's failure to floss her teeth and remove dental plaque regularly led to development of gingivitis and pyorrhea. Her dentist advised consulting a specialist who could treat her

    condition. Diagnosis: _____.

11. Imaging tests revealed a tumor in a section of Mr. Smith's pancreas. His physician told him that since it had not spread, he could hope for a cure with surgery. He had a pancreatoduodenectomy (Whipple procedure), which was successful.

    Diagnosis: _____.

12. Mr. Clark complained of pain during swallowing. His physician explained that the pain was caused by a failure of muscles in his lower esophagus to relax during swallowing.

    Diagnosis: _____.

5

L **Match the following pathologic diagnoses with their definitions.**

cholecystolithiasis (gallstones)	hemorrhoids	pancreatitis
cirrhosis	hiatal hernia	peptic ulcer
diverticulosis	ileus	ulcerative colitis
dysentery	intussusception	viral hepatitis
esophageal varices	irritable bowel syndrome	volvulus

1. protrusion of the upper part of the stomach through the diaphragm _____

2. painful, inflamed intestines caused by bacterial infection _____

3. swollen, twisted veins in the rectal region _____

4. open sore or lesion of the mucous membrane of the stomach or duodenum _____

5. loss of peristalsis _____

6. twisting of the intestine on itself _____

7. swollen, varicose veins on the surface of the distal portion of the esophagus _____

8. abnormal outpouchings in the intestinal wall _____

9. chronic inflammation of the colon with destruction of its inner surface _____

10. telescoping of the intestines _____

11. inflammation of the liver caused by type A, type B, or type C virus _____

12. inflammation of the pancreas _____

13. calculi in the sac that stores bile _____

14. chronic degenerative liver disease with scarring resulting from alcoholism or infectious

 hepatitis _____

15. gastrointestinal symptoms (diarrhea or constipation, abdominal pain, bloating) with no evidence

 of structural abnormalities _____

M **Complete the following terms from their meanings given below.**

1. membrane (peritoneal fold) that holds the intestines together: mes _____

2. removal of the gallbladder: _____ ectomy

3. black or dark brown, tarry stools containing blood: mel _____

4. high levels of pigment in the blood (jaundice): hyper _____

5. pertaining to under the tongue: sub _____

6. twisting of the intestine on itself: vol _____

7. organ under the stomach that produces insulin and digestive enzymes: pan _____

8. lack of appetite: an _____

9. swollen, twisted veins in the rectal region: _____ oids

10. new connection between two previously unconnected tubes: ana _____

11. absence of acid in the stomach: a _____

12. return of solids and fluids to the mouth from the stomach: gastro re _____ disease

13. removal of soft tissue hanging from the roof of the mouth: _____ ectomy

14. formation of stones: _____ genesis.

ANSWERS TO EXERCISES

A

1. colon
2. gallbladder
3. cecum
4. anus
5. jejunum
6. esophagus
7. ileum
8. liver
9. pharynx
10. sigmoid colon
11. duodenum
12. pancreas

B

See Figure 5-12 on page 149.

C

1. Villi. Papillae are nipple-like projections in the tongue where taste buds are located, and rugae are folds in the mucous membrane of the stomach and hard palate.
2. Parotid. The submandibular gland is under the lower jaw, and the sublingual gland is under the tongue.
3. Pyloric sphincter. The uvula is soft tissue hanging from the soft palate, and the lower esophageal sphincter is a ring of muscle between the esophagus and stomach.
4. Pulp. Dentin is the hard part of the tooth directly under the enamel and in the root, and enamel is the hard, outermost part of the tooth composing the crown.
5. Enzyme. A triglyceride is a large fat molecule, and an amino acid is a substance produced when proteins are digested.
6. Bilirubin. Glycogen is animal starch that is produced in liver cells from sugar, and melena is dark, tarry stools.
7. Insulin. Amylase and lipase are digestive enzymes produced by the exocrine cells of the pancreas.
8. Peristalsis. Deglutition is swallowing, and mastication is chewing.
9. Emulsification. Absorption is the passage of materials through the walls of the small intestine into the bloodstream, and anabolism is the process of building up proteins in a cell (protein synthesis).
10. Canine. An incisor is one of the four front teeth in the dental arch (not pointed or like a dog's tooth), and a molar is any of three large teeth just behind (distal to) the two premolar teeth.

D

1. lip
2. tongue
3. mouth
4. tooth
5. abdomen
6. sugar
7. fat
8. abnormal condition
9. gall, bile
10. removal, excision

E

1. sialadenectomy
2. pharyngeal
3. rectocele
4. hepatomegaly
5. palatoplasty
6. postprandial (post cibum—cib/o refers to meals or feeding)
7. proctoscopy
8. etiology
9. choledochotomy
10. dentibuccal
11. enteropathy
12. choledochojejunostomy
13. perianal
14. colostomy
15. submandibular
16. facial

F

1. proctologist
2. urologist
3. orthodontist
4. endodontist
5. oral surgeon
6. nephrologist
7. gastroenterologist
8. periodontist
9. colorectal surgeon

5

G

1. appendicitis
2. colitis
3. esophagitis
4. peritonitis (note that the e is dropped)
5. cholecystitis
6. ileitis
7. pancreatitis
8. gingivitis
9. hepatitis
10. stomatitis
11. sialadenitis
12. enterocolitis (when two combining forms for gastrointestinal organs are in a term, use the one that is closest to the mouth first)

H

1. hyperglycemia
2. cheilitis
3. parenteral
4. mucosa
5. defecation
6. glycogenolysis
7. mesentery
8. portal vein
9. anastomosis
10. biliary
11. gluconeogenesis
12. hyperbilirubinemia

I

1. hematochezia
2. anorexia
3. steatorrhea
4. melena
5. ascites
6. borborygmi (bowel sounds)
7. flatus
8. nausea
9. diarrhea
10. constipation
11. dysphagia
12. eructation

J

1. yellow-orange coloration of the skin and other tissues (hyperbilirubinemia)
2. a. any liver disease (hepatopathy—such as cirrhosis, hepatoma, or hepatitis), so that bilirubin is not processed into bile and cannot be excreted in feces

b. obstruction of bile flow, so that bile and bilirubin are not excreted and accumulate in the bloodstream

c. excessive hemolysis leading to overproduction of bilirubin and high levels in the bloodstream
3. cause is not known

K

1. esophageal cancer
2. anal fistula
3. dental caries
4. Crohn disease (Crohn's)
5. colonic polyps
6. oral leukoplakia
7. herpetic stomatitis
8. colorectal cancer
9. aphthous stomatitis
10. periodontal disease
11. pancreatic cancer
12. achalasia

L

1. hiatal hernia
2. dysentery
3. hemorrhoids
4. peptic ulcer
5. ileus
6. volvulus
7. esophageal varices
8. diverticulosis
9. ulcerative colitis
10. intussusception
11. viral hepatitis
12. pancreatitis
13. cholecystolithiasis (gallstones)
14. cirrhosis
15. irritable bowel syndrome

M

1. mesentery
2. cholecystectomy
3. melena
4. hyperbilirubinemia
5. sublingual
6. volvulus
7. pancreas
8. anorexia
9. hemorrhoids
10. anastomosis
11. achlorhydria
12. gastroesophageal reflux
13. uvulectomy
14. lithogenesis

5

PRONUNCIATION OF TERMS

To test your understanding of the terminology in this chapter, write the meaning of each term in the space provided. In addition, you may wish to cover the terms and write them by looking at your definitions. Make sure your spelling is correct. The page number after each term indicates where it is defined or used in the book, so you can easily check your responses. You will find complete definitions for all of these terms and their audio pronunciations on the Evolve website.

Pronunciation Guide

ā as in āpe	ă as in ăpple
ē as in ēven	ĕ as in ĕvery
ī as in īce	ĭ as in ĭnterest
ō as in ōpen	ŏ as in pŏt
ū as in ūnit	ŭ as in ŭnder

Vocabulary and Terminology

TERM	PRONUNCIATION	MEANING
absorption (150)	ăb-SŎRP-shŭn	_____
achlorhydria (158)	a-chlōr-HĪD-rē-ă	_____
amino acids (150)	ă-MĒ-nō ĂS-ĭdz	_____
amylase (150)	ĂM-ĭ-lās	_____
anastomosis (155)	ă-năs-tō-MŌ-sĭs	_____
anus (150)	Ā-nŭs	_____
appendectomy (153)	ăp-ĕn-DĔK-tō-mē	_____
appendicitis (153)	ă-pĕn-dĭ-SĪ-tĭs	_____
appendix (150)	ă-PĔN-dĭks	_____
bile (150)	bīl	_____
biliary (157)	BĬL-ē-ăr-ē	_____
bilirubin (150)	bĭl-ĭ-ROO-bĭn	_____
bowel (150)	BOW-ĕl	_____
buccal mucosa (153)	BŬK-ăl mū-KŌ-să	_____
canine teeth (150)	KĀ-nĭn tēth	_____
cecal (153)	SĒ-kăl	_____
cecum (150)	SĒ-kŭm	_____
celiac (153)	SĒ-lē-ăk	_____
cheilosis (154)	kī-LŌ-sĭs	_____
cholecystectomy (154)	kō-lĕ-sĭs-TĔK-tō-mē	_____
choledocholithiasis (158)	kō-lĕ-dō-kō-lĭ-THĪ-ă-sĭs	_____
choledochojejunostomy (156)	kō-lĕ-dō-kō-jĕ-jū-NŎS-tō-mē	_____
choledochotomy (154)	kō-lĕ-dō-KŎT-ō-mē	_____

5

TERM	PRONUNCIATION	MEANING
cholelithiasis (157)	kō-lē-lǐ-THĪ-ă-sǐs	
colon (150)	KŌ-lŏn	
colonic (154)	kō-LŎN-ǐk	
colonoscopy (154)	kō-lŏn-ŎS-kō-pē	
colostomy (154)	kŏ-LŎS-tō-mē	
common bile duct (150)	KŎM-ŏn bīl dŭkt	
defecation (150)	dĕf-ĕ-KĀ-shŭn	
deglutition (150)	dē-gloo-TĬSH-ŭn	
dentibuccal (155)	dĕn-tǐ-BŬK-ăl	
dentin (150)	DĚN-tǐn	
digestion (150)	di JES chun	
duodenal (155)	dū-ō-DĒ-năl or dū-ŎD-ĕ-năl	
duodenum (150)	dū-ō-DĒ-nŭm or dū-ŎD-ĕ-nŭm	
elimination (150)	ē-lǐm-ǐ-NĀ-shŭn	
emulsification (150)	ē-mŭl-sǐ-fǐ-KĀ-shŭn	
enamel (151)	ē-NĂM-ĕl	
endodontist (156)	ĕn-dō-DŎN-tǐst	
enterocolitis (155)	ĕn-tĕr-ō-kō-LĪ-tǐs	
enteroenterostomy (155)	ĕn-tĕr-ō-ĕn-tĕr-ŎS-tō-mē	
enzyme (151)	ĔN-zīm	
esophageal (156)	ĕ-sŏf-ă-JĒ-ăl	
esophagus (151)	ĕ-SŎF-ă-gŭs	
fatty acids (151)	FĂT-tē Ă-sǐdz	
facial (156)	FĀ-shŭl	
feces (151)	FĒ-sēz	
gallbladder (151)	GAWL-blă-dĕr	
gastrointestinal tract (140)	găs-trō-ǐn-TĔS-tǐn-ăl trăct	
gastrojejunostomy (156)	găs-trō-jĕ-jū-NŎS-tō-mē	
gastrostomy (156)	găs-TRŎS-tō-mē	
gingivitis (156)	jǐn-jǐ-VĪ-tǐs	
gluconeogenesis (158)	gloo-kō-nē-ō-JĔN-ĕ-sǐs	

5

TERM	PRONUNCIATION	MEANING
glucose (151)	GLOO-kōs	
glycogen (151)	GLĪ-kō-jĕn	
glycogenolysis (158)	glī-kō-jĕ-NŎL-ĭ-sĭs	
hepatoma (156)	hĕ-pă-TŌ-mă	
hepatomegaly (156)	hĕ-pă-tō-MĔG-ă-lē	
hydrochloric acid (151)	hī-drō-KLŎR-ĭk Ă-sĭd	
hyperbilirubinemia (157)	hī-pĕr-bĭl-ĭ-roo-bĭ-NĒ-mē-ă	
hyperglycemia (158)	hī-pĕr-glī-SĒ-mē-ă	
hypoglossal (156)	hī-pō-GLŎ-săl	
ileitis (156)	ĭl-ē-Ī-tĭs	
ileocecal sphincter (156)	ĭl-ē-ō-SĒ-kăl SFĬNK-tĕr	
ileostomy (156)	ĭl-ē-ŎS-tō-mē	
ileum (151)	ĬL-ē-ŭm	
incisor (151)	ĭn-SĪ-zŏr	
insulin (151)	ĬN-sŭ-lĭn	
jejunum (151)	jĕ-JOO-nŭm	
labial (156)	LĀ-bē-ăl	
laparoscopy (156)	lă-pă-RŎS-kō-pē	
lipase (151)	LĪ-pās	
lithogenesis (158)	lĭth-ō-JĔN-ĕ-sĭs	
liver (151)	LĬ-vĕr	
lower esophageal sphincter (151)	LŌW-ĕr ĕ-sŏf-ă-JĒ-ăl SFĬNK-tĕr	
mastication (151)	măs-tĭ-KĀ-shŭn	
mesentery (155)	MĔS-ĕn-tĕr-ē	
molar teeth (151)	MŌ-lăr tēth	
oral (157)	ŎR-ăl	
orthodontist (156)	ŏr-thō-DŎN-tĭst	
palate (151)	PĂL-ăt	
palatopharyngoplasty (157)	păl-ă-tō-fă-RĬNG-gō-plăs-tē	
palatoplasty (157)	PĂL-ă-tō-plăs-tē	
pancreas (151)	PĂN-krē-ăs	

5

TERM	PRONUNCIATION	MEANING
pancreatitis (157)	păn-krē-ă-TĪ-tĭs	_____
papillae (151)	pă-PĬL-ē	_____
parenteral (155)	pă-RĔN-tĕr-ăl	_____
parotid gland (151)	pă-RŎT-ĭd glănd	_____
perianal (153)	pĕ-rē-Ā-năl	_____
periodontist (156)	pĕr-ē-ō-DŎN-tĭst	_____
peritonitis (157)	pĕr-ĭ-tō-NĪ-tĭs	_____
peristalsis (152)	pĕr-ĭ-STĂL-sĭs	_____
pharyngeal (157)	făr-ăn-JĒ-ăl _or_ fă-RĬN-jē-ăl	_____
pharynx (152)	FĂR-ĭnks	_____
portal vein (152)	PŎR-tăl vān	_____
postprandial (158)	pōst-PRĂN-dē-ăl	_____
premolar teeth (141)	prē-MŌ-lăr tēth	_____
proctologist (157)	prŏk-TŎL-ō-jĭst	_____
protease (152)	PRŌ-tē-āse	_____
pulp (152)	pŭlp	_____
pyloric sphincter (152)	pī-LŎR-ĭk SFĬNK-tĕr	_____
pyloroplasty (157)	pī-LŎR-ō-plăs-tē	_____
pylorus (152)	pī-LŎR-ŭs	_____
rectocele (157)	RĔK-tō-sēl	_____
rectum (152)	RĔK-tŭm	_____
rugae (152)	ROO-gē	_____
saliva (152)	să-LĪ-vă	_____
salivary glands (152)	SĂL-ĭ-vār-ē glăndz	_____
sialadenitis (157)	sī-ăl-ă-dĕ-NĪ-tĭs	_____
sialolith (158)	sī-ĂL-ō-lĭth	_____
sigmoid colon (152)	SĬG-moyd KŌ-lŏn	_____
sigmoidoscopy (157)	sĭg-moyd-ŎS-kō-pē	_____
sphincter (152)	SFĬNK-tĕr	_____
steatorrhea (158)	stē-ă-tō-RĒ-ă	_____
stomach (152)	STŬM-ak	_____

TERM	PRONUNCIATION	MEANING
stomatitis (157)	stō-mă-TĪ-tĭs	_____
sublingual (156)	sŭb-LĬNG-wăl	_____
submandibular (156)	sŭb-măn-DĬB-ū-lăr	_____
triglycerides (153)	trī-GLĬ-sĕ-rīdz	_____
uvula (153)	Ū-vū-lă	_____
uvulectomy (157)	ū-vū-LĔK-tō-mē	_____
villi (153)	VĬL-ī	_____

Pathologic Terminology

TERM	PRONUNCIATION	MEANING
achalasia (162)	ăk-ă-LĀ-zē-ă	_____
anal fistula (164)	Ā-năl FĬS-tū-lă	_____
anorexia (159)	ăn-ō-RĔK-sē-ă	_____
aphthous stomatitis (161)	ĂF-thŭs stō-mă-TĪ-tĭs	_____
ascites (159)	ă-SĪ-tēz	_____
borborygmi (159)	bŏr-bō-RĬG-mē	_____
cholelithiasis (167)	kō-lĕ-lĭ-THĪ-a-sis	_____
cirrhosis (167)	sĭr-RŌ-sĭs	_____
colonic polyps (164)	kō-LŎN-ĭk pŏlĭps	_____
colorectal cancer (164)	kō-lō-RĔK-tăl KĂN-sĕr	_____
constipation (159)	cŏn-stĭ-PĀ-shŭn	_____
Crohn disease (164)	krōn dĭ-ZĒZ	_____
dental caries (161)	DĔN-tăl KĂR-ēz	_____
diarrhea (160)	dī-ăh-RĒ-ă	_____
diverticula (165)	dī-vĕr-TĬK-ū-lă	_____
diverticulitis (165)	dī-vĕr-tĭk-ū-LĪ-tĭs	_____
diverticulosis (165)	dī-vĕr-tĭk-ū-LŌ-sĭs	_____
dysentery (165)	DĬS-ĕn-tĕr-ē	_____
dysphagia (160)	dĭs-PHĀ-jē-ă	_____
eructation (160)	ē-rŭk-TĀ-shŭn	_____
esophageal cancer (162)	ĕ-sŏf-ă-JĒ-ăl KăN-sĕr	_____
esophageal varices (162)	ĕ-sŏf-ă-JĒ-ăl VĂR-ĭ-sēz	_____

5

TERM	PRONUNCIATION	MEANING
etiology (159)	ē-tē-ŎL-ō-jē	
flatus (160)	FLĀ-tŭs	
gastric cancer (162)	GĂS-trĭk KĂN-sĕr	
gastroesophageal reflux disease (162)	găs-trō-ĕ-sŏf-ă-JĒ-ăl RĒ-flŭx dĭ-ZĒZ	
hematochezia (160)	hē-mă-tō-KĒ-zē-ă	
hemorrhoids (165)	HĔM-ō-roydz	
hepatocellular carcinoma (169)	hĕ-păt-ō-SĔL-ū-lăr kăr-sĭ-NŌ-mă	
herpetic stomatitis (162)	hĕr-PĔT-ĭk stō-mă-TĪ-tĭs	
hiatal hernia (163)	hī-Ā-tăl HĔR-nē-ă	
icterus (160)	ĬK-tĕr-ŭs	
idiopathic (159)	ĭd-ē-ō-PĂTH-ĭk	
ileus (166)	ĬL-ē-ŭs	
inflammatory bowel disease (166)	ĭn-FLĂ-mă-tō-rē BOW-ĕl dĭ-ZĒZ	
inguinal hernia (163)	ĬNG-wĭ-năl HĔR-nē-ă	
intussusception (166)	ĭn-tŭs-sŭs-SĔP-shŭn	
irritable bowel syndrome (166)	ĬR-ĭ-tă-bl BOW-ĕl SĬN-drōm	
jaundice (160)	JAWN-dĭs	
lipoma (158)	lī-PŌ-mă	
melena (161)	MĔL-ĕ-nă *or* mĕ-LĒ-nă	
nausea (161)	NAW-zē-ă	
oral leukoplakia (162)	ŎR-ăl lū-kō-PLĀ-kē-ă	
pancreatic cancer (169)	păn-krē-Ă-tĭc KĂN-sĕr	
pancreatitis (169)	păn-krē-ă-TĪ-tĭs	
peptic ulcer (163)	PĔP-tĭc ŬL-sĕr	
periodontal disease (162)	pĕr-ē-ō-DŎN-tăl dĭ-ZĒZ	
pyorrhea (158)	pī-ŏr-RĒ-ă	
ulcerative colitis (166)	ŬL-sĕr-ă-tĭv kō-LĪ-tĭs	
viral hepatitis (169)	VĪ-răl hĕp-ă-TĪ-tĭs	
volvulus (167)	VŎL-vū-lŭs	

Note: A combination Review Sheet for this chapter and the next one is provided in Chapter 6 on page 213.

6

Additional Suffixes and Digestive System Terminology

Chapter Sections:

CHAPTER GOALS

- Define new suffixes and use them to form terms related to the digestive system.
- List and explain laboratory tests, clinical procedures, and abbreviations relevant to the digestive system.
- Apply your new knowledge to understanding medical terms in their proper context, such as in medical reports and records and in personal vignettes.

INTRODUCTION

This chapter gives you practice in word building, while not introducing a large number of new terms. It uses many familiar terms from Chapter 5, which should give you a breather after your hard work.

Study the suffixes presented next and complete the meanings of the terms. Checking the meanings of the terms with a dictionary may prove helpful and add another dimension to your understanding.

The information included under Laboratory Tests and Clinical Procedures and in the Abbreviations section relates to the gastrointestinal system and will be useful for work in clinical or laboratory medical settings.

The Practical Applications section gives you examples of medical language in context. Congratulate yourself as you decipher medical sentences, operative reports, and case studies.

SUFFIXES

Write the meaning of the medical term in the space provided.

SUFFIX	MEANING	TERMINOLOGY	MEANING
-ectasis, -ectasia	dilation, (dilatation), widening	cholangiectasis _____ *Cholangi/o means bile duct (vessel). This condition is secondary to bile duct obstruction.*	
-emesis	vomiting	hematemesis _____ *Bright red blood is vomited, often associated with esophageal varices or peptic ulcer.*	
-pepsia	digestion	dyspepsia _____	
-phagia	eating, swallowing	polyphagia _____ *Excessive appetite and uncontrolled eating.*	
		dysphagia _____	
-plasty	surgical repair	abdominoplasty _____ *This is commonly referred to as a "tummy tuck." Other surgical repairs are rhinoplasty and blepharoplasty.*	

 -ectasis, -ectasia

These suffixes are commonly used in respiratory system terminology in Chapter 12. Examples are bronchiectasis and atelectasis (a- = not, tel = complete), which is a collapsed lung.

 Dysphagia/Dysplasia/Dysphasia

Don't confuse **dysphagia**, which is difficulty in swallowing, with **dysplasia,** which is abnormal formation (plas/o = formation), or **dysphasia**, which is abnormal speech (phas/o = speech).

SUFFIX	MEANING	TERMINOLOGY	MEANING
-ptysis	spitting	hemo<u>ptysis</u> _____ _From the respiratory tract and lungs._	
-rrhage, -rrhagia	bursting forth (of blood)	hemo<u>rrhage</u> _____ _Loss of a large amount of blood in a short period._ gastro<u>rrhagia</u> _____	
-rrhaphy	suture	hernio<u>rrhaphy</u> _____ _Repair (as in stitching or suturing) of a hernia. Hernioplasty is a synonym. Tenorrhaphy (ten = tendon) is another common use of this suffix._	
-rrhea	flow, discharge	dia<u>rrhea</u> _____ _The embedded root rrh means flow or discharge._	
-spasm	involuntary contraction of muscles	pyloro<u>spasm</u> _____ broncho<u>spasm</u> _____ _A chief characteristic of bronchitis and asthma._	
-stasis	stopping, controlling	chole<u>stasis</u> _____ _Flow of bile from the liver to the duodenum is interrupted._	
-stenosis	narrowing, tightening	pyloric <u>stenosis</u> _____ _This is a congenital defect in newborns blocking the flow of food into the small intestine._	

6

Hemoptysis and Hematemesis

Hemoptysis is spitting up blood from the respiratory tract, a sign of bleeding and disease within the bronchial tubes and lungs. **Hematemesis** is vomiting blood, a sign of bleeding from the upper part of the gastrointestinal tract.

-rrhea

The suffix -rrhea is used to indicate flow or discharge of various substances:
- rhino<u>rrhea</u>-mucus from the nose
- meno<u>rrhea</u>-menstrual (men/o) blood from the uterine lining
- leuko<u>rrhea</u>-white, yellowish fluid from the vagina

Stenosis

Stenosis comes from the Greek meaning "narrowing." It is sometimes called a **stricture.** While this term is used in the gastrointestinal system to describe narrowing, as in bowel obstruction, biliary tract stenosis, and pyloric stenosis, there are other types of stenoses as well. These include:
- arterial stenosis
- heart valve stenosis
- spinal stenosis
- tracheal stenosis

SUFFIX	MEANING	TERMINOLOGY	MEANING
-tresia	opening	atresia _____ *Absence of a normal opening.*	
		esophageal atresia _____ *A congenital anomaly in which the esophagus does not connect with the stomach. A tracheoesophageal fistula often accompanies this abnormality (Figure 6-1).*	
		biliary atresia _____ *Congenital hypoplasia or nonformation of bile ducts causes neonatal cholestasis and jaundice.*	

Examples of suffixes that are used alone as separate terms are:

emesis (emetic)   If a child swallows poison, the physician may prescribe a drug to induce **emesis.** An example of an **emetic** is a strong solution of salt or ipecac syrup.

lysis   The disease caused **lysis** of liver cells.

spasm   Eating spicy foods can lead to **spasm** of gastric sphincters.

stasis   Overgrowth of bacteria within the small intestine can cause **stasis** of the intestinal contents.

stenosis   Projectile vomiting in an infant during feeding is a clinical sign of pyloric **stenosis.**

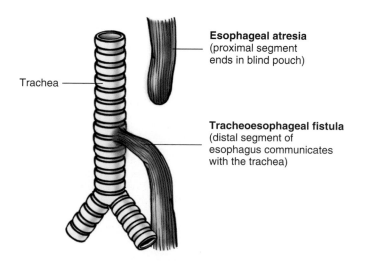

Esophageal atresia (proximal segment ends in blind pouch)

Trachea

Tracheoesophageal fistula (distal segment of esophagus communicates with the trachea)

FIGURE 6-1   Esophageal atresia with tracheoesophageal fistula.

TERMINOLOGY

Write the meaning of the terms in the spaces provided.

COMBINING FORM	MEANING	TERMINOLOGY	MEANING
bucc/o	_____	buccal _____	
cec/o	_____	cecal volvulus _____	
celi/o	_____	celiac disease _____	

*Damage to the lining of the small intestine occurring as a reaction to eating **gluten** (protein found in wheat, barley, and rye). Malabsorption and malnutrition result. Treatment consists of a lifelong gluten-free diet. It also is called **celiac sprue.***

cheil/o	_____	cheilosis _____	

Characterized by scales and fissures on the lips and resulting from a deficiency of vitamin B_2 (thiamine) in the diet.

chol/e	_____	cholelithiasis _____	
cholangi/o	_____	cholangitis _____	

In this term, one i is dropped. The most common cause of this condition is bacterial infection.

		cholangiocarcinoma _____	
cholecyst/o	_____	cholecystectomy _____	
choledoch/o	_____	choledochal _____	
		choledochectasia _____	
col/o	_____	colectomy _____	

*Surgeons perform **laparoscopic-assisted colectomy (LAC)** as an alternative to open colectomy to remove nonmetastatic colorectal carcinomas.*

colon/o	_____	colonoscopy _____	
dent/i	_____	dentalgia _____	
duoden/o	_____	duodenal _____	
enter/o	_____	gastroenteritis _____	
esophag/o	_____	esophageal atresia _____	

This congenital anomaly must be corrected surgically.

gastr/o	_____	gastrojejunostomy _____	
		gastrostomy _____	

*A gastrostomy is also called a **G tube** or "button." One type is a PEG (percutaneous endoscopic gastrostomy) tube, which is inserted (laparoscopically) through the abdomen into the stomach to deliver food and liquids when swallowing is impossible.*

6

COMBINING FORM	MEANING	TERMINOLOGY	MEANING
gingiv/o	_____	gingivectomy	_____
gloss/o	_____	glossectomy	_____
gluc/o	_____	gluconeogenesis	_____
glyc/o	_____	glycogen	_____
		A form of sugar stored in the liver.	
hepat/o	_____	hepatomegaly	_____
herni/o	_____	herniorrhaphy	_____
ile/o	_____	ileostomy	_____
jejun/o	_____	cholecystojejunostomy	_____
labi/o	_____	labiodental	_____
lingu/o	_____	sublingual	_____
lip/o	_____	lipase	_____
lith/o	_____	cholecystolithiasis	_____
odont/o	_____	periodontal membrane	_____
or/o	_____	oropharynx	_____
		The tonsils are located in the oropharynx.	
palat/o	_____	palatoplasty	_____
		Also called palatorrhaphy; this procedure corrects cleft (split) palate, a congenital anomaly.	
pancreat/o	_____	pancreatic	_____
		pancreatoduodenectomy	_____
		*Sometimes called a pancreaticoduodenectomy. This is a **Whipple procedure,** a surgical treatment for pancreatic cancer. See page 200.*	
proct/o	_____	proctosigmoidoscopy	_____
pylor/o	_____	pyloric stenosis	_____
rect/o	_____	rectal carcinoma	_____
sialaden/o	_____	sialadenectomy	_____
splen/o	_____	splenic flexure	_____
		*The downward bend in the transverse colon near the spleen. The **hepatic flexure** is the bend in the transverse colon near the liver.*	
steat/o	_____	steatorrhea	_____
stomat/o	_____	aphthous stomatitis	_____

6

LABORATORY TESTS AND CLINICAL PROCEDURES

Concentrate on learning the meanings in **bold** opposite the laboratory test or procedure. Additional information is provided to increase your understanding of terms.

LABORATORY TESTS

amylase and lipase tests

Tests for the levels of amylase and lipase enzymes in the blood.

Increased levels are associated with pancreatitis.

liver function tests (LFTs)

Tests for the presence of enzymes and bilirubin in blood.

LFTs are performed on blood serum (clear fluid that remains after blood has clotted). Examples of LFTs are tests for **ALT** (alanine transaminase) and **AST** (aspartate transaminase). ALT and AST are enzymes present in many tissues. **Levels are elevated in the serum of patients with liver disease.** High ALT and AST levels indicate damage to liver cells (as in hepatitis).

   Alkaline phosphatase (alk phos) is another enzyme that may be elevated in patients with liver, bone, and other diseases.

   Serum bilirubin levels are elevated in patients with liver disease and jaundice. A **direct bilirubin test** measures conjugated bilirubin. High levels indicate liver disease or biliary obstruction. An **indirect bilirubin test** measures unconjugated bilirubin. Increased levels suggest excessive hemolysis, as may occur in a newborn.

stool culture

Test for microorganisms present in feces.

Feces are placed in a growth medium and examined microscopically. (Figure 6-2A).

stool guaiac test or Hemoccult test

Test to detect occult (hidden) blood in feces.

This is an important screening test for colon cancer. **Guaiac** (GWĪ-ăk) is a chemical from the wood of trees. When added to a stool sample, it reacts with any blood present in the feces. See Figure 6-2B.

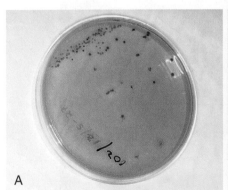
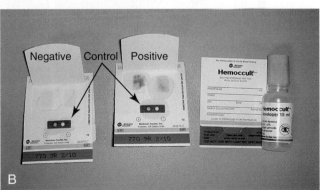

FIGURE 6-2   A, Stool culture. B, Stool guaiac test.

CLINICAL PROCEDURES

X-Ray Tests

X-ray imaging is used in many ways to detect pathologic conditions. In dental practice, x-ray images are commonly used to locate cavities (caries). Many of the x-ray tests listed here use a **contrast medium** (substance that x-rays cannot penetrate) to visualize a specific area of the digestive system. The contrast, because of its increased density relative to body tissue, allows organs and parts to be distinguished from one another on the film or screen.

lower gastrointestinal series (barium enema)	**X-ray images of the colon and rectum obtained after injection of barium into the rectum.** Radiologists inject barium (a contrast medium) by enema into the rectum. Figure 6-3A shows a barium enema study of a colon with diverticulosis.
upper gastrointestinal series	**X-ray images of the esophagus, stomach, and small intestine obtained after administering barium by mouth.** Often performed immediately after an upper gastrointestinal series, a **small bowel follow-through** study shows sequential x-ray pictures of the small intestine as barium passes through (Figure 6-3B). A **barium swallow** is a study of the esophagus.
cholangiography	**X-ray examination of the biliary system performed after injection of contrast into the bile ducts.** In **percutaneous transhepatic cholangiography,** the contrast medium is injected using a needle placed through the abdominal wall into the biliary vessels of the liver. In **endoscopic retrograde cholangiopancreatography (ERCP)** (Figure 6-4A), contrast medium is administered through an oral catheter (tube) and then passes through the esophagus, stomach, and duodenum and into bile ducts. This procedure helps diagnose problems involving the bile ducts, gallbladder, and pancreas.

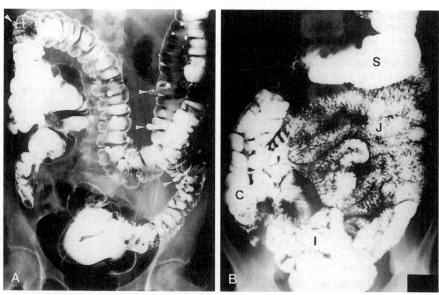

FIGURE 6-3   A, Barium enema. This x-ray image from a barium enema study demonstrates diverticulosis. The *arrowheads* point to the diverticula throughout the colon. Most patients with diverticula are asymptomatic, but complications (diverticulitis, perforated diverticulum, obstruction, or hemorrhage) may occur. **B,** An x-ray image of a **small-bowel follow-through** study demonstrating the normal appearance of the jejunum (J) in the upper left abdomen and of the ileum (I) in the right lower abdomen. Notice the contrast material within the stomach (S) and cecum (C).

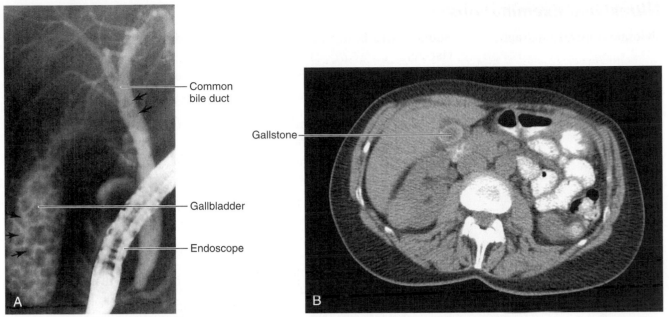

FIGURE 6-4   A, Endoscopic retrograde cholangiopancreatography (ERCP) showing choledocholithiasis in a patient with biliary colic (pain). Multiple stones are visible in the gallbladder and common bile duct. The stones *(arrows)* are seen as filling defects in the contrast-opacified gallbladder and duct. This patient was treated with open (performed via laparotomy) cholecystectomy and choledocholithotomy. **B, Computed tomography scan** with contrast showing large "porcelain stone" in the gallbladder. The patient was asymptomatic, but a therapeutic option with this type of stone is removal of the gallbladder *(using laparoscopy)* to prevent any future problems (such as cholecystitis or carcinoma of the gallbladder). *(B, Courtesy Radiology Department, Massachusetts General Hospital, Boston.)*

computed tomography (CT)	**A series of x-ray images are taken in multiple views (especially cross section).**

A **CT scan** uses a circular array of x-ray beams to produce the cross-sectional image based on differences in tissue densities. Use of contrast material allows visualization of organs and blood vessels and highlights differences in blood flow between normal and diseased tissues (Figure 6-4B and Figure 6-5A and B). **Tomography** (tom/o means cutting) produces a series of x-ray pictures showing multiple views of an organ. An earlier name for a CT scan is "CAT scan" (computerized axial tomography scan).

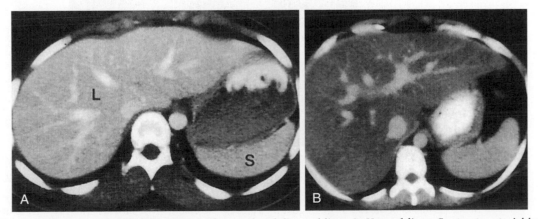

FIGURE 6-5   Computed tomography (CT) images of normal and diseased liver. **A, Normal liver.** Contrast material has been injected intravenously, making blood vessels appear bright. The liver (L) and spleen (S) are the same density on this CT image. **B, Fatty liver.** The radiodensity of the liver tissue is reduced because of the large volume of fat contained in the tissue, making it appear darker than normal. Excess fat can lead to inflammation of the liver and cirrhosis.

Ultrasound Examinations

abdominal ultrasonography	**Sound waves beamed into the abdomen produce an image of abdominal viscera.**
	Ultrasonography is especially useful for examination of fluid-filled structures such as the gallbladder.
endoscopic ultrasonography (EUS)	**Use of an endoscope combined with ultrasound to examine the organs of the gastrointestinal tract.**
	An endoscope is inserted through the mouth or rectum, and ultrasound images are obtained. This test is often used in assessing esophageal, pancreatic, and rectal cancer.

Magnetic Resonance Imaging

magnetic resonance imaging (MRI)	**Magnetic waves produce images of organs and tissues in all three planes of the body.**
	This technique does not use x-rays. It detects subtle differences in tissue composition, water content, and blood vessel density and can show sites of trauma, infection, or cancer. See Figure 6-6, which shows an MRI study of a patient with rectosigmoid carcinoma and polyps in the rectum. CT scanning would not have shown these lesions as clearly.

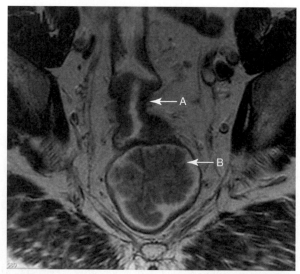

FIGURE 6-6 Rectal (MRI). A 68-year old man presented with rectal bleeding. MRI demonstrates (**A**) **colonic adenocarcinoma** in the rectosigmoid area as well as (**B**) **villous adenoma** in the rectum.

Nuclear Medicine Test

HIDA scan

Radioactive imaging procedure that tracks the production and flow of bile from the liver and gallbladder to the intestine.

HIDA stands for **h**epatobiliary **i**mino**d**iacetic **a**cid. **Cholescintigraphy** is another name for this test, which determines if the gallbladder is functioning properly.

Other Procedures

gastric bypass or bariatric surgery

Reducing the size of the stomach and diverting food to the jejunum (gastrojejunostomy).

This is **bariatric** (bar/o = weight; iatr/o = treatment) **surgery** for severe obesity. The **Roux-en-Y gastric bypass procedure** reduces the size of the stomach to a volume of 2 tablespoons and bypasses much of the small intestine (Figure 6-7). The name Roux-en-Y comes from the surgeon who first described it (César Roux) and the anastomosis of the duodenum and jejunum, which looks like the letter Y.

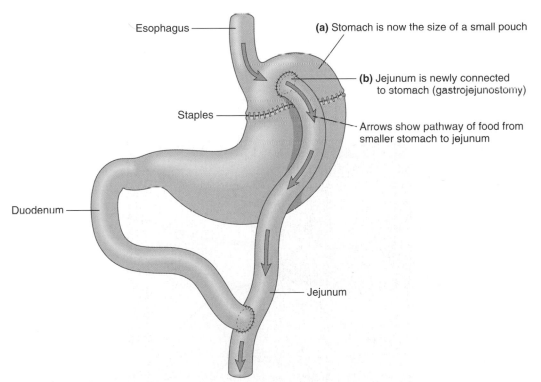

FIGURE 6-7   Gastric bypass. First (**a**) the stomach is stapled so that it is reduced in size to a small pouch. Next (**b**) a shortened jejunum is brought up to connect with the smaller stomach. This diverts food so that it has a shorter travel time through the intestine and less food is absorbed into the bloodstream.

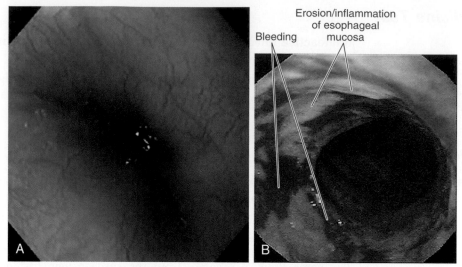

FIGURE 6-8 **A, Normal endoscopy of the esophagus. B, Esophagogastroduodenoscopy**. This endoscopic view shows severe esophagitis in a patient who had gastroesophageal reflux disease (GERD).

gastrointestinal endoscopy   **Visual examination of the gastrointestinal tract using an endoscope.**

A physician places a flexible fiberoptic tube through the mouth or the anus to view parts of the gastrointestinal tract. Examples are **esophagogastroduodenoscopy (EGD)** (Figure 6-8), **colonoscopy** (Figures 6-9 and 6-10), **sigmoidoscopy**, **proctoscopy**, and **anoscopy**.

Virtual colonoscopy (CT colonography) combines CT scanning and computer technology to enable physicians to examine the entire length of the colon by x-ray imaging in just minutes. Patients with abnormal findings require conventional colonoscopy afterward for further assessment or treatment, such as with biopsy or polypectomy.

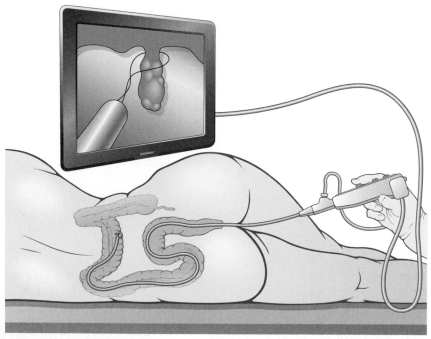

FIGURE 6-9 **Colonoscopy with polypectomy**. Before the procedure, the patient ingests agents to clean the bowel of feces. The patient is sedated, and the gastroenterologist advances the instrument in retrograde fashion, guided by images from a video camera on the tip of the colonoscope. When a polyp is located, a wire snare is passed through the endoscope and looped around the stalk. After the loop is gently tightened, an electrical current is applied to cut through the stalk. The polyp is removed (biopsy) for microscopic tissue examination.

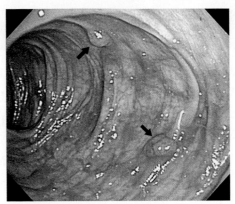

FIGURE 6-10   Colonoscopy case report. A 60-year-old man with a history of multiple and prominent colon adenomas (with some areas of high-grade dysplasia) underwent colonoscopy. The endoscope was passed through the anus and advanced to the cecum. Two pedunculated polyps (*arrows*) were found at the hepatic flexure. Polypectomy was performed using a hot snare. Resection and retrieval were complete.

laparoscopy	**Visual (endoscopic) examination of the abdomen with a laparoscope inserted through small incisions in the abdomen.** Laparoscopic cholecystectomy (see Figure 5-28, page 168) and laparoscopic appendectomy are performed by gastrointestinal and general surgeons. See the **In Person: Cholecystectomy** story of a woman who underwent laparoscopic cholecystectomy (see page 201).
liver biopsy	**Removal of liver tissue for microscopic examination.** A physician inserts a needle through the skin to remove a small piece of tissue for microscopic examination. The average sample is less than 1 inch long. The procedure helps doctors diagnose cirrhosis, chronic hepatitis, and tumors of the liver.
nasogastric intubation	**Insertion of a tube through the nose into the stomach.** Physicians use a nasogastric (NG) tube to remove fluid postoperatively and to obtain gastric or intestinal contents for analysis (Figure 6-11).
paracentesis (abdominocentesis)	**Surgical puncture to remove fluid from the abdomen.** This procedure is necessary to drain fluid (accumulated in ascites) from the peritoneal (abdominal) cavity.

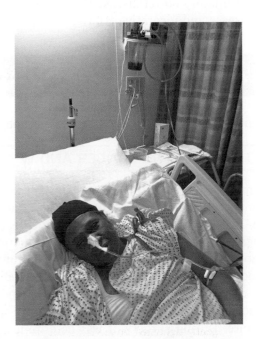

FIGURE 6-11   Nasogastric intubation. The nasogastric tube is suctioning secretions from the patient's stomach and intestines. The patient had a twisted blocked intestine (ileus), and the suction relieved pressure so that the intestine unwound and decompressed without surgery.

ABBREVIATIONS

AFP	alpha-fetoprotein—tumor marker for liver cancer	**J-tube**	jejunostomy tube—feeding tube
alk phos	alkaline phosphatase	**LAC**	laparoscopic-assisted colectomy
ALT, AST	alanine transaminase, aspartate transaminase—enzymes measured to evaluate liver function in blood	**LFTs**	liver function tests—alk phos, bilirubin, AST, ALT
		MRI	magnetic resonance imaging
BE	barium enema	**NASH**	nonalcoholic steatohepatitis (fatty liver)
BM	bowel movement	**NG tube**	nasogastric tube
BRBPR	bright red blood per rectum—hematochezia (Latin *per* means through)	**NPO**	nothing by mouth (Latin *nil per os*)
		PEG tube	percutaneous endoscopic gastrostomy tube—feeding tube
CD	celiac disease	**PEJ tube**	percutaneous endoscopic jejunostomy tube—feeding tube
CT	computed tomography	**PTHC**	percutaneous transhepatic cholangiography
EGD	esophagogastroduodenoscopy		
ERCP	endoscopic retrograde cholangiopancreatography	**PUD**	peptic ulcer disease
EUS	endoscopic ultrasonography	**TPN**	total parenteral nutrition
FOBT	fecal occult blood test		Intravenous TPN solutions typically contain sugar (dextrose), proteins (amino acids), electrolytes (sodium, potassium, chloride), and vitamins.
G tube	gastrostomy tube—feeding tube		
GB	gallbladder		
GERD	gastroesophageal reflux disease		
GI	gastrointestinal	**T-tube**	special tube (shaped like the letter T) placed in the bile duct for drainage into a small pouch (bile bag) on the outside of the body
HBV	hepatitis B virus		
IBD	inflammatory bowel disease (Crohn disease and ulcerative colitis)		

PRACTICAL APPLICATIONS

Answers to the questions about the case report are on page 209.

CASE REPORT: PANCREATIC CANCER AND WHIPPLE PROCEDURE

A 62-year-old man came to the ED [emergency department] with complaints of fatigue, weight loss, jaundice, and anorexia. Diagnostic studies including abdominal CT with contrast, ERCP, and EUS were performed. The CT scan showed a 4-cm mass at the head of the pancreas, and ERCP revealed evidence of bile duct obstruction; a stent was placed to open the duct. Examination of a tissue biopsy specimen obtained under US guidance confirmed a localized adenocarcinoma of the head of the pancreas.

Additional studies showed no evidence of hepatic or other metastases. Surgical treatment with a Whipple procedure was recommended. This procedure was performed and included pancreatoduodenectomy, choledochojejunostomy, and gastrojejunostomy. Lymph node removal and cholecystectomy were part of the operative procedure. During surgery, it was determined that the tumor was confined to the head of the pancreas. Despite removal of the tumor, the chance of recurrence is high, with a cure rate of only about 20%.

Questions about the Case Report

1. What caused the patient's jaundice?
   a. Excessive hemolysis
   b. Viral hepatitis
   c. Bile duct obstruction
   d. Cholelithiasis

2. What test identified mass as adenocarcinoma?
   a. Whipple procedure
   b. Biopsy with endoscopic ultrasonography
   c. CT scan with contrast
   d. ERCP

3. Which is included in a Whipple procedure?
   a. Removal of the pancreas (malignant area) and duodenum
   b. Removal of the gallbladder
   c. Removal of lymph nodes
   d. All of the above

4. What anastomosis was performed?
   a. Gallbladder and duodenum united.
   b. Common bile duct, pancreatic duct, and small intestine all connected together.
   c. Stomach and pancreas reconnected.
   d. Liver and pancreas connected to the stomach.

IN PERSON: CHOLECYSTECTOMY

This first-person narrative describes the symptoms and treatment of a woman with gallbladder stones.

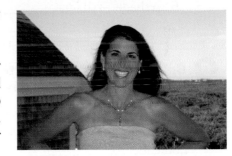

Everyone enjoys a little dessert after dinner, but when the ice cream or a creamy tart leads to pain, most would avoid it. I loved sweets, and despite the revenge they took on my waistline, I still would not pass up an ice cream cone—until my gallbladder decided it had had enough. After several late nights spent doubled over in pain, I tried to steer clear of fatty foods but could not resist the temptation of frozen yogurt.

With one hand, I pushed my cart through the supermarket; with the other hand, I fed myself some delicious low-fat (not nonfat) frozen yogurt. I never dreamed that the attendant at the quick service window actually gave me soft-serve ice cream. Within 10 minutes of eating the questionable yogurt, I broke out into a sweat; a wave of nausea took me, and a knifelike pain stabbed me in my right upper quadrant. It hurt even more when I pressed my hand on the area in an attempt to brace against the pain.

Several months earlier, after a similar painful episode, I had undergone an ultrasound of my gallbladder, and the surgeon then recommended cholecystectomy. The U/S showed multiple stones in my gallbladder. Most of the stones were just the right size to lodge in the common bile duct and cause blockage of the outflow of bile that occurs after a fatty meal. When I heard the ultrasound results, I swore off all fatty foods.

I just did not imagine that ice cream masquerading as "low-fat yogurt" would be the straw that broke the camel's back! Soon enough, I abandoned my shopping cart and apologized to the manager of the store for vomiting all over aisle 4. The unrelenting pain did not cease when I vomited—it only intensified. I have no idea how I made it home and into bed, but my husband found me several hours later in a deep sweat. I managed to call my surgeon and arrange for "semi-emergent" surgery the next morning.

Dr. Fernandez and his team performed a laparoscopic cholecystectomy and relayed to me as I came out of anesthesia that I no longer had a "bag of marbles" for a gallbladder. I had a gassy, distended feeling in my abdomen over the two weeks after surgery (carbon dioxide gas was injected into the abdomen before surgery to allow space between abdominal organs). I felt "tight as a drum" for the first few days, and then day by day it went away. My four tiny incisions healed just fine, and in about 2 weeks I was feeling back to "normal." Now I can eat ice cream to my heart's content, only suffering the padding on my waistline, not the stabbing pain just above. Without missing a beat, my liver now delivers the bile into my small intestine right after I eat a fatty meal. The bile emulsifies (breaks down) the fat. I just don't have a storage bag to hold bile in reserve.

I've had an appendectomy, my wisdom teeth removed, and now I gave up my gallbladder! How many more "useless" body parts are there to go?

Elizabeth Chabner Thompson is the CEO/Founder of BFFL Co, a company devoted to improving the patient experience. She is also a physician, ultramarathoner, and the proud mother of four children, ages 13 to 18.

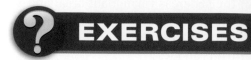 **EXERCISES**

Remember to check your answers carefully with the Answers to Exercises, pages 208 and 209.

A **Give the meanings of the following suffixes.**

1. -pepsia _____

2. -ptysis _____

3. -emesis _____

4. -phagia _____

5. -rrhea _____

6. -rrhage, -rrhagia _____

7. -rrhaphy _____

8. -plasty _____

9. -ectasis, -ectasia _____

10. -stenosis _____

11. -stasis _____

12. -spasm _____

13. -tresia _____

B **Build medical terms for the definitions that follow. Use the listed combining forms as appropriate to create terms.**

chol/e   gastr/o   herni/o
cholangi/o   hemat/o   palat/o
choledoch/o   hem/o   pylor/o

1. stoppage of bile (flow) _____

2. suture of a hernia _____

3. dilation of bile ducts _____

4. spitting up blood (from the respiratory tract) _____

5. vomiting blood (from the digestive tract) _____

6. surgical repair of roof of the mouth _____

7. narrowing of the pyloric sphincter _____

8. bursting forth of blood from the stomach _____

9. sudden, involuntary contraction of muscles at the distal region of the stomach

_____

10. bursting forth of blood _____

11. incision of the common bile duct _____

6

C **Give the meanings of the following terms.**

1. dysphagia _____

2. polyphagia _____

3. dyspepsia _____

4. biliary atresia _____

5. rhinorrhea _____

6. cholestasis _____

7. esophageal atresia _____

8. pyloroplasty _____

9. splenorrhagia _____

10. proctosigmoidoscopy _____

11. hemorrhage _____

12. cholangitis _____

D **Match the listed surgical procedures with the meanings that follow.**

abdominoplasty	colectomy	palatoplasty
cecostomy	gingivectomy	pancreatoduodenectomy
cholecystectomy	herniorrhaphy	paracentesis
cholecystojejunostomy	ileostomy	sphincterotomy

1. removal of the gallbladder _____

2. large bowel resection _____

3. suture of a weakened muscular wall (hernia) _____

4. new opening of the first part of the colon to the outside of the body _____

5. surgical repair of the abdomen _____

6. incision of a ring of muscles _____

7. removal of the pancreas and duodenum _____

8. opening of the third part of the small intestine to the outside of the body

_____

9. removal of gum tissue _____

10. anastomosis between the gallbladder and second part of the small intestine

_____

11. surgical puncture of the abdomen for withdrawal of fluid _____

12. surgical repair of the roof of the mouth _____

E **Use the given meanings to complete the following terms.**

1. discharge of fat: steat _____

2. difficulty in swallowing: dys _____

3. abnormal condition of gallstones: chole _____

4. pertaining to the cheek: _____ al

5. pertaining to lips and teeth: _____ dental

6. vomiting blood: hemat _____

7. enlargement of the liver: hepato _____

8. pertaining to under the tongue: sub _____

9. removal of the gallbladder: _____ ectomy

10. pertaining to the common bile duct: chole _____

11. hemorrhage from the stomach: gastro _____

F **Give the meanings of the following terms.**

1. cecal volvulus _____

2. aphthous stomatitis _____

3. celiac disease _____

4. lipase _____

5. cheilosis _____

6. oropharynx _____

7. glycogen _____

8. glossectomy _____

9. sialadenectomy _____

10. periodontal membrane _____

11. choledochectasia _____

12. cholangiocarcinoma _____

G **Match each listed laboratory test or clinical procedure with its description.**

abdominal ultrasonography	laparoscopy
barium enema	liver biopsy
CT scan of the abdomen	nasogastric intubation
endoscopic retrograde cholangiopancreatography	percutaneous transhepatic cholangiography
endoscopic ultrasonography	serum bilirubin
gastric bypass (bariatric surgery)	small bowel follow-through
gastrostomy (G tube)	stool culture
HIDA scan	stool guaiac (Hemoccult)

1. measurement of bile pigment in the blood _____

2. placement of feces in a growth medium for bacterial analysis _____

3. x-ray examination of the lower gastrointestinal tract _____

4. imaging of abdominal viscera using sound waves _____

5. test to reveal hidden blood in feces _____

6. sequential x-ray images of the small intestine _____

7. injection of contrast material through the skin into the liver, to obtain x-ray images of bile

   vessels _____

8. insertion of a tube through the nose into the stomach _____

9. transverse x-ray pictures of the abdominal organs _____

10. injection of contrast material through an endoscope for x-ray imaging of of the pancreas and

   bile ducts _____

11. reduction of stomach size and gastrojejunostomy _____

12. insertion of an endoscope and use of ultrasound imaging to visualize the organs of the

   gastrointestinal tract _____

13. percutaneous removal of liver tissue followed by microscopic examination

   _____

14. visual examination (endoscopic) of abdominal viscera through small abdominal incisions

   _____

15. new opening of the stomach to the outside of the body for feeding _____

16. radioactive imaging of the liver, gallbladder, and intestine _____

6

H **Give the meanings of the abbreviations in Column I. Then select the letter of the correct description from Column II.**

COLUMN I

1. TPN _____ _____
2. PUD _____ _____
3. EGD _____ _____
4. IBD _____ _____
5. BE _____ _____
6. BRBPR _____ _____
7. LFTs _____ _____
8. GERD _____ _____
9. HBV _____ _____
10. CT _____ _____

COLUMN II

A. Tests such as measurement of ALT, AST, alk phos, and serum bilirubin.
B. Heartburn is a symptom of this condition.
C. Includes Crohn disease and ulcerative colitis.
D. *H. pylori* causes this condition.
E. Intravenous injection of nutrition.
F. This is a lower gastrointestinal series.
G. X-ray procedure that produces a series of cross-sectional images.
H. This infectious agent causes chronic inflammation of the liver.
I. Hematochezia describes this gastrointestinal symptom.
J. Endoscopic visualization of the upper gastrointestinal tract.

I **Give the suffixes for the following terms.**

1. bursting forth (of blood) _____
2. flow, discharge _____
3. suture _____
4. dilation _____
5. narrowing (stricture) _____
6. vomiting _____
7. spitting _____
8. excision _____
9. digestion _____
10. eating, swallowing _____
11. hardening _____
12. stopping, controlling _____
13. surgical repair _____
14. opening _____
15. surgical puncture _____
16. involuntary contraction _____
17. new opening _____
18. incision _____

6

J **Circle the correct bold term in parentheses to complete each sentence.**

1. When Mrs. Smith began to have diarrhea and crampy abdominal pain, she consulted a **(urologist, nephrologist, gastroenterologist)** and worried that the cause of her symptoms might be **(inflammatory bowel disease, esophageal varices, achalasia).**

2. After taking a careful history and performing a thorough physical examination, Dr. Blakemore diagnosed Mr. Bean, a long-time drinker, with **(hemorrhoids, pancreatitis, appendicitis).** Mr. Bean had complained of sharp midepigastric pain and a change in bowel habits.

3. Many pregnant women cannot lie flat after eating without experiencing a burning sensation in their chest and throat. The usual cause of this symptom is **(volvulus, dysentery, gastroesophageal reflux).**

4. Mr. and Mrs. Cho brought their young infant son to the clinic after he had several bouts of projectile vomiting. The pediatric surgeon suspected a diagnosis of **(inguinal hernia, pyloric stenosis, ascites).**

5. Boris had terrible problems with his teeth. He needed not only a periodontist for his **(aphthous stomatitis, oral leukoplakia, gingivitis)** but also an **(endodontist, oral surgeon, orthodontist)** to straighten his teeth.

6. After 6 weeks of radiation therapy to her throat, Betty experienced severe esophageal irritation and inflammation. She complained to her doctor about her resulting **(dyspepsia, dysphagia, hematemesis).**

7. Steven, age 7 years, is brought to the clinic because of recurrent abdominal pain, occasional constipation and diarrhea, and weight loss. His pediatrician's diagnosis is **(lipase deficiency, dysentery, celiac disease)** and recommends a **(fat, gluten, sugar)**-free diet.

8. Chris had been a heavy alcohol drinker all of his adult life. His wife noticed worsening yellow discoloration of the whites of his eyes and skin. After a physical examination and blood tests, his family physician told him his **(colon, skin, liver)** was diseased. The yellow discoloration was **(jaundice, melena, flatus),** and his condition was **(cheilosis, cirrhosis, steatorrhea).**

9. When Carol was working as a phlebotomist, she accidentally cut her finger while drawing a patient's blood. Unfortunately the patient had **(pancreatitis, hemoptysis, hepatitis),** and HBV was transmitted to Carol. Blood tests and **(liver biopsy, gastrointestinal endoscopy, stool culture)** confirmed Carol's unfortunate diagnosis. Her doctor told her that her condition was chronic and that she might be a candidate for a **(bone marrow, liver, kidney)** transplant procedure in the future.

10. Operation Smile is a rescue project that performs surgical repair including **(herniorrhaphy, oral gingivectomy, palatoplasty)** on children with a congenital cleft in the roof of the mouth.

6

ANSWERS TO EXERCISES

A

1. digestion
2. spitting (from the respiratory tract)
3. vomiting
4. eating, swallowing
5. flow, discharge
6. bursting forth of blood
7. suture
8. surgical repair
9. dilation (dilatation), widening
10. narrowing, tightening
11. to stop; control
12. sudden, involuntary contraction of muscles
13. opening

B

1. cholestasis
2. herniorrhaphy
3. cholangiectasia
4. hemoptysis
5. hematemesis
6. palatoplasty
7. pyloric stenosis
8. gastrorrhagia
9. pylorospasm
10. hemorrhage
11. choledochotomy

C

1. difficulty in swallowing
2. excessive (much) eating
3. difficult digestion
4. biliary ducts are not open (congenital anomaly)
5. discharge of mucus from the nose
6. stoppage of flow of bile
7. esophagus is not open (closed off) at birth (congenital anomaly)
8. surgical repair of the pyloric sphincter
9. bursting forth of blood (hemorrhage) from the spleen
10. visual (endoscopic) examination of the rectum and sigmoid colon
11. bursting forth of blood
12. inflammation of bile duct (vessel)

D

1. cholecystectomy
2. colectomy
3. herniorrhaphy
4. cecostomy
5. abdominoplasty
6. sphincterotomy
7. pancreatoduodenectomy
8. ileostomy
9. gingivectomy
10. cholecystojejunostomy
11. paracentesis (abdominocentesis)
12. palatoplasty

E

1. steatorrhea
2. dysphagia
3. cholelithiasis
4. buccal
5. labiodental
6. hematemesis
7. hepatomegaly
8. sublingual
9. cholecystectomy
10. choledochal
11. gastrorrhagia

F

1. twisted intestine in the area of the cecum
2. inflammation of the mouth with small ulcers
3. autoimmune disorder in which villi in the lining of the small intestine are damaged, resulting from reaction to dietary glutens such as wheat, barley, and rye
4. enzyme to digest fat
5. abnormal condition of lips
6. the part of the throat near the mouth
7. storage form of sugar
8. removal of part or all of the tongue
9. removal of a salivary gland
10. membrane surrounding a tooth
11. dilation of the common bile duct
12. malignant tumor of bile vessels

G

1. serum bilirubin
2. stool culture
3. barium enema
4. abdominal ultrasonography
5. stool guaiac (Hemoccult)
6. small bowel follow-through
7. percutaneous transhepatic cholangiography (PTHC)
8. nasogastric intubation
9. CT scan of the abdomen
10. endoscopic retrograde cholangiopancreatography (ERCP)
11. gastric bypass (bariatric surgery)
12. endoscopic ultrasonography (EUS)
13. liver biopsy
14. laparoscopy (form of minimally invasive surgery)
15. gastrostomy (G tube)
16. HIDA scan

6

H

1. total parenteral nutrition: E
2. peptic ulcer disease: D
3. esophagoduodenoscopy: J
4. inflammatory bowel disease: C
5. barium enema: F
6. bright red blood per rectum: I
7. liver function tests: A
8. gastroesophageal reflux disease: B
9. hepatitis B virus: H
10. computed tomography: G

I

1. -rrhagia, -rrhage
2. -rrhea
3. -rrhaphy
4. -ectasis, -ectasia
5. -stenosis
6. -emesis
7. -ptysis
8. -ectomy
9. -pepsia
10. -phagia
11. -sclerosis
12. -stasis
13. -plasty
14. -tresia
15. -centesis
16. -spasm
17. -stomy
18. -tomy

J

1. gastroenterologist; inflammatory bowel disease
2. pancreatitis
3. gastroesophageal reflux
4. pyloric stenosis
5. gingivitis; orthodontist
6. dysphagia
7. celiac disease; gluten
8. liver; jaundice; cirrhosis
9. hepatitis; liver biopsy; liver
10. palatoplasty

Answers to Practical Applications

Case Report: Pancreatic Cancer and Whipple Procedure

1. c
2. b
3. d
4. b

6

PRONUNCIATION OF TERMS

To test your understanding of the terminology in this chapter, write the meaning of each term in the space provided. In addition, you may wish to cover the terms and write them by looking at your definitions. Make sure your spelling is correct. The page number after each term indicates where it is defined in the text, so you can easily check your responses. You will find complete definitions for all of these terms and their audio pronunciations on the Evolve website.

Pronunciation Guide

ā as in āpe	ă as in ăpple
ē as in ēven	ĕ as in ĕvery
ī as in īce	ĭ as in ĭnterest
ō as in ōpen	ŏ as in pŏt
ū as in ūnit	ŭ as in ŭnder

TERM	PRONUNCIATION	MEANING
abdominal ultrasonography (196)	ăb-DŎM-ĭn-ăl ŭl-tră-sō-NŎG-ră-fē	
abdominoplasty (188)	ăb-DŎM-ĭn-ō-plăs-tē	
amylase and lipase tests (193)	ă-mĭ-LĀS and LĪ-păs tests	
aphthous stomatitis (192)	ĂF-thŭs stō-mă-TĪ-tĭs	
atresia (190)	ā-TRĒ-zē-ă	
bariatric surgery (197)	bă-rē-Ă-trĭk SŬR-gĕr-ē	
biliary atresia (190)	BĬL-ē-ăr-ē ā-TRĒ-zē-ă	
bronchospasm (189)	BRŎN-kō-spăsm	
buccal (191)	BŬK-ăl	
cecal volvulus (191)	SĒ-kăl VŎL-vū-lŭs	
celiac disease (191)	SĒ-lē-ăk dĭ-ZĒZ	
cheilosis (191)	kī-LŌ-sĭs	
cholangiectasis (188)	kō-lăn-jē-ĔK-tă-sĭs	
cholangiocarcinoma (191)	kō-lăn-jē-ō-kăr-sĭ-NŌ-mă	
cholangitis (191)	kōl-ăn-JĪ-tĭs	
cholangiography (194)	kōl-ăn-jē-ŎG-ră-fē	
cholangiopancreatography (194)	kōl-ăn-jē-ō-păn-krē-ă-TŎG-ră-fē	
cholecystectomy (191)	kō-lē-sĭs-TĔK-tō-mē	
cholecystojejunostomy (192)	kō-lē-sĭs-tō-jĕ-jŭ-NŎS-tō-mē	
cholecystolithiasis (192)	kō-lē-sĭs-tō-lĭ-THĪ-ă-sĭs	
choledochal (191)	kō-lē-DŌK-ăl	

TERM	PRONUNCIATION	MEANING
choledochectasia (191)	kō-lē-dō-kĕk-TĀ-zē-ă	
cholelithiasis (191)	kō-lē-lĭ-THĪ-ă-sĭs	
cholestasis (189)	kō-lē-STĀ-sĭs	
colectomy (191)	kō-LĔK-tō-mē	
colonoscopy (191)	kō-lŏn-ŎS-kō-pē	
computed tomography (195)	kŏm-PŪ-tĕd tō-MŎG-ră-FĒ	
dentalgia (191)	dĕn-TĂL-jă	
diarrhea (189)	dī-ă-RĒ-ă	
duodenal (191)	doo-ō-DĒ-năl	
dyspepsia (188)	dĭs-PĔP-sē-ă	
dysphagia (188)	dĭs-FĀ-jē-ă	
endoscopic ultrasonography (196)	ĕn-dō-SKŎP-ĭk ŭl-tră-sō-NŎG-ră-fē	
esophageal atresia (190)	ĕ-sŏf-ă-JĒ-ăl ā-TRĒ-zē-ă	
gastric bypass (197)	GĂS-trĭk BĪ-păs	
gastroenteritis (191)	găs-trō-ĕn-tĕ-RĪ-tĭs	
gastrointestinal endoscopy (197)	găs-trō-ĭn-TĔS-tĭn-ăl ĕn-DŎS-kō-pē	
gastrojejunostomy (191)	găs-trō-jĕ-joo-NŎS-tō-mē	
gastrorrhagia (189)	găs-trō-RĂ-jă	
gastrostomy (191)	găs-TRŎS-tō-mē	
gingivectomy (192)	gĭn-gĭ-VĔK-tō-mē	
glossectomy (192)	glŏs-ĔK-tō-mē	
gluconeogenesis (192)	glū-kō-nē-ō-JĔN-ĕ-sĭs	
glycogen (192)	GLĪ-kō-jĕn	
hematemesis (188)	hē-mă-TĔM-ĕ-sĭs	
hemoptysis (189)	hē-MŎP-tĭ-sĭs	
hemorrhage (189)	HĔM-ŏr-ĭj	
hepatomegaly (192)	hĕp-ă-tō-MĔG-ă-lē	
herniorrhaphy (189)	hĕr-nē-ŎR-ă-fē	
HIDA scan (197)	HĪ-dă scăn	

6

TERM	PRONUNCIATION	MEANING
ileostomy (192)	ĭl-ē-ŎS-tō-mē	
labiodental (192)	lā-bē-ō-DĔN-tăl	
laparoscopy (197)	lă-păr-ŎS-kō-pē	
lipase (192)	LĪ-pās	
liver biopsy (197)	LĬ-vĕr BĪ-ŏp-sē	
liver function tests (193)	LĬ-vĕr FŬNG-shŭn tests	
lower gastrointestinal series (194)	LŌW-ĕr găs-trō-ĭn-TĔS-tĭ-năl SĔR-ēz	
magnetic resonance imaging (196)	măg-NĔT-ĭk RĔ-zō-năns ĬM-ă-gĭng	
nasogastric intubation (197)	nā-zō-GĂS-trĭk ĭn-too-BĀ-shŭn	
oropharynx (192)	ŏr-ō-FĂR-ĭnks	
palatoplasty (192)	PĂL-ă-tō-plăs-tē	
pancreatic (192)	păn-krē-ĂH-tĭk	
pancreatoduodenectomy (192)	păn-krē-ăh-tō-doo-ō-dĕ-NĔK-tō-mē	
paracentesis (197)	păr-ă-sĕn-TĒ-sĭs	
periodontal membrane (192)	pĕr-ē-ō-DŎN-tăl MĔM-brān	
polyphagia (188)	pŏl-ē-FĀ-jē-ă	
proctosigmoidoscopy (192)	prŏk-tō-sĭg-moyd-ŎS-kō-pē	
pyloric stenosis (189)	pī-LŎR-ĭk stĕ-NŌ-sĭs	
pylorospasm (189)	pī-LŎR-ō-spăzm	
rectal carcinoma (192)	RĔK-tăl kăr-sĭ-NŌ-mă	
sialadenectomy (192)	sī-ăl-ă-dĕ-NĔK-tō-mē	
splenic flexure (192)	SPLĔN-ĭk FLĔK-shŭr	
steatorrhea (192)	stē-ă-tō-RĒ-ă	
stool culture (193)	stool KŬL-chŭr	
stool guaiac (193)	stool GWĪ-ăk	
sublingual (192)	sŭb-LĬNG-wăl	
upper gastrointestinal series (194)	ŬP-ĕr găs-trō-ĭn-TĔS-tĭ-năl SĔR-ēz	

6

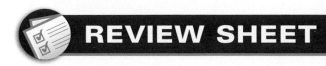 **REVIEW SHEET**

Write meanings for combining forms and suffixes in the spaces provided. Check your answers with information in Chapter 5 and this chapter or in the *Glossary (Medical Word Parts—English)* at the end of this book.

Combining Forms

COMBINING FORM	MEANING	COMBINING FORM	MEANING
abdomin/o		gastr/o	
amyl/o		gingiv/o	
an/o		gloss/o	
append/o, appendic/o		gluc/o, glyc/o	
bil/i		glycogen/o	
bilirubin/o		hem/o, hemat/o	
bucc/o		hepat/o	
cec/o		herni/o	
celi/o		idi/o	
cervic/o		ile/o	
cheil/o		pancreat/o	
chlorhydr/o		peritone/o	
chol/e		pharyng/o	
cholangi/o		proct/o	
cholecyst/o		prote/o	
choledoch/o		py/o	
cib/o		pylor/o	
cirrh/o		rect/o	
col/o, colon/o		sialaden/o	
dent/i		splen/o	
duoden/o		steat/o	
enter/o		stomat/o	
esophag/o		tonsill/o	
eti/o			

6

Suffixes

SUFFIX	MEANING	SUFFIX	MEANING
-ase	_____	-orexia	_____
-centesis	_____	-rrhage	_____
-chezia	_____	-rrhagia	_____
-ectasia	_____	-rrhaphy	_____
-ectasis	_____	-rrhea	_____
-ectomy	_____	-scopy	_____
-emesis	_____	-spasm	_____
-emia	_____	-stasis	_____
-genesis	_____	-stenosis	_____
-graphy	_____	-stomy	_____
-iasis	_____	-tomy	_____
-megaly	_____	-tresia	_____

6

evolve *Please visit the Evolve website for additional exercises, games, and images related to this chapter.*

Urinary System

Chapter Sections

CHAPTER GOALS

- Name essential organs of the urinary system and describe their locations and functions.
- Identify common pathologic conditions affecting the urinary system.
- Recognize how urinalysis is used and interpreted as a diagnostic test.
- Define urinary system–related combining forms, prefixes, and suffixes.
- List and explain laboratory tests, clinical procedures, and abbreviations that pertain to the urinary system.
- Understand medical terms in their proper contexts, such as medical reports and records.

INTRODUCTION

When foods containing proteins are used by cells in the body, nitrogenous waste products **(urea, creatinine,** and **uric acid)** are released into the bloodstream. The urinary system removes these nitrogenous wastes from the blood so that they do not accumulate and become harmful. As blood passes through the kidneys, the kidneys filter nitrogenous wastes to form **urine** (composed of water, salts, and acids). Urine leaves the body through the ureters, urinary bladder, and urethra. Every day, the kidneys process about 200 quarts of blood to filter out 2 quarts of urine.

Besides removing urea and other nitrogenous wastes from the blood, the kidneys maintain the proper balance of water, electrolytes, and acids in body fluids. **Electrolytes** such as **sodium (Na⁺)** and **potassium (K⁺)** are small molecules that conduct an electrical charge. Electrolytes are necessary for proper functioning of muscle and nerve cells. The kidney adjusts the amounts of water and electrolytes by secreting some substances into the urine and holding back others in the bloodstream for use in the body. This is an example of **homeostasis,** which is the body's ability to maintain an equilibrium within its internal environment. Home/o means sameness.

In addition to forming and excreting (eliminating) urine from the body, the kidneys secrete hormones such as **renin** (RĒ-nĭn) and **erythropoietin** (ĕ-rĭth-rō-POY-ĕ-tĭn). **Renin** raises blood pressure (to keep blood moving through the kidney). **Erythropoietin (EPO)** is a hormone that stimulates red blood cell production in the bone marrow.

The kidneys also secrete **calciferol,** an active form of vitamin D, necessary for the absorption of calcium from the intestine. In addition, the kidneys degrade and eliminate hormones such as insulin and parathyroid hormone from the bloodstream. Box 7-1 reviews the functions of the kidneys.

ANATOMY OF THE MAJOR ORGANS

The following paragraphs describe the organs of the urinary system. Label Figure 7-1 as you identify each organ.

The **kidney** [1] is one of two bean-shaped organs behind the abdominal cavity (retroperitoneal) on either side of the spine in the lumbar region. A cushion of adipose (fatty) tissue and fibrous connective tissue surrounds each kidney for protection. Each kidney (about the size of a fist) weighs about 4 to 6 ounces.

The kidneys consist of an outer **cortex** region (cortex means bark, as the bark of a tree) and an inner **medulla** region (medulla means marrow). The **hilum** is a depression on the medial border of the kidney. Blood vessels and nerves pass through the hilum.

The **ureter** [2] is one of two muscular tubes (16 to 18 inches long) lined with mucous membrane. Ureters carry urine in peristaltic waves from the kidneys to the urinary bladder.

The **urinary bladder** [3], a hollow, muscular sac, is a temporary reservoir for urine. The **trigone** is a triangular region at the base of the bladder where the ureters enter and the urethra exits.

Box 7-1 **FUNCTIONS OF THE KIDNEYS**
• **Remove nitrogenous wastes**: urea, creatinine, uric acid
• **Balance water and electrolytes** (sodium, potassium)
• **Release hormones**: renin, erythropoietin, calciferol
• **Degrade and eliminate hormones** from bloodstream

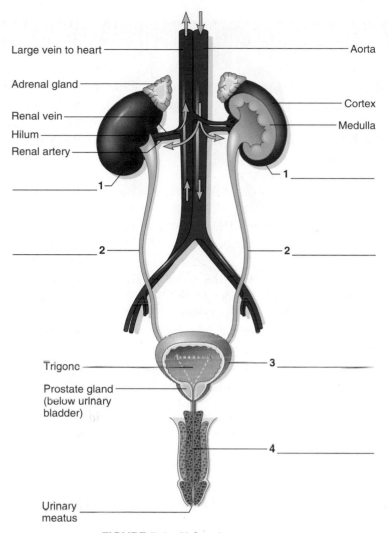

Large vein to heart

Adrenal gland

Renal vein

Hilum

Renal artery

Aorta

Cortex

Medulla

1 _____

1 _____

2 _____

2 _____

Trigone

Prostate gland
(below urinary
bladder)

3 _____

4 _____

Urinary
meatus

FIGURE 7-1 **Male urinary system.**

The **urethra** [4] is a tube that carries urine from the urinary bladder to the outside of the body. The process of expelling urine through the urethra is called **urination** or **voiding.** The external opening of the urethra is the **urinary meatus.** The female urethra, about $1\frac{1}{2}$ inches long, lies anterior to the vagina and vaginal meatus. The male urethra, about 8 inches long, extends downward through the prostate gland to the urinary meatus at the tip of the penis. Figure 7-2 illustrates the female urinary system. Compare it with Figure 7-1, which shows the male urinary system.

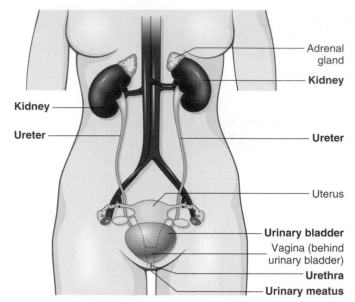

FIGURE 7-2 **Female urinary system.**

PHYSIOLOGY: HOW THE KIDNEYS PRODUCE URINE

Blood enters each kidney from the aorta by way of the right and left **renal arteries.** After the renal artery enters the kidney (at the hilum), it branches into smaller and smaller arteries. The smallest arteries are called **arterioles** (Figure 7-3A).

Because the arterioles are small, blood passes through them slowly but constantly. Blood flow through the kidney is so essential that the kidneys have their own special device for maintaining blood flow. If blood pressure falls in the vessels of the kidney, so that blood flow diminishes, the kidney produces **renin** and discharges it into the blood. Renin promotes the formation of a substance that stimulates the contraction of arterioles. This increases blood pressure and restores blood flow in the kidneys to normal.

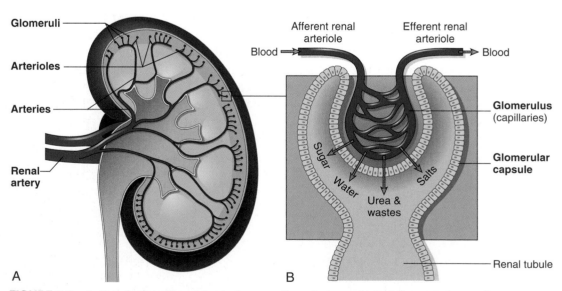

FIGURE 7-3 **A, Renal artery** branching to form smaller arteries and arterioles, and glomeruli. **B, Glomerulus** and **glomerular capsule.** Afferent arteriole carries blood toward (in this term, af- is a form of ad-) the glomerulus. Efferent arteriole carries blood away (ef- is a form of ex-) from the glomerulus.

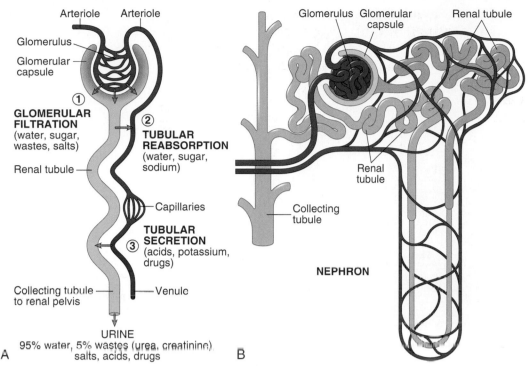

FIGURE 7-4 **A, Three steps in the formation of urine: (1) Glomerular filtration** of water, sugar, wastes (urea and creatinine), and sodium; **(2) Tubular reabsorption** of water, sugar, and sodium; and **(3) Tubular secretion** of acids, potassium, and drugs. **B,** A **nephron** is the combination of a glomerulus and a renal tubule.

Each arteriole in the cortex of the kidney leads into a mass of very tiny, coiled, and intertwined smaller blood vessels called **glomeruli** (see Figure 7-3A). Each **glomerulus** (singular) is a collection of tiny capillaries formed in the shape of a small ball. There are about 1 million glomeruli in the cortex region of each kidney.

The kidneys produce urine by **filtration.** As blood passes through the many glomeruli, the thin walls of each glomerulus (the filter) permit water, salts, sugar, and **urea** (with other nitrogenous wastes such as **creatinine** and **uric acid**) to leave the bloodstream. These materials collect in a tiny, cup-like structure, a **glomerular (Bowman) capsule,** that surrounds each glomerulus (Figure 7-3B). The walls of the glomeruli prevent large substances, such as proteins and blood cells, from filtering into the urine. These substances remain in the blood and normally do not appear in urine.

Attached to each glomerular capsule is a long, twisted tube called a **renal tubule** (Figure 7-3B; see also Figure 7-4). As water, sugar, salts, urea, and other wastes pass through the renal tubule, most of the water, all of the sugar, and almost all of the sodium return to the bloodstream through tiny capillaries surrounding each tubule. This active process of **reabsorption** ensures that the body retains essential substances such as sugar (glucose), water, and sodium while allowing waste products to be excreted in the urine. The final process in the formation of urine is **secretion** of some substances such as postassium, acids and drugs from the bloodstream into the renal tubule. Each renal tubule, now containing urine (95% water and 5% urea, creatinine, salts and acids) connects to a larger collecting tubule.

See Figure 7-4A, which reviews the steps involved in urine formation. Note that waste products may accumulate in the body as a result of kidney failure and may interfere with the function of vital organs, including the brain and heart. The combination of a glomerulus and a renal tubule forms a unit called a **nephron** (Figure 7-4B). Each kidney contains about 1 million nephrons.

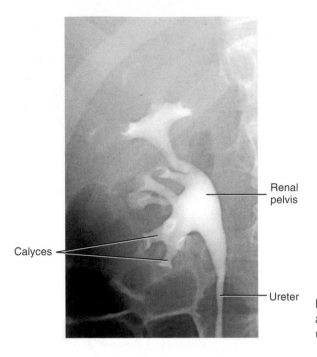

FIGURE 7-5   **Renal pelvis, calyces, and ureter** as seen on CT urogram (intravenous dye was used).

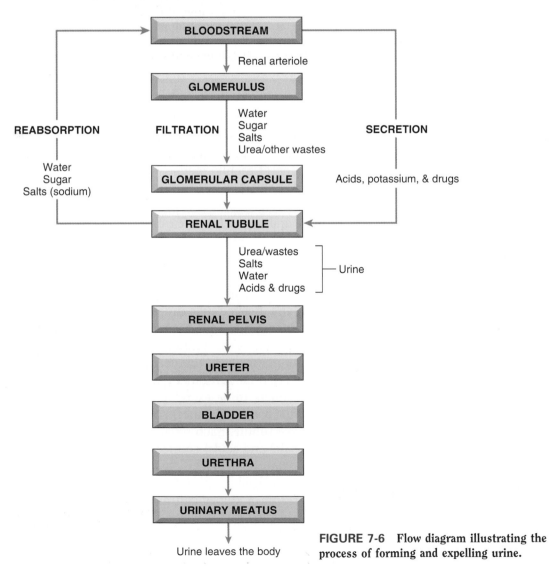

FIGURE 7-6   **Flow diagram illustrating the process of forming and expelling urine.**

All collecting tubules lead to the **renal pelvis,** a basin-like area in the central part of the kidney. Small, cup-like regions of the renal pelvis are called **calyces** or **calices** (singular: **calyx** or **calix**). Figure 7-5 is an x-ray image of a kidney showing the renal pelvis, calyces, and ureter.

The renal pelvis narrows into the **ureter,** which carries the urine to the **urinary bladder.** The bladder, a muscular sac, temporarily stores urine. Sphincter muscles control the exit area of the bladder to the **urethra.** As the bladder fills and pressure increases at its base, an individual notices a need to urinate and voluntarily relaxes sphincter muscles.

Study the diagram in Figure 7-6 tracing the process of urine formation and excretion.

VOCABULARY

arteriole	Small artery.
calciferol	Active form of vitamin D, secreted by the kidney.
calyx *or* **calix** (*plural:* **calyces** or **calices**)	Cup-like collecting region of the renal pelvis. The term comes from Greek, *kalux* meaning a cup or case surrounding a flower bud.
catheter	Tube for injecting or removing fluids.
cortex	Outer region of an organ; the renal cortex is the outer region of the kidney (**cortical** means pertaining to the cortex).
creatinine	Nitrogenous waste excreted in urine. **Creatinine clearance** is a measure of the efficiency of the kidneys in removing (clearing) creatinine from the blood. Creatinine is a product of muscle metabolism.
electrolyte	Chemical element that carries an electrical charge when dissolved in water. Electrolytes are necessary for functioning of muscles and nerves. The kidneys maintain the proper balance of electrolytes and water in the blood. Potassium (K^+) and sodium (Na^+) are electrolytes.
erythropoietin (EPO)	Hormone secreted by the kidney to stimulate the production of red blood cells by bone marrow. -Poietin means a substance that forms. EPO (Ē-pō) stimulates red blood cell production, and thus increases the amount of oxygen delivered to muscles. This enhances athletic endurance. However, use of EPO is a form of blood doping and is prohibited by the World Anti-Doping Authority (WADA).
filtration	Process whereby some substances, but not all, pass through a filter.
glomerular capsule	Enclosing structure surrounding each glomerulus. The glomerular capsule is also known as Bowman's capsule and it collects the material that is filtered from the blood through the walls of the glomerulus.
glomerulus (*plural:* **glomeruli)**	Tiny ball of capillaries (microscopic blood vessels) in the kidney.

Filtration of Blood Through the Kidney.

This process is maintained by output from the heart (25% of cardiac output goes to the kidneys) and adequate blood pressure to force blood through the glomerulus (filter). About 200 quarts (189 L) of fluid are filtered daily, but 98% to 99% of water and salts are returned to the blood. Only about 2 quarts (1500 mL) of urine are excreted daily

hilum	Depression in an organ where blood vessels and nerves enter and leave. Hilum comes from the Latin meaning a small thing. It is also used in the respiratory system to mark the depression in the lung where blood vessels, bronchus, and lymphatic vessels enter and leave.
kidney	One of two bean-shaped organs on either side of the backbone in the lumbar region; it filters nitrogenous wastes from the bloodstream to form urine.
meatus	Opening or canal.
medulla	Inner region of an organ. The renal medulla is the inner region of the kidney. The term comes from the Latin *medulla*, meaning marrow (inner part). The medullary cavity in long bones is the innermost part containing red and yellow marrow.
nephron	Combination of glomerulus and renal tubule where filtration, reabsorption, and secretion take place in the kidney. It is the functional unit of the kidney, each capable of forming urine by itself. There are about 1 million nephrons in a kidney.
nitrogenous waste	Substance containing nitrogen and excreted in urine. Examples of nitrogenous wastes are urea, uric acid, and creatinine.
potassium (K^+)	Electrolyte regulated by the kidney so that a proper concentration is maintained within the blood. Potassium is essential for allowing muscle contraction and conduction of nervous impulses.
reabsorption	Process whereby renal tubules return materials necessary to the body back into the bloodstream.
renal artery	Blood vessel that carries blood to the kidney.
renal pelvis	Central collecting region in the kidney.
renal tubule	Microscopic tube in the kidney where urine is formed after filtration.
renal vein	Blood vessel that carries blood away from the kidney and toward the heart.
renin	Hormone secreted by the kidney; it raises blood pressure by influencing vasoconstriction (narrowing of blood vessels).
sodium (Na^+)	Electrolyte regulated in the blood and urine by the kidneys; needed for proper transmission of nerve impulses, heart activity, and other metabolic functions. A common form of sodium is sodium chloride (table salt).
trigone	Triangular area in the urinary bladder.
urea	Major nitrogenous waste excreted in urine.
ureter	One of the two tubes leading from the kidneys to the urinary bladder.
urethra	Tube leading from the urinary bladder to the outside of the body.
uric acid	Nitrogenous waste excreted in the urine.
urinary bladder	Hollow, muscular sac that holds and stores urine.
urination (voiding)	Process of expelling urine; also called micturition.

7

TERMINOLOGY: STRUCTURES, SUBSTANCES, AND URINARY SIGNS AND SYMPTOMS

Write the meanings of the medical terms in the spaces provided.

STRUCTURES

COMBINING FORM	MEANING	TERMINOLOGY	MEANING
cali/o, calic/o	calyx (calix); cup-shaped	caliectasis _____	
		caliceal _____	
cyst/o	urinary bladder	cystitis _____	
		Bacterial infections often cause acute or chronic cystitis. In acute cystitis, the bladder contains blood as a result of mucosal hemorrhage (Figure 7-7).	
		cystectomy _____	
		cystostomy _____	
		An opening is made into the urinary bladder from the outside of the body. A catheter is placed into the bladder for drainage.	
glomerul/o	glomerulus	glomerular capsule _____	
meat/o	meatus	meatal stenosis _____	

7

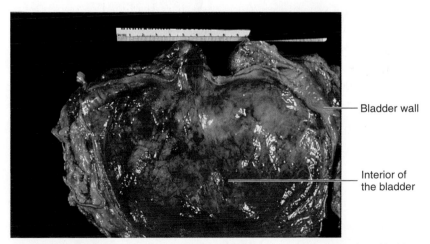

Bladder wall

Interior of the bladder

FIGURE 7-7   Acute cystitis. Notice that the mucosa of the bladder is red and swollen. Bladder and urinary tract infections are more common in women because of the shorter urethra, which allows easier bacterial colonization of the urinary bladder. They usually occur without a known cause but may be acquired during sexual intercourse ("honeymoon cystitis") or after surgical procedures and urinary catheterization.

COMBINING FORM	MEANING	TERMINOLOGY	MEANING
nephr/o	kidney	paranephric _____	
		nephropathy _____ *(ně-FRŎ-pă-thē)*	
		nephroptosis _____ *Downward displacement or dropping of a kidney when its anatomic supports are weakened.* **Nephropexy** *(-pexy means fixation) is an operation to put a "floating" kidney in place.*	
		nephrolithotomy _____ *Incision (percutaneous) into the kidney to remove a stone.*	
		hydronephrosis _____ *Obstruction of urine flow may be caused by renal calculi (Figure 7-8), compression of the ureter by tumor, or hyperplasia of the prostate gland at the base of the bladder in males.*	
		nephrostomy _____ *Surgical opening to the outside of the body (from the renal pelvis). This is necessary when a ureter becomes obstructed and the obstruction cannot be removed easily. The renal pelvis becomes distended with urine (hydronephrosis), making nephrostomy necessary.*	

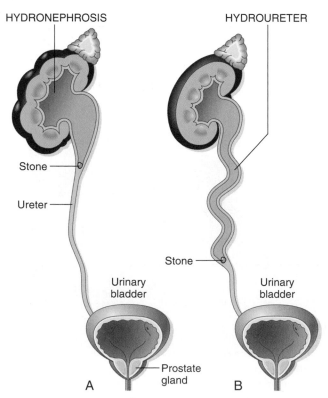

FIGURE 7-8 **A, Hydronephrosis** caused by a stone (obstruction) in the proximal part of a ureter. Notice the buildup of excess fluid in the kidney. **B, Hydroureter** with hydronephrosis caused by a stone in the distal part of the ureter.

COMBINING FORM	MEANING	TERMINOLOGY	MEANING
pyel/o	renal pelvis	pyelolithotomy _____ *Removal of a large calculus (stone) contributing to blockage of urine flow and development of infection. The renal pelvis is surgically opened.*	
ren/o	kidney	renal ischemia _____	
		renal colic _____ *Colic is intermittent spasms of pain caused by inflammation and distention of an organ. In renal colic, pain results from calculi in the kidney or ureter.*	
trigon/o	trigone (region of the bladder)	trigonitis _____	
ureter/o	ureter	ureteroplasty _____	
		ureteroileostomy _____ *After cystectomy, the urologic surgeon forms a pouch from a segment of the ileum, used in place of the bladder to carry urine from ureters out of the body (Figure 7-9). It is an **ileal conduit**.*	
urethr/o	urethra	urethritis _____	
		urethroplasty _____	
		urethral stricture _____ *A **stricture** is an abnormal narrowing of an opening or passageway.*	
vesic/o	urinary bladder	intravesical _____ *Do not confuse the term **vesical** with the term **vesicle**, which is a small blister on the skin.*	
		vesicoureteral reflux _____	

7

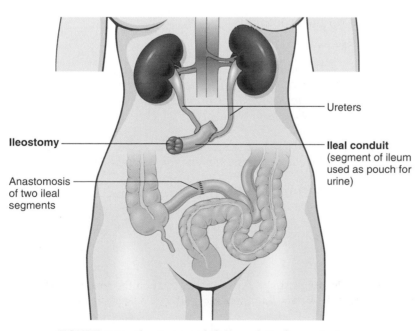

Ureters

Ileostomy

Ileal conduit
(segment of ileum used as pouch for urine)

Anastomosis of two ileal segments

FIGURE 7-9 Ileostomy and ileal conduit after cystectomy.

SUBSTANCES AND URINARY SIGNS AND SYMPTOMS

COMBINING FORM OR SUFFIX	MEANING	TERMINOLOGY	MEANING
albumin/o	albumin (a protein in the blood)	albuminuria	The suffix -uria means urine condition. This finding can indicate malfunction of the kidney as protein leaks out of damaged glomeruli. **Microalbuminuria** is leakage of very small amounts of albumin through the glomeruli.
azot/o	nitrogen	azotemia	This toxic condition is characteristic of uremia. It is indicated by an elevated **BUN (blood urea nitrogen)** test.
bacteri/o	bacteria	bacteriuria	Usually a sign of **urinary tract infection (UTI)**. The bacteria in the urine are cultured (grown in a special nutrient environment) and then tested with antibiotics to determine which will inhibit growth. This is known as **culture and sensitivity testing (C&S)**.
dips/o	thirst	polydipsia	Commonly, a sign of diabetes mellitus or diabetes insipidus. Polydipsia occurs when excessive urination (polyuria) signals the brain to cause thirst.
kal/o	potassium	hyperkalemia	Because potassium normally is excreted by the kidneys, it accumulates in blood when the kidneys fail.
ket/o, keton/o	ketone bodies (ketoacids and acetone)	ketosis	Often called **ketoacidosis,** because acids accumulate in the blood and tissues. The breath of a patient with ketosis has a sweet or "fruity" odor. This is produced by **acetone** (a ketone body) released from the blood in the lungs and exhaled through the mouth.
		ketonuria	
lith/o	stone	nephrolithiasis	
natr/o	sodium	hyponatremia	This condition can occur when water intake is excessive—primary polydipsia, or when athletes drink too much water in high-endurance events.
noct/o	night	nocturia	Frequent, excessive urination at night.
olig/o	scanty	oliguria	

7

COMBINING FORM OR SUFFIX	MEANING	TERMINOLOGY	MEANING
-poietin	substance that forms	erythropoietin _____	
py/o	pus	pyuria _____	
-tripsy	crushing	lithotripsy _____	
ur/o	urine (urea)	uremia _____	
		This toxic state results when nitrogenous waste accumulates abnormally in the blood.	
		enuresis ◣ _____	
		Literally, a condition (-esis) of being "in urine"; bed-wetting.	
		diuresis _____	
		Di- (from dia-) means complete. Caffeine and alcohol are well-known **diuretics**—*they induce increased excretion of urine (diuresis).*	
		antidiuretic hormone _____	
		This hormone from the pituitary gland normally acts on the renal tubules to promote water reabsorption. It is also called **vasopressin** *and is abbreviated* **ADH.**	
urin/o	urine	urinary incontinence _____	
		Incontinence literally means not (in-) able to hold (tin) together (con-). This is loss of control of the passage of urine from the bladder. **Stress incontinence** *occurs with strain on the bladder opening during coughing or sneezing.* **Urgency incontinence** *occurs with the inability to hold back urination when feeling the urge to void.*	
		urinary retention _____	
		This symptom results when the outflow of urine from the bladder is blocked.	
-uria	urination; urine condition	dysuria _____	
		anuria _____	
		Commonly caused by renal failure or urinary tract obstruction.	
		hematuria _____	
		Microhematuria *is hematuria that is visible only under a microscope, as opposed to* **gross hematuria,** *which can be seen with the naked eye.*	
		glycosuria _____	
		A sign of diabetes mellitus.	
		polyuria _____	
		A symptom of both diabetes insipidus and diabetes mellitus.	

7

Enuresis/Nocturia

Don't confuse enuresis, which is involuntary, with nocturia, which is voluntary, frequent urination at night.

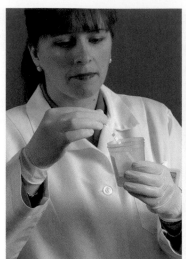
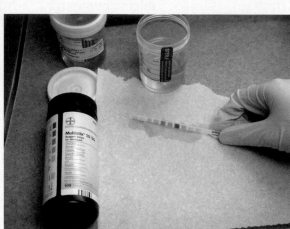

FIGURE 7-10 **Dipstick testing and urinalysis.**

URINALYSIS

Urinalysis is an examination of urine to determine the presence of abnormal elements that may indicate various pathologic conditions. It is an inexpensive, noninvasive test that provides valuable information not only about the contents of urine, but about diseases affecting the body as a whole. See Figure 7-10.

The following are some of the tests included in a urinalysis:

1. **Color**—Normal urine color is yellow (amber) or straw-colored. A colorless, pale urine indicates a large amount of water in the urine, whereas a smoky-red or brown color of urine indicates the presence of large amounts of blood. Foods such as beets and certain drugs also can produce a red coloration of urine.

2. **Appearance**—Normally, urine should be clear. Cloudy or **turbid** urine indicates a urinary tract infection with **pus (pyuria)** and **bacteria (bacteriuria).**

3. **pH**—Determination of pH reveals the chemical nature of urine. It indicates to what degree a solution is **acid** or **alkaline (basic)** (Figure 7-11). Normal urine is slightly acidic pH of 6.5. However, in some infections of the bladder, the urine pH may be alkaline, owing to the actions of bacteria in the urine that break down urea and release ammonia (an alkaline substance).

4. **Protein**—Small amounts of protein are normally found in the urine but not in sufficient quantity to produce a positive result by ordinary methods of testing. When urinary tests for protein become positive, **albumin** is usually responsible. Albumin is the major protein in blood plasma. If it is detected in urine **(albuminuria),** it may indicate a leak in the glomerular membrane, which allows albumin to enter the renal tubule and pass into the urine.

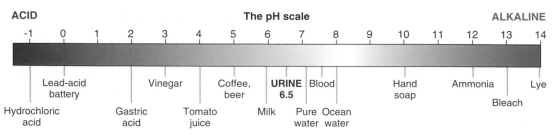

FIGURE 7-11 **The pH scale.** Pure water has a neutral pH.

Through more sensitive testing, smaller abnormal amounts of albumin may be detected, revealing **microalbuminuria,** when ordinary tests are negative. Microalbuminuria is recognized as the earliest sign of renal involvement in diabetes mellitus.

5. **Glucose**—Sugar is not normally found in the urine. In most cases, when it does appear **(glycosuria),** it indicates **diabetes mellitus.** In diabetes mellitus, there is excess sugar in the bloodstream (hyperglycemia), which leads to the "spilling over" of sugar into the urine. The renal tubules cannot reabsorb all the sugar that filters out through the glomerular membrane.

6. **Specific gravity**—The specific gravity of urine reflects the amounts of wastes, minerals, and solids in the urine. It is a comparison of the density of urine with that of water. The urine of patients with diabetes mellitus has a higher-than-normal specific gravity because of the presence of sugar.

7. **Ketone bodies**—Ketones (or **acetones,** a type of ketone body) are formed when fatty acids are broken down in the liver. Ketones accumulate in blood and urine when the body breaks down fat, instead of sugar, for fuel. **Ketonuria** occurs in diabetes mellitus when cells deprived of sugar must use up their available fat for energy. In starvation, when sugar is not available, ketonuria and ketosis (ketones in the blood) occur as fat is catabolized abnormally.

   Ketones in the blood are dangerous because they increase the acidity of the blood **(ketoacidosis).** If severe, this may lead to coma (unconsciousness) and death.

8. **Sediment and casts**—The presence of abnormal particles in the urine is a sign of a pathologic condition. Such particles, which may settle to the bottom of a urine sample as **sediment**, may include cells (epithelial, white, or red blood cells), bacteria, crystals, and **casts** (cylindrical structures of protein often containing cellular elements).

9. **Phenylketonuria (PKU)**—This is a rare condition in which a baby is born unable to break down an amino acid, phenylalanine. Resulting high blood levels of phenylalanine (phenylketones are detected in urine) can lead to mental retardation. Although the PKU test originally was performed on urine specimens, now it is done by pricking the newborn's heel to obtain a small blood sample. If phenylalanine is detected, the infant is fed a diet excluding phenylalanine. Affected children remain on this diet until adulthood.

10. **Bilirubin**—This pigment substance, which results from hemoglobin breakdown, may be present in the urine (bilirubinuria) of patients with liver disease. Urobilinogen, a breakdown product of bilirubin, also may be found in the urine.

PATHOLOGIC TERMINOLOGY: KIDNEY, BLADDER, AND ASSOCIATED CONDITIONS

KIDNEY

glomerulonephritis | **Inflammation of the glomeruli within the kidney.**

This condition can follow a streptococcal infection. It results in leaky glomeruli, hematuria, red blood cell casts, albuminuria, and when severe renal failure, and uremia. Drugs may be useful to control inflammation, and dialysis or renal transplantation may be necessary if uremia occurs.

interstitial nephritis

Inflammation of connective tissue that lies between the renal tubules.

Connective, supportive tissue lying between the renal tubules is made up of renal interstitial cells. **Interstitial cells** in any organ are found in addition to the essential, main functional cells, which make up the **parenchyma.** The parenchyma in the kidney consists of the glomeruli and the renal tubules (nephrons). Acute interstitial nephritis, an increasingly common disorder, may develop after use of NSAIDs (nonsteroidal anti-inflammatory drugs, such as aspirin and ibuprofen) and other drugs. It may be marked by fever, skin rash, and eosinophils in the blood and urine.

nephrolithiasis

Kidney stones (renal calculi).

Kidney stones usually are composed of uric acid or calcium salts. Stones often lodge in the ureter or bladder, as well as in the renal pelvis, and may require removal by **lithotripsy** (see page 234) or surgery.

nephrotic syndrome (nephrosis)

Group of clinical signs and symptoms caused by excessive protein loss in urine.

Nephrotic syndrome may follow glomerulonephritis or exposure to toxins or certain drugs, immune diseases, and other pathologic conditions, such as diabetes mellitus and cancer. Two important signs of nephrotic syndrome are **edema** (swelling caused by fluid in tissue spaces) and **hypoalbuminemia.** Both of these changes are caused by massive leakage of protein into urine.

polycystic kidney disease (PKD)

Multiple fluid-filled sacs (cysts) within and on the kidney.

There are two types of hereditary PKD. One type usually is **asymptomatic** (without symptoms) until middle age and then is marked by hematuria, urinary tract infections, nephrolithiasis, and renal failure. The other type of PKD occurs in infants or children and results in renal failure. Figure 7-12A shows polycystic kidney disease.

pyelonephritis

Inflammation of the lining of the renal pelvis and renal parenchyma.

The **parenchyma** of an organ is its essential and distinctive tissue. Nephrons make up the renal parenchyma. Bacterial infection in the urinary tract causes collections of pus to form in the kidney, often associated with bacteria spilling into the bloodstream. Urinalysis reveals pyuria. Treatment consists of antibiotics and surgical correction of any obstruction to urine flow.

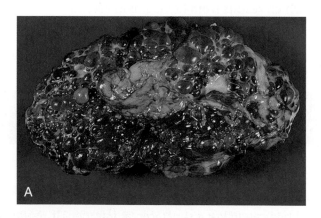

Tumor

FIGURE 7-12 **A, Polycystic kidney disease.** The kidneys contain masses of cysts. Typically, polycystic kidneys weigh 20 times more than their usual weight (150 to 200 grams). **B, Renal cell carcinoma.**

renal cell carcinoma (hypernephroma)	**Cancerous tumor of the kidney in adulthood.**

This tumor (see Figure 7-12B) accounts for 2% of all cancers in adults. Hematuria is the primary abnormal finding, and the tumor often metastasizes to bones and lungs. Nephrectomy or partial nephrectomy is the primary treatment.

renal failure — **Decrease in excretion of wastes results from impaired filtration function.**

A large number of conditions, including high blood pressure, infection, and diabetes, can lead to renal failure, which may be acute (ARF) or chronic (CRF), reversible or progressive, mild or severe. A newer classification of **chronic kidney disease (CKD)** stages its severity by the level of creatinine clearance and glomerular filtration rate (GFR), ranging from normal (stage 1) to end-stage renal failure (stage 5). See Spotlight on CKD stages on page 237.

renal hypertension — **High blood pressure resulting from kidney disease.**

Renal hypertension is a type of **secondary hypertension** (high blood pressure caused by an abnormal condition such as glomerulonephritis). However, the most common type of high blood pressure is **essential hypertension,** or **primary hypertension.** In essential hypertension there is no obvious underlying medical condition. Chronic essential hypertension can damage blood vessels potentially resulting in stroke, myocardial infarction (heart attack), heart failure, or renal failure.

Wilms tumor — **Malignant tumor of the kidney occurring in childhood.**

This tumor may be treated with surgery, radiation therapy, and chemotherapy.

URINARY BLADDER

bladder cancer — **Malignant tumor of the urinary bladder.**

Bladder cancer occurs more frequently in men (often smokers) and in persons older than 50 years of age, especially industrial workers exposed to dyes and leather-tanning agents. Signs and symptoms include gross (visible to the naked eye) or microscopic hematuria and dysuria. Cystoscopy with biopsy is the most common diagnostic procedure. Staging of the tumor is based on the depth to which the tumor invades the bladder wall and presence of metastasis. Superficial tumors are removed by electrocauterization (burning). Cystectomy, chemotherapy, and radiation therapy are treatments for disease that has spread deeply into the bladder wall, to regional lymph nodes, or to distant organs.

ASSOCIATED CONDITIONS

diabetes insipidus (DI) — **Antidiuretic hormone (ADH) is not secreted, or there is a resistance of the kidney to ADH.**

In DI, the kidney produces large amounts of dilute urine (polyuria). Lack of ADH prevents water from being reabsorbed into the blood through the renal tubules. Insipidus means tasteless, reflecting very dilute and watery urine, not sweet as in diabetes mellitus. The term **diabetes** comes from the Greek *diabainein,* meaning to pass through. Both types of diabetes (insipidus and mellitus) are marked by polyuria and polydipsia.

diabetes mellitus (DM) — **Insulin is not secreted adequately or tissues are resistant to its effects.**

The major signs and symptoms of diabetes mellitus are glycosuria, hyperglycemia, polyuria, and polydipsia. Without insulin, sugar cannot leave the bloodstream and is not available to body cells for energy. Sugar remains in the blood (hyperglycemia) and spills over into the urine (glycosuria). Mellitus means sweet, reflecting the content of the urine. The term diabetes, when used alone, refers to diabetes mellitus. See Chapter 18 for more information about diabetes mellitus.

LABORATORY TESTS AND CLINICAL PROCEDURES

LABORATORY TESTS

blood urea nitrogen (BUN)   **Measurement of urea levels in blood.**

Normally, the blood urea level is low because urea is excreted in the urine continuously. However, when the kidney is diseased or fails, urea accumulates in the blood (uremia), leading to unconsciousness and death.

creatinine clearance   **Measurement of the rate at which creatinine is cleared from the blood by the kidney.**

This is an important test to assess the functioning of the kidney. A blood sample is drawn and the creatinine concentration in blood is compared with the amount of creatinine excreted in the urine during a fixed time period. If the kidney is not functioning well in its job of clearing creatinine from the blood, the amount of creatinine in the blood will be high relative to the amount in urine. Creatinine clearance is a useful indicator of the **glomerular filtration rate (GFR),** which normally is 90 to 120 mL/minute.

CLINICAL PROCEDURES

X-Ray Studies

CT urography   **X-ray images obtained using computed tomography (CT) show multiple cross-sectional and other views of the kidney.**

CT scanners show multiple views of the kidney, taken with or without contrast material. Two main indications are to detect kidney stones and to evaluate patients with hematuria (Figure 7-13A).

kidneys, ureters, and bladder (KUB)   **X-ray examination (without contrast) of the kidneys, ureters, and bladder.**

A KUB study demonstrates the size and location of the kidneys in relation to other organs in the abdominopelvic region.

renal angiography   **X-ray examination (with contrast) of the blood vessels of the kidney.**

This procedure helps diagnose obstruction or constriction of blood vessels leading to the kidney. The same changes can be seen on CT and MRI urography.

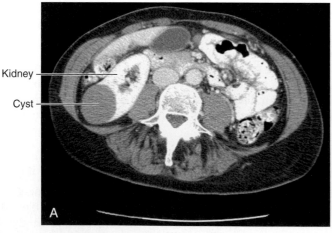
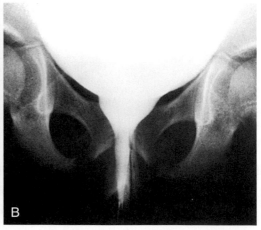

FIGURE 7-13 A, CT urography with contrast (axial view) shows a benign cyst on the kidney. It does not take up the contrast and is smooth and round. **B, Voiding cystourethrogram** showing a normal female urethra. *(Courtesy William H. Bush, Jr., MD, University of Washington, Seattle.)*

retrograde pyelogram (RP)	**X-ray image of the renal pelvis and ureters after injection of contrast through a urinary catheter into the ureters from the bladder.**
	This technique is useful in locating urinary stones and obstructions.
voiding cystourethrogram (VCUG)	**X-ray image (with contrast) of the urinary bladder and urethra obtained while the patient is voiding.** See Figure 7-13B.
	The bladder is filled with contrast material, followed by fluoroscopy (real-time x-ray imaging). Reflux of contrast into the ureters is abnormal and may occur with recurrent urinary tract infections.

Ultrasound Examination

ultrasonography	**Imaging of urinary tract structures using high-frequency sound waves.**
	Kidney size, tumors, hydronephrosis, polycystic kidney disease, and ureteral and bladder obstruction can be diagnosed using ultrasound techniques.

Radioactive Study

radioisotope scan	**Image of the kidney obtained after injecting a radioactive substance (radioisotope) into the bloodstream.**
	Pictures show the size and shape of the kidney **(renal scan)** and its functioning **(renogram).** These studies can indicate narrowing of blood vessels, diagnose obstruction, and determine the individual functioning of each kidney.

Magnetic Resonance Imaging

MRI urography	**Changing magnetic field produces images of the kidney and surrounding structures in three planes of the body.**
	The patient lies within a cylindrical magnetic resonance machine, and images are made of the pelvic and retroperitoneal regions using magnetic waves. This test is useful in visualizing tumor invasion of blood vessels, lymph nodes, and adjacent tissues.

OTHER PROCEDURES

cystoscopy	**Direct visualization of the urethra and urinary bladder with an endoscope (cystoscope).**
	The procedure can be performed in two ways. **Flexible cystoscopy** uses a thin fiberoptic cystoscope and is used for diagnosis and check-ups of the urinary bladder. **Rigid cystoscopy** uses a hollow metal tube, passed through the urethra and into the bladder. It is used to take biopsy samples, remove polyps, or perform laser treatments (Figure 7-14A and B).

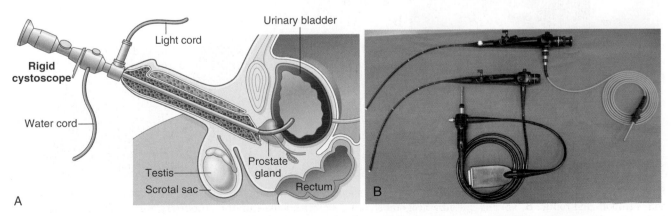

FIGURE 7-14   Cystoscopy. A, Rigid cystoscope in place within the urethra. **B, Flexible cystoscope.**

dialysis

Process of separating nitrogenous waste materials from the blood.

Dialysis is used to treat acute or chronic renal failure and some cases of drug use. There are two methods:

1. **Hemodialysis (HD)** uses an artificial kidney machine that receives waste-filled blood from the patient's bloodstream, filters it through an artificial porous membrane (dialyzer), and returns the dialyzed blood to the patient's body (Figure 7-15A). An **arteriovenous fistula** (communication between an artery and a vein) is created surgically to provide easy access for hemodialysis (Figure 7-15B).

2. **Peritoneal dialysis (PD)** uses a **catheter** to introduce fluid into the peritoneal (abdominal) cavity. Waste materials, such as urea, in the capillaries of the peritoneum pass out of the bloodstream and into the fluid. The fluid (with wastes) is then removed by catheter. When used to treat patients with chronic kidney disease, PD may be performed continuously by the patient without mechanical support (CAPD—continuous ambulatory PD; Figure 7-16) or with the aid of a mechanical apparatus used at night during sleep.

lithotripsy

Urinary tract stones are crushed.

The **extracorporeal method** uses shock waves directed toward the stone from the outside of the body (extra = outside, corpor/o = body). The patient receives light sedation or an anesthetic. Stones pass from the body in urine after the procedure. Abbreviation is **ESWL (extracorporeal shock wave lithotripsy).**

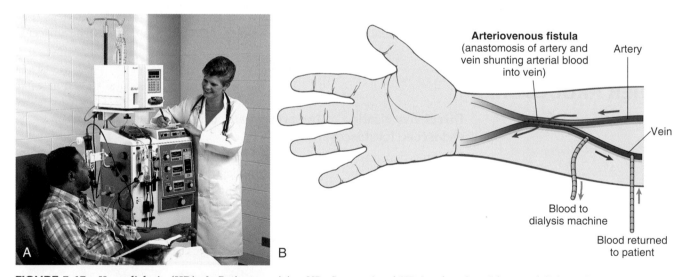

FIGURE 7-15   Hemodialysis (HD). A, Patient receiving HD. Conventional HD involves 3 to 4 hours of dialysis three times weekly. Newer alternative modalities include slower and longer dialysis, nocturnal HD, and daily short HD. **B, Arteriovenous fistula** for hemodialysis.

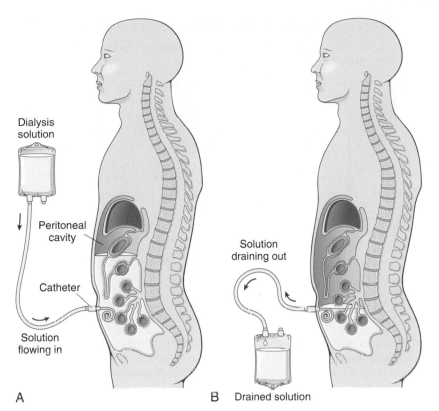

Dialysis
solution

Peritoneal
cavity

Catheter

Solution
flowing in

A

Solution
draining out

B Drained solution

FIGURE 7-16 **Continuous ambulatory peritoneal dialysis (CAPD). A,** The dialysis solution (dialysate) flows from a collapsible plastic bag through a catheter (Tenckhoff peritoneal catheter) into the patient's peritoneal cavity. The empty bag is then folded and inserted into undergarments. **B,** After 4 to 8 hours, the bag is unfolded, and the fluid is allowed to drain into it by gravity. The full bag is discarded, and a new bag of fresh dialysate is attached.

7

renal angioplasty	**Dilation of narrowed areas in renal arteries.**
	A balloon attached to a catheter is inserted into the artery and then inflated to enlarge the vessel diameter. Afterward, stents (metal-mesh tubes) may be inserted to keep the vessel open. This procedure is used to treat renal hypertension and to preserve renal function.
renal biopsy	**Removal of kidney tissue for microscopic examination.**
	Biopsy may be performed at the time of surgery (open) or through the skin (percutaneous, or closed). When the latter technique is used, the patient lies in the prone position; then, after administration of local anesthesia to the overlying skin and muscles of the back, the physician inserts a biopsy needle down into the kidney. Several specimens are obtained for examination by a pathologist.

DONOR

Right kidney

Left kidney

RECIPIENT

Adrenal gland

Donor's left kidney cradled in iliac fossa

Donor renal artery sutured to internal iliac artery

Ureter connected to recipient's bladder **(ureteroneo-cystostomy)**

A

B

FIGURE 7-17   Renal (kidney) transplantation. A, Left kidney of donor is removed for transplantation. **B,** Kidney is transplanted to the right pelvis (iliac fossa) of the recipient. The renal artery and vein of the donor kidney are joined to the recipient kidney's artery and vein, and the end of the donor ureter is connected to the recipient's bladder **(ureteroneocystostomy)**. The health of the donor is not affected by losing one kidney. In fact, the remaining kidney is able to take over full function.

renal transplantation	**Surgical transfer of a kidney from a donor to a recipient.**

Patients with renal failure may receive a kidney from a living donor, such as an identical twin (isograft) or other person (allograft), or from a patient at the time of death (cadaver transplant). Best results occur when the donor is closely related to the recipient—98% of transplanted kidneys survive for 1 year or longer (Figure 7-17). See the ***In Person: Kidney Transplant*** on page 240.

urinary catheterization	**Passage of a flexible, tubular instrument through the urethra into the urinary bladder.**

Catheters are used primarily for short- or long-term drainage of urine. A **Foley catheter** is an indwelling (left in the bladder) catheter held in place by a balloon inflated with liquid (Figure 7-18).

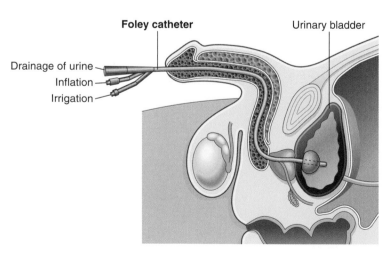

Foley catheter

Urinary bladder

Drainage of urine

Inflation

Irrigation

FIGURE 7-18   Foley catheter in place in the urinary bladder. The three-way catheter has three separate lumens: for drainage of urine, for inflation of balloons in the bladder, and for introduction of irrigating solutions into the bladder.

ABBREVIATIONS

ADH	antidiuretic hormone—vasopressin
AKI	acute kidney (renal) injury
BUN	blood urea nitrogen
CAPD	continuous ambulatory peritoneal dialysis
CKD	chronic kidney disease—a condition during which serum creatinine and BUN levels rise, which may result in impairment of all body systems
Cl⁻	chloride—an electrolyte excreted by the kidney
CrCl	creatinine clearance
CRF	chronic renal failure—progressive loss of kidney function
C&S	culture and sensitivity testing—to determine antibiotic effectiveness against bacteria grown from a patient's urine specimen
cysto	cystoscopic examination
eGFR	estimated glomerular filtration rate
ESWL	extracorporeal shock wave lithotripsy
HCO₃⁻	bicarbonate—an electrolyte conserved by the kidney
HD	hemodialysis
IC	interstitial cystitis—chronic inflammation of the bladder wall; not caused by bacterial infection and not responsive to conventional antibiotic therapy
IVP	intravenous pyelogram
K⁺	potassium—an electrolyte
KUB	kidney, ureter, and bladder
Na⁺	sodium—an electrolyte
PD	peritoneal dialysis
pH	potential hydrogen; scale to indicate degree of acidity or alkalinity
PKD	polycystic kidney disease
PUL	percutaneous ultrasound lithotripsy
RP	retrograde pyelography
sp gr	specific gravity
UA	urinalysis
UTI	urinary tract infection
VCUG	voiding cystourethrogram

7

CKD Stages

The five stages of **CKD** reflect increasing severity of kidney disease:

Stage 1: eGFR >90
Stage 2: eGFR 60-90
Stage 3: eGFR 30-60
Stage 4: eGFR 15-30
Stage 5: eGFR <15

PRACTICAL APPLICATIONS

Answers to the questions about the case report and the urinalysis findings are on page 248.

Urologic Case Report

The patient, a 50-year-old woman, presented to the clinic complaining of painless hematuria and clots in the urine. There had been no history of urolithiasis, pyuria, or previous hematuria. Nocturia had been present about 5 years earlier. Endoscopy revealed a carcinoma located about 2 cm from the left ureteral orifice. A metastatic workup was negative. Partial cystectomy was carried out and the lesion cleared. Bilateral pelvic lymphadenectomy revealed no positive nodes. No ileal conduit was necessary.

Questions about the Case Report

1. Urologic refers to which system of the body?
   a. Digestive
   b. Endocrine
   c. Excretory

2. What was the patient's reason for appearing at the clinic?
   a. Scanty urination
   b. Inability to urinate
   c. Blood in urine

3. Which of the following was a previous symptom?
   a. Excessive urination at night
   b. Blood in the urine
   c. Pus in the urine

4. What diagnostic procedure was carried out?
   a. Lithotripsy
   b. Cystoscopy
   c. Urinalysis

5. The patient's diagnosis was:
   a. Malignant tumor of the bladder
   b. Tumor in the proximal ureter
   c. Lymph nodes affected by tumor

6. Treatment was:
   a. Ureteroileostomy
   b. Removal of tumor and subtotal removal of the bladder
   c. Not necessary, because of negative lymph nodes

7

Urinalysis Findings

TEST	NORMAL	ABNORMAL
Color	Amber-yellow	Smoky-red (blood in urine): renal calculi; tumor; kidney disease; cystitis; urinary obstruction
Appearance	Clear	Cloudy (pyuria): urinary tract infection (UTI)
pH	4.6-8.0	Alkaline: UTI
Protein	None or small amount	Proteinuria: nephritis; renal failure
Glucose	None	Glycosuria: diabetes mellitus
Ketones	None	Ketonuria: diabetes mellitus
Bilirubin	None	Bilirubinuria: hepatitis or gallbladder disease
Specific gravity	1.003-1.030	High: renal calculi; diabetes mellitus Low: diabetes insipidus
Sediment	None	Casts: nephritis; renal disease

Name the appropriate test for detecting or evaluating each of the following.

1. Sugar in urine _____

2. Level of bile pigment in urine _____

3. Hematuria _____

4. Albumin in urine _____

5. Structures in the shape of renal tubules in urine _____

6. Chemical reaction of urine _____

7. Dilution or concentration of urine _____

8. Acetones in urine _____

9. Pus in urine _____

Urologic Case Study

A 22-year-old Brazilian fashion model comes to the ED [emergency department] with a history of fever, dysuria, and shaking chills. Results of her UA [urinalysis], with normal findings for comparison, are as follows:

TEST	UA RESULTS	NORMAL FINDINGS
Color	amber-yellow	amber-yellow
Appearance	turbid	clear
Specific gravity	1.040	1.003-1.030
pH	8.4	6.5 (range, 4.6-8.0)
Protein	neg	neg
Glucose	neg	neg
Ketones	neg	neg
Bili	neg	neg
WBC count	>100	0
Bacteria	bacilli (rods)	0
Sediment	WBC casts	none

What's the probable diagnosis?
a. Diabetes mellitus with glycosuria
b. Glomerulonephritis with staphylococcal infection
c. Nephrotic syndrome with albuminuria
d. Urinary tract infection with pyelonephritis

IN PERSON: KIDNEY TRANSPLANT

This first-person narrative was written by a kidney donor.

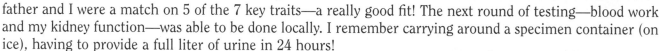

When my 64-year-old father-in-law announced to my wife and me that his kidney function was failing, it didn't really enter our minds that one of us might ultimately have a part to play in his survival. Five years later, dialysis was taking its toll on his organ systems, and there had been no success in obtaining a cadaveric kidney. Things had reached the point where he needed a kidney in short order, before his health deteriorated to the point where he would no longer be a candidate for transplantation.

My wife's blood type ruled out the possibility of her being a direct donor, so I volunteered to be tested. Turns out that her father and I were a match on 5 of the 7 key traits—a really good fit! The next round of testing—blood work and my kidney function—was able to be done locally. I remember carrying around a specimen container (on ice), having to provide a full liter of urine in 24 hours!

The results of those tests were favorable, and two weeks later I made the $3\frac{1}{2}$-hour drive to the transplant center at the University of Virginia in Charlottesville. While a transplant is really a team of two—donor and recipient—the entire process at UVA was very much individualized. A transplant coordinator (an experienced RN) was assigned specifically to our case, and I had a team of doctors and support staff dedicated exclusively to me, the donor. Similarly, there was a team that dealt only with my father-in-law as the recipient.

My visit involved some more in-depth blood tests and cardiac studies largely to determine that I was healthy enough for major surgery. My transplant team and I spent an entire afternoon discussing the implications of being a donor—the inherent risk in any surgery, potential implications for me and my family, the likely recovery time, and the possibility that, despite all of the up-front testing, the transplant might not be successful. The discussions that afternoon only reaffirmed that I was making the right decision. I had an opportunity to have a positive impact on someone else's life, with relatively little risk to my own health.

The events around the surgery itself were pretty straightforward. The surgery is a more involved procedure for the donor than for the recipient, so I was taken back first. A nurse started an IV and injected a mild sedative. From that point, my only memory is of one last hug for my wife and children, and then being shifted from the stretcher onto the operating table.

When I woke up in recovery, the news was all good. My surgery had gone well—four laparoscopic incisions through which the surgeons did most all of their work, and a lateral incision in my lower abdomen through which the kidney was removed. Equally important, my father-in-law had come through his surgery well and the kidney had immediately begun to function! I was discharged from the hospital on Sunday, and cleared to return home the next Friday, 8 days post-op.

As is typical following a major surgery, it took about 6 weeks for me to feel "normal" again. During those 6 weeks, I had weekly blood tests to chart the progress of my kidney function. I went back to UVA for a routine follow-up visit at the 6-week mark. I was recovering as expected, and my remaining kidney was actually growing in size and capacity. Blood tests continued on a monthly basis until I was officially "discharged" from the transplant center's care 6 months after the surgery.

Now, 8 years after the transplant, both my father-in-law and I continue to do well. As my mother-in-law likes to say, I donated a "rock star" kidney that has allowed our family to enjoy many visits and create many cherished memories that will last a lifetime. My two children, now 20 and 17, have enjoyed their grandfather's love and guidance during some very important years in their lives. This is especially meaningful to me, as I lost my father before my wife and I started our family, and our children missed out on an opportunity to know and love a wonderful man.

John Melson lives in Greensboro, North Carolina, with his wife and two wonderful children. He is a finance and marketing executive with a global textile firm and enjoys golf, tennis, and traveling. He is pictured with his father-in-law, Rod Beckwith.

EXERCISES

Remember to check your answers carefully with the Answers to Exercises, pages 247 and 248.

A Using the following terms, trace the path of urine from the renal arterioles (bloodstream) to the point at which urine leaves the body. The first answer is provided.

glomerular capsule   renal pelvis   ureter   urinary bladder
glomerulus   renal tubule   urethra   urinary meatus

1. *glomerulus* _____   5. _____

2. _____   6. _____

3. _____   7. _____

4. _____   8. _____

B Match the term in Column I with its definition or a term of similar meaning in Column II. Write the correct letter in the spaces provided.

COLUMN I

1. voiding _____
2. trigone _____
3. renal cortex _____
4. renal medulla _____
5. urea _____
6. erythropoietin _____
7. renin _____
8. electrolyte _____
9. hilum _____
10. calyx (calix) _____

COLUMN II

A. Hormone secreted by the kidney that stimulates formation of red blood cells
B. Notch on the surface of the kidney where blood vessels and nerves enter
C. Urination; micturition
D. Nitrogenous waste
E. Cup-like collecting region of the renal pelvis
F. Small molecule that carries an electric charge in solution
G. Inner region of the kidney
H. Hormone made by the kidney; increases blood pressure
I. Triangular area in the bladder
J. Outer section of the kidney

7

C Give the meanings of the following medical terms.

1. caliceal _____

2. uric acid _____

3. urinary meatal stenosis _____

4. cystocele _____

5. pyelolithotomy _____

6. trigonitis _____

7. ureteroileostomy _____

8. urethrostenosis _____

9. vesicoureteral reflux _____

10. creatinine _____

11. medullary _____

12. cortical _____

13. calciferol _____

D The following terms all contain the suffix -uria, meaning urination. Write their meanings in the spaces provided.

1. nocturia _____

2. dysuria _____

3. oliguria _____

4. polyuria _____

5. anuria _____

E In the following terms, -uria means urine condition (substance in the urine). What's in the urine?

1. pyuria _____   4. glycosuria _____

2. albuminuria _____   5. ketonuria _____

3. hematuria _____   6. bacteriuria _____

F Give the meanings of the following terms that relate to urinary signs and symptoms.

1. azotemia _____

2. polydipsia _____

3. urinary incontinence _____

4. enuresis _____

5. urinary retention _____

6. ketosis _____

G **Give short answers for the following.**

1. What is the difference between hematuria and uremia? _____

2. What is diuresis? _____

3. What is a diuretic? _____

4. What is antidiuretic hormone? _____

5. What is hyponatremia? _____

6. What is hyperkalemia? _____

7. What is PKU? _____

H **Match the listed terms, pertaining to urinalysis, with their meanings/descriptions that follow.**

albuminuria	hematuria	pyuria
bilirubinuria	ketonuria	sediment
glycosuria	pH	specific gravity

1. Abnormal particles present in the urine—cells, bacteria, casts, and crystals

    _____

2. Smoky-red color of urine caused by the presence of blood _____

3. Turbid (cloudy) urine caused by the presence of polymorphonuclear leukocytes and

    pus _____

4. Sugar in the urine; a sign of diabetes mellitus and a result of hyperglycemia

    _____

5. Urine test that reflects the acidity or alkalinity of the urine _____

6. High levels of acids and acetones accumulate in the urine as a result of abnormal fat

    breakdown _____

7. Dark pigment that accumulates in urine as a result of liver or gallbladder disease

    _____

8. Urine test that reflects the concentration of the urine _____

9. Leaky glomeruli can produce accumulation of protein in the urine _____

7

I **Describe the following abnormal conditions that affect the kidney.**

1. renal failure _____

2. polycystic kidney _____

3. interstitial nephritis _____

4. glomerulonephritis _____

5. nephrolithiasis _____

6. renal cell carcinoma _____

7. pyelonephritis _____

8. Wilms tumor _____

9. nephrotic syndrome _____

10. renal hypertension _____

J **Match the listed terms with their meanings/descriptions that follow.**

abscess   edema   renal colic
catheter   essential hypertension   secondary hypertension
diabetes insipidus   nephroptosis   stricture
diabetes mellitus

1. idiopathic high blood pressure _____

2. swelling, fluid in tissues _____

3. narrowed area in a tube _____

4. collection of pus _____

5. inadequate secretion of insulin or improper utilization of insulin leads to this condition

_____

6. high blood pressure caused by kidney disease or another disease _____

7. tube for withdrawing or giving fluid _____

8. inadequate secretion or resistance of the kidney to the action of antidiuretic hormone

_____

9. prolapse of a kidney _____

10. severe pain resulting from a stone that is blocking a ureter or a kidney

_____

7

K Give the meanings of the abbreviations in Column I. Then select the letter of the sentence in Column II that is the best association for each.

COLUMN I

1. CAPD_____ _____

2. BUN_____ _____

3. RP_____ _____

4. cysto_____ _____

5. UA_____ _____

6. UTI_____ _____

7. CKD_____ _____

8. K⁺_____ _____

9. VCUG_____ _____

10. HD_____ _____

COLUMN II

A. Bacterial invasion leads to this condition; acute cystitis is an example.

B. This electrolyte is secreted by renal tubules into the urine.

C. A machine removes nitrogenous wastes from the patient's blood.

D. High levels measured on this test lead to the suspicion of renal disease.

E. This endoscopic procedure is used to examine the interior of the urinary bladder.

F. Dialysate (fluid) is injected into the peritoneal cavity and then drained out.

G. Contrast is injected into the urinary bladder and ureters and x-ray pictures of the urinary tract are taken.

H. X-ray pictures of the urinary bladder and urethra are taken while the patient urinates.

I. The parts of this test include specific gravity, color, protein, glucose, and pH.

J. This condition includes mild to severe kidney failure.

L Match the listed procedures with their definitions/meanings that follow.

cystectomy   nephrectomy   ureterolithotomy
cystoscopy   nephrolithotomy   urethroplasty
cystostomy   nephrostomy   ureteroileostomy
lithotripsy

1. Excision of a kidney _____

2. Surgical incision into the kidney to remove a stone _____

3. Visual examination of the urinary bladder via endoscope _____

4. Crushing of stones _____

5. New opening of the ureters to a segment of ileum (in place of the bladder)

_____

6. Surgical repair of the urethra _____

7. Creation of an artificial opening into the kidney (via catheter) from the outside of the body

_____

8. Surgical formation of an opening from the bladder to the outside of the body

_____

9. Removal of the urinary bladder _____

10. Incision of a ureter to remove a stone _____

M **Circle the correct term to complete the following sentences.**

1. After diagnosis of renal cell carcinoma (made by renal biopsy), Dr. Davis advised Donna that **(nephrostomy, meatotomy, nephrectomy)** would be necessary.

2. Ever since Bill's condition of gout was diagnosed, he has been warned that uric acid crystals could accumulate in his blood and tissues, leading to **(pyuria, renal calculi, cystocele).**

3. The voiding cystourethrogram demonstrated blockage of urine flow from Jim's bladder and **(hydronephrosis, renal ischemia, azotemia).**

4. Narrowed arterioles in the kidney increase blood pressure, so **(urinary incontinence, urinary retention, nephrosclerosis)** is often associated with hypertension.

5. Eight-year-old Willy continually wet his bed at night while sleeping. His pediatrician instructed his mother to limit Willy's intake of fluids in the evening to discourage his **(nocturia, oliguria, enuresis).**

6. David's chronic type 1 diabetes eventually resulted in **(nephropathy, meatal stenosis, urolithiasis),** which led to renal failure.

7. After Sue's bilateral renal failure, her doctor advised dialysis and possible **(cystostomy, nephrolithotomy, renal transplantation).**

8. When Maria's left kidney stopped functioning, her contralateral kidney overdeveloped or **(metastasized, atrophied, hypertrophied)** to meet the increased workload.

9. A popular diet program recommends eating foods high in fats and protein. People on this diet check their urine for the presence of **(ketones, glucose, amino acids).**

10. Andrea's urinalysis revealed proteinuria, and her ankles began to swell, demonstrating pitting, a condition known as **(ascites, edema, stricture).** Her **(gastroenterologist, urologist, nephrologist)** diagnosed Andrea's condition as **(polycystic kidneys, nephrotic syndrome, bladder carcinoma)** and recommended drugs to heal leaky glomeruli and diuretics to reduce swelling.

7

ANSWERS TO EXERCISES

A

1. glomerulus
2. glomerular capsule
3. renal tubule
4. renal pelvis
5. ureter
6. urinary bladder
7. urethra
8. urinary meatus

B

1. C
2. I
3. J
4. G
5. D
6. A
7. H
8. F
9. B
10. E

C

1. pertaining to a calix (collecting cup of renal pelvis)
2. nitrogenous waste excreted in urine; high levels of uric acid in the blood are associated with gouty arthritis
3. narrowing of the urinary meatus
4. hernia of the urinary bladder
5. incision to remove a stone from the renal pelvis
6. inflammation of the trigone (triangular area in the bladder in which the ureters enter and urethra exits)
7. new opening between the ureter and the ileum (an anastomosis); urine then leaves the body through an ileostomy; this surgery (ileal conduit) is performed when the bladder has been removed
8. narrowing (narrowed portion) of the urethra
9. backflow of urine from the bladder into the ureter
10. nitrogenous waste produced as a result of muscle metabolism and excreted in the urine
11. pertaining to the inner, middle section (of the kidney)
12. pertaining to the outer section (of the kidney)
13. active form of vitamin D secreted by the kidneys

D

1. frequent urination at night
2. painful urination
3. scanty urination
4. excessive urination
5. no urination

E

1. pus
2. protein
3. blood
4. sugar
5. ketones or acetones
6. bacteria

F

1. excess nitrogenous waste in the bloodstream
2. condition of much thirst
3. inability to hold urine in the bladder
4. bedwetting
5. inability to release urine from the bladder
6. abnormal condition of ketone bodies (acids and acetones) in the blood and body tissues

G

1. Hematuria is the presence of blood in the urine, and uremia is a toxic condition of excess urea (nitrogenous waste) in the bloodstream. Hematuria is a symptomatic condition of the urine (-uria), and uremia is an abnormal condition of the blood (-emia).
2. Diuresis is the excessive production of urine (polyuria).
3. A diuretic is a drug or chemical (caffeine or alcohol) that causes diuresis to occur.
4. Antidiuretic hormone is a hormone produced by the pituitary gland that normally helps the renal tubules to reabsorb water back into the bloodstream. It works against diuresis to help retain water in the blood.
5. Hyponatremia is abnormally low levels of sodium in the bloodstream.
6. Hyperkalemia is abnormally high concentration of potassium in the blood. The major cause is chronic renal failure.
7. PKU is phenylketonuria. This occurs when there are high levels of phenylketones in urine and phenylalanine in the blood. The condition causes mental retardation in infants.

7

H

1. sediment
2. hematuria (blood in the urine)
3. pyuria (pus in the urine)
4. glycosuria (sugar in the urine)
5. pH
6. ketonuria (ketone bodies in the urine)
7. bilirubinuria (high levels of bilirubin in the urine)
8. specific gravity
9. albuminuria

I

1. kidney does not excrete wastes
2. multiple fluid-filled sacs form in and on the kidney
3. inflammation of the connective tissue (interstitium) lying between the renal tubules
4. inflammation of the glomerulus of the kidney (may be a complication after a streptococcal infection)
5. condition of kidney stones (renal calculi)
6. malignant tumor of the kidney in adults
7. inflammation of the renal pelvis and parenchyma of the kidney (caused by a bacterial infection, such as with *Escherichia coli,* that spreads to the urinary tract from the gastrointestinal tract)
8. malignant tumor of the kidney in children
9. group of symptoms (proteinuria, edema, hypoalbuminemia) that appears when the kidney is damaged by disease; also called nephrosis
10. high blood pressure caused by kidney disease

J

1. essential hypertension
2. edema
3. stricture
4. abscess
5. diabetes mellitus
6. secondary hypertension
7. catheter
8. diabetes insipidus
9. nephroptosis
10. renal colic

K

1. continuous ambulatory peritoneal dialysis: F
2. blood urea nitrogen: D
3. retrograde pyelogram: G
4. cystoscopy: E
5. urinalysis: I
6. urinary tract infection: A
7. chronic kidney disease: J
8. potassium: B
9. voiding cystourethrogram: H
10. hemodialysis: C

L

1. nephrectomy
2. nephrolithotomy
3. cystoscopy
4. lithotripsy
5. ureteroileostomy
6. urethroplasty
7. nephrostomy
8. cystostomy
9. cystectomy
10. ureterolithotomy

M

1. nephrectomy
2. renal calculi—don't confuse a calculus (stone) with dental calculus, which is an accumulation of dental plaque that has hardened
3. hydronephrosis
4. nephrosclerosis
5. enuresis
6. nephropathy
7. renal transplantation
8. hypertrophied
9. ketones
10. edema, nephrologist, nephrotic syndrome

Answers to Practical Applications

Urologic Case Report
1. c
2. c
3. a
4. b
5. a
6. b

Urinalysis Findings
1. glucose
2. bilirubin
3. color
4. protein
5. sediment
6. pH
7. specific gravity
8. ketones
9. appearance

Urologic Case Study
Correct diagnosis is d.

PRONUNCIATION OF TERMS

To test your understanding of the terminology in this chapter, write the meaning of each term in the space provided. In addition, you may wish to cover the terms and write them by looking at your definitions. Make sure your spelling is correct. The page number after each term indicates where it is defined or used in the book, so you can easily check your responses. You will find complete definitions for all of these terms and audio pronunciations on the Evolve website.

Pronunciation Guide

ā as in āpe	ă as in ăpple
ē as in ēven	ě as in ěvery
ī as in īce	ĭ as in ĭnterest
ō as in ōpen	ŏ as in pŏt
ū as in ūnit	ŭ as in ŭnder

TERM	PRONUNCIATION	MEANING
acetone (229)	ĂS-ě-tōn	
albuminuria (226)	ăl-bū-mĭn-Ū-rē-ă	
antidiuretic hormone (227)	ăn-tĭ-dī-ū-RĔ-tĭk HŎR-mōn	
anuria (227)	ăn-Ū-rē-ă	
arteriole (221)	ăr-TĒR-ē-ōl	
azotemia (226)	ă-zō-TĒ-mē-ă	
bacteriuria (226)	băk-te-rē-Ū-rē-ă	
calciferol (221)	căl-SĬ-fěr-ōl	
caliceal (223)	kā-lĭ-SĒ-ăl	
caliectasis (223)	kā-lē-ĔK-tă-sĭs	
calyx (calix); *plural*: calyces (calices) (221)	KĀ-lĭks; KĀ-lĭ-sēz	
catheter (221)	KĂ-thě-těr	
cortex (221)	KŎR-těks	
cortical (221)	KŎR-tĭ-kăl	
creatinine (221)	krē-ĂT-ĭ-nēn	
creatinine clearance (232)	krē-ĂT-ĭ-nēn KLĒR-ăns	
CT urography (232)	CT ū-RŎG-ră-fē	
cystectomy (232)	sĭs-TĔK-tō-mē	
cystitis (223)	sĭs-TĪ-tĭs	
cystoscopy (233)	sĭs-TŎS-kō-pē	
cystostomy (223)	sĭs-TŎS-tō-mē	
diabetes insipidus (231)	dī-ă-BĒ-tēz ĭn-SĬP-ĭ-dŭs	
diabetes mellitus (231)	dī-ă-BĒ-tēz MĔL-ĭ-tŭs	

7

TERM	PRONUNCIATION	MEANING
diuresis (227)	dī-ūr-RĒ-sĭs	
dysuria (227)	dĭs-Ū-rē-ă	
edema (230)	ĕ-DĒ-mă	
electrolyte (221)	ē-LĔK-trō-līt	
enuresis (227)	ĕn-ū-RĒ-sĭs	
erythropoietin (221)	ĕ-rĭth-rō-POY-ĕ-tĭn	
essential hypertension (231)	ē-SĔN-shŭl hī-pĕr-TĔN-shŭn	
filtration (231)	fĭl-TRĀ-shŭn	
glomerular capsule (221)	glō-MĔR-ū-lăr KĂP-sŭl	
glomerulonephritis (229)	glō-mĕr-ū-lō-nĕ-FRĪ-tĭs	
glomerulus; *plural*: glomeruli (221)	glō-MĔR-ū-lŭs; glō-MĔR-ū-lī	
glycosuria (227)	glī-kōs-Ū-rē-ă	
hematuria (227)	hēm-ă-TŪ-rē-ă	
hemodialysis (234)	hē-mō-dī-ĂL-ĭ-sĭs	
hilum (222)	HĪ-lŭm	
hydronephrosis (224)	hī-drō-nĕ-FRŌ-sĭs	
hyperkalemia (226)	hī-pĕr-kă-LĒ-mē-ă	
hyponatremia (226)	hī-pō-nă-TRĒ-mē-ă	
interstitial nephritis (230)	ĭn-tĕr-STĬ-shŭl nĕ-FRĪ-tĭs	
intravesical (225)	ĭn-tră-VĔS-ĭ-kăl	
ketonuria (226)	kē-tōn-Ū-rē-ă	
ketosis (226)	kē-TŌ-sĭs	
kidney (222)	KĬD-nē	
lithotripsy (234)	LĬTH-ō-trĭp-sē	
meatal stenosis (223)	mē-Ā-tăl stĕ-NŌ-sĭs	
meatus (222)	mē-Ā-tŭs	
medulla (222)	mĕ-DŪL-ă *or* mĕ-DŬL-ă	
medullary (222)	MĔD-ū-lăr-ē	
MRI urography (233)	MRI ū-RŎG-ră-fē	
nephrolithiasis (230)	nĕf-rō-lĭ-THĪ-ă-sĭs	
nephrolithotomy (224)	nĕf-rō-lĭ-THŎT-ō-mē	

7

TERM	PRONUNCIATION	MEANING
nephron (222)	NĔF-rŏn	
nephropathy (223)	nĕ-FRŎ-pă-thē	
nephroptosis (224)	nĕf-rŏp-TŌ-sĭs	
nephrostomy (224)	nĕ-FRŎS-tō-mē	
nephrotic syndrome (230)	nĕ-FRŎT-ĭk SĬN-drōm	
nitrogenous waste (222)	nĭ-TRŎJ-ĕ-nŭs wāst	
nocturia (226)	nŏk-TŪ-rē-ă	
oliguria (226)	ŏl-ĭ-GŪ-rē-ă	
parenchyma (230)	păr-ĔN-kĭ-mă	
paranephric (224)	pă-ră-NĔF-rĭk	
peritoneal dialysis (234)	pĕr-ĭ-tō-NĒ-ăl dī-ĂL-ĭ-sĭs	
phenylketonuria (229)	fĕ-nĭl-kē-tōn-UR-ē-ă	
polycystic kidney disease (230)	pŏl-ē-SĬS-tĭk KĬD-nē dĭ-ZĒZ	
polydipsia (226)	pŏl-ē-DĬP-sē-ă	
polyuria (227)	pŏl-ē-Ū-rē-ă	
potassium (222)	pō-TĂ-sē ŭm	
pyelolithotomy (225)	pī-ĕ-lo-lĭ-THŎT-ō-mē	
pyelonephritis (230)	pī-ĕ-lō-nĕf-RĪ-tĭs	
pyuria (227)	pī-Ū-rē-ă	
reabsorption (222)	rē-ăb-SŎRP-shŭn	
renal angiography (232)	RĒ-năl ăn-jē-ŎG-ră-fē	
renal angioplasty (235)	RĒ-năl ĂN-jē-ō-plăs-tē	
renal artery (222)	RĒ-năl ĂR-tĕ-rē	
renal calculi (230)	RĒ-năl KĂL-kū-lī	
renal cell carcinoma (231)	RĒ-năl sĕl kăr-sĭ-NŌ-mă	
renal colic (225)	RĒ-năl KŎL-ĭk	
renal failure (231)	RĒ-năl FĀL-ūr	
renal hypertension (231)	RĒ-năl hī-pĕr-TĔN-shŭn	
renal ischemia (225)	RĒ-năl ĭs-KĒ-mē-ă	
renal pelvis (222)	RĒ-năl PĔL-vĭs	
renal transplantation (236)	RĒ-năl trăns-plăn-TĀ-shŭn	

7

TERM	PRONUNCIATION	MEANING
renal tubule (222)	RĒ-năl TOO-būl	
renal vein (222)	RĒ-năl vān	
renin (222)	RĒ-nĭn	
retrograde pyelogram (233)	RĔ-trō-grād PĪ-ĕ-lō-grăm	
secondary hypertension (231)	SĔ-kŏn-dă-rē hī-pĕr-TĔN-shŭn	
sodium (222)	SŌ-dē-ŭm	
stricture (225)	STRĬK-shŭr	
trigone (222)	TRĪ-gōn	
trigonitis (225)	trī-gō-NĪ-tĭs	
urea (222)	ū-RĒ-ă	
uremia (227)	ū-RĒ-mē-ă	
ureter (222)	ū-RĒ-tĕr or ŪR-ĕ-tĕr	
ureteroileostomy (225)	ū-rē-tĕr-ō-ĭl-ē-ŎS-tō-mē	
ureteroneocystostomy (236)	ū-rē-tĕr-ō-nē-ō-sĭs-TŎS-tō-mē	
ureteroplasty (225)	ū-rē-tĕr-ō-PLĂS-tē	
urethra (222)	ū-RĒ-thră	
urethral stricture (225)	ū-RĒ-thrăl STRĬK-shŭr	
urethritis (225)	ū-rē-THRĪ-tĭs	
urethroplasty (225)	ū-rē-thrō-PLĂS-tē	
uric acid (222)	Ū-rĭk ĂS-ĭd	
urinalysis (228)	ū-rĭn-ĂL-ĭ-sĭs	
urinary bladder (222)	ŪR-ĭ-năr-ē BLĂ-dĕr	
urinary catheterization (236)	ŪR-ĭ-năr-ē kă-thĕ-tĕr-ĭ-ZĀ-shŭn	
urinary incontinence (227)	ŪR-ĭ-năr-ē ĭn-KŎN-tĭ-nĕns	
urinary retention (227)	ŪR-ĭ-năr-ē rē-TĔN-shŭn	
urination (222)	ūr-ĭ-NĀ-shŭn	
vesicoureteral reflux (225)	vĕs-ĭ-kō-ū-RĒ-tĕr-ăl RĒ-flŭks	
voiding (222)	VOY-dĭng	
voiding cystourethrogram (233)	VOY-dĭng sĭs-tō-ū-RĒ-thrō-grăm	
Wilms tumor (231)	wĭlmz TOO-mŭr	

7

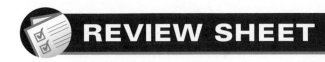

REVIEW SHEET

Write the meanings of the combining forms, suffixes, and prefixes in the spaces provided. Check your answers with the information in the chapter or in the *Glossary (Medical Word Parts—English)* at the end of this book.

Combining Forms

COMBINING FORM	MEANING	COMBINING FORM	MEANING
albumin/o		meat/o	
angi/o		natr/o	
azot/o		necr/o	
bacteri/o		nephr/o	
cali/o		noct/o	
calic/o		olig/o	
cyst/o		py/o	
dips/o		pyel/o	
glomerul/o		ren/o	
glycos/o		trigon/o	
hydr/o		ur/o	
isch/o		ureter/o	
kal/o		urethr/o	
ket/o		urin/o	
keton/o		vesic/o	
lith/o			

Suffixes

SUFFIX	MEANING	SUFFIX	MEANING
-ectasis		-pathy	
-ectomy		-plasty	
-emia		-poietin	
-esis		-ptosis	
-gram		-rrhea	
-lithiasis		-sclerosis	
-lithotomy		-stenosis	
-lysis		-stomy	
-megaly		-tomy	
-ole		-tripsy	
-osis		-uria	

7

Prefixes

PREFIX	MEANING	PREFIX	MEANING
a-, an-	_____	hypo-	_____
anti-	_____	peri-	_____
dia-	_____	poly-	_____
dys-	_____	retro-	_____
en-	_____		

Anatomic Terms

Match the locations/functions in Column I with the urinary system structures in Column II. Write the number of the correct structure in the blanks provided.

COLUMN I		COLUMN II
Tiny structure surrounding each glomerulus; receives filtered materials from blood.	_____	1. urethra
Tubes carrying urine from kidney to urinary bladder.	_____	2. cortex
Tubules leading from the glomerular capsule. Urine is formed there as water, sugar, and salts are reabsorbed into the bloodstream.	_____	3. glomerular capsule
		4. calices
Inner (middle) region of the kidney.	_____	5. renal pelvis
Muscular sac that serves as a reservoir for urine.	_____	6. glomerulus
Cup-like divisions of the renal pelvis that receive urine from the renal tubules.	_____	7. medulla
		8. renal tubules
Tube carrying urine from the bladder to the outside of the body.	_____	9. urinary bladder
Central urine-collecting basin in the kidney that narrows into the ureter.	_____	10. ureters
Collection of capillaries through which materials from the blood are filtered into the glomerular capsule.	_____	
Outer region of the kidney.	_____	

7

Give the medical terms for the following conditions related to urine or substances in urine.

1. sugar in urine _____

2. protein in urine _____

3. painful urination _____

4. scanty urination _____

5. bacteria in urine _____

6. excessive urination _____

7. blood in urine _____

8. ketones in urine _____

9. absence of urination _____

10. pus in urine _____

11. excessive urination at night _____

evolve *Please visit the Evolve website for additional exercises, games, and images related to this chapter.*

7

Female Reproductive System

CHAPTER GOALS

- Name and locate female reproductive organs and learn their combining forms.
- Explain how these organs and their hormones function in the normal processes of ovulation, menstruation, and pregnancy.
- Identify abnormal conditions of the female reproductive system and of the newborn.
- Describe important laboratory tests and clinical procedures used in gynecology and obstetrics, and recognize related abbreviations.
- Apply your new knowledge to understanding medical terms in their proper contexts, such as medical reports and records.

INTRODUCTION

Sexual reproduction is the union of the **ovum** (female sex cell) and the **sperm** (male sex cell). Each sex cell, known as a **gamete,** has half the number of chromosomes needed to create a new organism. In **fertilization,** nuclei of the two gamete unite to form a single nucleus with half of the chromosomes and genetic code from each parent.

Special organs called **gonads** in males and females produce the egg and sperm cells. The female gonads are the **ovaries,** and the male gonads are the **testes.** After an ovum leaves the ovary, it travels down one of two **fallopian tubes** leading to the **uterus** (womb). If **coitus** (copulation, sexual intercourse) has occurred and sperm cells travel into the fallopian tube, they can penetrate the ovum. This is **fertilization.** The fertilized ovum is then known as a **zygote.** After many cell divisions, a ball of cells forms, and the zygote is called an **embryo** (2 to 8 weeks) and finally a **fetus** (8 to 38 or 40 weeks). The period of development within the uterus is **gestation,** or **pregnancy.**

The female reproductive system consists of organs that produce **ova** (singular; ovum) and provide a place for the growth of the embryo. In addition, the female reproductive organs supply important hormones that contribute to the development of female secondary sex characteristics (body hair, breast development, structural changes in bones and fat).

The eggs, or ova, are present from birth in the female ovary but begin to mature and are released from the ovary in a 21- to 28-day cycle when secondary sex characteristics develop. The occurrence of the first cycle is called **menarche.** Menstrual cycles continue until **menopause,** when all eggs have been released, hormone production diminishes, and menstruation ends. If fertilization occurs during the years between menarche and menopause, the fertilized egg may grow and develop within the uterus. A new, blood vessel–rich organ called a **placenta** (connected to the embryo by the umbilical cord) develops to nourish the embryo, which implants in the uterine lining. Various hormones are secreted from the ovary and from the placenta to stimulate the expansion of the placenta. If fertilization does not occur, hormone changes result in shedding of the uterine lining, and bleeding, or **menstruation,** occurs.

The hormones of the ovaries, **estrogen** and **progesterone,** play important roles in the processes of menstruation and pregnancy, and in the development of secondary sex characteristics. The **pituitary gland,** located at the base of the brain, secretes other hormones that govern the reproductive functions of the ovaries, breasts, and uterus.

Gynecology is the study of the female reproductive system (organs, hormones, and diseases); **obstetrics** (Latin *obstetrix* means midwife) is a specialty concerned with pregnancy and the delivery of the fetus; and **neonatology** is the study of the care and treatment of the newborn.

ORGANS OF THE FEMALE REPRODUCTIVE SYSTEM

UTERUS, OVARIES, AND ASSOCIATED ORGANS

Label Figures 8-1 and 8-3 as you read the following description of the female reproductive system.

Figure 8-1 shows a side view of the female reproductive organs and their relationship to other organs in the pelvic cavity. The **ovaries** [1] (only one ovary is shown in this lateral view) are a pair of small almond-shaped organs located in the pelvis. The **fallopian tubes** [2] (only one is shown in this view) lead from each ovary to the **uterus** [3], which is a fibromuscular organ situated between the urinary bladder and the rectum. The uterus (womb) normally is the size and shape of a pear and is about 3 inches long in a nonpregnant

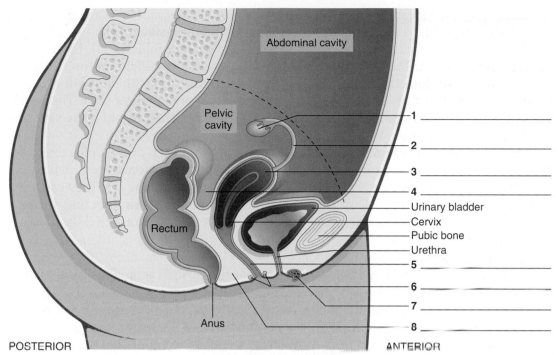

FIGURE 8-1   Organs of the female reproductive system, lateral view.

woman. Midway between the uterus and the rectum is a region in the abdominal cavity known as the **cul-de-sac** [4].

The **vagina** [5], a tubular structure, extends from the uterus to the exterior of the body. **Bartholin glands** [6] are two small, rounded glands on either side of the vaginal orifice. These glands produce a mucous secretion that lubricates the vagina. The **clitoris** [7] is an organ of sensitive, erectile tissue located anterior to the vaginal orifice and in front of the urethral meatus. The region between the vaginal orifice and the anus is the **perineum** [8].

The external genitalia of the female are collectively called the **vulva.** Figure 8-2 shows the various structures that are part of the vulva. The **labia majora,** the outer lips of the vagina, surround the smaller, inner lips, the **labia minora.** The **hymen,** a thin membrane partially covering the entrance to the vagina, is broken apart during the first episode of intercourse. The clitoris and Bartholin glands also are parts of the vulva.

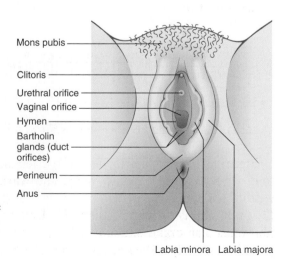

FIGURE 8-2   **Female external genitalia (vulva).** The mons pubis (Latin *mons*, mountain) is a pad of tissue overlying the pubic symphysis. After puberty it is covered with pubic hair.

Figure 8-3 shows an anterior view of the female reproductive system. Each **ovary** [1] is held in place on either side of the uterus by a **utero-ovarian ligament** [2].

Within each ovary are thousands of small sacs—the **ovarian follicles** [3]. Each follicle contains an **ovum** [4]. During **ovulation**, an ovum matures; its follicle ruptures through the surface and releases the ovum from the ovary. A ruptured follicle fills with a yellow, fat-like material. It is then called the **corpus luteum** [5], meaning yellow body. The corpus luteum secretes hormones (both estrogen and progesterone) that maintain the very first stages of pregnancy.

A **fallopian tube** [6] is about 5½ inches long and lies near each ovary. Collectively, the fallopian tubes, ovaries, and supporting ligaments are the **adnexa** (accessory structures) of the uterus. The finger-like ends of the fallopian tube are the **fimbriae** [7]. They catch the egg after its release from the ovary. **Cilia** (small hairs) line the fallopian tube and, through their motion, sweep the ovum along. It usually takes the ovum about 2 to 3 days to pass through the fallopian tube.

If sperm cells are present in the fallopian tube, fertilization may occur (Figure 8-4). If sperm cells are not present, the ovum remains unfertilized and eventually disintegrates.

The fallopian tubes, one on each side, lead into the **uterus** [8], a pear-shaped organ with muscular walls and a mucous membrane lining filled with a rich supply of blood vessels. The rounded upper portion of the uterus is the **fundus,** and the larger, central section is the **corpus** (body of the organ). The inner layer, a specialized epithelial mucosa of the uterus is the **endometrium** [9]; the middle, muscular layer of the uterine wall is the **myometrium** [10]; and the outer, membranous tissue layer is the **uterine serosa** [11], a lining that produces a watery, serum-like secretion. The outermost layer of an organ in the abdomen or thorax is known as a serosa.

The narrow, lowermost portion of the uterus is the **cervix** [12] (Latin *cervix* means neck). The cervical opening leads into a 3-inch-long muscular, mucosa-lined canal called the **vagina** [13], which opens to the outside of the body.

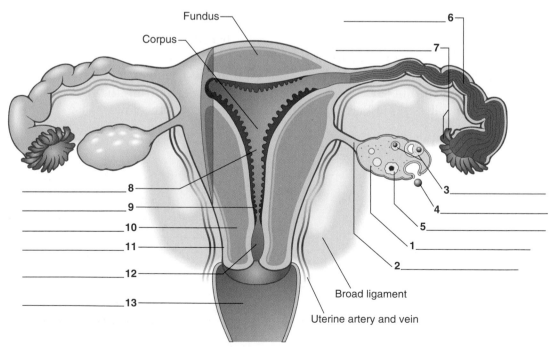

FIGURE 8-3 **Organs of the female reproductive system,** anterior view.

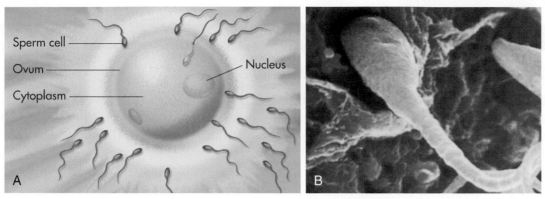

FIGURE 8-4   Fertilization. A, Once a single sperm cell has penetrated the ovum, others are prevented from entering. **B,** Electromicrograph showing a sperm cell penetrating an ovum.

THE BREAST (ACCESSORY ORGAN OF REPRODUCTION)

Label Figure 8-5 as you read the following description of breast structures.

The breasts, located on the upper anterior region of the chest, are composed mostly of **mammary glands.** The **glandular tissue** [1] contains milk glands or lobules that develop in response to hormones from the ovaries during puberty. The breasts also contain **fibrous** and **fatty tissue** [2], special **lactiferous** (milk-carrying) **ducts** [3], and **sinuses** (cavities) [4] that carry milk to the nipple, which has small openings for the ducts to release their milk. The breast nipple is the **mammary papilla** [5], and the dark pigmented area around the mammary papilla is the **areola** [6].

During pregnancy the hormones from the ovaries and the placenta stimulate glandular and other tissues in the breasts to their full development. After **parturition** (giving birth), hormones from the pituitary gland stimulate the normal secretion of milk **(lactation).**

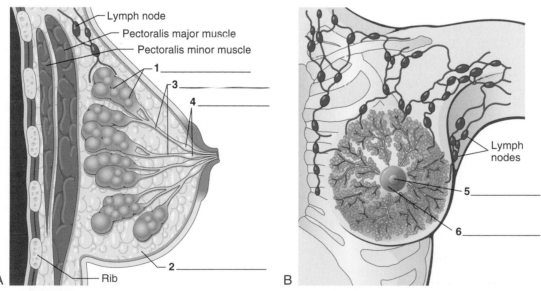

FIGURE 8-5   Views of the breast. A, Sagittal. **B,** Frontal. Notice the numerous lymph nodes.

MENSTRUATION AND PREGNANCY

MENSTRUAL CYCLE (FIGURE 8-6)

Menarche, or onset of menstruation with the first menstrual cycle, occurs at the time of puberty. An average menstrual cycle lasts for 28 days but may be shorter or longer, and cycles may be irregular in length. These days can be divided into four time periods, useful in describing the events of the cycle. The approximate time periods are as follows:

Days 1 to 5 (menstrual period)
Discharge of bloody fluid containing disintegrated endometrial cells, glandular secretions, and blood cells.

Days 6 to 12
After bleeding ceases, the endometrium begins to repair itself. The maturing follicle in the ovary releases **estrogen,** which aids in the repair. The ovum grows in the follicle during this period.

Days 13 and 14 (ovulatory period)
On about the 14th day of the cycle, the follicle ruptures and the egg leaves the ovary **(ovulation),** passing through the fallopian tube.

Days 15 to 28
The empty follicle fills with a yellow material and becomes the **corpus luteum.** The corpus luteum functions as an endocrine organ and secretes the hormone **progesterone** into the bloodstream. This hormone stimulates the building up of the lining of the uterus in anticipation of fertilization of the egg and pregnancy.

If fertilization does *not* occur, the corpus luteum in the ovary stops producing progesterone and regresses. At this time, lowered levels of progesterone and estrogen probably are responsible for some women's symptoms of depression, breast tenderness, and irritability before menstruation. The combination of these symptoms is known as **premenstrual syndrome (PMS).** After 2 days of decrease in hormones, the uterine endometrium breaks down, and the menstrual period begins (days 1 to 5).

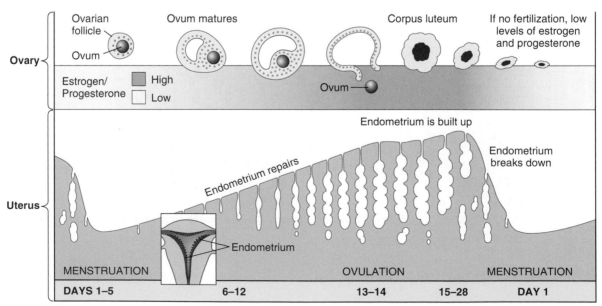

FIGURE 8-6 **The menstrual cycle.** *Tip:* Don't try to memorize this figure. Just get the big picture! In the **ovary,** as the ovum matures, hormone levels rise, culminating in ovulation (days 13 and 14). At the same time, in the **uterus,** the endometrium is building up in anticipation of pregnancy. If pregnancy does not occur, hormone levels drop and **menstruation** begins.

Note: Cycles vary in length, ranging from 21 to 42 days or longer. Ovulation typically occurs 14 days before the end of the cycle. A woman with a 42-day cycle ovulates on day 28, whereas a woman with a 21-day cycle ovulates on day 7.

PREGNANCY

If fertilization does occur in the fallopian tube, the fertilized egg travels to the uterus and implants in the uterine endometrium. The corpus luteum in the ovary continues to produce progesterone and estrogen. These hormones support the vascular and glandular development of the uterine lining.

The **placenta,** a vascular organ, now forms, attached to the uterine wall. The placenta is derived from maternal endometrium and from the **chorion,** the outermost membrane that surrounds the developing embryo. The **amnion,** the innermost of the embryonic membranes, holds the fetus suspended in an amniotic cavity surrounded by a fluid called the **amniotic fluid.** The amnion with its fluid also is known as the "bag of waters" or amniotic sac, which ruptures (breaks) during labor.

The maternal blood and the fetal blood never mix during pregnancy, but important nutrients, oxygen, and wastes are exchanged as the blood vessels of the fetus (coming from the umbilical cord) lie side by side with the mother's blood vessels in the placenta. Figure 8-7A and B shows implantation in the uterus and the embryo's relationship to the placenta and enveloping membranes (chorion and amnion).

As the placenta develops in the uterus, it produces its own hormone, **human chorionic gonadotropin (hCG).** When women test their urine with a pregnancy test kit, presence or absence of hCG confirms or rules out that they are pregnant. This hormone stimulates the corpus luteum to continue producing hormones until about the third month of pregnancy, when the placenta takes over the endocrine function and releases estrogen and progesterone. Progesterone maintains the development of the placenta. Low levels of progesterone can lead to spontaneous abortion in pregnant women and menstrual irregularities in nonpregnant women.

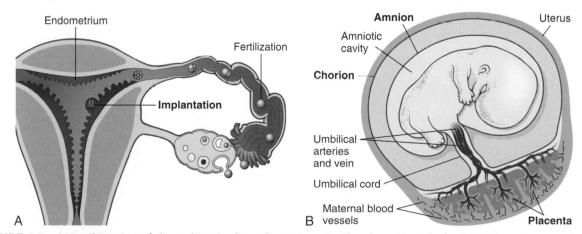

FIGURE 8-7 A, Implantation of the embryo in the endometrium. B, The placenta, with chorion and amnion membranes.

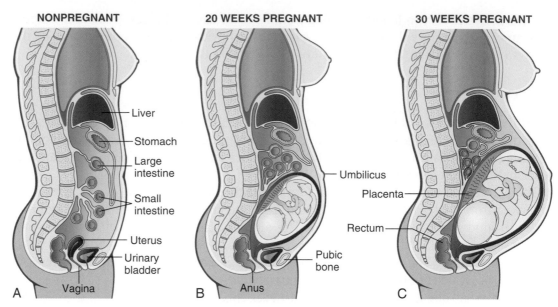

FIGURE 8-8   The growing uterus changes the pelvic anatomy during pregnancy, as shown here in sagittal section: **A,** nonpregnant woman, **B,** 20 weeks pregnant, **C,** 30 weeks pregnant.

The uterus normally lies within the pelvis. During pregnancy the uterus expands as the fetus grows, and the superior part rises out of the pelvic cavity to become an abdominal organ. By about 28 to 30 weeks, it occupies a large part of the abdominopelvic cavity and reaches the epigastric region (Figure 8-8).

The onset of true labor is marked by rhythmic contractions, dilation and thinning (effacement) of the cervix, and a discharge of bloody mucus from the cervix and vagina (the "show"). In a normal delivery position, the baby's head appears first (**cephalic presentation**). After vaginal delivery of the baby, the umbilical cord is cut and the placenta follows (Figure 8-9). Figure 8-10A and B shows photographs of a newborn and the placenta with attached cord, minutes after birth. The expelled placenta is the **afterbirth.**

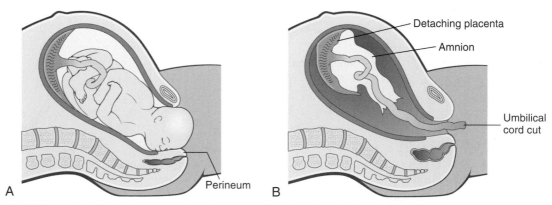

FIGURE 8-9   A, Cephalic presentation ("crowning") of the fetus during delivery from the vaginal (birth) canal. **B,** Usually within 15 minutes after parturition (birth), the placenta separates from the uterine wall. Forceful contractions expel the placenta and attached membranes, now called the **afterbirth.** The three phases of labor are (1) dilation of the cervix, (2) expulsion or birth of the infant, and (3) delivery of the placenta.

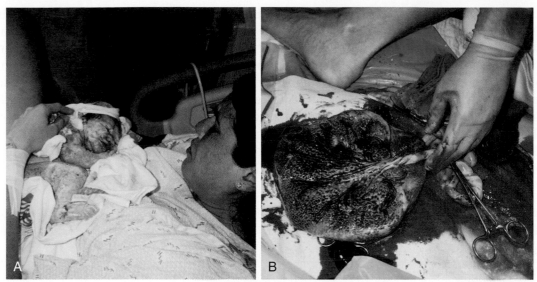

FIGURE 8-10   A, My newborn granddaughter, Beatrix Bess (Bebe) Thompson, and her mother, Dr. Elizabeth Chabner Thompson, minutes after Bebe's birth. Notice that Bebe's skin is covered with **vernix caseosa,** a mixture of a fatty secretion from fetal sebaceous (oil) glands and dead skin. The vernix protects the fetus's delicate skin from abrasions, chapping, and hardening as a result of being bathed in amniotic fluid. **B,** The **placenta and umbilical cord** just after expulsion from the uterus.

HORMONAL INTERACTIONS

The events of menstruation and pregnancy depend on hormones not only from the ovaries (estrogen and progesterone) but also from the **pituitary gland.** The pituitary gland secretes **follicle-stimulating hormone (FSH)** and **luteinizing hormone (LH)** after the onset of menstruation. As their levels rise in the bloodstream, FSH and LH stimulate maturation of the ovum and ovulation. After ovulation, LH in particular influences the maintenance of the corpus luteum and its production of estrogen and progesterone.

During pregnancy, the high levels of estrogen and progesterone from the ovary and placenta cause the pituitary gland to stop producing FSH and LH. Therefore, while a woman is pregnant, additional eggs do not mature and ovulation cannot occur. Oral contraceptives (birth control pills) work in the same way. ◣

Another female birth control method is an **IUD (intrauterine device).** A health care professional inserts the IUD, a small device designed to remain inside the uterus. It works by preventing implantation of the embryo. Birth control pills and an IUD do not protect a woman against sexually transmitted infections such as that caused by HIV. See page 290 for a table of contraceptive choices and their features.

When all of the ova are released and secretion of estrogen from the ovaries lessens, **menopause** begins. Menopause signals the gradual ending of menstrual cycles. Premature menopause occurs before age 40, whereas delayed menopause occurs after age 55. Artificial menopause occurs if the ovaries are removed by surgery or made nonfunctional as a result of radiation therapy or some forms of chemotherapy.

 How Do Birth Control Pills Work?

Birth control pills contain a combination of estrogen and progesterone or progesterone only. When taken as directed, they increase the levels of these hormones in the woman's bloodstream. High levels of estrogen and progesterone send a signal to the pituitary gland to shut down its secretion of follicle-stimulating hormone (FSH) and luteinizing hormone (LH). When these hormones are blocked, the ovaries will not release eggs, and pregnancy cannot occur. During pregnancy, levels of estrogen and progesterone also are high—and the ovaries will not release eggs then either! So birth control pills effectively fool the body into "thinking" that the woman is pregnant, and her ovaries stop producing eggs.

During menopause, when estrogen levels fall, the most common signs and symptoms are hot flashes (temperature regulation in the brain is disturbed), insomnia, and vaginal atrophy (lining of the vagina dries and thins, predisposing the affected woman to irritation and discomfort during sexual intercourse). **Hormone replacement therapy (HRT),** given orally or as a transdermal patch or vaginal ring, relieves these symptoms of menopause and delays the development of weak bones (osteoporosis). HRT use may be associated with an increased risk of breast cancer, endometrial cancer, stroke, or heart attack. This therapy should be used only after careful consideration of potential risks and benefits.

Table 8-1 reviews the various female hormones, including the sites where they are produced, their target organs, and their effect on the body.

TABLE 8-1	FEMALE HORMONES		
HORMONE	**PRODUCTION SITE(S)**	**TARGET ORGAN**	**EFFECT**
FSH	Pituitary gland	Ovary	Stimulates maturation of the ovum
LH	Pituitary gland	Ovary	Stimulates ovulation
Estrogen	Ovary Placenta (during pregnancy)	Uterus	Builds up the endometrial lining
Progesterone	Ovary (corpus luteum) Placenta (during pregnancy)	Uterus	Sustains uterine lining and placenta during pregnancy
hCG	Placenta	Ovary (corpus luteum)	Sustains pregnancy

FSH, follicle-stimulating hormone; hCG, human chorionic gonadotropin; LH, luteinizing hormone.

VOCABULARY

The following list reviews many of the new terms introduced in the text. Short definitions reinforce your understanding of the terms.

adnexa uteri	Fallopian tubes, ovaries, and supporting ligaments.
amnion	Innermost membranous sac surrounding the developing fetus.
areola	Dark-pigmented area surrounding the breast nipple.
Bartholin glands	Small mucus-secreting exocrine glands at the vaginal orifice (opening to outside of the body). Caspar Bartholin was a Danish anatomist who described the glands in 1637.
cervix	Lower, neck-like portion of the uterus.
chorion	Outermost layer of the two membranes surrounding the embryo; it forms the fetal part of the placenta.
clitoris	Organ of sensitive erectile tissue anterior to the opening of the female urethra.
coitus	Sexual intercourse; copulation. Pronunciation is KŌ-ĭ-tŭs.
corpus luteum	Empty ovarian follicle that secretes progesterone after release of the egg cell; literally means yellow (luteum) body (corpus).
cul-de-sac	Region in the lower abdomen, midway between the rectum and the uterus.

embryo	Stage in prenatal development from 2 to 8 weeks.
endometrium	Inner, mucous membrane lining of the uterus.
estrogen	Hormone produced by the ovaries; promotes female secondary sex characteristics.
fallopian tube	One of a pair of ducts through which the ovum travels to the uterus; also called an **oviduct.** The tubes were named for Gabriello Fallopia, an Italian anatomist.
fertilization	Union of the sperm cell and ovum from which the embryo develops.
fetus	Stage in prenatal development from 8 to 39 or 40 weeks.
fimbriae (*singular*: fimbria)	Finger- or fringe-like projections at the end of the fallopian tubes.
follicle-stimulating hormone (FSH)	Secreted by the pituitary gland to stimulate maturation of the egg cell (ovum).
gamete	Male or female sexual reproductive cell; sperm cell or ovum.
genitalia	Reproductive organs; also called genitals.
gestation	Period from fertilization of the ovum to birth.
gonad	Female or male reproductive organ that produces sex cells and hormones; ovary or testis.
gynecology	Study of the female reproductive organs including the breasts.
human chorionic gonadotropin (hCG)	Hormone produced by the placenta to sustain pregnancy by stimulating (-tropin) the ovaries to produce estrogen and progesterone.
hymen	Mucous membrane partially or completely covering the opening to the vagina.
labia	Lips of the vagina; labia majora are the larger, outermost lips, and labia minora are the smaller, innermost lips.
lactiferous ducts	Tubes that carry milk within the breast.
luteinizing hormone (LH)	Secreted by the pituitary gland to promote ovulation.
mammary papilla	Nipple of the breast. A **papilla** is any small nipple-shaped projection.
menarche	Beginning of the first menstrual period and ability to reproduce.
menopause	Gradual ending of menstruation.
menstruation	Monthly shedding of the uterine lining. The flow of blood and tissue normally discharged during menstruation is called the **menses** (Latin *mensis* means month).
myometrium	Muscle layer of the uterus.
neonatology	Branch of medicine that studies the disorders and care of the newborn (neonate).
obstetrics	Branch of medicine concerned with pregnancy and childbirth.
orifice	An opening.
ovarian follicle	Developing sac enclosing each ovum within the ovary. Only about 400 of these sacs mature in a woman's lifetime.
ovary	One of a pair of female organs (gonads) on each side of the pelvis. Ovaries are almond-shaped, about the size of large walnuts, and produce egg cells (ova) and hormones.

8

ovulation	Release of the ovum from the ovary.
ovum (*plural:* ova)	Mature egg cell (female gamete). Ova develop from immature egg cells called oocytes.
parturition	Act of giving birth.
perineum	In females, the area between the anus and the vagina.
pituitary gland	Endocrine gland at the base of the brain. It produces hormones that stimulate the ovaries. The pituitary gland also regulates other endocrine organs.
placenta	Vascular organ attached to the uterine wall during pregnancy. It permits the exchange of oxygen, nutrients, and fetal waste products between mother and fetus.
pregnancy	Condition in a female of having a developing embryo and fetus in her uterus for about 40 weeks.
progesterone	Hormone produced by the corpus luteum in the ovary and the placenta of pregnant women.
puberty	Point in the life cycle at which secondary sex characteristics appear and gametes are produced.
uterine serosa	Outermost layer surrounding the uterus.
uterus	Hollow, pear-shaped muscular female organ in which the embryo and fetus develop, and from which menstruation occurs. The upper portion is the fundus; the middle portion is the corpus; and the lowermost, neck-like portion is the cervix (see Figure 8-3, page 260).
vagina	Muscular, mucosa-lined canal extending from the uterus to the exterior of the body.
vulva	External female genitalia; includes the labia, hymen, clitoris, and vaginal orifice.
zygote	Stage in prenatal development from fertilization and implantation up to 2 weeks.

TERMINOLOGY

Write the meanings of the medical terms in the spaces provided.

COMBINING FORMS

COMBINING FORM	MEANING	TERMINOLOGY	MEANING
amni/o	amnion	amniocentesis _____	
		amniotic fluid _____ *Produced by fetal membranes and the fetus.*	
bartholin/o	Bartholin gland	bartholinitis _____ *A Bartholin cyst is a fluid-filled sac caused by blockage of a duct from the Bartholin gland. If bacterial infection occurs, an abscess may form.*	

COMBINING FORM	MEANING	TERMINOLOGY	MEANING
cervic/o	cervix, neck	endo<u>cervic</u>itis _____	
chori/o, chorion/o	chorion	<u>chorion</u>ic _____	
colp/o	vagina	<u>colp</u>oscopy _____	
culd/o	cul-de-sac	<u>culd</u>ocentesis _____ *A needle is placed through the posterior wall of the vagina and fluid is withdrawn for diagnostic purposes.*	
episi/o	vulva	<u>episi</u>otomy _____ *An incision through the skin of the perineum enlarges the vaginal orifice for delivery. The incision is repaired by* **perineorrhaphy.**	
galact/o	milk	<u>galact</u>orrhea _____ *Abnormal, persistent discharge of milk, commonly seen with pituitary gland tumors.*	
gynec/o	woman, female	<u>gynec</u>omastia _____ *Enlargement of breasts in a male. It often occurs with puberty or aging, or the condition can be drug-related.*	
hyster/o	uterus, womb	<u>hyster</u>ectomy _____ ***Total abdominal hysterectomy (TAH)** is removal of the entire uterus (including the cervix) through an abdominal incision (Figure 8-11). **Vaginal hysterectomy (VH)** is removal through the vagina. **Laparoscopic supracervical hysterectomy** (see Figure 8-11) is a partial hysterectomy that preserves the cervix.* <u>hyster</u>oscopy _____ *A gynecologist uses an endoscope (passed through the vagina and cervix) to view the uterine cavity.*	

8

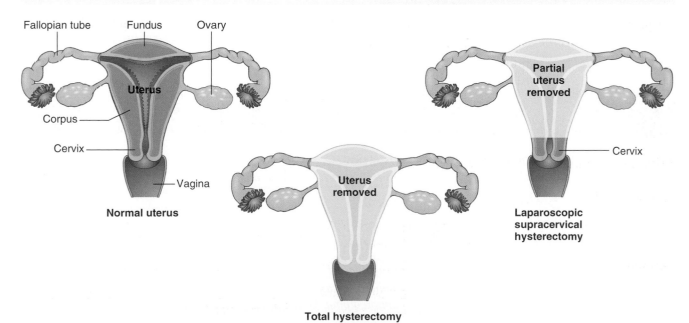

FIGURE 8-11 Normal uterus and hysterectomies. Total hysterectomy is removal of the entire uterus—fundus, corpus, and cervix. This may be performed via an abdominal incision or vaginally. **Laparoscopic supracervical hysterectomy** is removal of the top portion of the uterus (above the cervix), leaving the cervix intact. Three to five small incisions are made in the abdomen and the uterus is removed via laparoscope. Robotic hysterectomy (da Vinci surgery) is another option using small incisions, three-dimensional vision, and a magnified view of the surgical site.

COMBINING FORM	MEANING	TERMINOLOGY	MEANING
lact/o	milk	lactation _____ *The normal secretion of milk.*	
mamm/o	breast	inframammary _____ *Infra- means below.*	
		mammoplasty _____ *Includes reduction and augmentation (enlargement) operations.*	
mast/o	breast	mastitis _____ *Usually caused by streptococcal or staphylococcal infection.*	
		mastectomy _____ *Mastectomy procedures are discussed under carcinoma of the breast (see page 278).*	
men/o	menses, menstruation	amenorrhea _____ *Absence of menses for 6 months or for more than three of the patient's normal menstrual cycles.*	
		dysmenorrhea _____	
		oligomenorrhea _____ *Infrequent menstrual periods or scanty menses.*	
		menorrhagia _____ *Abnormally heavy or long menstrual periods.* **Fibroids** *(see page 276) are a leading cause of menorrhagia.*	
metr/o, metri/o	uterus	metrorrhagia _____ *Bleeding between menses. Possible causes of metrorrhagia include ectopic pregnancy, cervical polyps, and ovarian and uterine tumors.*	
		menometrorrhagia _____ *Excessive uterine bleeding during and between menstrual periods.*	
my/o, myom/o	muscle, muscle tumor	myometrium _____	
		myomectomy _____ *Removal of fibroids (myomas) from the uterus.*	
nat/i	birth	neonatal _____	
obstetr/o	pregnancy and childbirth	obstetrics _____ *From the Latin* obstetrix, *midwife.*	
o/o	egg	oogenesis _____	
		oocyte _____ *Immature ovum.*	
oophor/o	ovary	oophorectomy _____ *Oophor/o means to bear (phor/o) eggs (o/o). In a bilateral oophorectomy, both ovaries are removed.*	
ov/o	egg	ovum _____ *Mature egg cell.*	
ovari/o	ovary	ovarian _____	

8

COMBINING FORM	MEANING	TERMINOLOGY	MEANING
ovul/o	egg	anovulatory	
perine/o	perineum	perineorrhaphy	
phor/o	to bear	oophoritis	
salping/o	fallopian tubes	salpingectomy	
		Figure 8-12 shows a total hysterectomy with bilateral salpingo-oophorectomy (BSO).	
uter/o	uterus	uterine prolapse	
vagin/o	vagina	vaginal orifice	
		An orifice is an opening.	
		vaginitis	
		Bacteria and yeasts (usually Candida) commonly cause this infection. Use of antibiotic therapy may cause loss of normal vaginal bacteria, resulting in an environment allowing yeast to grow.	
vulv/o	vulva	vulvovaginitis	
		vulvodynia	
		Chronic pain (with no identifiable cause) that affects the vulvar area (labia, clitoris, and vaginal opening).	

SUFFIXES

SUFFIX	MEANING	TERMINOLOGY	MEANING
-arche	beginning	menarche	
-cyesis	pregnancy	pseudocyesis	
		Pseudo- means false. No pregnancy exists, but physical changes such as weight gain and amenorrhea occur.	
-gravida	pregnant	primigravida	
		A woman during her first pregnancy (primi- means first). Gravida also is used to designate a pregnant woman, often followed by a number to indicate the number of pregnancies (gravida 1, 2, 3).	

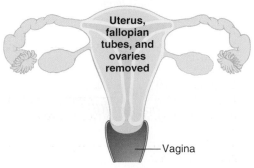

Uterus, fallopian tubes, and ovaries removed

Vagina

FIGURE 8-12   Total hysterectomy with bilateral salpingo-oophorectomy.

SUFFIX	MEANING	TERMINOLOGY	MEANING
-parous	bearing, bringing forth	primiparous _____ *An adjective describing a woman who has given birth to at least one child.* **Para** *also is used as a noun, often followed by a number to indicate the number of deliveries after the 20th week of gestation (para 1, para 2, para 3). When a woman arrives in the birthing facility, her gravidity and parity are important facts to include in the medical and surgical history. For example, G2P2 is medical shorthand for a woman who has had 2 pregnancies and 2 deliveries.*	
-rrhea	discharge	leukorrhea _____ *This vaginal discharge is normal or becomes more yellow (purulent or pus-containing) as a sign of infection.*	
		menorrhea _____	
-salpinx	fallopian (uterine) tube	pyosalpinx _____	
-tocia	labor, birth	dystocia _____	
		oxytocia _____ *Oxy- means sharp or quick. The pituitary gland releases* **oxytocin,** *which stimulates the pregnant uterus to contract (labor begins). It also stimulates milk secretion from mammary glands.*	
-version	act of turning	cephalic version _____ *The fetus turns so that the head is the body part closest to the cervix (version can occur spontaneously or can be performed by the obstetrician).* **Fetal presentation** *is the manner in which the fetus appears to the examiner during delivery. A* **breech presentation** *is buttocks first, or feet first in a footling breech; a* **cephalic presentation** *is head first.*	

PREFIXES

PREFIX	MEANING	TERMINOLOGY	MEANING
dys-	painful	dyspareunia _____ (dĭs-pă-ROO-nē-ă.) *Pareunia means sexual intercourse.*	
endo-	within	endometritis _____ *Usually caused by a bacterial infection.*	
in-	in	involution of the uterus _____ *Vol- means to roll. The uterus returns to its normal nonpregnant size.*	
intra-	within	intrauterine device _____ *Figure 8-13A shows an IUD.*	

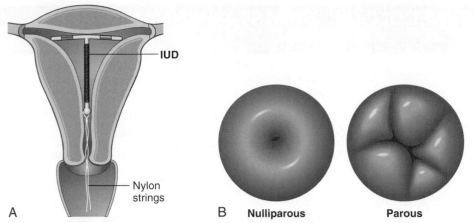

FIGURE 8-13   A, Intrauterine device (IUD) in place to prevent implantation of a fertilized egg. **B,** The cervix of a **nulliparous** woman (the os, or opening, is small and perfectly round) and the cervix of a **parous** woman (the os is wide and irregular). These views would be visible under **colposcopic examination**.

PREFIX	MEANING	TERMINOLOGY	MEANING
multi-	many	multipara	
		multigravida	
		A woman who has been pregnant more than once.	
nulli-	no, not, none	nulligravida	
		nullipara	
		Para 0. Figure 8-13B shows the cervix of a nulliparous woman and the cervix of a parous woman (who has had a vaginal delivery).	
pre-	before	prenatal	
primi-	first	primipara	
retro-	backward	retroversion	
		The uterus is abnormally tilted backward. This occurs in 30% of women.	

8

PATHOLOGY: GYNECOLOGIC, BREAST, PREGNANCY, AND NEONATAL

GYNECOLOGIC

Uterus

carcinoma of the cervix

Malignant cells within the cervix (cervical cancer).

Infection with **human papillomavirus (HPV)** is the most important cause of and risk factor for cervical cancer. Other factors that may act together with HPV to increase the risk of developing cervical cancer include cigarette smoking, having multiple sexual partners, and having a weakened immune system (e.g., patients with AIDS). HPV infection is one of the most common sexually transmitted infections in the world. Some types of HPV cause **genital warts** (benign growths on the vulva, cervix, vagina, or anus), whereas others cause cancer, especially HPV types 16 and 18.

Although most HPV infections do not progress to cervical cancer, the risk of developing cancer increases as Pap tests (see page 282) become abnormal and biopsies reveal **dysplasia** (abnormal cell growth), or more seriously, **carcinoma in situ (CIS),** a localized form of cancer (Figure 8-14). Local resection **(conization)** may be necessary to treat CIS and prevent development of invasive cancer. Figure 8-15 shows a normal cervix and one with cervical cancer.

Surgical treatment for cervical cancer requires **radical (complete) hysterectomy,** in which the entire uterus with ligaments, supportive tissues, and the top one third of the vagina are removed. Radiation therapy and chemotherapy are used to treat disease that has spread beyond the uterus, into the pelvis, and to distant organs.

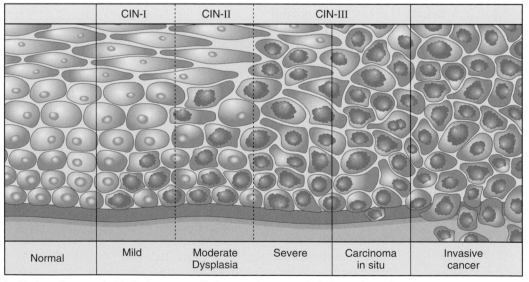

	CIN-I	CIN-II	CIN-III	
Normal	Mild	Moderate Dysplasia	Severe	Carcinoma in situ	Invasive cancer

FIGURE 8-14   Preinvasive neoplastic lesions are called **cervical intraepithelial neoplasia (CIN).** Pathologists diagnose such lesions from a **Pap test** (microscopic examination of cells scraped from cervical epithelium) and grade them as CIN I to CIN III.

HPV Vaccine

HPV vaccines are given in a series of three shots over 6 months to protect females and males against HPV infections. Girls can get this vaccine to prevent cervical cancer, vulvar and vaginal cancer, and genital warts. Boys get the vaccine to prevent anal cancer and genital warts.

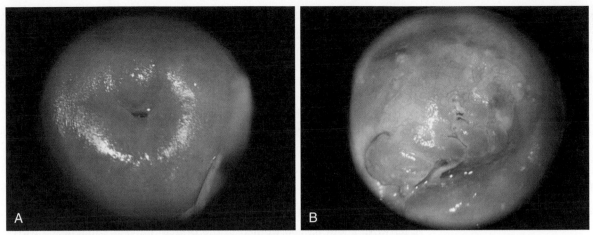

FIGURE 8-15   Normal cervix (A) and **cervix with cervical cancer** (B) as seen on **colposcopy**.

cervicitis	**Inflammation of the cervix.**

This condition can become chronic because the lining of the cervix is not renewed each month as is the uterine lining during menstruation.

Bacteria such as *Chlamydia trachomatis* and *Neisseria gonorrhoeae* commonly cause cervicitis. Acute cervicitis, marked by **cervical erosions** or ulcerations, appears as raw, red patches on the cervical mucosa. **Leukorrhea** (clear, white, or yellow pus-filled vaginal discharge) also is a sign of cervical erosion.

After the presence of malignancy has been excluded (by Pap test or biopsy), **cryocauterization** (destroying tissue by freezing) of the eroded area and treatment with antibiotics may be indicated.

carcinoma of the endometrium (endometrial cancer)	**Malignant tumor of the uterine lining (adenocarcinoma).**

The most common sign of endometrial cancer is postmenopausal bleeding. This malignancy occurs more often in women exposed to high levels of estrogen, either from exogenous estrogen (pills) or estrogen-producing tumors or with obesity (estrogen is produced by fat tissue) and in nulliparous women. Physicians perform endometrial biopsy, hysteroscopy, and **dilation** or **dilatation** (widening the cervical canal) and **curettage** (scraping the inner lining of the uterus) for diagnosis. When the cancer is confined to the uterus, surgery (hysterectomy and bilateral salpingo-oophorectomy) is curative. Radiation oncologists administer radiation therapy as additional treatment.

endometriosis	**Endometrial tissue located outside the uterus.**

Endometrial tissue may be found in ovaries, fallopian tubes, supporting ligaments or small intestine, causing inflammation and scar tissue. When the endometrium sheds and bleeds in its monthly cycle, it may cause dysmenorrhea and pelvic pain. Infertility (inability to become pregnant) and dyspareunia may also occur. Most cases are the result of growth of bits of menstrual endometrium that have passed backward through the **lumen** (opening) of the fallopian tube and into the peritoneal cavity. Often, when disease affects the ovaries, large blood-filled cysts (endometriomas, or "**chocolate cysts**") develop. Treatment ranges from symptomatic relief of pain and hormonal drugs that suppress the menstrual cycle to surgical removal of ectopic endometrial tissue and hysterectomy.

8

fibroids

Benign tumors in the uterus.

Fibroids, also called **leiomyomata** or **leiomyomas** (lei/o = smooth, my/o = muscle, and -oma = tumor), are composed of fibrous tissue and muscle. If fibroids grow too large and cause symptoms such as metrorrhagia, pelvic pain, or menorrhagia, hysterectomy or myomectomy is indicated. Fibroid ablation (destruction) without surgery may be accomplished by **uterine artery embolization (UAE),** in which tiny pellets (acting as emboli) are injected into a uterine artery, blocking the blood supply to fibroids, causing them to shrink. Figure 8-16A and B shows the location of uterine fibroids.

Ovaries

ovarian carcinoma (cancer)

Malignant tumor of the ovary (adenocarcinoma).

Each year, about 22,000 women in the United States are diagnosed with ovarian cancer. Two types of ovarian cancer are most common: **serous** (clear fluid) and **mucinous** (thick, pasty fluid) **cystic adenocarcinomas.** The tumor usually is discovered in an advanced stage as an abdominal mass and may produce few symptoms in its early stages. In most patients, the disease metastasizes beyond the ovary before diagnosis and often causes **ascites** (accumulation of fluid in the abdominal cavity). Treatment consists of total abdominal hysterectomy, bilateral salpingo-oophorectomy, and removal of the omentum, which often contains deposits of tumor, followed by chemotherapy. A protein marker produced by tumor cells, CA 125, can be measured in the bloodstream to assess effectiveness of treatment.

Inherited mutations (changes) in genes greatly increase the risk of developing ovarian and breast cancer. These mutations are **BRCA1** and **BRCA2** (short for breast cancer 1 and breast cancer 2). Women with a strong family history of ovarian cancer (with multiple members of the family affected) may seek genetic counseling to determine if they should be tested for these inherited defects. **Prophylactic** (preventive) **oophorectomy** significantly reduces the odds of developing ovarian cancer if a woman is at high risk.

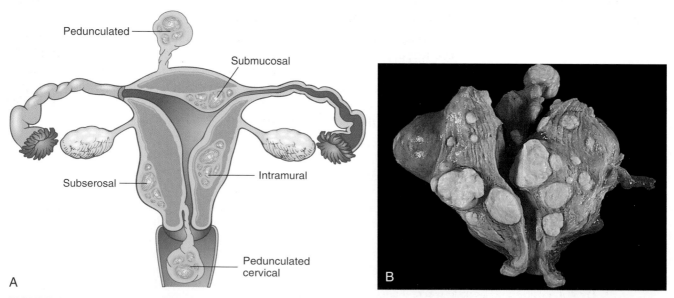

FIGURE 8-16   A, Location of uterine fibroids (leiomyomas). Pedunculated growths protrude on stalks. A **subserosal** mass lies under the serosal (outermost) layer of the uterus. A **submucosal** leiomyoma grows under the mucosal (innermost) layer. **Intramural** (mural means wall) masses arise within the muscular uterine wall. **B, Fibroids** shown after hysterectomy.

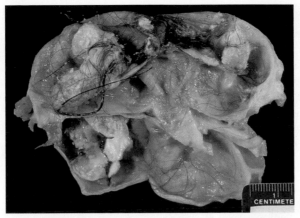

FIGURE 8-17   **Dermoid cyst of the ovary** with hair, skin, and teeth. *(Courtesy Dr. Elizabeth Chabner Thompson.)*

8

ovarian cysts	**Collections of fluid within sacs (cysts) in the ovary.**

Some cysts are benign and lined by typical cells of the ovary. These cysts originate in unruptured ovarian follicles (**follicular cysts**) or in follicles that have ruptured and have immediately been sealed (**luteal cysts**). Other cysts are malignant and lined with atypical or tumor cells (**cystadenocarcinomas**). Physicians decide to remove these cysts to distinguish between benign and malignant tumors.

Dermoid cysts contain a variety of cell types, including skin, hair, teeth, and cartilage, and arise from immature egg cells in the ovary. Because of the strange assortment of tissue types in the tumor (Figure 8-17), this tumor often is called a **benign cystic teratoma** (terat/o = monster) or a **mature teratoma.** Surgical removal of the cyst cures the condition. Cysts are bilateral 15% of the time.

Fallopian Tubes

pelvic inflammatory disease (PID)	**Inflammation and infection of organs in the pelvic region; salpingitis, oophoritis, endometritis, endocervicitis.**

The leading causes of PID are **sexually transmitted infections.** Repetitive episodes of these infections lead to formation of adhesions and scarring within the fallopian tubes. After PID, women have an increased risk of ectopic pregnancy and infertility. Signs and symptoms include fever, vaginal discharge, abdominal pain in the left and right lower quadrants (LLQ and RLQ), and tenderness to **palpation** (examining by touch) of the cervix. Antibiotics treat PID.

Sexually Transmitted Infections (STIs)

Examples of bacterial and viral STIs in women are:
- **gonorrhea** (gonococcal bacteria)
- **chlamydial infection** (chlamydial bacteria)
- **syphilis** (spirochete bacteria)
- **genital herpes** (herpes simplex virus—HSV)
- **HPV infection and genital warts** (human papillomavirus)

More information on STIs in women and men is on page 322.

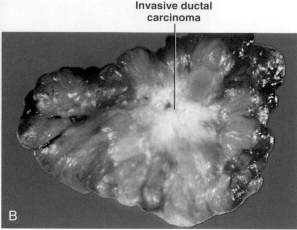

Invasive ductal
carcinoma

FIGURE 8-18   A, *Arrows* in **mammogram** point to invasive carcinoma of the breast. A dense white fragment of calcium is seen at 2 o'clock in the mass; calcifications like this frequently are a sign of cancer. **B,** Cut section of **invasive ductal carcinoma** of the breast.

Breast

**carcinoma of the breast
(breast cancer)**

Malignant tumor of the breast (arising from milk glands and ducts).

The most common type of breast cancer is **invasive ductal carcinoma.** Figure 8-18A shows the tumor on a mammogram. Figure 8-18B shows a cut section of an invasive ductal carcinoma. Other histopathologic (histo- means tissue) types are **lobular** and **medullary carcinoma** of the breast.

Breast cancer spreads first to lymph nodes in the axilla (armpit) adjacent to the affected breast and then to the skin and chest wall. From the lymph nodes it also may metastasize to other body organs, including bone, liver, lung, and brain. The diagnosis is first established by biopsy, either needle aspiration, or surgical removal of the specimen (solid mass or area of microcalcification). A **stereotactic core needle biopsy** is performed with the help of mammography for guidance.

For small primary tumors, the lump with immediately surrounding tissue can be removed (**lumpectomy**). To determine whether the tumor has spread to lymph nodes, a **sentinel node biopsy (SNB)** is performed. For this procedure, a blue dye or a radioisotope is injected into the tumor site and tracks to the axillary (underarm) lymph nodes. See Figure 8-19. After lumpectomy, radiation therapy to the breast and to any involved lymph nodes then follows, to kill remaining tumor cells.

An alternative surgical procedure is **mastectomy** (Figure 8-20A), which is removal of the entire breast. After either lumpectomy or mastectomy if lymph nodes are involved, adjuvant (aiding) chemotherapy is given to prevent recurrence of the tumor. Breast reconstruction is an option after mastectomy. See Figure 8-20B.

After surgery, further treatment may be indicated to prevent recurrence. To determine which treatment is best, it is important to test the breast cancer tumor for the presence of **estrogen receptors (ERs).** Two thirds of breast cancers are ER-positive (ER$^+$). These receptor proteins indicate that the tumor will respond to hormonal therapy. If metastases should subsequently develop, this information will be valuable in selecting further treatment. There are two types of drugs that block the effects of estrogen and thereby kill ER-positive breast cancer cells.

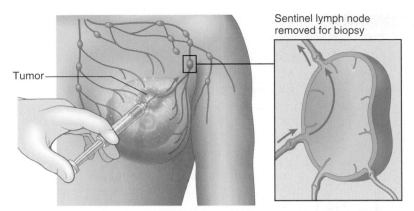

FIGURE 8-19   Sentinel node biopsy. After injection of dye or radioisotope, its path is visualized and the sentinel (first) lymph node is identified. It is the one most likely to contain a tumor if cells have left the breast. The sentinel node is removed and biopsied. If it is negative for tumor cells, the breast cancer has not spread.

Drugs of the first type directly block the ER reception. An example is **tamoxifen.** Drugs of the second type block the production of estrogen by inhibiting the enzyme, aromatase. These **aromatase inhibitors** are particularly useful in treating postmenopausal women. Examples are anastrozole (Arimidex) and letrozole (Femara).

A second receptor protein, **HER2,** is found in some breast cancers and signals a high risk of tumor recurrence. **Herceptin,** an antibody that binds to and blocks HER2, is effective in stopping growth when used with chemotherapy. A new drug (T-DMI), when combined with Herceptin is effective in treating HER2–positive advanced breast cancer. **Triple-negative tumors** lack estrogen, progesterone, and HER2 and are rapidly growing but respond well to chemotherapy.

Testing for hereditary mutations *BRCA1, BRCA2,* and *PALB2* (partner and localizer of *BRCA1* and *BRCA2*) is advised for women with a strong family history of breast cancer. Some women who test positively for the breast cancer genes elect to have prophylactic (preventive) bilateral mastectomy with reconstruction, to eliminate risk of developing a new breast cancer. See the ***In Person: Prophylactic Mastectomy*** story on page 291.

8

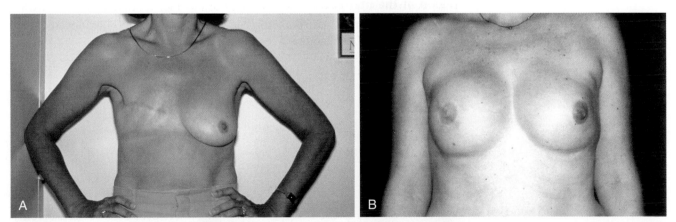

FIGURE 8-20   A, Surgical scar, mastectomy, right breast. A **modified radical mastectomy** removes the breast and axillary lymph nodes (usually 20 to 30 nodes). **B, Reconstruction of right breast after skin-sparing mastectomy.** A gel silicone implant was used. At a second operation, local tissue was manipulated to create the semblance of a nipple-areola complex. The procedure was completed by tattooing color around the nipple. In this patient, the left breast tissue was removed prophylactically and a silicone implant was inserted through an inframammary incision. *(A, Courtesy Dr. Elizabeth Chabner Thompson.)*

fibrocystic breast disease

Numerous small sacs of fluid surrounded by dense strands of fibrous tissue in the breast.

Women with this common benign condition notice a nodular (lumpy) consistency of the breast, often associated with premenstrual tenderness and fullness. Mammography and surgical biopsy are often indicated to differentiate fibrocystic changes from carcinoma of the breast.

PREGNANCY

abruptio placentae

Premature separation of the normally implanted placenta.

Abruptio placentae (Latin *ab*, away from; *ruptus*, ruptured) occurs because of trauma, such as a fall, or may be secondary to vascular insufficiency resulting from hypertension or preeclampsia (see page 281). Signs and symptoms of acute abruption include sudden searing (burning) abdominal pain and bleeding. It is an obstetric emergency.

ectopic pregnancy

Implantation of the fertilized egg in any site other than the normal uterine location.

The condition occurs in 1-2% of all pregnancies, and most of these occur in the fallopian tubes (**tubal pregnancy**). Rupture of the ectopic implant within the fallopian tube can lead to massive abdominal bleeding and death. Surgeons can remove the implant, or treatment with medication (methotrexate) can destroy it, thereby preserving the fallopian tube before rupture occurs. Other sites of ectopic pregnancy include the ovaries and abdominal cavity; whatever the location, ectopic pregnancy often constitutes a surgical emergency.

multiple gestations

More than one fetus inside the uterus.

Multiple births are increasing in the United States. This is because of assisted reproductive technology (ART) such as ovulation induction followed by intrauterine insemination (IUI) or in vitro fertilization (IVF). These pregnancies are at higher risk for preterm delivery, fetal growth restriction, high blood pressure, and diabetes.

placenta previa

Implantation of the placenta over the cervical opening or in the lower region of the uterus (Figure 8-21).

Maternal signs and symptoms include painless bleeding, hemorrhage, and premature labor. Cesarean delivery usually is recommended.

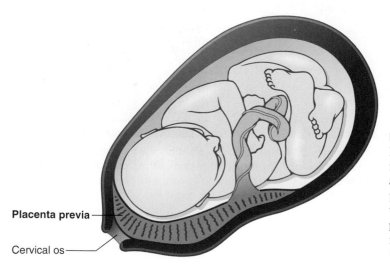

Placenta previa

Cervical os

FIGURE 8-21   Placenta previa. Previa means before or in the front of. Three forms of this abnormal implantation of the placenta are: **placenta accreta** (on the wall but not in muscle), **placenta increta** (in uterine muscle), and **placenta percreta** (attaching to another organ).

preeclampsia   **Abnormal condition associated with pregnancy, marked by high blood pressure, proteinuria, edema, and headache.**

Mild preeclampsia can be managed by bed rest and close monitoring of blood pressure. Women with severe preeclampsia need treatment with medications such as magnesium sulfate to prevent seizures, and the baby is delivered as quickly as possible. The Greek word *eklampein* means to shine forth, referring to the convulsions and hypertension—typically with visual symptoms of flashing lights—that accompany the condition. **Eclampsia** is the final and most severe phase of untreated preeclampsia. It often causes seizures and even death of the mother and baby.

NEONATAL

The following terms describe conditions or symptoms that can affect the newborn. The **Apgar score** (Figure 8-22) is a system of scoring an infant's physical condition at 1 and again 5 minutes after birth. **Heart rate, respiration, color, muscle tone,** and **response to stimuli** each are rated 0, 1, or 2. The maximum total score is 10. Infants with Apgar scores below 7 require immediate medical attention such as suctioning of the airways or oxygen to help breathing.

Down syndrome   **Chromosomal abnormality (trisomy 21) results in mental retardation, retarded growth, a flat face with a short nose, low-set ears, and slanted eyes.**

erythroblastosis fetalis   **Hemolytic disease in the newborn (HDN) caused by a blood group (Rh factor) incompatibility between the mother and the fetus.**

See explanation in Chapter 4, page 119.

hyaline membrane disease   **Acute lung disease commonly seen in the premature newborn.**

This condition, also called **respiratory distress syndrome of the newborn (RDS),** is caused by deficiency of **surfactant,** a protein necessary for proper lung function. Surfactant can be administered to the newborn to cure the condition. Hyaline refers to the shiny (hyaline means glassy) membrane that forms in the lung sacs.

SIGN	SCORE		
	0	**1**	**2**
Heart rate	Absent	Below 100	Over 100
Respiratory effort	Absent	Slow, irregular	Good, crying
Muscle tone	Limp	Some flexion of extremities	Active motion
Response to catheter in nostril (tested after oropharynx is clear)	No response	Grimace	Cough or sneeze
Color	Blue, pale	Body pink, extremities blue	Completely pink

FIGURE 8-22   Apgar scoring chart. This test is named for anesthesiologist Virginia Apgar (1909-1974), who devised it in 1953. Dr. Joseph Butterfield, in 1963, introduced an **"APGAR"** acronym as a mnemonic (memory device): **A**ppearance (color), **P**ulse (heart rate), **G**rimace (response to catheter in nostril), **A**ctivity (muscle tone), and **R**espiration (respiratory effort).

hydrocephalus	**Accumulation of fluid in the spaces of the brain.**
	In an infant with this condition, the entire head can enlarge because the bones of the skull do not completely fuse together at birth. Infants normally have a soft spot or **fontanelle** between the cranial bones that allows for some swelling during the birth of the baby. Hydrocephalus occurs because of a problem in the circulation of fluid within the brain and spinal cord, resulting in fluid accumulation.
meconium aspiration syndrome	**Abnormal inhalation of meconium produced by a fetus or newborn.**
	Meconium, a thick, sticky, greenish to black substance, is the first intestinal discharge (stools) from newborns. Intrauterine distress can cause its passage into amniotic fluid. Once the meconium has passed into the surrounding amniotic fluid, the fetus may breath meconium into its lungs. It can cause breathing problems due to inflammation in the baby's lungs after birth.
pyloric stenosis	**Narrowing of the opening of the stomach to the duodenum.**
	This condition may be present at birth and frequently is associated with Down syndrome. Surgical repair of the pyloric opening may be necessary.

CLINICAL TESTS AND PROCEDURES

CLINICAL TESTS

Pap test (Pap smear)	**Microscopic examination of stained cells removed from the vagina and cervix.**
	After inserting a vaginal **speculum** (instrument to hold apart the vaginal walls), the physician uses a small spatula to remove exfoliated (peeling and sloughing off) cells from the cervix and vagina (Figure 8-23). Microscopic analysis of the cell smear detects cervical or vaginal cellular abnormalities.
pregnancy test	**Blood or urine test to detect the presence of hCG.**

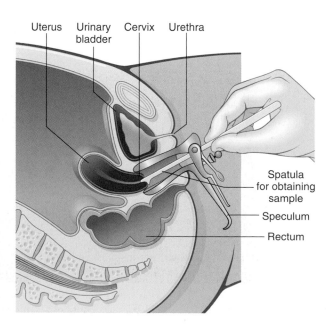

Uterus   Urinary   Cervix   Urethra
bladder

Spatula for obtaining sample

Speculum

Rectum

FIGURE 8-23 Method of obtaining a sample for a **Pap test.** The test is 95% accurate in diagnosing early carcinoma of the cervix. It was invented by and named for a Greek physician, Georgios Papanicolaou.

PROCEDURES

X-Ray Studies

hysterosalpingography (HSG)

X-ray imaging of the uterus and fallopian tubes after injection of contrast material.

This radiologic procedure is used to evaluate tubal patency (adequate opening) and uterine cavity abnormalities.

mammography

X-ray imaging of the breast.

Women are advised to have a baseline mammogram at 40 years of age for later comparison if needed. A mammogram every year is recommended for women older than 40, to screen for breast cancer. Figure 8-24 illustrates mammography.

A new method of mammography is **digital tomosynthesis.** In this procedure, an x-ray tube moves in an arc around the breast as several images are taken. These images are sent to a computer and clear, highly focused three-dimensional pictures are produced. In addition to being less painful, this procedure makes breast cancer easier to find in dense breast tissue.

Ultrasound Examination and Magnetic Resonance Imaging (MRI)

breast ultrasound imaging and breast MRI

Technologies using sound waves and a magnetic field to create images of breast tissue.

These imaging techniques confirm the presence of a mass and can distinguish a cystic from a solid mass. MRI is very useful in detecting masses in young women with dense breasts or in women with a strong family history of breast cancer and at high risk for this condition. Breast ultrasound imaging is useful to evaluate a specific area of cancer on a mammogram.

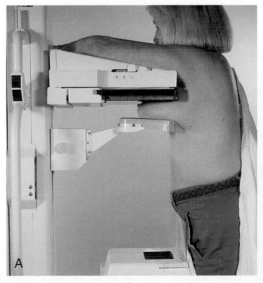
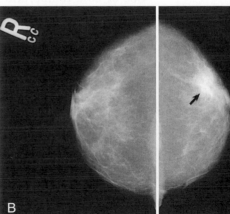
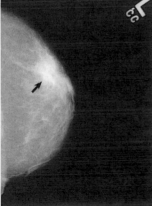

FIGURE 8-24   A, Mammography. The machine compresses the breast and x-ray pictures (*top to bottom* and *lateral*) are taken. **B, Mammograms** from a 63-year-old woman. The right breast is normal, and the left breast contains a carcinoma.

pelvic ultrasonography	**Recording images of sound waves as they bounce off organs in the pelvic region.**

This technique can evaluate fetal size and anatomy, as well as fetal and placental position. Uterine tumors and other pelvic masses, including abscesses, also are diagnosed by ultrasonography. **Transvaginal ultrasound** allows the radiologist a closer, sharper look at organs within the pelvis. The sound probe is placed in the vagina instead of over the pelvis or abdomen; this method is best used to evaluate fluid-filled cysts.

Gynecologic Procedures

aspiration	**Withdrawal of fluid from a cavity or sac with an instrument using suction.**

Aspiration needle biopsy is a valuable evaluation technique for patients with breast disease.

cauterization	**Destruction of tissue by burning.**

Destruction of abnormal tissue with chemicals (silver nitrate), or an electrically heated instrument. Cauterization is used to treat cervical dysplasia or cervical erosion. The **loop electrocautery excision procedure (LEEP)** (see Figure 8-26A) is used to further assess and often treat abnormal cervical tissue.

colposcopy	**Visual examination of the vagina and cervix using a colposcope.**

A colposcope is a lighted magnifying instrument resembling a small, mounted pair of binoculars. Gynecologists prefer colposcopy for pelvic examination when cervical dysplasia is present because it identifies the specific areas of abnormal cells. A biopsy specimen can then be taken for more accurate diagnosis (Figure 8-25).

conization	**Removal of a cone-shaped section (cone biopsy) of the cervix.**

The physician resects the tissue using a **LEEP (loop electrocautery excision procedure),** or with a carbon dioxide laser or surgical knife (scalpel). Figure 8-26A shows conization with LEEP, and Figure 8-26B shows the cone biopsy specimen removed surgically.

cryosurgery	**Use of cold temperatures to destroy tissue.**

A liquid nitrogen probe produces the freezing (cry/o means cold) temperature. Also called **cryocauterization.**

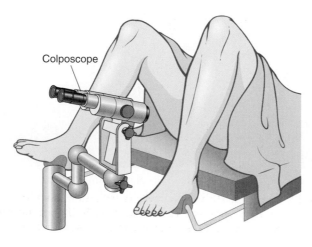

Colposcope

FIGURE 8-25 Colposcopy is used to evaluate a patient with an abnormal Pap test result. For this examination, the woman lies in the dorsal lithotomy position. This is the same position used to remove a urinary tract stone (lithotomy means incision to remove a stone).

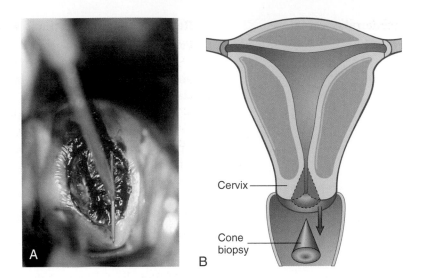

FIGURE 8-26 **A,** Cervical loop electrocautery excision procedure **(LEEP)** for cone biopsy. **B,** Surgical removal of **cone biopsy** specimen. (*A, Courtesy Dr. A. K. Goodman, Massachusetts General Hospital, Boston.*)

culdocentesis	**Needle aspiration of fluid from the cul-de-sac.**
	The physician inserts a needle through the vagina into the cul-de-sac. The presence of blood may indicate a ruptured ectopic pregnancy or ruptured ovarian cyst.
dilation (dilatation) and curettage (D&C)	**Widening the cervix and scraping off the endometrial lining of the uterus.**
	Dilation is accomplished by inserting a series of dilators of increasing diameter. A **curet** (metal loop at the end of a long, thin handle) is then used to sample the uterine lining. This procedure helps diagnose uterine disease and can temporarily halt prolonged or heavy uterine bleeding. When necessary, a D&C is used to remove the tissue during a spontaneous or therapeutic abortion (Figure 8-27).

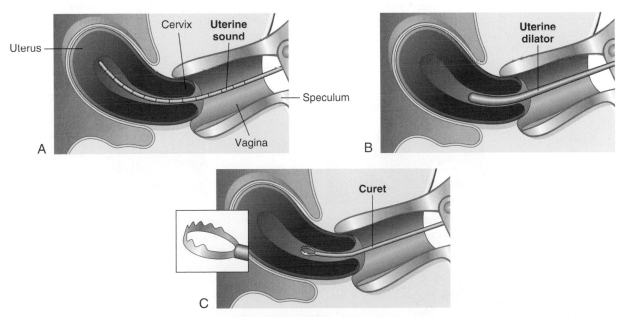

FIGURE 8-27 **Dilation and curettage (D&C) of the uterus. A,** The uterine cavity is explored with a **uterine sound** (a slender instrument used to measure the depth of the uterus) to prevent perforation during dilation. **B, Uterine dilators** (Hanks or Hagar) in graduated sizes are used to gradually dilate the cervix. **C,** The uterus is gently curetted and specimens are collected.

exenteration

Removal of internal organs within a cavity.

Pelvic exenteration is removal of the organs and adjacent structures of the pelvis.

laparoscopy

Visual examination of the abdominal cavity using an endoscope (laparoscope).

In this procedure, a form of **minimally invasive surgery (MIS),** small incisions (5 to 10 mm long) are made near the woman's navel for introduction of the laparoscope and other instruments. Uses of laparoscopy include inspection and removal of ovaries and fallopian tubes, diagnosis and treatment of endometriosis, and removal of fibroids. Laparoscopy also is used to perform subtotal (cervix is left in place) and total hysterectomies (Figure 8-28).

Morcellation (cutting up uterine tissue in the abdomen) is commonly performed when the uterus or fibroids are removed laparoscopically. It is contraindicated in situations of suspcious or pre-malignancy.

tubal ligation

Blocking the fallopian tubes to prevent fertilization from occurring.

This **sterilization** procedure (making an individual incapable of reproduction) is performed using laparoscopy or through a hysteroscope inserted via the cervical os (opening). **Ligation** means tying off and does not pertain solely to the fallopian tubes—which may be "tied" using clips or bands, or by surgically cutting or burning through the tissue.

Procedures Related to Pregnancy

abortion (AB)

Termination of pregnancy before the embryo or fetus can exist on its own.

Abortions are **spontaneous** or **induced.** Spontaneous abortions, commonly called "miscarriages," occur without apparent cause. Induced abortions can be **therapeutic** or **elective.** A therapeutic abortion is performed when the health of the pregnant woman is endangered. An elective abortion is performed at the request of the woman. Major methods for abortion include vaginal evacuation by D&C or vacuum aspiration (suction) and stimulation of uterine contractions by injection of saline (salt solution) into the amniotic cavity (in second-trimester pregnancies).

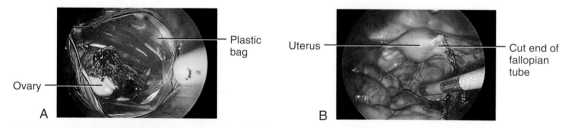

FIGURE 8-28 **Laparoscopic oophorectomy. A,** Notice the ovary placed in a plastic bag. The bag was inserted through the laparoscope and then opened, and the ovary was placed inside. **B,** Both are extracted through the laparoscope, leaving the uterus and the cut end of the fallopian tube. *(Courtesy Dr. A. K. Goodman, Massachusetts General Hospital, Boston.)*

amniocentesis	**Needle puncture of the amniotic sac to withdraw amniotic fluid for analysis** (Figure 8-29). The cells of the fetus, found in the fluid, are cultured (grown), and cytologic and biochemical studies are performed to check fetal chromosomes, concentrations of proteins and bilirubin, and fetal maturation.
cesarean section	**Surgical incision of the abdominal wall and uterus to deliver a fetus.** Indications for cesarean section include cephalopelvic disproportion (the baby's head is too big for the mother's birth canal), abruptio placentae or placenta previa, fetal distress (fetal hypoxia), and breech or shoulder presentation. The name comes from a law during the time of Julius Caesar requiring removal of the fetus before a deceased pregnant woman could be buried.
chorionic villus sampling (CVS)	**Sampling of placental tissues (chorionic villi) for prenatal diagnosis.** The sample of tissue is removed with a catheter inserted into the uterus. The procedure can be performed earlier than amniocentesis, at 10 or more weeks of gestation.
fetal monitoring	**Continuous recording of the fetal heart rate and maternal uterine contractions to assess fetal status and the progress of labor.**
in vitro fertilization (IVF)	**Egg and sperm cells are combined outside the body in a laboratory dish (in vitro) to facilitate fertilization.** After an incubation period of 3 to 5 days, the fertilized ova are injected into the uterus through the cervix. (Latin *in vitro* means in glass, as used for laboratory containers.) From 30% to 50% of all IVF procedures are now associated with **intracytoplasmic sperm injection (ICSI).** This is the direct injection of sperm into harvested ova.

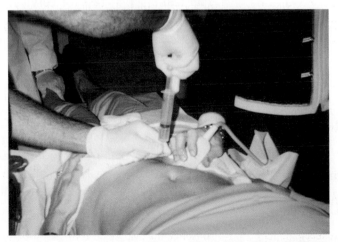

FIGURE 8-29   Amniocentesis. The obstetrician places a long needle through the pregnant woman's abdominal wall into the amniotic cavity. Needle placement (avoiding the fetus and the placenta) is guided by concurrent ultrasound imaging, performed using the transducer in the radiologist's hand. The yellow amniotic fluid is aspirated into the syringe attached to the needle. This procedure took place in the 16th week of pregnancy. The indication for the amniocentesis was a low alpha-fetoprotein (AFP) level. This finding suggested a higher risk of Down syndrome in the baby. Karyotype analysis (received 10 days later) showed normal chromosome configuration.

ABBREVIATIONS

AB	abortion	**GYN**	gynecology
AFP	alpha-fetoprotein—high levels in amniotic fluid of fetus or maternal serum indicate increased risk of neurologic birth defects in the infant.	**hCG** *or* **HCG**	human chorionic gonadotropin
		HDN	hemolytic disease of the newborn
		HPV	human papillomavirus
BRCA1 **BRCA2**	breast cancer 1 and 2—genetic mutations associated with increased risk for breast cancer	**HRT**	hormone replacement therapy
		HSG	hysterosalpingography
		IUD	intrauterine device; contraceptive
BSE	breast self-examination	**IVF**	in vitro fertilization
CA-125	protein marker elevated in ovarian cancer (normal range of values is 0 to 35 U/mL)	**LEEP**	loop electrocautery excision procedure
		LH	luteinizing hormone
C-section, CS	cesarean section	**LMP**	last menstrual period
CIN	cervical intraepithelial neoplasia	**multip**	multipara; multiparous
		OB	obstetrics
CIS	carcinoma in situ	**para 2-0-1-2**	a woman's reproductive history: 2 full-term infants, 0 preterm, 1 abortion, and 2 living children
CVS	chorionic villus sampling		
Cx	cervix		
D&C	dilation (dilatation) and curettage	**Pap test**	test for cervical or vaginal cancer
DCIS	ductal carcinoma in situ; a precancerous breast lesion that indicates a higher risk for invasive ductal breast cancer	**PID**	pelvic inflammatory disease
		PMS	premenstrual syndrome
		primip	primipara; primiparous
DUB	dysfunctional uterine bleeding	**SLN biopsy** *or* **SNB**	sentinel lymph node biopsy—blue dye or a radioisotope (or both) identifies the first lymph node draining the breast lymphatics
FHR	fetal heart rate		
FSH	follicle-stimulating hormone		
G	gravida (pregnant)		
GnRH	gonadotropin-releasing hormone—secreted by the hypothalamus to stimulate release of FSH and LH from the pituitary gland	**TAH-BSO**	total abdominal hysterectomy with bilateral salpingo-oophorectomy
		UAE	uterine artery embolization
		VH	vaginal hysterectomy

PRACTICAL APPLICATIONS

This section contains an actual operative report and brief excerpts from other medical records using words that you have studied in this and previous chapters. Explanations of more difficult terms are added in brackets.

OPERATIVE REPORT

Preoperative diagnosis: Menorrhagia, leiomyomata
Anesthetic: General
Material forwarded to laboratory for examination:
  A. Endocervical curettings
  B. Endometrial curettings
Operation performed: Dilation and curettage of the uterus
  With the patient in the dorsal lithotomy position [legs are flexed on the thighs, thighs flexed on the abdomen and abducted] and sterilely prepped and draped, manual examination of the uterus revealed it to be 6- to 8-week size, retroflexed; no adnexal masses noted. The anterior lip of the cervix was then grasped with a tenaculum [a hook-like surgical instrument for grasping and holding parts]. The cervix was dilated up to a #20 Hank's dilator. The uterus was sounded [depth measured] up to 4 inches. A sharp curettage of the endocervix showed only a scant amount of tissue. With a sharp curet, the uterus was curetted in a clockwise fashion with an irregularity noted in the posterior floor. A large amount of endometrial tissue was removed. The patient tolerated the procedure well.
Operative diagnosis: Leiomyomata uteri
Recommendation: Hysterectomy for myomectomy

SENTENCES USING MEDICAL TERMINOLOGY

1. *Mammogram report:* The breast parenchyma [essential tissue] is symmetric bilaterally. There are no abnormal masses or calcifications in either breast. The axillae are normal.

2. This is a 43-year-old gravida 3, para 2 with premature ovarian failure and now on HRT. She has history of endocervical atypia [cells are not normal or typical] secondary to chlamydial infection, which is now being treated.

3. The patient is a 40-year-old gravida 3, para 2 admitted for exploratory laparotomy to remove and evaluate a 10-cm left adnexal mass. Discharge diagnosis: (1) endometriosis, left ovary; (2) benign cystic teratoma [dermoid cyst], left ovary.

4. *History:* 51-year-old G3 P3; LMP early 40s; on HRT until age 49 when diagnosed with carcinoma of breast; treated with mastectomy and tamoxifen. Followed by ultrasounds showing slightly thickened 9-10 mm endometrium. No bleeding.
   Operative findings: office endometrial biopsy, scant tissue
   Clinical diagnosis: rule out hyperplasia

8

OPERATING ROOM SCHEDULE

The operating room schedule for one day in a large general hospital listed six different gynecologic procedures. Match the surgical procedures in Column I with the indications for surgery in Column II. Write the letter of the indication in the blanks provided. Answers are on page 302.

COLUMN I

1. Left oophorectomy _____

2. Vaginal hysterectomy with colporrhaphy _____

3. TAH-BSO, pelvic and periaortic lymphadenectomy _____

4. Exploratory laparotomy for uterine myomectomy _____

5. Conization of the cervix _____

6. Lumpectomy with SLN biopsy _____

COLUMN II

A. LLQ pain; ovarian mass on pelvic ultrasound
B. Fibroids
C. Endometrial carcinoma
D. Small invasive ductal carcinoma of the breast
E. Suspected cervical cancer
F. Uterine prolapse

CONTRACEPTIVE CHOICES

Review and compare the various birth control options available today.

METHOD	UNINTENDED PREGNANCY RATES: TYPICAL USE/ PERFECT USE
1. Abstinence—no sexual intercourse	0% / 0%
2. Cervical cap—inserted by doctor or nurse	16% / 9%
3. Condom—male	15% / 2%
4. Condom—female	21 / 5%
5. Diaphragm (with spermicide)	16% / 6%
6. Film and foam (with spermicide)	29% / 18%
7. Implant—inserted into upper arm; releases hormones; effective for 3 years	0.05% / 0.05%
8. Injectable—Depo-Provera given every 3 months	3% / 3%
9. Intrauterine device (IUD)	less than 1%
10. Oral contraceptives (birth control pills)	8% / 3%
11. Patch—applied to skin weekly	8% / 3%
12. Ring—inserted in vagina; effective for 1 month	8% / less than 1%
13. Sponge—used by women who have never given birth	16% / 9%
14. Suppositories—inserted in vagina (with spermicide)	29% / 15%
15. Withdrawal	27% / 4%

8

IN PERSON: PROPHYLACTIC MASTECTOMY

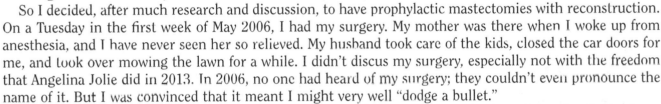

Whenever May rolls around, I think about my surgery and the decision I made many years ago to have prophylactic mastectomies. I grew up in a family of strong women. They were determined to work, play sports, and raise their families, except they all had breast cancer. It was a bump in the road for each one of them and, at age 36, I had 4 children, a wonderful career and a husband and abnormal mammograms. I had friends, holidays, and biopsies, and being a physician (radiation oncologist) and the daughter of a medical oncologist, I was worried about my own health.

When my mother tested negative for the BRCA gene, it did not relieve my anxiety. It just intensified it. What was causing the breast cancer in my family? Genetic counselors explained that only about 15% of breast cancer can be attributed to the BRCA genes; the rest are caused by other "faulty genes" or just changes in the breast cells.

I heard about a new procedure that physicians were pioneering—direct-to-implant breast reconstruction after mastectomy. One step and one surgery would drop my risk from 40% to close to 2% or 3%. I could preserve my anatomy and get rid of those breast cells that might kill me someday. It had a lot to do with my family and career. I did not want to have breast cancer.

So I decided, after much research and discussion, to have prophylactic mastectomies with reconstruction. On a Tuesday in the first week of May 2006, I had my surgery. My mother was there when I woke up from anesthesia, and I have never seen her so relieved. My husband took care of the kids, closed the car doors for me, and took over mowing the lawn for a while. I didn't discus my surgery, especially not with the freedom that Angelina Jolie did in 2013. In 2006, no one had heard of my surgery; they couldn't even pronounce the name of it. But I was convinced that it meant I might very well "dodge a bullet."

Nine years later, I smile when I see morning television shows talk about the "Angelina Effect"—implants and breast reconstruction, nipples, and risk reduction, all in the same story. It's wonderful that women can talk about their "faulty parts" without feeling shame. It's a great example for our daughters as well.

In March of 2015, Angelina wrote another op-ed discussing her oophorectomy and salpingectomy surgery (removal of both ovaries and both fallopian tubes). Women with BRCA genes have an increased risk not only for breast cancer but also for ovarian cancer. And this was the disease that took Angelina's mother's life. Ovarian cancer, unlike breast cancer, is often diagnosed at a very late stage. A majority of breast cancers are diagnosed at stage 1 or 2 or even at a "pre-cancer" DCIS [ductal carcinoma in situ] stage. Ovarian cancer, on the other hand, often is diagnosed after the cancer has already spread. Angelina also discussed another "taboo" subject: Removing ovaries and the fallopian tubes in a premenopausal woman (Angelina was 39 years old at the time of her surgery) sends her into early menopause. Hot flashes, skin changes, dryness (you know where) are hard topics to discuss in public. She put it out there, front and center, to destigmatize the subject for all women.

There is no history of ovarian cancer in my family, and we are BRCA-negative, so my genetic counselor did not recommend removing my ovaries and fallopian tubes. Rather, I have a pelvic ultrasound once a year and a blood test (CA-125) to make sure that nothing is abnormal.

Because of my decision to undergo prophylactic mastectomies, I know that my life has changed for the better. I don't have the fear of getting breast cancer. I also have decided to devote my life work to helping women recover with comfort, dignity, and grace after being blind-sided by the disease. Angelina Jolie says that knowledge is power! It behooves us to learn as much as we can to prevent disease and proactively take care of the fragile, precious thing we call our health.

Elizabeth Chabner Thompson is the CEO/Founder of BFFL Co, a company devoted to improving the patient experience. She is also a physician, ultramarathoner, and wife and the proud mother of four children, ages 13 to 18.

8

? EXERCISES

Remember to check your answers carefully with the Answers to Exercises, page 300.

A **Match the following terms for structures or tissues with their meanings below.**

amnion	fallopian tubes	perineum
areola	fimbriae	placenta
cervix	labia	uterine serosa
chorion	mammary papilla	vagina
clitoris	ovaries	vulva
endometrium		

1. inner lining of the uterus _____

2. area between the anus and the vagina in females _____

3. dark-pigmented area around the breast nipple _____

4. finger-like ends of the fallopian tube _____

5. ducts through which the egg travels into the uterus from the ovary _____

6. organ of sensitive erectile tissue in females; anterior to urethral orifice _____

7. nipple of the breast _____

8. vascular organ that attaches to the uterine wall during pregnancy _____

9. lower, neck-like portion of the uterus _____

10. innermost membrane around the developing embryo _____

11. outermost layer of the membranes around the developing embryo and forming part of the

    placenta _____

12. outermost layer surrounding the uterus _____

13. lips of the vulva _____

14. female gonads; producing ova and hormones _____

15. includes the perineum, labia and clitoris, and hymen; external genitalia _____

16. muscular, mucosa-lined canal extending from the uterus to the exterior of the body

    _____

B **Identify the following terms.**

1. fetus _____

2. lactiferous ducts _____

3. gametes _____

4. gonads _____

5. adnexa uteri _____

6. cul-de-sac _____

7. genitalia _____

8. Bartholin glands _____

9. ovarian follicle _____

10. corpus luteum _____

C **Match the listed terms with the descriptions/definitions that follow.**

coitus   human chorionic gonadotropin   myometrium
estrogen   luteinizing hormone   prenatal
fertilization   menarche   progesterone
follicle-stimulating hormone

1. hormone produced by the ovaries; promotes female secondary sex characteristics

    _____

2. hormone secreted by the pituitary gland to stimulate maturation of the egg cell (ovum)

    _____

3. sexual intercourse _____

4. before birth _____

5. beginning of the first menstrual period _____

6. hormone produced by the placenta to sustain pregnancy by stimulating the ovaries to produce

    estrogen and progesterone _____

7. muscle layer of the uterus _____

8. hormone produced by the corpus luteum in the ovary and the placenta of a pregnant woman

    _____

9. hormone produced by the pituitary gland to promote ovulation _____

10. union of the sperm cell and ovum from which the embryo develops _____

D **Supply definitions to complete the following sentences.**

1. galact/o and lact/o both mean _____.

2. colp/o and vagin/o both mean _____.

3. mamm/o and mast/o both mean _____.

4. metr/o, uter/o, and hyster/o all mean _____.

5. oophor/o and ovari/o both mean _____.

6. o/o, ov/o, and ovul/o all mean _____.

7. in- and endo- both mean _____.

8. -cyesis and -gravida both mean _____.

9. salping/o and -salpinx both mean _____.

10. episi/o and vulv/o both mean _____.

E **Match the listed terms with the meanings/descriptions that follow.**

bilateral salpingo-oophorectomy   lactation   oxytocin
cervicitis   neonatology   total hysterectomy
chorion   obstetrics   vulvovaginitis
culdocentesis

1. study of the newborn _____

2. hormone that stimulates the pregnant uterus to contract _____

3. secretion of milk _____

4. removal of the entire uterus _____

5. inflammation of the neck of the uterus _____

6. branch of medicine concerned with pregnancy and childbirth _____

7. outermost membrane surrounding the fetus _____

8. removal of both fallopian tubes and both ovaries _____

9. inflammation of the external female genitalia and vagina _____

10. needle puncture to remove fluid from the cul-de-sac _____

F **Give the meanings of the following signs and symptoms.**

1. amenorrhea _____

2. dysmenorrhea _____

3. leukorrhea _____

4. metrorrhagia _____

5. galactorrhea _____

6. menorrhagia _____

7. pyosalpinx _____

8. dyspareunia _____

9. menometrorrhagia _____

10. oligomenorrhea _____

G **State whether the following sentences are true or false, and explain your answers.**

1. After a total (complete) hysterectomy, a woman still has regular menstrual periods.

_____

2. After a total hysterectomy, a woman may still produce estrogen and progesterone.

_____

3. Birth control pills prevent pregnancy by keeping levels of estrogen and progesterone high.

_____

4. After a total hysterectomy with bilateral salpingo-oophorectomy, a doctor may advise hormone replacement therapy._____

5. Human papillomavirus can cause genital warts and ovarian cancer.

_____

6. A Pap test can detect cervical dysplasia. _____

7. Human chorionic gonadotropin is produced by the ovaries during pregnancy.

_____

8. Gynecomastia is a common condition in pregnant women.

_____

9. Treatment for endometriosis is uterine myomectomy.

_____

10. A gravida 3 para 2 is a woman who has given birth 3 times.

_____

11. A nulligravida is a woman who has had several pregnancies.

_____

12. Pseudocyesis is the same condition as a tubal pregnancy.

_____

13. Fibrocystic changes in the breast are a malignant condition.

_____

14. Cystadenomas occur in the ovaries.

_____

15. FSH and LH are ovarian hormones.

H Give the meanings of the following terms.

1. parturition _____

2. menopause _____

3. menarche _____

4. ovulation _____

5. gestation _____

6. anovulatory _____

7. dilatation _____

8. lactation _____

9. nulliparous _____

10. oophoritis _____

11. bartholinitis _____

12. vulvodynia _____

I Match the listed terms with the meanings/descriptions that follow.

abruptio placentae endometrial carcinoma multiple gestations
cervical carcinoma endometriosis placenta previa
cervicitis leiomyoma preeclampsia
cystadenocarcinoma

1. malignant tumor of the ovary _____

2. chlamydial infection causing inflammation in the lower, neck-like portion of the uterus

 _____

3. condition during pregnancy or shortly thereafter, marked by hypertension, proteinuria, and

 edema _____

4. uterine tissue located outside the uterus—for example, in the ovaries, cul-de-sac, fallopian

 tubes, or peritoneum _____

5. premature separation of a normally implanted placenta _____

6. placenta implantation over the cervical opening _____

7. more than one fetus inside the uterus _____

8. malignant condition that can be diagnosed by a Pap test, revealing dysplastic changes in cells

 _____

9. malignant condition of the inner lining of the uterus _____

10. benign muscle tumor in the uterus _____

8

J **Name the appropriate test or procedure for each of the following descriptions.**

1. Burning of abnormal tissue with chemicals or an electrically heated instrument:

   _____

2. Contrast material is injected into the uterus and fallopian tubes, and x-ray images are obtained:

   _____

3. Cold temperature is used to destroy tissue: _____

4. Visual examination of the vagina and cervix: _____

5. Widening the cervical opening and scraping the lining of the uterus:

   _____

6. Withdrawal of fluid by suction with a needle: _____

7. Process of recording x-ray images of the breast: _____

8. Removal of a cone-shaped section of the cervix for diagnosis or treatment of cervical dysplasia:

   _____

9. Surgical puncture to remove fluid from the cul-de-sac: _____

10. Echoes from sound waves create an image of structures in the pelvic region:

    _____

11. Blocking the fallopian tubes to prevent fertilization from occurring:

    _____

12. Visual examination of the abdominal cavity with an endoscope:

    _____

13. hCG is measured in the urine or blood: _____

14. Cells are scraped from the cervix or vagina for microscopic analysis:

    _____

15. Removal of internal gynecologic organs and adjacent structures in the pelvis:

    _____

8

K **Match the obstetric and neonatal terms with the descriptions that follow.**

abortion
Apgar score
cephalic version
cesarean section
erythroblastosis fetalis

fetal monitoring
fetal presentation
fontanelle
hyaline membrane disease

hydrocephalus
in vitro fertilization
meconium aspiration syndrome
pyloric stenosis

1. Turning the fetus so that the head presents during birth _____

2. The soft spot between the newborn's cranial bones _____

3. The evaluation of the newborn's physical condition _____

4. Premature termination of pregnancy _____

5. Removal of the fetus by abdominal incision of the uterus _____

6. Acute lung disease in the premature newborn: surfactant deficiency _____

7. Use of a machine to electronically record fetal heart rate during labor _____

8. Narrowing of the opening of the stomach to the small intestine in the infant _____

9. Hemolytic disease of the newborn _____

10. Accumulation of fluid in the spaces of a neonate's brain _____

11. Manner in which the fetus appears to the examiner during delivery _____

12. Thick, sticky green-black substance is discharged into the amniotic fluid, causing fetal lung problems _____

13. Union of the egg and sperm cell in a laboratory dish _____

L **Give medical terms for the following definitions. Pay careful attention to spelling.**

1. benign muscle tumors in the uterus _____

2. no menses _____

3. removal of an ovary _____

4. condition of female breasts (in a male) _____

5. ovarian hormone that sustains pregnancy _____

6. nipple-shaped elevation on the breast _____

M Give the meanings of the abbreviations in Column I. Then select the letter of the correct description from Column II.

COLUMN I

1. CIS _____ _____

2. FSH _____ _____

3. D&C _____ _____

4. multip _____ _____

5. C-section _____ _____

6. IVF _____ _____

7. Cx _____ _____

8. TAH-BSO _____ _____

9. primip _____ _____

10. OB _____

COLUMN II

A. This woman has given birth to more than one infant.

B. Egg and sperm cells are combined outside the body.

C. This woman has given birth for the first time.

D. Secretion from the pituitary gland stimulates the ovaries.

E. This procedure helps diagnose uterine disease.

F. Localized cancer growth.

G. Surgical procedure to remove the uterus, fallopian tubes, and ovaries.

H. Surgical delivery of an infant through an abdominal incision.

I. Branch of medicine dealing with pregnancy and delivery of infants.

J. Lower, neck-like region of the uterus.

N Match the following abbreviations in Column I with the best description in Column II.

COLUMN I

1. Pap test _____

2. HSG _____

3. AB _____

4. HPV _____

5. DCIS _____

6. HRT _____

COLUMN II

A. Precancerous lesion in the breast

B. X-ray record of the uterus and fallopian tubes

C. Hormones given to menopausal women

D. Diagnoses cervical and vaginal cancer

E. Termination of pregnancy; spontaneous or induced

F. Cause of cervical cancer

O Circle the term in parentheses that best completes the meaning of each sentence.

1. Dr. Hanson felt that it was important to do a (**culdocentesis, Pap test, amniocentesis**) once yearly on each of her GYN patients to screen for abnormal cells.

2. When Doris missed her period, her doctor checked for the presence of (**LH, IUD, hCG**) in Doris's urine to see if she was pregnant.

3. Ellen was 34 weeks pregnant and experiencing bad headaches and blurry vision, with a 10-pound weight gain in 2 days. Dr. Murphy told her to go to the obstetric emergency department because she suspected (**preeclampsia, pelvic inflammatory disease, fibroids**).

4. Fifty-two-year-old Sally noticed increasing pain, fullness, and swelling in her abdomen. She had a history of ovarian cancer, so her physician recommended **(sentinel node biopsy, pelvic ultrasonography, colposcopy)**.

5. Clara knew that she should not ignore her fevers and yellow vaginal discharge and the pain in her side. She had previous episodes of **(PMS, PID, HRT)** treated with IV antibiotics. She worried that she might have a recurrence.

6. After years of trying to become pregnant, Jill decided to speak to her **(hematologist, gynecologist, urologist)** about in vitro **(gestation, parturition, fertilization)**.

7. To harvest her ova, Jill's physician prescribed hormones to stimulate egg maturation and **(coitus, lactation, ovulation)**. Ova were surgically removed and fertilized with sperm cells in a Petri dish.

8. Next, multiple embryos were implanted into Jill's **(fallopian tube, vagina, uterus)**, and she received hormones to ensure the survival of at least one embryo.

9. The IVF was successful and after **(abdominal CT, ultrasound examination)**, Jill was told that she would have twins in 8½ months.

10. At 37 weeks, Jill went into labor. Under continuous **(chorionic villus sampling, culdocentesis, fetal monitoring)**, two healthy infants were delivered vaginally.

11. At age 41, Carol had a screening **(hysterosalpingogram, mammogram, conization)** of her breasts. The results showed tiny calcium deposits or calcifications, behind her **(areola, chorion, adnexa uteri)**. A core needle **(laparoscopy, colposcopy, biopsy)** was performed and showed cells that were an early sign of cancer called **(CIN, DCIS, DUB)**. Her surgical oncologist recommended **(lumpectomy, TAH-BSO, chorionic villus sampling)** to remove the calcifications and surrounding tissue as treatment.

8

ANSWERS TO EXERCISES

 A

1. endometrium
2. perineum
3. areola
4. fimbriae
5. fallopian tubes
6. clitoris
7. mammary papilla
8. placenta
9. cervix
10. amnion
11. chorion
12. uterine serosa
13. labia
14. ovaries
15. vulva
16. vagina

B

1. embryo from the third month (after 8 weeks) to birth
2. tubes that carry milk within the breast
3. sex cells; the egg and sperm cells
4. organs (ovaries and testes) in the female and male that produce gametes
5. ovaries, fallopian tubes, and supporting ligaments (accessory parts of the uterus)
6. region of the abdomen between the rectum and the uterus
7. reproductive organs (genitals)
8. small exocrine glands at the vaginal orifice that secrete a lubricating fluid
9. developing sac in the ovary that encloses the ovum
10. empty follicle that secretes progesterone after ovulation

 C

1. estrogen
2. follicle-stimulating hormone
3. coitus
4. prenatal
5. menarche
6. human chorionic gonadotropin
7. myometrium
8. progesterone
9. luteinizing hormone
10. fertilization

D

1. milk
2. vagina
3. breast
4. uterus

5. ovary
6. egg
7. in, within

8. pregnancy
9. fallopian tube
10. vulva (external female genitalia)

E

1. neonatology
2. oxytocin
3. lactation
4. total hysterectomy

5. cervicitis
6. obstetrics
7. chorion

8. bilateral salpingo-oophorectomy
9. vulvovaginitis
10. culdocentesis

F

1. no menstrual flow
2. painful menstrual flow
3. white discharge (normally from the vagina and also associated with cervicitis)
4. bleeding from the uterus at irregular intervals

5. abnormal discharge of milk from the breasts
6. profuse or prolonged menstrual periods occurring at regular intervals

7. pus in the fallopian (uterine) tubes
8. painful sexual intercourse
9. heavy bleeding at and between menstrual periods
10. scanty menstrual flow

G

1. False. Total hysterectomy means removal of the entire uterus so that menstruation does not occur.
2. True. Total hysterectomy does not mean that the ovaries have been removed.
3. True. Birth control pills contain estrogen and progesterone; high levels prevent ovulation and pregnancy.
4. True. This may be necessary to treat symptoms of estrogen loss (vaginal atrophy, hot flashes) and to prevent bone deterioration (osteoporosis).
5. False. HPV does produce genital warts but not ovarian cancer. In some cases, HPV infection may lead to cervical cancer.

6. True. A Pap test can detect abnormal changes in the cervix from cervical dysplasia to cervical intraepithelial neoplasia (CIN) and CIS (carcinoma in situ).
7. False. The hormone hCG is produced by the *placenta* during pregnancy.
8. False. Gynecomastia is a condition of increased breast development in *males*.
9. False. Myomectomy means removal of muscle tumors (fibroids). Endometriosis is abnormal location of uterine tissue outside the uterine lining.
10. False. A gravida 3 para 2 is a woman who has had two children and three pregnancies.

11. False. A nulligravida has had no pregnancies. A multigravida has had many pregnancies.
12. False. A pseudocyesis is a false pregnancy (no pregnancy occurs), and a tubal pregnancy is an example of ectopic pregnancy (pregnancy occurs in the fallopian tube, not in the uterus).
13. False. Fibrocystic changes in the breast are a benign condition.
14. True. Cystadenomas are glandular sacs lined with tumor cells; they occur in the ovaries.
15. False. FSH and LH are pituitary gland hormones. Estrogen and progesterone are secreted by the ovaries.

H

1. act of giving birth
2. gradual ending of menstrual function
3. beginning of the first menstrual period at puberty
4. release of the ovum from the ovary

5. pregnancy
6. pertaining to no ovulation (egg is not released from the ovary)
7. widening
8. natural secretion of milk

9. a woman who has never given birth
10. inflammation of the ovaries
11. inflammation of Bartholin glands
12. pain in the vulva

I

1. cystadenocarcinoma
2. cervicitis
3. preeclampsia
4. endometriosis

5. abruptio placentae
6. placenta previa
7. multiple gestations

8. cervical carcinoma
9. endometrial carcinoma
10. leiomyoma

8

J

1. cauterization
2. hysterosalpingography
3. cryosurgery or cryocauterization
4. colposcopy
5. dilation (dilatation) and curettage
6. aspiration
7. mammography
8. conization
9. culdocentesis
10. pelvic ultrasonography
11. tubal ligation
12. laparoscopy
13. pregnancy test
14. Pap test
15. pelvic exenteration

K

1. cephalic version
2. fontanelle
3. Apgar score
4. abortion
5. cesarean section
6. hyaline membrane disease (respiratory distress syndrome of the newborn)
7. fetal monitoring
8. pyloric stenosis
9. erythroblastosis fetalis
10. hydrocephalus
11. fetal presentation
12. meconium aspiration syndrome
13. in vitro fertilization

L

1. fibroids or leiomyomata
2. amenorrhea
3. oophorectomy
4. gynecomastia
5. progesterone
6. mammary papilla

M

1. carcinoma in situ: F
2. follicle-stimulating hormone: D
3. dilation (dilatation) and curettage: E
4. multipara: A
5. cesarean section: H
6. in vitro fertilization: B
7. cervix: J
8. total abdominal hysterectomy with bilateral salpingo-oophorectomy: G
9. primipara: C
10. obstetrics: I

N

1. D
2. B
3. E
4. F
5. A
6. C

O

1. Pap test
2. hCG
3. preeclampsia
4. pelvic ultrasonography
5. PID
6. gynecologist; fertilization
7. ovulation
8. uterus
9. ultrasound examination
10. fetal monitoring
11. mammogram; areola; biopsy; DCIS; lumpectomy

Answers to Practical Applications

Operating Room Schedule

1. A
2. F
3. C
4. B
5. E
6. D

PRONUNCIATION OF TERMS

To test your understanding of the terminology in this chapter, write the meaning of each term in the space provided. In addition, you may wish to cover the terms and write them by looking at your definitions. Make sure your spelling is correct. The page number after each term indicates where it is defined or used in the book, so you can easily check your responses. You will find complete definitions for all of these terms and audio pronunciations on the Evolve website.

Pronunciation Guide

ā as in āpe	ă as in ăpple
ē as in ēven	ĕ as in ĕvery
ī as in īce	ĭ as in ĭnterest
ō as in ōpen	ŏ as in pŏt
ū as in ūnit	ŭ as in ŭnder

Vocabulary and Terminology

TERM	PRONUNCIATION	MEANING
adnexa uteri (266)	ăd-NĔK-să Ū-tĕ rī	
amenorrhea (270)	āmĕn-ō-RĒ-ă	
amniocentesis (268)	ăm-nē-ō-sĕn-TĒ-sĭs	
amnion (266)	ĂM-nē-ŏn	
amniotic fluid (268)	ăm-nē-ŎT-ĭk FLOO-ĭd	
anovulatory (270)	ăn-ŎV-ū-lă-tōr-ē	
areola (266)	ă-RĒ-ō-lă	
Bartholin glands (266)	BĂR-thō-lĭn glăndz	
bartholinitis (268)	băr-thō-lĭ-NĪ-tĭs	
cephalic version (272)	sē-FĂL-lĭk VĔR-zhŭn	
cervix (266)	SĔR-vĭkz	
chorion (268)	KŎ-rē-ŏn	
chorionic (268)	kŏ-rē-ŎN-ĭk	
clitoris (266)	KLĬ-tō-rĭs	
coitus (266)	KŌ-ĭ-tŭs	
colposcopy (268)	kŏl-PŎS-kō-pē	
corpus luteum (266)	KŎR-pŭs LOO-tē-ŭm	
cul-de-sac (266)	KŬL-dē-săk	
culdocentesis (268)	kŭl-dō-sĕn-TĒ-sĭs	
dysmenorrhea (270)	dĭs-mĕn-ō-RĒ-ă	
dyspareunia (272)	dĭs-pă-ROO-nē-ă	

8

TERM	PRONUNCIATION	MEANING
dystocia (272)	dĭs-TŌ-sē-ă	
embryo (266)	ĔM-brē-ō	
endocervicitis (268)	ĕn-dō-sĕr-vĭs-SĪ-tĭs	
endometritis (272)	ĕn-dō-mĕ-TRĪ-tis	
endometrium (266)	ĕn-dō-MĒ-trē-ŭm	
episiotomy (268)	ĕ-pĭs-ē-ŎT-ō-mē	
estrogen (266)	ĔS-trō-jĕn	
fallopian tube (266)	fă-LŌ-pē-ăn tūb	
fertilization (266)	fĕr-tĭl-ĭ-ZĀ-shŭn	
fetal presentation (272)	FĒ-tăl prĕ-sĕn-TĀ-shŭn	
fetus (266)	FĒ-tŭs	
fimbriae (266)	FĬM-brē-ē	
follicle-stimulating hormone (266)	FŎL-lĭ-kl STĬM-ū-lā-tĭng HŌR-mōn	
galactorrhea (268)	gă-lăk-tō-RĒ-ă	
gamete (266)	GĂM-ēt	
genitalia (267)	jĕn-ĭ-TĀ-lē-ă	
gestation (267)	jĕs-TĀ-shŭn	
gonad (267)	GŌ-năd	
gynecology (267)	gī-nĕ-KŎL-ō-jē	
gynecomastia (269)	gī-nĕ-kō-MĂS-tē-ă	
human chorionic gonadotropin (267)	HŪ-măn kō-rē-ŎN-ĭk gō-nă-dō-TRŌ-pĭn	
hymen (267)	HĪ-mĕn	
hysterectomy (269)	hĭs-tĕr-ĔK-tō-mē	
hysteroscopy (269)	hĭs-tĕr-ŎS-kō-pē	
inframammary (269)	ĭn-fră-MĂM-ăr-ē	
intrauterine device (272)	ĭn-tră-Ū-tĕ-rĭn dĕ-VĪS	
involution (272)	ĭn-vō-LOO-shŭn	
labia (267)	LĀ-bē-ă	
lactation (269)	lăk-TĀ-shŭn	

8

TERM	PRONUNCIATION	MEANING
lactiferous ducts (267)	lăk-TĬ-fĕ-rŭs dŭkts	_____
leukorrhea (272)	loo-kō-RĒ-ă	_____
luteinizing hormone (267)	LOO-tē-nī-zĭng HŎR-mōn	_____
mammary papilla (267)	MĂM-ăr-ē pă-PĬL-ă	_____
mammoplasty (269)	MĂM-ō-plăs-tē	_____
mastectomy (270)	măs-TĔK-tō-mē	_____
mastitis (270)	măs-TĪ-tĭs	_____
menarche (267)	mĕ-NĂR-kē	_____
menometrorrhagia (270)	mĕn-ō-mĕl-rō-RĀ-jă	_____
menopause (267)	MĔN-ō-păwz	_____
menorrhea (272)	mĕn-ō-RĒ-ă	_____
menorrhagia (270)	mĕn-ō-RĀ-jă	_____
menstruation (267)	mĕn-strū-Ā-shŭn	_____
metrorrhagia (270)	mĕ-trō-RĀ-jă	_____
multigravida (273)	mŭl-tĭ-GRĂV-ĭ-dă	_____
multipara (273)	mŭl-TĬP-ă-ră	_____
myomectomy (270)	mī-ō-MĔK-tō-mē	_____
myometrium (267)	mī-ō-MĒ-trē-ŭm	_____
neonatal (270)	nē-ō-NĀ-tăl	_____
neonatology (267)	nē-ō-nā-TŎL-ō-jē	_____
nulligravida (273)	nŭl-lē-GRĂ-vĭ-dă	_____
nullipara (273)	nŭl-LĬP-ă-ră	_____
obstetrics (267)	ŏb-STĔT-rĭks	_____
oligomenorrhea (270)	ŏl-ĭ-gō-mĕn-ō-RĒ-ă	_____
oocyte (270)	ō-ō-SĪT	_____
oogenesis (270)	ō-ō-JĔN-ĕ-sĭs	_____
oophorectomy (270)	oo-fō-RĔK-tō-mē *or* ō-ŏf-ō-RĔK-tō-mē	_____
oophoritis (271)	ō-ŏf-ōr-Ī-tĭs	_____
orifice (267)	ŎR-ĭ-fĭs	_____
ovarian (170)	ō-VĀ-rē-ăn	_____

8

TERM	PRONUNCIATION	MEANING
ovarian follicle (267)	ō-VĀ-rē-ăn FŎL-lĭ-kl	
ovary (267)	Ō-vă-rē	
ovulation (267)	ŏv-ū-LĀ-shŭn	
ovum; ova (267)	Ō-vŭm; Ō-vă	
oxytocia (272)	ŏks-ē-TŌ-sē-ă	
oxytocin (272)	ŏks-ē-TŌ-sĭn	
parturition (267)	păr-tū-RĬSH-ŭn	
perineorrhaphy (270)	pĕ-rĭ-nē-ŎR-ră-fē	
perineum (267)	pĕ-rĭ-NĒ-ŭm	
pituitary gland (267)	pĭ-TOO-ĭ-tăr-ē glănd	
placenta (267)	plă-SĔN-tă	
pregnancy (267)	PRĔG-năn-sē	
prenatal (273)	prē-NĀ-tăl	
primigravida (271)	prī-mĭ-GRĂV-ĭ-dă	
primipara (273)	prī-MĬP-ă-ră	
primiparous (272)	prī-MĬP-ă-rŭs	
progesterone (268)	prō-JĔS-tĕ-rōn	
pseudocyesis (271)	sū-dō-sī-Ē-sĭs	
puberty (268)	PŪ-bĕr-tē	
pyosalpinx (272)	pī-ō-SĂL-pĭnks	
retroversion (273)	rĕ-trō-VĔR-zhŭn	
salpingectomy (271)	săl-pĭn-JĔK-tō-mē	
salpingitis (277)	săl-pĭn-JĪ-tĭs	
uterine prolapse (271)	Ū-tĕr-ĭn PRŌ-lăps	
uterine serosa (268)	Ū-tĕr-ĭn sē-RŌ-să	
uterus (268)	Ū-tĕr-ŭs	
vagina (268)	vă-JĪ-nă	
vaginal orifice (271)	VĂ-jĭ-năl ŎR-ĭ-fĭs	
vaginitis (271)	vă-jĭ-NĪ-tĭs	
vulva (268)	VŬL-vă	

8

TERM	PRONUNCIATION	MEANING
vulvodynia (271)	vŭl-vō-DĬ-nē-ă	_____
vulvovaginitis (271)	vŭl-vō-vă-jĭ-NĪ-tĭs	_____
zygote (268)	ZĪ-gōt	_____

Pathologic Conditions, Clinical Tests, and Procedures

TERM	PRONUNCIATION	MEANING
abortion (286)	ă-BŎR-shŭn	_____
abruptio placentae (280)	ă-BRŬP-shē-ō plă-SĔN-tā	_____
Apgar score (281)	ĂP-găr skōr	_____
aspiration (284)	ăs-pĬ-RĀ-shŭn	_____
carcinoma in situ (274)	kăr-sĭ-NO-mă ĭn SĪ-tū	_____
carcinoma of the breast (278)	kăr-sĭ-NŌ-mă of the brĕst	_____
carcinoma of the cervix (274)	kăr-sĭ-NŌ-mă of the SĔR-vĭks	_____
carcinoma of the endometrium (275)	kăr-sĭ-NŌ-mă of the ĕn-dō-MĒ-trē-ŭm	_____
cauterization (284)	kaw-tĕr-ĭ-ZĀ-shŭn	_____
cervical dysplasia (274)	SĔR-vĭ-kăl dĭs-PLĀ-zē-ă	_____
cervicitis (275)	sĕr-vĭ-SĪ-tĭs	_____
cesarean section (287)	sē-ZĀ-rē-ăn SĔK-shŭn	_____
chorionic villus sampling (287)	kō-rē-ŎN-ik VĬL-us SĂMP-lĭng	_____
colposcopy (284)	kōl-PŎS-kō-pē	_____
conization (284)	kō-nĭ-ZĀ-shŭn	_____
cryocauterization (284)	krī-ō-kaw-tĕr-ĭ-ZĀ-shŭn	_____
culdocentesis (285)	kŭl-dō-sĕn-TĒ-sĭs	_____
dermoid cysts (277)	DĔR-moyd sĭsts	_____
dilatation (285)	dĭ-lă-TĀ-shŭn	_____
dilation and curettage (285)	dī-LĀ-shŭn and kŭr-ĕ-TĂZH	_____
Down syndrome (281)	Dŏwn SĬN-drōm	_____
ectopic pregnancy (280)	ĕk-TŎP-ĭk PRĔG-năn-sē	_____

8

TERM	PRONUNCIATION	MEANING
endometriosis (275)	ĕn-dō-mē-trē-Ō-sĭs	
erythroblastosis fetalis (281)	ĕ-rĭth-rō-blăs-TŌ-sĭs fē-TĂ-lĭs	
exenteration (286)	ĕks-ĕn-tĕ-RĀ-shŭn	
fetal monitoring (287)	FĒ-tăl MŎN-ĭ-tŏ-rĭng	
fibrocystic breast disease (280)	fī-brō-SĬS-tĭk brĕst dĭ-ZĒZ	
fibroids (277)	FĪ-broydz	
hyaline membrane disease (281)	HĪ-ă-lĭn MĔM-brān dĭ-ZĒZ	
hydrocephalus (282)	hī-drō-SĔF-ă-lŭs	
hysterosalpingography (283)	hĭs-tĕr-ō-săl-pĭng-ŎG-ră-fē	
in vitro fertilization (287)	ĭn VĒ-trō fĕr-tĭl-ĭ-ZĀ-shŭn	
laparoscopy (286)	lă-pă-RŎS-kō-pē	
leiomyomas (276)	lī-ō-mī-Ō-măz	
mammography (283)	măm-MŎG-ră-fē	
meconium aspiration syndrome (282)	mĕ-KŌ-nē-ŭm ăs-pĭ-RĀ-shŭn SĬN-drōm	
multiple gestation (280)	MŬL-tĭ-pl jĕs-TĀ-shŭn	
ovarian carcinoma (276)	ō-VĀR-ē-an kăr-sĭ-NŌ-mă	
ovarian cysts (277)	ō-VĀR-ē-an sĭsts	
palpation (277)	păl-PĀ-shŭn	
Pap test (282)	păp tĕst	
pelvic inflammatory disease (277)	PĔL-vĭk ĭn-FLĂM-mă-tō-rē dĭ-ZĒZ	
pelvic ultrasonography (284)	PĔL-vĭk ŭl-tră-sŏn-ŎG-ră-fē	
placenta previa (280)	plă-SĔN-tă PRĒ-vē-ă	
preeclampsia (281)	prē-ē-KLĂMP-sē-ă	
pregnancy test (282)	PRĔG-năn-sē tĕst	
pyloric stenosis (282)	pī-LŎR-ĭk stĕ-NŌ-sĭs	
respiratory distress syndrome (281)	RĔS-pĭr-ă-tō-rē dĭs-STRĔS SĬN-drōm	
tubal ligation (286)	TOO-băl lī-GĀ-shŭn	

8

REVIEW SHEET

Write the meanings of the word parts in the spaces provided, and test yourself. Check your answers with the information in the chapter or in the *Glossary (Medical Word Parts—English)* at the end of the book.

Combining Forms

COMBINING FORM	MEANING	COMBINING FORM	MEANING
amni/o		myom/o	
bartholin/o		nat/i	
cephal/o		obstetr/o	
cervic/o		olig/o	
chori/o, chorion/o		o/o	
colp/o		oophor/o	
culd/o		ov/o	
episi/o		ovari/o	
galact/o		ovul/o	
gynec/o		perine/o	
hyster/o		phor/o	
lact/o		py/o	
mamm/o		salping/o	
mast/o		uter/o	
men/o		vagin/o	
metr/o, metri/o		vulv/o	
my/o			

Prefixes

PREFIX	MEANING	PREFIX	MEANING
bi-		oxy-	
dys-		peri-	
endo-		pre-	
in-		primi-	
intra-		pseudo-	
multi-		retro-	
nulli-		uni-	

8

Suffixes

SUFFIX	MEANING	SUFFIX	MEANING
-arche	_____	-plasty	_____
-cyesis	_____	-rrhagia	_____
-dynia	_____	-rrhaphy	_____
-ectomy	_____	-rrhea	_____
-flexion	_____	-salpinx	_____
-genesis	_____	-scopy	_____
-gravida	_____	-stenosis	_____
-itis	_____	-stomy	_____
-pareunia	_____	-tocia, -tocin	_____
-parous	_____	-tomy	_____
-plasia	_____	-version	_____

Diagnostic Procedures

Match the diagnostic procedures in Column I with their descriptions in Column II. Check your answers with the information in the chapter.

COLUMN I

1. needle aspiration _____

2. colposcopy _____

3. culdocentesis _____

4. hysterosalpingography _____

5. mammography _____

6. Pap test _____

7. pregnancy test _____

8. pelvic ultrasonography _____

COLUMN II

A. Uterus and fallopian tubes are imaged (x-ray procedure).

B. hCG is measured.

C. X-ray images are taken of the breast.

D. Procedure to biopsy breast tissue.

E. Removal of cervical and vaginal cells for analysis.

F. Fluid is obtained from the region between the rectum and the uterus.

G. Images of the region of the hip are obtained using sound waves.

H. Microscopic visual examination of the vagina and cervix.

8

Male Reproductive System

Chapter Sections:

CHAPTER GOALS

- Name, locate, and describe the functions of the organs of the male reproductive system.
- Define abnormal conditions and infectious diseases that affect the male reproductive system.
- Differentiate among several types of sexually transmitted infections.
- Define combining forms used to describe the structures of this system.
- Describe various laboratory tests and clinical procedures pertinent to disorders of the male reproductive system, and recognize related abbreviations.
- Apply your new knowledge to understanding medical terms in their proper contexts, such as medical reports and records.

INTRODUCTION

The male sex cell, the **spermatozoon** (sperm cell), is microscopic—in volume, only one third the size of a red blood cell and less than 1/100,000 the size of the female ovum. A relatively uncomplicated cell, the sperm is composed of a head region, containing nuclear hereditary material (chromosomes), and a tail region, consisting of a **flagellum** (hair-like process). The flagellum makes the sperm motile and makes it look somewhat like a tadpole. The spermatozoon cell contains relatively little food and cytoplasm, because it lives only long enough (3 to 5 days) to travel from its point of release from the male to where the egg cell lies within the female reproductive tract (fallopian tube). Only one spermatozoon out of approximately 300 million sperm cells released during a single **ejaculation** (ejection of sperm and fluid from the male urethra) can penetrate a single ovum and result in fertilization of the ovum. Figure 9-1 shows a diagram of a **sperm cell** and a photograph of **spermatozoa**.

If more than one egg is passing down the fallopian tube when sperm are present, multiple fertilizations are possible, and twins, triplets, quadruplets, and so on may occur. Twins resulting from the fertilization of separate ova by separate sperm cells are called **fraternal twins.** Fraternal twins, developing with separate placentas, can be of the same sex or different sexes and resemble each other no more than ordinary brothers and sisters. Fraternal twinning is hereditary; the daughters of mothers of twins can carry the gene.

Identical twins result from fertilization of a single egg cell by a single sperm. As the fertilized egg cell divides and forms many cells, it somehow splits, and each part continues separately to undergo further division, each producing an embryo. Most identical twins have one placenta and two amniotic sacs. Identical twins are always of the same sex and are very similar in form and feature.

The organs of the male reproductive system are designed to produce and release billions of spermatozoa throughout the lifetime of a male from puberty onward. In addition, the male reproductive system secretes a hormone called **testosterone.** Testosterone is responsible for the production of the bodily characteristics of the male (such as beard, pubic hair, and deeper voice) and for the proper development of male gonads **(testes)** and accessory organs **(prostate gland** and **seminal vesicles)** that secrete fluids to ensure the lubrication and viability of sperm.

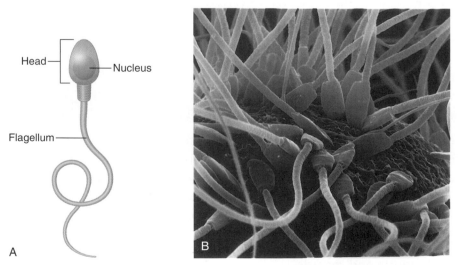

FIGURE 9-1 **A, Sperm cell. B,** Photograph of **spermatozoa.**

ANATOMY

Label Figure 9-2 as you study the following description of the anatomy of the male reproductive system.

Each male gonad is a **testis** [1]. There are two **testes** (plural) or **testicles** that develop in the abdomen at about the level of the kidneys before descending during embryonic development into the **scrotum** [2], a sac enclosing the testes on the outside of the body.

The scrotum, lying between the thighs, exposes the testes to a lower temperature than that of the rest of the body. This lower temperature is necessary for the adequate maturation and development of sperm **(spermatogenesis).** Located between the anus and the scrotum, at the floor of the pelvic cavity in the male, the **perineum** [3] is analogous to the perineal region in the female.

The interior of a testis is composed of a large mass of narrow, coiled tubules called the **seminiferous tubules** [4]. These tubules contain cells that manufacture spermatozoa. The seminiferous tubules are the **parenchymal tissue** of the testis, which means that they perform the essential work of the organ (formation of sperm). Other cells in the testis, lying adjacent to seminiferous tubules, are **interstitial cells.** They manufacture an important male hormone, **testosterone.**

All body organs contain **parenchyma**, which perform the essential functions of the organ. Organs also contain supportive, connective, and framework tissue, such as blood vessels, connective tissues, and sometimes muscle as well. This supportive tissue is called **stroma (stromal tissue).**

After formation, sperm cells move through the seminiferous tubules and collect in ducts that lead to a large tube, the **epididymis** [5], at the upper part of each testis. The spermatozoa

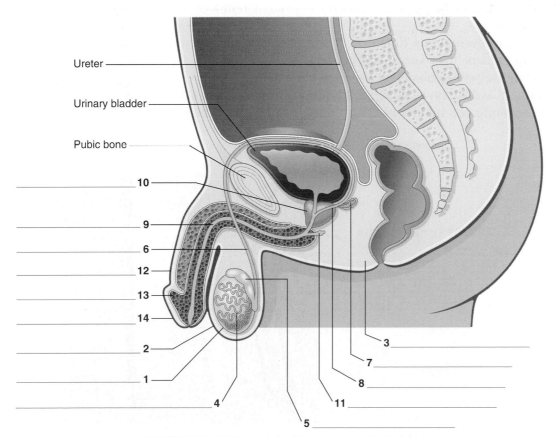

FIGURE 9-2   Male reproductive system, sagittal view.

mature, become motile in the epididymis, and are temporarily stored there. An epididymis runs down the length of each testicle (the coiled tube is about 16 feet long) and then turns upward again and becomes a narrow, straight tube called the **vas deferens** [6] or **ductus deferens.** Figure 9-3 shows the internal structure of a testis and the epididymis. The vas deferens is about 2 feet long and carries the sperm up into the pelvic region, at the level of the urinary bladder, merging with ducts from the **seminal vesicles** [7] to form the **ejaculatory duct** [8] leading toward the urethra. During a **vasectomy** or **sterilization** procedure, the urologist cuts and ties off each vas deferens by making an incision in the scrotum.

The seminal vesicles, two glands (only one is shown in Figure 9-2) located at the base of the bladder, open into the ejaculatory duct as it joins the **urethra** [9]. They secrete a thick, sugary, yellowish substance that nourishes the sperm cells and forms a portion of ejaculated semen. **Semen,** a combination of fluid (seminal fluid) and spermatozoa (sperm cells account for less than 1% of the semen volume), is ejected from the body through the urethra. In the male, as opposed to that in the female, the genital orifice combines with the urinary (urethral) opening.

The **prostate gland** [10] lies at the region where the vas deferens enters the urethra, almost encircling the upper end of the urethra. It secretes a milky white fluid that is a mixture of sugars, enzymes, and alkaline chemicals. As part of semen, this fluid is nutritious for sperm cells, and after ejaculation into the vagina, the alkaline chemicals promote the survival of sperm in the acidic environment of the vagina. Muscular tissue of the prostate aids in the expulsion of fluid during ejaculation. **Bulbourethral glands** [11], lying below the prostate gland, also secrete fluid into the urethra during ejaculation.

The urethra passes through the **penis** [12] to the outside of the body. The penis is composed of erectile tissue and at its tip expands to form a soft, sensitive region called the **glans penis** [13]. Ordinarily, a fold of skin called the **prepuce,** or **foreskin** [14], covers the glans penis. During a circumcision the foreskin is removed, leaving the glans penis visible at all times.

Erectile dysfunction (impotence) is the inability of the adult male to achieve an erection. Viagra (sildenafil), Cialis (tadalafil), and Stendra (avanafil) are drugs that increase blood flow to the penis, enhancing ability to have an erection.

The flow diagram in Figure 9-4 traces the path of spermatozoa from their formation in the seminiferous tubules of the testes to the outside of the body.

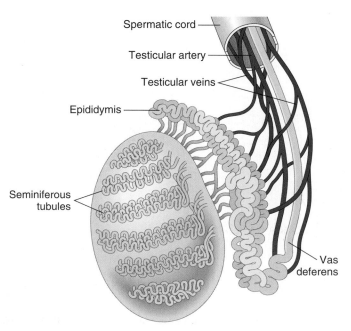

FIGURE 9-3   Internal structure of a testis and the epididymis.

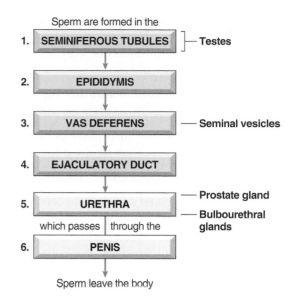

Sperm are formed in the

1. **SEMINIFEROUS TUBULES** ⎤— Testes

2. **EPIDIDYMIS**

3. **VAS DEFERENS** —— Seminal vesicles

4. **EJACULATORY DUCT**

5. **URETHRA** —— Prostate gland
—— Bulbourethral glands

which passes │ through the

6. **PENIS**

Sperm leave the body

FIGURE 9-4   The **passage of sperm** from the seminiferous tubules in the testes to the outside of the body.

VOCABULARY

This list reviews new terms introduced in the text. Short definitions reinforce your understanding.

bulbourethral glands	Pair of exocrine glands near the male urethra. They secrete fluid into the urethra. Also called **Cowper glands.**
ejaculation	Ejection of sperm and fluid from the male urethra.
ejaculatory duct	Tube through which semen enters the male urethra.
epididymis (*plural: epididymides*)	One of a pair of long, tightly coiled tubes above each testis. It stores and carries sperm from seminiferous tubules to the vas deferens.
erectile dysfunction	Inability of an adult male to achieve an erection; impotence.
flagellum	Hair-like projection on a sperm cell that makes it motile (able to move).
fraternal twins	Two infants resulting from fertilization of two separate ova by two separate sperm cells (Figure 9-5).
glans penis	Sensitive tip of the penis; comparable to the clitoris in the female.

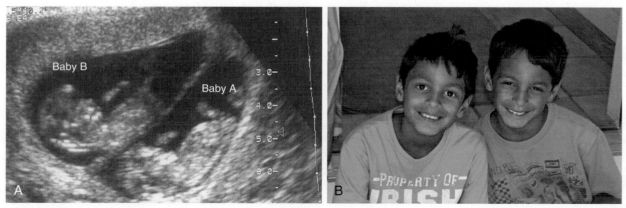

FIGURE 9-5   Fraternal twins. A, Notice the 6-week-old embryos in two separate amniotic sacs. **B,** Twins Marcos and Matheus Do Carmo are 10 years old. *(Courtesy Juliana Do Carmo.)*

9

identical twins	Two infants resulting from division of one fertilized egg into two distinct embryos. Conjoined ("Siamese") twins are incompletely separated identical twins.
interstitial cells of the testes	Specialized cells that lie adjacent to the seminiferous tubules in the testes. These cells produce testosterone and are also called **Leydig cells.**
parenchymal tissue	Essential distinctive cells of an organ. In the testis, the seminiferous tubules that produce sperm are parenchymal.
penis	Male external organ of reproduction.
perineum	External region between the anus and scrotum in the male.
prepuce	Foreskin; fold of skin covering the tip of the penis.
prostate gland	Exocrine gland at the base of the male urinary bladder. The prostate secretes fluid that contributes to semen during ejaculation. ✳ **HINT:** Don't confuse *prostate* with *prostrate,* which means lying down.
scrotum	External sac that contains the testes.
semen	Spermatozoa (sperm cells) and seminal fluid (prostatic and seminal vesicle secretions), discharged from the urethra during ejaculation.
seminal vesicles	Paired sac-like exocrine glands that secrete fluid (a major component of semen) into the vas deferens.
seminiferous tubules	Narrow, coiled tubules that produce sperm in the testes.
spermatozoon (*plural:* **spermatozoa)**	Sperm cell.
sterilization	Procedure that removes a person's ability to produce or release reproductive cells; removal of testicles, vasectomy, and oophorectomy are sterilization procedures.
stromal tissue	Supportive, connective tissue of an organ, as distinguished from its parenchyma. Also called **stroma.**
testis (*plural:* **testes)**	Male gonad **(testicle)** that produces spermatozoa and the hormone testosterone. *Remember:* Testis means one testicle, and testes are two testicles.
testosterone	Hormone secreted by the interstitial tissue of the testes; responsible for male sex characteristics.
vas deferens	Narrow tube (one on each side) carrying sperm from the epididymis toward the urethra. Also called **ductus deferens.**

 Perineum/Peritoneum

Don't confuse **perineum,** which is the area between the anus and scrotum in the male and the anus and vagina in females, with the **peritoneum,** which is the membrane surrounding the abdominal cavity!

 Semen/Sperm

Don't confuse *semen* with *sperm. Semen* is the thick, whitish secretion discharged from the urethra during ejaculation. **Sperm (spermatozoa)** are cells that develop in the testes. Semen contains sperm.

 Sterilization/Impotence

Don't confuse **sterilization,** which can be performed in men and women, with **impotence,** which is the inability of a male to sustain an erection or achieve ejaculation.

TERMINOLOGY

Write the meanings of the medical terms in the spaces provided.

COMBINING FORMS

COMBINING FORM	MEANING	TERMINOLOGY	MEANING
andr/o	male	androgen _____ *Testosterone is an androgen. The testes in males and the adrenal glands in both men and women produce androgens.*	
balan/o	glans penis (Greek *balanos,* means acorn)	balanitis _____ *An inflammation usually caused by overgrowth of organisms (bacteria and yeast) (Figure 9-6A).*	
cry/o	cold	cryogenic surgery _____ *Technique for prostate cancer treatment using freezing temperatures to destroy cancer cells.*	
crypt/o	hidden	cryptorchidism _____ *In this congenital condition, one or both testicles do not descend, by the time of birth, into the scrotal sac from the abdominal cavity (Figure 9-6B).*	
epididym/o	epididymis	epididymitis _____ *This is an inflammation usually caused by bacteria. Signs and symptoms are fever, chills, pain in the groin, and tender, swollen epididymis.*	
gon/o	seed (Greek *gone,* seed)	gonorrhea _____ *See page 322.*	
hydr/o	water, fluid	hydrocele _____ *See page 320.*	

9

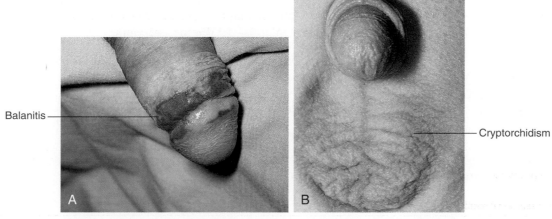

FIGURE 9-6   A, Balanitis. The **glans penis** (or **glans**) is the sensitive bulbous area at the distal end of the penis. **B, Cryptorchidism.**

COMBINING FORM	MEANING	TERMINOLOGY	MEANING
orch/o, orchi/o, orchid/o	testis, testicle	orchiectomy _____ *Castration in males. (Also called orchidectomy.)*	
		orchitis _____ *Caused by injury or by the mumps virus, which also infects the salivary glands.*	
pen/o	penis	penile _____ *-ile means pertaining to.*	
		penoscrotal _____	
prostat/o	prostate gland	prostatitis _____ *Bacterial (E. coli) prostatitis often is associated with urethritis and infection of the lower urinary tract.*	
		prostatectomy _____	
semin/i	semen, seed	seminiferous tubules _____ *The suffix -ferous means pertaining to bearing, or bearing or carrying.*	
sperm/o, spermat/o	spermatozoa, semen	spermolytic _____ *Noun suffixes ending in -sis, like -lysis, form adjectives by dropping the -sis and adding -tic.*	
		oligospermia _____	
		aspermia _____ *Lack of semen (sperm and fluid). One cause of aspermia is retrograde ejaculation (sperm flows backward into the urinary bladder) as a result of prostate surgery.*	
terat/o	monster (Greek *teras*, monster)	teratoma _____ *This tumor occurs in the testes or ovaries and is composed of different types of tissue, such as bone, hair, cartilage, and skin cells. Teratomas in the testes are malignant.*	
test/o	testis, testicle	testicular _____ *The term testis originates from a Latin term meaning witness. In ancient times men would take an oath with one hand on their testes, swearing by their manhood to tell the truth.*	
varic/o	varicose veins	varicocele _____ *A collection of varicose (swollen, twisted) veins above the testis. See page 320.*	
vas/o	vessel, duct; vas deferens	vasectomy _____ *See page 326. Remember: In this term, vas/o refers to the vas deferens, and not to any other vessel or duct.*	

9

Derivation of orchid/o

This combining form is derived from the Greek word *orchis* meaning testicle. The botanical name for orchid, the flower, is also derived from the same Greek word because of the fleshy tubers of the plant.

COMBINING FORM	MEANING	TERMINOLOGY	MEANING
zo/o	animal life	azoospermia _____ *Lack of spermatozoa in the semen. Causes include testicular dysfunction, chemotherapy, blockage of the epididymis, and vasectomy.*	

SUFFIXES

SUFFIX	MEANING	TERMINOLOGY	MEANING
-genesis	formation	spermato<u>genesis</u> _____	
-one	hormone	testoster<u>one</u> _____ *Ster/o indicates that this is a type of steroid compound. Examples of other steroids are estrogen, cortisol, and progesterone.*	
-pexy	fixation, put in place	orchio<u>pexy</u> _____ *A surgical procedure to correct cryptorchidism.*	
-stomy	new opening	vasovaso<u>stomy</u> _____ *Reversal of vasectomy; a urologist rejoins the cut ends of the vas deferens.*	

PATHOLOGIC CONDITIONS; SEXUALLY TRANSMITTED INFECTIONS

TUMORS AND ANATOMIC/STRUCTURAL DISORDERS

Testes

carcinoma of the testes (testicular cancer)

Malignant tumor of the testicles.

Testicular tumors are rare except in the 15- to 35-year-old age group. The most common tumor, a **seminoma,** arises from embryonic cells in the testes (Figure 9-7A). Nonseminomatous tumors are **embryonal carcinoma** (Figure 9-7B), **teratoma, choriocarcinoma,** and **yolk sac tumor.** Teratomas are composed of tissue such as bone, hair, cartilage, and skin cells (terat/o means monster).

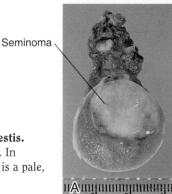
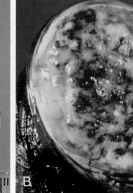

Seminoma

FIGURE 9-7   A, Seminoma of a testis. B, Embryonal carcinoma of a testis. In contrast with the seminoma, which is a pale, homogeneous mass, the embryonal carcinoma is a hemorrhagic mass.

Azoospermia/Aspermia

Azoospermia is semen without sperm cells, while **aspermia** is no semen at all.

If detected early, testicular cancers can be treated and cured with surgery (orchiectomy), radiotherapy, and chemotherapy. Tumors produce the proteins **human chorionic gonadotropin (hCG)** and **alpha-fetoprotein (AFP).** Serum levels of these proteins are used as **tumor markers** to determine success of treatment.

cryptorchidism; cryptorchism

Undescended testicles.

Orchiopexy is performed to bring the testes into the scrotum, if they do not descend on their own by the age of 1 or 2 years. Undescended testicles are associated with a high risk for sterility and increased risk of developing testicular cancer.

hydrocele

Sac of clear fluid in the scrotum.

Hydroceles (Figure 9-8) may be congenital or occur as a response to infection or tumors. Often idiopathic, they can be differentiated from testicular masses by ultrasound imaging. If the hydrocele does not resolve on its own, the sac fluid is aspirated using a needle and syringe, or hydrocelectomy may be necessary. In this procedure, the sac is surgically removed through an incision in the scrotum.

testicular torsion

Twisting of the spermatic cord (see Figure 9-8)**.**

The rotation of the spermatic cord cuts off blood supply to the testis. Torsion occurs most frequently in childhood. Surgical correction within hours of onset of symptoms can save the testis.

varicocele

Enlarged, dilated veins near the testicle.

Varicocele (see Figure 9-8) may be associated with oligospermia and azoospermia. Oligospermic men with varicocele and scrotal pain should have a varicocelectomy. In this procedure, the internal spermatic vein is ligated (the affected segment is cut out and the ends are tied off). On occasion, this leads to an increase in fertility.

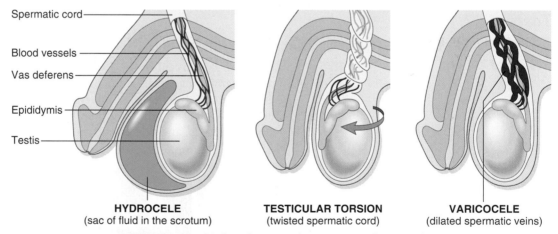

Spermatic cord

Blood vessels

Vas deferens

Epididymis

Testis

HYDROCELE
(sac of fluid in the scrotum)

TESTICULAR TORSION
(twisted spermatic cord)

VARICOCELE
(dilated spermatic veins)

FIGURE 9-8 Hydrocele, testicular torsion, and varicocele.

Testicular Cancer Detection

There may be no signs or symptoms of testicular cancer. Regular testicular self-examinations, however, can help identify growths earlier, when the chance for successful treatment is highest. A man should see a doctor if he detects any mass, pain, or swelling in the scrotum.

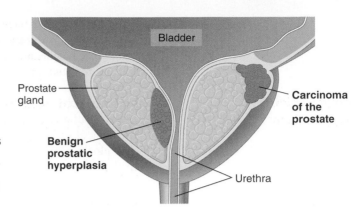

FIGURE 9-9 **The prostate gland with carcinoma and benign prostatic hyperplasia (BPH).** Carcinoma usually arises around the sides of the gland, whereas BPH occurs in the center of the gland. Because prostate cancers are located more peripherally, they can be palpated on digital rectal exam (DRE).

Prostate Gland

benign prostatic hyperplasia (BPH)

Benign growth of cells within the prostate gland.

BPH is a common condition in men older than 60 years of age. Urinary obstruction and inability to empty the bladder completely are symptoms. Figure 9-9 shows the prostate gland with BPH and with carcinoma. Surgical treatment by **transurethral resection of the prostate (TURP)** relieves the obstruction, but overgrowth of cells may recur over several years. In this procedure, an endoscope (resectoscope) is inserted into the penis and through the urethra. Prostatic tissue is removed by an electrical hot loop attached to the resectoscope (see page 325).

Several drugs to relieve BPH symptoms have been approved by the FDA. Finasteride (Proscar) inhibits production of a potent testosterone that promotes enlargement of the prostate. Other drugs, alpha blockers such as tamsulosin (Flomax), act by relaxing the smooth muscle of the prostate and the neck of the bladder.

Lasers also may be used to destroy prostatic tissue and relieve obstruction. A **laser TURP** or **GreenLight PVP** procedure uses a green light laser at the end of an endoscope (see page 325).

carcinoma of the prostate (prostate cancer)

Malignant tumor (adenocarcinoma) of the prostate gland.

This cancer commonly occurs in men who are older than 50 years. **Digital rectal examination (DRE)** (Figure 9-10) can detect the tumor at a later stage, but early detection depends on a **prostate-specific antigen (PSA) test.** PSA is a protein that is secreted by tumor cells into the bloodstream. PSA levels are elevated in patients with prostate cancer even at an early stage of tumor growth. The normal PSA level is 4.0 ng/mL or less.

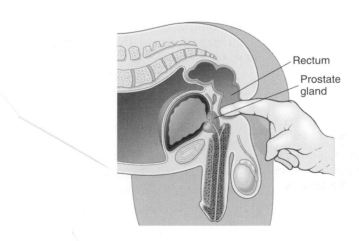

FIGURE 9-10   Digital .
prostate gland.

Diagnosis requires identification by a pathologist of abnormal prostate tissue in a prostate biopsy. Transrectal ultrasound (TRUS) guides the precise placement of the biopsy needle. Multiple needle biopsy specimens are taken through the rectal wall. Computed tomography (CT) detects lymph node metastases.

Treatment consists of surgery (prostatectomy), radiation therapy, and/or hormonal chemotherapy. Because prostatic cells are stimulated to grow in the presence of androgens, antiandrogen hormones slow tumor growth by depriving the cells of testosterone. Prostate cancer also is treated with leupron, a hormone that blocks pituitary stimulation of the testes and reduces the level of androgens in the bloodstream. Tumor cells also can be destroyed by brachytherapy (brachy = near), which means that radioactive seeds are implanted directly into the prostate gland. See the ***In Person: Prostate Cancer*** story on page 329.

Penis

hypospadias

Congenital abnormality in which the male urethral opening is on the undersurface of the penis, instead of at its tip.

Hypospadias (-spadias means the condition of tearing or cutting) occurs in 1 in every 300 live male births and can be corrected surgically (Figure 9-11A).

phimosis

Narrowing (stricture) of the opening of the prepuce over the glans penis.

This condition (phim/o = muzzle) can interfere with urination and cause secretions to accumulate under the prepuce, leading to infection. Treatment is by circumcision (cutting around the prepuce to remove it) (Figure 9-11B).

SEXUALLY TRANSMITTED INFECTIONS

9

Sexually transmitted infections (STIs) are infections transmitted by sexual or other genital contact. Also known as **sexually transmitted diseases (STDs)** or venereal diseases (from Latin Venus, the goddess of love), they occur in both men and women and are some of the most prevalent communicable diseases in the world.

chlamydial infection

Bacterial invasion (by *Chlamydia trachomatis*) of the urethra and reproductive tract.

Within 3 weeks after becoming infected, men may experience a burning sensation on urination and notice a white or clear discharge from the penis.

Infected women may notice a yellowish vaginal discharge (from the endocervix), but often the disease is asymptomatic. Antibiotics cure the infection, but if untreated, this STI can cause salpingitis (pelvic inflammatory disease [PID]) and infertility in women.

gonorrhea

Inflammation of the genital tract mucosa, caused by infection with gonococci (berry-shaped bacteria).

Other areas of the body, such as the eye, oral mucosa, rectum, and joints, may be affected as well. Signs and symptoms include dysuria and a yellow, mucopurulent (**purulent** means pus-filled) discharge from the male urethra (Figure 9-12A). The ancient Greeks mistakenly thought that this discharge was a leakage of semen, so they named the condition gonorrhea, meaning discharge of seed (gon/o = seed).

Many women carry the disease asymptomatically, whereas others have pain, vaginal and urethral discharge, and salpingitis (PID). As a result of sexual activity, men and women can acquire anorectal and pharyngeal gonococcal infections as well. Chlamydial infection and gonorrhea often occur together. When treating these infections, doctors give antibiotics for both and treat both partners.

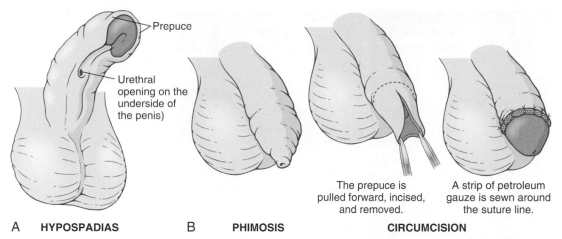

Prepuce

Urethral opening on the underside of the penis)

The prepuce is pulled forward, incised, and removed.

A strip of petroleum gauze is sewn around the suture line.

A   HYPOSPADIAS   B   PHIMOSIS   CIRCUMCISION

FIGURE 9-11   A, Hypospadias. Surgical repair involves elongating the urethra by using surrounding tissue or using a graft from tissue elsewhere in the body and bringing it to the exit at the tip of the penis. **B, Phimosis** and **circumcision** to correct the condition.

herpes genitalis

Infection of skin and genital mucosa, caused by the herpes simplex virus (HSV).

Most cases of herpes genitalis are caused by HSV type 2 (although some are caused by HSV type 1, which commonly is associated with oral infections such as cold sores or fever blisters). The usual clinical presentation is reddening of skin with formation of small, **fluid-filled blisters** and ulcers (Figure 9-12B). Initial episodes also may involve inguinal lymphadenopathy, fever, headache, and malaise. Remissions and relapse periods occur; no drug is known to be effective as a cure. Neonatal herpes affects infants born to women with active infection near the time of delivery. Gynecologists may deliver infants by cesarean section to prevent infection of these babies by HSV. Studies suggest that women with herpes genitalis are at a higher risk for developing vulvar and cervical cancer.

9

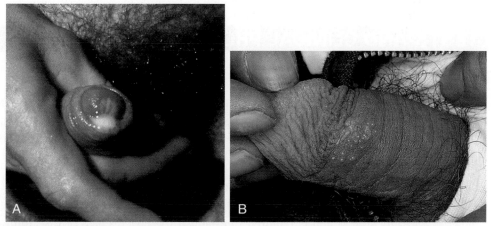

FIGURE 9-12   A, Gonorrhea. Discharge from the penis can be seen. **B, Herpes genitalis.** The classic blisters (vesicles) are evident.

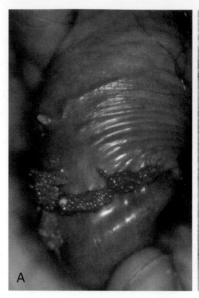
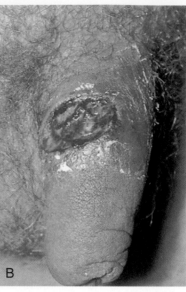

FIGURE 9-13   A, Genital warts. B, Primary syphilis with chancre on penis.

human papillomavirus (HPV) infection	**Infection of the skin and mucous membranes in the anogenital region by the human papillomavirus.**

Some types of HPV cause **genital warts** (see Figure 9-13A) and lead to cancer of the cervix as well as cancer in men. A vaccine is available for young girls and boys that protects against four types of HPV.

syphilis	**Chronic STI caused by a spirochete (spiral-shaped bacterium).**

A chancre (hard ulcer or sore) usually appears on the external genitalia a few weeks after bacterial infection (Figure 9-13B). Two to six months after the chancre disappears, secondary syphilis begins. Tertiary syphilis includes damage to the brain, spinal cord, and heart, which may appear years after the earlier symptoms disappear. Syphilis (which was so often fatal in early times that it was known as the "great pox"—versus the more familiar smallpox) can be congenital in the fetus if it is transmitted from the mother during pregnancy. Penicillin is effective for treatment in most cases.

LABORATORY TESTS AND CLINICAL PROCEDURES

LABORATORY TESTS

PSA test	**Measurement of levels of prostate-specific antigen (PSA) in the blood.**

PSA is produced by cells within the prostate gland. Elevated levels of PSA are associated with enlargement of the prostate gland and may be a sign of prostate cancer.

semen analysis	**Microscopic examination of ejaculated fluid.**

Sperm cells are counted and examined for motility and shape. The test is part of fertility studies and is required to establish the effectiveness of vasectomy. Men with sperm counts of less than 20 million/mL of semen usually are sterile (not fertile). Sterility can result in an adult male who becomes ill with mumps, an infectious disease affecting the testes (inflammation leads to deterioration of spermatozoa).

CLINICAL PROCEDURES

castration

Surgical excision of testicles or ovaries.

Castration may be performed to reduce production and secretion of hormones that stimulate growth of malignant cells (in breast cancer and prostate cancer). When a boy is castrated before puberty, he becomes a eunuch (Greek, *eune,* couch; *echein,* to guard). Male secondary sex characteristics fail to develop.

circumcision

Surgical procedure to remove the prepuce of the penis.

See Figure 9-11B, page 323.

digital rectal examination (DRE)

Finger palpation through the anal canal and rectum to examine the prostate gland.

See Figure 9-10, page 321.

photoselective vaporization of the prostate (GreenLight PVP)

Removal of tissue to treat benign prostatic hyperplasia (BPH) using a green light laser ("laser TURP").

This minimally invasive procedure in selected cases replaces TURP for treatment of BPH.

transurethral resection of the prostate (TURP)

Excision of benign prostatic hyperplasia using a resectoscope through the urethra.

This procedure treats benign prostatic hyperplasia (BPH). An electrical hot loop cuts the prostatic tissue; the bits of tissue (chips) are removed through the resectoscope (Figure 9-14).

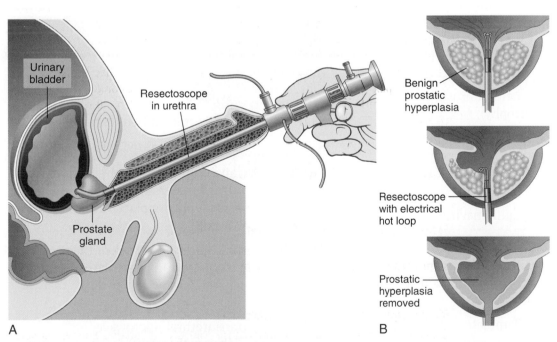

FIGURE 9-14   Transurethral resection of the prostate (TURP). A, The resectoscope contains a light, valves for controlling irrigating fluid, and an electrical loop that cuts tissue and seals blood vessels. **B,** The urologist uses a wire loop through the resectoscope to remove obstructing tissue one piece at a time. The pieces are carried by the fluid into the bladder and flushed out at the end of the operation.

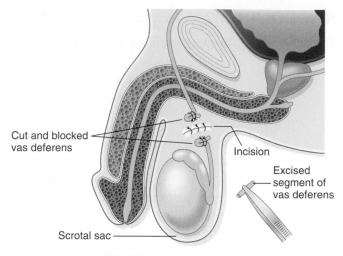

Cut and blocked
vas deferens

Incision

Excised
segment of
vas deferens

Scrotal sac

FIGURE 9-15 Vasectomy.

vasectomy   **Bilateral surgical removal of a part of the vas deferens.**

A urologist cuts the vas deferens, removes a piece, and performs a **ligation** (tying and binding off) of the free ends with sutures (Figure 9-15); this is repeated on the opposite side. The procedure is performed using local anesthesia and through an incision in the scrotal sac. Because spermatozoa cannot leave the body, the vasectomized man is sterile, but not castrated. Normal hormone secretion, sex drive, and potency (ability to have an erection) are intact. The body reabsorbs unexpelled sperm. In a small number of cases, a vasovasostomy can successfully reverse vasectomy.

9

ABBREVIATIONS

BPH	benign prostatic hyperplasia (also called benign prostatic hypertrophy)	**RPR**	rapid plasma reagin [test]; a test for syphilis
DRE	digital rectal examination	**STD**	sexually transmitted disease
ED	erectile dysfunction	**STI**	sexually transmitted infection
GU	genitourinary	**TRUS**	transrectal ultrasound [examination]; test to assess the prostate and guide precise placement of a biopsy needle
HPV	human papillomavirus		
HSV	herpes simplex virus		
NSU	nonspecific urethritis (not due to gonorrhea or chlamydial infection)	**TUIP**	transurethral incision of the prostate; successful in less enlarged prostates and less invasive than TURP
PID	pelvic inflammatory disease		
PIN	prostatic intraepithelial neoplasia; a precursor of prostate cancer	**TUMT**	transurethral microwave thermotherapy
PSA	prostate-specific antigen	**TUNA**	transurethral needle ablation; radiofrequency energy destroys prostate tissue
PVP	photoselective vaporization of the prostate; GreenLight PVP	**TURP**	transurethral resection of the prostate

PRACTICAL APPLICATIONS

Reproduced here from actual medical records is a case report on a patient with post-TURP complaints. Background data and explanations of more difficult terms are added in brackets. Answers to the questions are on page 327.

Also presented for your review is an actual surgical pathology report for a man diagnosed with prostate cancer, as well as a summary of current knowledge on anabolic steroids.

CASE REPORT: A MAN WITH POST-TURP COMPLAINTS

The patient is a 70-year-old man who underwent a TURP for BPH 5 years ago and now has severe obstructive urinary symptoms with a large postvoid residual.

On DRE, his prostate was found to be large, bulky, and nodular, with palpable extension to the left seminal vesicle. His PSA level was 15 ng/mL [normal is 0 to 4 ng/mL] and a bone scan was negative. A CT scan revealed bilateral external iliac adenopathy with lymph nodes measuring 1.5 cm on average [normal lymph node size is less than 1 cm]. A prostatic biopsy revealed a poorly differentiated adenocarcinoma.

This patient most likely has at least stage T3 N+ disease [extension into seminal vesicles and nodal metastases]. Recommendation is anti-testosterone hormonal drug treatment.

Questions about the Case Report

1. Five years previously, the patient had which type of surgery?
   a. Removal of testicles
   b. Perineal prostatectomy
   c. Partial prostatectomy (transurethral)

2. What was the reason for the surgery then?
   a. Cryptorchidism
   b. Benign overgrowth of the prostate gland
   c. Testicular cancer

3. What symptom does he have now?
   a. Burning pain on urination
   b. Urinary retention
   c. Premature ejaculation

4. What examination allowed the physician to feel the tumor?
   a. Palpation by a finger inserted into the rectum
   b. CT scan
   c. Prostate-specific antigen test

5. Where had the tumor spread?
   a. Testes
   b. Pelvic lymph nodes and left seminal vesicle
   c. Pelvic bone

6. What is likely to stimulate prostatic adenocarcinoma growth?
   a. Hormonal drug treatment
   b. Prostatic biopsy
   c. Testosterone secretion

7. Stage T3 N+ means that the tumor
   a. Is localized to the hip area
   b. Is confined to the prostate gland
   c. Has spread locally and beyond lymph nodes

8. Why is staging of tumors important?
   a. To classify the extent of spread of the tumor and to plan treatment
   b. To make the initial diagnosis
   c. To make an adequate biopsy of the tumor

SURGICAL PATHOLOGY REPORT: PROSTATE CANCER/HYPERPLASIA

Patient name: Bill Scott
DOB: 9/14/1942 (Age: 69)
Gender: M
Clinical Data: ?Nodule, right side of prostate; PSA 7.1
Specimen(s):
   A. Right side prostate biopsy
   B. Left side prostate biopsy
FINAL PATHOLOGIC DIAGNOSIS
   A. Needle biopsy of right side prostate gland (six cores)
      ADENOCARCINOMA, MODERATELY TO POORLY DIFFERENTIATED
      Gleason score 4 + 3 = 7
      Estimated tumor load, 10% of prostatic tissue
      Represented in both specimens A and B
   B. Needle biopsy of left side prostate gland
      BENIGN HYPERPLASIA

ABOUT ANABOLIC STEROIDS

Anabolic steroids are male hormones (androgens) that increase body weight and muscle size and may be used by doctors to increase growth in boys who do not mature physically as expected for their age. Steroids also may be used by athletes in an effort to increase strength and enhance performance; however, significant detrimental side effects of these drugs have been recognized:

- High levels of anabolic steroids cause acne, hepatic tumors, and sterility (testicular atrophy and oligospermia).
- In women, the androgenic effect of anabolic steroids leads to male hair distribution, deepening of the voice, amenorrhea, and clitoral enlargement.
- Anabolic steroid use also causes hypercholesterolemia, hypertension, jaundice (liver abnormalities), and salt and water retention (edema).

Gleason Score

The **Gleason score** (named after Dr. Donald Gleason, a pathologist who developed it in the 1960s) is based on the microscopic appearance of the prostate biopsy specimen. Cancers with a higher Gleason score are more aggressive and carry a worse prognosis. The pathologist assigns a grade (number) to the most common tumor cells and another to the next most common tumor cells. Adding these numbers together gives the Gleason score. The score is based on a scale from 1 to 5. More well-differentiated (closer to normal) cells are given a lower grade, and poorly differentiated (malignant) cells are given a higher grade.

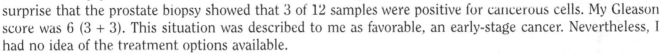

IN PERSON: PROSTATE CANCER

This is a first-person narrative of a man diagnosed with prostate cancer.

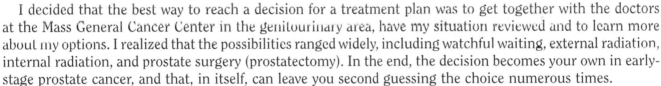

As with many men in their late 50s, the PSA prostate-related lab test was the first item I would always look at when having my annual physical. Over a few years, the PSA had been going up gradually, but nothing that seemed to indicate anything unusual. So it was a bit of a surprise when my primary care doctor suggested that it might be time to have a further medical review of the slowly increasing results. The PSA was 4.37 (4.0 or less is considered normal).

Being in good overall health, I expected the follow-up prostate exam and biopsy to be of a routine nature. It was with great surprise that the prostate biopsy showed that 3 of 12 samples were positive for cancerous cells. My Gleason score was 6 (3 + 3). This situation was described to me as favorable, an early-stage cancer. Nevertheless, I had no idea of the treatment options available.

I decided that the best way to reach a decision for a treatment plan was to get together with the doctors at the Mass General Cancer Center in the genitourinary area, have my situation reviewed and to learn more about my options. I realized that the possibilities ranged widely, including watchful waiting, external radiation, internal radiation, and prostate surgery (prostatectomy). In the end, the decision becomes your own in early-stage prostate cancer, and that, in itself, can leave you second guessing the choice numerous times.

After careful thought and review of the information with my physicians and family, I decided to pursue the internal radiation option, or brachytherapy, often referred to as implantation of radiation seeds. Even up to the time of the procedure, the question remained with me as to whether I was making the right choice: Should I wait a while and just see how things go, and would there be any of the unlikely side effects that are noted for this procedure? When the time came, I decided to go forward and had the procedure done at MGH. The entire medical team there made the process from start to completion as successful an event as one could hope for. The best news was that after the procedure, my PSA dropped to 2.5.

Now a year has passed, and I am happy to see that the PSA has continued downward. The long-term side effects of the brachytherapy procedure were related to urination and erectile dysfunction. While urination post-procedure was painful, discomfort dissipated within a week or so. Long term, managing the control of urination was an issue, but after a year it has definitely improved. Erectile dysfunction after any type of prostate procedure is an issue. I found it to be a major effect early on, but less as time progressed. There is still the required monitoring and checkups needed to see that nothing further develops from here on, but taking warning signs seriously, educating yourself, and making an informed decision with the help of the best medical team possible will make you feel good about your choices.

Kevin Mahoney is a U.S. veteran, now working as a program manager. He enjoys spending time with his family, including his wife, children, and grandchildren.

9

EXERCISES

Remember to check your answers carefully with those given in the Answers to Exercises, page 336.

A **Using the terms below, fill in the flow chart showing the passage of sperm.**

epididymis   penis   urethra
ejaculatory duct   seminiferous tubules   vas deferens

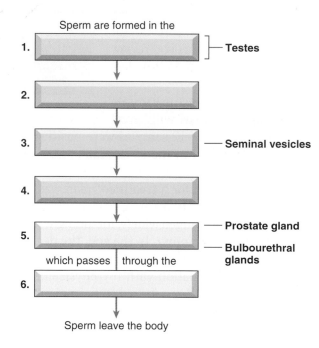

Sperm are formed in the

1. [   ]]— **Testes**

2. [   ]

3. [   ] — **Seminal vesicles**

4. [   ]

5. [   ] — **Prostate gland**
                  — **Bulbourethral**
which passes | through the   **glands**

6. [   ]

Sperm leave the body

B **Select from the list of terms to match the descriptions that follow.**

bulbourethral glands   scrotum   spermatozoon
epididymis   seminal vesicles   testis
prepuce   seminiferous tubules   vas deferens
prostate gland

1. one of a pair of long, tightly coiled tubes above each testis; carries and stores sperm _____

2. exocrine gland at the base of the male urinary bladder _____

3. narrow coiled tubules that produce sperm in the testes _____

4. sperm cell _____

5. foreskin _____

6. male gonad; produces testosterone and sperm cells _____

7. paired sac-like exocrine glands that secrete fluid into the vas deferens _____

8. external sac that contains the testes _____

9. narrow tube carrying sperm from the epididymis toward the urethra _____

10. pair of exocrine glands near the male urethra; Cowper glands _____

9

C **Select from the list of terms to match the descriptions that follow.**

ejaculation   fraternal twins   interstitial cells
ejaculatory duct   glans penis   parenchymal tissue
erectile dysfunction   identical twins   perineum
flagellum

1. hair-like projection on a sperm cell that makes it motile _____

2. sensitive tip of the penis _____

3. tube through which semen enters the urethra _____

4. two infants resulting from division of one fertilized egg into separate embryos _____

5. external region between the anus and scrotum _____

6. essential distinctive cells of an organ _____

7. two infants resulting from fertilization of two ova by two sperm cells _____

8. inability of an adult male to achieve erection; impotence _____

9. specialized cells that lie adjacent to the seminiferous tubules _____

10. ejection of sperm and fluid from the urethra _____

D **Match the listed terms with the descriptions that follow.**

aspermia   penis   stromal tissue
azoospermia   semen   testicle
impotence   sterilization   testosterone
oligospermia

1. male external organ of reproduction _____

2. sperm cells and seminal fluid _____

3. hormone secreted by interstitial cells of the testes _____

4. supportive connective tissue of an organ _____

5. lack of semen _____

6. lack of sperm cells in semen _____

7. procedure that removes a person's ability to produce or release reproductive cells _____

8. semen with a low concentration of sperm _____

9. male gonad _____

10. inability of a male to sustain or achieve an erection _____

9

E **Build medical terms for the following definitions. Parts of the words are given.**

1. inflammation of the testes: _____itis

2. inflammation of the tube that carries the spermatozoa to the vas deferens:

    _____itis

3. resection of the prostate gland: _____ectomy

4. inflammation of the prostate gland: _____itis

5. process of producing (the formation of) sperm cells: _____genesis

6. fixation of undescended testicle: orchio_____

7. inflammation of the glans penis: _____itis

8. condition of scanty sperm: _____spermia

9. lack of semen: a_____

10. pertaining to a testicle: _____ar

F **Answer true or false:**

1. _____ Cryogenic surgery uses cold temperatures to destroy tissue.

2. _____ Estrogen is an example of an androgen.

3. _____ Castration (orchiectomy or oophorectomy) is an example of sterilization.

4. _____ A teratoma is a benign tumor of the prostate gland.

5. _____ Spermolytic means formation of sperm.

6. _____ Balanitis is inflammation of a testicle.

7. _____ Azoospermia causes infertility.

8. _____ Aspermia can result from retrograde ejaculation.

9. _____ Seminiferous tubules are the interstitial cells of the testes.

10. _____ Testosterone is produced by the parenchymal tissue of the testes.

11. _____ Vasectomy produces impotence.

12. _____ Vasovasostomy is an anastomosis that can restore fertility (ability to reproduce offspring).

G Match the term in Column I with its meaning in Column II. Write the correct letter in the space provided.

COLUMN I

1. castration _____

2. semen analysis _____

3. ejaculation _____

4. purulent _____

5. vasectomy _____

6. circumcision _____

7. ligation _____

8. cryosurgery _____

9. seminoma _____

10. phimosis _____

COLUMN II

A. To tie off or bind
B. Removal of a piece of the vas deferens
C. Orchiectomy
D. Removal of the prepuce
E. Destruction of tissue by freezing
F. Pus-filled
G. Test of fertility (reproductive ability)
H. Ejection of sperm and fluid from the urethra
I. Narrowing (stricture) of the opening of the prepuce over the glans penis
J. Malignant tumor of the testis

H Select from the listed terms to fit the descriptions that follow.

adenocarcinoma of the
  prostate
benign prostatic
  hyperplasia

cryptorchidism
gonorrhea
herpes genitalis
human HPV infection

hydrocele
hypospadias
syphilis
varicocele

1. prostatic enlargement, nonmalignant _____

2. opening of the urethra on the undersurface of the penis _____

3. infection of skin and genital mucosa with HSV _____

4. malignant tumor of the prostate gland _____

5. enlarged, swollen veins near the testes _____

6. sexually transmitted disease with primary stage marked by formation of a chancre _____

7. infection of the skin and mucous membranes in the anogenital region by human

   papillomavirus _____

8. STI caused by berry-shaped bacteria and marked by inflammation of genital mucosa and

   mucopurulent discharge _____

9. undescended testicles _____

10. sac of clear fluid in the scrotum _____

I Spell out the abbreviations in Column I. Then match each abbreviation with its correct meaning from Column II.

COLUMN I

1. PSA _____ _____

2. BPH _____ _____

3. TURP _____ _____

4. TRUS _____ _____

5. DRE _____ _____

6. HSV _____ _____

7. STI _____ _____

COLUMN II

A. Manual diagnostic procedure to examine the prostate gland

B. Relieves symptoms of prostate gland enlargement

C. Etiologic agent of a sexually transmitted disease characterized by blister formation

D. Noncancerous enlargement of the prostate gland

E. Chlamydial infection, gonorrhea, and syphilis are examples of this general category of infections

F. Helpful procedure in guiding a prostatic biopsy needle

G. High serum levels of this protein indicate prostatic carcinoma

J Give the meanings of the following word parts.

1. -one _____

2. -stomy _____

3. semin/i _____

4. -cele _____

5. -pexy _____

6. -genesis _____

7. -plasia _____

8. prostat/o _____

9. orch/o _____

10. terat/o _____

11. gon/o _____

12. hydr/o _____

13. pen/o _____

14. balan/o _____

15. varic/o _____

16. vas/o _____

17. test/o _____

18. zo/o _____

19. crypt/o _____

20. andr/o _____

9

K **Match the listed surgical procedures with the following reasons for performing them.**

circumcision
hydrocelectomy
orchiectomy
orchiopexy

photoselective vaporization
of the prostate
radical (complete)
prostatectomy

varicocelectomy
vasectomy
vasovasostomy

1. carcinoma of the prostate gland _____

2. cryptorchidism _____

3. sterilization (hormones remain and potency is not impaired) _____

4. benign prostatic hyperplasia _____

5. abnormal collection of fluid in a scrotal sac _____

6. reversal of sterilization procedure _____

7. embryonal carcinoma of the testes _____

8. phimosis _____

9. ligation of swollen, twisted veins above the testes _____

L **Use the given definitions to complete the terms. Check your answers carefully.**

1. gland at the base of the urinary bladder in males: pro _____ gland

2. coiled tube on top of each testis: epi _____

3. essential tissue of an organ: par _____ tissue

4. foreskin: pre _____

5. bacterial infection that invades the urethra and reproductive tract of men and women and is the major cause of nonspecific urethritis in males and cervicitis in females:

   ch _____

6. ulcer that forms on genital organs after infection with syphilis: ch _____

7. androgen produced by the interstitial cells of the testis: test _____

8. fluid secreted by male reproductive glands and ejaculated with sperm: se _____

9. malignant tumor of the testis: sem _____

10. pertaining to the penis: pen _____

M **Circle the correct term(s) to complete the following sentences.**

1. When Fred was a newborn infant, his doctors could feel only one testicle within the scrotum and suggested close monitoring of his condition of **(gonorrhea, cryptorchidism, benign prostatic hyperplasia).**

2. Bob had many sexual partners, one of whom had been diagnosed with **(testosterone, phimosis, chlamydial infection)**, a highly communicable STI.

3. At age 65, Mike had some difficulty with urgency and discomfort when urinating. His doctor did a digital rectal examination to examine his **(prostate gland, urinary bladder, vas deferens).**

4. Just after Nick's birth, his parents had a difficult time deciding whether to have their infant son undergo (**TURP, castration, circumcision**).

5. Ted noticed a hard ulcer on his penis and made an appointment with his doctor, a (**gastroenterologist, gynecologist, urologist**). The doctor viewed a specimen of the ulcer under the microscope and did a blood test, which revealed that Ted had contracted (**gonorrhea, herpes genitalis, syphilis**), so the ulcer was a (**blister, chancre, seminoma**).

6. After his fifth child was born, Art decided to have a (**vasovasostomy, hydrocelectomy, vasectomy**) to prevent conception of another child. A/an (**nephrologist, urologist, abdominal surgeon**) performed the procedure to cut and ligate the (**urethra, epididymis, vas deferens**).

7. Twenty-six-year-old Lance noticed a hard testicular mass. His physician prescribed a brief trial with (**antibodies, antibiotics, pain killers**) to rule out (**epididymitis, testicular cancer, varicocele**). The mass remained and Lance underwent (**epididymectomy, orchiectomy, prostatectomy**). The mass was a (**seminoma, prostate cancer, hydrocele**).

8. Sarah and Steve had been trying to conceive a child for 7 years. Steve had a (**digital rectal examination, TURP, semen analysis**), which revealed 25% normal sperm count with 10% motility. He was told he had (**phimosis, azoospermia, oligospermia**).

9. To boost his sperm count, Steve was given (**estrogen, testosterone, progesterone**). As a side effect, this (**androgen, progestin, enzyme**) gave him a case of acne lasting several months.

10. Sarah eventually became pregnant. An ultrasound examination showed two embryos with two separate placentas and in separate (**peritoneal, scrotal, amniotic**) sacs. Sarah gave birth to two healthy (**identical, fraternal, perineal**) twin girls.

9

ANSWERS TO EXERCISES

A

1. seminiferous tubules
2. epididymis
3. vas deferens
4. ejaculatory duct
5. urethra
6. penis

B

1. epididymis
2. prostate gland
3. seminiferous tubules
4. spermatozoon
5. prepuce
6. testis
7. seminal vesicles
8. scrotum
9. vas deferens
10. bulbourethral (Cowper) glands

C

1. flagellum
2. glans penis
3. ejaculatory duct
4. identical twins
5. perineum
6. parenchymal tissue
7. fraternal twins
8. erectile dysfunction
9. interstitial cells
10. ejaculation

D

1. penis
2. semen
3. testosterone
4. stromal tissue
5. aspermia
6. azoospermia
7. sterilization
8. oligospermia
9. testicle
10. impotence

E

1. orchitis
2. epididymitis
3. prostatectomy
4. prostatitis
5. spermatogenesis
6. orchiopexy
7. balanitis
8. oligospermia
9. aspermia
10. testicular

F

1. True.
2. False. Estrogen is a female hormone. Androgens are male hormones. Testosterone is an androgen.
3. True.
4. False. Teratoma is a malignant tumor in the testis.
5. False. Spermolytic is destruction of sperm. Spermatogenesis is formation of sperm.
6. False. Balanitis is inflammation of the glans penis. Orchitis is inflammation of a testicle.
7. True.
8. True. Semen is discharged backward into the urinary bladder and not ejaculated.
9. False. Seminiferous tubules are the parenchymal tissue of the testes. The interstitial cells of the testis are the Leydig cells that secrete testosterone.
10. False. Testosterone is produced by the interstitial cells of the testis.
11. False. Vasectomy results in the inability of sperm to leave the body in semen. It does not affect erectile dysfunction and does not produce impotence.
12. True.

G

1. C
2. G
3. H
4. F
5. B
6. D
7. A
8. E
9. J
10. I

H

1. benign prostatic hyperplasia
2. hypospadias
3. herpes genitalis
4. adenocarcinoma of the prostate
5. varicocele
6. syphilis
7. HPV infection
8. gonorrhea
9. cryptorchidism
10. hydrocele

I

1. prostate-specific antigen: G
2. benign prostatic hyperplasia: D
3. transurethral resection of the prostate: B
4. transrectal ultrasound: F
5. digital rectal examination: A
6. herpes simplex virus: C
7. sexually transmitted infection: E

J

1. hormone
2. opening
3. semen, seed
4. hernia, swelling
5. fixation
6. formation
7. formation
8. prostate gland
9. testis
10. monster
11. seed
12. water
13. penis
14. glans penis
15. varicose veins
16. vessel, duct, vas deferens
17. testis, testicle
18. animal life
19. hidden
20. male

K

1. radical (complete) prostatectomy
2. orchiopexy
3. vasectomy
4. photoselective vaporization of the prostate
5. hydrocelectomy
6. vasovasostomy
7. orchiectomy
8. circumcision
9. varicocelectomy

L

1. prostate
2. epididymis
3. parenchymal
4. prepuce
5. chlamydia
6. chancre
7. testosterone
8. semen or seminal fluid
9. seminoma
10. penile

M

1. cryptorchidism
2. chlamydial infection
3. prostate gland
4. circumcision
5. urologist; syphilis; chancre
6. vasectomy; urologist; vas deferens
7. antibiotics; epididymitis; orchiectomy; seminoma
8. semen analysis; oligospermia
9. testosterone; androgen
10. amniotic; fraternal

Answers to Practical Applications

Case Report: A Man with Post-TURP Complaints

1. c
2. b
3. b
4. a
5. b
6. c
7. c
8. a

9

PRONUNCIATION OF TERMS

To test your understanding of the terminology in this chapter, write the meaning of each term in the space provided. In addition, you may wish to cover the terms and write them by looking at your definitions. Make sure your spelling is correct. The page number after each term indicates where it is defined or used in the book, so you can easily check your responses. You will find complete definitions for all of these terms and their audio pronunciations on the Evolve website.

Pronunciation Guide

ā as in āpe   ă as in ăpple
ē as in ēven   ĕ as in ĕvery
ī as in īce   ĭ as in ĭnterest
ō as in ōpen   ŏ as in pŏt
ū as in ūnit   ŭ as in ŭnder

TERM	PRONUNCIATION	MEANING
androgen (317)	ĂN-drō-jĕn	
aspermia (318)	ā-SPĔR-mē-ă	
azoospermia (319)	ā-zō-ō-SPĔR-mē-ă	
balanitis (317)	băl-ă-NĪ-tĭs	
benign prostatic hyperplasia (321)	bē-NĪN-prŏs-TĂT-ĭk hī-pĕr-PLĀ-zē-ă	
bulbourethral glands (315)	bŭl-bō-ū-RĒ-thrăl glăndz	
carcinoma of the prostate (321)	kăr-sĭ-NŌ-mă of the PRŎS-tāt	
carcinoma of the testes (319)	kăr-sĭ-NŌ-mă of the TĔS-tēz	
castration (325)	kăs-TRĀ-shŭn	
chancre (324)	SHĂNG-kĕr	
chlamydial infection (322)	klă-MĬD-ē-ăl ĭn-FEK-shŭn	
circumcision (325)	sĭr-kŭm-SĬZH-ŭn	
cryogenic surgery (317)	krī-ō-GĔN-ĭk SŬR-jĕr-ē	
cryptorchidism (317)	krĭp-TŎR-kĭdĭzm	
digital rectal exam (325)	DĬJ-ĕ-tăl RĔK-tăl ĕk-ZĂM	
ejaculation (315)	ē-jăk-ū-LĀ-shŭn	
ejaculatory duct (315)	ē-JĂK-ū-lă-tōr-ē dŭkt	
embryonal carcinoma (319)	ĕm-brē-ŌN-ăl kăr-sĭ-NŌ-mă	
epididymis (315)	ĕp-ĭ-DĬD-ĭ-mĭs	
epididymitis (317)	ĕp-ĭ-dĭd-ĭ-MĪ-tĭs	
erectile dysfunction (315)	ē-RĔK-tĭl dĭs-FŬNK-shŭn	

9

TERM	PRONUNCIATION	MEANING
flagellum (315)	flă-JĔL-ŭm	
fraternal twins (315)	fră-TĔR-năl twĭnz	
glans penis (315)	glănz PĒ-nĭs	
gonorrhea (322)	gŏn-ō-RĒ-ă	
herpes genitalis (323)	HĔR-pēz jĕn-ĭ-TĂL-ĭs	
human papillomavirus (324)	HŪ-măn păp-ĭ-LŌ-mă- vī-rŭs	
hydrocele (317)	HĪ-drō-sēl	
hypospadias (322)	hī-pō-SPĀ-dē-ăs	
identical twins (316)	ī-DĔN-tĭ-kăl twĭnz	
impotence (316)	ĬM-pō-tĕns	
interstitial cells of the testes (316)	ĭn-tĕr-STĬ-shŭl sĕlz of the TĔS-tĭs	
ligation (326)	lī-GĀ-shŭn	
oligospermia (318)	ŏl-ĭ-gō-SPĔR-mē-ă	
orchiectomy (318)	ŏr-kē-ĔK-tō-mē	
orchiopexy (319)	ŏr-kē-ō-PĔK sē	
orchitis (318)	ŏr-KĪ-tĭs	
parenchymal tissue (316)	pă-RĔNG-kĭ-măl TĬS-ū	
penile (318)	PĒ-nīl	
penis (316)	PĒ-nĭs	
penoscrotal (318)	pē-nō-SKRŌ-tăl	
perineum (316)	pĕr-ĭ-NĒ-ŭm	
phimosis (322)	fi-MŌ-sĭs	
photoselective vaporization of the prostate (325)	fō-tō-sĕ-LĔK-tĭv vā-pŏr-ĭ-ZĀ-shŭn of the PRŎS-tāt	
prepuce (316)	PRĒ-pŭs	
prostatectomy (318)	prŏs-tă-TĔK-tō-mē	
prostate gland (316)	PRŎS-tāt glănd	
prostatitis (318)	prŏs-tă-TĪ-tĭs	
purulent (322)	PŪR-ū-lĕnt	
scrotum (316)	SKRŌ-tŭm	

9

TERM	PRONUNCIATION	MEANING
semen (316)	SĒ-mĕn	
semen analysis (324)	SĒ-mĕn ă-NĂL-ĭ-sĭs	
seminal vesicles (316)	SĔM-ĭn-ăl VĔS-ĭ-klz	
seminiferous tubules (316)	sĕ-mĭ-NĬF-ĕr-ŭs TOOB-ūlz	
seminoma (319)	sĕ-mĭ-NŌ-mă	
spermatogenesis (319)	spĕr-mă-tō-JĔN-ĕ-sĭs	
spermatozoa (316)	spĕr-mă-tō-ZŌ-ă	
spermatozoon (316)	spĕr-mă-tō-ZŌ-ĕn	
spermolytic (318)	spĕr-mō-LĬT-ĭk	
sterilization (316)	stĕr-ĭ-lĭ-ZĀ-shŭn	
stromal tissue (316)	STRŌ-măl TĬS-ū	
syphilis (324)	SĬF-ĭ-lĭs	
teratoma (318)	tĕr-ă-TŌ-mă	
testicular (318)	tĕs-TĬK-ū-lăr	
testicular torsion (320)	tĕs-TĬK-ū-lăr TŎR-shŭn	
testis (316)	TĔS-tĭs	
testosterone (316)	tĕs-TŎS-tĕ-rōn	
transurethral resection of the prostate (325)	trănz-ū-RĒ-trăl rē-SĔK-shun of the PRŎS-tāt	
varicocele (318)	VĀR-ĭ-kō-sēl	
vas deferens (316)	văs DĔF-ĕr-ĕnz	
vasectomy (326)	vă-SĔK-tō-mē	
vasovasostomy (319)	vă-zō-vă-ZŎS-tō-mē	

REVIEW SHEET

Write the meanings of the word parts in the spaces provided. Check your answers with the information in the chapter or in the **Glossary (Medical Word Parts—English)** at the end of the book.

Combining Forms

COMBINING FORM	MEANING	COMBINING FORM	MEANING
andr/o		pen/o	
balan/o		prostat/o	
cry/o		semin/i	
crypt/o		sperm/o	
epididym/o		spermat/o	
gon/o		terat/o	
hydr/o		test/o	
orch/o		varic/o	
orchi/o		vas/o	
orchid/o		zo/o	

Suffixes

SUFFIX	MEANING	SUFFIX	MEANING
-cele		-one	
-ectomy		-pexy	
-gen		-plasia	
-genesis		-rrhea	
-genic		-stomy	
-lysis		-tomy	
-lytic		-trophy	

evolve *Please visit the Evolve website for additional exercises, games, and images related to this chapter.*

Nervous System

Chapter Sections:

CHAPTER GOALS

- Name, locate, and describe the major organs of the nervous system and their functions.
- Learn nervous system combining forms and use them with suffixes and prefixes.
- Define pathologic conditions affecting the nervous system.
- Describe nervous system–related laboratory tests, clinical procedures, and abbreviations.
- Apply your new knowledge to understanding medical terms in their proper contexts, such as medical reports and records.

INTRODUCTION

The nervous system is one of the most complex of all human body systems. More than 100 billion nerve cells operate constantly all over the body to coordinate the activities we do consciously and voluntarily, as well as those that occur unconsciously or involuntarily. We speak, move muscles, hear, taste, see, and think. Our glands secrete hormones, and we respond to danger, pain, temperature, and touch. All of these functions comprise only a small number of the many activities controlled by the nervous system.

Fibers exiting from microscopic **nerve cells** (**neurons**) are collected into macroscopic bundles called **nerves,** which carry electrical messages all over the body. External stimuli, as well as internal chemicals such as **acetylcholine,** activate the cell membranes of nerve cells, which results in electrical discharges of these cells. These electrical discharges, **nervous impulses**, may then traverse the length of the associated nerves. External **receptors** (sense organs) as well as internal receptors in muscles and blood vessels receive these impulses and may in turn transmit impulses to the complex network of nerve cells in the brain and spinal cord. Within this central part of the nervous system, impulses are recognized, interpreted, and finally relayed to other nerve cells that extend out to all parts of the body, such as muscles, glands, and internal organs.

GENERAL STRUCTURE OF THE NERVOUS SYSTEM

The nervous system is classified into two major divisions: the **central nervous system (CNS)** and the **peripheral nervous system (PNS).** The central nervous system consists of the **brain** and **spinal cord.** The peripheral nervous system consists of **cranial nerves** and **spinal nerves, plexuses,** and **peripheral nerves** throughout the body (Figure 10-1). Cranial nerves carry impulses between the brain and the head and neck. The one exception is the tenth cranial nerve, called the **vagus nerve.** It carries messages to and from the neck, chest, and abdomen. Figure 10-2 shows cranial nerves, their functions, and the parts of the body that they carry messages to and from. Spinal nerves carry messages between the spinal cord and the chest, abdomen, and extremities.

A **plexus** ▨ is a large network of nerves in the peripheral nervous system. The cervical, brachial (brachi/o means arm), and lumbosacral plexuses are examples that include cervical, lumbar, and sacral nerves. Figure 10-1 illustrates the relationship of the brain and spinal cord to the spinal nerves and plexuses.

The spinal and cranial nerves are composed of nerves that help the body respond to changes in the outside world. They include sense **receptors** for sight (eye), hearing and balance (ear), smell (olfactory), and touch (skin sensation) and **sensory (afferent) nerves** that carry messages related to changes in the environment *toward* the spinal cord and brain. In addition, **motor (efferent) nerves** travel *from* the spinal cord and brain to muscles of the body, telling them how to respond. For example, when you touch a hot stove, temperature and pain receptors in the skin stimulate afferent nerves, which carry messages toward the spinal cord and brain. Instantaneously, the message is conveyed to efferent nerve cells in the spinal cord, which then activate voluntary muscles to pull your hand away from the stove.

◤ **Plexus**

There are other **plexuses** in the body—networks of intersecting blood vessels (vascular) and lymphatic vessels.
- Lymphatic plexus is an interconnecting network of lymph vessels.
- Rectal plexus is a plexus of veins in the rectal region.
- Vertebral plexus is a plexus of veins related to the backbone.

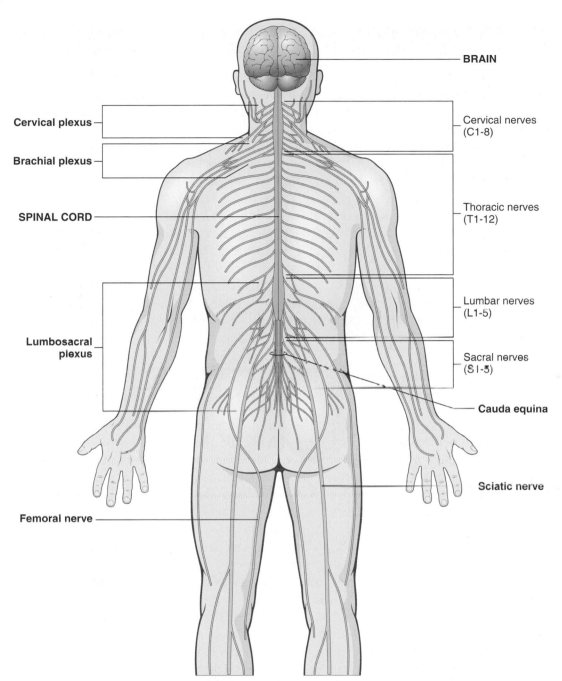

FIGURE 10-1   The brain and the spinal cord, spinal nerves, and spinal plexuses. The **femoral nerve** is a lumbar nerve leading to and from the thigh (femur). The **sciatic nerve** is a nerve beginning in a region of the hip. The **cauda equina** (Latin for "horse's tail") is a bundle of spinal nerves below the end of the spinal cord.

In addition to the spinal and cranial nerves (whose functions are mainly voluntary and involved with sensations of smell, taste, sight, hearing, and muscle movements), the peripheral nervous system also contains a large group of nerves that function involuntarily or automatically, without conscious control. These peripheral nerves belong to the **autonomic nervous system.** This system of nerve fibers carries impulses *away from* the CNS to the glands, heart, blood vessels, and involuntary muscles found in the walls of tubes like the intestines and hollow organs like the stomach and urinary bladder.

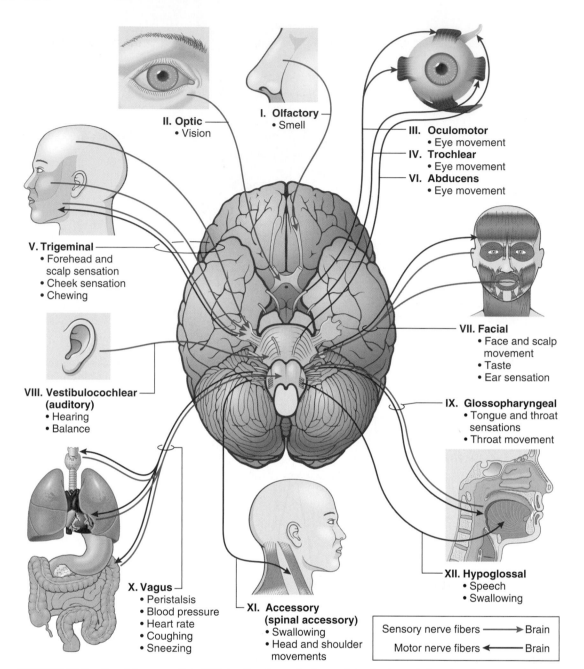

FIGURE 10-2   Cranial nerves (I to XII) leading from the base of the brain and showing the parts of the body they affect. **Sensory** or **afferent** nerves are colored *blue* and carry messages *toward* the brain. **Motor** or **efferent** nerves are colored *red* and carry messages *from* the brain to muscles and organs. Some nerves (mixed) carry both sensory and motor fibers. Don't try to memorize this figure! Just get the big picture: Cranial nerves carry messages to and from the brain to all parts of head and neck and also (in the case of the vagus nerve) to other parts of the body.

Some autonomic nerves are **sympathetic** nerves and others are **parasympathetic** nerves. The sympathetic nerves stimulate the body in times of stress and crisis. They increase heart rate and forcefulness, dilate (relax) airways so more oxygen can enter, and increase blood pressure. In addition, sympathetic neurons stimulate the adrenal glands to secrete epinephrine (adrenaline), while also inhibiting intestinal contractions to slow digestion. The parasympathetic nerves normally act as a balance for the sympathetic nerves.

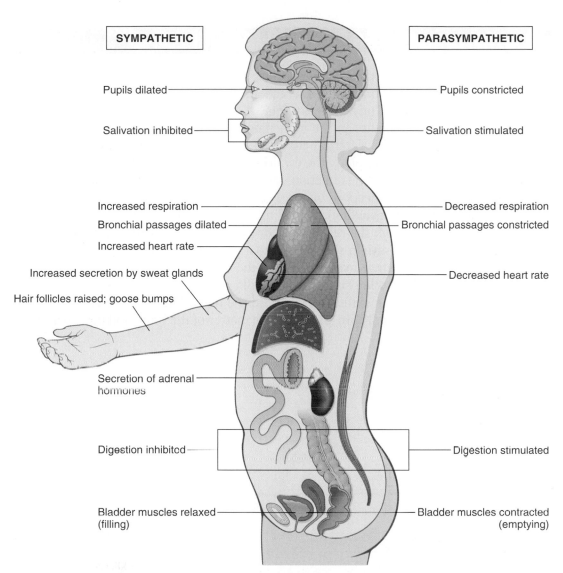

FIGURE 10-3   Actions of parasympathetic and sympathetic nerves.

Parasympathetic nerves slow down heart rate, lower blood pressure, and stimulate intestinal contractions to clear the rectum. Figure 10-3 shows the differences in actions between the sympathetic and parasympathetic nerves.

Figure 10-4 summarizes the divisions of the central and peripheral nervous systems.

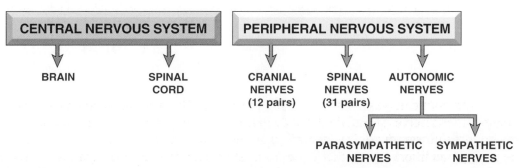

FIGURE 10-4   Divisions of the central nervous system (CNS) and peripheral nervous system (PNS). The autonomic nervous system is a part of the peripheral nervous system.

NEURONS, NERVES, AND GLIAL CELLS

A neuron is an individual nerve cell, a microscopic structure. Impulses pass along the parts of a nerve cell in a definite manner and direction. The parts of a neuron are pictured in Figure 10-5; label it as you study the following.

A **stimulus** begins an impulse in the branching fibers of the neuron, which are called **dendrites** [1]. A change in the electrical charge of the dendrite membranes is thus begun, and the nervous impulse moves along the dendrites like the movement of falling dominoes. The impulse, traveling in only one direction, next reaches the **cell body** [2], which contains the **cell nucleus** [3]. Small collections of nerve cell bodies outside the brain and spinal cord are called **ganglia** (*singular*: **ganglion**). Extending from the cell body is the **axon** [4], which carries the impulse away from the cell body. Axons can be covered with a fatty tissue called myelin. The purpose of this **myelin sheath** [5] is to insulate the axon and speed transmission of the electrical impulse. Demyelination is loss of the myelin insulating the nerve fiber and is characteristic of multiple sclerosis, an acquired illness affecting the CNS.

The myelin sheath gives a white appearance to the nerve fiber—hence the term white matter, as in parts of the spinal cord and the white matter of the brain and most peripheral

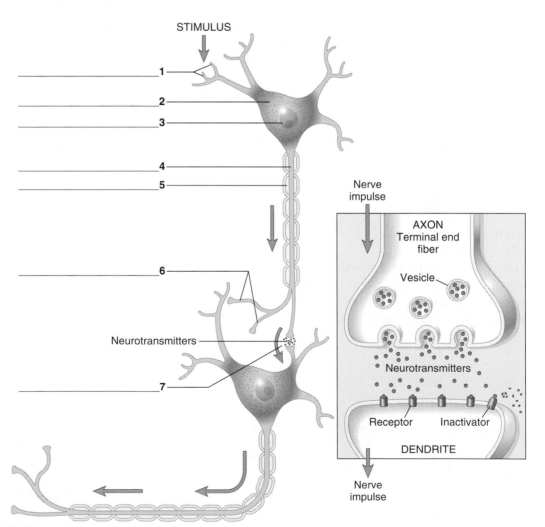

FIGURE 10-5 Parts of a neuron and the pathway of a nervous impulse. Neurons are the **parenchymal** (essential) **cells** of the nervous system. The *boxed drawing* shows what happens in a synapse: Vesicles store neurotransmitters in the terminal end fibers of axons. Receptors on the dendrites pick up the neurotransmitters. Inactivators end the activity of neurotransmitters when they have finished their job.

nerves. The gray matter of the brain and spinal cord is composed of the cell bodies of neurons that appear gray because they are not covered by a myelin sheath.

The nervous impulse passes through the axon to leave the cell via the **terminal end fibers** [6] of the neuron. The space where the nervous impulse jumps from one neuron to another is called the **synapse** [7]. The transfer of the impulse across the synapse depends on the release of a chemical substance, called a **neurotransmitter,** by the neuron that brings the impulse to the synapse. See the boxed diagram in Figure 10-5. Tiny sacs (vesicles) containing the neurotransmitter are located at the ends of neurons, and they release the neurotransmitter into the synapse. **Acetylcholine, norepinephrine, epinephrine (adrenaline), dopamine, serotonin,** and **endorphins** are examples of neurotransmitters.

Whereas a neuron is a microscopic structure within the nervous system, a **nerve** is macroscopic, able to be seen with the naked eye. A nerve consists of a bundle of dendrites and axons that travel together like strands of rope. Peripheral nerves that carry impulses *to* the brain and spinal cord from stimulus receptors like the skin, eye, ear, and nose are **afferent** or **sensory nerves;** those that carry impulses *from* the CNS to organs that produce responses, such as muscles and glands, are **efferent** or **motor nerves.**

Neurons and nerves are the **parenchyma** of the nervous system. Parenchyma is the essential distinguishing tissue of an organ. In the brain and spinal cord, neurons, which conduct electrical impulses, are the parenchymal tissue. **Stroma** of an organ is the connective and supportive tissue of an organ. The stromal tissue of the central nervous system consists of the **glial (neuroglial) cells,** which make up its supportive framework and help it ward off infection. Glial cells do not transmit impulses. They are far more numerous than neurons and can reproduce.

There are four types of supporting or glial cells (see Figure 10-6). **Astrocytes (astroglial cells)** are star-like in appearance (astr/o means star) and transport water and salts between capillaries and neurons. **Microglial cells** are small cells with many branching processes (dendrites). As phagocytes, they protect neurons in response to inflammation. **Oligodendroglial cells (oligodendrocytes)** have few (olig/o means few or scanty) dendrites. These cells form the myelin sheath in the CNS. By contrast, **ependymal cells** (Greek *ependyma* means upper garment) line membranes within the brain and spinal cord where CSF is produced and circulates.

Glial cells, particularly the astrocytes, are associated with blood vessels and regulate the passage of potentially harmful substances from the blood into the nerve cells of the brain. This protective barrier between the blood and brain cells is called the **blood-brain barrier (BBB).** This barrier consists of special lining (endothelial) cells, which along with astrocytes separate capillaries from nerve cells. Delivery of chemotherapeutic drugs to treat brain tumors is thus difficult, because the BBB blocks drug access to brain tissues. Figure 10-6 illustrates glial cells.

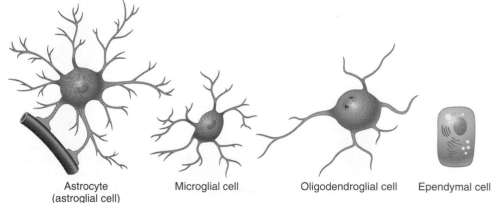

FIGURE 10-6   Glial cells (neuroglial cells). These are the supportive, protective, and connective tissue cells of the CNS. Glial cells are **stromal** (framework) **tissue,** whereas neurons carry nervous impulses.

Astrocyte (astroglial cell)   Microglial cell   Oligodendroglial cell   Ependymal cell

THE BRAIN

The brain controls body activities. In the human adult, it weighs about 3 pounds and has many different parts, all of which control different aspects of body functions.

The largest part of the brain is the "thinking" area, or **cerebrum.** On the surface of the cerebrum, nerve cells lie in sheets, which make up the **cerebral cortex.** These sheets, arranged in folds called **gyri,** are separated from each other by grooves known as **sulci.** The brain is divided in half, a right side and a left side, which are called **cerebral hemispheres.** Each hemisphere is subdivided into four major lobes named for the cranial (skull) bones that overlie them. Figure 10-7 shows these lobes—frontal, parietal, occipital, and temporal—as well as gyri and sulci.

The cerebrum has many functions. It is responsible for thought, judgment, memory, association, and discrimination. In addition, sensory impulses are received through afferent cranial nerves, and when registered in the cortex, they are the basis for perception. Cranial nerves carry motor impulses from the cerebrum to muscles and glands, and these produce movement and activity. Figure 10-7 shows the location of some of the centers in the cerebral cortex that control speech, vision, smell, movement, hearing, and thought processes.

In the middle of the cerebrum are spaces, or canals, called **ventricles** (pictured in Figure 10-8). They contain a watery fluid that flows throughout the brain and around the spinal cord. This fluid is **cerebrospinal fluid (CSF),** and it protects the brain and spinal cord from shock by acting like a cushion. CSF usually is clear and colorless and contains lymphocytes, sugar, and proteins. Spinal fluid can be withdrawn for diagnosis or relief of pressure on the brain; this is called a **lumbar puncture (LP).** For this procedure, a hollow needle is

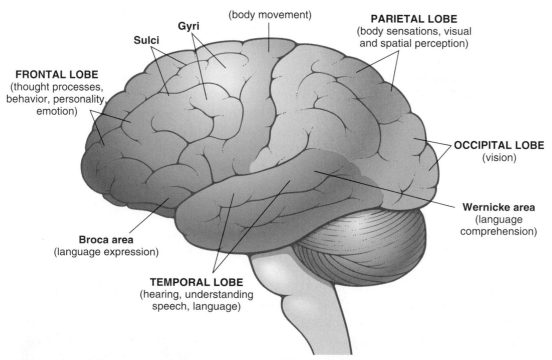

FIGURE 10-7 Left cerebral hemisphere (lateral view). **Gyri** (convolutions) and **sulci** (fissures) are indicated. Notice the lobes of the cerebrum and the functional centers that control speech, vision, movement, hearing, thinking, and other processes. Neurologists believe that the two hemispheres have different abilities. The **left brain** is more concerned with language, mathematical functioning, reasoning, and analytical thinking. The **right brain** is more active in spatial relationships, art, music, emotions, and intuition.

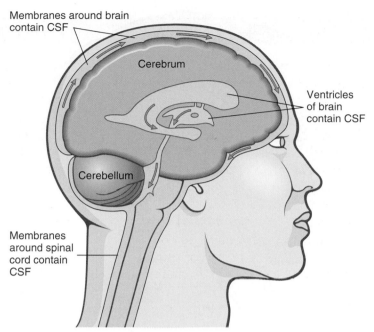

Membranes around brain contain CSF

Cerebrum

Ventricles of brain contain CSF

Cerebellum

Membranes around spinal cord contain CSF

FIGURE 10-8 **Circulation of cerebrospinal fluid (CSF) in the brain (ventricles) and around the spinal cord.** CSF is formed within the ventricles and circulates between the membranes around the brain and within the spinal cord. CSF empties into the bloodstream through the membranes surrounding the brain and spinal cord.

inserted into the lumbar region of the spinal column below the region where the nervous tissue of the spinal cord ends, and CSF is withdrawn.

Two other important parts of the brain are the **thalamus** and the **hypothalamus** (Figure 10-9). The thalamus acts like a triage center. It decides what is important and what is not, selectively processing and relaying sensory information to the cerebral cortex. The thalamus also plays a major role in maintaining levels of awareness and consciousness. The hypothalamus (below the thalamus) contains neurons that control body temperature, sleep, appetite, sexual desire, and emotions such as fear and pleasure. The hypothalamus also regulates the release of hormones from the pituitary gland at the base of the brain and integrates the activities of the sympathetic and parasympathetic nervous systems.

The following structures within the brain lie in the back and below the cerebrum and connect the cerebrum with the spinal cord: **cerebellum, midbrain, pons,** and **medulla oblongata**. The midbrain, pons and medulla are part of the **brainstem.** See Figure 10-9.

The **cerebellum** functions to coordinate voluntary movements and to maintain balance and posture.

The **midbrain** is the uppermost portion of the brainstem. It contains pathways connecting the cerebrum with lower portions of the brain and structures involved with seeing and hearing.

The **pons** is a part of the brainstem that literally means bridge. It contains nerve fiber tracts that connect the cerebellum and cerebrum with the rest of the brain. Nerves affecting the face and eye movement are located here.

The **medulla oblongata,** also in the brainstem, connects the spinal cord with the rest of the brain. Nerve tracts cross from right to left and left to right in the medulla oblongata. For example, nerve cells that control movement of the left side of the body are found in the right half of the cerebrum. These cells send out axons that cross over (decussate) to the opposite side of the brain in the medulla oblongata and then travel down the spinal cord.

10

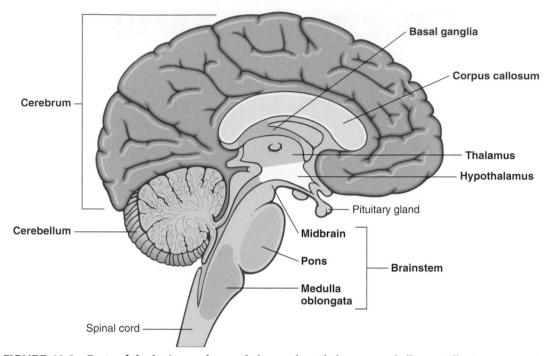

FIGURE 10-9 **Parts of the brain: cerebrum, thalamus, hypothalamus, cerebellum, midbrain, pons, and medulla oblongata.** Note the location of the pituitary gland below the hypothalamus. The **basal ganglia** (a group of cells) regulate intentional movements of the body. The **corpus callosum** lies in the center of the brain and connects the two hemispheres (halves).

In addition, the medulla oblongata contains three important vital centers that regulate internal activities of the body:

1. **Respiratory center**—controls muscles of respiration in response to chemicals or other stimuli
2. **Cardiac center**—slows the heart rate when the heart is beating too rapidly
3. **Vasomotor center**—affects (constricts or dilates) the muscles in the walls of blood vessels, thus influencing blood pressure

Figure 10-9 shows the locations of the thalamus, hypothalamus, cerebellum, pons, and medulla oblongata. Table 10-1 reviews the functions of these parts of the brain.

TABLE 10-1	FUNCTIONS OF THE PARTS OF THE BRAIN
STRUCTURE	**FUNCTION(S)**
Cerebrum	Thinking, personality, sensations, movements, memory
Thalamus	Relay station ("triage center") for sensory impulses; control of awareness and consciousness
Hypothalamus	Body temperature, sleep, appetite, emotions; control of the pituitary gland
Cerebellum	Coordination of voluntary movements and balance
Pons and Midbrain	Connection of nerve and nerve fiber pathways including those to the eyes and face
Medulla oblongata	Nerve fibers cross over, left to right and right to left; contains centers to regulate heart, blood vessels, and respiratory system

THE SPINAL CORD AND MENINGES

SPINAL CORD

The **spinal cord** is a column of nervous tissue extending from the medulla oblongata to the second lumbar vertebra within the vertebral column. Below the end of the spinal cord is the **cauda equina** (Latin for "horse's tail"), a fan of nerve fibers (see Figure 10-1, page 345). The spinal cord carries all the nerves to and from the limbs and lower part of the body, and it is the pathway for impulses going to and from the brain. A cross-sectional view of the spinal cord (Figure 10-10) reveals an inner region of **gray matter** (containing cell bodies and dendrites) and an outer region of **white matter** (containing the nerve fiber tracts with myelin sheaths) conducting impulses to and from the brain.

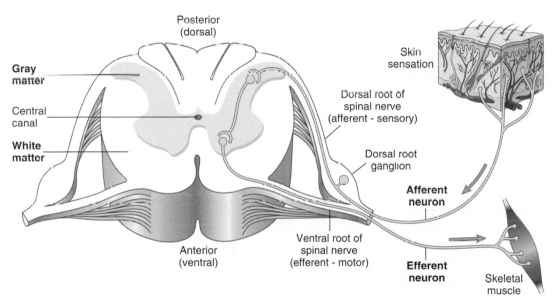

FIGURE 10-10   The spinal cord, showing gray and white matter (transverse view). **Afferent neurons** bring impulses from a sensory receptor (such as the skin) into the spinal cord. **Efferent neurons** carry impulses from the spinal cord to effector organs (such as skeletal muscle). The central canal is the space through which CSF travels.

MENINGES

The **meninges** are three layers of connective tissue membranes that surround the brain and spinal cord. Label Figure 10-11 as you study the following description of the meninges.

The outermost membrane of the meninges is the **dura mater** [1]. This thick, tough membrane contains channels (dural sinuses) that contain blood. The **subdural space** [2] is below the dural membrane. The second layer surrounding the brain and spinal cord is the **arachnoid membrane** [3]. The arachnoid (spider-like) membrane is loosely attached to the other meninges by web-like fibers, so there is a space for fluid between the fibers and the third membrane. This is the **subarachnoid space** [4], containing CSF. The third layer of the meninges, closest to the brain and spinal cord, is the **pia mater** [5]. It contains delicate (Latin *pia*) connective tissue with a rich supply of blood vessels. Most physicians refer to the pia and arachnoid membranes together as the pia-arachnoid.

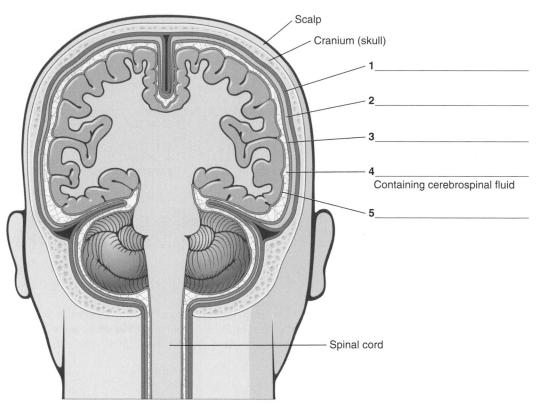

Scalp

Cranium (skull)

1 _____

2 _____

3 _____

4 _____
Containing cerebrospinal fluid

5 _____

Spinal cord

FIGURE 10-11 **The meninges,** posterior view.

VOCABULARY

This list reviews the new terms introduced in the text. Short definitions reinforce your understanding of the terms. Refer to the Pronunciation of Terms section for help with unfamiliar or more difficult words.

acetylcholine	Neurotransmitter chemical released at the ends of nerve cells.
afferent nerve	Carries messages *toward* the brain and spinal cord (sensory nerve). Afferent comes from *af-* (a form of *ad-,* meaning toward) and *-ferent* (meaning carrying).
arachnoid membrane	Middle layer of the three membranes (meninges) that surround the brain and spinal cord. The Greek *arachne* means spider.
astrocyte	Type of glial (neuroglial) cell that transports water and salts from capillaries.
autonomic nervous system	Nerves that control involuntary body functions of muscles, glands, and internal organs.
axon	Microscopic fiber that carries the nervous impulse along a nerve cell.
blood-brain barrier	Protective separation between the blood and brain cells. This makes it difficult for substances (such as anticancer drugs) to penetrate capillary walls and enter the brain.
brainstem	Posterior portion of the brain that connects the cerebrum with the spinal cord; includes the midbrain, pons, and medulla oblongata.
cauda equina	Collection of spinal nerves below the end of the spinal cord.
cell body	Part of a nerve cell that contains the nucleus.
central nervous system (CNS)	The brain and the spinal cord.
cerebellum	Posterior part of the brain that coordinates muscle movements and maintains balance.
cerebral cortex	Outer region of the cerebrum, containing sheets of nerve cells; gray matter of the brain.
cerebrospinal fluid (CSF)	Circulates throughout the brain and spinal cord.
cerebrum	Largest part of the brain; responsible for voluntary muscular activity, vision, speech, taste, hearing, thought, and memory.
cranial nerves	Twelve pairs of nerves that carry messages to and from the brain with regard to the head and neck (except the vagus nerve).
dendrite	Microscopic branching fiber of a nerve cell that is the first part to receive the nervous impulse.
dura mater	Thick, outermost layer of the meninges surrounding and protecting the brain and spinal cord. Latin for "hard mother."
efferent nerve	Carries messages *away from* the brain and spinal cord; motor nerve. Efferent comes from *ef-* (meaning away from) and *-ferent* (meaning to carry).
ependymal cell	Glial cell that lines membranes within the brain and spinal cord and helps form cerebrospinal fluid.

10

ganglion (*plural*: **ganglia**)	Collection of nerve cell bodies in the peripheral nervous system.
glial cell (**neuroglial cell**)	Supportive and connective nerve cell that does not carry nervous impulses. Examples are astrocytes, microglial cells, ependymal cells, and oligodendrocytes. Glial cells can reproduce themselves, as opposed to neurons.
gyrus (*plural*: **gyri**)	Sheet of nerve cells that produces a rounded ridge on the surface of the cerebral cortex; convolution.
hypothalamus	Portion of the brain beneath the thalamus; controls sleep, appetite, body temperature, and secretions from the pituitary gland.
medulla oblongata	Part of the brain just above the spinal cord; controls breathing, heartbeat, and the size of blood vessels; nerve fibers cross over here.
meninges	Three protective membranes that surround the brain and spinal cord.
microglial cell	Phagocytic glial cell that removes waste products from the central nervous system.
midbrain	Uppermost portion of the brainstem.
motor nerve	Carries messages away from the brain and spinal cord to muscles and organs; efferent nerve.
myelin sheath	Covering of white fatty tissue that surrounds and insulates the axon of a nerve cell. Myelin speeds impulse conduction along axons.
nerve	Macroscopic cord-like collection of fibers (axons and dendrites) that carry electrical impulses.
neuron	Nerve cell that carries impulses throughout the body; parenchyma of the nervous system.
neurotransmitter	Chemical messenger released at the end of a nerve cell. It stimulates or inhibits another cell, which can be a nerve cell, muscle cell, or gland cell. Examples of neurotransmitters are acetylcholine, norepinephrine, dopamine, and serotonin.
oligodendroglial cell	Glial cell that forms the myelin sheath covering axons. Also called oligodendrocyte.
parasympathetic nerves	Involuntary, autonomic nerves that regulate normal body functions such as heart rate, breathing, and muscles of the gastrointestinal tract.
parenchyma	Essential, distinguishing tissue of any organ or system. The parenchyma of the nervous system includes the neurons and nerves that carry nervous impulses. Parenchymal cells of the liver are hepatocytes, and parenchymal tissue of the kidney includes the nephrons, where urine is formed. Note the pronunciation: păr-ĔN-kĭ-mă.
peripheral nervous system	Nerves outside the brain and spinal cord: cranial, spinal, and autonomic nerves.
pia mater	Thin, delicate inner membrane of the meninges.
plexus (*plural*: **plexuses**)	Large, interlacing network of nerves. Examples are lumbosacral, cervical, and brachial (brachi/o means arm) plexuses. The term originated from the Indo-European *plek*, meaning to weave together.
pons	Part of the brain anterior to the cerebellum and between the medulla and the rest of the midbrain (Latin *pons* means bridge). It is a bridge connecting various parts of the brain.

10

receptor	Organ that receives a nervous stimulus and passes it on to afferent nerves. The skin, ears, eyes, and taste buds are receptors.
sciatic nerve	Nerve extending from the base of the spine down the thigh, lower leg, and foot. **Sciatica** is pain or inflammation along the course of the nerve.
sensory nerve	Carries messages toward the brain and spinal cord from a receptor; afferent nerve.
spinal nerves	Thirty-one pairs of nerves arising from the spinal cord.
stimulus (*plural*: **stimuli**)	Agent of change (light, sound, touch, pressure, and pain) in the internal or external environment that evokes a response.
stroma	Connective and supporting tissue of an organ. Glial cells make up the stromal tissue of the brain.
sulcus (*plural*: **sulci**)	Depression or groove in the surface of the cerebral cortex; fissure.
sympathetic nerves	Autonomic nerves that influence bodily functions involuntarily in times of stress.
synapse	Space through which a nervous impulse travels between nerve cells or between nerve and muscle or glandular cells. From the Greek *synapsis*, a point of contact.
thalamus	Main relay center of the brain. It conducts impulses between the spinal cord and the cerebrum; incoming sensory messages are relayed through the thalamus to appropriate centers in the cerebrum. Latin *thalamus* means room. The Romans, who named this structure, thought this part of the brain was hollow, like a little room.
vagus nerve	Tenth cranial nerve (cranial nerve X); its branches reach to the larynx, trachea, bronchi, lungs, aorta, esophagus, and stomach. Latin *vagus* means wandering. Unlike the other cranial nerves, the vagus leaves the head and "wanders" into the abdominal and thoracic cavities.
ventricles of the brain	Canals in the brain that contain cerebrospinal fluid. Ventricles are also found in the heart—they are the two lower chambers of the heart.

10

TERMINOLOGY

This section is divided into terms that describe organs and structures of the nervous system and those that relate to neurologic signs and symptoms. Write the meanings of the medical terms in the spaces provided.

ORGANS AND STRUCTURES

COMBINING FORM	MEANING	TERMINOLOGY	MEANING
cerebell/o	cerebellum	<u>cerebell</u>ar _____	
cerebr/o	cerebrum	<u>cerebr</u>ospinal fluid _____	
		<u>cerebr</u>al cortex _____ *Cortical means pertaining to the cortex or outer area of an organ.*	

COMBINING FORM	MEANING	TERMINOLOGY	MEANING
dur/o	dura mater	subdural hematoma _____	
		Remember: Hematomas are not tumors of blood, but are collections of blood.	
		epidural hematoma _____	
		Figure 10-12 shows subdural, epidural, and intracerebral hematomas.	
encephal/o	brain	encephalitis _____	
		encephalopathy _____	
		Chronic traumatic encephalopathy *(CTE) is a progressive degenerative disease associated with repetitive brain trauma (concussion).*	
		anencephaly _____	
		A congenital brain malformation; not compatible with life and may be detected with amniocentesis or ultrasonography of the fetus.	
gli/o	glial cells	glioblastoma _____	
		This is a highly malignant tumor (-blast means immature). Gliomas are tumors of glial (neuroglial) cells.	
lept/o	thin, slender	leptomeningeal _____	
		The pia and arachnoid membranes are known as the leptomeninges because of their thin, delicate structure.	
mening/o, meningi/o	membranes, meninges	meningeal _____	
		meningioma _____	
		Slowly growing, benign tumor.	
		myelomeningocele _____	
		Neural tube defect caused by failure of the neural tube to close during embryonic development. This abnormality occurs in infants born with spina bifida. See page 363.	

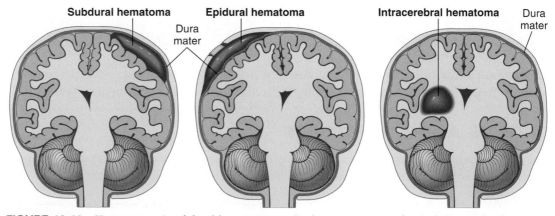

FIGURE 10-12 Hematomas. A **subdural hematoma** results from the tearing of veins between the dura and arachnoid membranes. It often is the result of blunt trauma, such as from blows to the head in boxers or in elderly patients who have fallen out of bed. An **epidural hematoma** occurs between the skull and the dura as the result of a ruptured meningeal artery, usually after a fracture of the skull. An **intracerebral hematoma** is caused by bleeding directly into brain tissue, such as can occur in the case of uncontrolled hypertension (high blood pressure).

COMBINING FORM	MEANING	TERMINOLOGY	MEANING
my/o	muscle	myoneural _____	
myel/o	spinal cord (means bone marrow in other contexts)	myelopathy _____	
		poliomyelitis _____ *Polio-* means gray matter. This viral disease affects the gray matter of the spinal cord, leading to paralysis of muscles that rely on the damaged neurons. Effective vaccines developed in the 20th century have made "polio" relatively uncommon.	
neur/o	nerve	neuropathy _____	
		polyneuritis _____	
pont/o	pons	cerebellopontine _____ *The suffix -ine means pertaining to.*	
radicul/o	nerve root (of spinal nerves)	radiculopathy _____ ***Sciatica*** *is a radiculopathy affecting the sciatic nerve root in the back. A herniated disk is a common cause leading to pain, weakness, or numbness down the leg. See* **In Person: Sciatica** *story on page 379.*	
		radiculitis _____ *This condition often results in pain and loss of function.*	
thalam/o	thalamus	thalamic _____	
thec/o	sheath (refers to the meninges)	intrathecal injection _____ *Chemicals, such as chemotherapeutic drugs, can be delivered into the subarachnoid space.*	
vag/o	vagus nerve (10th cranial nerve)	vagal _____ *This cranial nerve has branches to the head and neck, as well as to the chest.*	

SIGNS AND SYMPTOMS

COMBINING FORM OR SUFFIX	MEANING	TERMINOLOGY	MEANING
alges/o, -algesia	sensitivity to pain	analgesia _____	
		hypalgesia _____ *Diminished sensation to pain. (Notice that the o in hypo- is dropped.) Hyperalgesia is increased sensitivity to pain.*	

myel/o and my/o

Don't confuse these combining forms. **Myel/o** means spinal cord or bone marrow, while **my/o** means muscle. Another pair to watch out for is **pyel/o** (renal pelvis of the kidney) and **py/o** (pus).

Neuropathies

Neuropathies are diseases of peripheral nerves. They can affect motor, sensory, and autonomic functions. **Polyneuropathies** affect many nerves, while **mononeuropathies** affect individual nerves.

10

COMBINING FORM OR SUFFIX	MEANING	TERMINOLOGY	MEANING
-algia	pain (see page 377 for information on pain medications)	neuralgia _____ *Trigeminal neuralgia involves flashes of pain radiating along the course of the trigeminal nerve (fifth cranial nerve).* cephalgia _____ *Headaches may result from vasodilation (widening) of blood vessels in tissues surrounding the brain or from tension in neck and scalp muscles.*	
caus/o	burning	causalgia _____ *Intense burning pain following injury to a sensory nerve.*	
comat/o	deep sleep (coma)	comatose _____ *A **coma** is a state of unconsciousness from which the patient cannot be aroused. Semicomatose refers to a stupor (unresponsiveness) from which a patient can be aroused. In an irreversible coma (brain death), there is complete unresponsitivity to stimuli, no spontaneous breathing or movement, and a flat electroencephalogram (EEG) tracing.*	
esthesi/o, -esthesia	feeling, nervous sensation	anesthesia _____ *Lack of normal sensation (e.g., absence of sense of touch or pain). Two common types of regional anesthesia are spinal and epidural (caudal) blocks (Figure 10-13).* ***Anesthetics** are agents that reduce or eliminate sensation. General and local anesthetics are listed in Table 21-2, page 889.* hyperesthesia _____ *A light touch with a pin may provoke increased sensation. Diminished sensitivity to pain is called hypesthesia.* paresthesia _____ *Par- (from para-) means abnormal. Paresthesias include tingling, burning, and "pins and needles" sensations.*	
kines/o, kinesi/o -kinesia, -kinesis, -kinetic	movement	bradykinesia _____ hyperkinesis _____ *Amphetamines (CNS stimulants) are used to treat hyperkinesia in children, but the mechanism of their action is not understood.* dyskinesia _____ *Condition marked by involuntary, spasmodic movements. **Tardive** (occurring late) **dyskinesia** may develop in people who receive certain antipsychotic drugs for extended periods.* akinetic _____	
-lepsy	seizure	epilepsy _____ *See page 365.* narcolepsy _____ *Sudden, uncontrollable compulsion to sleep (narc/o = stupor, sleep). Amphetamines and stimulant drugs are prescribed to prevent attacks.*	

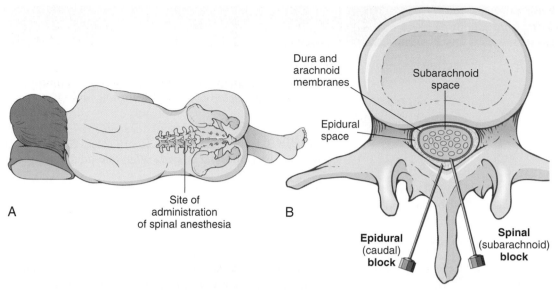

FIGURE 10-13 A, Positioning of a patient for spinal anesthesia. B, Cross-sectional view of the spinal cord showing injection sites for **epidural** and **spinal blocks (anesthesia).** Epidural (caudal) anesthesia is achieved by injecting an agent into the epidural space and is commonly used in obstetrics. Spinal anesthesia is achieved by injecting a local anesthetic into the subarachnoid space. Patients may experience loss of sensation and paralysis of feet, legs, and abdomen.

COMBINING FORM OR SUFFIX	MEANING	TERMINOLOGY	MEANING
lex/o	word, phrase	dyslexia	
		This is a developmental reading disorder occurring when the brain does not properly recognize, process, and interpret language.	
-paresis	weakness	hemiparesis	
		Affects either right or left side (half) of the body. **Paresis** *also is used by itself to mean partial paralysis or weakness of muscles.*	
-phasia	speech	aphasia	
		Difficulty with speech. **Motor** *(also called Broca or expressive)* **aphasia** *is present when the patient knows what he or she wants to say but cannot say it. The patient with* **sensory aphasia** *has difficulty understanding language and may pronounce (articulate) words easily but use them inappropriately.*	
-plegia	paralysis (loss or impairment of the ability to move parts of the body)	hemiplegia	
		Affects the right or left half of the body and results from a stroke or other brain injury. The hemiplegia is contralateral to the brain lesion because motor nerve fibers from the right half of the brain cross to the left side of the body (in the medulla oblongata).	
		paraplegia	
		Originally, the term paraplegia meant a stroke (paralysis) on one side (para-). Now, however, the term means paralysis of both legs and the lower part of the body caused by injury or disease of the spinal cord or cauda equina.	
		quadriplegia	
		Quadri- means four. All four extremities are affected. Injury is at the cervical level of the spinal cord.	

10

COMBINING FORM OR SUFFIX	MEANING	TERMINOLOGY	MEANING
-praxia	action	apraxia _____ _Movements and behavior are not purposeful. A patient with motor apraxia cannot use an object or perform a task. Motor weakness is not the cause._	
-sthenia	strength	neurasthenia _____ _Nervous exhaustion and fatigue, often following depression._	
syncop/o	to cut off, cut short	syncopal _____ **_Syncope_** _(SĬN-kō-pē) means fainting; sudden and temporary loss of consciousness caused by inadequate flow of blood to the brain. The term comes from a Greek word meaning cutting into pieces—thus, a fainting spell meant one's strength was "cut off."_ ✱ **HINT:** _Syncopal means pertaining to fainting and is an adjective. A patient can experience a syncopal episode._	
tax/o	order, coordination	ataxia _____ _Condition of decreased coordination. Persistent unsteadiness on the feet can be caused by a disorder involving the cerebellum._	

PATHOLOGY

The bones of the skull, the vertebral column, and the meninges, containing CSF, provide a hard box with an interior cushion around the brain and spinal cord. In addition, glial cells surrounding neurons form a blood-brain barrier that prevents many potentially harmful substances in the bloodstream from gaining access to neurons. However, these protective factors are counterbalanced by the extreme sensitivity of nerve cells to oxygen deficiency (brain cells die in a few minutes when deprived of oxygen).

Neurologic disorders may be classified in the following categories:

- Congenital
- Degenerative, movement, and seizure
- Infectious (meningitis and encephalitis)
- Neoplastic (tumors)
- Traumatic
- Vascular (stroke)

CONGENITAL DISORDERS

hydrocephalus

Abnormal accumulation of fluid (CSF) in the brain.

If circulation of CSF in the brain or spinal cord is impaired, fluid accumulates under pressure in the ventricles of the brain. To relieve pressure on the brain, a catheter (shunt) can be placed from the ventricle of the brain into the peritoneal space (ventriculoperitoneal shunt) or right atrium of the heart so that the CSF is continuously drained from the brain.

Hydrocephalus also can occur in adults as a result of tumors and infections.

spina bifida

Congenital defects in the lumbar spinal column caused by imperfect union of vertebral parts (neural tube defect).

In **spina bifida occulta,** the vertebral defect is covered over with skin and evident only on x-ray or other imaging examination. **Spina bifida cystica** is a more severe form, with cyst-like protrusions. In **meningocele,** the meninges protrude to the outside of the body, and in **myelomeningocele** (or meningomyelocele), both the spinal cord and meninges protrude (Figure 10-14A and B).

The etiology of neural tube defects is unknown. Defects originate in the early weeks of pregnancy as the spinal cord and vertebrae develop. Prenatal diagnosis is helped by imaging methods and testing maternal blood samples for alpha-fetoprotein.

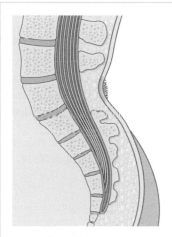 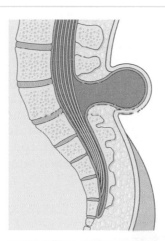 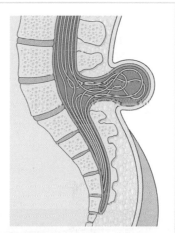

SPINA BIFIDA OCCULTA
Posterior vertebrae have not fused. No herniation of the spinal cord or meninges. There may be visible signs on the skin such as a mole, dimple, or patch of hair.

SPINA BIFIDA CYSTICA WITH MENINGOCELE
External protruding sac contains meninges and CSF.

SPINA BIFIDA CYSTICA WITH MYELOMENINGOCELE
External sac contains meninges, CSF, and the spinal cord. Often associated with hydrocephalus and paralysis.

A

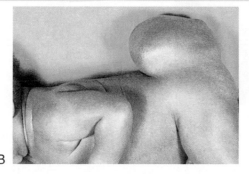

B

FIGURE 10-14   A, Spina bifida (neural tube defects). **B, Spina bifida cystica** with **myelomeningocele.**

DEGENERATIVE, MOVEMENT, AND SEIZURE DISORDERS

Alzheimer disease (AD) (Alzheimer's)

Brain disorder marked by gradual and progressive mental deterioration (dementia), personality changes, and impairment of daily functioning.

Characteristics of AD include confusion, memory failure, disorientation, restlessness, and speech disturbances. Anxiety, depression, and emotional disturbances can occur as well. The disease sometimes begins in middle life with slight defects in memory and behavior, but can worsen after the age of 70. On autopsy there is atrophy of the cerebral cortex and widening of the cerebral sulci, especially in the frontal and temporal regions (Figure 10-15A and B). Microscopic examination shows **senile plaques** resulting from degeneration of neurons and **neurofibrillary tangles** (bundles of fibrils in the cytoplasm of a neuron) in the cerebral cortex. Deposits of **amyloid** (a protein) occur in neurofibrillary tangles, senile plaques, and blood vessels. The cause of AD remains unknown, although genetic factors may play a role. A mutation on chromosome 14 has been linked to familial cases. There is as yet no effective treatment.

amyotrophic lateral sclerosis (ALS)

Degenerative disorder of motor neurons in the spinal cord and brainstem.

ALS manifests in adulthood. Signs and symptoms are weakness and atrophy of muscles in the hands, forearms, and legs; difficulty in swallowing and talking and dyspnea develop as the throat and respiratory muscles become affected. Etiology (cause) and cure for ALS both are unknown.

A famous baseball player, Lou Gehrig, became a victim of this disease in the mid-1900s, so the condition became known as **Lou Gehrig disease.**

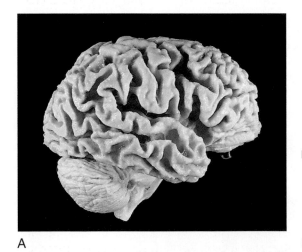

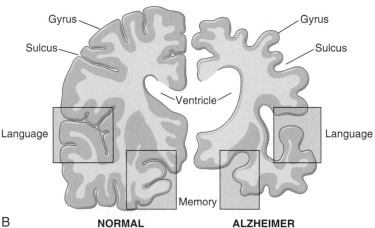

FIGURE 10-15   A, Alzheimer disease. Generalized loss of brain parenchyma (neuronal tissue) results in narrowing of the cerebral gyri and widening of the sulci. **B,** Cross-sectional comparison of a normal brain and a brain from a person with Alzheimer disease.

epilepsy

Chronic brain disorder characterized by recurrent seizure activity.

Seizures are abnormal, sudden discharges of electrical activity within the brain. Seizures often are symptoms of underlying brain pathologic conditions, such as brain tumors, meningitis, vascular disease, or scar tissue from a head injury. **Tonic-clonic seizures (grand mal** or **ictal events)** are characterized by a sudden loss of consciousness, falling down, and then tonic contractions (stiffening of muscles) followed by clonic contractions (twitching and jerking movements of the limbs). These convulsions often are preceded by an **aura,** which is a peculiar sensation experienced by the affected person before onset of a seizure. Dizziness, numbness, and visual or olfactory (sense of smell) disturbances are examples of an aura. **Absence seizures** are a form of seizure consisting of momentary clouding of consciousness and loss of awareness of the person's surroundings. These include **petit mal seizures** in children. Drug therapy (anticonvulsants) is used for control of epileptic seizures. After seizures, there may be neurologic symptoms such as weakness called **postictal events.**

In **temporal lobe epilepsy,** seizures begin in the temporal lobe (on each side of the brain near the ears) of the brain. The most common type of seizure is a **complex partial seizure.** Complex means impaired consciousness and partial indicates not generalized. Commonly these patients have seizures that cause them to pause in whatever they are doing, become confused, and have memory problems.

The term epilepsy comes from the Greek epilepsis, meaning a laying hold of. The Greeks thought a victim of a seizure was laid hold of by some mysterious force. The word ictal originates from the Latin ictus, meaning a blow or a stroke.

Huntington disease (Huntington's)

Hereditary disorder marked by degenerative changes in the cerebrum leading to abrupt involuntary movements and mental deterioration.

In this genetic condition, symptoms typically begin in adulthood and include personality changes, along with choreic (meaning dance-like) movements (uncontrollable, irregular, jerking movements of the arms and legs and facial grimacing). It is also known as **Huntington's chorea.**

The genetic defect in patients with Huntington disease is located on chromosome 4. Patients can be tested for the gene; however, no cure exists, and management is symptomatic.

multiple sclerosis (MS)

Destruction of the myelin sheath on neurons in the CNS and its replacement by plaques of sclerotic (hard) tissue.

One of the leading causes of neurologic disability in persons 20 to 40 years of age, MS is a chronic disease often marked by long periods of stability (remission) and worsening (relapse). **Demyelination** (loss of myelin insulation) prevents the conduction of nerve impulses through the axon. See figure 10-16A. Demyelination causes paresthesias, muscle weakness, unsteady **gait** (manner of walking), and paralysis. There may be visual (blurred and double vision) and speech disturbances as well. Areas of scarred myelin (plaques) can be seen on MRI scans of the brain (Figure 10-16B). Etiology is unknown but probably involves an autoimmune disease of lymphocytes reacting against myelin. Drugs that are commonly used to treat MS are corticosteroids (to reduce inflammation), interferons (to slow the rate of progression of MS symptoms), and drugs such as glatiramer that block the immune system's attack on myelin.

Epilepsy and Seizures

Epilepsy is a brain disorder in which at least two or more seizures appear spontaneously and recurrently. Having a single seizure does not mean that the affected person has epilepsy.

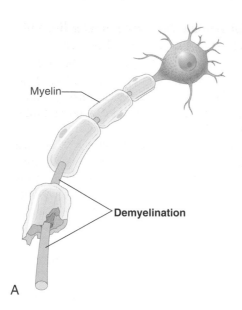

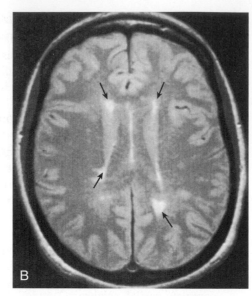

FIGURE 10-16 **Multiple sclerosis. A, Demyelination** of a nerve cell. **B,** This MRI scan shows multiple abnormal white areas that correspond to MS plaques (*arrows*). The plaques are scar tissue that forms when myelin sheaths are destroyed.

myasthenia gravis (MG)

Autoimmune neuromuscular disorder characterized by weakness of voluntary muscles.

MG is a chronic autoimmune disorder. Antibodies block the ability of acetylcholine (neurotransmitter) to transmit the nervous impulse from nerve to muscle cell. Onset of symptoms usually is gradual. Brainstem signs are prominent and include ptosis of the upper eyelid, double vision (diplopia), and facial weakness. Respiratory paralysis is the main clinical concern. Therapy to reverse symptoms includes anticholinesterase drugs, which inhibit the enzyme that breaks down acetylcholine. Immunosuppressive therapy is used, including medications such as corticosteroids (prednisone) and other immunosuppressive drugs. **Thymectomy** is also a method of treatment and is beneficial to many patients.

palsy

Paralysis (partial or complete loss of motor function).

Cerebral palsy is partial paralysis and lack of muscular coordination caused by loss of oxygen (hypoxia) or blood flow to the cerebrum during pregnancy or in the perinatal period. **Bell palsy** (or Bell's palsy) (Figure 10-17) is paralysis on one side of the face. The likely cause is a viral infection, and therapy is directed against the virus (antiviral drugs) and nerve swelling (corticosteriods).

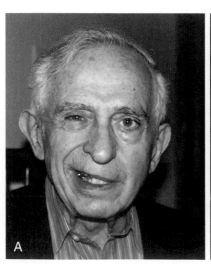

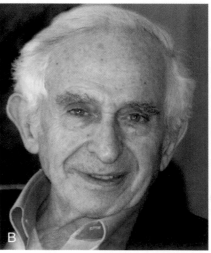

FIGURE 10-17 **A, Bell palsy.** Notice the paralysis on the left side of this man's face: The eyelid does not close properly, the forehead is not wrinkled as would be expected, and there is clear paralysis of the lower face. **B,** The palsy spontaneously resolved after 6 months.

**Parkinson disease
(Parkinson's)**

Degeneration of neurons in the basal ganglia, occurring in later life and leading to tremors, weakness of muscles, and slowness of movement.

This slowly progressive condition is caused by a deficiency of **dopamine,** a neurotransmitter made by cells in the basal ganglia (see Figure 10-9). Motor disturbances include stooped posture, shuffling gait, and muscle stiffness (rigidity). Other signs are a typical "pill-rolling" tremor of hands and a characteristic mask-like lack of facial expression. See Figure 10-18.

Therapy with drugs such as levodopa plus carbidopa (Sinemet) to increase dopamine levels in the brain is **palliative** (relieving symptoms but not curative). Many patients may have clinical features of Parkinson's (parkinsonism) and yet not have the disease itself. They would not benefit from antiparkinsonian medication. Implantation of fetal brain tissue containing dopamine-producing cells is an experimental treatment but has produced uncertain results.

**Tourette syndrome
(Tourette's)**

Involuntary, spasmodic, twitching movements; uncontrollable vocal sounds; and inappropriate words.

These involuntary movements, usually beginning with twitching of the eyelid and muscles of the face with verbal outbursts, are called **tics.** Although the cause of Tourette syndrome is not known, it is associated with either an excess of dopamine or a hypersensitivity to dopamine. Psychological problems do not cause Tourette syndrome, but physicians have had some success in treating it with the antipsychotic drug haloperidol (Haldol), antidepressants, and mood stabilizers.

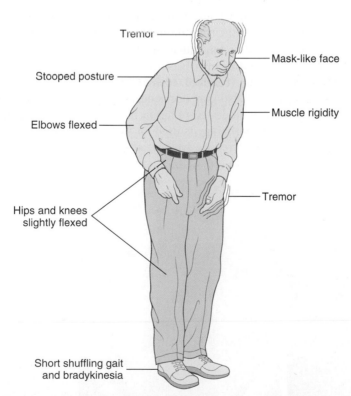

FIGURE 10-18 Primary symptoms of Parkinson disease are tremors in hands, arms, legs, jaw, and face; rigidity or stiffness of limbs and trunk; bradykinesia (shuffling gait), stooped posture, and masklike facies.

INFECTIOUS DISORDERS

herpes zoster (shingles)

Viral infection affecting peripheral nerves.

Blisters and pain spread along peripheral nerves (see Figure 10-19A) and are caused by inflammation due to a herpesvirus **(herpes zoster),** the same virus that causes chickenpox (varicella). Reactivation of the chickenpox virus (herpes varicella-zoster), which remains in the body after the person had chickenpox, occurs. Painful blisters follow the underlying route of cranial or spinal nerves around the trunk of the body; zoster means girdle. Zostavax is a vaccine to prevent shingles. It is recommended for people 60 years of age and older.

meningitis

Inflammation of the meninges; leptomeningitis.

This condition can be caused by bacteria (pyogenic meningitis) or viruses (aseptic or viral meningitis). Signs and symptoms are fever and signs of meningeal irritation, such as headache, photophobia (sensitivity to light), and a stiff neck. Lumbar punctures are performed to examine CSF. Physicians use antibiotics to treat the more serious pyogenic form, and antivirals for the viral form.

human immunodeficiency virus (HIV) encephalopathy

Brain disease and dementia occurring with AIDS.

Many patients with AIDS develop neurologic dysfunction. In addition to encephalitis and dementia (loss of mental functioning), some patients develop brain tumors and other infections.

NEOPLASTIC DISORDERS

brain tumor

Abnormal growth of brain tissue and meninges.

Most primary brain tumors arise from glial cells **(gliomas)** or the meninges **(meningiomas).** Types of gliomas include **astrocytoma** (Figure 10-19B), **oligodendroglioma,** and **ependymoma.** The most malignant form of astrocytoma is **glioblastoma multiforme** (-blast means immature) (see Figure 10-19B). Tumors can cause swelling **(cerebral edema)** and hydrocephalus. If CSF pressure is increased, swelling also may occur near the optic nerve (at the back of the eye). Other symptoms include severe headache and new seizures. Gliomas are removed surgically, and radiotherapy is used for tumors that are not completely resected. Steroids are given to reduce swelling after surgery.

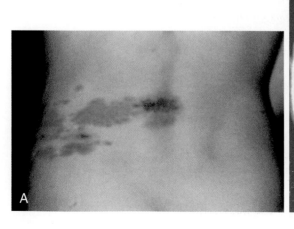
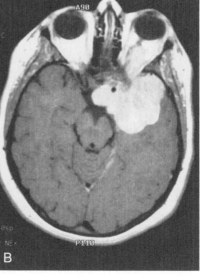

FIGURE 10-19 A, Shingles. B, Glioblastoma as seen on MRI.

Meningiomas usually are benign and surrounded by a capsule, but they may cause compression and distortion of the brain.

Tumors in the brain also may be single or multiple metastatic growths. Most arise from the lung, breast, skin (melanoma), kidney, and gastrointestinal tract and spread to the brain.

TRAUMATIC DISORDERS

cerebral concussion

Type of traumatic brain injury caused by a blow to the head.

There is usually no evidence of structural damage to brain tissue, and loss of consciousness may not occur. Rest is very important after a concussion because it allows the brain to heal. Doctors recommend avoiding demanding mental and physical activities.

cerebral contusion

Bruising of brain tissue resulting from direct trauma to the head.

A cerebral contusion may be associated with a fracture of the skull, as well as with edema and an increase in intracranial pressure. Subdural and epidural hematomas occur (see Figure 10-12), leading to permanent brain injury with altered memory or speech or development of epilepsy.

VASCULAR DISORDERS

cerebrovascular accident (CVA)

Disruption in the normal blood supply to the brain; stroke.

This condition, also known as a **cerebral infarction,** is the result of impaired oxygen supply to the brain. There are three types of strokes (Figure 10-20):

1. **Thrombotic**—blood clot **(thrombus)** in the arteries leading to the brain, resulting in occlusion (blocking) of the vessel. Atherosclerosis leads to this common type of stroke as blood vessels become blocked over time. Before total occlusion occurs, a patient may experience symptoms that point to the gradual occlusion of blood vessels. These short episodes of neurologic dysfunction are known as **transient ischemic attacks (TIAs).**

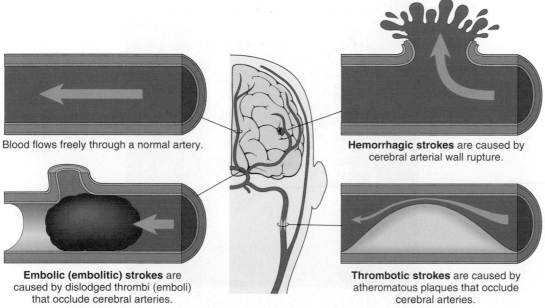

Blood flows freely through a normal artery.

Hemorrhagic strokes are caused by cerebral arterial wall rupture.

Embolic (embolitic) strokes are caused by dislodged thrombi (emboli) that occlude cerebral arteries.

Thrombotic strokes are caused by atheromatous plaques that occlude cerebral arteries.

FIGURE 10-20   Three types of strokes: embolic, hemorrhagic, and thrombotic.

2. **Embolic**—an **embolus** (a dislodged thrombus) travels to cerebral arteries and occludes a small vessel. This type of stroke occurs very suddenly.

3. **Hemorrhagic**—a blood vessel, such as the cerebral artery, breaks and bleeding occurs. This type of stroke can be fatal and results from advancing age, atherosclerosis, or high blood pressure, all of which result in degeneration of cerebral blood vessels. With small hemorrhages, the body reabsorbs the blood and the patient makes good recovery with only slight disability. In a younger patient, cerebral hemorrhage usually is caused by mechanical injury associated with skull fracture or rupture of an arterial **aneurysm** (weakened area in the vessel wall that balloons and may eventually burst). See Figure 10-21.

The major risk factors for stroke are hypertension, diabetes, smoking, and heart disease. Other risk factors include obesity, substance abuse (cocaine), and elevated cholesterol levels.

Thrombotic strokes are treated with antiplatelet or anticoagulant (clot-dissolving) therapy. **Tissue plasminogen activator (tPA)** may be started shortly after the onset of a stroke. Surgical intervention with carotid endarterectomy (removal of the atherosclerotic plaque along with the inner lining of the affected carotid artery) also is possible.

migraine

Severe, recurring, unilateral, vascular headache.

Prodromal symptoms are known as an **aura** (peculiar sensations that precede the onset of illness). Symptoms of aura are temporary visual and sensory disturbances, including flashes of light and zigzag lines. Sensitivity to sound (phonophobia) and light (photophobia) are associated with the migraine itself. Migraine pain is believed to be related to dilation of the blood vessels. Treatment to prevent a migraine attack includes medications such as sumatriptan succinate (Imitrex) that target serotonin receptors on blood vessels and nerves. Drugs of this type reduce inflammation and restrict dilation of blood vessels.

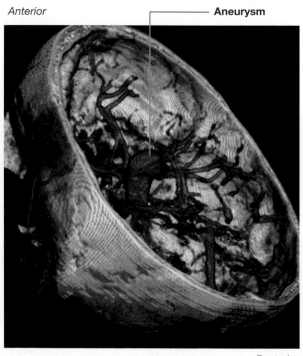

Anterior — Aneurysm

Posterior

FIGURE 10-21 Cerebral aneurysm.

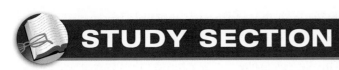

STUDY SECTION

The following list reviews the new terms used in the Pathology section. Practice spelling each term and know its meaning.

absence seizure	Form of seizure consisting of momentary clouding of consciousness and loss of awareness of surroundings.
aneurysm	Enlarged, weakened area in an arterial wall, which may rupture, leading to hemorrhage and CVA (stroke).
astrocytoma	Malignant tumor of astrocytes (glial brain cells).
aura	Peculiar symptom or sensation occurring before the onset (prodromal) of an attack of migraine or an epileptic seizure.
dementia	Mental decline and deterioration.
demyelination	Destruction of myelin on axons of neurons (as in multiple sclerosis).
dopamine	CNS neurotransmitter, deficient in patient with Parkinson disease.
embolus	Clot of material that travels through the bloodstream and suddenly blocks a vessel.
gait	Manner of walking.
ictal event	Pertaining to a sudden, acute onset, as with the convulsions of an epileptic seizure.
occlusion	Blockage.
palliative	Relieving symptoms but not curing them.
thymectomy	Removal of the thymus gland (a lymphocyte-producing gland in the chest); used as treatment for myasthenia gravis.
TIA	Transient ischemic attack. TIAs can occur with all three types of strokes: thrombolytic, embolic, and even hemorrhagic (if minor.) They are characterized by a limited time course of neurologic deficits.
tic	Involuntary movement of a small group of muscles, as of the face; characteristic of Tourette syndrome.
tonic-clonic seizure	Major (grand mal) convulsive seizure marked by sudden loss of consciousness, stiffening of muscles, and twitching and jerking movements.

LABORATORY TESTS AND CLINICAL PROCEDURES

LABORATORY TESTS

cerebrospinal fluid analysis   **Samples of CSF are examined.**

CFS analysis measures protein, glucose, and red (RBC) and white (WBC) blood cells as well as other chemical contents of the CSF. CSF analysis also can detect tumor cells (by cytology), bacteria, and viruses. These studies are used to diagnose infection, tumors, or multiple sclerosis.

CLINICAL PROCEDURES

X-Ray Tests

cerebral angiography   **X-ray imaging of the arterial blood vessels in the brain after injection of contrast material.**

Contrast is injected into the femoral artery (in the thigh), and x-ray motion pictures are taken. These images diagnose vascular disease (aneurysm, occlusion, hemorrhage) in the brain.

computed tomography (CT) of the brain	**Computerized x-ray technique that generates multiple images of the brain and spinal cord.**

Contrast material may be injected intravenously to highlight abnormalities. The contrast leaks through the **blood-brain barrier** from blood vessels into the brain tissue and shows tumors, aneurysms, bleeding, brain injury, skull fractures, and blood clots. Operations are performed using the CT scan as a local road map. CT scans also are particularly useful for visualizing blood and bone.

Magnetic Resonance Techniques

magnetic resonance imaging (MRI)	**Magnetic field and pulses of radiowave energy create images of the brain and spinal cord.**

MRI is better than CT at evaluation of brain parenchyma. It is excellent for viewing brain damage related to infection, inflammation or tumors. It also is used to look for causes of headaches, to help diagnose a stroke, and detect bleeding problems and head injury. Contrast material may be used to enhance images. **Magnetic resonance angiography (MRA)** produces images of blood vessels using magnetic resonance techniques.

Radionuclide Studies

positron emission tomography (PET) scan	**Radioactive glucose is injected and then detected in the brain to image the metabolic activity of cells.**

PET scans provide valuable information about the function of brain tissue in patients, to detect malignancy and to evaluate brain abnormalities in Alzheimer disease, stroke, schizophrenia, and epilepsy (Figure 10-22). Combined **PET-CT scanners** provide images that pinpoint the location of abnormal metabolic activity within the brain.

Ultrasound Examination

Doppler ultrasound studies	**Sound waves detect blood flow in the carotid and intracranial arteries.**

The carotid artery carries blood to the brain. These studies detect occlusion in blood vessels.

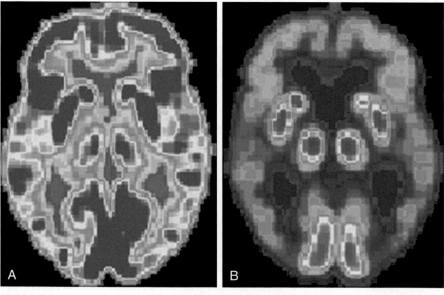

FIGURE 10-22   PET scans. A, Normal brain. B, Brain affected by Alzheimer disease. *Red* and *yellow areas* indicate high neural activity. *Blue* and *purple* indicate low neural activity.

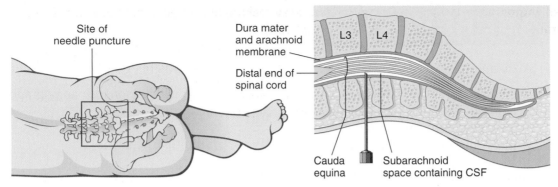

FIGURE 10-23   **Lumbar puncture.** The patient lies laterally, with the knees drawn up to the abdomen and the chin brought down to the chest. This position increases the spaces between the vertebrae. The lumbar puncture needle is inserted between the third and fourth (or the fourth and fifth) lumbar vertebrae and then is advanced to enter the subarachnoid space.

Other Procedures

electroencephalography (EEG)	**Recording of the electrical activity of the brain.** EEG demonstrates seizure activity resulting from brain tumors, other diseases, and injury to the brain. It can also help define diffuse cortical dysfunction (encephalopathies).
lumbar puncture (LP)	**CSF is withdrawn from between two lumbar vertebrae for analysis** (Figure 10-23). A device to measure the pressure of CSF may be attached to the end of the needle after it has been inserted. Injection of intrathecal medicines may be administered as well. Some patients experience headache after LP. An informal name for this procedure is "spinal tap."
stereotactic radiosurgery	**Use of a specialized instrument to locate and treat targets in the brain.** The stereotactic instrument is fixed onto the skull and guides the insertion of a needle by three-dimensional measurement. A **Gamma Knife** (high-energy radiation beam) is used to treat deep and often inaccessible intracranial brain tumors and abnormal blood vessel masses (**arteriovenous malformations**) without surgical incision. **Proton stereotactic radiosurgery (PSRS)** delivers a uniform dose of proton radiation to a target and spares surrounding normal tissue (Figure 10-24 A and B).

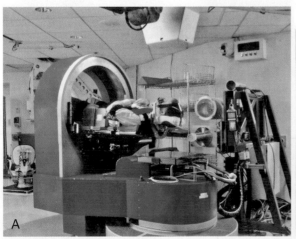
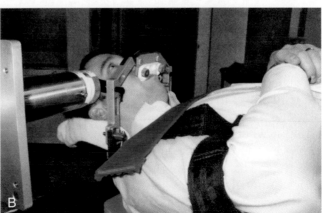

FIGURE 10-24   **A,** Patient in position on **stereotactic proton unit, ready to take an alignment x-ray. B, Stereotactic frame** holds the patient's head in place for treatment with proton beam radiosurgery. (*Courtesy Department of Radiation Therapy, Massachusetts General Hospital, Boston.*)

10

ABBREVIATIONS

AD	Alzheimer disease
AFP	alpha-fetoprotein; elevated levels in amniotic fluid and maternal blood are associated with congenital malformations of the nervous system, such as anencephaly and spina bifida
ALS	amyotrophic lateral sclerosis—Lou Gehrig disease
AVM	arteriovenous malformation; congenital tangle of arteries and veins in the cerebrum
BBB	blood-brain barrier
CNS	central nervous system
CSF	cerebrospinal fluid
CTE	chronic traumatic encephalopathy
CVA	cerebrovascular accident
EEG	electroencephalography
GABA	gamma-aminobutyric acid (neurotransmitter)
ICP	intracranial pressure (normal pressure is 5 to 15 mm Hg)
LP	lumbar puncture
MAC	monitored anesthetic care

MG	myasthenia gravis
MRA	magnetic resonance angiography
MRI	magnetic resonance imaging
MS	multiple sclerosis
½ P	hemiparesis
PCA	patient-controlled analgesia
PET	positron emission tomography
PNS	peripheral nervous system
PSRS	proton stereotactic radiosurgery
Sz	seizure
TBI	traumatic brain injury
TENS	transcutaneous electrical nerve stimulation; technique using a battery-powered device to relieve acute and chronic pain
TIA	transient ischemic attack; temporary interference with the blood supply to the brain
TLE	temporal lobe epilepsy
tPA	tissue plasminogen activator; a clot-dissolving drug used as therapy for stroke

PRACTICAL APPLICATIONS

CASE STUDY: A PATIENT'S ACCOUNT OF ULNAR NERVE NEUROPATHY

I am definitely not one of those ambidextrous people. I am a true righty, so the "experiment" of making me a lefty out of necessity didn't go so well. Over the past decade, I had slowly lost sensation in my right pinky, and a fair amount of function, in my right hand. You might think that I should have taken care of treating it when it initially presented itself with an electric shock down my arm from hitting my "funny bone" over and over. The "funny bone," of course, is not a bone at all. It is the ulnar nerve, which runs across the medial and posterior aspect of the elbow as it travels to the hand. See Figure 10-25. After multiple injuries to my elbow, my pinky just became useless and numb.

As a physician, I realized that my ulnar nerve had become entrapped and scarred from repeated injury. Over the years, I tolerated this situation because other nerves had remain unaffected, providing sensation and function to my hand. It was only when I saw myself in a video (my hand looked like a claw) that I recognized how compromised the function of the hand had become.

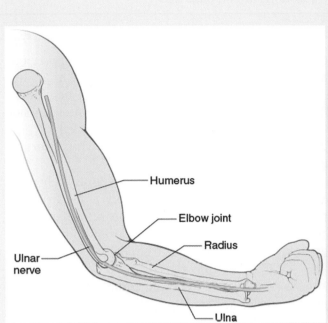

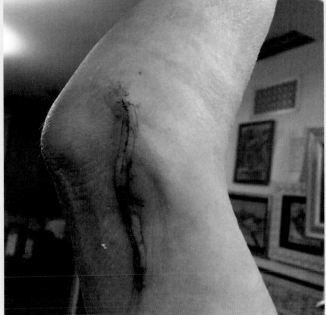

FIGURE 10-25 Pathway of ulnar nerve running behind the elbow joint (median epicondyle of the humerus) and toward the hand.

FIGURE 10-26 Post-operative scar from ulnar nerve surgery.

During an exam by an orthopedic elbow specialist, testing revealed poor sensation and atrophy of my right hand muscles. My grip strength was also affected and was now actually stronger on my left rather than my right.

Surgery was scheduled immediately with hopes of halting atrophy and clawing of my hand and regaining sensation in my pinky. My surgeon performed an Eaton procedure. He moved the scarred ulnar nerve from its vulnerable path and placed sutures to hold the ulnar nerve in its new place under the fascia (connective tissue) of my elbow. He created a little "curtain" with the fascia to keep the nerve from moving again. This ultimately allowed the nerve to take a "short cut" on the way to my hand while taking tension off the injured nerve and keeping it away from the bony prominence of the elbow.

When I awoke from the anesthesia, I could immediately tell that something was different about my hand. I had tingling in my previously numb fingers and soon had a warm sensation and even sweating in my palm. These findings demonstrated the return of the autonomic function of the nerve, something that had also been affected by the long-standing injury.

My arm was in a sling until my post op appointment. Figure 10-26 shows my arm and scar just after the 2 week post operative check. A compression sleeve prevented swelling and reminded me not to use my arm too much.

At 3 months post surgery I was back to my usual routine typing, writing, and using my hand. Sensation gradually returned to my pinky and the function in my hand improved as well but very slowly. Injured nerves can regenerate, as long as they are not cut or completely crushed. The nerve heals from proximal to distal (starting at the elbow and working toward the tip of the finger). Doctors quote the statistic a millimeter a day, or roughly an inch per month. The feeling in my pinky is still not normal, but it is improving, and it's encouraging to notice the progress. The muscles in my hand are also getting stronger. The true test will be to check my grip strength when I return for my 6 month follow-up appointment.

I am grateful for the brisk action and skilled surgery that was possible before my ulnar nerve was permanently damaged. I am also thankful that the body can heal itself when provided the appropriate help. I had become so used to the numb feeling and I had no idea of what I had been missing!

10

Answers to the following case report and case study questions are on page 389.

CASE REPORT: CEREBRAL INFARCTION

This patient was admitted on January 14 with a history of progressive right hemiparesis for the previous 1 to 2 months; fluctuating numbness of the right arm, thorax, and buttocks; jerking of the right leg; periods of speech arrest; diminished comprehension in reading; and recent development of a hemiplegic gait. He is suspected of having a left parietal tumor [the parietal lobes of the cerebrum are on either side under the roof of the skull].

Examinations done before hospitalization included skull films, EEG, and CSF analysis, which were all normal. After admission, an MRI was abnormal in the left parietal region, as was the EEG.

An MRA study to assess cerebral blood vessels was attempted, but the patient became progressively more restless and agitated after sedation, so the procedure was stopped. During the recovery phase from the sedation, the patient was alternately somnolent [sleepy] and violent, but it was later apparent that he had developed almost a complete aphasia and right hemiplegia.

In the next few days, he became more alert, although he remained dysarthric [from the Greek *arthroun*, to utter distinctly] and hemiplegic.

MRI and MRA with the patient under general anesthesia on January 19 showed complete occlusion of the left internal carotid artery with cross-filling of the left anterior and middle cerebral arteries from the right internal carotid circulation.

Final diagnosis: Left CVA caused by left internal carotid artery occlusion.

[Figure 10-27 shows the common carotid arteries and their branches within the head and brain.]

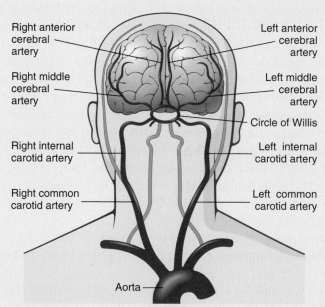

FIGURE 10-27 Common carotid arteries and their branches.

Questions about the Case Report

1. The patient was admitted with a history of:
   a. Right-sided paralysis caused by a previous stroke
   b. Paralysis on the left side of his body
   c. Increasing paresis on the right side of his body

2. The patient also had experienced periods of:
   a. Aphasia and dyslexia
   b. Dysplastic gait
   c. Apraxia and aphasia

3. After his admission to the hospital, where did the MRI show an abnormality?
   a. Right posterior region of the brain
   b. Left and right sides of the brain
   c. Left side of the brain

4. What test determined the final diagnosis?
   a. EEG for both sides of the brain
   b. CSF analysis and cerebral angiography
   c. MRI and MRA

5. What was the final diagnosis?
   a. Stroke; ischemic injury to tissue in the left cerebrum caused by blockage of an artery
   b. Cross-filling of blood vessels from the left to the right side of the brain
   c. Cerebral palsy on the left side of the brain with cross-filling of two cerebral arteries

10

PAIN MEDICATIONS

Pain is a major symptom in many medical conditions. Both the area of injury and how the brain deals with it affect the sensations of pain. Medications to relieve pain (analgesics) act in different ways:

- **Nonsteroidal anti-inflammatory drugs (NSAIDs)** relieve pain by stopping inflammation. Examples are nonprescription drugs such as ibuprofen (Advil, Motrin, Excedrin), aspirin (Anacin, Ascriptin, Bufferin), and naproxen (Aleve). Other NSAIDs that require a prescription are Toradol (ketorolac) and Feldene (piroxicam).
- **Acetaminophen (Tylenol)** relieves fever and mild pain but is not an anti-inflammatory drug. It is not clear how acetaminophen works.
- **Narcotics** relieve pain by affecting receptors in the brain to control the perception of pain. Examples are morphine, codeine, oxycodone, and hydrocodone. Combinations of narcotics and acetaminophen are Vicodin (acetaminophen with hydrocodone) and Percocet (acetaminophen with oxycodone).

NEUROPATHIC PAIN WITH A CASE STUDY

Neuropathic pain is a unique type of pain that accompanies illnesses and trauma. Patients may describe this pain as:

- radiating or spreading
- an electric shock–like sensation
- hot or burning
- shooting, piercing, darting, or stabbing (lancinating)

- abnormal skin sensations (paresthesias): numbness, tingling, "pins and needles"
- pain to light touch
- extreme sensitivity to ordinary, innocuous stimuli
- often independent of movement

Case Study:

A 68-year-old man awoke one morning with severe pain in his right shoulder. On turning his head or lifting his shoulder, he experienced extreme discomfort and lancinating pain. The pain was a sharp, burning pain that moved across his shoulder and down into his right arm. Finding a comfortable position lying down was difficult. A cervical MRI study showed no bone abnormalities, whereas a neurologic examination provided evidence of damage to multiple peripheral nerves. He developed weakness of his shoulder muscles and was unable to lift his right arm. Final diagnosis was brachial plexus neuritis [also known as Parsonage-Turner syndrome]. The cause of the condition is unknown, but it may be related to a flu vaccination he received 2 weeks previously. Treatment consisted of pain medication and physical therapy to rehabilitate weakened muscles in his arm and shoulder.

Questions about the Case Study

1. The cervical MRI study showed:
   a. Damage to the vertebrae in the neck
   b. Nerve entrapment in the upper spine
   c. Damage to multiple peripheral nerves
   d. Normal vertebrae in the neck

2. Lancinating pain is:
   a. Pain to light touch
   b. Characterized by paresthesia
   c. Stabbing, piercing, shooting
   d. Characterized by numbness and tingling

3. The patient's diagnosis is best described as:
   a. Inflammation of cervical nerve roots affecting his shoulder and arm
   b. Inflammation of a network of nerves in his shoulder that control muscles in his arm
   c. First stages of a heart attack, marked by radiating arm pain
   d. Autoimmune disorder affecting voluntary muscles in his shoulder and arm

IN PERSON: SCIATICA

This is a first-person account of a woman in her mid-forties living with sciatica.

Eight years ago, I wouldn't have believed that reaching into a laundry basket could change my my life. But in January 2009, it did.

I had gotten my first-ever backache a few days earlier, after a long car trip. A Google search instructed me to apply ice for the first 48 hours and then heat, if the pain persisted. My husband took over the kids' school day routine while I recuperated. That third morning, I could hear my younger son rifling around for his favorite sweatshirt; I knew it was at the foot of my bed waiting to be sorted. In the instant it took to reach into the laundry basket for that sweatshirt, my back went from dull ache to a crippling pain that radiated all the way down my left leg, to the tip of my left foot.

An MRI scan confirmed the diagnosis: spinal disc herniation, protruding onto the nerve roots affecting the sciatic nerve, and causing my leg pain. Surgery being presented as a last resort, I embarked on a crash course of physical therapy, NSAIDs, oral steroids, muscle relaxants, epidural steroid injections, and lots and lots of patience. I saw gradual improvement for about three months, to the point that I was able to resume a modified daily routine.

Then, the improvement stopped. Conventional treatment had run its course. I was at the "last resort" stage. So I "cried uncle" and requested a surgical consult. The surgeon ordered a follow-up MRI, which showed good news: There had been much improvement to the herniation. To my surprise, the MRI also revealed nerve roots supplying the sciatic nerve were now free and clear of impingement. If the nerve was back to normal, why was I still in such pain? Because, it turns out, the nerve was injured by its ordeal. Not uncommon, I was reassured. This development took the surgical option off the table. After all, the goal of the surgery would have been to relieve the affected nerve from compression by the protruding disc. In my case, even the relieved nerve was causing problems, and that meant not surgery, but more patience. The wait began: to see whether the the nerve would repair itself—I was told that could take years—or worse, whether I was facing permanent nerve damage

Three years later the verdict seems clear: my sciatic nerve sustained what appears to be permanent damage. To this day, I have not regained full use of my left leg. Along with chronic, dull pain, there are also paresthesias—simultaneous burning and numbness along the path of the sciatic nerve accompanied by constant, involuntary muscle spasms. I've lost my Achilles jerk reflex, and so unresponsive is my left foot that I can't feel it hit the ground when I'm walking.

In those critical first months, I thought my options were either resolving the herniation with surgery or resolving it without surgery. It never once occurred to me that, four years later, the injury would remain unresolved.

There's always a new treatment, or specialist, or drug that shows promise or really worked for a friend of a friend. Until recently, it felt like I was giving up hope if I didn't pursue each lead. Now I'm focusing more on adapting to my new circumstances than on finding a "cure." I don't want my whole life to revolve around sciatica. I found a medication that reduces the chronic pain to more of an annoyance than a crisis (with occasional flare-ups).

I missed my old life and wanted it back. At the risk of sounding like a late-night pharmaceutical ad, I'm not giving up; I'm going on.

AUTHOR'S NOTE: Everyone's experience with sciatica is unique. I recently experienced the condition myself, resulting from a L4-L5 disk herniation. After 7 months of pain radiating down my right leg, I had microdiskectomy surgery, which fortunately alleviated my pain and sciatica.

10

EXERCISES

Remember to check your answers carefully with the Answers to Exercises, page 387.

A **Match the listed neurologic structures with the descriptions/definitions that follow.**

astrocyte   dendrite   neuron
axon   meninges   oligodendroglial cell
cauda equina   myelin sheath   plexus
cerebral cortex

1. microscopic fiber leading from the cell body that carries the nervous impulse along a nerve cell

   _____

2. large, interlacing network of nerves _____

3. three protective membranes surrounding the brain and spinal cord _____

4. microscopic branching fiber of a nerve cell that is the first part to receive the nervous impulse

   _____

5. outer region of the largest part of the brain; composed of gray matter _____

6. glial cell that transports water and salts between capillaries and nerve cells _____

7. glial cell that produces myelin _____

8. a nerve cell that transmits a nerve impulse _____

9. collection of spinal nerves below the end of the spinal cord at the level of the second lumbar

   vertebra _____

10. fatty tissue that surrounds the axon of a nerve cell _____

B **Give the meanings of the following terms.**

1. dura mater _____

2. central nervous system _____

3. peripheral nervous system _____

4. arachnoid membrane _____

5. hypothalamus _____

6. synapse _____

7. sympathetic nerves _____

8. medulla oblongata _____

9. pons _____

10. cerebellum _____

10

11. thalamus _____

12. ventricles of the brain _____

13. brainstem _____

14. cerebrum _____

15. ganglion _____

C **Match the following terms with the meanings or associated terms below.**

glial cells	neurotransmitter	sensory nerves
gyri	parenchymal cell	subarachnoid space
motor nerves	pia mater	sulci

1. innermost meningeal membrane _____

2. carry messages away from (efferent) the brain and spinal cord to muscles and glands

_____

3. carry messages toward (afferent) the brain and spinal cord from receptors _____

4. grooves in the cerebral cortex _____

5. contains cerebrospinal fluid _____

6. elevations in the cerebral cortex _____

7. chemical that is released at the end of a nerve cell and stimulates or inhibits another cell

(example: acetylcholine) _____

8. essential cell of the nervous system; a neuron _____

9. connective and supportive (stromal) tissue _____

D **Circle the correct boldface term for the given definition.**

1. disease of the brain **(encephalopathy, myelopathy)**

2. part of the brain that controls muscular coordination and balance **(cerebrum, cerebellum)**

3. collection of blood above the dura mater **(subdural hematoma, epidural hematoma)**

4. inflammation of the pia and arachnoid membranes **(leptomeningitis, causalgia)**

5. condition of absence of a brain **(hypalgesia, anencephaly)**

6. inflammation of the gray matter of the spinal cord **(poliomyelitis, polyneuritis)**

7. pertaining to the membranes around the brain and spinal cord **(cerebellopontine, meningeal)**

8. disease of nerve roots (of spinal nerves) **(neuropathy, radiculopathy)**

9. hernia of the spinal cord and meninges **(myelomeningocele, meningioma)**

10. pertaining to the tenth cranial nerve **(thalamic, vagal)**

10

E Give the meanings of the following terms.

1. cerebral cortex _____

2. intrathecal _____

3. polyneuritis _____

4. thalamic _____

5. myelopathy _____

6. meningioma _____

7. glioma _____

8. subdural hematoma _____

F Match the listed neurologic symptoms with the definitions/descriptions that follow.

aphasia	dyslexia	narcolepsy
ataxia	hemiparesis	neurasthenia
bradykinesia	hyperesthesia	paraplegia
causalgia	motorapraxia	syncope

1. reading disorder _____

2. condition of decreased coordination _____

3. condition of slow movement _____

4. condition of increased sensation _____

5. seizure of sleep; uncontrollable compulsion to sleep _____

6. difficulty with speech _____

7. inability to perform a task _____

8. weakness in the right or left half of the body _____

9. severe burning pain due to nerve injury _____

10. paralysis in the lower part of the body _____

11. fainting _____

12. nervous exhaustion (lack of strength) and fatigue _____

G Give the meanings of the following terms.

1. analgesia _____

2. motor aphasia _____

3. paresis _____

4. quadriplegia _____

5. asthenia _____

10

6. comatose _____

7. paresthesia _____

8. hyperkinesis _____

9. anesthesia _____

10. causalgia _____

11. akinetic _____

12. hypalgesia _____

13. dyskinesia _____

14. migraine _____

H **Match the listed neurologic pathology terms with the descriptions that follow. The terms in boldface are clues!**

Alzheimer disease	Huntington disease	myasthenia gravis
amyotrophic lateral sclerosis	hydrocephalus	Parkinson disease
Bell palsy	multiple sclerosis	myelomeningocele
epilepsy		

1. Destruction of myelin sheath (demyelination) and its replacement by **hard** plaques:

   _____

2. Sudden, transient disturbances of brain function cause **seizures**: _____

3. The **spinal** column is imperfectly joined (a **split** in a vertebra occurs), and part of the meninges and spinal cord can herniate out of the spinal cavity: _____

4. **Atrophy** of muscles and paralysis caused by damage to motor neurons in the spinal cord and brainstem: _____

5. Patient displays bizarre, abrupt, involuntary, **dance**-like movements, as well as decline in mental functions: _____

6. Cerebrospinal **fluid** accumulates in the **head** (in the ventricles of the brain): _____

7. **Loss of muscle strength** due to the inability of a neurotransmitter (acetylcholine) to transmit impulses from nerve cells to muscle cells: _____

8. Degeneration of nerves in the basal ganglia occurring in later life, leading to tremors, shuffling gait, and muscle stiffness; **dopamine** (neurotransmitter) is deficient in the brain:

   _____

9. Deterioration of mental capacity **(dementia)**; autopsy shows cerebral cortex atrophy, widening of cerebral sulci, and microscopic neurofibrillary tangles: _____

10. Unilateral facial **paralysis**: _____

10

I Give the meanings of the following terms for abnormal conditions.

1. astrocytoma _____

2. pyogenic meningitis _____

3. Tourette syndrome _____

4. cerebral contusion _____

5. cerebrovascular accident _____

6. cerebral concussion _____

7. herpes zoster _____

8. cerebral embolus _____

9. cerebral thrombosis _____

10. cerebral hemorrhage _____

11. cerebral aneurysm _____

12. HIV encephalopathy _____

J Match the term in Column I with the letter of its description or meaning in Column II.

COLUMN I

1. ataxia _____
2. aura _____
3. transient ischemic attack _____
4. tonic-clonic seizure _____
5. herpes zoster _____
6. palliative _____
7. dopamine _____
8. occlusion _____
9. absence seizure _____
10. glioblastoma multiforme _____

COLUMN II

A. relieving, but not curing
B. virus that causes chickenpox and shingles
C. uncoordinated gait
D. neurotransmitter
E. peculiar sensation experienced by patient before onset of seizure
F. malignant brain tumor of immature glial cells
G. major epileptic seizure; ictal event
H. blood flow to the brain stops for a brief period of time
I. minor epileptic seizure
J. blockage

K Describe what happens in the following two procedures.

1. MRI of the brain: _____

2. stereotactic radiosurgery with Gamma Knife: _____

_____

10

L Match these easily confused terms for neurologic pathology with the meanings/descriptions that follow.

analgesia ataxia neurasthenia
anesthesia dyskinesia paresis
aphasia dyslexia paresthesia
apraxia hyperkinesia

1. lack of nerve strength _____

2. inability to speak _____

3. inability to perform purposeful actions _____

4. condition of insensitivity to pain _____

5. condition of loss of sensation _____

6. sensations of tingling, numbness, or "pins and needles" _____

7. lack of coordination _____

8. excessive movement _____

9. abnormal, involuntary, spasmodic movements _____

10. developmental reading disorder _____

11. partial paralysis _____

M Spell out the abbreviations in Column I, and then select the letter of the best association from Column II for each.

COLUMN I

1. EEG _____ _____

2. PET _____ _____

3. AFP _____ _____

4. MS _____ _____

5. MRI _____ _____

6. LP _____ _____

7. CVA _____ _____

8. AD _____ _____

9. TIA _____ _____

10. CSF _____ _____

COLUMN II

A. Gradually progressive dementia.

B. Stroke; embolus, hemorrhage, and thrombosis are etiologic factors.

C. Intrathecal medications can be administered through this procedure.

D. This fluid is analyzed for abnormal blood cells, chemicals, and protein.

E. Procedure to diagnose abnormal electrical activity in the brain.

F. Neurologic symptoms and/or signs due to temporary interference of blood supply to the brain.

G. High levels in amniotic fluid and maternal blood are associated with spina bifida.

H. Diagnostic procedure that allows excellent visualization of soft tissue in the brain.

I. Radioactive materials, such as glucose, are taken up by the brain, and images recorded.

J. Destruction of the myelin sheath in the CNS occurs with plaques of hard scar tissue.

10

N **Circle the boldface terms that complete the meanings of the sentences.**

1. Maria had such severe headaches that she could find relief only with strong analgesics. Her condition of **(spina bifida, migraine, epilepsy)** was debilitating.

2. Paul was in a coma after his high-speed car accident. His physicians were concerned that he had suffered a **(palsy, myelomeningocele, contusion and subdural hematoma)** as a result of the accident.

3. Dick went to the emergency department complaining of dizziness, nausea, and headache. The physician, suspecting increased ICP, prescribed corticosteroids, and Dick's symptoms disappeared. They returned, however, when the steroids were discontinued. A/an **(MRI study of the brain, electroencephalogram, CSF analysis)** revealed a large brain lesion. It was removed surgically and determined to be a/an **(embolus, glioblastoma multiforme, migraine)**.

4. Dorothy felt weakness in her hand and numbness in her arm, and noticed blurred vision, all signs of **(herpes zoster, meningitis, TIA)**. Her physician requested **(myelography, MRA, lumbar puncture)** to assess any damage to cerebral blood vessels and possible stroke.

5. When Bill noticed ptosis and muscle weakness in his face, he reported these symptoms to his doctor. The doctor diagnosed his condition as **(Tourette syndrome, Huntington disease, myasthenia gravis)** and prescribed **(dopamine, anticonvulsants, anticholinesterase drugs)**, which relieved his symptoms.

6. To rule out bacterial **(epilepsy, encephalomalacia, meningitis)**, Dr. Phillips, a pediatrician, requested that a/an **(EEG, PET scan, LP)** be performed on the febrile (feverish) child.

7. Eight-year-old Barry reversed his letters and had difficulty learning to read and write words. His family physician diagnosed his problem as **(aphasia, dyslexia, ataxia)**.

8. After his head hit the steering wheel during a recent automobile accident, Clark noticed **(hemiparesis, paraplegia, hyperesthesia)** on the left side of his body. A head CT scan revealed **(narcolepsy, neurasthenia, subdural hematoma)**.

9. For her 35th birthday, Elizabeth's husband threw her a surprise party. She was so startled by the crowd that she experienced a weakness of muscles and loss of consciousness. Friends placed her on her back in a horizontal position with her head low to improve blood flow to her brain. She soon recovered from her **(myoneural, syncopal, hyperkinetic)** episode.

10. Near his 65th birthday, Edward began having difficulty remembering recent events. Over the next 5 years, he developed **(dyslexia, dementia, seizures)** and was diagnosed with **(multiple sclerosis, myasthenia gravis, Alzheimer disease)**.

11. Elderly Mrs. Smith had been taking an antipsychotic drug for 5 years when she began exhibiting lip smacking and darting movements of her tongue. Her doctor described her condition as **(radiculitis, tardive dyskinesia, hemiparesis)** and discontinued her drug. The condition, acquired after use of the drug, would be considered **(iatrogenic, congenital, ictal)**.

⊙ Complete the spelling of the following terms based on their meanings.

1. part of the brain that controls sleep, appetite, temperature, and secretions of the pituitary gland:

   hypo _____

2. pertaining to fainting: syn _____

3. abnormal tingling sensations: par _____

4. slight paralysis: par _____

5. inflammation of a spinal nerve root: _____ itis

6. inability to speak correctly: a _____

7. movements and behavior that are not purposeful: a _____

8. lack of muscular coordination: a _____

9. developmental reading disorder: dys _____

10. excessive movement: hyper _____

11. paralysis in one half (right or left) of the body: _____ plegia

12. paralysis in the lower half of the body: _____ plegia

13. paralysis in all four limbs: _____ plegia

14. nervous exhaustion and fatigue: neur _____

ANSWERS TO EXERCISES

A

1. axon
2. plexus
3. meninges
4. dendrite
5. cerebral cortex
6. astrocyte
7. oligodendroglial cell
8. neuron
9. cauda equina
10. myelin sheath

B

1. outermost meningeal layer surrounding the brain and spinal cord
2. brain and the spinal cord
3. nerves outside the brain and spinal cord; cranial, spinal, and autonomic nerves
4. middle meningeal membrane surrounding the brain and spinal cord
5. part of the brain below the thalamus; controls sleep, appetite, body temperature, and secretions from the pituitary gland
6. space through which a nervous impulse is transmitted from a nerve cell to another nerve cell or to a muscle or gland cell
7. autonomic nerves that influence body functions involuntarily in times of stress
8. part of the brain just above the spinal cord that controls breathing, heartbeat, and the size of blood vessels
9. part of the brain anterior to the cerebellum and between the medulla and the upper parts of the brain; connects these parts of the brain
10. posterior part of the brain that coordinates voluntary muscle movements
11. part of the brain below the cerebrum; relay center that conducts impulses between the spinal cord and the cerebrum
12. canals in the interior of the brain that are filled with CSF
13. lower portion of the brain that connects the cerebrum with the spinal cord (includes the pons and the medulla)
14. largest part of the brain; controls voluntary muscle movement, vision, speech, hearing, thought, memory
15. collection of nerve cell bodies outside the brain and spinal cord

10

C

1. pia mater
2. motor nerves
3. sensory nerves
4. sulci
5. subarachnoid space
6. gyri
7. neurotransmitter
8. parenchymal cell
9. glial cells

D

1. encephalopathy
2. cerebellum
3. epidural hematoma
4. leptomeningitis
5. anencephaly
6. poliomyelitis
7. meningeal
8. radiculopathy
9. myelomeningocele
10. vagal

E

1. outer region of the cerebrum (contains gray matter)
2. pertaining to within a sheath
3. inflammation of many nerves
4. pertaining to the thalamus
5. disease of the spinal cord
6. tumor of the meninges
7. tumor of neuroglial cells (a brain tumor)
8. mass of blood below the dura mater (outermost meningeal membrane)

F

1. dyslexia
2. ataxia
3. bradykinesia
4. hyperesthesia
5. narcolepsy
6. aphasia
7. motor apraxia
8. hemiparesis
9. causalgia
10. paraplegia
11. syncope
12. neurasthenia

G

1. lack of sensitivity to pain
2. difficulty in speaking (patient cannot articulate words but can understand speech and knows what she or he wants to say)
3. weakness and partial loss of movement
4. paralysis in all four extremities (damage is to the cervical part of the spinal cord)
5. no strength (weakness)
6. pertaining to coma (loss of consciousness from which the patient cannot be aroused)
7. condition of abnormal sensations (prickling, tingling, burning)
8. excessive movement
9. condition of no sensation or nervous feeling
10. severe burning pain from injury to peripheral nerves
11. pertaining to without movement
12. diminished sensation to pain
13. impairment of the ability to perform voluntary movements
14. recurrent vascular headache with severe pain of unilateral onset and photophobia (sensitivity to light)

H

1. multiple sclerosis
2. epilepsy
3. myelomeningocele
4. amyotrophic lateral sclerosis
5. Huntington disease
6. hydrocephalus
7. myasthenia gravis
8. Parkinson disease
9. Alzheimer disease
10. Bell palsy

I

1. tumor of neuroglial brain cells (astrocytes)
2. inflammation of the meninges (bacterial infection with pus formation)
3. involuntary spasmodic, twitching movements (tics), uncontrollable vocal sounds, and inappropriate word
4. bruising of brain tissue as a result of direct trauma to the head
5. disruption of the normal blood supply to the brain; stroke or cerebral infarction
6. traumatic brain injury caused by a blow to the head
7. neurologic condition caused by infection with herpes zoster virus; blisters form along the course of peripheral nerves
8. blockage of a blood vessel in the cerebrum caused by material from another part of the body that suddenly occludes the vessel
9. blockage of a blood vessel in the cerebrum caused by the formation of a clot within the vessel
10. collection of blood in the brain (can cause a stroke)
11. widening of a blood vessel (artery) in the cerebrum; the aneurysm can burst and lead to a CVA
12. brain disease (dementia and encephalitis) caused by infection with AIDS virus

J

1. C	5. B	8. J
2. E	6. A	9. I
3. H	7. D	10. F
4. G		

K

1. use of magnetic waves to create an image (in frontal, transverse, or sagittal plane) of the brain

2. an instrument (stereotactic) is fixed onto the skull and locates a target by three-dimensional measurement; gamma radiation or proton beams are used to treat deep brain lesions

L

1. neurasthenia	5. anesthesia	9. dyskinesia
2. aphasia	6. paresthesia	10. dyslexia
3. apraxia	7. ataxia	11. paresis
4. analgesia	8. hyperkinesia	

M

1. electroencephalography: E	5. magnetic resonance imaging: H	8. Alzheimer disease: A
2. positron emission tomography: I	6. lumbar puncture: C	9. transient ischemic attack: F
3. alpha-fetoprotein: G	7. cerebrovascular accident: B	10. cerebrospinal fluid: D
4. multiple sclerosis: J		

N

1. migraine	5. myasthenia gravis; anticholinesterase drugs	8. hemiparesis; subdural hematoma
2. contusion and subdural hematoma	6. meningitis; LP	9. syncopal
3. MRI of the brain; glioblastoma multiforme	7. dyslexia	10. dementia; Alzheimer disease
4. TIA; MRA		11. tardive dyskinesia; iatrogenic

O

1. hypothalamus	6. aphasia	11. hemiplegia
2. syncopal	7. apraxia	12. paraplegia
3. paresthesias	8. ataxia	13. quadriplegia
4. paresis	9. dyslexia	14. neurasthenia
5. radiculitis	10. hyperkinesis	

Answers to Practical Applications

Case Report: Cerebral Infarction

1. c
2. a
3. c
4. c
5. a

Neuropathic Pain and Case Study

1. d
2. c
3. b

10

PRONUNCIATION OF TERMS

To test your understanding of the terminology in this chapter, write the meaning of each term in the space provided. In addition, you may wish to cover the terms and write them by looking at your definitions. Make sure your spelling is correct. The page number after each term indicates where it is defined or used in the book, so you can easily check your responses. You will find complete definitions for all of these terms and their audio pronunciations on the Evolve website.

Pronunciation Guide

ā as in āpe	ă as in ăpple
ē as in ēven	ĕ as in ĕvery
ī as in īce	ĭ as in ĭnterest
ō as in ōpen	ŏ as in pŏt
ū as in ūnit	ŭ as in ŭnder

Vocabulary and Combining Forms and Terminology

TERM	PRONUNCIATION	MEANING
acetylcholine (355)	ăs-ĕ-tĭl-KŌ-lēn	_____
afferent nerve (355)	ĂF-fĕr-ĕnt nĕrv	_____
akinetic (360)	ă-kĭ-NĔT-ĭk	_____
analgesia (359)	ăn-ăl-JĒ-zē-ă	_____
anencephaly (359)	ăn-ĕn-SĔF-ă-lē	_____
anesthesia (360)	ăn-ĕs-THĒ-zē-ă	_____
aphasia (361)	ă-FĀ-zē-ă	_____
apraxia (362)	Ā-PRĂK-sē-ă	_____
arachnoid membrane (355)	ă-RĂK-noyd MĔM-brān	_____
astrocyte (355)	ĂS-trō-sīt	_____
ataxia (362)	ă-TĂK-sē-ă	_____
autonomic nervous system (355)	ăw-tō-NŌM-ĭk NĔR-vŭs SĬS-tĕm	_____
axon (355)	ĂK-sŏn	_____
blood-brain barrier (355)	blŭd-BRĀN BĂ-rē-ĕr	_____
bradykinesia (360)	BRĀ-dē-kĭ-NĒ-zē-ă	_____
brainstem (355)	BRĀN-stĕm	_____
cauda equina (355)	KĂW-dă ĕ-KWĪ-nă	_____
causalgia (360)	kăw-ZĂL-jă	_____
cell body (355)	sĕl BŎD-ē	_____
central nervous system (355)	SĔN-trăl NĔR-vŭs SĬS-tĕm	_____
cephalgia (360)	sĕ-FĂL-jă	_____
cerebellar (357)	sĕr-ĕ-BĔL-ăr	_____

10

TERM	PRONUNCIATION	MEANING
cerebellopontine (359)	sĕr-ĕ-bĕl-ō-PŎN-tēn	
cerebellum (355)	sĕr-ĕ-BĔL-ŭm	
cerebral cortex (355)	sĕ-RĒ-brăl (p. or SĔR-ĕ-brăl) KŎR-tĕks	
cerebrospinal fluid (355)	sĕ-rē-brō-SPĪ-năl FLOO-ĭd	
cerebrum (355)	sĕ-RĒ-brŭm	
coma (360)	KŌ-mă	
comatose (360)	KŌ-mă-tōs	
cranial nerves (355)	KRĀ-nē-ăl nĕrvz	
dendrite (355)	DĔN-drīt	
dura mater (355)	DŪR-ă MĂ-tĕr	
dyslexia (361)	dĭs-LĔK-sē-ă	
dyskinesia (360)	dĭs-kĭ-NĒ-zē-ă	
efferent nerve (355)	ĔF-fĕr-ĕnt nĕrvz	
encephalitis (358)	ĕn-sĕf-ă-LĪ-tĭs	
encephalopathy (358)	ĕn-sĕf-ă-LŎP-ă-thē	
ependymal cell (355)	ĕp-ĔN-dĭ-măl sĕl	
epidural hematoma (358)	ĕp-ĕ-DŪ-răl hē-mă-TŌ-mă	
ganglion (356)	GĂNG-lē-ŏn	
glial cell (355)	GLĒ-ăl sĕl	
glioblastoma (358)	glē-ō-blă-STŌ-mă	
gyrus; gyri (356)	JĪ-rŭs; JĪ-rē	
hemiparesis (361)	hĕm-ē-pă-RĒ-sĭs	
hemiplegia (361)	hĕm-ē-PLĒ-jă	
hypalgesia (359)	hīp-ăl-GĒ-zē-ă	
hyperesthesia (360)	hī-pĕr-ĕs-THĒ-zē-ă	
hyperkinesis (360)	hī-pĕr-kĭ-NĒ-sĭs	
hypothalamus (356)	hī-pō-THĂL-ă-mŭs	
intrathecal injection (359)	ĭn-tră-THĒ-kăl ĭn-JĔK-shun	
leptomeningeal (358)	lĕp-tō-mĕn-ĭn-JĒ-ăl	
medulla oblongata (356)	mĕ-DŪL-ă (or mĕ-DŬL-ă) ŏb-lŏn-GĂ-tă	

10

TERM	PRONUNCIATION	MEANING
meningeal (358)	mĕ-NĬN-jē-ăl *or* mĕ-nĭn-JĒ-ăl	
meninges (356)	mĕ-NĬN-jēz	
meningioma (358)	mĕ-nĭn-jē-Ō-mă	
microglial cell (356)	mī-krō-GLĒ-ăl sĕl	
midbrain (351)	MĬD-brān	
motor nerve (356)	MŌ-tĕr nĕrv	
myelin sheath (356)	MĪ-ĕ-lĭn shēth	
myelomeningocele (358)	mī-ĕ-lō-mĕ-NĬN-gō-sēl	
myelopathy (359)	mī-ĕ-LŌP-ă-thē	
myoneural (359)	mī-ō-NŪR-ăl	
narcolepsy (360)	NĂR-kō-lĕp-sē	
nerve (356)	nĕrv	
neuralgia (360)	nūr-ĂL-jă	
neurasthenia (362)	nūr-ăs-THĒ-nē-ă	
neuroglial cells (349)	nūr-ō-GLĒ-ăl cells	
neuron (356)	NŪR-ŏn	
neuropathy (359)	nūr-ŎP-ă-thē	
neurotransmitter (356)	nūr-ō-trănz-MĬT-ĕr	
oligodendroglial cell (356)	ŏl-ĭ-gō-dĕn-drō-GLĒ-ăl sĕl	
paraplegia (361)	păr-ă-PLĒ-jă	
parasympathetic nerves (356)	păr-ă-sĭm-pă-THĔT-ĭk nĕrvz	
parenchyma (356)	păr-ĔN-kĭ-mă	
paresis (361)	pă-RĒ-sĭs	
paresthesia (360)	păr-ĕs-THĒ-zē-ă	
peripheral nervous system (356)	pĕ-RĬF-ĕr-ăl NĔR-vŭs SĬS-tĕm	
pia mater (356)	PĒ-ă MĂ-tĕr	
plexus (356)	PLĔK-sŭs	
poliomyelitis (359)	pō-lē-ō-mī-ĕ-LĪ-tĭs	
polyneuritis (359)	pŏl-ē-nŭ-RĪ-tĭs	
pons (356)	pŏnz	
quadriplegia (361)	kwŏd-rĭ-PLĒ-jă	

TERM	PRONUNCIATION	MEANING
radiculitis (359)	ră-dĭk-ū-LĪ-tĭs	_____
radiculopathy (359)	ră-dĭk-ū-LŎP-ă-thē	_____
receptor (357)	rē-SĔP-tŏr	_____
sciatic nerve (357)	sī-ĂT-ĭk nĕrv	_____
sciatica (357)	sī-ĂT-ĭ-kăh	_____
sensory nerve (357)	SĔN-sō-rē nĕrv	_____
spinal nerves (357)	SPĪ-năl nĕrvz	_____
stimulus (357)	STĬM-ū-lŭs	_____
stroma (357)	STRŌ-mă	_____
subdural hematoma (358)	sŭb-DŪ-răl hē-mă-TŌ-mă	_____
sulcus; sulci (357)	SŬL-kŭs; SŬL-sī	_____
sympathetic nerves (357)	sĭm-pă-THĔT-ĭk nĕrvz	_____
synapse (357)	SĬN-ăps	_____
syncopal (362)	SĬN-kō-păl	_____
syncope (362)	SĬN-kō-pē	_____
thalamic (359)	THĂL-ă-mĭk _or_ thă-LĂM-ĭk	_____
thalamus (357)	THĂL-ă-mŭs	_____
trigeminal neuralgia (360)	trī-GĔM-ĭn-ăl nūr-ĂL-jă	_____
vagal (359)	VĀ-găl	_____
vagus nerve (357)	VĀ-gŭs nĕrv	_____
ventricles of the brain (357)	VĔN-trĭ-kulz of the brān	_____

Pathology, Laboratory Tests, and Clinical Procedures

TERM	PRONUNCIATION	MEANING
absence seizure (371)	ĂB-sĕns SĒ-zhŭr	_____
Alzheimer disease (364)	ĂLZ-hī-mĕr dĭ-ZĒZ	_____
amyotrophic lateral sclerosis (364)	ā-mī-ō-TRŌ-fĭk LĂ-tĕr-ăl sklĕ-RŌ-sĭs	_____
aneurysm (371)	ĂN-ūr-ĭ-zĭm	_____
astrocytoma (371)	ăs-trō-sī-TŌ-mă	_____
aura (371)	ĀW-ră	_____

TERM	PRONUNCIATION	MEANING
Bell palsy (366)	bĕl PĂL-zē	
brain tumor (368)	BRĀN TŪ-mŏr	
cerebral angiography (371)	sĕ-RĒ-brăl ăn-jē-ŎG-ră-fē	
cerebral concussion (369)	sĕ-RĒ-brăl kŏn-KŬS-shŭn	
cerebral contusion (369)	sĕ-RĒ-brăl kŏn-TOO-shŭn	
cerebral hemorrhage (370)	sĕ-RĒ-brăl HĔM-ōr-ĭj	
cerebral palsy (366)	sĕ-RĒ-brăl (or SĔR-ĕ-brăl) PĂL-zē	
cerebrospinal fluid analysis (371)	sĕ-rē-brō-SPĪ-năl FLOO-ĭd ă-NĂL-ĭ-sĭs	
cerebrovascular accident (369)	sĕ-rē-brō-VĂS-kū-lăr ĂK-sĭ-dĕnt	
computed tomography (372)	kŏm-PŪ-tĕd tō-MŎG-ră-fē	
dementia (371)	dĕ-MĔN-shē-ă	
demyelination (371)	dē-mī-ĕ-lĭ-NĀ-shun	
dopamine (371)	DŌ-pă-mēn	
Doppler ultrasound studies (372)	DŎP-lĕr ŬL-tră-sound STŬ-dēz	
electroencephalography (373)	ĕ-lĕk-trō-ĕn-sĕf-ă-LŎG-ră-fē	
embolus (371)	ĔM-bō-lŭs	
epilepsy (365)	ĔP-ĭ-lĕp-sē	
gait (371)	GĀT	
glioblastoma (368)	glē-ō-blăs-TŌ-mă	
herpes zoster (368)	HĔR-pēz ZŎS-tĕr	
HIV encephalopathy (368)	HIV ĕn-sĕf-ă-LŎP-ă-thē	
Huntington disease (365)	HŬN-ting-tŏn dĭ-ZĒZ	
hydrocephalus (362)	hī-drō-SĔF-ă-lŭs	
ictal event (371)	ĬK-tăl ē-VĔNT	
lumbar puncture (373)	LŬM-băr PŬNK-shŭr	
magnetic resonance imaging (372)	măg-NĔT-ĭk RĒ-zō-năns ĬM-ă-jĭng	
meningitis (368)	mĕn-ĭn-JĪ-tĭs	
meningocele (363)	mĕ-NĬN-gō-sĕl	

10

TERM	PRONUNCIATION	MEANING
migraine (370)	MĪ-grān	
multiple sclerosis (365)	MŬL-tǐ-pl sklě-RŌ-sǐs	
myasthenia gravis (366)	mī-ăs-THĒ-nē-ă GRĂ-vǐs	
occlusion (371)	ō-KLŪ-zhŭn	
palliative (371)	PĂ-lē-ă-tǐv	
palsy (366)	PAWL-zē	
Parkinson disease (367)	PĂR-kǐn-sŭn dǐ-ZĒZ	
positron emission tomography (372)	PŎS-ǐ-trŏn ē-MĬ-shŭn tō-MŎG-ră-fē	
shingles (368)	SHĬNG-ŭlz	
spina bifida (363)	SPĪ-nă BĬF-ǐ-dă	
stereotactic radiosurgery (373)	stě-rē-ō-TĂK-tǐk ra-dē-ō-SŬR-gěr ē	
thrombus (369)	THRŎM-bŭs	
tic (371)	TĬK	
tonic-clonic seizure (371)	TŎN-ǐk-KLŎ-nǐk SĒ-zhŭr	
Tourette syndrome (367)	tŭ-RĚT SĬN-drōm	
transient ischemic attack (369)	TRĂN-zē-ěnt ǐs-KĒ-mǐk ă-TĂK	

10

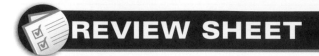

REVIEW SHEET

Write the meanings of the word parts in the spaces provided. Check your answers with the information in the chapter or in the *Glossary (Medical Word Parts—English)* at the end of the book.

Combining Forms

COMBINING FORM	MEANING	COMBINING FORM	MEANING
alges/o		lex/o	
angi/o		mening/o, meningi/o	
caus/o		my/o	
cephal/o		myel/o	
cerebell/o		narc/o	
cerebr/o		neur/o	
comat/o		olig/o	
crani/o		pont/o	
cry/o		radicul/o	
dur/o		spin/o	
encephal/o		syncop/o	
esthesi/o		tax/o	
gli/o		thalam/o	
hydr/o		thec/o	
kines/o, kinesi/o		troph/o	
lept/o		vag/o	

Prefixes

PREFIX	MEANING	PREFIX	MEANING
a-, an-		micro-	
dys-		para-	
epi-		polio-	
hemi-		poly-	
hyper-		quadri-	
hypo-		sub-	
intra-			

Suffixes

SUFFIX	MEANING	SUFFIX	MEANING
-algesia	_____	-ose	_____
-algia	_____	-paresis	_____
-blast	_____	-pathy	_____
-cele	_____	-phagia	_____
-esthesia	_____	-phasia	_____
-gram	_____	-plegia	_____
-graphy	_____	-praxia	_____
-ine	_____	-ptosis	_____
-itis	_____	-sclerosis	_____
kinesia, -kinesis	_____	-sthenia	_____
-kinetic	_____	-tomy	_____
-lepsy	_____	-trophy	_____
-oma	_____		

Match the neurologic pathology terms and abbreviations in Column I with the descriptions/definitions in Column II.

COLUMN I		COLUMN II
1. Alzheimer	_____	A. destruction of myelin sheath on neurons in CNS
2. ALS	_____	B. stroke; disruption in normal blood supply to the brain
3. epilepsy	_____	C. shingles; viral infection affecting peripheral nerves
4. MS	_____	D. progressive dementia; memory failure; senile plaques and neurofibrillary tangles
5. Parkinson's	_____	E. brain tumor; malignant astrocytoma
6. herpes zoster	_____	F. degeneration of neurons in basal ganglia; tremors, bradykinesia, and shuffling gait
7. glioblastoma multiforme	_____	G. recurrent seizure disorder; tonic-clonic and absence types
8. CVA	_____	H. degeneration of motor neurons in spinal cord and brain stem; weakness and muscle atrophy

10

BOOKS WITH NEUROLOGIC TOPICS

The following list of books may be of interest to you. They deal with fictional characters or actual individuals who are coping with neurologic illnesses. Oliver Sachs, M.D., the late professor of neurology at the NYU School of Medicine, has written extensively about neurological case histories, including *The Man Who Mistook his Wife for a Hat*. Please contact me with your comments and other suggestions of good reads!

Alzheimer Disease

Elegy for Iris by John Bayley (story of novelist Iris Murdoch; written by her husband who becomes her caretaker).

Amyotrophic Lateral Sclerosis

I Choose to Live: A Journey Through Life with ALS by William Sinton (a story of coping with this disease).

Tuesdays with Morrie by Mitch Albom (written by a student who spends time with his former teacher and learns valuable life lessons).

Cerebral Palsy

My Left Foot by Christy Brown (Born in Dublin with cerebral palsy, this is his autobiography (later made into a film).

Epilepsy

The Spirit Catches You and You Fall Down by Anne Fadiman (story of the Hmong people and how they deal with epilepsy after coming to the United States).

The Spiral Staircase: My Climb out of Darkness by Karen Armstrong (how author Karen Armstrong deals with temporal lobe epilepsy).

The Idiot by Fydor Dostoevsky (Russian novel whose main character, Prince Myshkin, like Dostoevsky himself, suffers from epilepsy).

Huntington Disease

Saturday by Ian McEwan (a novel whose primary character suffers from this disease).

Parkinson Disease

Life in the Balance by Thomas Grayboys and Peter Zheutlin (prominent Boston cardiologist deals with this disease).

Stroke

My Stroke of Insight by Jill Brotle Taylor, PhD (a brain scientist, who had a stroke at age 37, writes about it).

---

evolve *Please visit the Evolve website for additional exercises, games, and images related to this chapter.*

Cardiovascular System

Chapter Sections:

CHAPTER GOALS

- Name the parts of the heart and associated blood vessels and their functions in the circulation of blood.
- Trace the pathway of blood through the heart.
- Identify and describe major pathologic conditions affecting the heart and blood vessels.
- Define combining forms that relate to the cardiovascular system.
- Describe important laboratory tests and clinical procedures pertaining to the cardiovascular system, and recognize relevant abbreviations.
- Apply your new knowledge to understand medical terms in their proper context, such as in medical reports and records.

INTRODUCTION

Body cells are dependent on a constant supply of nutrients and oxygen. When the supplies are delivered and then chemically combined, they release the energy necessary to do the work of each cell. How does the body ensure that oxygen and food will be delivered to all of its cells? The cardiovascular system, consisting of the heart (a powerful muscular pump) and blood vessels (fuel line and transportation network), performs this important work. This chapter explores terminology related to the heart and blood vessels.

BLOOD VESSELS AND THE CIRCULATION OF BLOOD

BLOOD VESSELS

There are three types of blood vessels in the body: **arteries, veins, and capillaries.**

Arteries are large blood vessels that carry blood away from the heart. Their walls are lined with connective tissue, muscle tissue, and elastic fibers, with an innermost layer of epithelial cells called **endothelium.** Endothelial cells, found in all blood vessels, secrete factors that affect the size of blood vessels, reduce blood clotting, and promote the growth of blood vessels. Because arteries carry blood away from the heart, they must be strong enough to withstand the high pressure of the pumping action of the heart. Their elastic walls allow them to expand as the heartbeat forces blood into the arterial system throughout the body.

Smaller branches of arteries are **arterioles.** Arterioles are thinner than arteries and carry the blood to the tiniest of blood vessels, the capillaries.

Capillaries have walls that are only one endothelial cell in thickness. These delicate, microscopic vessels carry nutrient-rich, oxygenated blood from the arteries and arterioles to the body cells. Their thin walls allow passage of oxygen and nutrients out of the bloodstream and into cells. There, the nutrients are burned in the presence of oxygen (catabolism) to release energy. At the same time, waste products such as carbon dioxide and water pass out of cells and into the thin-walled capillaries. Waste-filled blood then flows back to the heart in small **venules,** which combine to form larger vessels called veins.

Veins have thinner walls compared with arteries. They conduct blood (that has given up most of its oxygen) toward the heart from the tissues. Veins have little elastic tissue and less connective tissue than that typical of arteries, and blood pressure in veins is extremely low compared with pressure in arteries. In order to keep blood moving back toward the heart, veins have **valves** that prevent the backflow of blood and keep the blood moving in one direction. Muscular action also helps the movement of blood in veins. Figure 11-1 illustrates the differences in blood vessels. Figure 11-2 reviews their characteristics and relationship to one another.

Blood Vessels and Blood

What color is blood? Blood is bright red in arteries (contains oxygen) and dark red (maroon) in veins (contains carbon dioxide). From the outside of the body, blood in veins *appears* blue because the color reflects off the skin.

How much blood is in the body? The average adult has about 5 quarts (4.7 liters) of blood in his or her body.

What is the length of all the blood vessels? The total length of all the blood vessels in the body is 60,000 miles!

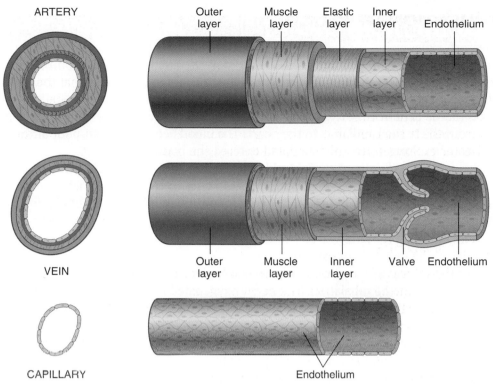

FIGURE 11-1 Blood vessels. Observe the differences in thickness of walls among an artery, a vein, and a capillary. All three vessels are lined with endothelium. Endothelial cells actively secrete substances that prevent clotting and regulate the tone of blood vessels. Examples of endothelial secretions are endothelium-derived relaxing factor (EDRF) and endothelin (a vasoconstrictor).

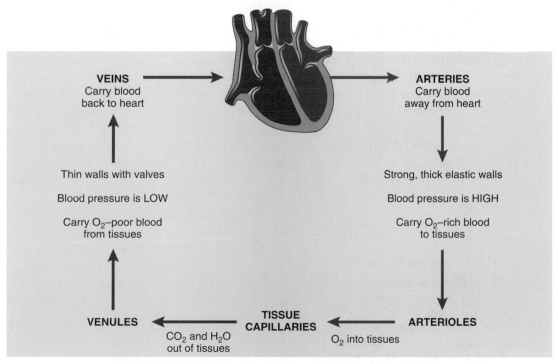

FIGURE 11-2 Relationship and characteristics of blood vessels.

CIRCULATION OF BLOOD

Arteries, arterioles, veins, venules, and capillaries, together with the heart, form a circulatory system for the flow of blood. Figure 11-3 is a more detailed representation of the entire circulatory system. Refer to it as you read the following paragraphs. (Note that the bracketed numbers in the following paragraphs correspond with those in Figure 11-3.)

Blood that is deficient in oxygen flows through two large veins, the **venae cavae** [1], on its way from the tissue capillaries to the heart. The blood became oxygen-poor at the tissue capillaries when oxygen left the blood and entered the body cells.

Oxygen-poor blood enters the **right side of the heart** [2] and travels through that side and into the **pulmonary artery** [3], a vessel that divides in two: one branch leading to the left lung, the other to the right lung. The arteries continue dividing and subdividing within the lungs, forming smaller and smaller vessels (arterioles) and finally reaching the **lung capillaries** [4]. The pulmonary artery is unusual in that it is the only artery in the body that carries blood deficient in oxygen.

While passing through the lung (pulmonary) capillaries, blood absorbs the oxygen that entered the body during inhalation. The newly oxygenated blood next returns immediately to the heart through **pulmonary veins** [5]. The pulmonary veins are unusual in that they are the only veins in the body that carry oxygen-rich **(oxygenated)** blood. The circulation of blood through the vessels from the heart to the lungs and then back to the heart again is the **pulmonary circulation.**

Oxygen-rich blood enters the **left side of the heart** [6] from the pulmonary veins. The muscles in the left side of the heart pump the blood out of the heart through the largest

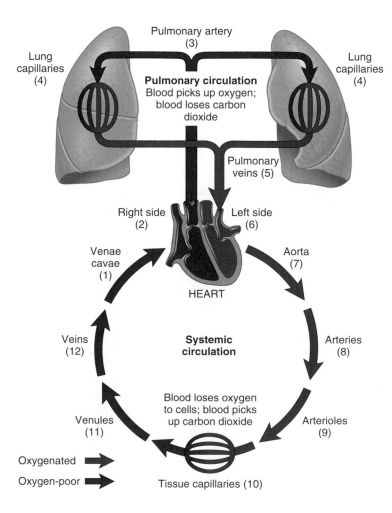

FIGURE 11-3 Schematic diagram of the **pulmonary circulation** (blood flow from the heart to lung capillaries and back to the heart) and **systemic circulation** (blood flow from the heart to tissue capillaries and back to the heart).

single artery in the body, the **aorta** [7]. The aorta moves up at first (ascending aorta) but then arches over dorsally and runs downward (descending aorta) just in front of the vertebral column. The aorta divides into numerous branches called **arteries** [8] that carry the oxygenated blood to all parts of the body. The names of some of these arterial branches will be familiar to you: brachial (brachi/o means arm), axillary, splenic, gastric, and renal arteries. The **carotid** arteries supply blood to the head and neck.

The relatively large arterial vessels branch further to form smaller **arterioles** [9]. The arterioles, still containing oxygenated blood, branch into smaller **tissue capillaries** [10], which are near the body cells. Oxygen leaves the blood and passes through the thin capillary walls to enter the body cells. There, food is broken down, in the presence of oxygen, and energy is released.

This chemical process also releases **carbon dioxide (CO_2)** as a waste product. Carbon dioxide passes out from the cell into the tissue capillaries at the same time that oxygen enters. Thus the blood returning to the heart from tissue capillaries through **venules** [11] and **veins** [12] is filled with carbon dioxide but is depleted of oxygen.

As this oxygen-poor blood enters the heart from the venae cavae, the circuit is complete. The pathway of blood from the heart to the tissue capillaries and back to the heart is the **systemic circulation.**

Figure 11-4 shows the aorta, selected arteries, and pulse points. The **pulse** is the beat of the heart as felt through the walls of arteries.

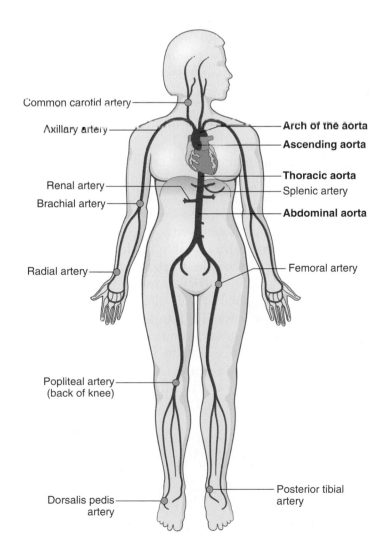

FIGURE 11-4   The aorta and arteries. *Solid gold dots* indicate pulse points in arteries. These are areas in which the **pulse** expansion and contraction of a superficial artery can be felt.

ANATOMY OF THE HEART

The human heart weighs less than a pound, is roughly the size of an adult fist, and lies in the thoracic cavity, just behind the breastbone in the mediastinum (between the lungs).

The heart is a pump consisting of four chambers: two upper chambers called **atria** (*singular*: **atrium**) and two lower chambers called **ventricles.** It is actually a double pump, bound into one organ and synchronized very carefully. Blood passes through each pump in a definite pattern. Pump station number one, on the right side of the heart, sends oxygen-deficient blood to the lungs, where the blood picks up oxygen and releases its carbon dioxide. The newly oxygenated blood returns to the left side of the heart to pump station number two and does not mix with the oxygen-poor blood in pump station number one. Pump station number two then forces the oxygenated blood out to all parts of the body. At the body tissues, the blood loses its oxygen, and on returning to the heart, to pump station number one, blood poor in oxygen (rich in carbon dioxide) is sent out to the lungs to begin the cycle anew.

Label Figure 11-5 as you learn the names of the parts of the heart and the vessels that carry blood to and from it.

Oxygen-poor blood enters the heart through the two largest veins in the body, the **venae cavae.** The **superior vena cava** [1] drains blood from the upper portion of the body, and the **inferior vena cava** [2] carries blood from the lower part of the body.

The venae cavae bring oxygen-poor blood that has passed through all of the body to the **right atrium** [3], the thin-walled upper right chamber of the heart. The right atrium contracts to force blood through the **tricuspid valve** [4] (cusps are the flaps of the valves) into the **right ventricle** [5], the lower right chamber of the heart. The cusps of the tricuspid valve form a one-way passage designed to keep the blood flowing in only one direction. As the right ventricle contracts to pump oxygen-poor blood through the **pulmonary valve** [6] into the **pulmonary artery** [7], the tricuspid valve stays shut, thus preventing blood from pushing back into the right atrium. The pulmonary artery then branches to carry oxygen-deficient blood to each lung.

The blood that enters the lung capillaries from the pulmonary artery soon loses its large quantity of carbon dioxide into the lung tissue, and the carbon dioxide is expelled. At the same time, oxygen enters the capillaries of the lungs and is brought back to the heart via the **pulmonary veins** [8]. The newly oxygenated blood enters the **left atrium** [9] of the heart from the pulmonary veins. The walls of the left atrium contract to force blood through the **mitral valve** [10] into the **left ventricle** [11].

The left ventricle has the thickest walls of all four heart chambers (three times the thickness of the right ventricular wall). It must pump blood with great force so that the blood travels through arteries to all parts of the body. The left ventricle propels the blood through the **aortic valve** [12] into the **aorta** [13], which branches to carry blood all over the body. The aortic valve closes to prevent return of aortic blood to the left ventricle.

In Figure 11-6, notice that the four chambers of the heart are separated by partitions called **septa** (*singular*: **septum**). (Label Figure 11-6 as you read these paragraphs.) The **interatrial septum** [1] separates the two upper chambers (atria), and the **interventricular septum** [2], a muscular wall, lies between the two lower chambers (ventricles).

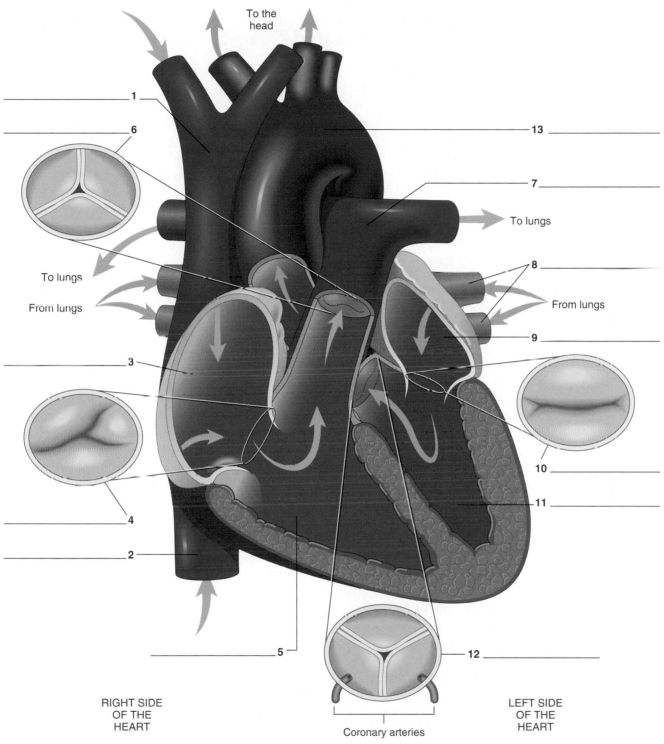

To the head

1

6

To lungs

From lungs

3

To lungs

From lungs

13

7

To lungs

8

9

10

11

4

2

5

12

RIGHT SIDE
OF THE
HEART

Coronary arteries

LEFT SIDE
OF THE
HEART

11

FIGURE 11-5 **Structure of the heart.** *Blue arrows* indicate oxygen-poor blood flow. *Red arrows* show oxygenated blood flow.

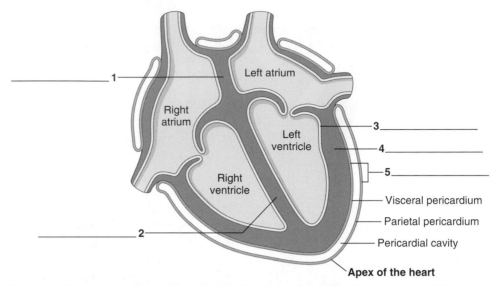

FIGURE 11-6   The septa (walls of the heart) and the pericardium. Note that the **apex of the heart** is the conical (shaped like a cone) lower tip of the heart.

Figure 11-6 shows the three layers of the heart. The **endocardium** [3], a smooth layer of endothelial cells, lines the interior of the heart and heart valves. The **myocardium** [4], the middle, muscular layer of the heart wall, is its thickest layer. The **pericardium** [5], a fibrous and membranous sac, surrounds the heart. It is composed of two layers, the **visceral pericardium,** adhering to the heart, and the **parietal** (parietal means wall) **pericardium,** lining the outer fibrous coat. The **pericardial cavity** (between the visceral and the parietal pericardial layers) normally contains 10 to 15 mL of pericardial fluid, which lubricates the membranes as the heart beats.

Figure 11-7 reviews the pathway of blood through the heart.

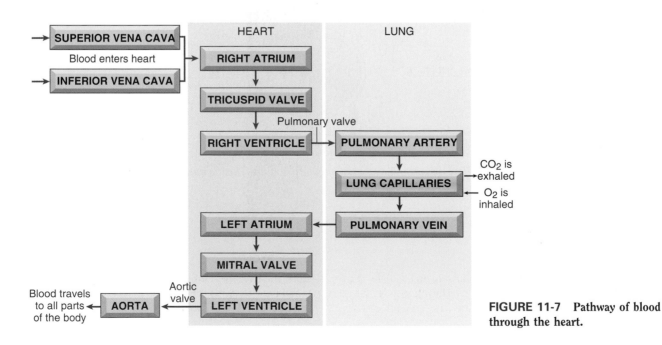

FIGURE 11-7   Pathway of blood through the heart.

PHYSIOLOGY OF THE HEART

HEARTBEAT AND HEART SOUNDS

There are two phases of the heartbeat: **diastole** (relaxation) and **systole** (contraction). Diastole occurs when the ventricle walls relax and blood flows into the heart from the venae cavae and the pulmonary veins. The tricuspid and mitral valves open in diastole, as blood passes from the right and left atria into the ventricles. The pulmonary and aortic valves close during diastole (Figure 11-8).

Systole occurs next, as the walls of the right and left ventricles contract to pump blood into the pulmonary artery and the aorta. Both the tricuspid and the mitral valves are closed during systole, thus preventing the flow of blood back into the atria (see Figure 11-8).

This diastole-systole cardiac cycle occurs between 70 and 80 times per minute (100,000 times a day). The heart pumps about 3 ounces of blood with each contraction. This means that about 5 quarts of blood are pumped by the heart in 1 minute (75 gallons an hour and about 2000 gallons a day).

Closure of the heart valves is associated with audible sounds, such as "lubb-dubb," which can be heard on listening to a normal heart with a stethoscope. The "lubb" is associated with closure of the tricuspid and mitral valves at the beginning of systole, and the "dubb" with the closure of the aortic and pulmonary valves at the end of systole. The "lubb" sound is called the first heart sound (S1) and the "dubb" is the second heart sound (S2), because the normal cycle of the heartbeat starts with the beginning of systole. Sometimes the flow of blood through the valves can produce an abnormal swishing sound known as a **murmur.**

CONDUCTION SYSTEM OF THE HEART

What keeps the heart at its perfect rhythm? Although the heart has nerves that affect its rate, they are not primarily responsible for its beat. The heart starts beating in the embryo before it is supplied with nerves, and continues to beat in experimental animals even when the nerve supply is cut.

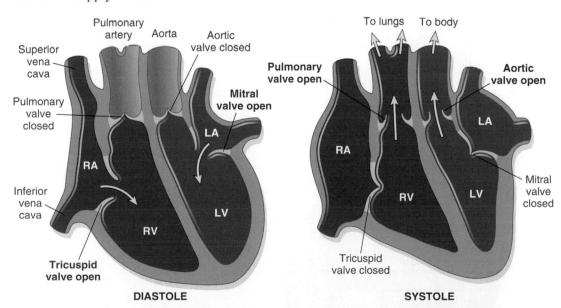

FIGURE 11-8   Phases of the heartbeat: diastole and systole. During diastole, the tricuspid and mitral valves are open as blood enters the ventricles. During systole, the pulmonary and aortic valves are open as blood is pumped to the pulmonary artery and aorta. LA, left atrium; LV, left ventricle; RA, right atrium; RV, right ventricle.

Label Figure 11-9 as you read the following. Primary responsibility for initiating the heartbeat rests with a small region of specialized muscle tissue in the posterior portion of the right atrium, where an electrical impulse originates. This is the **sinoatrial node (SA node),** or **pacemaker** [1] of the heart. The current of electricity generated by the pacemaker causes the walls of the atria to contract and force blood into the ventricles.

Almost like ripples in a pond of water when a stone is thrown, the wave of electricity passes from the pacemaker to another region of the myocardium. This region is within the interatrial septum and is the **atrioventricular node (AV node)** [2]. The AV node immediately sends the excitation wave to a bundle of specialized muscle fibers called the **atrioventricular bundle,** or **bundle of His** [3]. Within the interventricular septum, the bundle of His divides into the **left bundle branch** [4] and the **right bundle branch** [5], which form the conduction myofibers that extend through the ventricle walls and contract on stimulation. Thus systole occurs and blood is pumped away from the heart. A short rest period follows, and then the pacemaker begins the wave of excitation across the heart again.

The record used to detect these electrical changes in heart muscle as the heart beats is an **electrocardiogram** (**ECG** or **EKG**). The normal ECG tracing shows five waves, or **deflections,** that represent the electrical changes as a wave of excitation spreads through the heart. The deflections are called **P, QRS,** and **T** waves. Figure 11-10 illustrates P, QRS, and T waves on a normal ECG tracing.

Heart rhythm (originating in the SA node and traveling through the heart) is called **normal sinus rhythm (NSR).** Sympathetic nerves speed up the heart rate during conditions of emotional stress or vigorous exercise. Parasympathetic nerves slow the heart rate when there is no need for extra pumping.

BLOOD PRESSURE

Blood pressure is the force that the blood exerts on the arterial walls. This pressure is measured with a **sphygmomanometer** (Figure 11-11).

The sphygmomanometer consists of a rubber bag inside a cloth cuff that is wrapped around the upper arm, just above the elbow. The rubber bag is inflated with air using a

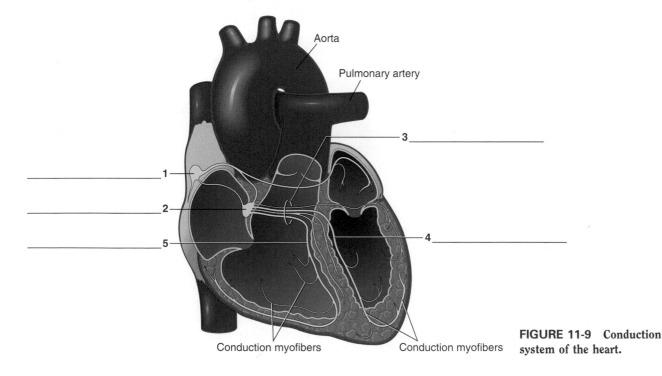

Aorta

Pulmonary artery

3 _____

1 _____

2 _____

5 _____

4 _____

Conduction myofibers   Conduction myofibers

FIGURE 11-9 Conduction system of the heart.

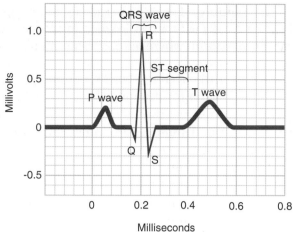

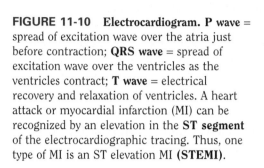

FIGURE 11-10 Electrocardiogram. P wave = spread of excitation wave over the atria just before contraction; **QRS wave** = spread of excitation wave over the ventricles as the ventricles contract; **T wave** = electrical recovery and relaxation of ventricles. A heart attack or myocardial infarction (MI) can be recognized by an elevation in the **ST segment** of the electrocardiographic tracing. Thus, one type of MI is an ST elevation MI **(STEMI)**.

hand bulb pump. As the bag is pumped up, the pressure within it increases and is measured on a recording device attached to the cuff.

The brachial artery in the upper arm is compressed by the air pressure in the bag. When there is sufficient air pressure in the bag to stop the flow of blood, the pulse in the lower arm (where the observer is listening with a stethoscope) drops.

Air is then allowed to escape from the bag and the pressure is lowered slowly, allowing the blood to begin to make its way through the gradually opening artery. At the point when the person listening with the stethoscope first hears the sounds of the pulse beats, the reading on the device attached to the cuff shows the higher, systolic blood pressure (pressure in the artery when the left ventricle is contracting to force the blood into the aorta and other arteries).

As air continues to escape, the sounds become progressively louder. Finally, when a change in sound from loud to soft occurs, the observer makes note of the pressure on the recording device. This is the diastolic pressure (pressure in the artery when the ventricles relax and the heart fills, receiving blood from the venae cavae and pulmonary veins).

Blood pressure is expressed as a fraction—for example, 120/80 mm Hg, in which the upper number (120) is the systolic pressure and the lower number (80) is the diastolic pressure. Hypertension, or high blood pressure, is defined as blood pressure greater than 140/90 mm Hg. New guidelines for treatment of hypertension (HTN) in patients over age 60 are 150/90. Both the systolic and diastolic components of hypertension are associated with increased risk of heart attack and stroke.

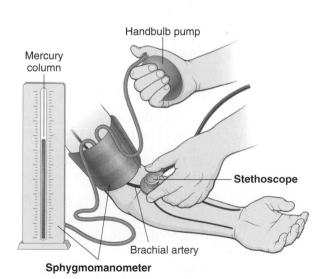

FIGURE 11-11 Measurement of blood pressure with a sphygmomanometer and stethoscope.

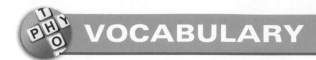

VOCABULARY

This list reviews new terms introduced in the text. Short definitions reinforce your understanding of the terms. See page 451 of this chapter for pronunciation of terms.

aorta	Largest artery in the body.
apex of the heart	Lower tip of the heart.
arteriole	Small artery.
artery	Largest type of blood vessel; carries blood away from the heart to all parts of the body. Notice that artery and away begin with an "a."
atrioventricular bundle (bundle of His)	Specialized muscle fibers connecting the atria with the ventricles and transmitting electrical impulses between them. His is pronounced "hiss."
atrioventricular node (AV node)	Specialized tissue in the wall between the atria. Electrical impulses pass from the pacemaker (SA node) through the AV node and the atrioventricular bundle or bundle of His toward the ventricles.
atrium (*plural*: **atria**)	One of two upper chambers of the heart.
capillary	Smallest blood vessel. Materials pass to and from the bloodstream through the thin capillary walls.
carbon dioxide (CO₂)	Gas (waste) released by body cells, transported via veins to the heart, and then to the lungs for exhalation.
coronary arteries	Blood vessels that branch from the aorta and carry oxygen-rich blood to the heart muscle.
deoxygenated blood	Blood that is oxygen-poor.
diastole	Relaxation phase of the heartbeat. (From Greek *diastole,* dilation.)
electrocardiogram	Record of the electricity flowing through the heart. The electricity is represented by waves or deflections called P, QRS, or T.
endocardium	Inner lining of the heart.
endothelium	Innermost lining of blood vessels.
mitral valve	Valve between the left atrium and the left ventricle; bicuspid valve.
murmur	Abnormal swishing sound caused by improper closure of the heart valves.
myocardium	Muscular, middle layer of the heart.
normal sinus rhythm	Heart rhythm originating in the sinoatrial node with a rate in patients at rest of 60 to 100 beats per minute.
oxygen	Gas that enters the blood through the lungs and travels to the heart to be pumped via arteries to all body cells.
pacemaker (sinoatrial node)	Specialized nervous tissue in the right atrium that begins the heartbeat. An artificial cardiac pacemaker is an electronic apparatus implanted in the chest to stimulate heart muscle that is weak and not functioning.
pericardium	Double-layered membrane surrounding the heart.

11

pulmonary artery	Artery carrying oxygen-poor blood from the heart to the lungs.
pulmonary circulation	Flow of blood from the heart to the lungs and back to the heart.
pulmonary valve	Valve positioned between the right ventricle and the pulmonary artery.
pulmonary vein	One of two pairs of vessels carrying oxygenated blood from the lungs to the left atrium of the heart.
pulse	Beat of the heart as felt through the walls of the arteries.
septum (*plural*: **septa**)	Partition or wall dividing a cavity; such as between the right and left atria (interatrial septum) and right and left ventricles (interventricular septum).
sinoatrial node (SA node)	Pacemaker of the heart.
sphygmomanometer	Instrument to measure blood pressure.
systemic circulation	Flow of blood from body tissue to the heart and then from the heart back to body tissues.
systole	Contraction phase of the heartbeat. (From Greek *systole*, contraction.)
tricuspid valve	Located between the right atrium and the right ventricle; it has three (tri-) leaflets, or cusps.
valve	Structure in veins or in the heart that temporarily closes an opening so that blood flows in only one direction.
vein	Thin-walled vessel that carries blood from body tissues and lungs back to the heart. Veins contain valves to prevent backflow of blood.
vena cava (*plural*: **venae cavae**)	Largest vein in the body. The superior and inferior venae cavae return blood to the right atrium of the heart.
ventricle	One of two lower chambers of the heart.
venule	Small vein.

 # TERMINOLOGY

Write the meaning of the medical term in the space provided.

COMBINING FORM	MEANING	TERMINOLOGY	MEANING
angi/o	vessel	angiogram _____	
		angioplasty _____	
aort/o	aorta	aortic stenosis _____	
arter/o, arteri/o	artery	arteriosclerosis _____	
		arterial anastomosis _____ *From the Greek* anastomoien, *providing a mouth.*	
		arteriography _____	
		endarterectomy _____ *See page 433.*	

COMBINING FORM	MEANING	TERMINOLOGY	MEANING
ather/o	yellowish plaque, fatty substance (Greek *athere* means porridge)	atheroma _____	
		The suffix -oma means mass or collection. Atheromas are collections of plaque that protrude into the **lumen** *(opening) of an artery, weakening the muscle lining.*	
		atherosclerosis _____	
		The major form of arteriosclerosis in which deposits of yellow plaque (atheromas) containing cholesterol and lipids are found within the lining of the artery (Figure 11-12).	
		atherectomy _____	
atri/o	atrium, upper heart chamber	atrial _____	
		atrioventricular _____	
brachi/o	arm	brachial artery _____	
cardi/o	heart	cardiomegaly _____	
		cardiomyopathy _____	
		One type of cardiomyopathy is **hypertrophic cardiomyopathy**— *abnormal thickening of heart muscle, usually in the left ventricle. The ventricle has to work harder to pump blood. The condition may be inherited or develop over time because of high blood pressure or aging. Often the cause is unknown (idiopathic).*	
		bradycardia _____	
		Slower than 60 beats per minute. Normal pulse is about 60 to 80 beats per minute. Brady- means slow.	
		tachycardia _____	
		Faster than 100 beats per minute. Supraventricular tachycardia (SVT) involves rapid beats coming from the atria (above the ventricles) and causing palpitation (abnormal sensations in the chest). Tachy- means fast.	
		cardiogenic shock _____	
		Results from failure of the heart in its pumping action. **Shock** *is circulatory failure associated with inadequate delivery of oxygen and nutrients to body tissues.*	
cholesterol/o	cholesterol (a lipid substance)	hypercholesterolemia _____	
		Statins *are drugs that work by blocking a key enzyme in the production of cholesterol by the liver.*	
coron/o	heart	coronary arteries _____	
		These arteries come down over the top of the heart like a crown (corona); see Figure 11-23A, page 428.	

---

ather/o, arteri/o, arthr/o

These three combining forms are easily confused.

    ather/o = yellowish plaque
    arteri/o = artery
    arthr/o = joint

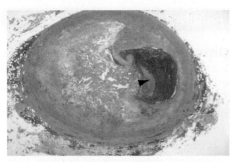

FIGURE 11-12 Atherosclerosis. *Arrow* points to accumulated plaque in lumen of an artery. *(Courtesy Sid Murphree, MD, Department of Pathology, University of Texas Southwestern Medical School, Dallas, Texas.)*

COMBINING FORM	MEANING	TERMINOLOGY	MEANING
cyan/o	blue	cyanosis	
		This bluish discoloration of the skin indicates diminished oxygen content of the blood.	
myx/o	mucus	myxoma	
		A benign tumor derived from connective tissue, with cells embedded in soft mucoid stromal tissue. These rare tumors occur most frequently in the left atrium.	
ox/o	oxygen	hypoxia	
		Inadequate oxygen in tissues. **Anoxia** is an extreme form of hypoxia.	
pericardi/o	pericardium	pericardiocentesis	
phleb/o	vein	phlebotomy	
		A phlebotomist is trained in opening veins for phlebotomy.	
		thrombophlebitis	
		Often shortened to phlebitis. If the affected vein is deep within a muscle, the condition is **deep vein thrombosis (DVT)**.	
rrhythm/o	rhythm	arrhythmia	
		Dysrhythmia is also used to describe an abnormal heart rhythm. Notice that one "r" is dropped.	
sphygm/o	pulse	sphygmomanometer	
		A sphygmomanometer measures pressure.	
steth/o	chest	stethoscope	
		A misnomer because the examination is by ear, not by eye. **Auscultation** means listening to sounds within the body, typically using a stethoscope.	
thromb/o	clot	thrombolysis	

11

COMBINING FORM	MEANING	TERMINOLOGY	MEANING
valvul/o, valv/o	valve	valvuloplasty _____ _A balloon-tipped catheter dilates a cardiac valve._	
		mitral valvulitis _____ _Commonly associated with rheumatic fever, an inflammatory disease caused by inadequate treatment of a streptococcal infection. An autoimmune reaction occurs, leading to inflammation and damage to heart valves. (See Figure 11-19, page 422.)_	
		valvotomy _____	
vas/o	vessel	vasoconstriction _____ _Constriction means to tighten or narrow._	
		vasodilation _____	
vascul/o	vessel	vascular _____	
ven/o, ven/i	vein	venous _____ _A venous cutdown is a small surgical incision to permit access to a collapsed vein. An intravenous infusion is delivery of fluids into a vein._	
		venipuncture _____ _This procedure is performed for phlebotomy or to start an intravenous infusion._	
ventricul/o	ventricle, lower heart chamber	interventricular septum _____	

PATHOLOGY: THE HEART AND BLOOD VESSELS

HEART

arrhythmias	**Abnormal heart rhythms (dysrhythmias).**

Arrhythmias are problems with the conduction or electrical system of the heart. More than 4 million Americans have recurrent cardiac arrhythmias.

Examples of cardiac arrhythmias are:

1. bradycardia and heart block (atrioventricular block)

Failure of proper conduction of impulses from the SA node through the AV node to the atrioventricular bundle (bundle of His).

Damage to the SA node may cause its impulses to be too weak to activate the AV node and impulses fail to reach the ventricles. The heart beats slowly and bradycardia results. If the failure occurs only occasionally, the heart misses a beat in a rhythm at regular intervals (partial heart block). If no impulses reach the AV node from the SA node, the ventricles contract slower than the atria and are not coordinated. This is complete heart block.

Right and left bundle branch block (RBBB and LBBB) are common types of heart block. They involve delay or failure of impulses traveling through the right and left bundle branches to the ventricles.

Implantation of an artificial **cardiac pacemaker** overcomes arrhythmias and keeps the heart beating at the proper rate. The pacemaker power source is a generator that contains a computer and lithium battery. It is implanted under the skin just below the collarbone, with leads (wires) to both chambers, usually on the right side of the heart. A newer type of pacemaker, called a **biventricular pacemaker,** treats delays and abnormalities in ventricular contractions (dysynergy) and also can relieve symptoms and improve quality of life in patients with congestive heart failure. It reduces exacerbations of heart failure that require hospital admission (Figure 11-13C).

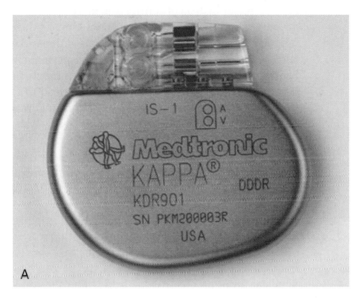

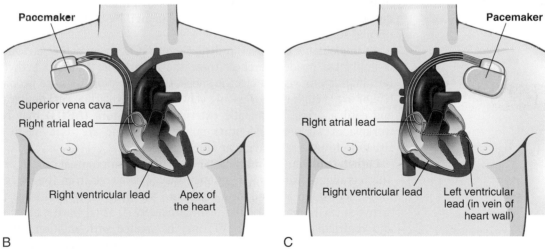

FIGURE 11-13   **A, A dual-chamber, rate-responsive pacemaker** (*actual size shown*) is designed to detect body movement and automatically increase or decrease paced heart rates based on levels of physical activity. **B, Cardiac pacemaker** with leads in the right atrium and right ventricle enable it to sense and pace in both heart chambers. **C, Biventricular pacemaker** with leads in the right atrium and the right and left ventricles to synchronize ventricular contractions.

How Does a Pacemaker Work?

The pacemaker leads (wires) detect the heart's own electrical activity and transmit that information to the generator (computer). The computer analyzes the heart's signals and decides when and where to pace. If the rate is slow, the generator emits a signal to stimulate contraction and increase the rate. Pacemakers with multiple leads can pace the atrium and ventricle in proper sequence. Rate-responsive pacemakers have sensors that detect body movement and breathing to then determine the best heart rate.

2. flutter — **Rapid but regular contractions, usually of the atria.**

Heart rate may reach up to 300 beats per minute. Atrial flutter often is symptomatic of heart disease and frequently requires treatment such as medication, electrical cardioversion, or catheter ablation (see below under fibrillation).

3. fibrillation — **Very rapid, random, inefficient, and irregular contractions of the heart (350 beats or more per minute).**

Atrial fibrillation (AF) is the most common type of cardiac arrhythmia, affecting 5% to 10% of 70- to 80-year-old people and greater than 15% of individuals in their 80s. Electrical impulses move randomly throughout the atria, causing the atria to quiver instead of contracting in a coordinated rhythm. Common symptoms are **palpitations** (uncomfortable sensations in the chest from missed heartbeats), fatigue, and shortness of breath. Patients with **paroxysmal AF** (irregular heartbeats occur periodically and episodically) and **permanent** or **persistent AF** (irregular heartbeats continue indefinitely) are at a much greater risk for stroke. This is because ineffective atrial contractions can lead to the formation of blood clots in the left atrial appendage (the area where clots form) that may travel to the brain. Also, sometimes AF can make the heart beat very fast for long periods of time, leading to weakening of the heart muscle.

The risk for stroke with AF can be reduced by 80% with the use of anticoagulants (blood thinners such as warfarin) and new oral anticoagulants called **NOACs** (**no**vel **antic**oagulants). Examples of NOACs are apixaban (Eliquis), dabiatran (Pradaxa), and rivaroxaban (Xarelto).

In **ventricular fibrillation (VF)**, electrical impulses move randomly throughout the ventricles. This life-threatening situation may result in sudden cardiac death or **cardiac arrest** (sudden stoppage of heart movement) unless help is provided immediately. If treatment is immediate, VF can be interrupted with **defibrillation** (application of an electrical shock). Defibrillation stops electrical activity in the heart for a brief moment so that normal rhythm takes over. Medications such as **digoxin, beta blockers,** and **calcium channel blockers** convert fibrillation to normal sinus rhythm.

An **implantable cardioverter-defibrillator (ICD)** is a small electrical device that is implanted inside the chest (near the collarbone) to sense arrhythmias and terminate them with an electric shock. Candidates for ICDs are people who have had or are at high risk for having ventricular tachycardia, ventricular fibrillation, and cardiac arrest. **Automatic external defibrillators (AEDs)** may be found in workplaces, airports, and other public places and are used in an emergency situation to reverse ventricular fibrillation.

Catheter ablation is a minimally invasive treatment to treat cardiac arrhythmias. The technique, using radiofrequency energy delivered from the tip of a catheter inserted through a blood vessel and into the heart, destroys tissue that causes arrhythmias. Supraventricular tachycardia (SVT), atrial flutter, atrial fibrillation, and ventricular tachycardia (VT) may be treated with ablation when clinically indicated. This procedure may provide a permanent cure in many clinical situations.

Palpitation/Palpation

Don't confuse **palpitation** with **palpation,** which means to touch, feel, or examine with the hands and fingers.

congenital heart disease   **Abnormalities in the heart at birth.**

The following conditions are congenital anomalies resulting from some failure in the development of the fetal heart.

1. **coarctation of the aorta (CoA)**

   Narrowing (coarctation) of the aorta.

   Figure 11-14A shows coarctation of the aorta. Surgical treatment consists of removal of the constricted region and end-to-end anastomosis of the aortic segments.

2. **patent ductus arteriosus (PDA)**

   Passageway (ductus arteriosus) between the aorta and the pulmonary artery remains open (patent) after birth.

   The ductus arteriosus normally closes after birth, but in this congenital condition it remains open (see Figure 11-14B), resulting in the flow of oxygenated blood from the aorta into the pulmonary artery. PDA occurs in premature infants, causing cyanosis, fatigue, and rapid breathing. Although the defect often closes on its own within months after birth, treatment may be necessary if patency continues. Treatments include use of a drug (indomethacin) to promote closure; surgery via catheterization (with coil embolization to "plug" the ductus); and ligation (tying off) performed through a small incision between the ribs.

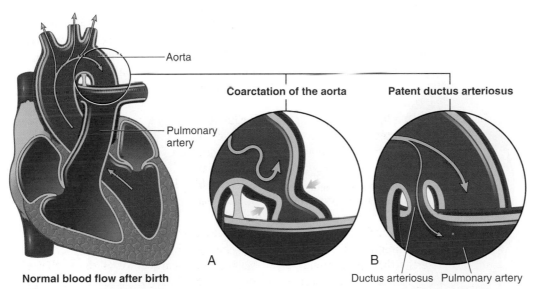

FIGURE 11-14   A, Coarctation of the aorta. Localized narrowing of the aorta reduces the supply of blood to the lower part of the body. **B, Patent ductus arteriosus.** The ductus arteriosus fails to close after birth, and blood from the aorta flows through it into the pulmonary artery.

3. septal defects

Small holes in the wall between the atria (atrial septal defects) or the ventricles (ventricular septal defects). Figure 11-15A shows a ventricular septal defect.

Although many septal defects close spontaneously, others require open heart surgery to close the hole between heart chambers. Septal defects are closed while maintaining a general circulation by means of a **heart-lung machine.** This machine, connected to the patient's circulatory system, relieves the heart and lungs of pumping and oxygenation functions during heart surgery.

Alternatively, septal defects may be repaired with a less invasive catheter technique using a device (Amplatzer device) in the defect to close it.

4. tetralogy of Fallot
(fă-LŌ)

Congenital malformation involving four (tetra-) distinct heart defects.

The condition, named for Etienne Fallot, the French physician who described it in 1888, is illustrated in Figure 11-15B. The four defects are:

- **Pulmonary artery stenosis.** Pulmonary artery is narrow or obstructed.
- **Ventricular septal defect.** Large hole between two ventricles lets venous blood pass from the right to the left ventricle and out to the aorta without oxygenation.
- **Shift of the aorta to the right.** Aorta overrides the interventricular septum. Oxygen-poor blood passes from the right ventricle to the aorta.
- **Hypertrophy of the right ventricle.** Myocardium works harder to pump blood through a narrowed pulmonary artery.

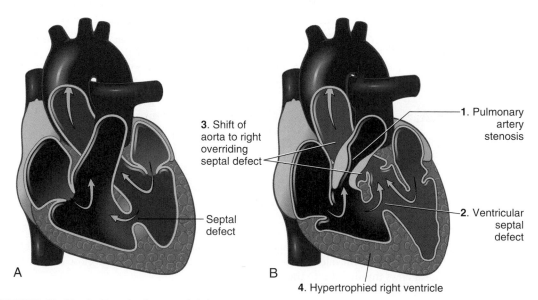

FIGURE 11-15 A, Ventricular septal defect. A hole in the ventricular septum causes blood to flow from the left ventricle to the right and into the lings via the pulmonary artery. **B, Tetralogy of Fallot** showing the four defects. The flow of blood is indicated by the *arrows.*

An infant with this condition is described as a "blue baby" because of the extreme degree of **cyanosis** present at birth. Surgery for tetralogy of Fallot includes a patch closure of the ventricular septal defect and removing obstruction to the outflow at the pulmonary artery.

Other congenital conditions such as **transposition of the great arteries (TGA)** (pulmonary artery arises from the left ventricle and the aorta from the right ventricle) cause cyanosis and hypoxia as well. Surgical correction of TGA involves an arterial switch procedure (pulmonary artery and aorta are reconnected in their proper positions).

congestive heart failure (CHF)

Heart is unable to pump its required amount of blood.

There are two types of congestive heart failure: systolic and diastolic. In **systolic CHF,** left ventricular dysfunction results in a low ejection fraction (the amount of blood that leaves the left ventricle). Less blood is pumped from the heart. In **diastolic CHF,** the heart can contract normally but is "stiff" or less compliant when relaxed or filling with blood. Fluid backs up in the lungs and other parts of the body. The most common cause of diastolic CHF is hypertension.

Symptoms of CHF include shortness of breath, exercise intolerance, and fluid retention. **Pulmonary edema** (fluid accumulation in the lungs) and swelling or edema in the legs, feet, and ankles are common. Treatment includes lowering dietary intake of sodium and the use of diuretics to promote fluid loss.

Angiotensin-converting enzyme (ACE) inhibitors (type I), beta blockers, spironolactone (increases excretion of water and sodium by the kidney), and **digoxin** also are used.

If drug therapy and lifestyle changes fail to control congestive heart failure, heart transplantation may be the only treatment option. While waiting for a transplant, patients may need a device to assist the heart's pumping. A **left ventricular assist device (LVAD)** is a booster pump implanted in the abdomen, with a cannula (tube) inserted into the left ventricle. It pumps blood out of the heart to all parts of the body. LVAD may be used either as a "bridge to transplant" or as a "destination" therapy when heart transplantation is not possible. Because of the severe shortage of donor hearts, research efforts are directed at developing total artificial hearts.

coronary artery disease (CAD)

Disease of the arteries surrounding the heart.

The coronary arteries are a pair of blood vessels that arise from the aorta and supply oxygenated blood to the heart. After blood leaves the heart via the aorta, a portion is at once led back over the surface of the heart through the coronary arteries.

CAD usually is the result of **atherosclerosis.** This is the deposition of fatty compounds on the inner lining of the coronary arteries (any other artery can be similarly affected). The ordinarily smooth lining of the artery becomes roughened as the atherosclerotic plaque collects in the artery.

11

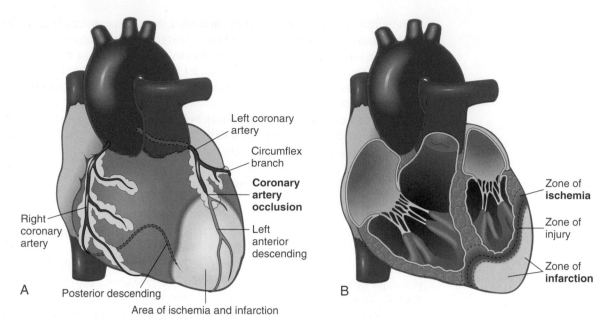

Left coronary
artery

Circumflex
branch

**Coronary
artery
occlusion**

Left
anterior
descending

Right
coronary
artery

A   Posterior descending

Area of ischemia and infarction

Zone of
ischemia

Zone of
injury

Zone of
infarction

B

FIGURE 11-16   **A, Ischemia** and **infarction** produced by coronary artery occlusion. **B,** Internal view of the heart showing an area damaged by **myocardial infarction.**

The plaque first causes plugging of the coronary artery. Next, the roughened lining of the artery may rupture or cause abnormal clotting of blood, leading to **thrombotic occlusion** (blocking of the coronary artery by a clot). Blood flow is decreased (**ischemia**) or stopped entirely, leading to death (**necrosis**) of a part of the myocardium. This sequence of events constitutes a **myocardial infarction,** or heart attack, and the area of dead myocardial tissue is known as an infarct. The infarcted area is eventually replaced by scar tissue. Figure 11-16 shows coronary arteries branching from the aorta and illustrates coronary artery occlusion leading to ischemia and infarction of heart muscle. Figure 11-17 is a photograph of myocardium after an acute myocardial infarction.

Acute coronary syndromes (ACSs) are conditions caused by myocardial ischemia. These conditions are **unstable angina** (chest pain at rest or chest pain of increasing frequency) and **myocardial infarction** (Figure 11-18).

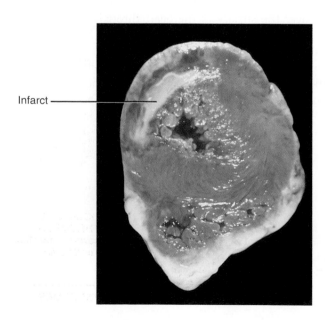

Infarct

FIGURE 11-17   **Acute myocardial infarction (MI),** 5 to 7 days old. The infarct is visible as a well-demarcated, pale yellow lesion in the posterolateral region of the left ventricle. The border of the infarct is surrounded by a dark red zone of acute inflammation.

Patients with ACSs benefit from early angiography (x-ray imaging of coronary arteries) and PCI (percutaneous coronary intervention with a balloon catheter and stents) or CABG (coronary artery bypass grafting) to improve blood flow to the heart muscle (revascularization). Drugs used to treat ACSs are anticoagulants and antiplatelet agents such as aspirin and clopidogrel (Plavix), prasugrel (Effient), and ticagrelor (Brilinta).

For acute attacks of angina, **nitroglycerin** is given sublingually (under the tongue). This drug, one of several called **nitrates,** is a vasodilator that increases coronary blood flow and lowers blood pressure. Nitrates also produce venodilation to reduce venous return and decrease myocardial oxygen consumption, both of which help decrease the work of the heart.

Physicians advise patients to avoid risk factors such as smoking, obesity, and lack of exercise, and they prescribe effective drugs to prevent CAD and ACSs. These drugs include **aspirin** (to prevent clumping of platelets), **beta blockers** (to reduce the force and speed of the heartbeat and to lower blood pressure), **ACE inhibitors** (to reduce high blood pressure and the risk of future heart attack even if the patient is not hypertensive), **calcium channel blockers** (to relax muscles in blood vessels), and **statins** (to lower cholesterol levels).

Cardiac surgeons perform an open heart operation called **coronary artery bypass grafting (CABG)** to treat CAD by replacing clogged vessels. Interventional cardiologists perform **percutaneous coronary intervention (PCI),** in which catheterization with balloons and stents opens clogged coronary arteries.

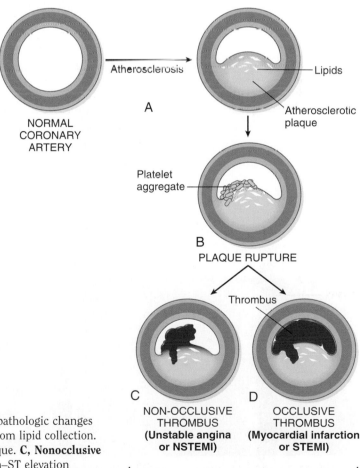

FIGURE 11-18 **Acute coronary syndromes:** sequence of pathologic changes leading to cardiac event. **A, Atherosclerotic plaque** forms from lipid collection. **B, Plaque rupture,** causing platelet aggregation on the plaque. **C, Nonocclusive thrombus** forms, causing **unstable angina** or **NSTEMI** (non–ST elevation myocardial infarction). **D,** Alternatively, formation of an **occlusive thrombus** leads to a **myocardial infarction** or **STEMI** (ST elevation myocardial infarction).

endocarditis	**Inflammation of the inner lining of the heart.**

Damage to the heart valves from infection **(bacterial endocarditis)** produces lesions called **vegetations** (resembling cauliflower) that break off into the bloodstream as **emboli** (material that travels through the blood). The emboli can lodge in other vessels, leading to a **transient ischemic attack (TIA),** or a stroke, or in small vessels of the skin, where multiple pinpoint hemorrhages known as **petechiae** (from the Italian *petechio*, a flea bite) form. Antibiotics can cure bacterial endocarditis.

hypertensive heart disease	**High blood pressure affecting the heart.**

This condition results from narrowing of arterioles, which leads to increased pressure in arteries. The heart is affected (left ventricular hypertrophy) because it pumps more vigorously to overcome the increased resistance in the arteries.

mitral valve prolapse (MVP)	**Improper closure of the mitral valve.**

This condition occurs because the mitral valve enlarges and prolapses into the left atrium during systole. The physician hears a midsystolic click on **auscultation** (listening with a stethoscope) and occasionally, **mitral regurgitation** (backflow of blood into the left atrium). Most people with MVP live normal lives, but severely prolapsed valves can be associated with severe mitral regurgitation and on rare occasions may become infected (endocarditis).

murmur	**Extra heart sound, heard between normal beats.**

Murmurs are heard with the aid of a stethoscope and usually are caused by a valvular defect or disease that disrupts the smooth flow of blood in the heart. They also are heard in cases of interseptal defects, in which blood flows abnormally between chambers through holes in the septa. Functional murmurs are not caused by valve or septal defects and do not seriously endanger a person's health.

A **bruit** (brū-Ē) is a murmur heard on auscultation. A **thrill,** which is a vibration felt on palpation of the chest, often accompanies a murmur.

pericarditis	**Inflammation of the membrane (pericardium) surrounding the heart.**

In most instances, pericarditis results from pulmonary infection. Bacteria and viruses cause the condition, or the etiology may be idiopathic. Malaise, fever, and chest pain occur, and auscultation often reveals a **pericardial friction rub** (heard as a scraping or grating sound). Compression of the heart caused by collection of fluid in the pericardial cavity is **cardiac tamponade** (tăm-pō-NŎD). Treatment includes anti-inflammatory drugs and other agents to manage pain. If the pericarditis is infective, antibiotics or antifungals are prescribed, depending on the microorganisms detected in specimens obtained by pericardiocentesis.

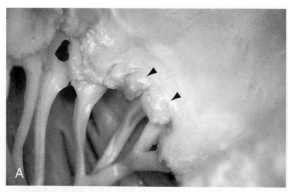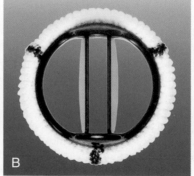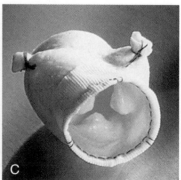

FIGURE 11-19 **A,** Acute rheumatic **mitral valvulitis** with chronic rheumatic heart disease. Small vegetations are visible along the line of closure of the mitral valve leaflet (*arrows*). Previous episodes of rheumatic valvulitis have caused fibrous thickening and fusion of the chordae tendineae of the valves. **B, Artificial heart valve. C, Porcine xenograft** valve. A xenograft valve (Greek *xen/o* means stranger) is tissue that is transferred from an animal of one species (pig) to one of another species (human).

rheumatic heart disease

Heart disease caused by rheumatic fever.

Rheumatic fever is a childhood disease that follows a streptococcal infection with sore throat (pharyngitis). The heart valves can be damaged by inflammation and scarred with **vegetations,** so that they do not open and close normally (Figure 11-19A). Repeat streptococcal infection is thought to be required to produce heart disease, so children with a history of rheumatic fever are treated with monthly penicillin injections given intramuscularly until the age of 21.

Mitral stenosis, atrial fibrillation, and congestive heart failure, caused by weakening of the myocardium, also can result from rheumatic heart disease. Treatment consists of reduced activity, drugs to control arrhythmia, surgery to repair a damaged valve, and anticoagulant therapy to prevent emboli from forming. Artificial and porcine (pig) valve implants can replace deteriorated heart valves (Figure 11-19B and C).

BLOOD VESSELS

aneurysm

Local widening (dilation) of an arterial wall.

An aneurysm (Greek *aneurysma,* widening) usually is caused by atherosclerosis and hypertension or a congenital weakness in the vessel wall. Aneurysms are common in the aorta but may occur in peripheral vessels as well. The danger of an aneurysm is rupture and hemorrhage. Treatment depends on the vessel involved, the site, and the health of the patient. In aneurysms of small vessels in the brain (**berry aneurysms**), treatment is occlusion of the vessel with small clips. For larger arteries, such as the aorta, a stent graft may be sewn within the affected vessel. Figure 11-20A shows an abdominal aortic aneurysm (called "**AAA**"), and Figure 11-20B illustrates a stent graft in place. Note that the graft is anastomosed to the normal portion of the aorta, and the aneurysm sac is closed around the graft to prevent fistula formation from graft to bowel.

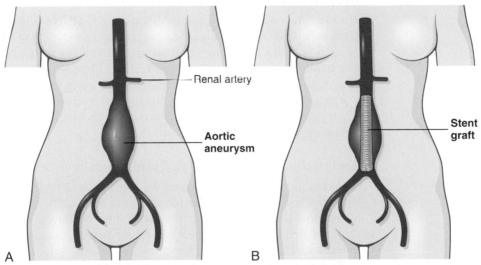

FIGURE 11-20   A, Abdominal aortic aneurysm (AAA). A **dissecting aortic aneurysm** is a splitting or dissection of the wall of the aorta by blood entering a tear or hemorrhage within the walls of the vessel. **B, Stent graft in place.** This stent graft procedure is an **endovascular aneurysm repair or EVAR.**

Aortic Aneurysms and Marfan Syndrome

Aortic aneurysms are often associated with **Marfan syndrome,** a genetic disorder marked by long, thin fingers, great arm span, ocular lens dislocation, and loose joints. Abraham Lincoln is thought to have had Marfan syndrome, and the syndrome also has been diagnosed in basketball and volleyball players who have died suddenly as a result of ruptured aortic aneurysms.

deep vein thrombosis (DVT)	**Blood clot (thrombus) forms in a large vein, usually in a lower limb.**

This condition may result in a **pulmonary embolism** (clot travels to the lung) if not treated effectively. Examples of anticoagulants (blood-thinning drugs) are warfarin (Coumadin) and new oral anticoagulants (NOACs). They are used to prevent DVTs and pulmonary emboli (PEs) ◥.

hypertension (HTN)	**High blood pressure.**

Most high blood pressure is **essential hypertension,** with no identifiable cause. In adults, a blood pressure of 140/90 mm Hg or greater is considered high. Diuretics, ACE inhibitors, calcium channel blockers, and beta-blockers, are used to treat essential hypertension. Losing weight, limiting sodium (salt) intake, stopping smoking, and reducing fat in the diet also can reduce blood pressure.

In **secondary hypertension,** the increase in pressure is caused by another associated lesion, such as glomerulonephritis, pyelonephritis, or disease of the adrenal glands.

peripheral arterial disease (PAD)	**Blockage of arteries carrying blood to the legs, arms, kidneys and other organs.**

Any artery can be affected, such as the **carotid** (neck), **femoral** (thigh), or **popliteal** (back of the knee). A sign of PAD in the lower extremities is **intermittent claudication** (absence of pain or discomfort in a leg at rest, but pain, tension, and weakness after walking has begun). Treatment is exercise, avoidance of nicotine (which causes vessel constriction), and control of risk factors such as hypertension, hyperlipidemia, and diabetes. Surgical treatment includes endarterectomy and bypass grafting (from the normal proximal vessel around the diseased area to a normal vessel distally).

Percutaneous treatments include balloon angioplasty, atherectomy, and stenting. **Embolic protection devices** are parachute-like filters used to capture embolic debris during stenting.

Raynaud's (rā-NŌZ) **disease (Raynaud's)**	**Recurrent episodes of pallor and cyanosis primarily in fingers and toes.**

This is a rare disorder of unknown cause that affects blood flow in arteries. Raynaud's is sometimes called a disease, phenomenon, or syndrome. It is marked by brief episodes of intense constriction and vasospasm of arterioles in young, otherwise healthy women. See Figure 11-21. Episodes can be triggered by cold temperatures, emotional stress, or cigarette smoking and caffeine.

Raynaud's can be controlled by protecting the body from cold and avoiding other triggers. Medications that increase blood flow to the hands and feet may relieve symptoms.

varicose veins	**Abnormally swollen and twisted veins, usually occurring in the legs.**

This condition is caused by damaged valves that fail to prevent the backflow of blood (Figure 11-22A to C). The blood then collects in the veins, which distend to many times their normal size. Because of the slow flow of blood in the varicose veins and frequent injury to the vein, thrombosis may occur as well. **Hemorrhoids** (piles) are varicose veins near the anus.

Physicians now treat varicose veins with sclerotherapy (injections with sclerosing solution) or laser and pulsed-light treatments to seal off veins. Surgical interventions such as vein stripping and ligation are used less frequently.

◥ **Warfarin (Coumadin) and NOACs**

While the oral anticoagulant **warfarin** is used to prevent or treat thromboembolic diseases, treatment with warfarin requires careful monitoring and is complicated by drug-drug or drug-food interactions. New oral anticoagulants (NOACs) such as apixaban (Eliquis), edoxaban (Savaysa), dabigatran (Pradaxa), and rivaroxaban (Xarelto) address these limitations and have been approved recently by the Food and Drug Administration (FDA) for anticoagulation in non-valvular atrial fibrillation and for the prevention and treatment of DVTs and PEs.

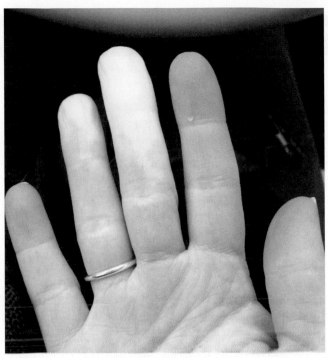

FIGURE 11-21 Raynaud's disease.

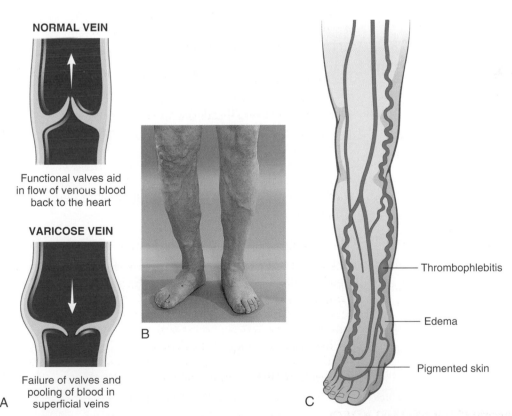

FIGURE 11-22 **A,** Valve function in normal vein and varicose vein. **B,** Varicose veins. **C,** The slow flow in veins increases susceptibility to **thrombophlebitis** (clot formation), **edema,** and **pigmented skin** (blood pools in the lower parts of the leg and fluid leaks from distended small capillaries). If a thrombus becomes loosened from its place in the vein, it can travel to the lungs **(pulmonary embolism)** and block a blood vessel there.

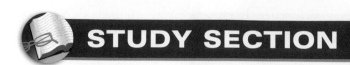
STUDY SECTION

Practice spelling each term and know its meaning.

acute coronary syndromes (ACSs)	Unstable angina and myocardial infarction (heart attack), which are consequences of plaque rupture in coronary arteries.
angina (pectoris)	Chest pain resulting from myocardial ischemia. Stable angina occurs predictably with exertion; unstable angina is chest pain that occurs more often and with less exertion.
angiotensin-converting enzyme (ACE) inhibitor	Antihypertensive drug that blocks the conversion of angiotensin I to angiotensin II, causing blood vessels to dilate. It prevents heart attacks, CHF, stroke, and death. See Table 21-6 on page 893 for names of ACE inhibitors and other cardiovascular drugs.
auscultation	Listening for sounds in blood vessels or other body structures, typically using a stethoscope.
beta blocker	Drug used to treat angina, hypertension, and arrhythmias. It blocks the action of epinephrine (adrenaline) at receptor sites on cells, slowing the heartbeat and reducing the workload on the heart.
biventricular pacemaker	Device enabling ventricles to beat together (in synchrony) so that more blood is pumped out of the heart.
bruit	Abnormal blowing or swishing sound heard during auscultation of an artery or organ.
calcium channel blocker	Drug used to treat angina and hypertension. It dilates blood vessels by blocking the influx of calcium into muscle cells lining vessels.
cardiac arrest	Sudden, unexpected stoppage of heart action, often leading to sudden cardiac death.
cardiac tamponade	Pressure on the heart caused by fluid in the pericardial space.
claudication	Pain, tension, and weakness in a leg after walking has begun, but absence of pain at rest.
digoxin	Drug that treats arrhythmias and strengthens the heartbeat.
embolus (*plural*: **emboli**)	Clot or other substance that travels to a distant location and suddenly blocks a blood vessel.
infarction	Area of dead tissue.
nitrates	Drugs used in the treatment of angina. They dilate blood vessels, increasing blood flow and oxygen to myocardial tissue.
nitroglycerin	Nitrate drug used in the treatment of angina.
occlusion	Closure of a blood vessel due to blockage.
palpitations	Uncomfortable sensations in the chest related to cardiac arrhythmias, such as premature ventricular contractions (PVCs).
patent	Open.
pericardial friction rub	Scraping or grating noise heard on auscultation of the heart; suggestive of pericarditis.
petechiae	Small, pinpoint hemorrhages.
statins	Drugs used to lower cholesterol in the bloodstream.
thrill	Vibration felt over an area of turmoil in blood flow (as a blocked artery).
vegetations	Clumps of platelets, clotting proteins, microorganisms, and red blood cells on diseased heart valves.

11

LABORATORY TESTS AND CLINICAL PROCEDURES

LABORATORY TESTS

BNP test

Measurement of BNP (brain natriuretic peptide) in blood.

BNP is elevated in patients with heart failure, and it is useful in the diagnosis of CHF in patients with dyspnea who come to the emergency department. Its presence also identifies patients at risk for complications when presenting with acute coronary syndromes (e.g., myocardial infarction, unstable angina). It is secreted when the heart becomes overloaded, and it acts as a diuretic to help heart function return to normal. Cardiologists also measure NT-proBNP levels to assess the degree of heart failure. NT stands for N-terminal.

The reference to brain in this term originates from the initial identification of the protein in the brain of a pig.

cardiac biomarkers

Chemicals are measured in the blood as evidence of a heart attack.

Damaged heart muscle releases chemicals into the bloodstream. The substances tested for are **troponin-I (cTnI)** and **troponin-T (cTnT)**. Troponin is a heart muscle protein released into circulation after myocardial injury.

C-reactive protein **(CRP)** is a biomarker of inflammation. High-sensitivity CRP **(IIs-CRP)** is useful in predicting risk for heart attack, stroke, or other major heart disease.

lipid tests (lipid profile)

Measurement of cholesterol and triglycerides (fats) in a blood sample.

High levels of lipids are associated with atherosclerosis. The general guideline for total cholesterol in the blood is less than 200 mg/dL. **Saturated fats** (of animal origin, such as milk, butter, and meats) increase cholesterol in the blood, whereas **polyunsaturated fats** (of vegetable origin, such as corn and safflower oil) decrease blood cholesterol.

Treatment of hyperlipidemia includes proper diet (low-fat, high-fiber intake) and exercise. Niacin (a vitamin) also helps reduce lipids. Drug therapy includes **statins,** which reduce the risk of heart attack, stroke, and cardiovascular death. Statins lower cholesterol by reducing its production in the liver. Examples are simvastatin (Zocor), atorvastatin (Lipitor), pravastatin (Pravachol), and rosuvastatin (Crestor).

lipoprotein electrophoresis

Lipoproteins (combinations of fat and protein) are physically separated and measured in a blood sample.

Examples of lipoproteins are **low-density lipoprotein (LDL)** and **high-density lipoprotein (HDL).** High levels of LDL are associated with atherosclerosis. The National Guideline for LDL is less than 130 mg/dL in normal persons and less than 70 mg/dL in patients with CAD, PAD, and diabetes mellitus. High levels of HDL protect adults from atherosclerosis. Factors that increase HDL are exercise and alcohol consumption in moderation.

CLINICAL PROCEDURES: DIAGNOSTIC

X-Ray and Electron Beam Tests

angiography

X-ray imaging of blood vessels after injection of contrast material.

Arteriography is x-ray imaging of arteries after injection of contrast via a catheter into the aorta or an artery.

11

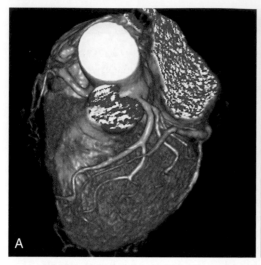

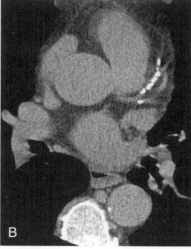

FIGURE 11-23 **A, Computed tomography angiography (CTA) showing coronary arteries.** High radiation exposure is a drawback to the use of CTA. **B, Electron beam computed tomography** showing significant calcification (*white areas*) in the coronary arteries, indicating advanced coronary artery disease. (**A,** *Courtesy Massachusetts General Hospital, Boston.*)

computed tomography angiography (CTA)	**Three-dimensional x-ray images of the heart and coronary arteries using computed tomography (64-slice CT scanner).**

This newer technique takes hundreds of images of the heart per second. Cross-sectional images are assembled by computer into a three-dimensional picture. It is less invasive than angiography (contrast material is injected into a small peripheral vein with a small needle) and provides excellent views of the coronary arteries for diagnosis of coronary artery disease (Figure 11-23A).

digital subtraction angiography (DSA)

Video equipment and a computer produce x-ray images of blood vessels.

After taking an initial x-ray picture and storing it in a computer, physicians inject contrast material and take a second image of that area. The computer compares the two images and subtracts digital data for the first from the second, leaving an image of vessels with contrast.

electron beam computed tomography (EBCT *or* EBT)

Electron beams and CT identify calcium deposits in and around coronary arteries to diagnose early CAD.

A coronary artery calcium score ◣ is derived to indicate future risk of heart attack and stroke (see Figure 11-23B).

Ultrasound Examination

Doppler ultrasound studies

Sound waves measure blood flow within blood vessels.

An instrument focuses sound waves on blood vessels, and echoes bounce off red blood cells. The examiner can hear various alterations in blood flow caused by vessel obstruction. **Duplex ultrasound** combines Doppler and conventional ultrasound to allow physicians to image the structure of blood vessels and measure the speed of blood flow. Carotid artery occlusion, aneurysms, varicose veins, and other vessel disorders can be diagnosed with duplex ultrasound.

◣ **Coronary Artery Calcium Score**

0-99   low risk
100-399   intermediate risk
>400   high risk
A calcium score >400 is associated with a nearly 25% chance of a heart attack or stroke occurring within 10 years.

| echocardiography (ECHO) | **Echoes generated by high-frequency sound waves produce images of the heart** (Figure 11-24A). |

ECHOs show the structure and movement of the heart. In **transesophageal echocardiography (TEE),** a transducer placed in the esophagus provides ultrasound and Doppler information (Figure 11-24B). This technique detects cardiac masses, prosthetic valve function, aneurysms, and pericardial fluid.

Nuclear Cardiology

| positron emission tomography (PET) scan | **Images show blood flow and myocardial function following uptake of radioactive glucose.** |

PET scanning can detect CAD, myocardial function, and differences between ischemic heart disease and cardiomyopathy.

| technetium Tc 99m sestamibi scan | **Technetium Tc 99m sestamibi injected intravenously is taken up in cardiac tissue, where it is detected by scanning.** |

This scan is used in persons who have had an MI, to assess the amount of damaged heart muscle. It also is used with an exercise tolerance test (**ETT-MIBI**). Sestamibi is a radioactive tracer compound used to define areas of poor blood flow in heart muscle.

| thallium 201 scan | **Concentration of radioactive thallium is measured to give information about blood supply to the heart muscle.** |

Thallium studies show the viability of heart muscle. Infarcted or scarred myocardium shows up as "cold spots."

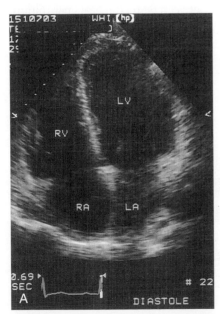

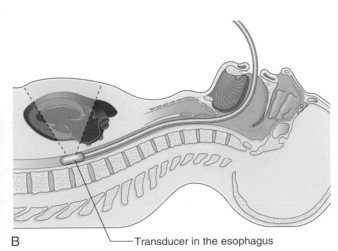

Transducer in the esophagus

FIGURE 11-24   A, Echocardiogram. Notice that in this view, the ventricles are above the atria. **B, Transesophageal echocardiography.**

Magnetic Resonance Imaging (MRI)

cardiac MRI	**Images of the heart are produced using radiowave energy in a magnetic field.**

These images in multiple planes give information about left and right ventricular function, wall thickness, and fibrosis, aneurysms, cardiac output, and patency of peripheral and coronary arteries. The magnetic waves emitted during MRI could interfere with implanted pacemakers because of their metal content and heat generation, so it is currently contraindicated for a patient with a pacemaker to undergo cardiac MRI. However, new MRI-safe pacemakers have been approved. **Magnetic resonance angiography (MRA)** is a type of MRI that gives highly detailed images of blood vessels. Physicians use MRA to view arteries and blockage inside arteries. **Gadolinium** is the most common contrast agent used for MRI procedures.

Other Diagnostic Procedures

cardiac catheterization	**Thin, flexible tube is guided into the heart via a vein or an artery.**

This procedure detects pressures and patterns of blood flow in the heart. Contrast may be injected and x-ray images taken of the heart and blood vessels (Figure 11-25). This procedure may be used in diagnosis and treatment of heart conditions (see under percutaneous coronary intervention [PCI] on page 433).

At the time of catheterization, the interventional cardiologist also may perform **intravascular ultrasound (IVUS)** to evaluate the severity of vessel narrowing. It also measures fractional flow reserve (FFR) to determine the impact of the coronary artery blockage on blood flow.

electrocardiography (ECG)	**Recording of electricity flowing through the heart.**

Continuous monitoring of a patient's heart rhythm in hospitals is performed via **telemetry** (electronic transmission of data—tele/o means distant). Sinus rhythm begins in the SA node, and the normal rate is between 60 to 100 beats per minute. Figure 11-26 shows ECG strips for normal sinus rhythm and several types of dysrhythmias (abnormal rhythms).

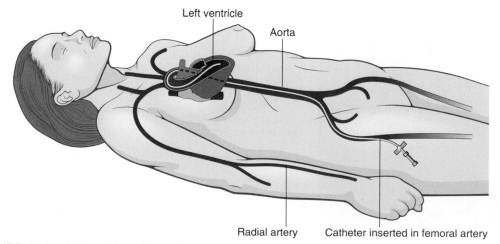

Left ventricle

Aorta

Radial artery   Catheter inserted in femoral artery

FIGURE 11-25 Left-sided cardiac catheterization. The catheter is passed retrograde (backward) from the femoral artery into the aorta and then into the left ventricle. Catheterization also is performed using the radial artery by an increasing number of interventional cardiologists. For right-sided cardiac catheterization, the cardiologist inserts a catheter through the femoral vein and advances it to the right atrium and right ventricle and into the pulmonary artery.

Holter monitoring	**An ECG device is worn during a 24-hour period to detect cardiac arrhythmias.**
	Rhythm changes are correlated with symptoms recorded in a diary.
stress test	**Exercise tolerance test (ETT) determines the heart's response to physical exertion (stress).**
	A common protocol uses 3-minute stages at set speeds and elevations of a treadmill. Continual monitoring of vital signs and ECG rhythms is important in the diagnosis of CAD and left ventricular function.

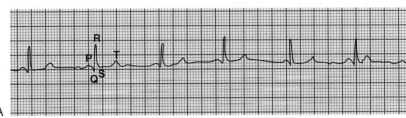

A

Normal sinus rhythm. Notice the regularity of the P, QRS, and T waves.

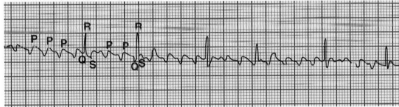

B

Atrial flutter. Notice the rapid atrial rate (P wave) compared with the slower ventricular rate (QRS)

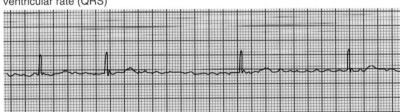

C

Atrial fibrillation. P waves are replaced by irregular and rapid fluctuations. There are no effective atrial contractions.

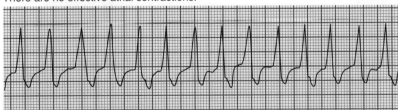

D

Ventricular tachycardia. Ventricular rate may be as high as 250 beats per minute. The rhythm is regular, but the atria are not contributing to ventricular filling and blood output is poor.

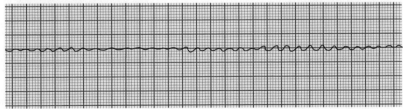

E

Ventricular fibrillation. Notice the abnormal, irregular waves. Ventricles in fibrillation cannot pump blood effectively. Circulation stops and sudden cardiac death follows if fibrillation is not reversed.

FIGURE 11-26   ECG rhythm strips showing normal sinus rhythm and dysrhythmias (arrhythmias).

CLINICAL PROCEDURES: TREATMENT

catheter ablation

Brief delivery of radiofrequency energy to destroy areas of heart tissue that may be causing arrhythmias

A catheter is guided through a vein in the leg to the vena cava and into the heart. The abnormal electrical pathway is located and ablated (destroyed) using energy emitted from the catheter. See Figure 11-27A.

coronary artery bypass grafting (CABG)

Arteries and veins are anastomosed to coronary arteries to detour around blockages.

Internal mammary (breast) and radial (arm) arteries and saphenous (leg) vein grafts are used to keep the myocardium supplied with oxygenated blood (Figure 11-27B). Cardiac surgeons perform minimally invasive CABG surgery using smaller incisions instead of the traditional sternotomy to open the chest. Vein and artery grafts are removed endoscopically through small incisions as well.

Although most operations are performed with a heart-lung machine ("on pump"), an increasing number are performed "off pump" with a beating heart. See *In Person: Coronary Artery Bypass Surgery,* page 438.

defibrillation

Brief discharges of electricity are applied across the chest to stop dysrhythmias (ventricular fibrillation).

For patients at high risk for sudden cardiac death from ventricular dysrhythmias, an **implantable cardioverter-defibrillator (ICD)** or **automatic implantable cardioverter-defibrillator (AICD)** is placed in the upper chest.

Cardioversion is another technique using lower energy to treat atrial fibrillation, atrial flutter, and supraventricular tachycardia.

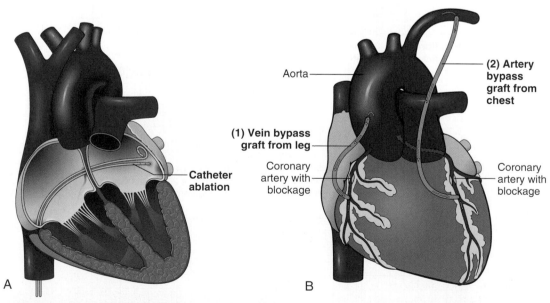

FIGURE 11-27   A, Catheter ablation. SVT, atrial flutter, AF, and VT may be treated with ablation when clinically indicated. **B, Coronary artery bypass grafting (CABG)** surgery with anastomosis of vein and arterial grafts. **(1)** A section of a vein is removed from the leg and anastomosed (upside down because of its directional valves) to a coronary artery, to bypass an area of arteriosclerotic blockage. **(2)** An internal mammary artery is grafted to a coronary artery to bypass a blockage.

endarterectomy	**Surgical removal of plaque from the inner layer of an artery.**

Fatty deposits (atheromas) and thromboses are removed to open clogged arteries. **Carotid endarterectomy** is a procedure to remove plaque buildup in the carotid artery to reduce risk of stroke.

extracorporeal circulation

Heart-lung machine diverts blood from the heart and lungs while the heart is repaired.

Blood leaves the body, enters the heart-lung machine, where it is oxygenated, and then returns to a blood vessel (artery) to circulate through the bloodstream. The machine uses the technique of **extracorporeal membrane oxygenation (ECMO).**

heart transplantation

Donor heart is transferred to a recipient.

While waiting for a transplant, a patient may need a **left ventricular assist device (LVAD),** which is a booster pump implanted in the chest or abdomen with cannulae (flexible tubes) from the left ventricle to the ascending aorta.

percutaneous coronary intervention (PCI)

Balloon-tipped catheter is inserted into a coronary artery to open the artery; stents are put in place.

An interventional cardiologist places the catheter in the femoral or radial artery and then threads it up the aorta into the coronary artery. **Stents** (expandable slotted metal tubes that serve as permanent scaffolding devices) create wide lumens and make restenosis less likely. **Drug-eluting stents (DESs)** are coated with polymers that elute (release) anti-inflammatory and antiproliferative drugs to prevent scar tissue formation leading to restenosis (Figure 11-28). Other devices are bioabsorbable vascular scaffolds (BVSs), made of dissolvable material, and drug-coated balloons (DCBs) that release paclitaxel.

PCI techniques include percutaneous transluminal coronary angioplasty (PTCA), stent placement, laser angioplasty (a small laser on the tip of a catheter vaporizes plaque), and atherectomy.

11

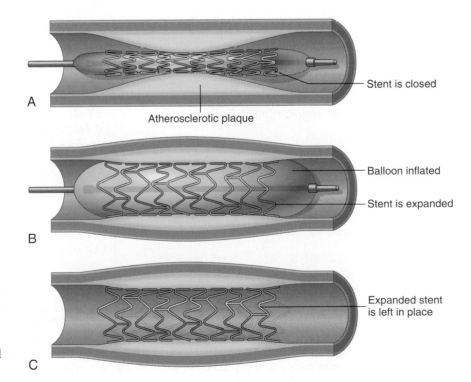

FIGURE 11-28 Placement of an intracoronary artery drug-eluting stent. A, The stent is positioned at the site of the lesion. **B,** The balloon is inflated, expanding the stent and compressing the plaque. **C,** When the balloon is withdrawn, the stent supports the artery and releases a drug to reduce the risk of restenosis. Stents are stainless-steel scaffolding devices that help hold open arteries, such as the coronary, renal, and carotid arteries.

A — Stent is closed — Atherosclerotic plaque

B — Balloon inflated — Stent is expanded

C — Expanded stent is left in place

thrombolytic therapy	**Drugs to dissolve clots are injected into the bloodstream of patients with coronary thrombosis.**
	Tissue plasminogen activator (**tPA**) and **streptokinase** restore blood flow to the heart and limit irreversible damage to heart muscle. The drugs are given within 12 hours after the onset of a heart attack. Thrombolytic agents reduce the mortality rate in patients with myocardial infarction by 25%.
transcatheter aortic valve replacement (TAVR)	**Placement of a balloon-expandable aortic heart valve into the body via a catheter.**
	The catheter is guided into the heart through the femoral artery, and a stent valve device is inserted using the catheter. This is a newer, minimally invasive catheter-based technology used to treat aortic stenosis.

ABBREVIATIONS

AAA	abdominal aortic aneurysm	**BP**	blood pressure
ACE inhibitor	angiotensin-converting enzyme inhibitor	**CABG**	coronary artery bypass grafting
ACLS	advanced cardiac life support; CPR plus drugs and defibrillation	**CAD**	coronary artery disease
		CCU	coronary care unit
ACS	acute coronary syndrome	**Cath**	catheterization
ADP	adenosine diphosphate; ADP blockers are used to prevent cardiovascular-related death, heart attack, and strokes and after all stent procedures	**CHF**	congestive heart failure
		CK	creatine kinase; enzyme released after injury to skeletal or heart muscles.
		CoA	coarctation of the aorta
AED	automatic external defibrillator	**CPR**	cardiopulmonary resuscitation
AF, a-fib	atrial fibrillation	**CRT**	cardiac resynchronization therapy; biventricular pacing
AICD	automatic implantable cardioverter-defibrillator	**CTNI** or **cTnI**; **CTNT** or **cTnT**	cardiac troponin-I and cardiac troponin-T; troponin is a protein released into the bloodstream after myocardial injury
AMI	acute myocardial infarction		
ARB	angiotensin II receptor blocker		
ARVD	arrhythmogenic right ventricular dysplasia	**DES**	drug-eluting stent
AS	aortic stenosis	**DSA**	digital subtraction angiography
ASD	atrial septal defect	**DVT**	deep vein thrombosis
AV, A-V	atrioventricular	**ECG;** also seen as **EKG**	electrocardiography
AVR	aortic valve replacement		
BBB	bundle branch block	**ECHO**	echocardiography
BNP	brain natriuretic peptide; elevated in congestive heart failure	**ECMO**	extracorporeal membrane oxygenation

EF	ejection fraction; measure of the amount of blood that pumps out of the heart with each beat
EPS	electrophysiology study; electrode catheters are inserted into veins and threaded into the heart and electrical conduction is measured (tachycardias are provoked and analyzed)
ETT	exercise tolerance test
ETT-MIBI	exercise tolerance test combined with a radioactive tracer (sestamibi) scan
EVAR	endovascular aneurysm repair
FFR	fractional flow reserve
HDL	high-density lipoprotein; high blood levels are associated with lower incidence of coronary artery disease
hsCRP	high-sensitivity C-reactive protein; biomarker for inflammation in prediction of heart attack risk
HTN	hypertension (high blood pressure)
IABP	intra-aortic balloon pump; used to support patients in cardiogenic shock
ICD	implantable cardioverter-defibrillator
IVUS	intravascular ultrasound
LAD	left anterior descending (coronary artery)
LDL	low-density lipoprotein
LMWH	low-molecular-weight heparin
LV	left ventricle
LVAD	left ventricular assist device
LVH	left ventricular hypertrophy
MI	myocardial infarction
MUGA	multiple-gated acquisition scan; a radioactive test of heart function
MVP	mitral valve prolapse
NOAC	novel anticoagulant drug
NSR	normal sinus rhythm
NT-proBNP	N-terminal pro-peptide of BNP
NSTEMI	non–ST elevation myocardial infarction
PAC	premature atrial contraction
PAD	peripheral arterial disease
PCI	percutaneous coronary intervention
PDA	patent ductus arteriosus; posterior descending artery
PE	pulmonary embolus
PVC	premature ventricular contraction
SA, S-A node	sinoatrial node
SCD	sudden cardiac death
SOB	shortness of breath
SPECT	single photon emission computed tomography; used for myocardial imaging with sestamibi scans
STEMI	ST elevation myocardial infarction
SVT	supraventricular tachycardia; rapid heartbeats arising from the atria and causing palpitations, SOB, and dizziness
TAVR	transcatheter aortic valve replacement
TEE	transesophageal echocardiography
TEVAR	thoracic endovascular aneurysm repair
TGA	transposition of the great arteries
tPA	tissue-type plasminogen activator; a drug used to prevent thrombosis
UA	unstable angina; chest pain at rest or of increasing frequency
VF	ventricular fibrillation
VSD	ventricular septal defect
VT	ventricular tachycardia
WPW	Wolff-Parkinson-White syndrome; an abnormal ECG pattern often associated with paroxysmal tachycardia

11

PRACTICAL APPLICATIONS

Answers to Practical Applications are found on page 451.

OPERATING ROOM SCHEDULE: GENERAL HOSPITAL

Match the operative treatment in Column I with the appropriate surgical indication (diagnosis) in Column II.

COLUMN I

1. coronary artery bypass grafting _____

2. left carotid endarterectomy _____

3. sclerosing injections and laser treatment _____

4. LV aneurysmectomy _____

5. atrial septal defect repair _____

6. left ventricular assist device _____

7. pericardiocentesis _____

8. aortic valve replacement _____

9. pacemaker implantation _____

10. femoral-popliteal bypass grafting _____

COLUMN II

A. Congestive heart failure
B. Cardiac tamponade (fluid in the space surrounding the heart)
C. Atherosclerotic occlusion of a main artery leading to the head
D. Congenital hole in the wall of the upper chamber of the heart
E. Disabling angina and extensive coronary atherosclerosis despite medical therapy
F. Peripheral vascular disease
G. Heart block
H. Varicose veins
I. Protrusion of the wall of a lower heart chamber
J. Aortic stenosis

NEW AND IMPORTANT CARDIOVASCULAR DRUGS

Antiplatelet agents: These drugs are used after stent placement or after ACS (acute coronary syndromes).
• clopidrogrel (Plavix)
• prasugrel (Effient)
• ticagrelor (Brilinta)

NOACs (new oral anticoagulant agents): These drugs are used to prevent strokes related to atrial fibrillation and clot formation.
• apixaban (Eliquis)
• dabidatran (Pradoxa)
• edoxaban (Savaysa
• rivaroxaban (Xarelto)

LCZ696: Exciting new combination drug to treat heart failure. It has outperformed traditional angiotensin-converting enzyme (ACE) inhibitors in a major clinical trial and has been shown to reduce mortality due to heart failure.
• valsartan/sacubritril (LCZ696)

CLINICAL CASES: WHAT'S YOUR DIAGNOSIS?

Case 1: A 24-year-old woman with a history of palpitations [heartbeat is unusually strong, rapid, or irregular, so that patient is aware of it] and vague chest pains enters the hospital. With the patient supine, you hear a midsystolic click that is followed by a grade 3/6 [moderately loud—6/6 is loud and 1/6 is quiet] honking murmur.

1. Your diagnosis is:
   a. Tetralogy of Fallot
   b. Mitral valve prolapse
   c. Raynaud's disease
   d. Congestive heart failure

Case 2: Mr. Smith was admitted to the telemetry unit for cardiac monitoring after an episode of chest pain. His cardiac enzymes (troponin-T, and troponin-I) were slightly elevated, and the ECG showed elevation in the ST segment. An angiogram reveals plaque blocking the LAD. PCI with DES is recommended.

1. What did the ECG reveal?
   a. NSTEMI and unstable angina
   b. Aortic aneurysm
   c. CHF
   d. STEMI

2. Your diagnosis for this patient is:
   a. Heart attack
   b. Rheumatic heart disease
   c. Unstable angina
   d. Patent ductus arteriosus

3. What treatment is recommended?
   a. Coronary artery bypass grafting
   b. Catheterization with drug-eluting stent placement
   c. Defibrillation and cardioversion
   d. Thrombolytic drugs

Case 3: A 42-year-old female runner recovering from an upper respiratory infection comes to the ED complaining of chest pain that is sharp and constant, worse when she is lying down and decreased with sitting up and leaning forward. Serum troponin levels rule out an acute MI. The ED physician auscultates a pericardial friction rub.

1. What's your diagnosis for this patient?
   a. Myocardial ischemia
   b. Unstable angina and NSTEMI
   c. Endocarditis
   d. Pericarditis

2. The danger of this condition is the risk for progression to:
   a. Cardiac tamponade
   b. Aneurysm
   c. Pulmonary embolism
   d. Claudication

11

IN PERSON: CORONARY ARTERY BYPASS SURGERY

Possible heart attack? You have to be kidding. I had none of the supposed symptoms—shortness of breath or chest pain. Instead, I had bouts of atrial fibrillation off and on for several months. I got tired easily, and I could feel my blood pressure drop. After lying down for about an hour, I was fine, so in November 2010 I decided to get it checked out.

My cardiologist decided to do a stress test. He put me on a treadmill, which seemed like an eternity, and then did some ultrasound on me. I work out every day on a treadmill and a recumbent bike, so the test on the treadmill wasn't that difficult, although I loved the words "just a couple of seconds to go."

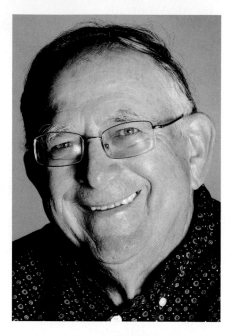

The cardiologist at Johns Hopkins told me after the stress test that it appeared that I had a slight blockage of an artery. No problem, I thought.

Angioplasty was recommended. During angioplasty, a catheter was inserted up my right arm and, although I was lightly sedated, I still felt it, particularly when the doctor hit a problem and had to make a slight correction. I was certain that they would put in a stent and I'd be home by the weekend. "No," said my doctor. "You have three blockages and will need bypass surgery." I thought he must be talking about someone else. That can't be me!

The blockages did not require immediate surgery. After all, I was pain free and asymptomatic. Still, I asked for an early date for surgery and it was set for January 11, 2011. (That was 1/11/11. How odd.)

The triple coronary artery bypass opened me up like a beached tuna and made me an official member of the "zipper club." The atrial fibrillation was fixed with radiofrequency ablation.

After surgery I had to lie on my back, which meant minimal sleep for a week. Lasix (a diuretic) was my biggest problem, along with a dozen pills I had to take far too often. According to my surgeon, who visited me a day later, things went well, and I was up and walking the hallways of Hopkins with the help of a nurse and a walker.

I went home in a week. The toughest part of the ordeal, oddly enough, was trying to get to the bathroom in time and the bumpy ride home. Those bumps made me hold that pillow [for abdominal support] as close as I could. Ouch.

After I returned home, two nurses came for home care, and they were fabulous. I lost about 20 pounds before the surgery and another 17 pounds afterwards. I went from 210 pounds to around 173 pounds.

Nowadays, I eat no red meat, nothing with butter, and as little fat and salt as possible. In other words, I eat fish primarily. I work out every day (between 30 and 60 minutes), and I have regular checkups with my cardiologist.

I was lucky that the atrial fibrillation alerted my physicians to a deeper problem that may have resulted in a heart attack or even death. Secondly, I was fortunate to have some true professionals on hand to get me through the darkest days of my life. Many people who had bypass surgery told me I would have more energy after surgery due to my new plumbing. That occurred within 6-7 months after my surgery.

Stan Ber was born in Maine, is a graduate of Bowdoin College. He retired from his career as a sports editor and columnist for the Columbia Flier and Howard County Times in December 2014 after 44 years. He was inducted into the Howard County's Sports Hall of Fame in 2009 and has been recognized by the Maryland State Legislature.

11

? EXERCISES

Remember to check your answers carefully with the Answers to Exercises, page 448.

A Match the listed structures with the descriptions that follow.

aorta   inferior vena cava   superior vena cava
arteriole   mitral valve   tricuspid valve
atrium   pulmonary artery   ventricle
capillary   pulmonary vein   venule

1. valve that lies between the right atrium and the right ventricle _____

2. smallest blood vessel _____

3. carries oxygenated blood from the lungs to the heart _____

4. largest artery in the body _____

5. brings oxygen-poor blood into the heart from the upper parts of the body _____

6. upper chamber of the heart _____

7. carries oxygen-poor blood to the lungs from the heart _____

8. small artery _____

9. valve that lies between the left atrium and the left ventricle _____

10. brings blood from the lower half of the body to the heart _____

11. small vein _____

12. lower chamber of the heart _____

B Trace the path of blood through the heart. Begin as the blood enters the right atrium from the venae cavae (and include the valves within the heart).

1. *right atrium* _____   7. _____

2. _____   8. _____

3. _____   9. _____

4. _____   10. _____

5. _____   11. _____

6. *capillaries of the lung* _____   12. *aorta* _____

11

C **Complete the following sentences.**

1. The pacemaker of the heart is the _____.

2. The sac-like membrane surrounding the heart is the _____.

3. The wall of the heart between the right and the left atria is the _____.

4. The relaxation phase of the heartbeat is called _____.

5. Specialized conductive tissue in the wall between the ventricles is the _____.

6. The inner lining of the heart is the _____.

7. The contractive phase of the heartbeat is called _____.

8. A gas released as a metabolic product of catabolism is _____.

9. Specialized conductive tissue at the base of the wall between the two upper heart chambers
   is the _____.

10. The inner lining of the pericardium, adhering to the outside of the heart, is the

    _____.

11. An abnormal heart sound due to improper closure of heart valves is a _____.

12. The beat of the heart as felt through the walls of arteries is called the _____.

D **Complete the following terms using the given definitions.**

1. hardening of arteries: arterio _____

2. disease condition of heart muscle: cardio _____

3. enlargement of the heart: cardio _____

4. inflammation of a vein: phleb _____

5. condition of rapid heartbeat: _____ cardia

6. condition of slow heartbeat: _____ cardia

7. high levels of cholesterol in the blood: hyper _____

8. surgical repair of a valve: valvulo _____

9. condition of deficient oxygen: hyp _____

10. pertaining to an upper heart chamber: _____ al

11. narrowing of the mitral valve: mitral _____

12. breakdown of a clot: thrombo _____

E **Give the meanings of the following terms.**

1. cyanosis _____

2. phlebotomy _____

3. arterial anastomosis _____

4. cardiogenic shock _____

5. atheroma _____

6. arrhythmia _____

7. sphygmomanometer _____

8. stethoscope _____

9. mitral valvulitis _____

10. atherosclerosis _____

11. vasoconstriction _____

12. vasodilation _____

F **Match the following pathologic conditions of the heart with their meanings below.**

atrial septal defect	endocarditis	mitral valve prolapse
coarctation of the aorta	fibrillation	patent ductus arteriosus
congestive heart failure	flutter	pericarditis
coronary artery disease	hypertensive heart disease	tetralogy of Fallot

1. inflammation of the inner lining of the heart _____

2. rapid but regular atrial or ventricular contractions _____

3. small hole between the upper heart chambers; congenital anomaly _____

4. improper closure of the valve between the left atrium and ventricle during systole

   _____

5. blockage of the arteries surrounding the heart leading to ischemia _____

6. high blood pressure affecting the heart _____

7. rapid, random, ineffectual, and irregular contractions of the heart _____

8. inflammation of the sac surrounding the heart _____

9. inability of the heart to pump its required amount of blood _____

10. congenital malformation involving four separate heart defects _____

11. congenital narrowing of the large artery leading from the heart _____

12. a duct between the aorta and the pulmonary artery, which normally closes soon after birth,

   remains open _____

11

G **Give the meanings of the following terms.**

1. heart block _____

2. cardiac arrest _____

3. palpitations _____

4. artificial cardiac pacemaker _____

5. thrombotic occlusion _____

6. angina _____

7. myocardial infarction _____

8. necrosis _____

9. infarction _____

10. ischemia _____

11. nitroglycerin _____

12. digoxin _____

13. bruit _____

14. thrill _____

15. acute coronary syndromes _____

16. pericardial friction rub _____

17. deep vein thrombosis _____

18. biventricular pacemaker _____

11

H Match the following terms with their descriptions.

aneurysm	essential hypertension	Raynaud's disease
auscultation	murmur	rheumatic heart disease
claudication	peripheral arterial disease	secondary hypertension
emboli	petechiae	vegetations

1. lesions that form on heart valves after damage by infection _____

2. clots that travel to and suddenly block a blood vessel _____

3. small, pinpoint hemorrhages _____

4. an extra heart sound, heard between normal beats and caused by a valvular defect or condition

    that disrupts the smooth flow of blood through the heart _____

5. listening with a stethoscope _____

6. heart disease caused by rheumatic fever _____

7. high blood pressure in arteries when the etiology is idiopathic _____

8. high blood pressure related to kidney disease _____

9. episodes of pallor numbness, and cyanosis in fingers and toes caused by a temporary

    constriction of arterioles _____

10. local widening of an artery _____

11. pain, tension, and weakness in a limb after walking has begun _____

12. blockage of arteries in the lower extremities; etiology is atherosclerosis _____

I Give short answers for the following.

1. Types of drugs used to treat acute coronary syndromes include _____

    _____.

2. When damaged valves in veins fail to prevent the backflow of blood, a condition (swollen, twisted

    vein) that results is _____.

3. Swollen, twisted veins in the rectal region are called _____.

4. Name the four defects in tetralogy of Fallot from their descriptions:

    a. narrowing of the artery leading to the lungs from the heart _____

    b. gap in the wall between the ventricles _____

    c. the large vessel leading from the left ventricle moves over the interventricular septum

        _____

    d. excessive development of the wall of the right lower heart chamber _____

        _____

11

J **Select from the list of cardiac tests and procedures to complete the definitions that follow.**

angiography (arteriography)	defibrillation	lipid tests (profile)
cardiac biomarkers	echocardiography	lipoprotein electrophoresis
cardiac MRI	electrocardiography	stress test
coronary artery bypass grafting	endarterectomy	thallium 201 scan

1. surgical removal of plaque from the inner lining of an artery _____

2. application of brief electrical discharges across the chest to stop ventricular fibrillation and pulseless ventricular tachycardia _____

3. measurement of levels of fatty substances (cholesterol and triglycerides) in the bloodstream

   _____

4. measurement of the heart's response to physical exertion (patient monitored while jogging on a treadmill) _____

5. measurement of troponin-T and troponin-I after myocardial infarction

   _____

6. injection of contrast into vessels and x-ray imaging _____

7. recording of the electricity in the heart _____

8. intravenous injection of a radioactive substance and measurement of its accumulation in heart muscle _____

9. use of echoes from high-frequency sound waves to produce images of the heart

   _____

10. separation of HDL and LDL from a blood sample _____

11. anastomosis of vessel grafts to existing coronary arteries to maintain blood supply to the myocardium _____

12. beaming of magnetic waves at the heart to produce images of its structure

   _____

11

K **Give the meanings for the following terms.**

1. digital subtraction angiography _____

2. heart transplantation _____

3. ETT-MIBI _____

4. Doppler ultrasound _____

5. Holter monitoring _____

6. thrombolytic therapy _____

7. extracorporeal circulation _____

8. cardiac catheterization _____

9. percutaneous coronary intervention _____

10. drug-eluting stent _____

11. electron beam computed tomography _____

12. CT angiography _____

L **Identify the following cardiac dysrhythmias from their abbreviations.**

1. AF _____

2. VT _____

3. VF _____

4. PVC _____

5. PAC _____

M **Identify the following abnormal cardiac conditions from their abbreviations.**

1. CHF _____

2. VSD _____

3. MI _____

4. PDA _____

5. MVP _____

6. AS _____

7. CAD _____

8. ASD _____

11

N Match the listedabbreviations for cardiac tests and procedures with the explanations/descriptions that follow.

BNP   ECMO   LDL
CRT   ETT   LVAD
cTnI or cTnT   ETT-MIBI   RFA
ECHO   ICD   TEE

1. cardiac serum enzyme test for myocardial infarction _____

2. booster pump implanted in the abdomen with a cannula leading to the heart as a "bridge to transplant" _____

3. ultrasound imaging of the heart using transducer within the esophagus_____

4. device implanted in the chest that senses and corrects arrhythmias by shocking the heart

   _____

5. catheter delivery of a high-frequency current to damage a small portion of the heart muscle and reverse an abnormal heart rhythm _____

6. procedure to determine the heart's response to physical exertion (stress) _____

7. cardiac imaging using high-frequency sound waves pulsed through the chest wall and bounced off heart structures _____

8. radioactive test of heart function with stress test _____

9. technique using heart-lung machine to divert blood from the heart and lungs while the heart is being repaired _____

10. biventricular pacing to correct serious abnormal ventricular rhythms _____

11. lipoprotein sample is measured _____

12. brain chemical measured to identify patients at risk for complications after MI and with CHF

   _____

O Spell the terms correctly from its definition.

1. pertaining to the heart: _____ ary

2. not a normal heart rhythm: arr _____

3. abnormal condition of blueness: _____ osis

4. relaxation phase of the heartbeat: _____ tole

5. chest pain: _____ pectoris

6. inflammation of a vein: _____ itis

7. widening of a vessel: vaso _____

8. enlargement of the heart: cardio _____

9. hardening of arteries with fatty plaque: _____ sclerosis

10. swollen veins in the rectal region: _____ oids

P **Match the listed terms for cardiovascular procedures with the meanings/descriptions that follow.**

aneurysmorrhaphy	catheter ablation	pericardiocentesis
atherectomy	embolectomy	STEMI
BNP test	endarterectomy	thrombolytic therapy
CABG	PCI	valvotomy

1. incision of a heart valve _____

2. removal of a clot that has traveled into a blood vessel and suddenly caused occlusion

_____

3. coronary artery bypass grafting (to relieve ischemia) _____

4. surgical puncture to remove fluid from the pericardial space _____

5. insertion of a balloon-tipped catheter and stents into a coronary artery _____

6. removal of the inner lining of an artery to make it wider _____

7. suture (repair) of a ballooned-out portion of an artery _____

8. removal of plaque from an artery _____

9. type of acute coronary syndrome _____

10. use of streptokinase and tPA to dissolve clots _____

11. brief delivery of radiofrequency energy to destroy areas of heart tissue for treating arrhythmias

_____

12. measures a peptide elevated in patients with heart failure _____

11

Q **Select the boldface terms that best complete each sentence.**

1. Bill was having pain in his chest that radiated up his neck and down his arm. He called his family physician, who thought Bill should report to the local hospital's emergency department (ED) immediately. The first test performed in the ED was a/an **(stress test, ECG, CABG)**.

2. Dr. Kelly explained to the family that their observation of the bluish color of baby Charles's skin helped her make the diagnosis of a/an **(thrombotic, aneurysmal, septal)** defect in the baby's heart, which needed immediate attention.

3. Mr. Duggan had a fever of unknown origin. When the doctors completed an echocardiogram and saw vegetations on his mitral valve, they suspected **(bacterial endocarditis, hypertensive heart disease, angina)**.

4. Claudia's fingers turned white or bluish whenever she went out into the cold or became stressed. Her physician thought it might be wise to evaluate her for **(varicose veins, Raynaud's, intermittent claudication)**.

5. Daisy's heart felt like it was skipping beats every time she drank coffee. Her physician suggested that she wear a/an **(Holter monitor, LVAD, CABG)** for 24 hours to assess the nature of the arrhythmia.

6. Paola's father and grandfather died of heart attacks. Her physician tells her that she has inherited a tendency to accumulate fats in her bloodstream. Blood tests reveal high levels of **(enzymes, lipids, nitroglycerin)**. Discussing her family history with her **(gynecologist, hematologist, cardiologist)**, she understands that she has familial **(hypocholesterolemia, hypercholesterolemia, cardiomyopathy)**.

7. While exercising, Bernard experienced a pain (cramp) in his calf muscle. The pain disappeared when he was resting. After performing **(Holter monitoring, Doppler ultrasound, echocardiography)** on his leg to assess blood flow, Dr. Shaw found **(stenosis, fibrillation, endocarditis)**, indicating poor circulation. She recommended a daily exercise program, low-fat diet, careful foot care, and antiplatelet drug therapy to treat Bernard's intermittent **(palpitations, hypertension, claudication)**.

8. Carol noticed that her 6-week-old son Louis had a slightly bluish or **(jaundiced, cyanotic, diastolic)** coloration to his skin. She consulted a pediatric **(dermatologist, hematologist, cardiologist)**, who performed **(echocardiography, PET scan, endarterectomy)** and diagnosed Louis's condition as **(endocarditis, congestive heart disease, tetralogy of Fallot)**.

9. Seventy-eight-year-old John Smith has had coronary artery disease and high blood pressure for the past 10 years. His history included an acute heart attack, or **(MI, PDA, CABG)**. He often was tired and complained of **(dyspnea, nausea, migraine headaches)** and swelling in his ankles. His physician diagnosed his condition as **(aortic aneurysm, congestive heart failure, congenital heart disease)** and recommended restricted salt intake, diuretics, and an **(ACE inhibitor, antibiotic, analgesic)**.

10. Sarah had a routine checkup that included **(auscultation, vasoconstriction, vasodilation)** of her chest with a **(catheter, stent, stethoscope)** to listen to her heart. Her physician noticed a midsystolic murmur characteristic of **(DVT, MVP, LDL)**. An echocardiogram confirmed the diagnosis.

ANSWERS TO EXERCISES

A

1. tricuspid valve	5. superior vena cava	9. mitral valve
2. capillary	6. atrium	10. inferior vena cava
3. pulmonary vein	7. pulmonary artery	11. venule
4. aorta	8. arteriole	12. ventricle

B

1. right atrium	5. pulmonary artery	9. mitral valve
2. tricuspid valve	6. capillaries of the lung	10. left ventricle
3. right ventricle	7. pulmonary veins	11. aortic valve
4. pulmonary valve	8. left atrium	12. aorta

C

1. sinoatrial (SA) node	6. endocardium	10. visceral pericardium (the outer lining is the parietal pericardium)
2. pericardium	7. systole	
3. interatrial septum	8. carbon dioxide (CO_2)	11. murmur
4. diastole	9. atrioventricular (AV) node	12. pulse
5. atrioventricular bundle or bundle of His		

D

1. arteriosclerosis
2. cardiomyopathy
3. cardiomegaly
4. phlebitis
5. tachycardia
6. bradycardia
7. hypercholesterolemia
8. valvuloplasty
9. hypoxia
10. atrial
11. mitral stenosis
12. thrombolysis

E

1. bluish discoloration of the skin owing to deficient oxygen in the blood
2. incision of a vein
3. new connection between arteries
4. circulatory failure due to poor heart function
5. mass of yellowish plaque (fatty substance)
6. abnormal heart rhythm
7. instrument to measure blood pressure
8. instrument to listen to sounds within the chest
9. inflammation of the mitral valve
10. hardening of arteries with a yellowish, fatty substance (plaque)
11. narrowing of a vessel
12. widening of a vessel

F

1. endocarditis
2. flutter
3. atrial septal defect
4. mitral valve prolapse
5. coronary artery disease
6. hypertensive heart disease
7. fibrillation
8. pericarditis
9. congestive heart failure
10. tetralogy of Fallot
11. coarctation of the aorta
12. patent ductus arteriosus

G

1. failure of proper conduction of impulses through the AV node to the atrioventricular bundle (bundle of His)
2. sudden unexpected stoppage of heart action
3. uncomfortable sensations in the chest associated with arrhythmias
4. battery-operated device that is placed in the chest and wired to send electrical current to the heart to establish a normal sinus rhythm
5. blockage of a vessel by a clot
6. chest pain resulting from insufficient oxygen being supplied to the heart muscle (ischemia)
7. area of necrosis (tissue death in the heart muscle; heart attack)
8. abnormal condition of death (dead tissue)
9. damage or death of tissue due to deprivation of oxygen
10. blood is held back from an area of the body
11. nitrate drug used in the treatment of angina
12. drug that treats arrhythmias and strengthens the heartbeat
13. abnormal sound (murmur) heard on auscultation
14. vibration felt on palpation of the chest
15. consequences of plaque rupture in coronary arteries; MI and unstable angina
16. scraping or grating noise on auscultation of heart; indicates pericarditis
17. clot formation in a large vein, usually in lower limb
18. device enabling ventricles to beat in synchrony; cardiac resynchronization therapy

H

1. vegetations
2. emboli
3. petechiae
4. murmur
5. auscultation
6. rheumatic heart disease
7. essential hypertension
8. secondary hypertension
9. Raynaud's disease
10. aneurysm
11. claudication
12. peripheral arterial disease

I

1. beta blockers, ACE inhibitors, statins, aspirin, calcium channel blockers
2. varicose veins
3. hemorrhoids
4. a. pulmonary artery stenosis
   b. ventricular septal defect
   c. shift of the aorta to the right
   d. hypertrophy of the right ventricle

J

1. endarterectomy
2. defibrillation
3. lipid tests (profile)
4. stress test
5. cardiac biomarkers
6. angiography (arteriography)
7. electrocardiography
8. thallium 201 scan
9. echocardiography
10. lipoprotein electrophoresis
11. coronary artery bypass grafting
12. cardiac MRI

11

1. Video equipment and a computer produce x-ray pictures of blood vessels by taking two pictures (without and with contrast) and subtracting the first image (without contrast) from the second.
2. A donor heart is transferred to a recipient.
3. Exercise tolerance test combined with a radioactive tracer scan.
4. An instrument that focuses sound waves on a blood vessel to measure blood flow.
5. A compact version of an electrocardiograph is worn during a 24-hour period to detect cardiac arrhythmias.

6. Treatment with drugs (streptokinase and tPA) to dissolve clots after a heart attack.
7. A heart-lung machine is used to divert blood from the heart and lungs during surgery. The machine oxygenates the blood and sends it back into the bloodstream.
8. A catheter (tube) is inserted into an artery or vein and threaded into the heart chambers. Contrast can be injected to take x-ray pictures, patterns of blood flow can be detected, and blood pressures can be measured.

9. A balloon-tipped catheter is inserted into a coronary artery to open the artery; stents are put in place.
10. Stents are expandable slotted tubes that are placed in arteries during PCI. They release polymers that prevent plaque from reforming.
11. Electron beams and CT identify calcium deposits in and around coronary arteries to diagnose CAD.
12. X-ray images of the heart and coronary arteries obtained using CT technology.

L

1. atrial fibrillation
2. ventricular tachycardia
3. ventricular fibrillation

4. premature ventricular contraction
5. premature atrial contraction

M

1. congestive heart failure
2. ventricular septal defect
3. myocardial infarction

4. patent ductus arteriosus
5. mitral valve prolapse
6. aortic stenosis

7. coronary artery disease
8. atrial septal defect

1. cTnI or cTnT: cardiac troponin-I and troponin-T
2. LVAD: left ventricular assist device
3. TEE: transesophageal echocardiography
4. ICD: implantable cardioverter-defibrillator

5. RFA: radiofrequency catheter ablation
6. ETT: exercise tolerance test
7. ECHO: echocardiography
8. ETT-MIBI: exercise tolerance test with sestamibi scan

9. ECMO: extracorporeal membrane oxygenation
10. CRT: cardiac resynchronization therapy
11. LDL: low-density lipoprotein; high levels indicate risk for CAD
12. BNP: brain natriuretic peptide

O

1. coronary
2. arrhythmia
3. cyanosis
4. diastole

5. angina pectoris
6. phlebitis
7. vasodilation

8. cardiomegaly
9. atherosclerosis
10. hemorrhoids

P

1. valvotomy
2. embolectomy
3. CABG
4. pericardiocentesis
5. PCI

6. endarterectomy
7. aneurysmorrhaphy
8. atherectomy
9. STEMI (ST segment elevation myocardial infarction)

10. thrombolytic therapy
11. catheter ablation
12. BNP test

Q

1. ECG
2. septal
3. bacterial endocarditis
4. Raynaud's
5. Holter monitor
6. lipids; cardiologist; hypercholesterolemia

7. Doppler ultrasound; stenosis; claudication
8. cyanotic; cardiologist; echocardiography; tetralogy of Fallot

9. MI; dyspnea; congestive heart failure; ACE inhibitor
10. auscultation; stethoscope; MVP

Answers to Practical Applications

Operating Room Schedule

1. E	5. D	8. J
2. C	6. A	9. G
3. H	7. B	10. F
4. I		

Clinical Cases: What's Your Diagnosis?

Case 1	Case 2	Case 3
1. b	1. d	1. d
	2. a	2. a
	3. b	

PRONUNCIATION OF TERMS

To test your understanding of the terminology in this chapter, write the meaning of each term in the space provided. In addition, you may wish to cover the terms and write them by looking at your definitions. Make sure your spelling is correct. The page number after each term indicates where it is defined or used in the book, so you can easily check your responses. You will find complete definitions for all of these terms and their audio pronunciations on the Evolve website.

Pronunciation Guide

ā as in āpe	ă as in ăpple
ē as in ēven	ĕ as in ĕvery
ī as in īce	ĭ as in ĭnterest
ō as in ōpen	ŏ as in pŏt
ū as in ūnit	ŭ as in ŭnder

Vocabulary and Terminology

TERM	PRONUNCIATION	MEANING
angiogram (411)	ĂN-jē-ō-grăm	
angioplasty (411)	ĂN-jē-ō-plăs-tē	
anoxia (413)	ă-NŎK-sē-ă	
aorta (410)	ā-ŌR-tă	
aortic stenosis (411)	ā-ŌR-tĭk stĕ-NŌ-sĭs	
apex of the heart (410)	Ā-pĕks of the hărt	
arrhythmia (413)	ā-RĬTH-mē-ă	
arterial anastomosis (411)	ăr-TĒ-rē-ăl ă-năs-tō-MŌ-sĭs	
arteriography (411)	ăr-tē-rē-ŎG-ră-fē	
arteriole (410)	ăr-TĒ-rē-ōl	
arteriosclerosis (411)	ăr-tē-rē-ō-sklĕ-RŌ-sĭs	
artery (410)	ĂR-tĕ-rē	
atherectomy (412)	ă-thĕ-RĔK-tō-mē	
atheroma (412)	ăth-ĕr-Ō-mă	
atherosclerosis (412)	ăth-ĕr-ō-sklĕ-RŌ-sĭs	

11

TERM	PRONUNCIATION	MEANING
atrial (412)	Ā-trē-ăl	_____
atrioventricular bundle (410)	ā-trē-ō-věn-TRĬK-ū-lăr BŬN-dl	_____
atrioventricular node (410)	ā-trē-ō-věn-TRĬK-ū-lăr nōd	_____
atrium; atria (410)	Ā-trē-ŭm; Ā-trē-ă	_____
brachial artery (412)	BRĀ-kē-ăl ĂR-tě-rē	_____
bradycardia (412)	brād-ē-KĂR-dē-ă	_____
bundle of His (410)	BŬN-dl of Hĭss	_____
capillary (410)	KĂP-ĭ-lăr-ē	_____
carbon dioxide (410)	KĂR-bŏn dī-ŎK-sīd	_____
cardiogenic shock (412)	kăr-dē-ō-JĔN-ĭk shŏk	_____
cardiomegaly (412)	kăr-dē-ō-MĔG-ă-lē	_____
cardiomyopathy (412)	kăr-dē-ō-mī-ŎP-ă-thē	_____
coronary arteries (410)	KŎR-ō-năr-ē ĂR-tě-rēz	_____
cyanosis (413)	sī-ă-NŌ-sĭs	_____
deoxygenated blood (410)	dē-ŎK-sĭ-jě-NĀ-těd blŭd	_____
diastole (410)	dī-ĂS-tō-lē	_____
electrocardiogram (410)	ě-lěk-trō-KĂR-dē-ō-grăm	_____
endocardium (410)	ěn-dō-KĂR-dē-ŭm	_____
endothelium (410)	ěn-dō-THĒ-lē-um	_____
hypercholesterolemia (412)	hī-pěr-kō-lěs-těr-ŏl-Ē-mē-ă	_____
hypoxia (413)	hī-PŎK-sē-ă	_____
interventricular septum (414)	ĭn-těr-věn-TRĬK-ū-lăr SĔP-tŭm	_____
mitral valve (410)	MĪ-trăl vălv	_____
mitral valvulitis (414)	MĪ-trăl văl-vū-LĪ-tĭs	_____
myocardium (410)	mī-ō-KĂR-dē-ŭm	_____
myxoma (413)	mĭk-SŌ-mă	_____
normal sinus rhythm (410)	NŎR-măl SĪ-nus RĬ-thěm	_____
oxygen (410)	ŎK-sĭ-jěn	_____
pacemaker (410)	PĀS-mā-kěr	_____
pericardiocentesis (413)	pěr-ĭ-kăr-dē-ō-sěn-TĒ-sĭs	_____
pericardium (410)	pěr-ĭ-KĂR-dē-ŭm	_____

11

TERM	PRONUNCIATION	MEANING
phlebotomy (413)	flĕ-BŎT-ō-mē	
pulmonary artery (410)	PŬL-mō-nĕr-ē ĂR-tĕr-ē	
pulmonary circulation (410)	PŬL-mō-nĕr-ē sĕr-kū-LĀ-shŭn	
pulmonary valve (411)	PŬL-mō-nĕr-ē vălv	
pulmonary vein (411)	PŬL-mō-nĕr-ē vān	
pulse (411)	pŭls	
septum; septa (411)	SĔP-tŭm; SĔP-tă	
sinoatrial node (411)	sī-nō-Ā-trē-ăl nōd	
sphygmomanometer (411)	sfĭg-mō-mă-NŎM-ĕ-tĕr	
stethoscope (413)	STĔTH-ō-skōp	
systemic circulation (411)	sĭs-TĔM-ĭk sĕr-kū-LĀ-shŭn	
systole (411)	SĬS-tō-lē	
tachycardia (412)	tăk-ē-KĂR-dē-ă	
thrombolysis (413)	thrŏm-BŎL-ĭ-sĭs	
thrombophlebitis (413)	thrŏm-bō-flĕ-BĪ-tĭs	
tricuspid valve (411)	trī-KŬS-pĭd vălv	
valve (411)	vălv	
valvotomy (414)	văl-VŎT-ō-mē	
valvuloplasty (414)	văl-vū-lō-PLĂS-tē	
vascular (414)	VĂS-kū-lăr	
vasoconstriction (414)	văz-ō-kōn-STRĬK-shŭn	
vasodilation (414)	văz-ō-dī-LĀ-shŭn	
vein (411)	vān	
vena cava; venae cavae (411)	VĒ-nă KĀ-vă; VĒ-nē KĀ-vē	
venipuncture (414)	vĕ-nĭ-PŬNK-chŭr	
venous (414)	VĒ-nŭs	
ventricle (411)	VĔN-trĭ-kl	
venule (411)	VĔN-ūl	

11

Pathology, Laboratory Tests, and Clinical Procedures

TERM	PRONUNCIATION	MEANING
ACE inhibitor (426)	ĀCE ĭn-HĬB-ĭ-tŏr	
acute coronary syndromes (426)	ă-KŪT kŏr-ō-NĂR-ē SĬN-drōmz	
aneurysm (423)	ĂN-ū-rĭzm	
angina (426)	ăn-JĪ-nă *or* ĂN-jĭ-nă	
angiography (427)	ăn-jē-ŎG-ră-fē	
atrioventricular block (414)	ā-trē-ō-vĕn-TRĬK-ū-lăr blŏk	
atrial fibrillation (416)	Ā-trē-ăl fĭb-rĭ-LĀ-shŭn	
auscultation (426)	ăw-skŭl-TĀ-shŭn	
beta blocker (426)	BĀ-tă BLŎK-ĕr	
biventricular pacemaker (426)	bī-vĕn-TRĬK-ū-lăr PĀS-mā-kĕr	
BNP test (427)	BNP tĕst	
bruit (426)	BRŪ-ē	
calcium channel blocker (426)	KĂL-sē-ŭm CHĂ-nĕl BLŎK-ĕr	
cardiac arrest (426)	KĂR-dē-ăk ā-RĔST	
cardiac catheterization (430)	KĂR-dē-ăk kăth-ĕ-tĕr-ĭ-ZĀ-shŭn	
cardiac MRI (430)	KĂR-dē-ăk MRI	
cardiac biomarkers (427)	KĂR-dē-ăk BĪ-ō-mar-kerz	
cardiac tamponade (426)	KĂR-dē-ăk tăm-pō-NŎD	
cardioversion (432)	kăr-dē-ō-VĔR-zhŭn	
catheter ablation (432)	KĂTH-ĕ-tĕr ăb-LĀ-shŭn	
claudication (426)	klăw-dĕ-KĀ-shŭn	
coarctation of the aorta (417)	kō-ărk-TĀ-shŭn of the ā-ŎR-tă	
computed tomography angiography (428)	kŏm-PŪ-tĕd tō-MŎG-ră-fē ăn-jē-ŎG-ră-fē	
congenital heart disease (417)	kŏn-GĔN-ĭ-tăl hărt dĭ-ZĒZ	
congestive heart failure (419)	kŏn-GĔS-tĭv hărt FĀL-ŭr	
coronary artery disease (419)	kŏr-ō-NĂR-ē ĂR-tĕ-rē dĭ-ZĒZ	
coronary artery bypass grafting (432)	kŏr-ō-NĂR-ē ĂR-tĕ-rē BĪ-păs GRĂF-tĭng	
deep vein thrombosis (424)	dēp vān thrŏm-BŌ-sĭs	
defibrillation (432)	dē-fĭb-rĭ-LĀ-shun	

TERM	PRONUNCIATION	MEANING
digoxin (426)	dĭ-JŎK-sĭn	
digital subtraction angiography (428)	DĬJ-ĭ-tăl sŭb-TRĂK-shŭn ăn-jē-ŎG-ră-fē	
Doppler ultrasound (428)	DŎP-lĕr ŬL-tră-sŏnd	
dysrhythmia (414)	dĭs-RĬTH-mē-ă	
echocardiography (429)	ĕk-ō-kăr-dē-ŎG-ră-fē	
electrocardiography (430)	ē-lĕk-trō-kăr-dē-ŎG-ră-fē	
electron beam computed tomography (428)	ē-LĔK-trŏn bēm kŏm-PŪ-tĕd tō-MŎG-ră-fē	
embolus; emboli (426)	ĔM-bō-lŭs; ĔM-bō-lī	
endarterectomy (433)	ĕnd ăr-tĕr-ĔK-tō-mē	
endocarditis (422)	ĕn-dō-kăr-DĪ-tĭs	
extracorporeal circulation (433)	ĕks-tră-kŏr-PŎR-ē-ăl sĕr-kū-LĀ shŭn	
fibrillation (416)	fĭb-rĭ-LĀ-shŭn	
flutter (416)	FLŬ-tĕr	
heart block (414)	hărt blŏk	
heart transplantation (433)	hărt trănz-plăn-TĀ-shŭn	
hemorrhoids (425)	HĔM-ō-roydz	
Holter monitoring (431)	HŌL-tĕr MŎN-ĭ-tĕ-rĭng	
hypertension (424)	hī-pĕr-TĔN-shŭn	
hypertensive heart disease (422)	hī-pĕr-TĔN-sĭv hărt dĭ-ZĒZ	
implantable cardioverter-defibrillator (416)	ĭm-PLĂNT-ă-bŭl kăr-dē-ō-VĔR-tĕr dē-FĬB-rĭ-lă-tŏr	
infarction (426)	ĭn-FĂRK-shŭn	
ischemia (425)	ĭs-KĒ-mē-ă	
left ventricular assist device (419)	lĕft vĕn-TRĬ-kū-lăr ă-SĬST dē-VĪS	
lipid tests (427)	LĬ-pĭd tĕsts	
lipoprotein electrophoresis (427)	lī-pō-PRŌ-tēn ē-lĕk-trō-fŏr-Ē-sĭs	
mitral stenosis (423)	MĪ-trăl stĕ-NŌ-sĭs	
mitral valve prolapse (422)	MĪ-trăl vălv PRŌ-laps	
murmur (422)	MŬR-mĕr	

11

TERM	PRONUNCIATION	MEANING
myocardial infarction (420)	mī-ō-KĂR-dē-ăl ĭn-FĂRK-shŭn	
nitrates (426)	nī-TRĀTZ	
nitroglycerin (426)	nī-trō-GLĬS-ĕr-ĭn	
occlusion (426)	ŏ-KLŪ-jŭn	
palpitations (426)	păl-pĭ-TĀ-shŭnz	
patent (426)	PĀ-tĕnt	
patent ductus arteriosus (417)	PĀ-tĕnt DŬK-tŭs ăr-tēr-ē-Ō-sŭs	
percutaneous coronary intervention (433)	pĕr-kū-TĀ-nē-ŭs KŎR-ō-năr-ē ĭn-tĕr-VĔN-shŭn	
pericardial friction rub (426)	pĕr-ĭ-KĂR-dē-ăl FRĬK-shŭn rŭb	
pericarditis (420)	pĕr-ĭ-kăr-DĪ-tĭs	
peripheral arterial disease (422)	pĕ-RĬ-fĕr-ăl ăr-TĒ-rē-ăl dĭ-ZĒZ	
petechiae (426)	pĕ-TĒ-kē-ē	
positron emission tomography (429)	pŏs-ĭ-tron ē-MĬSH-un tō-MŎG-ră-fē	
Raynaud's disease (424)	rā-NŌZ dĭ-ZĒZ	
rheumatic heart disease (423)	roo-MĂT-ik hărt dĭ-ZĒZ	
septal defects (418)	SĔP-tăl DĒ-fĕkts	
statins (426)	STĂ-tĭnz	
stress test (431)	STRĔS tĕst	
telemetry (430)	tĕl-ĔM-ĕ-trē	
tetralogy of Fallot (418)	tĕ-TRĂL-ō-jē of fă-LŌ	
technetium Tc99m sestamibi scan (429)	tĕk-NĒ-shē-ŭm Tc99m sĕs-tă-MĬ-bē skăn	
thallium 201 scan (429)	THĂL-ē-um 201 skăn	
thrill (426)	thrĭl	
thrombolytic therapy (434)	thrŏm-bō-LĬ-tĭk THĔ-ră-pē	
thrombotic occlusion (420)	thrŏm-BŎT-ĭk ŏ-KLŪ-zhĕn	
transcatheter aortic valve replacement (434)	trănz-KĂTH-ĕ-tĕr ā-ŎR-tĭk valve rē-PLĀS-mĕnt	
varicose veins (424)	VĂR-ĭ-kōs vānz	
vegetations (426)	vĕj-ĕ-TĀ-shŭnz	

11

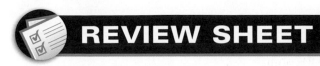

REVIEW SHEET

Write the meanings of each word part in the space provided. Check your answers with the information in the chapter or in the **Glossary (Medical Word Parts—English)** at the end of the book.

Combining Forms

COMBINING FORM	MEANING	COMBINING FORM	MEANING
aneurysm/o		ox/o	
angi/o		pericardi/o	
aort/o		phleb/o	
arter/o, arteri/o		pulmon/o	
ather/o		rrhythm/o	
atri/o		sphygm/o	
axill/o		steth/o	
brachi/o		thromb/o	
cardi/o		valv/o	
cholesterol/o		valvul/o	
coron/o		vas/o	
cyan/o		vascul/o	
isch/o		ven/o, ven/i	
my/o		ventricul/o	
myx/o			

Suffixes

SUFFIX	MEANING	SUFFIX	MEANING
-constriction		-oma	
-dilation		-osis	
-emia		-plasty	
-graphy		-sclerosis	
-lysis		-stenosis	
-megaly		-tomy	
-meter			

Prefixes

PREFIX	MEANING	PREFIX	MEANING
a-, an-	_____	hypo-	_____
brady-	_____	inter-	_____
de-	_____	peri-	_____
dys-	_____	tachy-	_____
endo-	_____	tetra-	_____
hyper-	_____	tri-	_____

Use the listed cardiovascular anatomy terms to complete the accompanying chart.

aorta
inferior vena cava
left atrium
left ventricle

lung capillaries
mitral valve
pulmonary artery
pulmonary vein

right atrium
right ventricle
superior vena cava
tricuspid valve

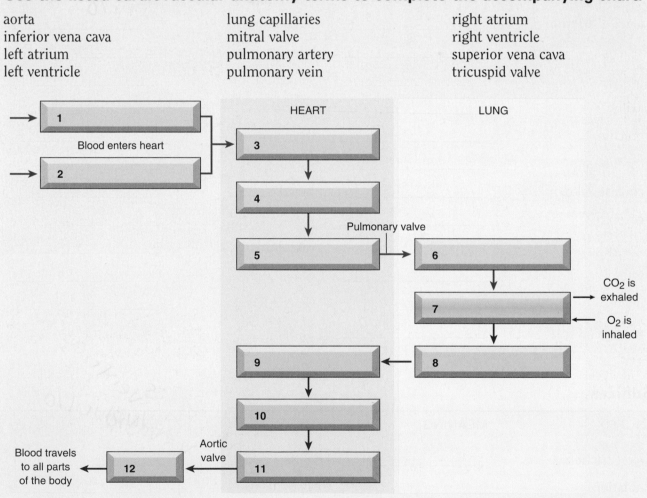

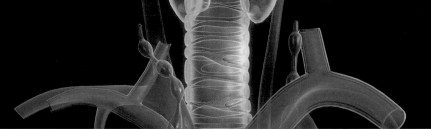

Respiratory System

CHAPTER GOALS

- Name the organs of the respiratory system and their location and function.
- Identify pathologic conditions that affect the respiratory system.
- Learn medical terms that pertain to respiration.
- Describe important clinical procedures related to the respiratory system, and recognize relevant abbreviations.
- Apply your new knowledge to understanding medical terms in their proper contexts, such as medical reports and records.

INTRODUCTION

We usually think of **respiration** as the mechanical process of breathing, the exchange of air between the lungs and the external environment. This exchange of air at the lungs is called **external respiration.** In external respiration, oxygen is inhaled (inhaled air contains about 21% oxygen) into the air spaces (sacs) of the lungs and immediately passes into tiny blood vessels (capillaries) surrounding the air spaces. Simultaneously, carbon dioxide, a gas produced when oxygen and food combine in cells, passes from the capillary blood vessels into the air spaces of the lungs to be exhaled.

Whereas external respiration occurs between the outside environment and the capillary blood of the lungs, another form of respiration occurs simultaneously between the individual body cells and the tiny capillary blood vessels that surround them. This is **internal (cellular) respiration,** which involves an exchange of gases at the level of the cells within all organs of the body. Here, oxygen passes out of the capillaries into tissue cells. At the same time, carbon dioxide passes from tissue cells into the capillaries to travel to the lungs for exhalation.

ANATOMY AND PHYSIOLOGY OF RESPIRATION

Label Figure 12-1 as you read the following paragraphs.

Air enters the body via the **nose** [1] through two openings called nostrils or **nares.** Air then passes through the **nasal cavity** [2], lined with a mucous membrane and fine hairs **(cilia)** to help filter out foreign bodies, as well as to warm and moisten the air. **Paranasal sinuses** [3] are hollow, air-containing spaces within the skull that communicate with the nasal cavity. They, too, have a mucous membrane lining. Besides producing mucus, a lubricating fluid, the sinuses lighten the bones of the skull and help produce sound.

After passing through the nasal cavity, the air next reaches the **pharynx (throat).** There are three divisions of the pharynx. The first is the **nasopharynx** [4]. It contains the **pharyngeal tonsils,** or **adenoids** [5], which are collections of lymphatic tissue. They are more prominent in children and, if enlarged, can obstruct air passageways. Below the nasopharynx and closer to the mouth is the second division of the pharynx, the **oropharynx** [6]. The **palatine tonsils** [7], two rounded masses of lymphatic tissue, are in the oropharynx. The third division of the pharynx, the **laryngopharynx** [8], serves as a common passageway for food from the mouth and air from the nose. It divides into the **larynx (voice box)** [9] and the **esophagus** [10].

The esophagus leads into the stomach and carries food to be digested. The larynx contains the vocal cords and is surrounded by pieces of cartilage for support and to keep the airway open. The thyroid cartilage is the largest and in men is commonly referred to as the Adam's apple. As expelled air passes the vocal cords, they vibrate to produce sounds. The tension of the vocal cords determines the high or low pitch of the voice.

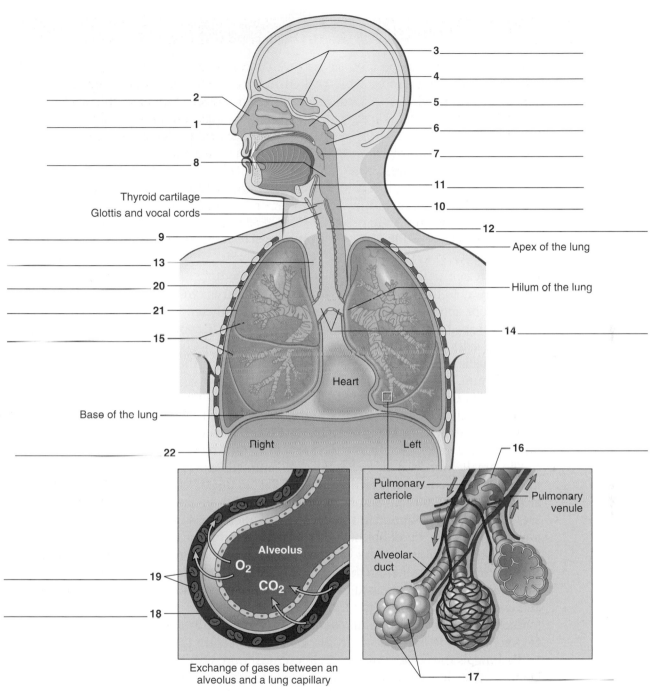

Thyroid cartilage
Glottis and vocal cords

Apex of the lung

Hilum of the lung

Base of the lung

Heart

Right   Left

Pulmonary
arteriole

Pulmonary
venule

Alveolar
duct

Alveolus

O_2

CO_2

Exchange of gases between an
alveolus and a lung capillary

FIGURE 12-1 Organs of the respiratory system.

Because food entering from the mouth and air entering from the nose mix in the pharynx, what prevents food or drink from entering the larynx and respiratory system during swallowing? Even if a small quantity of solid or liquid matter finds its way into the air passages, aspirated food can cause irritation in the lungs and breathing can stop. The **epiglottis** [11], a flap of cartilage attached to the root of the tongue, prevents choking or aspiration of food. It acts as a lid over the opening of the larynx. During swallowing, when food and liquid move through the throat, the epiglottis closes over the larynx, preventing material from entering the lungs. Figure 12-2 shows the larynx from a superior view.

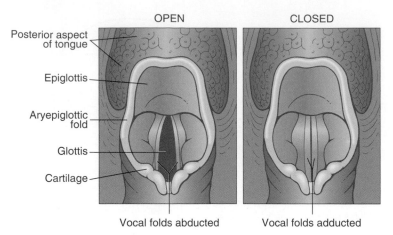

FIGURE 12-2   The larynx, viewed from above (superior view).

On its way to the lungs, air passes through the larynx to the **trachea (windpipe)** [12], a vertical tube about 4½ inches long and 1 inch in diameter. The trachea is kept open by 16 to 20 C-shaped rings of cartilage separated by fibrous connective tissue that stiffen the front and sides of the tube.

The **mediastinum** [13] is a space in the center of the chest. In the region of the mediastinum, the trachea divides into two branches, the right and left **bronchial tubes,** or **bronchi** [14] (*singular:* **bronchus**). The bronchi are tubes composed of delicate epithelium surrounded by cartilage rings and a muscular wall. Each bronchus leads to a separate **lung** [15], where it divides and subdivides into smaller and finer tubes, somewhat like the branches of a tree.

The small bronchial branches are the **bronchioles.** Each **terminal bronchiole** [16] narrows into alveolar ducts, which end in collections of air sacs called **alveoli** [17] (*singular:* **alveolus**). About 300 million alveoli are estimated to be present in both lungs. The total area of the alveoli is approximately the size of a tennis court. Each alveolus is lined with a one-cell-thick layer of epithelium. This very thin wall permits an exchange of gases between the alveolus and the **capillary** [18] surrounding it. Blood flowing through the capillary accepts oxygen from the alveolus while depositing carbon dioxide into the alveolus. **Erythrocytes** [19] in the blood carry oxygen away from the lungs to all parts of the body and carbon dioxide back to the lungs for exhalation.

Each lung is covered by a double-layered membrane called the **pleura.** The outer layer of this membrane, nearer the ribs, is the **parietal pleura** [20], and the inner layer, closer to the lung, is the **visceral pleura** [21]. A serous (thin, watery fluid) secretion moistens the pleura and facilitates movements of the lungs within the chest (thorax).

The two lungs are not quite mirror images of each other. The slightly larger right lung is divided into three **lobes,** whereas the smaller left lung has two lobes. One lobe of the lung can be removed without significantly compromising lung function. The uppermost part of the lung is the **apex,** and the lower area is the **base.** The **hilum** of the lung is the midline region in which blood vessels, nerves, lymphatic tissue, and bronchial tubes enter and exit.

The lungs extend from the collarbone to the **diaphragm** [22] in the thoracic cavity. The diaphragm is a muscular partition separating the thoracic from the abdominal cavity and aiding in the process of breathing. It contracts and descends with each **inhalation (inspiration)** and relaxes and ascends with each **exhalation (expiration).** The downward movement of the diaphragm enlarges the area in the thoracic cavity, decreasing internal air pressure, so that air flows into the lungs to equalize the pressure. When the lungs are full, the diaphragm relaxes and elevates, making the area in the thoracic cavity smaller,

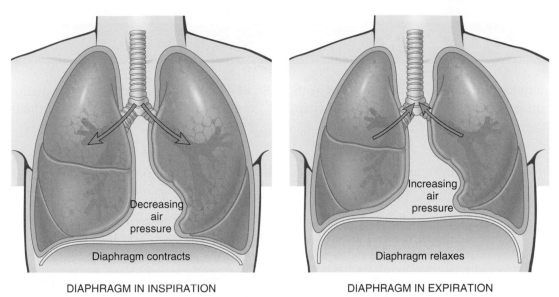

Decreasing
air
pressure

Diaphragm contracts

DIAPHRAGM IN INSPIRATION

Increasing
air
pressure

Diaphragm relaxes

DIAPHRAGM IN EXPIRATION

FIGURE 12-3   Position of the diaphragm during inspiration (inhalation) and expiration (exhalation).

thus increasing air pressure in the chest. Air then is expelled out of the lungs to equalize the pressure; this is **exhalation (expiration).**

Figure 12-3 shows the position of the diaphragm in inspiration and in expiration.

Figure 12-4 is a flow diagram of the pathway of air from the nose, where air enters the body, to the capillaries of the lungs, where oxygen enters the bloodstream.

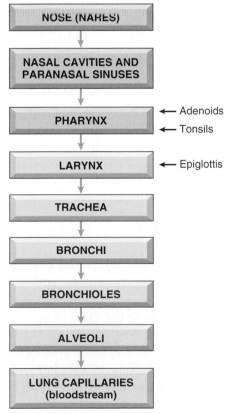

NOSE (NARES)

NASAL CAVITIES AND
PARANASAL SINUSES

PHARYNX   ← Adenoids
← Tonsils

LARYNX   ← Epiglottis

TRACHEA

BRONCHI

BRONCHIOLES

ALVEOLI

LUNG CAPILLARIES
(bloodstream)

FIGURE 12-4   Pathway of air from the nose to the capillaries of the lungs.

VOCABULARY

This list reviews terminology introduced in the preceding section. Short definitions and additional information will reinforce your understanding. Refer to the Pronunciation of Terms on page 496 for help with difficult or unfamiliar words.

adenoids	Lymphatic tissue in the nasopharynx; pharyngeal tonsils.
alveolus (*plural:* **alveoli**)	Air sac in the lung.
apex of the lung	Tip or uppermost portion of the lung. An apex is the tip of a structure. **Apical** means pertaining to or located at the apex. The apex of the heart is at the bottom of the heart.
base of the lung	Lower portion of the lung; from the Greek *basis*, foundation. **Basilar** means located at or in the base.
bronchioles	Smallest branches of the bronchi. Terminal bronchioles lead to alveolar ducts.
bronchus (*plural:* **bronchi**)	Branch of the trachea (windpipe) that is a passageway into the lung; bronchial tube.
carbon dioxide (CO₂)	Gas produced by body cells when oxygen and carbon atoms from food combine; exhaled through the lungs.
cilia	Thin hairs attached to the mucous membrane epithelium lining the respiratory tract. They clear bacteria and foreign substances from the lung. Cigarette smoke impairs the function of cilia.
diaphragm	Muscle separating the chest and abdomen. It contracts to pull air into the lungs and relaxes to push air out.
epiglottis	Lid-like piece of cartilage that covers the larynx, preventing food from entering the larynx and trachea during swallowing.
expiration	Breathing out (exhalation).
glottis	Slit-like opening to the larynx.
hilum of the lung	Midline region where the bronchi, blood vessels, and nerves enter and exit the lungs. **Hilar** means pertaining to (at) the hilum.
inspiration	Breathing in (inhalation).
larynx	Voice box; containing the vocal cords.
lobe	Division of a lung.
mediastinum	Region between the lungs in the chest cavity. It contains the trachea, heart, lymph nodes, aorta, esophagus, and bronchial tubes.
nares	Openings through the nose carrying air into the nasal cavities.
oxygen (O₂)	Gas that makes up 21 percent of the air. It passes into the bloodstream at the lungs and travels to all body cells.
palatine tonsil	One of a pair of almond-shaped masses of lymphatic tissue in the oropharynx (palatine means pertaining to the roof of the mouth).
paranasal sinus	One of the air cavities in the bones near the nose.
parietal pleura	Outer layer of pleura lying closer to the ribs and chest wall.

12

pharynx	Throat; including the nasopharynx, oropharynx, and laryngopharynx.
pleura	Double-layered membrane surrounding each lung.
pleural cavity	Space between the folds of the pleura.
pulmonary parenchyma	Essential parts of the lung, responsible for respiration; bronchioles and alveoli.
respiration	Process of moving air into and out of the lungs; breathing
trachea	Windpipe.
visceral pleura	Inner layer of pleura lying closer to the lung tissue.

TERMINOLOGY

Write the meanings of the medical terms in the spaces provided.

COMBINING FORMS

COMBINING FORM	MEANING	TERMINOLOGY	MEANING
adenoid/o	adenoids	adenoidectomy _____	
		adenoid hypertrophy _____	
alveol/o	alveolus, air sac	alveolar _____	
bronch/o bronchi/o	bronchial tube, bronchus	bronchospasm _____ *This tightening of the bronchus is a chief characteristic of asthma and bronchitis.*	
		bronchiectasis _____ *Caused by weakening of the bronchial wall from infection.*	
		bronchodilator _____ *This drug causes dilation, or enlargement, of the opening of a bronchus to improve ventilation to the lungs. An example is albuterol, delivered via an inhaler.*	
		bronchopleural _____ *A **bronchopleural fistula** is an abnormal connection between the bronchial tube and the pleural cavity (space). Occurring as a result of lung disease or surgical complication, this can cause an air leak into the pleural space.*	
bronchiol/o	bronchiole, small bronchus	bronchiolitis _____ *This is an acute viral infection occurring in infants younger than 18 months of age.*	
capn/o	carbon dioxide	hypercapnia _____	
coni/o	dust	pneumoconiosis _____ *See page 474.*	

12

COMBINING FORM	MEANING	TERMINOLOGY	MEANING
cyan/o	blue	cyanosis	
		Caused by deficient oxygen in the blood.	
epiglott/o	epiglottis	epiglottitis	
		Characterized by fever, sore throat, and an erythematous, swollen epiglottis.	
laryng/o	larynx, voice box	laryngeal	
		laryngospasm	
		Spasm of laryngeal muscles that closes the larynx.	
		laryngitis	
lob/o	lobe of the lung	lobectomy	
		Figure 12-5 shows four different types of pulmonary resections.	

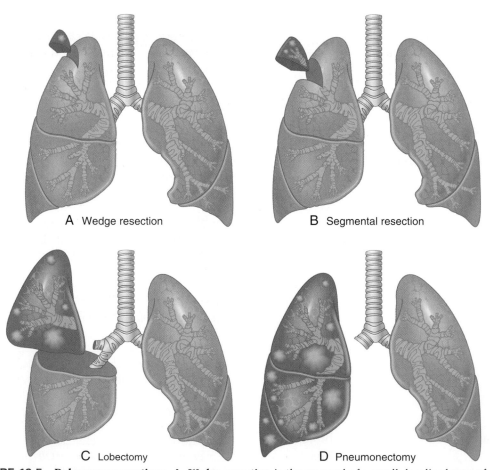

A Wedge resection B Segmental resection

C Lobectomy D Pneumonectomy

FIGURE 12-5 Pulmonary resections. A, Wedge resection is the removal of a small, localized area of diseased tissue near the surface of the lung. Pulmonary function and structure are relatively unchanged after healing. **B, Segmental resection** is the removal of a bronchiole and its alveoli (one or more lung segments). The remaining lung tissue expands to fill the previously occupied space. **C, Lobectomy** is the removal of an entire lobe of the lung. After lobectomy, the remaining lung increases in size to fill the space in the thoracic cavity. **D, Pneumonectomy** is the removal of an entire lung. Techniques such as removal of ribs and elevation of the diaphragm are used to reduce the size of the empty thoracic space.

COMBINING FORM	MEANING	TERMINOLOGY	MEANING
mediastin/o	mediastinum	mediastinoscopy _____ *An endoscope is inserted through an incision in the chest.*	
nas/o	nose	paranasal sinuses _____ *Para- means near in this term.*	
		nasogastric intubation _____	
orth/o	straight, upright	orthopnea _____ *An abnormal condition in which breathing (-pnea) is easier in the upright position. A major cause of orthopnea is congestive heart failure (the lungs fill with fluid when the patient is lying flat). Physicians assess the degree of orthopnea by the number of pillows a patient requires to sleep comfortably (e.g., two-pillow orthopnea).*	
ox/o	oxygen	hypoxia _____ *Tissues have a decreased amount of oxygen, and cyanosis can result.*	
pector/o	chest	expectoration _____ *Clearing of secretions from the airway by coughing or spitting. This sputum can contain mucus, blood, cellular debris, pus, and microorganisms.*	
pharyng/o	pharynx, throat	pharyngeal _____	
phon/o	voice	dysphonia _____ *Hoarseness or other voice impairment.*	
phren/o	diaphragm	phrenic nerve _____ *The motor nerve to the diaphragm.*	
pleur/o	pleura	pleurodynia _____ *The suffix -dynia means pain. The intercostal muscles or pleura are inflamed, causing pain during breathing.*	
		pleural effusion _____ *An **effusion** is the escape of fluid from blood vessels or lymphatics into a cavity or into tissue spaces.*	

12

COMBINING FORM	MEANING	TERMINOLOGY	MEANING
pneum/o, pneumon/o	air, lung	pneumothorax _____ *The suffix -thorax means chest. Because of a hole in the lung, air accumulates in the pleural cavity, between the layers of the pleura (Figure 12-6).*	
		pneumonectomy _____	
pulmon/o	lung	pulmonary _____	
rhin/o	nose	rhinoplasty _____	
		rhinorrhea _____ *Commonly known as "runny nose."*	
sinus/o	sinus, cavity	sinusitis _____	
spir/o	breathing	spirometer _____	
		expiration _____ *Note that the s is omitted (when it's preceded by an x).*	
		respiration _____ ***Cheyne-Stokes respirations*** *are marked by rhythmic changes in the depth of breathing (rapid breathing and then absence of breathing). The pattern occurs every 45 seconds to 3 minutes. The cause may be heart failure or brain damage, both of which affect the respiratory center in the brain.*	

12

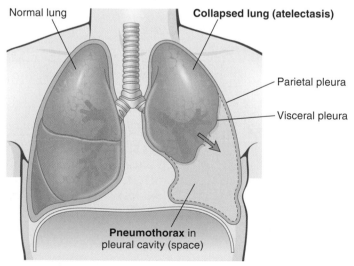

FIGURE 12-6   Pneumothorax. Air gathers in the pleural cavity, causing the lung to collapse. When this happens, the lung cannot fill up with air, breathing becomes more difficult, and the body gets less oxygen. Onset of pneumothorax is marked by sudden, sharp chest pain with difficulty breathing.

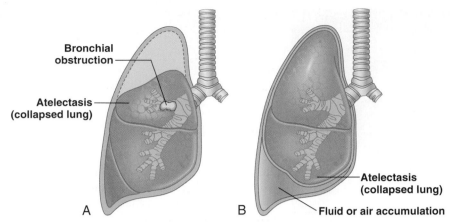

FIGURE 12-7 **Two forms of atelectasis. A, Bronchial obstruction** prevents air from reaching distal airways, and alveoli collapse. The most frequent cause is blockage of a bronchus by a mucous or mucopurulent (pus-containing) plug, as might occur postoperatively. **B, Accumulations of fluid, blood, or air within the pleural cavity collapse the lung.** This can occur with congestive heart failure (poor circulation leads to fluid buildup in the pleural cavity), pneumonia, trauma, or a pneumothorax.

COMBINING FORM	MEANING	TERMINOLOGY	MEANING
tel/o	complete	atelectasis	
		Collapsed lung; incomplete expansion (-ectasis) of a lung (Figure 12-7). Atelectasis may occur after surgery when a patient experiences pain and does not take deep breaths, preventing full expansion of the lungs.	
thorac/o	chest	thoracotomy	
		thoracic	
tonsill/o	tonsils	tonsillectomy	
		The oropharyngeal (palatine) tonsils are removed.	
trache/o	trachea, windpipe	tracheotomy	
		tracheal stenosis	
		Injury to the trachea from trauma, a burn, or serious infection can cause scarring and contraction that obstructs the flow of air. For example, having an endotracheal tube in place for a prolonged period may lead to tracheal injury or the formation of scar tissue.	

SUFFIXES

SUFFIX	MEANING	TERMINOLOGY	MEANING
-ema	condition	empyema	
		Em- at the beginning of this term means in. Empyema (pyothorax) is a collection of pus in the pleural cavity.	
-osmia	smell	anosmia	

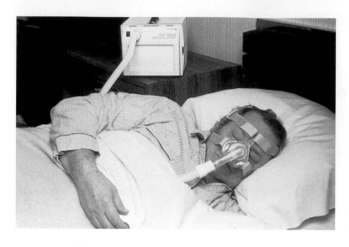

FIGURE 12-8 This man is sleeping with a **nasal CPAP (continuous positive airway pressure)** mask in place. The pressure supplied by air coming from the compressor opens the oropharynx and nasopharynx.

SUFFIX	MEANING	TERMINOLOGY	MEANING
-pnea	breathing	apnea	
		Sleep apnea is sudden cessation of breathing during sleep. It can result in hypoxia, leading to cognitive impairment, hypertension, and arrhythmias. Obstructive sleep apnea (OSA) involves narrowing or occlusion in the upper airway. Continuous positive airway pressure (CPAP) is gentle ventilatory support used to keep the airways open (Figure 12-8).	
		dyspnea	
		Dys- means abnormal here and is associated with shortness of breath (SOB). Paroxysmal (sudden) nocturnal (at night) dyspnea may be experienced by patients with congestive heart failure when they recline in bed. Patients often describe the sensation as "air hunger."	
		hyperpnea	
		An increase in the depth of breathing, occurring normally with exercise and abnormally with any condition in which the supply of oxygen is inadequate.	
		tachypnea	
		Tachy- means fast. Excessively rapid and shallow breathing; hyperventilation.	
-ptysis	spitting	hemoptysis	
		Blood is coughed up from the bronchial tubes and lungs; occurs with bronchitis or pneumonia, but also with tuberculosis, cancer, bronchiectasis, and pulmonary embolism.	
-sphyxia	pulse	asphyxia	
		This condition, literally meaning lack of pulse, is severe hypoxia leading to hypoxemia, hypercapnia, loss of consciousness, and death.	
-thorax	pleural cavity, chest	hemothorax	
		pyothorax	
		Empyema of the chest.	

PATHOLOGY

DIAGNOSTIC TERMS

auscultation

Listening to sounds within the body.

This procedure, performed with a stethoscope, is used chiefly for listening to the passage of air into and out of the lungs and listening to heart sounds. It is helpful to diagnose conditions of the lungs, pleura, heart, and abdomen, as well as to determine the condition of the fetus during pregnancy.

percussion

Tapping on a surface to determine the difference in the density of the underlying structure.

Tapping over a solid organ produces a dull sound without resonance. Percussion over an air-filled structure, such as the lung, produces a resonant, hollow note. When the lungs or the pleural space are filled with fluid and become more dense, as in pneumonia, resonance is replaced by dullness.

pleural rub

Scratchy sound produced by pleural surfaces rubbing against each other.

Pleural rub (also called a **friction rub**) occurs when the pleurae are roughened and thickened by inflammation, infection, scarring, or neoplastic cells. It is heard on auscultation and can be felt by placing the fingers on the chest wall.

rales (crackles)

Fine crackling sounds heard on auscultation (during inhalation) when there is fluid in the alveoli.

These popping or clicking sounds can be heard in patients with pneumonia, bronchiectasis, or acute bronchitis. The French word *rale* means rattle.

rhonchi (*singular*: **rhonchus**)

Loud rumbling sounds heard on auscultation of bronchi obstructed by sputum.

These coarse rumbling sounds resemble snoring and are usually caused by secretions in larger bronchial tubes.

sputum

Material expelled from the bronchi, lungs, or upper respiratory tract by spitting.

Purulent (containing pus) sputum often is green or brown. It results from infection and may be seen with asthma. Blood-tinged sputum is suggestive of tuberculosis or malignancy. For a **sputum culture,** the specimen is maintained in a nutrient medium to promote growth of a pathogen. **Culture and sensitivity (C&S)** testing identifies the sputum pathogen and determine which antibiotic will be effective in destroying or reducing its growth.

stridor

Strained, high-pitched sound heard on inspiration caused by obstruction in the pharynx or larynx.

Common causes of stridor include throat abscess, airway injury, croup, allergic reaction, or epiglottitis and laryngitis.

wheezes

Continuous high-pitched whistling sounds produced during breathing.

Wheezes are heard when air is forced through narrowed or obstructed airways. Patients with asthma or emphysema commonly experience wheezing as bronchi narrow and tighten.

12

UPPER RESPIRATORY DISORDERS

croup

Acute viral infection of infants and children with obstruction of the larynx, accompanied by barking cough and stridor.

The most common causative agents are influenza viruses or **respiratory syncytial virus (RSV).**

diphtheria

Acute infection of the throat and upper respiratory tract caused by the diphtheria bacterium *(Corynebacterium).*

Inflammation occurs, and a leathery, opaque membrane (Greek *diphthera*, leather membrane) forms in the pharynx andtrachea.

Immunity to diphtheria (by production of antibodies) is induced by the administration of weakened toxins (antigens) beginning between the sixth and eighth weeks of life. These injections usually are given as combination vaccines with pertussis and tetanus toxins and so are called **DPT** injections.

epistaxis

Nosebleed.

Epistaxis is a Greek word meaning a dropping. It commonly results from irritation of nasal mucous membranes, trauma, vitamin K deficiency, clotting abnormalities, blood-thinning medications (such as aspirin and warfarin), or hypertension.

pertussis

Whooping cough; highly contagious bacterial infection of the pharynx, larynx, and trachea caused by *Bordetella pertussis.*

Pertussis is characterized by **paroxysmal** (violent, sudden) spasms of coughing that ends in a loud "whooping" inspiration.

BRONCHIAL DISORDERS

12

asthma

Chronic bronchial inflammatory disorder with airway obstruction due to bronchial edema and constriction and increased mucus production.

Associated signs and symptoms of asthma are dyspnea, wheezing, and cough. Etiology can involve allergy or infection. Triggers for asthmatic attacks include exercise, strong odors, cold air, stress, allergens (e.g., tobacco smoke, pet dander, dust, molds, pollens, foods), and medications (aspirin, beta blockers).
Asthma treatments are:

- Fast-acting agents for acute symptoms; example is an albuterol inhaler **(bronchodilator).**
- Long-acting agents for long-term control; examples are glucocorticoids (inhaled), oral steroids (anti-inflammatory drugs), and leukotriene blockers such as montelukast (Singulair).

Other conditions, such as gastroesophageal reflux disease (GERD), sinusitis, and allergic rhinitis, can exacerbate asthma.

bronchiectasis

Chronic dilation of a bronchus, usually secondary to infection.

This condition is caused by chronic infection with loss of elasticity of the bronchi. Secretions puddle and do not drain normally. Signs and symptoms are cough, fever, and expectoration of foul-smelling, **purulent** (pus-containing) sputum. Treatment is **palliative** (noncurative) and includes antibiotics, mucolytics, bronchodilators, respiratory therapy, and surgical resection if other therapies are not effective.

chronic bronchitis

Inflammation of bronchi persisting over a long time; type of chronic obstructive pulmonary disease (COPD).

Infection and cigarette smoking are etiologic factors. Signs and symptoms include excessive secretion of often infected mucus, a productive cough, and obstruction of respiratory passages. Chronic bronchitis and emphysema (lung disease in which air exchange at the alveoli is severely impaired) are types of **chronic obstructive pulmonary disease (COPD)**.

cystic fibrosis (CF)

Inherited disorder of exocrine glands resulting in thick mucinous secretions in the respiratory tract that do not drain normally.

This is a genetic disorder caused by a mutation in a gene. It can be diagnosed by newborn screening blood test, sweat test, and genetic testing. CF affects the epithelium (lining cells) of the respiratory tract, leading to chronic airway obstruction, infection, bronchiectasis, and sometimes respiratory failure. It also involves exocrine glands, such as the pancreas (insufficient secretion of digestive enzymes leads to poor growth) and sweat glands (salty tasting skin). There is no known cure, but therapy includes antibiotics, aerosolized medications, chest physiotherapy, and replacement of pancreatic enzymes. A new medication called ivacaftor (Kalydeco) helps prevent the buildup of thick mucus in the lungs. Lung transplantation becomes necessary for some patients. It can restore lung function and prolong life.

LUNG DISORDERS

atelectasis

Collapsed lung; incomplete expansion of alveoli, (Figure 12-7, page 469).

In atelectasis, the bronchioles and alveoli (pulmonary parenchyma) resemble a collapsed balloon.

emphysema

Hyperinflation of air sacs with destruction of alveolar walls (Figure 12-9A and B).

Loss of elasticity and the breakdown of alveolar walls result in expiratory flow limitation. There is a strong association between cigarette smoking and emphysema. As a result of the destruction of lung parenchyma, including blood vessels, pulmonary artery pressure rises and the right side of the heart must work harder to pump blood. This leads to right ventricular hypertrophy and right heart failure **(cor pulmonale)**.

Emphysema and chronic bronchitis are both forms of **COPD**.

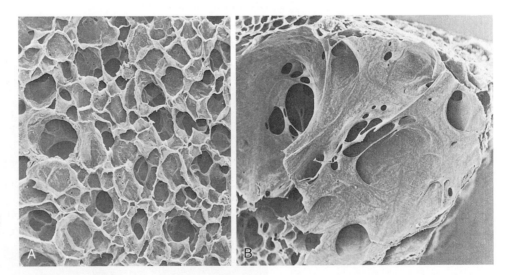

FIGURE 12-9 A, Normal lung tissue. B, Emphysema. Notice the overinflation of air sacs and destruction of alveolar walls.

Atelectasis: Common Causes
- Bronchial obstruction—by secretions or tumor
- Complications following surgery—poor breathing ability
- Chest wounds—air (pneumothorax), fluid (pleural effusion), or blood (hemothorax) accumulate in the pleural cavity

lung cancer

Malignant tumor arising from the lungs and bronchi (Figure 12-10).

This group of cancers, often associated with cigarette smoking, is the most frequent fatal malignancy. Lung cancers are divided into two general categories: **non–small cell lung cancer (NSCLC)** and **small cell lung cancer (SCLC).**

NSCLC accounts for 90% of lung cancers and comprises three main types: adenocarcinoma (derived from mucus-secreting cells), squamous cell carcinoma (derived from the lining cells of the upper airway), and large cell lung cancer. When lung cancer is diagnosed, physicians assess the *stage* of the tumor (determined by its size, lymph node involvement, and any distant areas of spread) to prepare a protocol for treatment.

For localized tumors, surgery may be curative. Staging of NSCLC by assessing mediastinal lymph nodes is critical. If nodes are negative and there are no other medical problems, the patient is a good candidate for surgery. If nodes are positive, multimodality treatment (chemotherapy and irradiation), with or without surgery, may be an option. Doctors treat metastatic disease (to liver, brain, and bones) with palliative chemotherapy and/or radiation therapy.

In some patients, often nonsmokers, NSCLC may be caused by a mutation (change) in epithelial lung tissue. An example is a mutation in the epidermal growth factor receptor (EGFR), which is sensitive to treatment with EGFR inhibitors (Iressa and Tarceva). This is an example of targeted drug therapy for cancer. Examples of tumors treatable by interfering with mutated gene products are increasing.

SCLC derives from small, round cells ("oat" cells) found in pulmonary epithelium. It grows rapidly early and quickly spreads outside the lung. Treatment with surgery, radiation therapy, and/or chemotherapy may lead to remissions.

pneumoconiosis

Abnormal condition caused by dust in the lungs, with chronic inflammation, infection, and bronchitis (Figure 12-11A).

Various forms are named according to the type of dust particle inhaled: **anthracosis**—coal (anthrac/o) dust (black lung disease); **asbestosis**—asbestos (asbest/o) particles (in shipbuilding and construction trades); **silicosis**—silica (silic/o = rocks) or glass (grinder's disease).

12

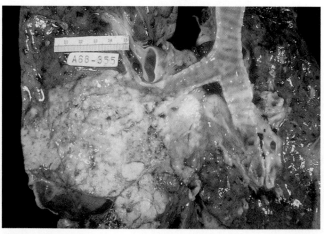

FIGURE 12-10 Lung cancer. The gray-white tumor tissue is infiltrating the substance of the lung. This tumor was identified as a squamous cell carcinoma. Squamous cell carcinomas arise in major bronchi and spread to local hilar lymph nodes.

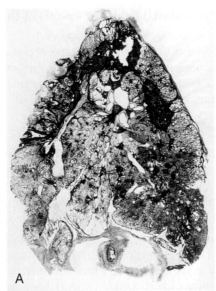

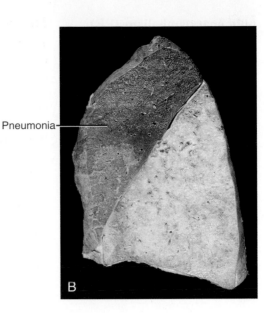

Pneumonia

A

B

FIGURE 12-11 **A, Anthracosis** or black lung disease. Notice the dark black deposits of coal dust throughout the lung. **B, Lobar pneumonia** (at autopsy). Notice that the condition affects a lobe of the lung. The patient's signs and symptoms included fever, chills, cough, dark sputum, rapid shallow breathing, and hypoxia. If diagnosis is made early, antibiotic therapy is successful.

pneumonia	**Acute inflammation and infection of alveoli, which fill with pus or products of the inflammatory reaction.** Etiologic agents are pneumococci, staphylococci, and other bacteria, fungi, or viruses. Infection damages alveolar membranes so that an **exudate** (fluid, blood cells, and debris) consolidates the alveoli (sacs become "glued" together, making air exchange less effective). An **infiltrate** is a fluid-filled area within the lungs as seen on a chest x-ray or CT scan. **Lobar pneumonia** (see Figure 12-11B) involves an entire lobe of a lung. **Bronchopneumonia** is a limited form of infection that produces patchy consolidation (abscesses) in the lung parenchyma. Treatment includes appropriate antibiotics and, if necessary, oxygen and mechanical ventilation in severe cases. See ***In Person: Recurring Pneumonia***, page 486. **Community-acquired pneumonia** results from a contagious respiratory infection, caused by a variety of viruses and bacteria (including pneumococci and *Mycoplasma* bacteria). It usually is treated at home with oral antibiotics. **Hospital-acquired pneumonia** or **nosocomial pneumonia** is acquired during hospitalization (Greek *nosokomeion* means hospital). For example, patients may contract pneumonia while on mechanical ventilation or as a hospital-acquired infection. **Aspiration pneumonia** is caused by material, such as food or vomitus, lodging in bronchi or lungs. It is a danger in the elderly, Alzheimer disease patients, stroke victims, and people with esophageal reflux and feeding tubes. X-ray images of a normal chest and one with pneumonia are on page 478.
pulmonary abscess	**Large collection of pus (bacterial infection) in the lungs.**
pulmonary edema	**Fluid in the air sacs and bronchioles.** This condition most often is caused by the inability of the heart to pump blood (congestive heart failure). Blood backs up in the pulmonary blood vessels, and fluid seeps out into the alveoli and bronchioles. Acute pulmonary edema requires immediate medical attention, including drugs (diuretics), oxygen in high concentrations, and keeping the patient in a sitting position (to decrease venous return to the heart).

12

pulmonary embolism (PE)	**Clot or other material lodges in vessels of the lung** (Figure 12-12A and B).

The clot (embolus) travels from distant veins, usually in the legs. Occlusion can produce an area of dead (necrotic) tissue; this is a **pulmonary infarction.** PE often causes acute pleuritic chest pain (pain on inspiration) and may be associated with blood in the sputum, fever, and respiratory insufficiency. CT angiography is the primary diagnostic tool for pulmonary emboli.

pulmonary fibrosis	**Formation of scar tissue in the connective tissue of the lungs.**

This condition can be primary (idiopathic) or secondary as the result of chronic inflammation or irritation caused by tuberculosis, pneumonia, or pneumoconiosis.

sarcoidosis	**Chronic inflammatory disease in which small nodules (granulomas) develop in lungs, lymph nodes, and other organs.**

The cause of sarcoidosis is unknown. Bilateral hilar lymphadenopathy or lung involvement is visible on chest x-ray in most cases. Many patients are asymptomatic and retain adequate pulmonary function. Sarcoidosis may affect the brain, heart, liver, and other organs. Other patients have more active disease and impaired pulmonary function. Glucocorticoids are used to prevent progression of the illness.

tuberculosis (TB)	**Infectious disease caused by _Mycobacterium tuberculosis_; lungs usually are involved, but any organ in the body may be affected.**

Rod-shaped bacteria called **bacilli** invade the lungs, producing small tubercles (from Latin _tuber,_ a swelling) of infection. Early TB usually is asymptomatic and detected on routine chest x-ray studies. Signs and symptoms of advanced disease are cough, weight loss, night sweats, hemoptysis, and pleuritic pain. Antituberculosis chemotherapy (isoniazid, rifampin) is effective in most cases. Immunocompromised patients are particularly susceptible to antibiotic-resistant TB. It is important and often necessary to treat TB with several drugs at the same time to prevent drug resistance.

The PPD skin test (see page 482) is given to most hospital and medical employees because TB is highly contagious. A positive PPD test, indicates exposure to TB, and treatment with isoniazid will be necessary even in the absence of lung infection.

PLEURAL DISORDERS

mesothelioma	**Rare malignant tumor arising in the pleura.**

Mesotheliomas are derived from mesothelium, which forms the lining of the pleural surface. These tumors usually are caused by asbestos exposure.

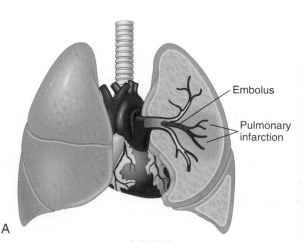
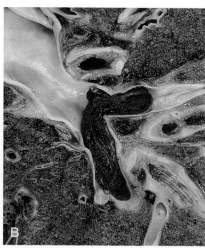

Embolus

Pulmonary infarction

A

B

FIGURE 12-12 Pulmonary embolism (A and B).

pleural effusion	**Abnormal accumulation of fluid in the pleural space (cavity).** Two types of pleural effusions are **exudates** (fluid from tumors and infections) and **transudates** (fluid from congestive heart failure, pulmonary embolism, or cirrhosis).
pleurisy (pleuritis)	**Inflammation of the pleura.** This condition causes pleurodynia and dyspnea and, in chronic cases, pleural effusion.
pneumothorax	**Collection of air in the pleural space.** Pneumothorax may occur in the course of a pulmonary disease (emphysema, carcinoma, tuberculosis, or lung abscess) when a break in the lung surface releases air into the pleural space. This allows communication between an alveolus or bronchus and the pleural cavity. It may also follow trauma and perforation of the chest wall or prolonged high-flow oxygen delivered by a respirator in an intensive care unit (ICU). **Pleurodesis** (-desis means to bind) is the artificial production of adhesions between the parietal and visceral pleura for treatment of persistent pneumothorax and severe pleural effusion. This is accomplished by using talc powder or drugs, such as antibiotics, that cause irritation and scarring of the pleura.

STUDY SECTION

12

Practice spelling each term and know its meaning.

anthracosis	Coal dust accumulates in the lungs.
asbestosis	Asbestos particles accumulate in the lungs.
bacilli (*singular:* **bacillus**)	Rod-shaped bacteria.
chronic obstructive pulmonary disease (COPD)	Chronic condition of persistent obstruction of air flow through bronchial tubes and lungs. COPD is caused by smoking, air pollution, chronic infection, and, in a minority of cases, asthma. Patients with predominant **chronic bronchitis** COPD may be referred to as "blue bloaters" (cyanotic, stocky build), whereas those with predominant **emphysema** may be called "pink puffers" (short of breath, but with near-normal blood oxygen levels, and no change in skin color).
cor pulmonale	Failure of the right side of the heart to pump a sufficient amount of blood to the lungs because of underlying lung disease.
exudates	Fluid, cells, and other substances (pus) that filter from cells or capillaries ooze into lesions or areas of inflammation.
hydrothorax	Collection of fluid in the pleural cavity.
infiltrate	Collection of fluid or other material within the lung, as seen on a chest film, CT scan, or other radiologic image.
palliative	Relieving symptoms, but not curing the disease.
paroxysmal	Pertaining to a sudden occurrence, such as a spasm or seizure; oxysm/o means sudden.
pulmonary infarction	Area of necrosis (death of lung tissue).
purulent	Containing pus.
silicosis	Disease due to silica or glass dust in the lungs; occurs in mining occupations.

CLINICAL PROCEDURES

X-RAY TESTS

chest x-ray (CXR)

Radiographic image of the thoracic cavity (chest film).

Chest x-rays are taken in the frontal (coronal) plane as posteroanterior (PA) or anteroposterior (AP) views and in the sagittal plane as lateral views. Figure 12-13A and B shows a normal chest film and an x-ray film of the chest with pneumonia.

computed tomography (CT) scan of the chest

Computer-generated series of x-ray images show thoracic structures in cross section and other planes.

This test is for diagnosis of lesions difficult to assess by conventional x-ray studies, such as those in the lungs, mediastinum, and pleura.

    CT pulmonary angiography (CTPA) is the combination of CT scanning and angiography. It is useful to examine the pulmonary circulation in the diagnosis of a pulmonary embolism.

MAGNETIC RESONANCE IMAGING

magnetic resonance imaging (MRI) of the chest

Magnetic waves create detailed images of the chest in frontal, lateral (sagittal), and cross-sectional (axial) planes.

This test is helpful in defining mediastinal tumors (such as those of Hodgkin disease) difficult to assess by CT scan.

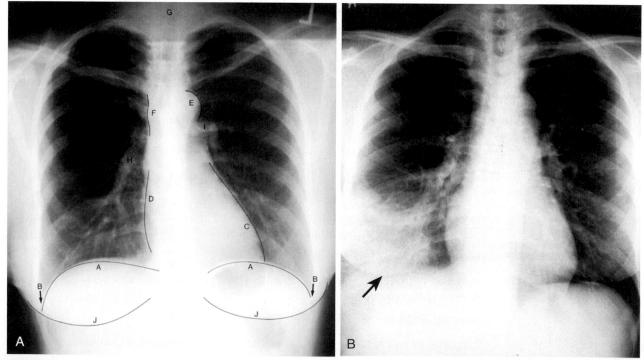

FIGURE 12-13   A, A normal chest x-ray appearance. The image is taken from the **posteroanterior (PA)** view (x-ray passes from back to front). The *backward L* in the upper corner is placed on the film to indicate the left side of the patient's chest. A, Diaphragm; B, costophrenic angle; C, left ventricle; D, right atrium; E, aortic arch; F, superior vena cava; G, trachea; H, right bronchus; I, left bronchus; J, breast shadows. Air-filled lung spaces appear black. **B, Pneumonia** of the right lung shown on an x-ray image of the chest.

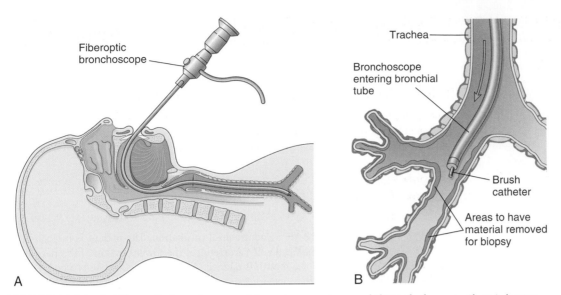

FIGURE 12-14   A, Fiberoptic bronchoscopy. A bronchoscope is passed through the nose, throat, larynx, and trachea into a bronchus. **B,** A **bronchoscope,** with brush catheter, in place in a bronchial tube.

NUCLEAR MEDICINE TESTS

positron emission tomography (PET) scan of the lung	**Radioactive glucose is injected, and images reveal metabolic activity in the lungs.** This scanning technique can identify malignant tumors, which have higher metabolic activity. It is also used to assess small nodules seen on a CT scan.
ventilation-perfusion (V/Q) scan	**Detection device records radioactivity in the lung after intravenous injection of a radioisotope and inhalation of a small amount of radioactive gas (xenon).** This test can identify areas of the lung not receiving adequate air flow (ventilation) or blood flow (perfusion) as well as areas where there is a mismatch in air flow (V) and blood flow (Q). Air flow without matched blood flow suggests a pulmonary embolus.

OTHER PROCEDURES

bronchoscopy	**Fiberoptic endoscope examination of the bronchial tubes.** A physician places the bronchoscope through the throat, larynx, and trachea into the bronchi for diagnosis, biopsy, or collection of secretions. In **bronchoalveolar lavage (bronchial washing),** fluid is injected and withdrawn. In **bronchial brushing**, a brush is inserted through the bronchoscope and is used to scrape off tissue (Figure 12-14). **Endobronchial ultrasound (EBUS)** is performed during bronchoscopy to diagnose and stage lung cancer. An EBUS-guided forceps biopsy allows for sampling of small (<3 cm) peripheral lesions endoscopically.

12

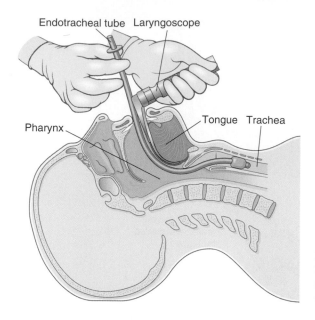

FIGURE 12-15   Endotracheal intubation. The patient is in a supine position; the head is hyperextended, the lower portion of the neck is flexed, and the mouth is opened. A **laryngoscope** is used to hold the airway open, to expose the vocal cords, and as a guide for placing the tube into the trachea.

endotracheal intubation	**Placement of a tube through the mouth into the pharynx, larynx, and trachea to establish an airway** (Figure 12-15).
	This procedure also allows the patient to be placed on a mechanical **ventilator** (an apparatus that moves air into and out of the lungs).
laryngoscopy	**Visual examination of the voice box.**
	A lighted, flexible endoscope is passed through the mouth or nose into the larynx.
lung biopsy	**Removal of lung tissue followed by microscopic examination.**
	Specimens may be obtained by bronchoscopy, thoracotomy (open-lung biopsy), needle biopsy through the chest wall, or video-assisted thoracoscopic surgery (VATS).
mediastinoscopy	**Endoscopic visual examination of the mediastinum.**
	An incision is made above the breastbone (suprasternal) for inspection and biopsy of lymph nodes in the underlying space (mediastinum).
pulmonary function tests (PFTs)	**Tests that measure the ventilation mechanics of the lungs: airway function, lung volume, and the capacity of the lungs to exchange oxygen and carbon dioxide efficiently.** See Figure 12-16.

PFTs are used for many reasons: (1) to evaluate patients with shortness of breath (SOB); (2) to monitor lung function in patients with known respiratory disease; (3) to evaluate disability; and (4) to assess lung function before surgery. A **spirometer** measures the volume and rate of air passing into and out of the lung.

PFTs determine if lung disease is obstructive, restrictive, or both. In **obstructive lung disease,** airways are narrowed, which results in resistance to air flow during breathing. A hallmark PFT abnormality in obstructive disease is decreased expiratory flow rate or **FEV_1** (forced expiratory volume in the first second of expiration). Examples of obstructive lung diseases are asthma, COPD, bronchiectasis, cystic fibrosis, and bronchiolitis.

In **restrictive lung disease,** expansion of the lung is limited by disease that affects the chest wall, pleura, or lung tissue itself. A hallmark PFT abnormality in restrictive disease is decreased **total lung capacity (TLC).** Examples of lung conditions that stiffen and scar the lung are pulmonary fibrosis, radiation damage to the lung, and pneumoconiosis. Other causes of restrictive lung disease are neuromuscular conditions that affect the lung, such as myasthenia gravis, muscular dystrophy, and diaphragmatic weakness and paralysis.

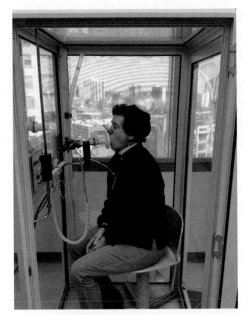

FIGURE 12-16   An individual undergoing a **pulmonary function test**.

The ability of gas to diffuse across the alveolar-capillary membrane is assessed by determining the diffusion capacity of the lung for carbon monoxide (**DL$_{CO}$**). A patient breathes in a small amount of carbon monoxide (CO), and the length of time it takes the gas to enter the bloodstream is measured.

thoracentesis

Surgical puncture to remove fluid from the pleural space.

This procedure is used to obtain pleural fluid for diagnosis or to therapeutically drain a pleural effusion (Figure 12 17).

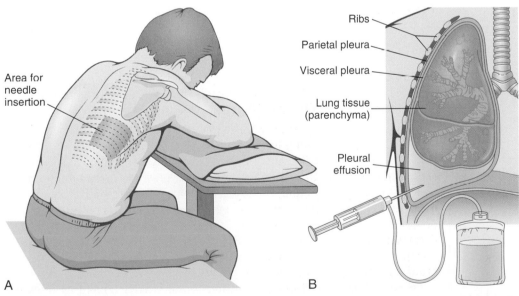

FIGURE 12-17   Thoracentesis. A, The patient is sitting in the correct position for the procedure; it allows the chest wall to be pulled outward in an expanded position. **B,** The needle is inserted close to the base of the effusion so that gravity can help with drainage, but it is kept as far away from the diaphragm as possible. The needle is inserted above the appropriate rib to avoid the neurovascular structures that run beneath each rib.

thoracotomy	**Large surgical incision of the chest.** The incision is large, cutting into bone, muscle, and cartilage. It is necessary for lung biopsies and resections (lobectomy and pneumonectomy).
thoracoscopy (thorascopy)	**Visual examination of the chest via small incisions and use of an endoscope.** **Video-assisted thoracic surgery (VATS)** allows the surgeon to view the chest from a video monitor. The thorascope (thoracoscope) is equipped with a camera that magnifies the image on the monitor. Thoracoscopy can diagnose and treat conditions of the lung, pleura, and mediastinum.
tracheostomy	**Surgical creation of an opening into the trachea through the neck.** A tube is inserted to create an airway. The tracheostomy tube may be permanent as well as an emergency device (Figure 12-18). A **tracheotomy** is the incision necessary to create a tracheostomy.
tuberculin test	**Determines past or present tuberculous infection based on a positive skin reaction.** Examples are the **Heaf test** and the **tine test,** using purified protein derivative **(PPD)** applied with multiple punctures of the skin, and the **Mantoux test,** using PPD given by intraepidermal injection.
tube thoracostomy	**A flexible, plastic chest tube is passed into the pleural space through an opening in the chest.** This procedure is used to continuously remove air (pneumothorax), fluid (pleural effusion), or pus (empyema). See Figure 12-19.

12

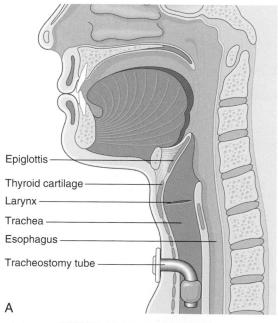

Epiglottis
Thyroid cartilage
Larynx
Trachea
Esophagus
Tracheostomy tube

A

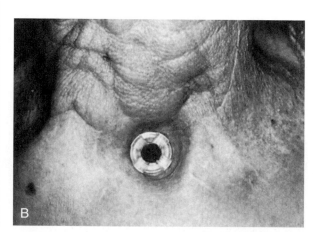

B

FIGURE 12-18 **A, Tracheostomy tube** in place. **B, Healed tracheostomy** after laryngectomy.

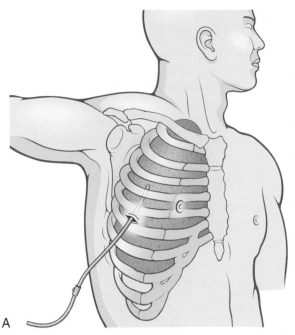
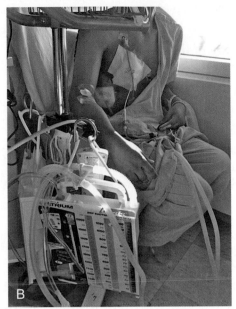

FIGURE 12-19 A, Tube thoracostomy. B, A patient with two thoracostomy tubes draining a pleural effusion from two different areas of the chest.

ABBREVIATIONS

ABGs	arterial blood gases
AFB	acid-fast bacillus—the type of organism that causes tuberculosis
ARDS	acute respiratory distress syndrome—severe, sudden lung injury caused by acute illness
BAL	bronchoalveolar lavage
Bronch	bronchoscopy
CF	cystic fibrosis
CO$_2$	carbon dioxide
COPD	chronic obstructive pulmonary disease—airway obstruction associated with emphysema and chronic bronchitis
CPAP	continuous positive airway pressure
CPR	cardiopulmonary resuscitation—three basic steps (CAB): C, *c*irculation restored by external cardiac compression; A, *a*irway opened by tilting the head; B, *b*reathing restored by mouth-to-mouth breathing
C&S	culture and sensitivity testing (of sputum)
CTPA	computed tomography pulmonary angiography
CXR	chest x-ray [film]
DL$_{CO}$	diffusion capacity of the lung for carbon monoxide
DOE	dyspnea on exertion
DPT	diphtheria, pertussis, tetanus—toxoids for vaccination of infants, to provide immunity to these diseases
FEV$_1$	forced expiratory volume in 1 second
FVC	forced vital capacity—amount of gas that can be forcibly and rapidly exhaled after a full inspiration
ICU	intensive care unit
LLL	left lower lobe (of lung)
LUL	left upper lobe (of lung)
MAC	*Mycobacterium avium* complex—the cause of a noncontagious lung infection related to tuberculosis
MDI	metered-dose inhaler—used to deliver aerosolized medications to patients
NSCLC	non–small cell lung cancer
O$_2$	oxygen

12

OSA	obstructive sleep apnea
PaCO₂	carbon dioxide partial pressure—measure of the amount of carbon dioxide in arterial blood
PaO₂	oxygen partial pressure—a measure of the amount of oxygen in arterial blood
PCP	*Pneumocystis* pneumonia—a type of pneumonia seen in patients with AIDS or other immunosuppression
PE	pulmonary embolism
PEP	positive expiratory pressure—mechanical ventilator strategy in which the patient takes a deep breath and then exhales through a device that resists air flow (helps refill underventilated areas of the lung)
PEEP	positive end-expiratory pressure—common mechanical ventilator setting in which airway pressure is maintained above atmospheric pressure
PFTs	pulmonary function tests
PND	paroxysmal nocturnal dyspnea
PPD	purified protein derivative—substance used in a tuberculosis test
RDS	respiratory distress syndrome—in the newborn infant; marked by dyspnea and cyanosis and related to absence of surfactant (lubricating substance that permits normal expansion of lungs); also called hyaline membrane disease
RLL	right lower lobe (of lung)

RML	right middle lobe (of lung)
RSV	respiratory syncytial virus—common cause of bronchiolitis, bronchopneumonia, and the common cold, especially in children (in tissue culture, forms syncytia or giant cells, so that cytoplasm flows together)
RUL	right upper lobe (of lung)
RV	residual volume—amount of air remaining in lungs at the end of maximal expiration
SABA	short-acting beta agonist (for relief of asthma symptoms)
SCLC	small cell lung cancer
SOB	shortness of breath
TB	tuberculosis
TLC	total lung capacity—volume of gas in the lungs at the end of maximal inspiration; equals VC plus RV
URI	upper respiratory infection
V_T	tidal volume—amount of air inhaled and exhaled during a normal ventilation
VATS	video-assisted thoracic surgery (thoracoscopy)
VC	vital capacity—equals inspiratory reserve volume plus expiratory reserve volume plus tidal volume
V/Q scan	ventilation-perfusion scan—radioactive test of lung ventilation and blood perfusion throughout the lung capillaries (lung scan)

PRACTICAL APPLICATIONS

CASE STUDY: TARGETED THERAPY FOR LUNG CANCER

In 2008, Sarah Broom was a 35-year-old literature instructor and poet living in New Zealand. Married with two young sons, she was pregnant with her third child when she noticed shortness of breath accompanied by a persistent cough. An x-ray of her lungs during her 7th month of pregnancy showed a large mass in

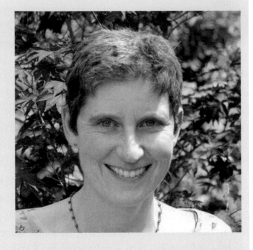

one lung. After a cesarean section (her daughter was born safely), she had a biopsy and other tests, which revealed NSCLC-advanced lung cancer. Sarah was a nonsmoker.

The doctors in New Zealand told her that her care would be palliative and that she had only a few months to live.

Sarah was desperate to explore every option, and through a personal connection, she sent her biopsy slides to the MGH Cancer Center in Boston. The slides were analyzed using cutting edge technology, and her tumor was found to have a mutation called EML4-ALK, which occurs in only 5% of lung cancers. The doctors at MGH knew of a new drug called crizotinib that was being evaluated to treat lung cancers with this specific mutation. Finding a specific mutation in a tumor and targeting that mutation with particular drug is a cutting edge approach to cancer treatment.

Sarah was given the new drug—and her tumors shrunk! She was in remission for over 2 years. In 2010, the tumors returned, and Sarah traveled back to Boston for further drug treatment, which was not successful. She developed brain metastases.

Her doctors in Boston knew of one more targeted therapy drug called ceritinib that was still in clinical trials and therefore would not be available for patients. However, through coordinated and persistent efforts, the pharmaceutical company (Novartis) allowed her advance, compassionate access to the drug, and it worked for 2 years! Because it was seen that this drug was effective against lung cancer in patients with relapsed disease, the FDA has now given the drug rapid approval.

In April 2013, Sarah lost her battle with lung cancer. But her case serves as an example of the importance of exploring all options and remaining open to new cancer treatments, such as targeted therapy.

CASE REPORT

A 22-year-old man who was a known heroin abuser was admitted to an emergency department comatose, with shallow respirations. Routine laboratory studies and chest x-ray studies were done after the patient was aroused. He was then transferred to the ICU. He complained of left-sided chest pain. Examination of the chest film showed three fractured ribs on the right and a large right pleural effusion. Further questioning of a friend revealed that he had fallen and struck the corner of a table after injecting heroin.

The diagnosis was traumatic hemothorax secondary to rib fractures, and a chest tube was inserted into the right pleural space. No blood could be obtained despite maneuvering of the tube. Another chest x-ray showed that the tube was correctly placed in the right pleural space, but the fractured ribs and pleural effusion were on the left. The radiologist then realized that he had reversed the first film. A second tube was inserted into the left pleural space, and 1500 mL [6 to 7 cups] of blood was evacuated.

X-RAY AND BRONCHOSCOPY REPORTS

1. *CXR*: Complete opacification of left hemithorax with deviation of mediastinal structures of right side. Massive pleural effusion.

2. *Chest tomograms*: Mass most compatible with LUL bronchogenic carcinoma. Possible left paratracheal adenopathy or direct involvement of mediastinum.

3. *Bronchoscopy*: Larynx, trachea, **carina** [area of bifurcation or forking of the trachea], and left lung all within normal limits. On the right side there was irregularity and roughening of the bronchial mucosa on the lateral aspect of the bronchial wall. This irregularity extended into the RUL, and the apical and posterior segments [divisions of lobes of the lung] each contained inflamed irregular mucosa. Conclusion: Suspicious for infiltrating tumor, but may be nonspecific inflammation. Bronchial washings, brushings, and bxs [biopsies] taken. Bronchial biopsy diagnosis: squamous cell carcinoma. Washings and brushings showed no malignant cells.

IN PERSON: RECURRENT PNEUMONIA

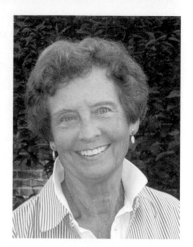

While growing up in West Virginia in the 1940s and 50s, I was frighteningly aware of the prevalence of lung diseases. With coal mining at its peak, large numbers of miners suffered and died from black lung disease. Tuberculosis was not uncommon, and neither was pneumonia. Little did I imagine, then or in 1999, when I first contracted the disease, that recurring pneumonia would become my most troublesome medical issue.

As bitter cold temperatures persisted during the winter of 1999, I was not particularly concerned about a lingering cold and cough. But when I developed a low-grade fever and decreased energy, a chest x-ray confirmed that I had pneumonia in my left lung (lower lobe). My doctor prescribed a one-week course of antibiotics and reassured me that the diagnosis was not unusual. I quickly improved and a follow-up x-ray showed that the pneumonia had cleared. My doctor then suggested that I receive the pneumonia vaccine, which produces antibodies against many types of pneumococcal bacteria. End of story. Or so I thought.

In October of 2001, at age 60, I began training to run the Boston Marathon. A few days after a long training run in January of 2002, I could not stop coughing. Once again, a low-grade fever and rather marked fatigue set in. The thought of pneumonia did not cross my mind initially. But, when symptoms didn't improve, a visit to my doctor and a chest x-ray confirmed my second diagnosis of pneumonia, again in my left lower lobe. I felt some relief when my physician, a pulmonologist and a serious runner himself, assured me that cold weather training had not caused the pneumonia. After a course of antibiotics, a follow-up chest CT performed in May showed no abnormal result, and bronchoscopy ruled out any malignancy. Relieved, I assumed I was finished with pneumonia.

However, pneumonia wasn't finished with me. I had periods where I went almost 6 years without a recurrence, but over and over, despite pulmonary function tests that were normal and trials of steroids, I seem to always end up with pneumonia when I develop even the slightest "cold."

With all the information, gathered and evaluated by experts, what happens next? At this point, the doctors conclude that my pneumonia is probably idiopathic. They suggest that I have a follow-up CT scan and additional testing when pneumonia episodes actually occur. They also caution me about exposure around children and hospitalized patients. I asked my lung specialist if he thought this pneumonia puzzle would ever be resolved. His reply was, "Something is going on that we will eventually understand. We just haven't figured it out yet." Unsettling and stress producing as this has been, I know I am fortunate to be dealing with an illness that has, so far, responded to medication. Still, every time I get cold signs and symptoms, I worry. And I never take good health for granted.

Brenda Melson's professional career was in teaching, counseling, and college advising.

❓ EXERCISES

Remember to check your answers carefully with the Answers to Exercises, page 494.

Ⓐ Match the listed anatomic structures with the descriptions that follow.

adenoids   epiglottis   paranasal sinuses
alveoli   hilum   parietal pleura
bronchi   larynx   pharynx
bronchioles   mediastinum   trachea
cilia   palatine tonsils   visceral pleura

1. outer fold of pleura lying closer to the ribs _____.

2. collections of lymph tissue in the nasopharynx _____.

3. windpipe _____.

4. lid-like piece of cartilage that covers the voice box _____.

5. branches of the windpipe that lead into the lungs _____.

6. region between the lungs in the chest cavity _____.

7. air-containing cavities in the bones around the nose _____.

8. thin hairs attached to the mucous membrane lining the respiratory tract

   _____.

9. inner fold of pleura closer to lung tissue _____.

10. throat _____.

11. air sacs of the lung _____.

12. voice box _____.

13. smallest branches of bronchi _____.

14. collections of lymph tissue in the oropharynx _____.

15. midline region of the lungs where bronchi, blood vessels, and nerves enter and exit the lungs

   _____.

Ⓑ Complete the following sentences.

1. The apical part of the lung is the _____.

2. The gas that passes into the bloodstream at the lungs is _____.

3. Breathing in air is called _____.

4. Divisions of the lungs are known as _____.

12

5. The gas produced by cells and exhaled through the lungs is _____.

6. The space between the visceral and the parietal pleura is the _____.

7. Breathing out air is called _____.

8. The essential tissues of the lung that perform its main function are pulmonary

_____.

9. The exchange of gases in the lung is _____ respiration.

10. The exchange of gases at the tissue cells is _____ respiration.

C **Give meanings for the following terms relating to respiratory disorders and structures.**

1. bronchiectasis _____

2. pleuritis _____

3. pneumothorax _____

4. anosmia _____

5. laryngectomy _____

6. nasopharyngitis _____

7. phrenic _____

8. alveolar _____

9. glottis _____

10. tracheal stenosis _____

D **Complete the medical terms for the following respiratory symptoms.**

1. excessive carbon dioxide in the blood: hyper _____

2. breathing is easiest or possible only in an upright position: _____ pnea

3. difficult breathing: _____ pnea

4. condition of blueness of skin: _____ osis

5. spitting up blood: hemo _____

6. deficiency of oxygen: hyp _____

7. condition of pus in the pleural cavity: pyo _____ *or* em _____

8. hoarseness; voice impairment: dys _____

9. blood in the pleural cavity: hemo _____

10. nosebleed: epi _____

12

E **Give the meanings of the following medical terms.**

1. rales (crackles) _____

2. auscultation _____

3. sputum _____

4. percussion _____

5. rhonchi _____

6. pleural rub _____

7. purulent _____

8. paroxysmal nocturnal dyspnea _____

9. hydrothorax _____

10. pulmonary infarction _____

11. stridor _____

12. wheeze _____

F **Match the lung pathology terms with the descriptions that follow.**

asbestosis	croup	infiltrate
asthma	cystic fibrosis	lung cancer
atelectasis	diphtheria	pertussis
chronic bronchitis	emphysema	sarcoidosis

1. Acute infectious disease of the throat caused by *Corynebacterium*: _____

2. Acute respiratory syndrome in children and infants that is marked by obstruction of the larynx
   and stridor: _____

3. Hyperinflation of air sacs with destruction of alveolar walls: _____

4. Inflammation of tubes that lead from the trachea, present over a long period of time:

   _____

5. Chronic inflammatory disorder characterized by airway obstruction: _____

6. Lung or a portion of a lung is collapsed: _____

7. Malignant neoplasm originating in a lung or bronchus: _____

8. Whooping cough: _____

9. A collection of fluid or other material within the lung as seen on chest film, CT scan, or other
   radiologic study: _____

10. Inherited disease of exocrine glands; mucous secretions lead to airway obstruction:

    _____

11. Type of pneumoconiosis; dust particles are inhaled: _____

12. Inflammatory disease in which small nodules form in lungs and lymph nodes: _____

12

G Use the listed terms and abbreviations to complete the sentences that follow.

CPAP	fibrosis	PaO$_2$
DL$_{CO}$	obstructive lung disease	palliative
exudate	OSA	restrictive lung disease
FEV$_1$	PaCO$_2$	rhonchi

1. Sarah had a pulmonary function test in which she inhaled as much air as she could and the air that she expelled in the first second was measured. The result of this PFT is a/an

   _____.

2. Dr. Smith heard loud _____ when he auscultated Kate's chest. Her bronchial tubes were obstructed with thick mucous secretions.

3. Karl was asked to breathe in a small amount of carbon monoxide and then blood samples were taken to detect the gas in his bloodstream. This PFT assesses how well gases can diffuse across the alveolar membrane, and the result of the test is called _____.

4. Formation of scar tissue in the connective tissue of the lungs is pulmonary

   _____.

5. A purulent _____ consists of white blood cells, microorganisms (dead and alive), and other debris.

6. Myasthenia gravis and muscular dystrophy are examples of neuromuscular conditions that produce _____.

7. Chronic bronchitis and asthma are examples of _____.

8. Patients with a small pharyngeal airway that closes during sleep may experience

   _____.

9. With nasal _____, positive pressure (air coming from a compressor) opens the oropharynx and nasopharynx, preventing obstructive sleep apnea.

10. Doctors realized that they could not cure Jean's adenocarcinoma of the lung. They used _____ measures to relieve her uncomfortable symptoms.

11. During an apneic period, a patient experiences severe hypoxemia (decreased _____) and hypercapnia (increased _____).

H Give the meanings of the following medical terms.

1. pulmonary abscess _____

2. pulmonary edema _____

3. pneumoconiosis _____

4. pneumonia _____

5. pulmonary embolism _____

12

6. tuberculosis _____

7. pleural effusion _____

8. pleurisy _____

9. anthracosis _____

10. mesothelioma _____

11. adenoid hypertrophy _____

12. pleurodynia _____

13. expectoration _____

14. tachypnea _____

I **Match the clinical procedure or abbreviation with its description.**

bronchoalveolar lavage   laryngoscopy   tracheostomy
bronchoscopy   mediastinoscopy   tube thoracostomy
CT pulmonary angiography   pulmonary function tests tuberculin tests
endotracheal intubation   thoracentesis   V/Q scan

1. Placement of a tube through the mouth into the trachea to establish an airway:

   _____

2. Injection or inhalation of radioactive material and recording images of its distribution in the

   lungs: _____

3. Tine and Mantoux tests: _____

4. Puncture of the chest wall to obtain fluid from the pleural cavity: _____

5. Tests that measure the ventilation mechanics of the lung: _____

6. Creation of an opening into the trachea through the neck to establish an airway:

   _____

7. Visual examination of the bronchi: _____

8. Injection of fluid into the bronchi, followed by withdrawal of the fluid for examination:

   _____

9. Insertion of an endoscope into the larynx to view the voice box: _____

10. Combination of computer-generated x-ray images and recording (with contrast) of blood flow in

    the lung: _____

11. Visual examination of the area between the lungs: _____

12. Continuous drainage of the pleural spaces from a chest tube placed through a small skin

    incision: _____

12

J Spell out the following abbreviations and then select the letter of the description that is the best definition for each.

COLUMN I

1. DOE _____ ____

2. PND _____ ____

3. VATS _____ ____

4. CPR _____ ____

5. NSCLC _____ ____

6. ARDS _____ ____

7. COPD _____ ____

8. PFTs _____ ____

9. PPD _____ ____

10. DPT _____ ____

COLUMN II

A. Patients with congestive heart failure and pulmonary edema experience this symptom when they recline in bed.

B. Chronic bronchitis and emphysema are examples.

C. Substance used in the test for tuberculosis.

D. Adenocarcinoma and squamous cell carcinoma are types.

E. Visual examination of the chest via endoscope and a video monitor.

F. Injection in an infant to provide immunity.

G. A spirometer is used for these respiratory tests.

H. This symptom means that a patient has difficulty breathing and becomes short of breath when exercising.

I. Three basic steps: A, airway opened by tilting the head; B, breathing restored by mouth-to-mouth breathing; C, circulation restored by external cardiac compressions.

J. A group of symptoms resulting in acute respiratory failure.

K Match the respiratory system procedures with their meanings.

laryngectomy   rhinoplasty   thoracotomy
lobectomy   thoracentesis   tonsillectomy
pneumonectomy   thoracoscopy (thorascopy)

1. removal of lymph tissue in the oropharynx _____

2. surgical puncture of the chest to remove fluid from the pleural space _____

3. surgical repair of the nose _____

4. incision of the chest _____

5. removal of the voice box _____

6. removal of a region of a lung _____

7. endoscopic examination of the chest _____

8. pulmonary resection _____

12

L **Circle the boldface terms that best complete the meaning of each sentence.**

1. Ruth was having difficulty taking a deep breath, and her chest x-ray showed accumulation of fluid in her pleural spaces. Dr. Smith ordered **(PPD, tracheotomy, thoracentesis)** to relieve the pressure on her lungs.

2. Dr. Wong used her stethoscope to perform **(percussion, auscultation, thoracentesis)** on the patient's chest.

3. Before making a decision to perform surgery on Mrs. Hope, an 80-year-old woman with lung cancer, her physicians ordered **(COPD, bronchoscopy, PFTs)** to determine the functioning of her lungs.

4. Sylvia produced yellow-colored sputum and had a high fever. Her physician told her that she probably had **(pneumonia, pulmonary embolism, pneumothorax)** and needed antibiotics.

5. The night before her thoracotomy for lung biopsy, Mrs. White was told by her anesthesiologist that he would place a/an **(thoracostomy tube, mediastinoscope, endotracheal tube)** down her throat to keep her airway open during surgery.

6. Early in her pregnancy, Sonya had a routine **(PET scan, CXR, MRI)** that revealed a/an **(epiglottic, alveolar, mediastinal)** mass in the area between her lungs. After delivery of her child, the mass was removed, and biopsy revealed a malignant thymoma (tumor of the thymus gland).

7. Five-year-old Seth was allergic to cats and experienced wheezing, coughing, and difficult breathing at night when he was trying to sleep. After careful evaluation by a **(cardiologist, pulmonologist, neurologist)**, his parents were told that Seth had **(pleurisy, sarcoidosis, asthma)** involving inflammation of his **(nasal passages, pharynx, bronchial tubes)**.

8. Six-year-old Daisy had a habit of picking her nose. During the winter months, heat in her family's house caused drying of her nasal **(mucus, mucous, pleural)** membranes. She had frequent bouts of **(epistaxis, croup, stridor)**.

9. Seventy-five-year-old Beatrice had been a pack-a-day smoker all of her adult life. Over the previous 3 months she noticed a persistent cough, weight loss, blood in her sputum **(hemoptysis, hematemesis, asbestosis)**, and dyspnea. A chest CT scan revealed a mass. Biopsy confirmed the diagnosis of **(tuberculosis, pneumoconiosis, adenocarcinoma)**, which is a type of **(small cell, non–small cell, lymph node)** lung cancer.

10. Carrie's lungs were normal at birth, but thick bronchial secretions soon blocked her **(arterioles, venules, bronchioles)**, which became inflamed. She was losing weight, and tests revealed inadequate amounts of pancreatic enzymes necessary for digestion of fats and proteins. Her pediatrician diagnosed her hereditary condition as **(chronic bronchitis, asthma, cystic fibrosis)**.

12

ANSWERS TO EXERCISES

A

1. parietal pleura
2. adenoids
3. trachea
4. epiglottis
5. bronchi

6. mediastinum
7. paranasal sinuses
8. cilia
9. visceral pleura
10. pharynx

11. alveoli
12. larynx
13. bronchioles
14. palatine tonsils
15. hilum

B

1. uppermost part
2. oxygen
3. inspiration; inhalation
4. lobes

5. carbon dioxide
6. pleural cavity
7. expiration; exhalation

8. parenchyma
9. external
10. internal

C

1. chronic dilation of a bronchus
2. inflammation of pleura
3. air in the chest (pleural cavity)
4. lack of sense of smell

5. removal of the voice box
6. inflammation of the nose and throat

7. pertaining to the diaphragm
8. pertaining to an air sac
9. opening to the larynx
10. narrowing of the windpipe

D

1. hypercapnia
2. orthopnea
3. dyspnea
4. cyanosis

5. hemoptysis
6. hypoxia
7. pyothorax; empyema

8. dysphonia
9. hemothorax
10. epistaxis

E

1. fine crackling sounds heard during inhalation when there is fluid in the alveoli
2. listening to sounds within the body
3. material expelled from the respiratory tract by deep coughing and spitting
4. tapping on the surface to determine the underlying structure
5. loud rumbling sounds on auscultation of chest; bronchi obstructed by sputum

6. scratching sound produced by pleural surfaces rubbing against each other (caused by inflammation or tumor cells)
7. pus-filled
8. sudden attack of difficult breathing associated with lying down at night (caused by congestive heart failure and pulmonary edema as the lungs fill with fluid)

9. fluid in the pleural cavity
10. area of dead tissue in the lung
11. strained, high-pitched inspirational sound
12. continuous high-pitched whistling sound produced during breathing when air is forced through a narrow space; heard in asthma

F

1. diphtheria
2. croup
3. emphysema
4. chronic bronchitis

5. asthma
6. atelectasis
7. lung cancer
8. pertussis

9. infiltrate
10. cystic fibrosis
11. asbestosis
12. sarcoidosis

G

1. FEV_1 (forced expiratory volume in first second)
2. rhonchi
3. DL_{CO} (diffusion capacity of the lung for carbon monoxide)

4. fibrosis
5. exudate
6. restrictive lung disease
7. obstructive lung disease
8. OSA: obstructive sleep apnea

9. CPAP: continuous positive airway pressure
10. palliative
11. PaO_2, $PaCO_2$

12

H

1. collection of pus in the lungs
2. swelling, fluid collection in the air sacs and bronchioles
3. abnormal condition of dust in the lungs
4. acute inflammation and infection of alveoli; they become filled with fluid and blood cells
5. floating clot or other material blocking the blood vessels of the lung
6. an infectious disease caused by rod-shaped bacilli and producing tubercles (nodes) of infection
7. collection of fluid in the pleural cavity
8. inflammation of pleura
9. abnormal condition of coal dust in the lungs (black lung disease)
10. malignant tumor arising in the pleura; composed of mesothelium (epithelium that covers the surfaces of membranes such as pleura and peritoneum)
11. excessive growth of cells in the adenoids (lymph tissue in the nasopharynx)
12. pain of the pleura (irritation of pleural surfaces leads to intercostal pain)
13. coughing up of material from the chest
14. rapid breathing; hyperventilation

I

1. endotracheal intubation
2. V/Q scan
3. tuberculin tests
4. thoracentesis
5. pulmonary function tests
6. tracheostomy
7. bronchoscopy
8. bronchoalveolar lavage
9. laryngoscopy
10. CT pulmonary angiography
11. mediastinoscopy
12. tube thoracostomy

J

1. dyspnea on exertion: H
2. paroxysmal nocturnal dyspnea: A
3. video-assisted thoracic surgery: E
4. cardiopulmonary resuscitation: I
5. non–small cell lung cancer: D
6. acute (adult) respiratory distress syndrome: J
7. chronic obstructive pulmonary disease: B
8. pulmonary function tests: G
9. purified protein derivative: C
10. diphtheria, pertussis, and tetanus: F

K

1. tonsillectomy
2. thoracentesis
3. rhinoplasty
4. thoracotomy
5. laryngectomy
6. lobectomy
7. thoracoscopy (thorascopy)
8. pneumonectomy

L

1. thoracentesis
2. auscultation
3. PFTs
4. pneumonia
5. endotracheal tube
6. CXR; mediastinal
7. pulmonologist; asthma; bronchial tubes
8. mucous; epistaxis
9. hemoptysis; adenocarcinoma; non–small cell
10. bronchioles; cystic fibrosis

12

PRONUNCIATION OF TERMS

To test your understanding of the terminology in this chapter, write the meaning of each term in the space provided. In addition, you may wish to cover the terms and write them by looking at your definitions. Make sure your spelling is correct. The page number after each term indicates where it is defined or used in the book, so you can easily check your responses. You will find complete definitions for all of these terms and their audio pronunciations on the Evolve website.

Pronunciation Guide

ā as in āpe	ă as in ăpple
ē as in ēven	ĕ as in ĕvery
ī as in īce	ĭ as in ĭnterest
ō as in ōpen	ŏ as in pŏt
ū as in ūnit	ŭ as in ŭnder

Vocabulary and Terminology

TERM	PRONUNCIATION	MEANING
adenoidectomy (465)	ăd-ĕ-noyd-ĔK-tō-mē	_____
adenoid hypertrophy (465)	ĂD-ĕ-noyd hī-PĔR-trō-fē	_____
adenoids (464)	ĂD-ĕ-noydz	_____
alveolar (465)	ăl-VĒ-ō-lăr	_____
alveolus; alveoli (464)	ăl-VĒ-ō-lŭs; ăl-VĒ-ō-lī	_____
anosmia (469)	ăn-ŎS-mē-ă	_____
apex of the lung (464)	Ā-pĕks of the lŭng	_____
apical (464)	Ā-pĭ-kăl	_____
apnea (470)	ĂP-nē-ă	_____
asphyxia (470)	ăs-FĬK-sē-ă	_____
atelectasis (469)	ă-tĕ-LĔK-tă-sĭs	_____
base of the lung (464)	bās of the lŭng	_____
bronchiectasis (465)	brŏng-kē-ĔK-tă-sĭs	_____
bronchioles (464)	BRŎNG-kē-ōlz	_____
bronchiolitis (465)	brŏng-kē-ō-LĪ-tĭs	_____
bronchodilator (465)	brŏng-kō-DĪ-lā-tĕr	_____
bronchopleural (465)	brŏng-kō-PLOO-răl	_____
bronchospasm (465)	BRŎNG-kō-spăzm	_____
bronchus; bronchi (464)	BRŎNG-kŭs; BRŎNG-kī	_____
carbon dioxide (464)	KĂR-bŏn dī-ŎK-sīd	_____
cilia (464)	SĬL-ē-ă	_____
cyanosis (466)	sī-ă-NŌ-sĭs	_____
diaphragm (464)	DĪ-ă-frăm	_____

12

TERM	PRONUNCIATION	MEANING
dysphonia (467)	dĭs-FŌ-nē-ă	
dyspnea (470)	DĬSP-nē-ă	
empyema (469)	ĕm-pī-Ē-mă	
epiglottis (464)	ĕp-ĭ-GLŎT-ĭs	
epiglottitis (466)	ĕp-ĭ-glŏ-TĪ-tĭs	
expectoration (467)	ĕk-spĕk-tō-RĀ-shŭn	
expiration (464)	ĕks-pĭr-RĀ-shŭn	
glottis (464)	GLŎ-tĭs	
hemoptysis (470)	hē-MŎP-tĭ-sĭs	
hemothorax (470)	hē-mō-THŌ-răks	
hilum of the lung (464)	HĪ-lŭm of the lŭng	
hilar (464)	HĪ-lăr	
hypercapnia (465)	hī-pĕr-KĂP-nē-ă	
hyperpnea (470)	hī-PĔRP-nē-ă	
hypoxia (467)	hī-PŎK-sē-ă	
inspiration (464)	ĭn-spĭ-RĀ-shŭn	
laryngeal (466)	lă-RĬN-jē-ăl *or* lăr-ĭn-JĒ-ăl	
laryngospasm (466)	lă-RĬNG-gō-spăzm	
laryngitis (466)	lă-rĭn-JĪ-tĭs	
larynx (464)	LĂR-ĭnks	
lobectomy (466)	lō-BĔK-tō-mē	
mediastinoscopy (467)	mē-dē-ă-stī-NŎS-kō-pē	
mediastinum (464)	mē-dē-ă-STĪ-nŭm	
nares (464)	NĀ-rēz	
nasogastric intubation (467)	nā-zō-GĂS-trĭk ĭn-too-BĀ-shŭn	
orthopnea (467)	ŏr-THŎP-nē-ă	
oxygen (464)	ŎKS-ĭ-jĕn	
palatine tonsil (464)	PĂL-ĭ-tīn TŎN-sĭl	
paranasal sinus (464)	pă-ră-NĀ-zăl SĪ-nŭs	
parietal pleura (464)	pă-RĪ-ĕ-tăl PLOO-ră	
pharyngeal (467)	fă-RĬN-jē-ăl *or* făr-ĭn-JĒ-ăl	

12

TERM	PRONUNCIATION	MEANING
pharynx (465)	FĂR-ĭnkz	
phrenic nerve (467)	FRĔN-ĭk nĕrv	
pleura (465)	PLOOR-ă	
pleural cavity (465)	PLOOR-ăl KĂ-vĭ-tē	
pleurodynia (467)	ploor-ō-DĬN-ē-ă	
pneumonectomy (468)	nū-mō-NĔK-tō-mē	
pneumothorax (468)	nū-mō-THŌ-răks	
pulmonary (468)	PŬL-mō-nār-ē	
pulmonary parenchyma (465)	pŭl-mō-NĀR-ē pă-RĔN-kĭ-mă	
pyothorax (470)	pī-ō-THŌ-răks	
respiration (465)	rĕs-pĭ-RĀ-shĕn	
rhinoplasty (468)	RĪ-nō-plăs-tē	
rhinorrhea (468)	rī-nō-RĒ-ăh	
sinusitis (468)	sī-nū-SĪ-tĭs	
spirometer (468)	spī-RŎM-ĕ-tĕr	
tachypnea (470)	tăk-ĬP-nē-ă	
thoracic (469)	thōr-RĂ-sĭk	
thoracotomy (469)	thōr-ră-KŎT-ō-mē	
tonsillectomy (469)	tŏn-sĭ-LĔK-tō-mē	
trachea (465)	TRĀ-kē-ă	
tracheal stenosis (469)	TRĀ-kē-ăl stĕ-NŌ-sĭs	
tracheotomy (469)	trā-kē-ŎT-ō-mē	
visceral pleura (465)	VĬS-ĕr-ăl PLOOR-ă	

Pathologic Conditions, Laboratory Tests, and Clinical Procedures

TERM	PRONUNCIATION	MEANING
anthracosis (477)	ăn-thră-KŌ-sĭs	
asbestosis (477)	ăs-bĕs-TŌ-sĭs	
asthma (472)	ĂZ-mă	
atelectasis (473)	ă-tĕ-LĔK-tă-sĭs	
auscultation (471)	ăw-skŭl-TĀ-shŭn	

TERM	PRONUNCIATION	MEANING
bacilli (477)	bă-SĬL-ī	
bronchoalveolar lavage (479)	BRŎNG-kō-ăl-vē-Ō-lar lă-VĂJ	
bronchiectasis (470)	brŏng-kē-ĔK-tă-sĭs	
bronchoscopy (479)	brŏng-KŎS-kō-pē	
chronic bronchitis (472)	KRŎ-nĭk brŏng-KĪ-tĭs	
chronic obstructive pulmonary disease (475)	KRŎ-nĭk ŏb-STRŬK-tĭv PŬL-mō-nă-rē dĭ-ZĒZ	
computed tomography (478)	kŏm-PŪ-tĭd tō-MŎG-ră-fē	
cor pulmonale (477)	kŏr pŭl-mō-NĂ-lē	
croup (472)	kroop	
cystic fibrosis (473)	SĬS-tĭk fī-BRŌ-sĭs	
diphtheria (472)	dĭf-THĔR-ē-ă	
emphysema (473)	ĕm-fĭ-ZĒ-mă	
endotracheal intubation (480)	ĕn-dō-TRĀ-kē-ăl ĭn-tū-BĀ-shŭn	
epistaxis (472)	ĕp-ĭ-STĂK-sĭs	
exudate (477)	ĔK-sū-dāt	
hydrothorax (477)	hī-drō-THŎR-ăks	
infiltrate (477)	ĬN-fĭl-trāt	
laryngoscopy (480)	lăr-ĭng-GŎS-kō-pē	
lung biopsy (480)	lŭng BĪ-ŏp-sē	
lung cancer (474)	lŭng KĂN-sĕr	
magnetic resonance imaging of the chest (499)	măg-NĔ-tĭk RĔ-zō-năns ĬM-ă-gĭng of the chĕst	
mediastinoscopy (480)	mē-dē-ă-stī-NŎS-kō-pē	
mesothelioma (476)	mĕz-ō-thē-lē-Ō-mă	
obstructive lung disease (480)	ŏb-STRŬK-tĭv lŭng dĭ-ZĒZ	
palliative (477)	PĂL-ē-ă-tĭv	
paroxysmal (477)	păr-ŏk-SĬZ-măl	
percussion (471)	pĕr-KŬSH-ŭn	
pertussis (472)	pĕr-TŬS-ĭs	
pleural effusion (477)	PLOOR-ăl ĕ-FŪ-zhŭn	
pleural rub (471)	PLOOR-ăl rŭb	

12

TERM	PRONUNCIATION	MEANING
pleurisy (477)	PLOOR-ĭ-sē	_____
pneumoconiosis (474)	nū-mō-kō-nē-Ō-sĭs	_____
pneumonia (475)	nū-MŌ-nē-ă	_____
pneumothorax (477)	nū-mō-THŎR-ăks	_____
positron emission tomography (479)	PŎS-ĭ-trŏn ē-MĬ-shŭn tō-MŎG-ră-fē	_____
pulmonary abscess (475)	PŬL-mō-nă-rē ĂB-sĕs	_____
pulmonary edema (475)	PŬL-mō-nă-rē ĕ-DĒ-mă	_____
pulmonary embolism (476)	PŬL-mō-nă-rē ĔM-bō-lĭzm	_____
pulmonary fibrosis (476)	PŬL-mō-nă-rē fī-BRŌ-sĭs	_____
pulmonary function tests (480)	PŬL-mō-nă-rē FŬNK-shŭn tĕsts	_____
pulmonary infarction (477)	PŬL-mō-nă-rē ĭn-FĂRK-shŭn	_____
purulent (477)	PŪ-rū-lĕnt	_____
rales (471)	răhlz	_____
restrictive lung disease (480)	rē-STRĬK-tĭv lŭng dĭ-ZĒZ	_____
rhonchi (471)	RŎNG-kī	_____
sarcoidosis (476)	săr-koy-DŌ-sĭs	_____
silicosis (477)	sĭ-lĭ-KŌ-sĭs	_____
sputum (471)	SPŪ-tŭm	_____
sputum culture (471)	SPŪ-tŭm KŬL-chŭr	_____
stridor (471)	STRĪ-dŏr	_____
thoracentesis (471)	thō-ră-sĕn-TĒ-sĭs	_____
thoracotomy (469)	thō-ră-KŎ-tō-mē	_____
thoracoscopy (thorascopy) (482)	thō-ră-KŎS-kō-pē (thō-RĂS-kō-pē)	_____
tracheostomy (482)	trā-kē-ŎS-tō-mē	_____
tuberculin test (482)	too-BĔR-kū-lĭn tĕst	_____
tuberculosis (476)	too-bĕr-kū-LŌ-sĭs	_____
tube thoracostomy (482)	toob thŏr-ă-KŎS-tō-mē	_____
ventilation-perfusion scan (479)	vĕn-tĭ-LĀ-shŭn pĕr-FŪ-zhŭn scăn	_____
wheezes (471)	WĒZ-ĕz	_____

12

REVIEW SHEET

Write the meanings of the word parts in the spaces provided. Check your answers with the information in the chapter or in the *Glossary (Medical Word Parts—English)* at the end of the book.

Combining Forms

COMBINING FORM	MEANING	COMBINING FORM	MEANING
adenoid/o		pector/o	
alveol/o		pharyng/o	
bronch/o		phon/o	
bronchi/o		phren/o	
bronchiol/o		pleur/o	
capn/o		pneum/o	
coni/o		pneumon/o	
cyan/o		pulmon/o	
epiglott/o		py/o	
hydr/o		rhin/o	
laryng/o		sinus/o	
lob/o		spir/o	
mediastin/o		tel/o	
nas/o		thorac/o	
or/o		tonsill/o	
orth/o		trache/o	
ox/o			

Suffixes

SUFFIX	MEANING	SUFFIX	MEANING
-algia		-oxia	
-capnia		-phonia	
-centesis		-plasty	
-dynia		-pnea	
-ectasis		-ptysis	
-ectomy		-rrhea	
-ema		-scopy	
-lysis		-sphyxia	
-osmia		-stenosis	

12

SUFFIX	MEANING	SUFFIX	MEANING
-stomy	_____	-tomy	_____
-thorax	_____	-trophy	_____

Prefixes

PREFIX	MEANING	PREFIX	MEANING
a-, an-	_____	hyper-	_____
brady-	_____	hypo-	_____
dys-	_____	para-	_____
em-	_____	per-	_____
eu-	_____	re-	_____
ex-	_____	tachy-	_____

Label the following lung abnormalities: atelectasis, pleural effusion, pneumothorax, and pulmonary edema.

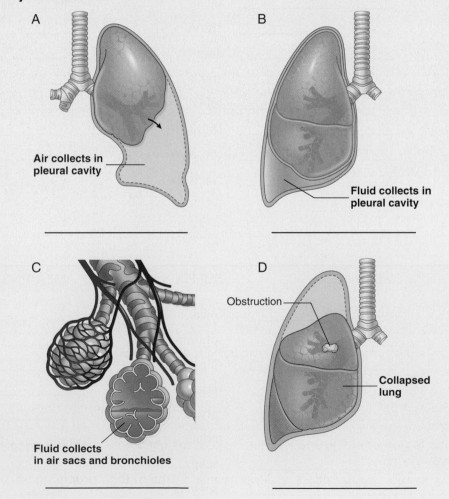

A

Air collects in
pleural cavity

_____

B

Fluid collects in
pleural cavity

_____

C

Fluid collects
in air sacs and bronchioles

_____

D

Obstruction

Collapsed
lung

_____

12

Blood System

Chapter Sections:

CHAPTER GOALS

- Identify terms relating to the composition, formation, and function of blood.
- Differentiate among the four major blood types.
- Identify terms related to blood clotting.
- Build words and recognize combining forms used in blood system terminology.
- Identify various pathologic conditions affecting blood.
- Describe various laboratory tests and clinical procedures used with hematologic disorders, and recognize relevant abbreviations.
- Apply your new knowledge to understanding medical terms in their proper contexts, such as medical reports and records.

INTRODUCTION

The primary function of blood is to maintain a constant environment for the other living tissues of the body. Blood transports nutrients, gases, and wastes to and from the cells of the body. Nutrients from food, digested in the stomach and small intestine, pass into the bloodstream through the lining cells of the small intestine. Blood then carries these nutrients to all body cells. Oxygen enters the body through the air sacs of the lungs. Red blood cells then transport the oxygen to cells throughout the body. Blood also helps remove the waste products released by cells. It carries gaseous waste (such as carbon dioxide) to the lungs to be exhaled. It carries chemical waste, such as urea, to the kidneys to be excreted in the urine.

Blood transports chemical messengers called hormones from their sites of secretion in glands, such as the thyroid or pituitary, to distant sites where they regulate growth, reproduction, and energy production. These hormones are discussed later in the endocrine chapter, page 747.

Finally, blood contains proteins, white blood cells and antibodies that fight infection, and platelets (thrombocytes) and other proteins that help the blood to clot.

COMPOSITION AND FORMATION OF BLOOD

Blood is composed of **cells,** or formed elements, suspended in a clear, straw-colored liquid called **plasma.** The cells normally constitute 45% of the blood volume and include **erythrocytes** (red blood cells), **leukocytes** (white blood cells), and **platelets** or **thrombocytes** (clotting cells). The remaining 55% of blood is plasma, a solution of water, proteins, sugar, salts, hormones, lipids, and vitamins.

CELLS

Beginning at birth, all blood cells originate in the marrow cavity of bones. Both the red blood cells that carry oxygen and the white blood cells that fight infection arise from the same blood-forming or **hematopoietic stem cells.** Under the influence of proteins in the blood and bone marrow, stem cells change their size and shape to become specialized, or **differentiated.** In this process, the cells change in size from large (immature cells) to small (mature forms), and the cell nucleus shrinks (in red cells, the nucleus actually disappears). Figure 13-1 illustrates these changes in the formation of blood cells. Use Figure 13-1 as a reference as you learn the names of mature blood cells and their earlier forms.

ERYTHROCYTES

As a red blood cell matures (from erythroblast to erythrocyte), it loses its nucleus and assumes the shape of a biconcave disk. This shape (a depressed or hollow surface on each side of the cell, resembling a cough drop with a thin central portion) allows for a large surface area so that absorption and release of gases (oxygen and carbon dioxide) can take place (Figure 13-2A and B). Red cells contain the unique protein **hemoglobin,** composed of **heme** (iron-containing pigment) and **globin** (protein). Hemoglobin enables the erythrocyte to carry oxygen. The combination of oxygen and hemoglobin (oxyhemoglobin) produces the bright red color of blood.

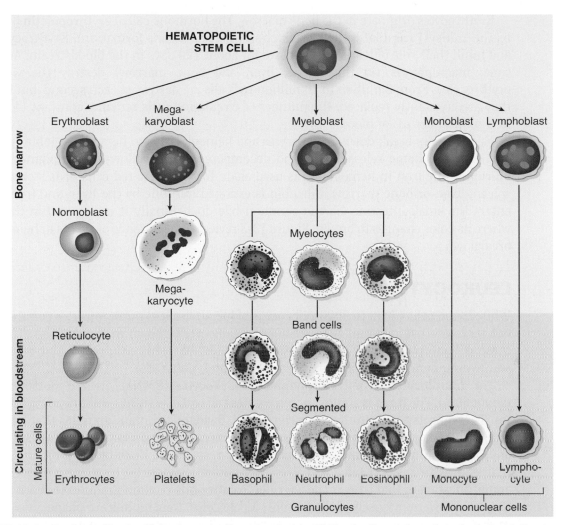

FIGURE 13-1   Stages in blood cell development (hematopoiesis). All blood cells originate from **hematopoietic stem cells.** Progenitor cells are derived from hematopoietic stem cells. Myeloid progenitor cells give rise to **erythroblasts, megakaryoblasts, myeloblasts** and **monoblasts.** Lymphoid progenitor cells give rise to **lymphoblasts.** Notice that the suffix **-blast** indicates immature forms of all cells. **Band cells** are identical to **segmented granulocytes** except that the nucleus is U-shaped and it does not have distinct nuclear lobes.

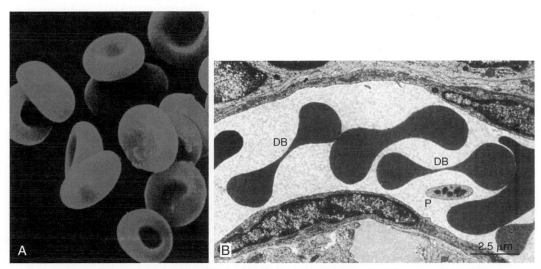

FIGURE 13-2   A, Normal erythrocytes (red blood cells). **B, Electron micrograph showing erythrocytes within a capillary.** Note the classic biconcave or "dumbbell" shape (DB) seen when the erythrocyte is cut through its thin central zone. A platelet (P) is seen as well.

Erythrocytes originate in the bone marrow. The hormone called **erythropoietin** (secreted by the kidneys) stimulates their production (**-poiesis** means formation). Erythrocytes live and fulfill their role of transporting gases for about 120 days in the bloodstream. After this time, **macrophages** (in the spleen, liver, and bone marrow) destroy the worn-out erythrocytes. From 2 million to 10 million red cells are destroyed each second, but because they are constantly replaced, the number of circulating cells remains constant (4 million to 6 million per µL of blood).

Macrophages break down erythrocytes and hemoglobin into heme and globin (protein) portions. The heme releases iron and decomposes into a yellow-orange pigment called **bilirubin.** The iron in hemoglobin is used again to form new red cells or is stored in the spleen, liver, or bone marrow. Bilirubin is excreted into bile by the liver, and from bile it enters the small intestine via the common bile duct. Finally it is excreted in the stool, where its color changes to brown. Figure 13-3 reviews the sequence of events in hemoglobin breakdown.

LEUKOCYTES

White blood cells (7000 to 9000 cells per µ of blood) are less numerous than erythrocytes, but there are five different types of mature leukocytes, shown in Figure 13-4. These are three polymorphonuclear granulocytic leukocytes (basophil eosinophil, and neutrophil) and two mononuclear leukocytes (lymphocyte and monocyte).

The **granulocytes,** or **polymorphonuclear leukocytes (PMNs),** are the most numerous (about 60%). The three granulocytic leukocytes end with the suffix -phil (meaning attraction to). This reflects their affinity for various dyes. **Basophils** contain granules that stain dark blue with a basic (alkaline) dye. These granules contain heparin (an anticlotting substance) and histamine (a chemical released in allergic responses). **Eosinophils** contain granules that stain with eosin, a red acidic dye. These granules increase in allergic responses and engulf substances that trigger the allergies. **Neutrophils** contain granules that are neutral; they do not stain intensely and show only a pale color. Neutrophils are **phagocytes (phag/o** means to eat or swallow) that accumulate at sites of infection, where they ingest and destroy bacteria. Figure 13-5 shows phagocytosis by a neutrophil.

Specific proteins called **colony-stimulating factors** (CSFs) promote the growth of granulocytes in bone marrow. **G-CSF** (granulocyte CSF) and **GM-CSF** (granulocyte-macrophage CSF) are given to restore granulocyte production in cancer patients. **Erythropoietin,** like CSFs, can be produced by recombinant DNA techniques. It stimulates red blood cell production (erythropoiesis).

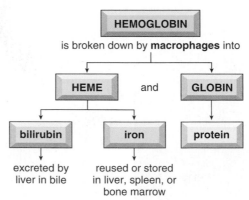

FIGURE 13-3   The breakdown of hemoglobin.

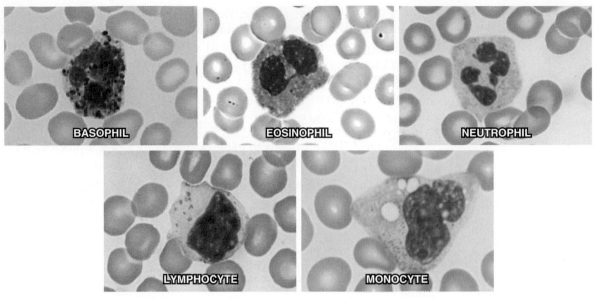

FIGURE 13-4 Leukocytes.

Although all granulocytes are **polymorphonuclear** (they have multilobed nuclei), the term **polymorphonuclear granulocytes ("polys")** most often refers to neutrophils, which are the most numerous of the granulocytes.

Mononuclear (containing one large nucleus) **leukocytes** do not have large numbers of granules in their cytoplasm, but they may have a few granules. These are **lymphocytes** and **monocytes** (see Figure 13-1). Lymphocytes are made in bone marrow and lymph nodes and circulate both in the bloodstream and in the parallel circulating system, the lymphatic system.

Lymphocytes play an important role in the **immune response** that protects the body against infection. They can directly attack foreign matter and, in addition, make **antibodies** that neutralize and can lead to the destruction of foreign **antigens** (bacteria and viruses). **Monocytes** are phagocytic cells that also fight disease. As **macrophages**, they move from the bloodstream into tissues and dispose of dead and dying cells and other tissue debris by phagocytosis.

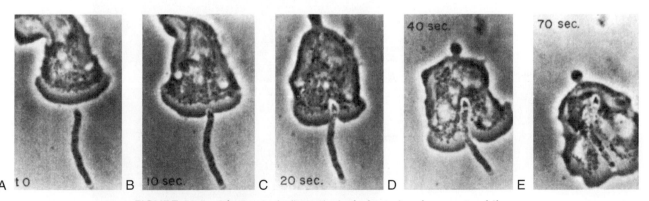

FIGURE 13-5 **Phagocytosis** (ingestion) of a bacterium by a neutrophil.

TABLE 13-1	LEUKOCYTES	
LEUKOCYTE	**NORMAL PERCENTAGE IN BLOOD**	**FUNCTION**
Granulocytes		
Basophil	0-1	Responds to allergens; releases histamine and heparin
Eosinophil	1-4	Responds to parasitic infections and is a phagocyte in allergic reactions
Neutrophil	50-70	Major role in fighting bacterial infection; phagocyte
Mononuclear Cells		
Lymphocyte	20-40	Controls the immune response; makes antibodies to antigens
Monocyte	3-8	Phagocytic cell that becomes a macrophage and digests bacteria and tissue debris

Table 13-1 reviews the different types of leukocytes, their numbers in the blood, and their functions.

PLATELETS (THROMBOCYTES)

Platelets, actually blood cell fragments, are formed in bone marrow from giant cells with multilobed nuclei called **megakaryocytes** (Figure 13-6A and B). The main function of platelets is to help blood to clot. Specific terms related to blood clotting are discussed later in this chapter.

PLASMA

Plasma, the liquid part of the blood, consists of water, dissolved proteins, sugar, wastes, salts, hormones, and other substances. The four major plasma proteins are **albumin, globulins, fibrinogen,** and **prothrombin** (the last two are clotting proteins).

Albumin maintains the proper proportion (and concentration) of water in the blood. Because albumin cannot pass easily through capillary walls, it remains in the blood and

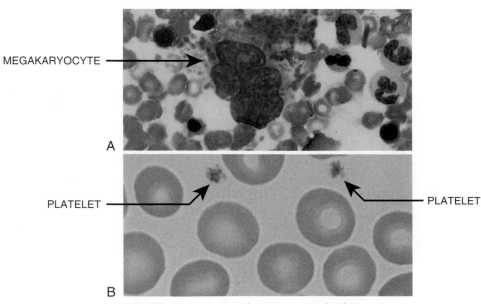

MEGAKARYOCYTE

A

PLATELET

PLATELET

B

FIGURE 13-6   A, Megakaryocyte. B, Platelets.

carries smaller molecules bound to its surface. It attracts water from the tissues back into the bloodstream and thus opposes the water's tendency to leave the blood and leak out into tissue spaces. **Edema** (swelling) results when too much fluid from blood "leaks" out into tissues. This happens in a mild form when a person ingests too much salt (water is retained in the blood and seeps out into tissues) and in a severe form when a person is burned in a fire. In this situation, albumin escapes from capillaries as a result of the burn injury. Then water cannot be held in the blood; it escapes through the skin, and blood volume drops.

Globulins are another component of blood and one of the plasma proteins. There are alpha, beta, and gamma globulins. The gamma globulins are **immunoglobulins,** which are antibodies that bind to and sometimes destroy antigens (foreign substances). Examples of immunoglobulin antibodies are **IgG** (found in high concentration in plasma) and **IgA** (found in breast milk, saliva, tears, and respiratory mucus). Other immunoglobulins are **IgM, IgD,** and **IgE.** Immunoglobulins are separated from other plasma proteins by **electrophoresis.** In this process, an electrical current passes through a solution of plasma. The different proteins in plasma separate as they migrate at different speeds to the source of the electricity.

Plasmapheresis (-apheresis means removal) is the process of separating plasma from cells and then removing the plasma from the patient. In plasmapheresis, the entire blood sample is spun in a centrifuge machine, and the plasma, being lighter in weight than the cells, moves to the top of the sample.

Figure 13-7 reviews the composition of blood.

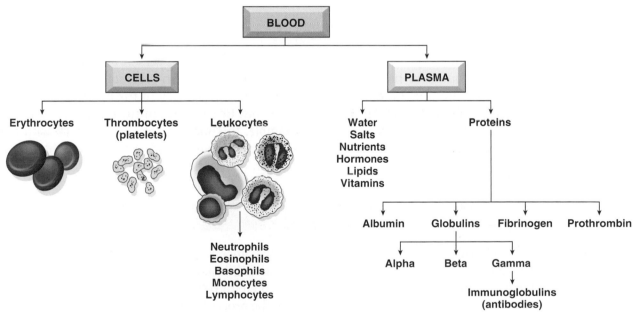

FIGURE 13-7   The composition of blood.

TABLE 13-2	BLOOD TYPES		
TYPE	**PERCENTAGE IN POPULATION**	**RED CELL ANTIGENS**	**SERUM ANTIBODIES**
A	41	A	Yes (anti-B)
B	10	B	Yes (anti-A)
AB	4	A and B	No (anti-A or anti-B)
O	45	No A and B	Yes (anti-A and anti-B)

BLOOD TYPES

Transfusions of whole blood (cells and plasma) are used to replace blood lost after injury, during surgery, or in severe shock. A patient who is severely anemic and needs only red blood cells will receive a transfusion of **packed red cells** (whole blood with most of the plasma removed). Human blood falls into four main types: A, B, AB, and O. These types are based on the antigens on red blood cells and the antibodies found in each person's serum (Table 13-2).

There are harmful effects of transfusing blood from a donor of one blood type into a recipient who has blood of another blood type. Therefore, before blood is transfused, both the blood donor and the blood recipient are tested, to make sure that the transfused blood will be compatible with the recipient's blood type. ◣ During transfusion, if blood is not compatible, then **hemolysis** (breakdown of red blood cells) occurs. This may be followed by excessive clotting in blood vessels (**disseminated intravascular coagulation,** or **DIC**), which is a life-threatening condition.

Besides A and B antigens, many other antigens are located on the surface of red blood cells. One of these is called the **Rh factor** (named because it was first found in the blood of a rhesus monkey). The term Rh positive (Rh+) refers to a person who is born with the Rh antigen on his or her red blood cells. An Rh negative (Rh−) person does not have the Rh antigen. See Chapter 4, page 120, for more information about the Rh factor. In clinical practice, blood types are named to indicate both Rh and ABO antigen status. If a woman has an A+ (A positive) blood type, for example, this means that she was born with both A antigen and Rh antigen on her red blood cells. If a man has a B− (B negative) blood type, this means he was born with the B antigen on his red blood cells but not Rh antigen.

BLOOD CLOTTING

Blood clotting, or **coagulation,** is a complicated process involving many different substances and chemical reactions. The final result (usually taking less than 15 minutes) is the formation of a **fibrin clot** from the plasma protein **fibrinogen.** The suffix -gen means giving rise to. Platelets are important in beginning the process following injury to tissues or blood vessels. The platelets become sticky and collect, or aggregate, at the site of injury. Then, in combination with tissue and protein clotting factors, plus calcium, vitamin K, prothrombin, and thrombin, fibrinogen is converted to fibrin to form a clot (Figure 13-8). One of the important clotting factors is factor VIII. It is missing in some people who are born with hemophilia. Other hemophiliacs are missing factor IX.

Why is Type O the "Universal Donor" Blood Type?

Type O blood does not contain A or B red cell antigens and therefore will not react with antibodies in any recipient's bloodstream. Anti-A and anti-B antibodies present in type O blood become diluted in the recipient's bloodstream and do not cause an adverse reaction.

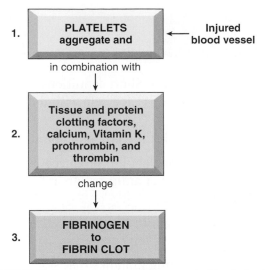

FIGURE 13-8 The sequence of events in blood clotting.

The fibrin threads form the clot by trapping red blood cells (Figure 13-9 shows a red blood cell trapped by fibrin threads). Then the clot retracts into a tight ball, leaving behind a clear fluid called **serum.** Normally, clots (thrombi) do not form in blood vessels unless the vessel is damaged or the flow of blood is impeded. **Anticoagulant substances** in the blood inhibit blood clotting, so clots do not form. **Heparin,** produced by tissue cells (especially in the liver), is an example of an anticoagulant. Other drugs such as **warfarin (Coumadin)** are given to patients with thromboembolic diseases to prevent the formation of clots. **Newer oral anticoagulants (NOACs)** work by inhibiting blood clotting factors such as thrombin.

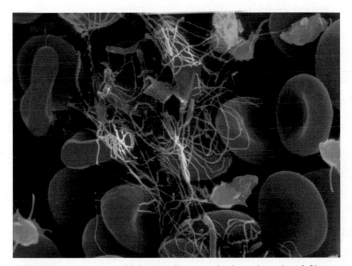

FIGURE 13-9 A red blood cell enmeshed in threads of fibrin.

13

VOCABULARY

This list reviews many of the new terms introduced in the text. Short definitions reinforce your understanding of the terms. Refer to the Pronunciation of Terms on page 541 for help with difficult or unfamiliar words.

albumin	Protein in blood; maintains the proper amount of water in the blood.
antibody (Ab)	Specific protein (immunoglobulin) produced by lymphocytes in response to bacteria, viruses, or other antigens. An antibody is specific to an antigen and inactivates it.
antigen	Substance (usually foreign) that stimulates the production of an antibody.
basophil	White blood cell containing granules that stain blue; associated with release of histamine and heparin.
bilirubin	Orange-yellow pigment in bile; formed by the breakdown of hemoglobin when red blood cells are destroyed.
coagulation	Blood clotting.
colony-stimulating factor (CSF)	Protein that stimulates growth of white blood cells (granulocytes).
differentiation	Change in structure and function of a cell as it matures; specialization.
electrophoresis	Method of separating serum proteins by electrical charge.
eosinophil	White blood cell containing granules that stain red; associated with allergic reactions.
erythroblast	Immature red blood cell.
erythrocyte	Red blood cell. There are about 5 million per microliter (μL) or cubic millimeter (mm^3) of blood.
erythropoietin (EPO)	Hormone secreted by the kidneys; stimulates red blood cell formation.
fibrin	Protein that forms the basis of a blood clot.
fibrinogen	Plasma protein that is converted to fibrin in the clotting process.
globulin	Plasma protein; alpha, beta, and gamma (immune) globulins are examples.
granulocyte	White blood cell with numerous dark-staining granules: eosinophil, neutrophil, and basophil.
hematopoietic stem cell	Cell in the bone marrow that gives rise to all types of blood cells.
hemoglobin	Blood protein containing iron; carries oxygen in red blood cells.
heparin	Anticoagulant found in blood and tissue cells.
immune reaction	Response of the immune system to foreign invasion.
immunoglobulin	Protein (a globulin) with antibody activity; examples are IgG, IgM, IgA, IgE, IgD. Immun/o means protection.

leukocyte	White blood cell.
lymphocyte	Mononuclear leukocyte that produces antibodies.
macrophage	Monocyte that migrates from the blood to tissue spaces. As a phagocyte, it engulfs foreign material and debris. In the liver, spleen, and bone marrow, macrophages destroy worn out red blood cells.
megakaryocyte	Large platelet precursor cell found in the bone marrow.
monocyte	Leukocyte with one large nucleus. It is a cell that engulfs foreign material and debris. Monocytes become macrophages as they leave the blood and enter body tissues.
mononuclear	Pertaining to a cell (leukocyte) with a single round nucleus; lymphocytes and monocytes are mononuclear leukocytes.
myeloblast	Immature bone marrow that gives rise to granulocytes.
neutrophil	Granulocytic leukocyte formed in bone marrow. It is a phagocytic tissue-fighting cell. Also called a **polymorphonuclear leukocyte.**
plasma	Liquid portion of blood; contains water, proteins, salts, nutrients, lipids, hormones, and vitamins.
plasmapheresis	Removal of plasma from withdrawn blood by centrifuge. Collected cells are retransfused back into the donor. Fresh-frozen plasma or salt solution is used to replace withdrawn plasma.
platelet	Small blood fragment that collects at sites of injury to begin the clotting process.
polymorphonuclear	Pertaining to a white blood cell with a multilobed nucleus; neutrophil.
prothrombin	Plasma protein; converted to thrombin in the clotting process.
reticulocyte	Immature erythrocyte. A network of strands (reticulin) is seen after staining the cell with special dyes.
Rh factor	Antigen on red blood cells of Rh-positive (Rh+) individuals. The factor was first identified in the blood of a <u>rh</u>esus monkey.
serum	Plasma minus clotting proteins and cells. Clear, yellowish fluid that separates from blood when it is allowed to clot. It is formed from plasma, but does not contain protein-coagulation factors.
stem cell	Unspecialized cell that gives rise to mature, specialized forms. A **hematopoietic stem cell** is the progenitor for all different types of blood cells.
thrombin	Enzyme that converts fibrinogen to fibrin during coagulation.
thrombocyte	Platelet.

13

TERMINOLOGY

Write the meanings of the medical terms in the spaces provided.

COMBINING FORMS

COMBINING FORM	MEANING	TERMINOLOGY	MEANING
bas/o	base (*alkaline, the opposite of acid*)	basophil _____ *The suffix -phil means attraction to. Granules in basophils are attracted to a basic dye.*	
chrom/o	color	hypochromic _____ *Hypochromic anemia is marked by a decreased concentration of hemoglobin in red blood cells.*	
coagul/o	clotting	anticoagulant _____	
		coagulopathy _____	
cyt/o	cell	cytology _____	
eosin/o	red, dawn, rosy	eosinophil _____	
erythr/o	red	erythroblast _____ *-blast means immature.*	
granul/o	granules	granulocyte _____	
hem/o	blood	hemolysis _____ *Destruction or breakdown of red blood cells. See hemolytic anemia, page 518.*	
hemat/o	blood	hematocrit _____ *The suffix -crit means to separate. The hematocrit gives the percentage of red blood cells in a volume of blood. See page 523.*	
hemoglobin/o	hemoglobin	hemoglobinopathy _____	
is/o	same, equal	anisocytosis _____ *An abnormality of red blood cells; they are of unequal (anis/o) size; -cytosis means an increase in the number of cells.*	
kary/o	nucleus	megakaryocyte _____	
leuk/o	white	leukopenia _____	
mon/o	one, single	monocyte _____ *The cell has a single, rather than a multilobed, nucleus.*	
morph/o	shape, form	morphology _____	

COMBINING FORM	MEANING	TERMINOLOGY	MEANING
myel/o	bone marrow	myeloblast _____ *The suffix -blast indicates an immature or embryonic cell.*	
		myelodysplasia _____ *This is a preleukemic condition.*	
neutr/o	neutral (neither base nor acid)	neutropenia _____ *This term refers to neutrophils.*	
nucle/o	nucleus	polymorphonuclear _____	
phag/o	eat, swallow	phagocyte _____	
poikil/o	varied, irregular	poikilocytosis _____ *Irregularity in the shape of red blood cells. Poikilocytosis occurs in certain types of anemia.*	
sider/o	iron	sideropenia _____	
spher/o	globe, round	spherocytosis _____ *In this condition, the erythrocyte has a round shape, making the cell fragile and easily able to be destroyed.*	
thromb/o	clot	thrombocytopenia _____	

SUFFIXES

SUFFIX	MEANING	TERMINOLOGY	MEANING
-apheresis	removal, a carrying away	plasmapheresis _____ *A centrifuge spins blood to remove plasma from the other parts of blood.*	
		leukapheresis _____	
		plateletpheresis _____ *Note that the a of apheresis is dropped in this term. Platelets are removed from the donor's blood (and used in a patient), and the remainder of the blood is reinfused into the donor.*	
-blast	immature or embryonic cell	monoblast _____	

Don't Confuse -apheresis with -phoresis

The suffix **-apheresis** refers to the removal of blood from a donor with a portion separated and retained and the remainder reinfused into the donor (see page 524). The suffix **-phoresis** indicates transmission (as in **electrophoresis,** the transmission of electricity to separate substances).

SUFFIX	MEANING	TERMINOLOGY	MEANING
-cytosis	abnormal condition of cells (increase in cells)	macrocytosis _____ *Macrocytes are erythrocytes that are larger (macro-) than normal.* microcytosis _____ *In this condition, the erythrocytes are smaller (micro-) than normal. Table 13-3 reviews terms related to abnormalities of red blood cell morphology.*	
-emia	blood condition	leukemia _____ *See page 520.*	
-gen	giving rise to; producing	fibrinogen _____ *Fibrin is a protein that forms the basis of a blood clot.*	
-globin	protein	hemoglobin _____	
-globulin		immunoglobulin _____	
-lytic	pertaining to destruction	thrombolytic therapy _____ *Used to dissolve clots.*	
-oid	derived or originating from	myeloid _____	
-osis	abnormal condition	thrombosis _____	
-penia	deficiency	granulocytopenia _____ pancytopenia _____	
-phage	eat, swallow	macrophage _____ *A large phagocyte that destroys worn-out red blood cells and foreign material.*	
-philia	attraction for (an increase in cell numbers)	eosinophilia _____ neutrophilia _____	
-phoresis	carrying, transmission	electrophoresis _____	
-poiesis	formation	hematopoiesis _____ erythropoiesis _____ **Erythropoietin** *is produced by the kidneys to stimulate erythrocyte formation.* myelopoiesis _____	
-stasis	stop, control	hemostasis _____	

13

TABLE 13-3	ABNORMALITIES OF RED BLOOD CELL MORPHOLOGY
ABNORMALITY	**DESCRIPTION**
Anisocytosis	Cells are **unequal** in size
Hypo**chromia**	Cells have reduced **color** (less hemoglobin)
Macrocytosis	Cells are **large**
Microcytosis	Cells are **small**
Poikilocytosis	Cells are **irregularly shaped**
Spherocytosis	Cells are **spherical** (loss of normal concave shape)

PATHOLOGY

Any abnormal or pathologic condition of the blood generally is referred to as a blood **dyscrasia** (disease). The blood dyscrasias discussed in this section are organized in the following order: diseases of red blood cells, disorders of blood clotting, diseases of white blood cells, and disease of the bone marrow.

DISEASES OF RED BLOOD CELLS

anemia

Deficiency in erythrocytes or hemoglobin.

The most common type of anemia is **iron deficiency anemia**; it is caused by a lack of iron, which is required for hemoglobin production (Figure 13-10).

Other types of anemia include:

1. aplastic anemia

Failure of blood cell production in the bone marrow.

The cause of most cases of aplastic anemia is unknown (idiopathic), but some have been linked to benzene exposure and rarely to antibiotics such as chloramphenicol. **Pancytopenia** occurs when stem cells fail to produce leukocytes, platelets, and erythrocytes. Blood transfusions prolong life, allowing the marrow time to resume its normal functioning, and antibiotics control infections. Bone marrow transplantation and regimens of drugs that inhibit the immune system are successful treatments in cases in which spontaneous recovery is unlikely.

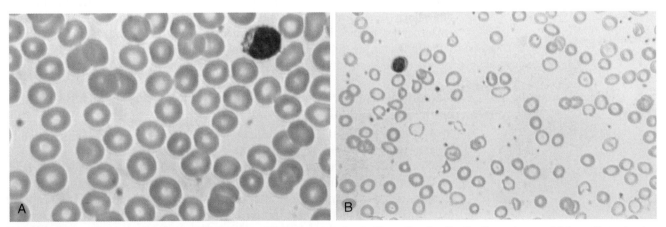

FIGURE 13-10   Normal red blood cells and iron deficiency anemia. A, Normal red cells. Erythrocytes are fairly uniform in size and shape. The red cells are normal in hemoglobin content (normochromic) and size (normocytic). **B, Iron deficiency anemia.** Many erythrocytes are small (**microcytic**) and have increased central pallor (**hypochromic**). Red cells in this slide show variation in size (**anisocytosis**) and shape (**poikilocytosis**).

13

13

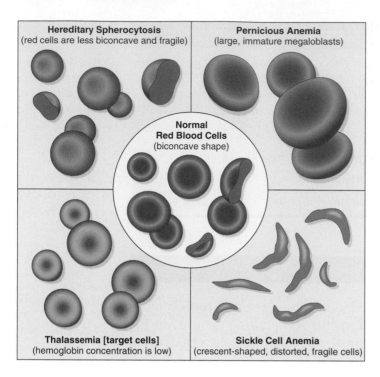

Hereditary Spherocytosis
(red cells are less biconcave and fragile)

Pernicious Anemia
(large, immature megaloblasts)

**Normal
Red Blood Cells**
(biconcave shape)

Thalassemia [target cells]
(hemoglobin concentration is low)

Sickle Cell Anemia
(crescent-shaped, distorted, fragile cells)

FIGURE 13-11 Normal red blood cells and the abnormal cells in several types of anemia.

2. hemolytic anemia	**Reduction in red cells due to excessive destruction.**

One example of hemolytic anemia is **congenital spherocytic anemia (hereditary spherocytosis).** Instead of their normal biconcave shape, erythrocytes become spheroidal. This rounded shape makes them fragile and easily destroyed (hemolysis). Shortened red cell survival results in increased reticulocytes in blood as the bone marrow compensates for hemolysis of mature erythrocytes. Because the spleen destroys red cells, removal of the spleen usually improves this anemia. Figure 13-11 shows the altered shape of erythrocytes in hereditary spherocytosis.

3. pernicious anemia	**Lack of mature erythrocytes caused by inability to absorb vitamin B_{12} into the bloodstream.**

Vitamin B_{12} is necessary for the proper development and maturation of erythrocytes. Although vitamin B_{12} is a common constituent of food (liver, kidney, sardines, egg yolks, oysters), it cannot be absorbed into the bloodstream without the aid of a special substance called **intrinsic factor,** which normally is found in gastric juice. People with pernicious anemia lack this factor in their gastric juice, and the result is unsuccessful maturation of red blood cells, with an excess of large, immature, and poorly functioning cells in the bone marrow and large, often oval red cells (macrocytes) in the circulation. Treatment is injection or oral administration of vitamin B_{12} for life. Figure 13-11 illustrates cells in pernicious anemia. Pernicious means ruinous or hurtful.

4. sickle cell anemia	**Hereditary disorder of abnormal hemoglobin producing sickle-shaped erythrocytes and hemolysis.**

The crescent, or sickle, shape of the erythrocyte (see Figure 13-11) is caused by an abnormal type of hemoglobin (hemoglobin S) in the red cell. The distorted, fragile erythrocytes cannot pass through small blood vessels normally. This leads to thrombosis and infarction (local tissue death from ischemia). Signs and symptoms are arthralgias, acute attacks of abdominal pain, and ulcerations of the extremities. The genetic defect (presence of the hemoglobin S gene) is particularly prevalent among people of African or Hispanic ancestry and appears with different degrees of severity. Persons with the sickle cell trait inherit just one gene for the disorder and usually do not have symptoms.

5. thalassemia

Inherited disorder of abnormal hemoglobin production leading to hypochromia.

A defect in a gene affects production of **globin,** the protein that is the major component of hemoglobin. This condition, usually occurring in persons of Mediterranean or Asian background, manifests in varying forms and degrees of severity and usually leads to hypochromic anemia with diminished hemoglobin content in red cells (see Figure 13-11). *Thalassa* is a Greek word meaning sea.

hemochromatosis

Excess iron deposits throughout the body.

Common signs and symptoms may include skin pigmentation, joint pain, and fatigue. Without timely treatment, serious problems such as cirrhosis, diabetes, and cardiac failure may occur. This condition can be hereditary. See ***In Person: Hereditary Hemochromatosis,*** page 530.

polycythemia vera

General increase in red blood cells (erythremia).

Blood consistency is viscous (thick) because of greatly increased numbers of erythrocytes. The bone marrow is hyperplastic, and leukocytosis and thrombocytosis commonly accompany the increase in red blood cells. Treatment consists of reduction of red cell volume to normal levels by phlebotomy (removal of blood from a vein) and by suppressing blood cell production with myelotoxic drugs.

DISORDERS OF BLOOD CLOTTING

hemophilia

Excessive bleeding caused by hereditary lack of factors VIII and IX necessary for blood clotting.

Although the platelet count of a hemophiliac patient is normal, deficiency in clotting factors (factor VIII or IX) results in a prolonged coagulation time. Patients with clotting factor deficiencies often bleed into weight-bearing joints, especially ankles and knees. See Figure 13-12. Treatment consists of administration of the deficient factors.

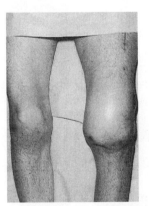

FIGURE 13-12   Lower limbs of a male with **hemophilia** showing the effect of recurrent hemorrhage into the left knee. *(Courtesy Dr. G. Dolan, University Hospital, Nottingham, UK.)*

Why Hemophilia Mainly Affects Males

Because the genes for factors VIII and IX are on the X chromosome, hemophilia mainly affects males. Males only have one X chromosome. In females, hemophilia rarely occurs because typically one of their two X chromosomes is normal and it compensates for the defective gene if it is on the other X chromosome.

purpura

Multiple pinpoint hemorrhages and accumulation of blood under the skin.

Hemorrhages into the skin and mucous membranes produce red-purple discoloration of the skin. **Petechiae** are tiny purple or red flat spots appearing on the skin as a result of hemorrhages. **Ecchymoses** are larger, blue or purplish patches on the skin (bruises) (Figure 13-13). Purpura can result from having too few platelets (thrombocytopenia). The cause may be immunologic, meaning that the body produces an antiplatelet factor that harms its own platelets. **Autoimmune thrombocytopenic purpura** is a condition in which the patient makes an antibody that destroys platelets. Bleeding time is prolonged; splenectomy (the spleen is the site of platelet destruction) and drug therapy with glucocorticoids are common treatments.

DISEASES OF WHITE BLOOD CELLS

leukemia

Increase in cancerous white blood cells (leukocytes).

Acute leukemias have common clinical characteristics: abrupt onset of signs and symptoms—fatigue, fever, bleeding, bone pain, lymphadenopathy, splenomegaly, and hepatomegaly. If the disease has spread to the spinal canal, headache and vomiting also may occur. In addition, because normal blood cells are crowded out, patients have little defense against infection.

Four types of leukemia are:

1. **Acute myeloid (myelocytic) leukemia (AML).** Immature granulocytes (myeloblasts) predominate. Platelets and erythrocytes are diminished because of infiltration and replacement of the bone marrow by large numbers of myeloblasts (Figure 13-14A).

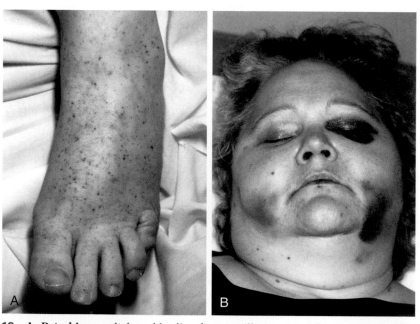

FIGURE 13-13 **A, Petechiae** result from bleeding from capillaries or small arterioles. **B, Ecchymoses** are larger and more extensive than petechiae.

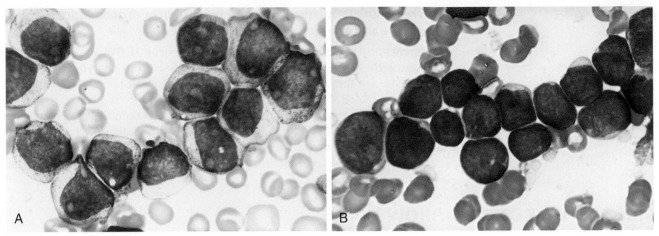

FIGURE 13-14   Acute leukemia. A, Acute myeloid leukemia (AML). Myeloblasts (immature granulocytes) predominate. There are large cells with small granules in their cytoplasm. AML affects primarily adults. A majority of patients achieve remission with intensive chemotherapy, but relapse is common. Hematopoietic stem cell transplantation may be a curative therapy. **B, Acute lymphoid leukemia (ALL).** Lymphoblasts (immature lymphocytes) predominate. ALL is a disease of children and young adults. Most children are cured with chemotherapy. *(Courtesy Dr. Robert W. McKenna, Department of Pathology, University of Texas Southwestern Medical School, Dallas.)*

2. **Acute lymphoid leukemia (ALL).** Immature lymphocytes (lymphoblasts) predominate. This form is seen most often in children and adolescents; onset is sudden (see Figure 13-14B).
3. **Chronic myeloid (myelocytic) leukemia (CML).** Both mature and immature granulocytes are present in large numbers in the marrow and blood. This is a slowly progressive illness with which patients (often adults older than 55) may live for many years without encountering life-threatening problems. New therapies (such as the drug Gleevec) target abnormal proteins responsible for malignancy and produce long-term control.
4. **Chronic lymphoid (lymphocytic) leukemia (CLL).** Abnormal numbers of relatively mature lymphocytes predominate in the marrow, lymph nodes, and spleen. This most common form of leukemia usually occurs in the elderly and follows a slowly progressive course. It often does not require immediate treatment.

All forms of leukemia are treated with chemotherapy, using drugs that prevent cell division and selectively injure rapidly dividing cells. Effective treatment can lead to a **remission** (disappearance of signs and symptoms of disease). **Relapse** occurs when disease symptoms and signs reappear, necessitating further treatment.

Transplantation of normal bone marrow from donors of similar tissue type is successful in restoring normal bone marrow function in some patients with acute leukemia. This procedure is performed after high-dose chemotherapy, which is administered to eliminate the leukemic cells.

granulocytosis

Abnormal increase in granulocytes in the blood.

An increase in neutrophils in the blood may occur in response to infection or inflammation of any type. **Eosinophilia** is an increase in eosinophilic granulocytes, seen in certain allergic conditions, such as asthma, or in parasitic infections (tapeworm, pinworm). **Basophilia** is an increase in basophilic granulocytes seen in certain types of leukemia.

13

mononucleosis | **Infectious disease marked by increased numbers of mononuclear leukocytes and enlarged cervical lymph nodes.**

This disease is transmitted by the **Epstein-Barr virus (EBV).** Lymphadenitis is present, with fever, fatigue, asthenia (weakness), and pharyngitis. Atypical lymphocytes are present in the blood, liver, and spleen (leading to hepatomegaly and splenomegaly).

Mononucleosis usually is transmitted by direct oral contact (salivary exchange during kissing) and affects primarily young adults. No treatment is necessary for EBV infections. Antibiotics are not effective for self-limited viral illnesses. Rest during the period of acute symptoms and slow return to normal activities are advised.

DISEASE OF BONE MARROW CELLS

multiple myeloma | **Malignant neoplasm of bone marrow.**

Malignant cells, lymphocytes called plasma cells, produce antibodies that destroy bone tissue and cause of immunoglobulins, including **Bence Jones protein,** an immunoglobulin fragment found in urine. The condition leads to osteolytic lesions, hypercalcemia, anemia, renal damage, and increased susceptibility to infection. Treatment is with analgesics, radiotherapy, various doses of chemotherapy, and special orthopedic supports. Drugs such as thalidomide and Velcade (bortezomib) are **palliative** (relieving symptoms) and stop disease progression, which improves the outlook for this disease. **Autologous bone marrow transplantation** (ABMT), in which the patient serves as his or her own donor for stem cells, may lead to prolonged remission.

13 | LABORATORY TESTS AND CLINICAL PROCEDURES

LABORATORY TESTS

antiglobulin (Coombs) test | **Test for the presence of antibodies that coat and damage erythrocytes.**

This test determines the presence of antibodies in infants of Rh-negative women or in patients with autoimmune hemolytic anemia.

bleeding time | **Time required for blood to stop flowing from a tiny puncture wound.**

Normal time is 8 minutes or less. Either the Simplate or the Ivy method is used. Platelet disorders and the use of aspirin prolong bleeding time.

coagulation time | **Time required for venous blood to clot in a test tube.**

Normal time is less than 15 minutes.

complete blood count (CBC) | **Determination of numbers of blood cells, hemoglobin concentration, hematocrit, and red cell values—MCH, MCV, MCHC** (see Abbreviations).

erythrocyte sedimentation rate (ESR) | **Speed at which erythrocytes settle out of plasma.**

Venous blood is collected into an anticoagulant, and the blood is placed in a tube in a vertical position. The distance that the erythrocytes sink in a given period of time is the sedimentation rate. The rate increases with infections, joint inflammation, and tumor, which increase the fibrinogen content of the blood. Also called sed rate for short.

hematocrit (Hct)	**Percentage of erythrocytes in a volume of blood.** A sample of blood is spun in a centrifuge so that the erythrocytes fall to the bottom of the sample.
hemoglobin test (H, Hg, Hgb, HGB)	**Total amount of hemoglobin in a sample of peripheral blood.**
platelet count	**Number of platelets per cubic millimeter (mm³) or microliter (μL) of blood.** Platelets normally average between 150,000 and 350,000 per mm³ (cu mm) or μL.
prothrombin time (PT)	**Test of the ability of blood to clot.** Prothrombin is one of the clotting factors (factor II) made by the liver. This test is used to monitor (follow) patients taking anticoagulant drugs. Another blood clotting test, **partial thromboplastin time (PTT)**, measures other clotting factors. Both PT and PTT are often done at the same time to check for bleeding problems.
red blood cell count (RBC)	**Number of erythrocytes per cubic millimeter (mm³) or microliter (μL) of blood.** The normal number is 4 million to 6 million per mm³ (or μL).
red blood cell morphology	**Microscopic examination of a stained blood smear to determine the shape of individual red cells.** Abnormal morphology includes anisocytosis, poikilocytosis, and sickle cells.
white blood cell count (WBC)	**Number of leukocytes per cubic millimeter (mm³) or microliter (μL) of blood.** Automated counting devices record numbers within seconds. Normal number of leukocytes averages between 5000 and 10,000 per mm³ (or μL).
white blood cell differential [count]	**Percentages of different types of leukocytes in the blood.** Some instruments can produce an automated differential count, but otherwise the cells are stained and counted under a microscope by a technician. Percentages of neutrophils, eosinophils, basophils, monocytes, lymphocytes, and immature cells (bands) are determined. See page 528 for the normal differential values. The term **shift to the left** describes an increase in immature neutrophils in the blood.

13

Shift to the Left

The phrase **"shift to the left"** derives from the early practice of reporting percentages of each WBC type across the top of a page, starting with blasts (immature cells) on the left and more mature cells on the right. An increase in immature neutrophils (as seen with severe infection) would be seen in the left-hand column of the reporting form. This "shift to the left" indicates an infection and reflects the body's effort to fight it by making more neutrophils.

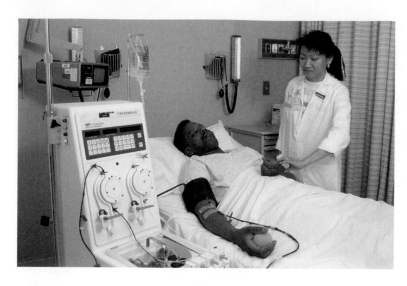

FIGURE 13-15 Leukapheresis. This machine is an automated blood cell separator that removes large numbers of white blood cells and returns red cells, platelets, and plasma to the patient.

CLINICAL PROCEDURES

apheresis

Separation of blood into component parts and removal of a select portion from the blood.

This procedure can remove toxic substances or autoantibodies from the blood and can collect blood cells. Leukapheresis, plateletpheresis, and plasmapheresis are examples (Figure 13-15). If plasma is removed from the patient and fresh plasma is given, the procedure is termed **plasma exchange.**

blood transfusion

Whole blood or cells are taken from a donor and infused into a patient.

Appropriate testing to ensure a match of red blood cell type (A, B, AB, or O) is essential. Tests also are performed to detect the presence of hepatitis and the acquired immunodeficiency syndrome (AIDS) virus (HIV). **Autologous transfusion** is the collection and later reinfusion of a patient's own blood or blood components. **Packed cells** are a preparation of red blood cells separated from liquid plasma and administered in severe anemia to restore levels of hemoglobin and red cells without overdiluting the blood with excess fluid.

bone marrow biopsy

Microscopic examination of a core of bone marrow removed with a needle.

This procedure is helpful in the diagnosis of blood disorders such as anemia, pancytopenias, and leukemia. Bone marrow also may be removed by brief suction produced by a syringe, which is termed a **bone marrow aspiration.** See Figure 13-16.

hematopoietic stem cell transplantation

Peripheral stem cells from a compatible donor are administered to a recipient.

Patients with malignancies, such as AML, ALL, CLL, CML, lymphoma and multiple myeloma, are candidates for this treatment. First the donor is treated with a drug that mobilizes stem cells into the blood. Then stem cells are removed from the donor, a process like leukapheresis in Figure 13-15. Meanwhile, the patient (recipient) undergoes a conditioning process in which radiation and chemotherapy drugs are administered to kill malignant marrow cells and inactivate the patient's immune system so that subsequently infused stem cells will not be rejected. A cell suspension containing the donor's stem cells, which will repopulate the bone marrow, is then given through a vein to the recipient. In **autologous stem cell transplantation,** the patient's own stem cells are collected, stored, and reinfused after potent chemotherapy. See ***In Person: Autologous Stem Cell Transplant,*** page 531.

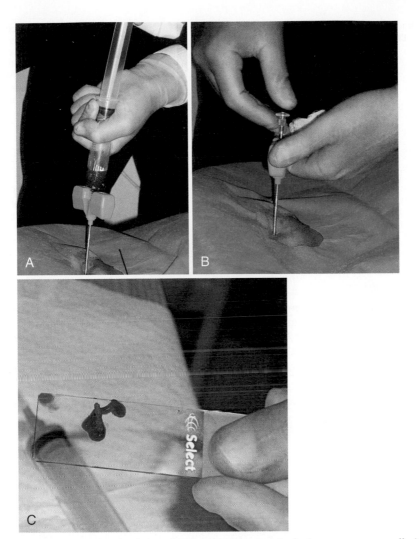

FIGURE 13-16   Bone marrow aspiration and biopsy. A, Placement of a bone marrow needle into the iliac crest (upper portion of hipbone) and aspiration of liquid bone marrow. **B,** Trephine needle is then inserted and anchored in the bone. **C,** A solid piece of bone marrow (biopsy sample) is then extracted through the needle.

Bone marrow transplantation follows the same procedure, except that bone marrow cells are used rather than peripheral stem cells (Figure 13-17). Problems encountered subsequently may include serious infection, **graft-versus-host disease (GVHD),** and relapse of the original disease despite the treatment.

In GVHD, the immunocompetent cells in the donor's tissue recognize the recipient's tissues as foreign and attack them. Because the recipient patient is totally immunosuppressed, his or her immune system cannot defend against the attack. Intensive prophylaxis (prevention) with **immunosuppressive drugs** is standard for patients undergoing **allogeneic transplants** (see Figure 13-17). These drugs include cyclosporine, methotrexate, glucocorticoids, sirolimus (Rapamune), and mycophenolate.

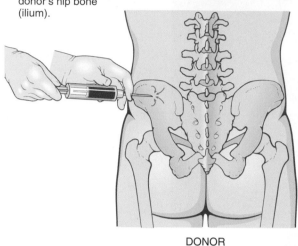

1. Stem cells from the donor's circulating blood are collected in a transfer bag, or marrow cells are aspirated from the donor's hip bone (ilium).

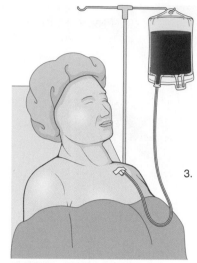

2. Stem cells or marrow cells are mixed with an anticlotting agent and strained to remove bits of bone and fat.

3. Stem cells or marrow cells are given intravenously via a catheter implanted in the upper chest and leading to a central vein.

DONOR   PATIENT

FIGURE 13-17 **Hematopoietic stem cell and bone marrow transplantation.** These procedures constitute **allogeneic** (all/o means other, different) **transplantation,** in which a relative or an unrelated person with a close or identical HLA (human leukocyte antigen) type is the donor. It carries a high rate of morbidity (disease) and mortality (death) because of complications of incompatibility such as GVHD (graft-versus-host disease). In an **autologous transplantation,** stem cells or bone marrow cells are removed from the patient during a remission phase and given back to the patient after intensive chemotherapy (drug treatment).

ABBREVIATIONS

13

Ab	antibody
ABMT	autologous bone marrow transplantation—patient serves as his or her own donor for stem cells
ABO	four main blood types—A, B, AB, and O
ALL	acute lymphoid leukemia
AML	acute myeloid leukemia
ANC	absolute neutrophil count—total WBC times a measure of the number of bands and segs present in the blood; an ANC less than 1500 cells/uL is neutropenia
ASCT	autologous stem cell transplantation
bands	immature white blood cells (granulocytes)
baso	basophils
BMT	bone marrow transplantation
CBC	complete blood count
CLL	chronic lymphoid leukemia
CML	chronic myeloid leukemia

DIC	disseminated intravascular coagulation—bleeding disorder marked by reduction in blood clotting factors due to their use and depletion for intravascular clotting
diff	differential count (white blood cells)
EBV	Epstein-Barr virus; cause of mononucleosis
eos	eosinophils
EPO	erythropoietin
ESR	erythrocyte sedimentation rate
Fe	iron
G-CSF	granulocyte colony-stimulating factor—promotes neutrophil production
GM-CSF	granulocyte-macrophage colony-stimulating factor—promotes myeloid progenitor cells with differentiation to granulocytes
g/dL	gram per deciliter (1 deciliter = one tenth of a liter; 1 liter = 1.057 quarts)

GVHD	graft-versus-host disease—immune reaction of donor's cells to recipient's tissue	**μL**	microliter—one millionth of a liter; 1 liter = 1.057 quarts
HCL	hairy cell leukemia—abnormal lymphocytes accumulate in bone marrow, leading to anemia, thrombocytopenia, neutropenia, and infection	**MDS**	myelodysplastic syndrome— preleukemic condition (anemia, cytopenias, and possible transformation to AML)
Hct	hematocrit	**mm³**	cubic millimeter—one millionth of a liter; 1 liter = 1.057 quarts
Hgb, HGB	hemoglobin	**mono**	monocyte
H and H	hemoglobin and hematocrit	**polys, PMNs, PMNLs**	polymorphonuclear leukocytes; neutrophils, eosinophils, basophils
HLA	human leukocyte antigen	**PT, pro time**	prothrombin time
IgA, IgD, IgE, IgG, IgM	immunoglobulins	**PTT**	partial thromboplastin time
ITP	idiopathic thrombocytopenic purpura	**RBC**	red blood cell; red blood cell count
lymphs	lymphocytes	**sed rate**	erythrocyte sedimentation rate
MCH	mean corpuscular hemoglobin— average amount of hemoglobin per cell	**segs**	segmented, mature white blood cells (neutrophils)
MCHC	mean corpuscular hemoglobin concentration—average concentration of hemoglobin in a single red cell; when MCHC is low, the cell is hypochromic	**SMAC**	Sequential Multiple Analyzer Computer—an automated chemistry system that determines substances in serum
MCV	mean corpuscular volume—average volume or size of a single red blood cell; when MCV is high, the cells are macrocytic, and when low, the cells are microcytic	**WBC**	white blood cell; white blood cell count
		WNL	within normal limits

13

PRACTICAL APPLICATIONS

The cases presented here are based on data from actual medical records. Use the table of normal values to help you decide on a probable diagnosis in each case. Answers to the questions are on page 540.

Normal Laboratory Values

WBC 4500-11,000/mm³ or μL		**RBC**	M:	4.5-6.0 million per mm³ *or* μL
Differential			F:	4.0-5.5 million per mm³ *or* μL
Segs (polys)	54-62%	**Hct**	M:	40-50%
Lymphs	20-40%		F:	37-47%
Eos	1-3%	**Hgb**	M:	14-16 g/dL
Baso	0-1%		F:	12-14 g/dL
Mono	3-7%	**Platelets** 150,000-350,000/mm³ *or* μL		

FIVE SHORT CLINICAL CASES

1. A 65-year-old woman visits her physician complaining of shortness of breath and swollen ankles. Lab tests reveal that her hematocrit is 18.0 and her hemoglobin 5.8. Her blood smear shows macrocytes and her blood level of vitamin B_{12} is very low. What is a likely diagnosis?
   a. Aplastic anemia
   b. Hemochromatosis
   c. Pernicious anemia

2. A 22-year-old college student visits the clinic with a fever, complaining of a sore throat. Blood tests show a WBC of 28,000 per mm³ with 95% myeloblasts (polys are 5%). Platelet count is 15,000 per mm³, hemoglobin is 10 g/dL, and hematocrit is 22.5. What is your diagnosis?
   a. Chronic lymphoid leukemia
   b. Acute myeloid leukemia
   c. Thalassemia

3. A 35-year-old woman goes to her physician complaining of spots on her legs and bleeding gums. On examination, she has tiny purple spots covering her legs and evidence of dried blood in her mouth. Her CBC shows hemoglobin 14 g/dL, hematocrit 42%, WBC 5000/mm³ with normal differential [count], and platelet count 4000/mm³ (with megakaryocytes in bone marrow). What is your diagnosis?
   a. Sickle cell anemia
   b. Hemolytic anemia
   c. Autoimmune thrombocytopenic purpura

4. A 55-year-old man is admitted to the hospital after a motorcycle crash. He sustained right hemopneumothorax (blood and air in the chest cavity) requiring placement of a chest tube. His admission hemoglobin was 11.4 g/dL and his hematocrit was 33.7%. On the third day of hospitalization, his hemoglobin dropped to 7.5 g/dL and his hematocrit fell to 22.4%. What do you think his physician should order?
   a. Bone marrow aspiration and biopsy
   b. Transfusion of packed red blood cells
   c. Leukapheresis

5. A 45-year-old woman has recently been traveling internationally and comes to the ED complaining of diarrhea, vomiting, and severe abdominal pain lasting for the previous 2 weeks. Her total WBC was elevated. Stool cultures reveal a parasitic infection. Which element of the differential do you expect to be elevated?
   a. Eosinophils
   b. Monocytes
   c. Segs (polys)

CASE REPORT

Four-year-old Sally has been running a low-grade fever for several weeks, with recurrent sore throat, earache, and cough. Her mother takes her to the family physician, who diagnoses her condition as otitis. Sally continues to be fatigued and anorexic. Her mother then notices bruising on her legs and arms. The family physician finally orders blood tests and an antibiotic drug. Peripheral blood tests reveal Hgb 7.4, platelet count 40,000, and WBC count 85,000 with 90% lymphoblasts. A bone marrow biopsy is ordered.

1. What's the likely diagnosis for this patient?
   a. AML
   b. CLL
   c. ALL
   d. CML

2. The probable cause of Sally's ecchymoses is:
   a. Neutropenia
   b. Thrombocytopenia
   c. Anorexia
   d. Otitis

3. The likely explanation for Sally's fatigue is:
   a. Anemia
   b. Sore throat and cough
   c. Thrombocytopenia
   d. Neutropenia

4. Treatment for Sally's condition is likely to be:
   a. Prolonged antibiotic therapy
   b. Intravenous feeding
   c. Surgery to repair the bone marrow
   d. Chemotherapy

13

IN PERSON: HEREDITARY HEMOCHROMATOSIS

When I was 71, my primary care physician diagnosed, somewhat by accident, that I had hemochromatosis—an unhealthy buildup of iron in my blood. Since I was borderline anemic at a regular spring check-up, she ordered a follow-up blood test to see if I might have iron deficiency anemia. Much to her surprise, I actually had a high ferritin (protein that stores iron) concentration of 250 [ng per milliliter], whereas in iron deficiency, the ferritin would be abnormally low. The normal range in women is 10 to 150.

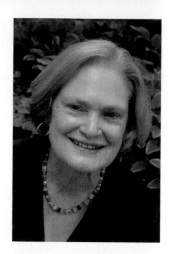

I was referred to a hematologist, who told me that the gene mutations that cause hemochromatosis probably evolved around the time of Charlemagne, 950 AD. As he explained, in the 10th century those gene mutations served a survival purpose, especially for Northern Europeans who had little iron in their diets. The genetic abnormality allowed the retention of healthy levels of iron. Today, however, we regularly consume plenty of iron. As my hematologist said, "Everything is fortified with iron." If one happens to have one of the associated genetic mutations, the blood condition of hemochromatosis may result. My hematologist sent a sample of my blood for genetic testing. The results showed that I have a mutation in one copy of the hemochromatosis gene *H63D*. He e-mailed me some additional information: "In your case, there is evidence for some hepatic iron accumulation based on your ferritin level. It is not severe, far from it, but I think we should arrange for two phlebotomies, a month or so apart, to bring your ferritin level to under 100."

As I learned, the treatment for hemochromatosis, at least the mild case that I have, is phlebotomy, the drawing down of the volume of the blood, a pint at a time. The reason that this treatment is effective is that it removes iron along with the blood. I had the two phlebotomy procedures that summer, and the desired goal was reached: My ferritin level dropped to 88. The treatment was easy, exactly like donating blood, and effective. I now will be tested every 6 months to check on the blood ferritin concentration, and to have phlebotomies when necessary.

I also learned from my hematologist that untreated hemochromatosis can result in iron buildup in the liver, heart, or brain, potentially resulting in serious disease. Women with hemochromatosis typically do not become symptomatic until mid-life, since menstruation and childbirth result in natural blood loss. I now wonder whether my father, who died at age 62 of liver disease, could have had hemochromatosis and perhaps have been the carrier of the gene mutation that I have. As my hematologist told me, if one has untreated hemochromatosis and consumes even small amounts of alcohol, the outcome could be cirrhosis. I'm very grateful to my alert doctor, who diagnosed my case before I had any symptoms or illness. And I am grateful that my siblings do not have the mutation, and that our children, who are adopted, have not inherited this condition.

Carolyn Peter

13

IN PERSON: AUTOLOGOUS STEM CELL TRANSPLANT

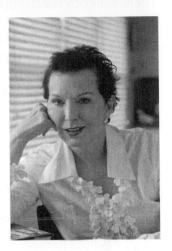

I was scheduled for a stem cell transplant to cure my recurrent primary central nervous system lymphoma, or PCNSL, a rare type of brain cancer. Until around 15 years ago, stem cell transplants depended upon bone marrow from which to harvest the cells. Since then, scientists have discovered that there are actually more cells available in peripheral (circulating) blood than in marrow. I was given two medicines, Mozobil and Neupogen, aimed at stimulating enough stem cells to be collected from that peripheral source. In a peripheral autologous blood stem cell transplant, stem cells are collected from the circulating blood by apheresis, in which blood is withdrawn through a sterile needle, and passed through a machine that harvests stem cells into a container, while the remaining blood components are then transferred back into the patient's bloodstream. The fraction containing the blood stem cells is then frozen until needed for transplantation. Because patients get their own cells back, no chance exists for immune mismatch or graft-versus-host problems.

On the first day of stem cell collection, I produced half of the total stem cells I would need for my treatment. By the end of the third day of collection, I had reached the magic number of stem cells needed, and was able to go home to wait for the hospital to schedule me for the transplant. A representative phoned 2 days later, laying out the next 5 weeks for me: I'd be admitted in 11 days to the transplant division, where I would remain, they hoped, for no more than a month. My (presumably clean) stem cells were safely stored in a freezer while I was to undergo intensive chemotherapy meant to destroy any lurking cancer cells in my brain (and of course, benign others in the medicine's "take-no-prisoners" path).

I was glad when the date arrived, and my husband Dennis moved me into my next month's home on the eighth floor of the hospital. What I had failed to understand is the nature of an autologous stem cell transplant, at least for primary CNS lymphoma. I was to be blasted, rendered helpless, with a trio of chemo agents able to pass through the blood-brain barrier, but not ordinarily available for treatment-as-a-threesome due to their combined viciousness: busulfan, thiotepa (mustard gas–related), and cyclophosphamide (also a nitrogen mustard alkylating agent). I could risk receiving these killers because my uncontaminated stem cells were stored in the freezer. They would eventually replace my currently circulating blood that was being saturated with chemotherapy agents.

After 9 days, my white blood count was as low as it could go: I was at ground zero, "my second birthday." The blood we'd collected with the help of Mozobil and company was slowly thawed, for a few hours, and soon I was given a transfusion of my previously frozen blood, swarming with stem cells. Before long, I felt so sick I thought I was dying. Wearing diapers that had to be changed every 20 minutes, having rectal samples taken from my chafed, sometimes bloody "toilet skin" (as the nurse called it), being forced to sit up every minute, even at night, so that I could put the suction tube down my throat to keep from drowning in the rope-like mucositis, which ulcerated the membranes lining my digestive system—I could go on and on.

But as I'd been promised, nearly 5 weeks post-admission for the life-giving stem cell transplant, I was deemed ready to go home. For a month, however, our house operated like a medical office. That first week, I kept down half a shake a day. When I returned for my first checkup, I had to stay an extra 5 hours for a hydration infusion. Four days later, my red blood count was low and I needed a transfusion. By the second week, I'd started eating Cheerios with milk throughout the day, and my weight at least stabilized. I no longer looked like a skeleton.

At 100 days post-transplant, we could make love again. I worried that Dennis would find my scrawniness a turnoff, but he accepted my new "boy's body" and enthusiastically helped me recapture my faith in our oneness. After all, we'd been through the battle and needed now to smell the perennial flowers. Turns out they're as colorful as ever.

Laura Claridge Oppenheimer is a writer with Farrar, Straus and Giroux,
currently working on a biography of publisher Blanche Knopf.

13

❓ EXERCISES

Remember to check your answers carefully with the Answers to Exercises, page 539.

Ⓐ Match the cells with their definitions.

basophil	hematopoietic stem cell	neutrophil
eosinophil	lymphocyte	platelet
erythrocyte	monocyte	

1. mononuclear white blood cell (agranulocyte) formed in lymph tissue; it is a phagocyte and the

   precursor of a macrophage _____

2. thrombocyte or cell fragment that helps blood clot _____

3. cell in the bone marrow that gives rise to different types of blood cells _____

4. mononuclear leukocyte formed in lymph tissue; produces antibodies _____

5. leukocyte with dense, reddish granules having an affinity for red acidic dye; associated with

   allergic reactions _____

6. red blood cell _____

7. leukocyte (polymorphonuclear granulocyte) formed in the bone marrow; granules do not stain

   intensely and have a pale color _____

8. leukocyte (granulocyte) with dark-staining blue granules; releases histamine and heparin

   _____

Ⓑ Give the meanings of the following terms.

1. coagulation _____

2. granulocyte _____

3. mononuclear _____

4. polymorphonuclear _____

5. globulin _____

6. erythroblast _____

7. megakaryocyte _____

8. macrophage _____

9. hemoglobin _____

10. plasma _____

11. myeloblast _____

C Match the listed terms with the descriptions/definitions that follow.

albumin   colony-stimulating factor   globulin
antibody   differentiation   heparin
antigen   erythropoietin   plasma
bilirubin   fibrinogen   serum

1. liquid portion of blood _____

2. orange-yellow pigment produced from hemoglobin when red blood cells are destroyed

   _____

3. plasma protein converted to fibrin in clotting process _____

4. proteins in plasma; separated into alpha, beta, and gamma types _____

5. hormone secreted by the kidneys to stimulate bone marrow to produce red blood cells

   _____

6. substance (usually foreign) that stimulates production of an antibody _____

7. protein in blood that maintains the proper amount of water in the blood _____

8. specific protein produced by lymphocytes in response to antigens in the blood _____

9. anticoagulant found in blood and tissue cells _____

10. plasma minus clotting proteins and cells _____

11. change in structure and function of a cell as it matures _____

12. protein that stimulates growth of white blood cells _____

D Give short answers for the following.

1. Name four types of plasma proteins. _____

   _____

2. What is the Rh factor? _____

3. What is hemolysis? _____

4. A person with type A blood has _____ antigens and _____ antibodies in his or her blood.

5. A person with type B blood has _____ antigens and _____ antibodies in his or her blood.

6. A person with type O blood has _____ antigens and _____ antibodies in his or her blood.

7. A person with type AB blood has _____ antigens and _____ antibodies in his or her blood.

8. Can you transfuse blood from a type A donor into a type B recipient? _____ Why or why not?

   _____

9. Can you transfuse blood from a type AB donor into a type O recipient? Why or why not?

   _____

10. What is electrophoresis? _____

13

11. What is an immunoglobulin? _____

12. What is differentiation? _____

13. What is plasmapheresis? _____

14. Why is a person with type O blood the universal donor? _____

E **Match the listed terms related to clotting with the descriptions/definitions that follow.**

coagulation	heparin	thrombin
fibrin	prothrombin	warfarin (Coumadin)
fibrinogen	serum	

1. anticoagulant substance found in liver cells, blood, and tissues _____

2. protein thread that forms the basis of a blood clot _____

3. plasma protein that is converted to thrombin in the clotting process _____

4. plasma minus clotting proteins and cells _____

5. drug given to patients to prevent formation of clots _____

6. plasma protein that is converted to fibrin in the clotting process _____

7. process of clotting _____

8. enzyme that helps convert fibrinogen to fibrin _____

F **Divide the following terms into component parts and give the meanings of the complete terms.**

1. anticoagulant _____

2. hemoglobinopathy _____

3. cytology _____

4. leukopenia _____

5. morphology _____

6. megakaryocyte _____

7. sideropenia _____

8. phagocyte _____

9. myelopoiesis _____

10. plateletpheresis _____

11. monoblast _____

12. myelodysplasia _____

13. hemostasis _____

14. thrombolytic (therapy) _____

15. hematopoiesis _____

13

G Match the hematology terms with their meanings.

coagulopathy   leukapheresis   thrombocytopenia
eosinophilia   myeloid   thrombosis
hematocrit   neutropenia

1. derived in bone marrow _____

2. deficiency of a type of white blood cell _____

3. percentage of red blood cells in a volume of blood _____

4. increase in a type of white blood cell (seen in allergies) _____

5. abnormal condition of clot formation _____

6. separation of white blood cells from a blood sample _____

7. disease of clotting process _____

8. deficiency of platelets _____

H Match the listed terms concerning red blood cells with the descriptions/definitions that follow.

anemia   hemoglobin   microcytosis
anisocytosis   hemolysis   poikilocytosis
erythropoiesis   hypochromic   polycythemia vera
hematocrit   macrocytosis   spherocytosis

1. any irregularity in the shape of red blood cells _____

2. oxygen-containing protein in red blood cells _____

3. formation of red blood cells _____

4. deficiency in numbers of red blood cells _____

5. destruction of red blood cells _____

6. pertaining to reduction of hemoglobin in red blood cells _____

7. variation in size of red blood cells _____

8. abnormal numbers of round, rather than normally biconcave-shaped, red blood cells

   _____

9. increase in number of small red blood cells _____

10. general increase in numbers of red blood cells; erythremia _____

11. increase in numbers of large red blood cells _____

12. separation of blood so that the percentage of red blood cells in relation to the volume of a blood

    sample is measured _____

13

I Describe the problem in each of the following forms of anemia.

1. iron deficiency anemia _____

2. pernicious anemia _____

3. sickle cell anemia _____

4. aplastic anemia _____

5. thalassemia _____

J Give the meanings of the following terms for blood dyscrasias.

1. purpura _____

2. granulocytosis _____

3. hemophilia _____

4. hemochromatosis _____

5. multiple myeloma _____

6. mononucleosis _____

K Match the term in Column I with its meaning in Column II. Write the letter of the meaning in the space provided.

COLUMN I

1. relapse _____

2. remission _____

3. palliative _____

4. Bence Jones protein _____

5. ecchymoses _____

6. pancytopenia _____

7. apheresis _____

8. eosinophilia _____

9. petechiae _____

10. packed cells _____

COLUMN II

A. Deficiency of all blood cells
B. Immunoglobulin fragment found in the urine of patients with multiple myeloma
C. Increase in numbers of granulocytes; seen in allergic conditions
D. Large blue or purplish patches on skin (bruises)
E. Symptoms of the disease return
F. Tiny purple or flat red spots on skin occurring as a result of small hemorrhages
G. Symptoms of the disease disappear
H. Separation of blood into its parts
I. Preparation of erythrocytes separated from plasma
J. Relieving but not curing

13

L **Match the laboratory test or clinical procedure with its description.**

antiglobulin (Coombs) test   erythrocyte sedimentation rate   platelet count
autologous transfusion   hematocrit   red blood cell count
bleeding time   hematopoietic stem cell   red blood cell morphology
bone marrow biopsy   transplantation   white blood cell differential
coagulation time

1. microscopic examination of a stained blood smear to determine the shape of individual red
   blood cells _____

2. percentage of red blood cells in a volume of blood _____

3. determines the number of clotting cells per mm^3 or µL of blood _____

4. time required for venous blood to clot in a test tube _____

5. speed at which erythrocytes settle out of plasma _____

6. percentages of different types of leukocytes in the blood _____

7. test for the presence of antibodies that coat and damage erythrocytes _____

8. peripheral stem cells from a compatible donor are infused into a recipient's vein to repopulate
   the bone marrow _____

9. time required for blood to stop flowing from a small puncture wound _____

10. microscopic examination of a core of bone marrow removed with a needle _____

    _____

11. number of erythrocytes per mm^3 or µL of blood _____

12. blood is collected from and later reinfused into the same patient _____

M **Circle the boldface terms that best complete the meaning of the sentences.**

1. Gary, a 1-year-old African American child, was failing to gain weight normally. He seemed pale
   and without energy. His blood tests showed a decreased hemoglobin (5.0 g/dL) and decreased
   hematocrit (16.5%). After a blood smear revealed abnormally shaped red cells, the physician
   told Gary's parents that their son had **(iron deficiency anemia, hemophilia, sickle cell anemia)**.

2. While in the hospital, Mr. Klein was told he had an elevated **(red blood cell, white blood cell,
   platelet)** count with a "shift to the left." This was information that confirmed his diagnosis of a
   systemic infection.

3. While Mr. Chen was taking warfarin (Coumadin), a blood thinner, his physician made sure to
   check his **(prothrombin time, hematocrit, sed rate)**.

4. Sixty-one-year-old Barbara's laboratory tests showed abnormal proteins in her plasma and Bence
   Jones protein in her urine. She had osteopenia and a fracture in one of her ribs. Her oncologist
   diagnosed her condition as **(mononucleosis, thrombocytopenic purpura, multiple myeloma)**.
   He prescribed analgesics and drugs such as thalidomide and bortezomib (Velcade).

5. Bobby was diagnosed at a very early age with a bleeding disorder called **(hemophilia,
   thalassemia, eosinophilia)**. He needed factor VIII regularly, especially after even the slightest
   traumatic injury.

13

6. Juan was a 9-year-old boy who suddenly noticed many black and blue marks all over his legs. He had a fever and was tired all the time. The physician did a blood test that revealed pancytopenia. A bone marrow biopsy confirmed the diagnosis of (**acute lymphoid leukemia, polycythemia vera, aplastic anemia**).

7. Alice and her friends had been staying up late for weeks, cramming for exams. She developed a sore throat and swollen lymph nodes in her neck and felt fatigued all the time. Dr. Smith did a blood test, and the results showed lymphocytosis and antibodies to EBV in the bloodstream. His diagnosis was (**leukapheresis, lymphocytopenia, mononucleosis**).

8. Susan was experiencing heavy menstrual periods (**menorrhea, menorrhagia, hemoptysis**). Because of the bleeding, she frequently felt tired and weak and probably was sideropenic. Her physician performed blood tests that revealed her problem as (**thrombocytopenia, pernicious anemia, iron deficiency anemia**).

9. Dr. Harris examined a highly allergic patient and sent a blood sample to a specialist, a (**pulmonary, cardiovascular, hematologic**) pathologist. The specialist stained the blood smear and found an abundance of leukocytes with dense, reddish granules. She made the diagnosis of (**basophilia, eosinophilia, neutrophilia**).

10. George's blood cell counts had been falling in recent weeks. His scheduled laparotomy was canceled because blood tests revealed (**pancytopenia, plasmapheresis, myelopoiesis**). Bone marrow biopsy determined that the cause was (**hyperplasia, hypoplasia, differentiation**) of all cellular elements.

N Spell out the abbreviations in Column I, and then select the best description for each from the definitions in Column II.

COLUMN I

1. Hgb _____ _____
2. GVHD _____ _____
3. ALL _____ _____
4. PT _____ _____
5. CML _____ _____
6. EPO _____ _____
7. IgA, IgE, IgD _____ _____
8. CLL _____ _____
9. Hct _____ _____
10. AML _____ _____

COLUMN II

A. Blood protein that transports oxygen to tissues.
B. Malignant condition of white blood cells; immature granulocytes (myeloblasts) predominate.
C. Malignant condition of white blood cells; immature lymphocytes predominate.
D. Test used to follow patients who are taking certain anticoagulants.
E. Percentage of red cells in blood volume.
F. Malignant condition of white blood cells in which both mature and immature granulocytes are present; a slowly progressive illness.
G. Immune reaction of donor's cells/tissue to recipient's cells/tissue; a possible outcome of hematopoietic stem cell or bone marrow transplantation.
H. Proteins containing antibodies.
I. Malignant condition of white blood cells in which relatively mature lymphocytes predominate in lymph nodes, spleen, and bone marrow; usually seen in elderly patients.
J. Hormone that stimulates the growth of red blood cells.

13

ANSWERS TO EXERCISES

A

1. monocyte
2. platelet
3. hematopoietic stem cell
4. lymphocyte
5. eosinophil
6. erythrocyte
7. neutrophil
8. basophil

B

1. blood clotting
2. white blood cell with numerous, dark-staining granules (neutrophil, basophil, and eosinophil)
3. pertaining to a leukocyte with a single round nucleus; monocytes and lymphocytes are mononuclear leukocytes
4. pertaining to a white blood cell with a multilobed nucleus; neutrophil
5. plasma protein; alpha, beta, and gamma (immune) globulins are examples
6. immature red blood cell
7. large platelet precursor (forerunner) cell found in bone marrow
8. monocyte that migrates from blood to tissue spaces; phagocyte that engulfs foreign material and ingests red blood cells
9. blood protein containing iron; carries oxygen in erythrocytes
10. liquid portion of blood
11. immature bone marrow cell that gives rise to granulocytes

C

1. plasma
2. bilirubin
3. fibrinogen
4. globulin
5. erythropoietin
6. antigen
7. albumin
8. antibody
9. heparin
10. serum
11. differentiation
12. colony-stimulating factor

D

1. albumin, globulins, fibrinogen, and prothrombin
2. an antigen normally found on red blood cells of Rh+ individuals
3. destruction or breakdown of red blood cells
4. A; anti-B
5. B; anti-A
6. no A or B; anti-A and anti-B
7. A and B; no anti-A and no anti-B
8. no; A antigens will react with the anti-A antibodies in the type B recipient's bloodstream
9. no; A and B antigens will react with the anti-A and anti-B antibodies in the type O recipient's bloodstream
10. a method of separating serum proteins by electrical charge
11. protein with antibody activity; IgG, IgH, IgE
12. change in structure and function of a cell as it matures; specialization
13. removal by centrifuge of plasma from withdrawn blood
14. type O blood does not contain A or B antigens and therefore will not react with antibodies in any recipient's blood

E

1. heparin
2. fibrin
3. prothrombin
4. serum
5. warfarin (Coumadin)
6. fibrinogen
7. coagulation
8. thrombin

F

1. anti/coagul/ant—a substance that prevents clotting
2. hemoglobin/o/pathy—disease (abnormality) of hemoglobin
3. cyt/o/logy—study of cells
4. leuk/o/penia—deficiency of white (blood) cells
5. morph/o/logy—study of the shape or form (of cells)
6. mega/kary/o/cyte—cell with a large (mega-) nucleus (kary); platelet precursor
7. sider/o/penia—deficiency of iron
8. phag/o/cyte—cell that eats or swallows other cells
9. myel/o/poiesis—formation of bone marrow
10. platelet/pheresis—separation of platelets from the rest of the blood
11. mon/o/blast—immature monocyte
12. myel/o/dys/plasia—abnormal (ineffective) production of myeloid cells in bone marrow. Myeloid progenitor cells give rise to erythrocytes, granulocytes, and platelets
13. hem/o/stasis—controlling or stopping the flow of blood
14. thromb/o/lytic (therapy)—pertaining to treatment using drugs to destroy clots
15. hemat/o/poiesis—formation of blood cells

13

G

1. myeloid
2. neutropenia
3. hematocrit
4. eosinophilia
5. thrombosis
6. leukapheresis
7. coagulopathy
8. thrombocytopenia

H

1. poikilocytosis
2. hemoglobin
3. erythropoiesis
4. anemia
5. hemolysis
6. hypochromic
7. anisocytosis
8. spherocytosis
9. microcytosis
10. polycythemia vera
11. macrocytosis
12. hematocrit

I

1. lack of iron leading to insufficient hemoglobin production
2. lack of mature erythrocytes caused by inability to absorb vitamin B_{12} into the bloodstream (intrinsic factor is missing in gastric juice, so B_{12} is not absorbed)
3. hereditary disorder of abnormal hemoglobin producing sickle-shaped erythrocytes and hemolysis
4. failure of blood cell production in bone marrow
5. inherited disorder of abnormal hemoglobin production leading to hypochromia

J

1. multiple pinpoint hemorrhages and accumulation of blood under the skin (cause is deficiency of platelets)
2. abnormal increase in granulocytes in the blood (eosinophilia and basophilia)
3. excessive bleeding caused by hereditary lack of blood clotting factors
4. excessive iron deposits throughout the body
5. malignant neoplasm of bone marrow
6. infectious disease marked by increased numbers of mononuclear leukocytes and enlarged cervical lymph nodes

K

1. E
2. G
3. J
4. B
5. D
6. A
7. H
8. C
9. F
10. I

L

1. red blood cell morphology
2. hematocrit
3. platelet count
4. coagulation time
5. erythrocyte sedimentation rate
6. white blood cell differential
7. antiglobulin (Coombs) test
8. hematopoietic stem cell transplantation
9. bleeding time
10. bone marrow biopsy
11. red blood cell count
12. autologous transfusion

M

1. sickle cell anemia
2. white blood cell
3. prothrombin time
4. multiple myeloma
5. hemophilia
6. aplastic anemia
7. mononucleosis
8. menorrhagia; iron deficiency anemia
9. hematologic; eosinophilia
10. pancytopenia; hypoplasia

N

1. hemoglobin: A
2. graft-versus-host disease: G
3. acute lymphoid leukemia: C
4. prothrombin time: D
5. chronic myeloid (myelocytic) leukemia: F
6. erythropoietin: J
7. immunoglobulins: H
8. chronic lymphoid leukemia: I
9. hematocrit: E
10. acute myeloid (myelocytic) leukemia: B

Answers to Practical Applications

Five Short Clinical Cases

1. c
2. b
3. c
4. b
5. a

Case Report

1. c
2. b
3. a
4. d

13

PRONUNCIATION OF TERMS

To test your understanding of the terminology in this chapter, write the meaning of each term in the space provided. In addition, you may wish to cover the terms and write them by looking at your definitions. Make sure your spelling is correct. The page number after each term indicates where it is defined or used in the book, so you can easily check your responses. You will find complete definitions for all of these terms and their audio pronunciations on the Evolve website.

Pronunciation Guide

ā as in āpe	ă as in ăpple
ē as in ēven	ĕ as in ĕvery
ī as in īce	ĭ as in ĭnterest
ō as in ōpen	ŏ as in pŏt
ū as in ūnit	ŭ as in ŭnder

Vocabulary and Terminology

TERM	PRONUNCIATION	MEANING
albumin (512)	ăl-BŪ-mĭn	
anisocytosis (514)	ăn-ī-sō-sī-TŌ-sĭs	
antibody (512)	ĂN-tĭ-bŏd-ē	
anticoagulant (514)	ăn-tĭ-cō-ĂG-ū-lănt	
antigen (512)	ĂN-tĭ-jĕn	
basophil (512)	BĀ-sō-fĭl	
bilirubin (512)	bĭl-ĭ-ROO-bĭn	
coagulation (512)	kō-ăg-ū-LĀ-shŭn	
coagulopathy (514)	kō-ăg-ū-LŎP-ă-thē	
colony-stimulating factor (512)	KŎL-ō-nē STĬM-ū-lā-tĭng FĂK-tŏr	
cytology (514)	sī-TŎL-ō-jē	
differentiation (512)	dĭf-ĕr-ĕn-shē-Ā-shŭn	
electrophoresis (512)	ē-lĕk-trō-fō-RĒ-sis	
eosinophil (512)	ē-ō-SĬN-ō-fĭl	
eosinophilia (516)	ē-ō-sĭn-ō-FĬL-ē-ă	
erythroblast (512)	ĕ-RĬTH-rō-blăst	
erythrocyte (512)	ĕ-RĬTH-rō-sīt	
erythropoiesis (516)	ĕ-rĭth-rō-poy-Ē-sĭs	
erythropoietin (512)	ĕ-rĭth-rō-POY-ĕ-tĭn	
fibrin (512)	FĪ-brĭn	
fibrinogen (512)	fī-BRĬN-ō-jĕn	
globulin (512)	GLŎB-ū-lĭn	
granulocyte (514)	GRĂN-ū-lō-sīt	
granulocytopenia (516)	grăn-ū-lō-sī-tō-PĒ-nē-ă	
hematopoiesis (516)	hē-mă-tō-poy-Ē-sĭs	

13

TERM	PRONUNCIATION	MEANING
hematopoietic stem cell (512)	hē-mă-tō-poy-EH-tĭk stĕm sĕl	_____
hemoglobin (512)	HĒ-mō-glō-bĭn	_____
hemoglobinopathy (514)	hē-mō-glō-bĭn-ŎP-ă-thē	_____
hemolysis (512)	hē-MŎL-ĭ-sĭs	_____
hemostasis (516)	hē-mō-STĀ-sĭs	_____
heparin (512)	HĔP-ă-rĭn	_____
hypochromic (514)	hī-pō-KRŌ-mĭk	_____
immune reaction (512)	ĭm-MŪN rē-ĂK-shŭn	_____
immunoglobulin (512)	ĭm-ū-nō-GLŎB-ū-lĭn	_____
leukapheresis (515)	loo-kă-fĕ-RĒ-sĭs	_____
leukocyte (513)	LOO-kō-sīt	_____
leukopenia (514)	loo-kō-PĒ-nē-ă	_____
lymphocyte (513)	LĬM-fō-sīt	_____
macrocytosis (516)	măk-rō-sī-TŌ-sĭs	_____
macrophage (513)	MĂK-rō-făj	_____
megakaryocyte (513)	mĕg-ă-KĀR-ē-ō-sīt	_____
microcytosis (516)	mī-krō-sī-TŌ-sĭs	_____
monoblast (515)	MŎN-ō-blăst	_____
monocyte (513)	MŎN-ō-sīt	_____
mononuclear (513)	mŏn-ō-NŪ-klē-ăr	_____
morphology (514)	mŏr-FŎL-ō-jē	_____
myeloblast (513)	MĪ-ĕ-lō-blăst	_____
myelodysplasia (515)	mī-ĕ-lō-dĭs-PLĀ-zhē-ă	_____
myeloid (516)	MĪ-ĕ-loyd	_____
myelopoiesis (516)	mī-ĕ-lō-poy-Ē-sĭs	_____
neutropenia (515)	noo-trō-PĒ-nē-ă	_____
neutrophil (513)	NOO-trō-fĭl	_____
neutrophilia (516)	noo-trō-FĬL-ē-ă	_____
pancytopenia (516)	păn-sī-tō-PĒ-nē-ă	_____
phagocyte (515)	FĂG-ō-sīt	_____
plasma (513)	PLĂZ-mă	_____
plasmapheresis (513)	plăz-mă-fĕ-RĒ-sĭs	_____
platelet (513)	PLĀT-lĕt	_____
plateletpheresis (515)	plāt-lĕt-fĕ-RĒ-sĭs	_____

13

TERM	PRONUNCIATION	MEANING
poikilocytosis (515)	poy-kĭ-lō-sī-TŌ-sĭs	
polymorphonuclear (513)	pŏl-ē-mŏr-fō-NOO-klē-ăr	
prothrombin (513)	prō-THRŎM-bĭn	
reticulocyte (513)	rĕ-TĬK-ū-lō-sīt	
Rh factor (513)	R-h FĂK-tŏr	
serum (513)	SĔ-rŭm	
sideropenia (515)	sĭd-ĕr-ō-PĒ-nē-ă	
spherocytosis (517)	sfĕr-ō-sī-TŌ-sĭs	
stem cell (513)	STĔM sĕl	
thrombin (513)	THRŎM-bĭn	
thrombocyte (513)	THRŎM-bō-sīt	
thrombocytopenia (515)	thrŏm-bō-sī-tō-PĒ-nē-ă	
thrombolytic therapy (516)	thrŏm-bō-LI-tĭk THĔR-ă-pē	
thrombosis (516)	thrŏm-BŌ-sĭs	

Pathology, Laboratory Tests, and Clinical Procedures

TERM	PRONUNCIATION	MEANING
acute lymphoid leukemia (521)	ă-KŪT LĬM-fŏyd loo-KĒ-mē-ă	
acute myeloid leukemia (520)	ă-KŪT MĪ-ĕ-lŏyd loo-KĒ-mē-ă	
anemia (517)	ă-NĒ-mē-ă	
antiglobulin test (522)	ăn-tē-GLŎB-ū-lĭn tĕst	
apheresis (524)	ă-fĕ-RĒ-sĭs	
aplastic anemia (517)	ā-PLĂS-tĭk ă-NĒ-mē-ă	
autologous transfusion (524)	ăw-TŎL-ō-gŭs trăns-FŪ-zhŭn	
bleeding time (522)	BLĒ-dĭng tīm	
blood transfusion (524)	blŭd trăns-FŪ-zhŭn	
bone marrow biopsy (524)	bōn MĂ-rō BĪ-ŏp-sē	
chronic lymphoid leukemia (521)	KRŎ-nĭk LĬM-fŏyd loo-KĒ-mē-ă	
chronic myeloid leukemia (521)	KRŎ-nĭk MĪ-ĕ-lŏyd loo-KĒ-mē-ă	
coagulation time (522)	kō-ăg-ū-LĀ-shŭn tīm	
complete blood count (522)	kŏm-PLĒT blŭd kount	

TERM	PRONUNCIATION	MEANING
dyscrasia (517)	dĭs-KRĀ-zē-ă	
ecchymoses (520)	ĕk-kĭ-MŌ-sēs	
erythrocyte sedimentation rate (522)	ĕ-RĬTH-rō-sīt sĕd-ĭ-mĕn-TĀ-shŭn rāt	
granulocytosis (521)	grăn-ū-lō-sī-TŌ-sis	
hematocrit (523)	hē-MĂT-ō-krĭt	
hematopoietic stem cell transplant (524)	hē-mă-tō-poy-Ĕ-tĭk stĕm sĕl TRĂNS-plănt	
hemochromatosis (519)	hē-mō-krō-mă-TŌ-sĭs	
hemoglobin test (523)	HĒ-mō-glō-bĭn tĕst	
hemolytic anemia (518)	hē-mō-LĬ-tĭk ă-NĒ-mē-ă	
hemophilia (519)	hē-mō-FĬL-ē-ă	
intrinsic factor (518)	ĭn-TRĬN-sĭk FĂK-tŏr	
leukemia (520)	loo-KĒ-mē-ă	
mononucleosis (522)	mŏ-nō-noo-klē-Ō-sĭs	
multiple myeloma (522)	MŬL-tĭ-pl mī-ĕ-LŌ-mă	
palliative (522)	PĂL-ē-ă-tĭv	
pernicious anemia (518)	pĕr-NĬSH-ŭs ă-NĒ-mē-ă	
petechiae (520)	pĕ-TĒ-kē-ā	
platelet count (523)	PLĀT-lĕt kount	
polycythemia vera (519)	pŏl-ē-sī-THĒ-mē-ă VĔR-ă	
prothrombin time (523)	prō-THRŎM-bĭn tīm	
purpura (520)	PŬR-pū-ră	
red blood cell count (523)	rĕd blŭd sĕl kount	
red blood cell morphology (523)	rĕd blŭd sĕl mŏr-FŎL-ō-jē	
relapse (521)	RĒ-lăps	
remission (521)	rē-MĬSH-ŭn	
sickle cell anemia (518)	SĬK-l sĕl ă-NĒ-mē-ă	
thalassemia (519)	thăl-ă-SĒ-mē-ă	
white blood cell count (523)	wīt blŭd sĕl kount	
white blood cell differential (523)	wīt blŭd sĕl dĭ-fĕr-ĔN-shŭl	

13

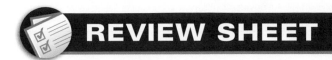

REVIEW SHEET

Write the meanings of the word parts in the spaces provided. Check your answers with the information in the chapter or in the Glossary *(Medical Word Parts—English)* at the end of the book.

Combining Forms

COMBINING FORM	MEANING	COMBINING FORM	MEANING
bas/o		leuk/o	
chrom/o		kary/o	
coagul/o		mon/o	
cyt/o		morph/o	
eosin/o		myel/o	
erythr/o		neutr/o	
fibrin/o		nucle/o	
granul/o		phag/o	
hem/o		poikil/o	
hemat/o		sider/o	
hemoglobin/o		spher/o	
is/o		thromb/o	

Suffixes

SUFFIX	MEANING	SUFFIX	MEANING
-apheresis		-osis	
-blast		-penia	
-cytosis		-phage	
-emia		-philia	
-gen		-phoresis	
-globin		-plasia	
-globulin		-poiesis	
-lytic		-stasis	
-oid			

13

Prefixes

PREFIX	MEANING	PREFIX	MEANING
a-, an-		micro-	
anti-		mono-	
hypo-		pan-	
macro-		poly-	
mega-			

Components of blood: Study Figure 13-7, page 509, and fill in the blank boxes.

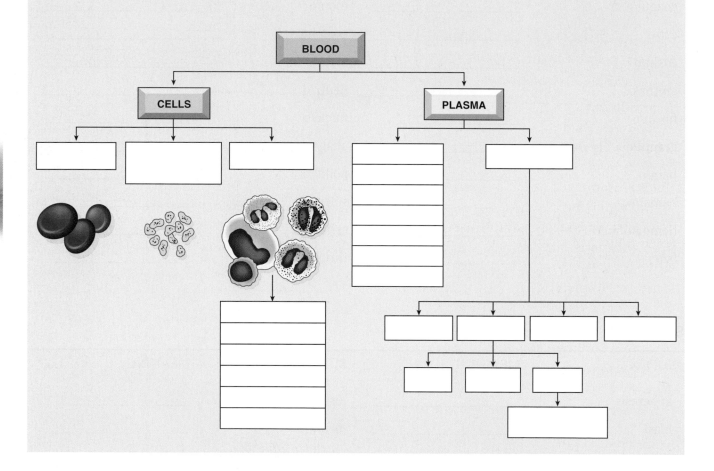

13

Lymphatic and Immune Systems

Chapter Sections

CHAPTER GOALS

- Identify the structures of the lymphatic and immune systems and understand how the systems work.
- Learn basic terminology, combining forms, and other word parts related to these systems.
- Recognize terms describing pathologic conditions involving components of the lymphatic and immune systems.
- Identify laboratory tests, clinical procedures, and abbreviations relating to the lymphatic and immune systems.
- Apply your new knowledge to understanding medical terms in their proper contexts, such as medical reports and records.

INTRODUCTION

The lymphatic system and the immune system are considered together in this chapter because aspects of their functions in the body are very closely related.

Lymph is a clear, watery fluid that surrounds body cells and flows in a system of thin-walled lymph vessels (the lymphatic system) that extends throughout the body.

Lymph differs from blood, but it has a close relationship to the blood system. Lymph fluid does not contain erythrocytes or platelets, but it is rich in two types of white blood cells (leukocytes): **lymphocytes** and **monocytes**. The liquid part of lymph is similar to blood plasma in that it contains water, salts, sugar, and wastes of metabolism such as urea and creatinine, but it differs in that it contains less protein. Lymph actually originates from the blood. It is the same fluid that filters out of tiny blood capillaries into the spaces between cells. This fluid that surrounds body cells is called **interstitial fluid**. Interstitial fluid passes continuously into specialized thin-walled vessels called **lymph capillaries**, which are found coursing through tissue spaces (Figure 14-1). The fluid in the lymph capillaries, now called **lymph** instead of interstitial fluid, passes through larger lymphatic vessels and through clusters of lymph tissues (**lymph nodes**), finally reaching large lymphatic vessels in the upper chest. Lymph enters these large lymphatic vessels, which then empty into the bloodstream. Figure 14-2 illustrates schematically the relationship between the blood and the lymphatic systems. Table 14-1 reviews the differences between lymph and blood.

The lymphatic system has several functions. First, it is a drainage system to transport needed proteins and fluid that have leaked out of the blood capillaries (and into the interstitial fluid) back to the bloodstream via the veins. Second, the lymphatic vessels in the intestines absorb lipids (fats) from the small intestine and transport them to the bloodstream.

A third function of the lymphatic system relates to the **immune system:** the defense of the body against foreign organisms such as bacteria and viruses. Lymphocytes and monocytes, originating in bone marrow, lymph nodes, and organs such as the spleen and thymus gland, protect the body by producing antibodies and by mounting a cellular attack on foreign cells and organisms.

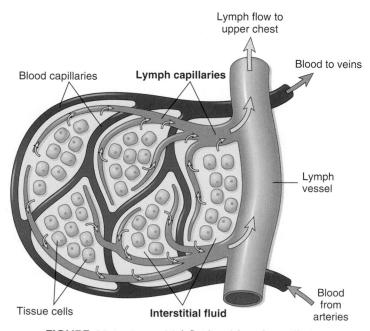

FIGURE 14-1   Interstitial fluid and lymph capillaries.

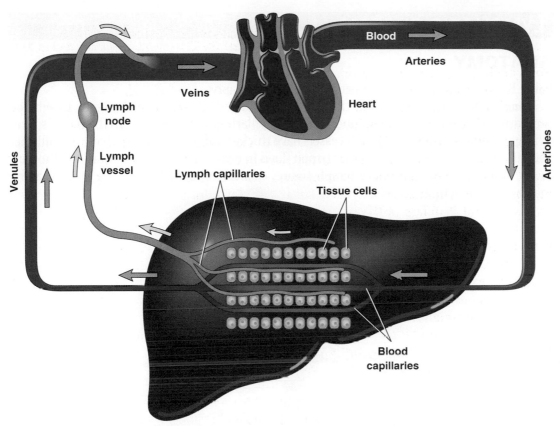

FIGURE 14-2   Relationship between the circulatory systems of blood and lymph.

14

TABLE 14-1	LYMPH AND BLOOD
LYMPH (colorless)	**BLOOD** (red)
NO PUMP Fluid moved along by muscle movement and valves	**PUMP** Heart pumps blood through blood vessels
WHITE BLOOD CELLS Lymphocytes Monocytes	**ALL BLOOD CELLS** Erythrocytes (give blood its red color) Leukocytes Platelets
INTERSTITIAL FLUID Water Less protein and other plasma components Lipids (fats) from small intestine	**PLASMA** Water Proteins Salts, nutrients, lipids, and wastes

LYMPHATIC SYSTEM

ANATOMY

Label Figure 14-3A as you read the following paragraphs.

Lymph capillaries [1] begin at the spaces around cells throughout the body. Like blood capillaries, they are thin-walled tubes. Lymph capillaries carry lymph from the tissue spaces to larger **lymph vessels** [2]. Lymph vessels have thicker walls than those of lymph capillaries and, like veins, contain valves so that lymph flows in only one direction, toward the thoracic cavity. Collections of stationary lymph tissue, called **lymph nodes** [3], are located along the path of the lymph vessels.

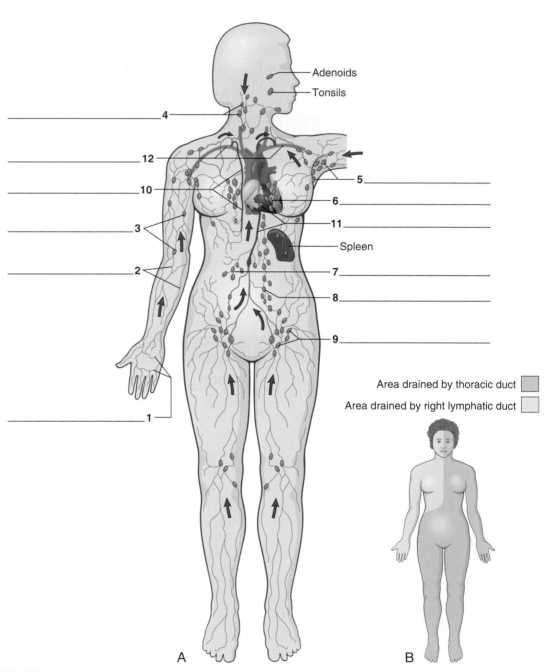

Adenoids

Tonsils

Spleen

Area drained by thoracic duct

Area drained by right lymphatic duct

A   B

FIGURE 14-3 Lymphatic system. A, Label the figure according to the descriptions in the text. **B,** Note the **different regions of the body drained by the right lymphatic duct and the thoracic duct.**

Major sites of lymph node concentration are shown in Figure 14-3A. These are the **cervical** (neck) [4], **axillary** (armpit) [5], **mediastinal** (chest) [6], **mesenteric** (intestinal) [7], **paraaortic** (lumbar) [8], and **inguinal** (groin) [9] regions. Remember that **tonsils** are masses of lymph tissue in the throat near the back of the mouth (oropharynx), and **adenoids** are enlarged lymph tissue in the part of the throat near the nasal passages (nasopharynx).

Lymph vessels all lead toward the thoracic cavity and empty into two large ducts in the upper chest. These are the **right lymphatic duct** [10] and the **thoracic duct** [11]. The thoracic duct drains the lower body and the left side of the head, whereas the right lymphatic duct drains the right side of the head and the chest (a much smaller area) (see Figure 14-3B). Both ducts carry the lymph into **large veins** [12] in the neck, where the lymph then enters the bloodstream.

Lymph nodes not only produce lymphocytes but also filter lymph and trap substances from infectious, inflammatory, and cancerous lesions. Special cells called **macrophages**, located in lymph nodes (as well as in the spleen, liver, and lungs), swallow (phagocytose) foreign substances. When bacteria are present in lymph nodes that drain a particular area of the body, the nodes become swollen with collections of cells and their engulfed debris and become tender. Lymph nodes also fight disease when specialized lymphocytes called **B lymphocytes (B cells)**, which are present in the nodes, produce antibodies. Other lymphocytes present in nodes are **T lymphocytes (T cells)**. They attack bacteria and foreign cells by accurately recognizing a cell as foreign and destroying it. T cells also help B cells make antibodies. See Figure 14-4 for an illustration of a lymph node. B cells mature in bone marrow, whereas T cells originate in the thymus gland.

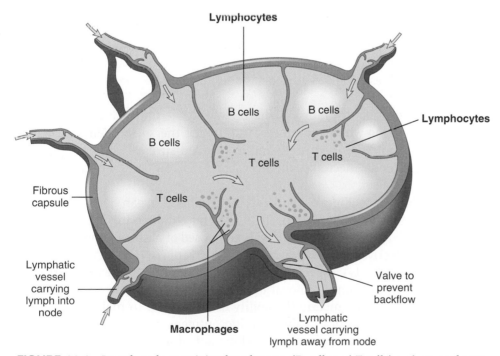

FIGURE 14-4   **Lymph node** containing **lymphocytes (B cells** and **T cells)** and **macrophages.**

14

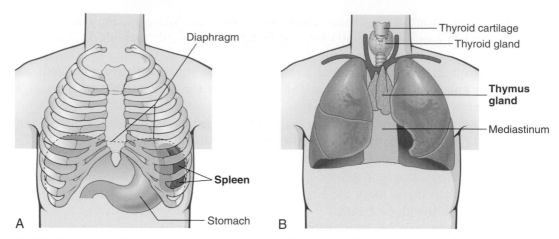

FIGURE 14-5 **A, Spleen** and adjacent structures. **B, Thymus gland** in its location in the mediastinum between the lungs.

SPLEEN AND THYMUS GLAND

The spleen and the thymus gland are specialized organs that also are a part of the lymphatic system.

The **spleen** (Figure 14-5A) is located in the left upper quadrant of the abdomen, next to the stomach. Although the spleen is not essential to life, it has several important functions:

1. **Destruction of old erythrocytes by macrophages.** In the slow-moving circulation of the spleen, red cell breakdown liberates hemoglobin, which is converted to bilirubin in the liver and then is excreted into the bile.
2. **Filtration of microorganisms and other foreign material from the blood.**
3. **Activation of lymphocytes.** Activated B lymphocytes (B cells) produce antibodies. Activated T lymphocytes (T cells) attack foreign materials.
4. **Storage of blood**, especially erythrocytes and platelets.

The spleen is susceptible to injury. A sharp blow to the upper abdomen (as from the impact of a car's steering wheel) may cause rupture of the spleen. Massive hemorrhage can occur when the spleen is ruptured, and immediate surgical removal (splenectomy) may be necessary. After splenectomy, the liver, bone marrow, and lymph nodes take over the functions of the spleen.

The **thymus gland** (see Figure 14-5B) is a lymphatic organ located in the upper mediastinum between the lungs. During fetal life and childhood it is quite large, but it becomes smaller with age. The thymus gland is composed of nests of lymphoid cells resting on a platform of connective tissue. It plays an important role in the body's ability to protect itself from disease (immunity), especially in fetal life and during the early years of growth. It is known that a thymectomy (removal of the thymus gland) performed in an animal during the first weeks of life impairs the ability of the animal to make antibodies and to produce immune cells that fight against foreign antigens such as bacteria and viruses. Thus, the thymus gland is important in development of an effective immune system in childhood.

Early in development, in the thymus, lymphocytes learn to recognize and accept the body's own antigens as "self" or friendly. This acceptance of "self" antigens is called **tolerance.** When the tolerance process fails, immune cells react against normal cells, resulting in various pathologic conditions (autoimmune disease). See page 558, under **autoimmune disease** (aut/o = self).

IMMUNE SYSTEM

The immune system is specialized to defend the body against **antigens** (such as toxins, bacterial proteins, or foreign blood cells). This system includes **leukocytes** such as **neutrophils, monocytes,** and **macrophages,** which are phagocytes found in blood and tissues throughout the body. In addition, **lymphoid organs,** such as the lymph nodes, spleen, thymus gland, tonsils, and adenoids, produce **lymphocytes** and **antibodies.**

NATURAL AND ADAPTIVE IMMUNITY

Immunity is the body's ability to resist foreign organisms and toxins that damage tissues and organs. **Natural immunity is resistance present at birth.** It is not dependent on previous exposure to an antigen (infectious agent). An example of natural immunity is the body's handling of a bacterial infection. White blood cells respond immediately to the intruding antigens. **Neutrophils** travel to the infected area and ingest bacteria. Other white blood cells, such as **monocytes, macrophages,** and **lymphocytes (NK** or **natural killer cells),** also participate in the body's natural immunity against infection. Typically, there is no immunological memory (ability to remember antigens on pathogens) with natural immunity.

In addition to natural immunity, a healthy person can develop **adaptive immunity.** This is the body's ability to **recognize** and **remember** specific antigens in an immune response. **Lymphocytes (T and B cells)** are part of adaptive immunity. **T cells recognize** and **remember** specific antigens and produce stronger attacks each time the antigen is encountered. **B cells** secrete **antibodies** against antigens. Think of what happens when you have a cold or the flu: You are exposed to a viral antigen. Your B cells secrete antibodies, which not only destroy the virus but remain in the blood so that when the virus reappears, at a later time, you have adaptive immunity to it! Another example of adaptive immunity is that achieved with **vaccination.** You are given an injection of a killed virus (for example, poliovirus) that doesn't make you ill, but stimulates your B cells to secrete antibodies against that virus, so that if you are exposed to it at a later time, you will have adaptive immunity.

In certain instances, more immediate adaptive immunity is necessary. Poisons (toxins) that rapidly cause major damage (for example, snake venom) can be counteracted by giving ready-made antibodies, called **antitoxins,** produced in another organism. Injections of other ready-made antibodies, such as **immunoglobulins,** can boost your adaptive immunity before you travel to a foreign country. Infants acquire adaptive immunity when they receive **maternal antibodies** through the placenta, before birth, or in breast milk. Figure 14-6 reviews the general differences between natural and adaptive immunity.

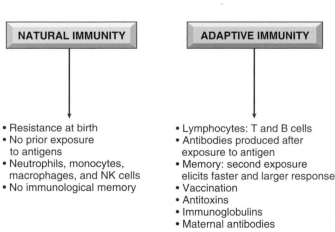

FIGURE 14-6   Types of immunity.

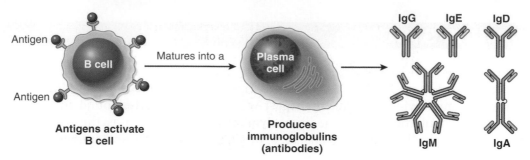

FIGURE 14-7   Humoral immunity: B cell, plasma cell, and immunoglobulins.

Adaptive immunity has two components: **humoral immunity** and **cell-mediated immunity.** Humoral immunity involves **B cells (B lymphocytes),** whereas cell-mediated immunity involves **T cells (T lymphocytes).** In **humoral immunity, B cells** produce **antibodies** after exposure to specific antigens (viruses and bacteria). This is what happens: The B cell matures into another cell called a **plasma cell.** It is the plasma cell that produces antibodies called **immunoglobulins,** which block the effects of antigens. Examples of immunoglobulins **(Ig = immunoglobulin)** are **IgM, IgA, IgG, IgE,** and **IgD.** One maternal immunoglobulin, **IgG,** crosses the placenta to provide immunity for newborns. Another, **IgE,** is important in allergic reactions and in fighting parasitic infections. Figure 14-7 reviews the relationship of a B cell, plasma cell, and immunoglobulins in humoral immunity.

Cell-mediated immunity does not involve antibodies. Rather, it involves several types of **T cells** with different functions. For example, **cytotoxic T cells (CD8+ T cells)** attach to antigens and directly kill them. Cytotoxic cells also secrete **cytokines (interferons and interleukins),** which aid other cells in antigen destruction. **Helper T cells (CD4+ T cells)** assist B cells in making antibodies and they stimulate T cells to attack antigens. **Suppressor T cells** (also called **regulatory T cells,** or **Tregs**) inhibit both B and T cells and prevent them from attacking the body's own good cells. Figure 14-8 reviews the types of T cells in cell-mediated immunity.

The adaptive immune system is helped by a number of other proteins and cells found in circulating blood. One of these is the **complement system,** a group of proteins that helps antibodies kill their target. Another warrior is the **dendritic cell,** which initiates adaptive immunity by presenting antigens to T and B cells, showing them precisely what they need to counteract. A number of cell types can present antigens to T cells, but dendritic cells are especially efficient at this task. Figure 14-9 reviews the roles of B cells, T cells, complement, and dendritic cells.

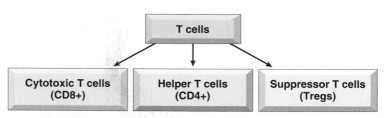

FIGURE 14-8   Cell-mediated immunity: Types of T cells.

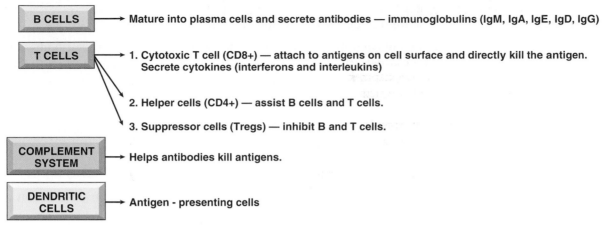

FIGURE 14-9   Functions of B cells, T cells, complement, and dendritic cells.

IMMUNOTHERAPY

Immunotherapy is the use of antibodies, B cells (producing antibodies), and T cells to treat disease such as cancer. Types of immunotherapy are:

Monoclonal antibodies (MoAb)—These are antibodies created in a laboratory by special reproductive (cloning) techniques. They are designed to attack specific cancer cells. An example of monoclonal antibody therapy is use of the drug rituximab (Rituxan), made to kill malignant lymphoma cells. The antibody may be chemically linked to various toxins or radioactive particles and delivered to tumor cells, to enhance the killing effect.

Vaccines—These preparations contain antigens (proteins) from a patient's tumor cells. When they are injected, they stimulate the patient's own T cells to recognize and kill the cancerous cells. Vaccines may be injected or given orally or as a nasal spray.

Transfer of immune cells—In bone marrow transplantation, T lymphocytes from a donor can replace a patient's immune system with new cells that recognize tumor cells as foreign and kill them.

Monoclonal antibody therapy and transfer of immune cells are passive immunotherapy (immune agents are given to the patient), whereas vaccination is active immunotherapy (the patient's own immune system is stimulated to do the work).

 ## VOCABULARY

This list reviews many of the new terms introduced in the text. Short definitions reinforce your understanding of the terms. Refer to the Pronunciation of Terms on page 575 for help with unfamiliar or difficult words.

adaptive immunity	The ability to recognize and remember specific antigens and mount an attack on them. Humoral (B cells) and cell-mediated immunity (T cells) are examples.
adenoids	Mass of lymphatic tissue in the nasopharynx.
antibody	Protein produced by B cells to destroy antigens.
antigen	Substance that the body recognizes as foreign; evokes an immune response. Most antigens are proteins or protein fragments found on the surface of bacteria, viruses, or organ transplant tissue cells.

axillary nodes	Lymph nodes in the armpit (underarm).
B cell (B lymphocyte)	Lymphocyte that matures into a plasma cell to secrete antibodies. The B refers to the bursa of Fabricius, an organ in birds in which B cell differentiation and growth were first noted to occur.
cell-mediated immunity	T cells (cytotoxic, helper and suppressor) respond to antigens and destroy them; a type of adaptive immunity.
cervical nodes	Lymph nodes in the neck region.
complement system	Set of proteins in the blood that help antibodies kill their target.
cytokines	Proteins secreted by cytotoxic T cells to aid in antigen destruction. Examples are interferons and interleukins.
cytotoxic T cell	Lymphocyte that directly kills antigens; called (CD8+) T cell.
dendritic cell	Antigen-presenting cell. Shows T and B cells what to attack.
helper T cell	Lymphocyte that aids B cells and stimulates T cells. Also called (CD4+) T cell.
humoral immunity	B cells produce antibodies after exposure to specific antigens; type of adaptive immunity.
immunity	Body's ability to resist foreign organisms and toxins that damage tissues and organs. This includes natural immunity and adaptive immunity. The word immunity comes from Latin *immunis,* meaning exempt or protected from.
immunoglobulins	Antibodies such as IgA, IgE, IgG, IgM, and IgD; secreted by plasma cells (mature B cells) in response to the presence of an antigen.
immunotherapy	Use of immune cells, antibodies, or vaccines to treat or prevent disease.
inguinal nodes	Lymph nodes in the groin region.
interferons	Proteins (cytokines) secreted by T cells and other cells to aid and regulate the immune response.
interleukins	Proteins (cytokines) that stimulate the growth of B and T lymphocytes.
interstitial fluid	Fluid in the spaces between cells. This fluid becomes lymph when it enters lymph capillaries.
lymph	Thin, watery fluid found within lymphatic vessels and collected from tissues throughout the body. Latin *lympha* means clear spring water.
lymph capillaries	Tiniest lymphatic vessels.
lymphoid organs	Lymph nodes, spleen, and thymus gland.
lymph node	Collection of stationary solid lymphatic tissue along lymph vessels; contains cells (lymphocytes and macrophages) that fight infection.
lymph vessel	Carrier of lymph throughout the body; lymphatic vessels empty lymph into veins in the upper part of the chest.
macrophage	Large phagocyte found in lymph nodes and other tissues of the body. Phag/o means to eat or swallow.
mediastinal nodes	Lymph nodes in the area between the lungs in the thoracic (chest) cavity.

14

mesenteric nodes	Lymph nodes in the mesentery (intestinal region).
monoclonal antibody	Antibody produced in a laboratory to attack antigens and to destroy cells; useful in immunotherapy.
natural immunity	Protection that an individual is born with to fight infection such as neutrophils, monocytes, macrophages, and NK cells. It is not antigen specific and does not elicit memory.
paraaortic nodes	Lymph nodes near the aorta in the lumbar (waist) area of the body.
plasma cell	Lymphocyte that secretes antibodies. It matures from B lymphocytes.
right lymphatic duct	Lymphatic vessel in the chest that drains lymph from the upper right part of the body. It empties lymph into a large vein in the neck.
spleen	Organ in the left upper quadrant of the abdomen that destroys worn-out red blood cells, activates lymphocytes, and stores blood.
suppressor T cell	Lymphocyte that inhibits the activity of B and T cells. Also called a **Treg (regulatory T cell).**
T cell (T lymphocyte)	Lymphocyte that acts directly on antigens to destroy them or produce chemicals (cytokines) such as interferons and interleukins that are toxic to antigens.
tolerance	The ability of T lymphocytes to recognize and accept the body's own antigens as "self" or friendly. Once tolerance is established, the immune system will not react against the body.
thoracic duct	Large lymphatic vessel that drains lymph from the lower and left side of the body (head, neck, arm, and chest). It empties lymph into large veins in the neck.
thymus gland	Lymphoid organ in the mediastinum that conditions T cells to react to foreign cells and aids in the immune response.
tonsils	Masses of lymphatic tissue in the back of the oropharynx.
toxin	Poison; a protein produced by certain bacteria, animals, or plants.
vaccination	Exposure of an individual to a foreign protein (antigen) that provokes an immune response. The response will destroy any cell that possesses the antigen on its surface and will protect against infection. The term comes from the Latin *vacca*, cow—the first inoculations were given with organisms that caused the disease cowpox to produce immunity to smallpox.
vaccine	Weakened or killed microorganisms, toxins, or other proteins given to induce immunity to infection or disease.

14

TERMINOLOGY

Write the meanings of the medical terms in the spaces provided.

COMBINING FORMS

COMBINING FORM	MEANING	TERMINOLOGY	MEANING
immun/o	protection	autoimmune disease _____	
		Examples are rheumatoid arthritis and systemic lupus erythematosus. These are chronic, disabling diseases caused by the abnormal production of antibodies against normal body tissues. Signs and symptoms are inflammation of joints, skin rash, and fever. Glucocorticoid drugs (prednisone) and other immunosuppressants (azathioprine, methotrexate) are effective as treatment but make patients susceptible to infection.	
		immunoglobulin _____	
		immunosuppression _____	
		This may occur because of exposure to drugs (corticosteroids) or as the result of disease (AIDS and cancer). Immunosuppressed patients are susceptible to infection with fungi, Pneumocystis bacteria, and other pathogens.	
lymph/o	lymph	lymphopoiesis _____	
		lymphedema _____	
		Interstitial fluid collects within the spaces between cells as a result of obstruction of lymphatic vessels and nodes. Radiation therapy may destroy lymphatics and produce lymphedema, as in breast cancer treatment (Figure 14-10).	
		lymphocytopenia _____	
		lymphocytosis _____	
		lymphoid _____	
		The suffix -oid means resembling or derived from. Lymphoid organs include lymph nodes, spleen, and thymus gland.	

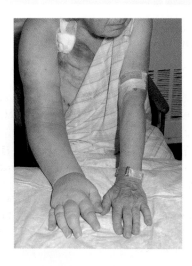

FIGURE 14-10 Lymphedema of right arm secondary to mastectomy, lymphadenectomy, and radiotherapy.

COMBINING FORM	MEANING	TERMINOLOGY	MEANING
lymphaden/o	lymph node (gland)	lymphadenopathy _____	
		lymphadenitis _____	
splen/o	spleen	splenomegaly _____	
		Note that the combining form for spleen contains only one e.	
		splenectomy _____	
		asplenia _____	
		The condition may be congenital or result from surgical removal.	
		hypersplenism _____	
		A syndrome marked by splenomegaly and often associated with blood cell destruction, anemia, leukopenia, and thrombocytopenia.	
thym/o	thymus gland	thymectomy _____	
tox/o	poison	toxic _____	

PREFIXES

PREFIX	MEANING	TERMINOLOGY	MEANING
ana-	again, anew	anaphylaxis _____	
		The suffix -phylaxis means protection. This is an unusual hypersensitivity to previously encountered foreign proteins or other antigens. Vasodilation and a decrease in blood pressure can be life-threatening.	
inter-	between	interstitial fluid _____	
		The suffix -stitial means pertaining to standing or positioned.	

PATHOLOGIC CONDITIONS

IMMUNODEFICIENCY

Some immunodeficiency disorders are present at birth. An example is **severe combined immunodeficiency disease (SCID).** Affected infants are born with a deficiency of B cells and T cells, resulting in a lack of immunity. The thymus is small, and children have little or no protection against infection.

acquired immunodeficiency syndrome (AIDS)	**Group of clinical signs and symptoms associated with suppression of the immune system and marked by opportunistic infections, secondary neoplasms, and neurologic problems.** AIDS is caused by the **human immunodeficiency virus (HIV)**. HIV destroys **helper T cells** (also known as **CD4+ cells,** containing the CD4 protein antigen). This disrupts the immune response, allowing infections to occur. Infectious diseases associated with AIDS are called **opportunistic infections** because HIV lowers resistance and allows infection by bacteria and parasites that are easily otherwise contained by normal defenses. Table 14-2 lists many of these opportunistic infections; use the table as a reference.

14

TABLE 14-2	OPPORTUNISTIC INFECTIONS ASSOCIATED WITH AIDS
INFECTION	**DESCRIPTION**
candidiasis	Yeast-like fungus *(Candida)*, normally present in the mouth, skin, intestinal tract, and vagina, overgrows, causing infection of the mouth (thrush), respiratory tract, and skin.
cryptococcal infection (Crypto)	Yeast-like fungus *(Cryptococcus)* causes lung, brain, and blood infections. Pathogen is found in pigeon droppings and nesting places, air, water, and soil.
cryptosporidiosis	Parasitic infection of the gastrointestinal tract and brain and spinal cord. The pathogen, *Cryptosporidium*, is a one-celled organism commonly found in farm animals.
cytomegalovirus (CMV) infection	Virus causes enteritis and retinitis (inflammation of the retina at the back of the eye). Found in saliva, semen, cervical secretions, urine, feces, blood, and breast milk, but usually causes disease only when the immune system is compromised.
herpes simplex	Viral infection causes small blisters on the skin of the lips or nose or on the genitals. Herpes simplex virus also can cause encephalitis.
histoplasmosis (Histo)	Fungal infection caused by inhalation of dust contaminated with *Histoplasma capsulatum*; causes fever, chills, and lung infection. Pathogen is found in bird and bat droppings.
***Mycobacterium avium-intracellulare* (MAI) complex infection**	Bacterial disease manifesting with fever, malaise, night sweats, anorexia, diarrhea, weight loss, and lung and blood infections.
***Pneumocystis* pneumonia (PCP)**	One-celled organism causes lung infection, with fever, cough, and chest pain. Pathogen is found in air, water, and soil and is carried by animals. Infection is treated with trimethoprim-sulfamethoxazole (Bactrim), a combination of several antibiotics, or pentamidine. Aerosolized pentamidine, which is inhaled, can prevent occurrence of PCP.
toxoplasmosis (Toxo)	Parasitic infection involving the central nervous system (CNS) and causing fever, chills, visual disturbances, confusion, hemiparesis (slight paralysis in half of the body), and seizures. Pathogen *(Toxoplasma)* is acquired by eating uncooked lamb or pork, unpasteurized dairy products, or raw eggs or vegetables.
tuberculosis (TB)	Bacterial disease (caused by *Mycobacterium tuberculosis*) involving the lungs, brain, and other organs. Signs and symptoms are fever, cough, loss of weight, anorexia, and blood in sputum.

Malignancies associated with AIDS are **Kaposi sarcoma** (a cancer arising from the lining cells of capillaries that produces dark-purplish skin nodules) and **lymphoma** (cancer of lymph nodes). **Wasting syndrome**, marked by weight loss and decrease in muscular strength, appetite, and mental activity, also may occur with AIDS (Figure 14-11A and B).

Persons who were exposed to HIV and now have antibodies in their blood against this virus are **HIV-positive.** HIV is found in blood, semen, vaginal and cervical secretions, saliva, and other body fluids. Transmission of HIV may occur by three routes: sexual contact, blood inoculation (through sharing of contaminated needles, accidental needlesticks, or contact with contaminated blood or blood products), and passage of the virus from infected mothers to their newborns. Table 14-3 summarizes the common routes of transmission of HIV.

14

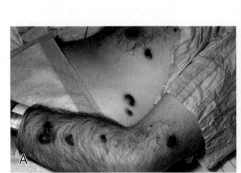
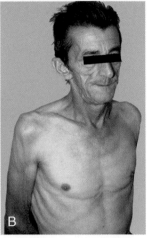

FIGURE 14-11   A, Kaposi sarcoma. B, Wasting syndrome.

HIV-infected patients may remain asymptomatic for as long as 10 years. Signs and symptoms associated with HIV infection are lymphadenopathy, neurologic disease, oral thrush (fungal infection), night sweats, fatigue, and evidence of opportunistic infections.

Some drugs that are used to treat AIDS are inhibitors of the viral enzyme called **reverse transcriptase (RT).** After invading the helper T cell (carrying the CD4+ antigen), HIV releases reverse transcriptase to help it grow and multiply inside the cell. Examples of **reverse transcriptase inhibitors (RTIs)** are zidovudine and lamivudine (Epivir). A second class of anti HIV drugs is the **protease inhibitors**. These drugs inhibit another viral enzyme called protease. HIV needs protease to reproduce. Use of combinations of protease inhibitors (nelfinavir, amprenavir) and RTIs is called **HAART (highly active antiretroviral therapy)**. This treatment has in many cases abolished evidence of viral infection in affected people.

14

TABLE 14-3	COMMON ROUTES OF TRANSMISSION OF AIDS VIRUS
ROUTE	**PEOPLE AFFECTED**
Receptive oral and anal intercourse	Men and women
Receptive vaginal intercourse	Women
Sharing of needles and equipment (users of intravenous drugs)	Men and women
Contaminated blood (for transfusion) or blood products	Men and women (with hemophilia)
From mother—in utero or by breast feeding	Neonates

HYPERSENSITIVITY

allergy

Abnormal hypersensitivity acquired by exposure to an antigen.

Allergic (all/o = other) reactions occur when a sensitized person, who has previously been exposed to an agent **(allergen),** reacts violently to a subsequent exposure. This reaction varies in intensity from **allergic rhinitis** or hay fever (caused by pollen or animal dander) to **systemic anaphylaxis,** in which an extraordinary hypersensitivity reaction occurs throughout the body, leading to fall in blood pressure (hypotension), shock, respiratory distress, and edema (swelling) of the larynx. Anaphylaxis can be life-threatening, but the patient usually survives if the airways are kept open and treatment is given immediately (epinephrine and antihistamines).

Other allergies include **asthma** (pollens, dust, molds), **hives** (caused by food or drugs), and **atopic dermatitis** (rash from soaps, cosmetics, chemicals). Atopic means related to **atopy,** a hypersensitivity or allergic state arising from an inherited predisposition. A person who is atopic is prone to allergies (Figure 14-12).

MALIGNANCIES

lymphoma

Malignant tumor of lymph nodes and lymph tissue.

There are many types of lymphoma, varying according to the particular cell type and degree of differentiation. Some examples are:

Hodgkin lymphoma—Malignant tumor of lymphoid tissue in the spleen and lymph nodes. This disease is characterized by **lymphadenopathy** (lymph nodes enlarge), splenomegaly, fever, weakness, and loss of weight and appetite. The diagnosis often is made by identifying a type of malignant cell (**Reed-Sternberg cell**) in the lymph nodes. If disease is localized, the treatment may be radiotherapy or chemotherapy. If the disease is more widespread, chemotherapy is given alone. There is a very high probability of cure with available treatments. Figure 14-13 illustrates staging of Hodgkin lymphoma.

14

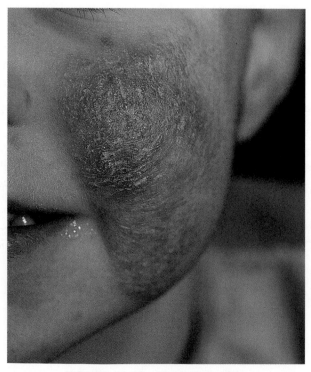

FIGURE 14-12   Atopic dermatitis.

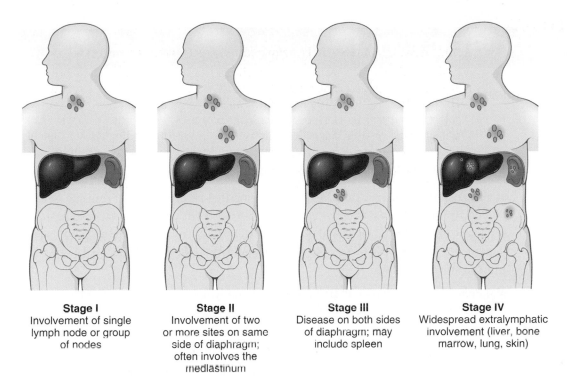

Stage I
Involvement of single lymph node or group of nodes

Stage II
Involvement of two or more sites on same side of diaphragm; often involves the mediastinum

Stage III
Disease on both sides of diaphragm; may include spleen

Stage IV
Widespread extralymphatic involvement (liver, bone marrow, lung, skin)

FIGURE 14-13   Staging of Hodgkin lymphoma involves assessing the extent of spread of the disease. Lymph node biopsies, laparotomy with liver and lymph node biopsies, and splenectomy may be necessary for staging.

14

Non-Hodgkin lymphomas—These include **follicular lymphoma** (composed of collections of small lymphocytes in a follicle or nodule arrangement) and **large cell lymphoma** (composed of large lymphocytes that infiltrate nodes and tissues diffusely). Non-Hodgkin lymphomas are mostly B cell lymphomas and rarely T cell malignancies. Chemotherapy may cure or stop the progress of this disease.

multiple myeloma

Malignant tumor of bone marrow cells.

This is a tumor composed of **plasma cells** (antibody-producing B lymphocytes) associated with high levels of one of the specific immunoglobulins, usually IgG. **Waldenström macroglobulinemia** is another disorder of malignant B cells. This disease involves B cells that produce large quantities of IgM (a globulin of high molecular weight). Increased IgM concentration impairs the passage of blood through capillaries in the brain and eyes, causing a hyperviscosity syndrome (thickening of the blood).

thymoma

Malignant tumor of the thymus gland.

Often thymoma is associated with a neuromuscular disorder, myasthenia gravis. Many patients with thymoma have other associated autoimmune disorders such as systemic lupus erythematosus, rheumatoid arthritis, and red cell aplasia.

Surgery is the principal method of treating thymoma; postoperative radiation therapy is used for patients with evidence of spread of the tumor.

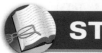 **STUDY SECTION**

Practice spelling each term and know its meaning.

allergen	Substance capable of causing a specific hypersensitivity reaction in the body; a type of antigen.
anaphylaxis	Exaggerated or unusual hypersensitivity to foreign protein or other substance.
atopy	Hypersensitive or allergic state involving an inherited predisposition. From the Greek *atopia,* meaning strangeness.
CD4+ cells	Helper T cells that carry the CD4 protein antigen on their surface. HIV binds to CD4 and infects and kills T cells bearing this protein. AIDS patients have an inadequate number of CD4+ cells.
Hodgkin lymphoma	Malignant tumor of lymphoid tissue in spleen and lymph nodes; Reed-Sternberg cells are often found on microscopic analysis.
human immunodeficiency virus (HIV)	Virus (retrovirus) that causes AIDS.
Kaposi sarcoma	Malignant lesion associated with AIDS; arises from the lining of capillaries and appears as red, purple, brown, or black skin nodules.
non-Hodgkin lymphomas	Group of malignant tumors involving lymphoid tissue. Examples are follicular lymphoma and large cell lymphoma.
opportunistic infections	Infectious diseases associated with AIDS; they occur because HIV infection lowers the body's resistance and allows infection by bacteria and parasites that normally are easily contained.
protease inhibitor	Drug that treats AIDS by blocking the production of protease, a proteolytic enzyme that helps create new viral pieces for HIV.
reverse transcriptase inhibitor (RTI)	Drug that treats AIDS by blocking reverse transcriptase, an enzyme needed to make copies of HIV.
wasting syndrome	Weight loss, decrease in muscular strength, appetite, and mental activity; associated with AIDS.

14

LABORATORY TESTS AND CLINICAL PROCEDURES

LABORATORY TESTS

CD4+ cell count	**Measures the number of CD4+ T cells (helper T cells) in the bloodstream of patients with AIDS.**
	A normal count usually is between 500 and 1500 CD4+ cells per mm^3. If the CD4+ count falls below 250 to 200, it is recommended to start treatment with anti-HIV drugs.
ELISA	**Screening test to detect anti-HIV antibodies in the bloodstream.**
	Antibodies to HIV begin to appear within 2 weeks of infection with HIV. If the result of this test is positive, it is confirmed with a **Western blot** test, which is more specific. ELISA is an abbreviation for <u>e</u>nzyme-<u>l</u>inked <u>i</u>mmuno<u>s</u>orbent <u>a</u>ssay.

immunoelectrophoresis	**Test that separates immunoglobulins (IgM, IgG, IgE, IgA, IgD).**
	This procedure detects the presence of abnormal levels of antibodies in patients with conditions such as multiple myeloma and Waldenström macroglobulinemia.
viral load test	**Measurement of the amount of AIDS virus (HIV) in the bloodstream.**
	Two viral load tests are a PCR (polymerase chain reaction) assay and an NASBA (nucleic acid sequence–based amplification) test.

CLINICAL PROCEDURES

computed tomography (CT) scan	**X-ray imaging produces cross-sectional and other views of anatomic structures.**
	These x-ray views show abnormalities of lymphoid organs, such as lymph nodes, spleen, and thymus gland.

ABBREVIATIONS

14

AIDS	acquired immunodeficiency syndrome	**HSV**	herpes simplex virus
CD4+ cell	helper T cell	**IgA, IgD, IgE, IgG, IgM**	immunoglobulins
CD8+ cell	cytotoxic T cell		
CMV	cytomegalovirus—causes opportunistic AIDS-related infection	**IL1 to IL38**	interleukins
Crypto	*Cryptococcus*—causes opportunistic AIDS-related infection	**KS**	Kaposi sarcoma
		MAI	*Mycobacterium avium-intracellulare* (MAI) complex—group of pathogens that cause lung and systemic disease in immunocompromised patients
ELISA	enzyme-linked immunosorbent assay—test to detect anti-HIV antibodies		
G-CSF	granulocyte colony-stimulating factor—cytokine that promotes neutrophil production	**MoAb**	monoclonal antibody
		NHL	non-Hodgkin lymphoma
GM-CSF	granulocyte-macrophage colony-stimulating factor—cytokine secreted by macrophages to promote growth of myeloid progenitor cells and their differentiation to granulocytes	**PCP**	*Pneumocystis* pneumonia—opportunistic AIDS-related infection
		PI	protease inhibitor
		RTI	reverse transcriptase inhibitor—for example, zidovudine (Retrovir) or lamivudine (Epivir)
HAART	highly active antiretroviral therapy—use of combinations of drugs that are effective against AIDS	**SCID**	severe combined immunodeficiency disease
Histo	histoplasmosis—fungal infection seen in AIDS patients	**Treg**	regulatory T cell (suppressor T cell)
HIV	human immunodeficiency virus—causes AIDS	**Toxo**	toxoplasmosis—parasitic infection associated with AIDS

IN PERSON: HODGKIN LYMPHOMA

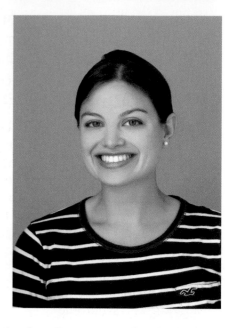

When I began noticing persistent back pain and fatigue in 2006, my doctor and I didn't take the symptoms seriously until 2007, when I noticed I was losing weight and short of breath. I saw a lung specialist, who took a chest x-ray and discovered a mass the size of a grapefruit in my mediastinum. Immediately, my stress level went sky high, and being 25 in New York City on my own (my family was in California and my mother was going through metastatic breast cancer treatment), I felt afraid and alone.

I was scheduled for a PET-CT scan and visited a friend who was a radiation oncologist. She was alarmed by my symptoms and appearance and through her father, a medical oncologist, immediately put me in contact with a cancer specialist. The results from the PET-CT plus bronchoscopy with a biopsy, and a bone marrow biopsy confirmed that I had Stage 2B Hodgkin lymphoma with "bulky disease" [large tumor mass] in my mediastinum. This diagnosis was really scary for me. But watching my mother go through her difficult battle with breast cancer made me realize that if I emulated her positive attitude, it would make life easier for my entire family.

The treatment was six cycles of chemotherapy. After two cycles, enough of my hair started falling out that I shaved my head. A Powerport was installed in my upper chest so that I could receive the chemotherapy more quickly and with less pain. Because I was so young, I received hormones to put my body into temporary menopause, to preserve my fertility.

Three months into my treatment a PET-CT showed that the mass was still large, and it was likely that I would need radiation to my chest after the chemotherapy. By the time that I was finishing my chemotherapy, I was having a difficult time coping with the ongoing side effects and time in the hospital. Nevertheless, I rallied and traveled to Boston for 4 weeks of proton [powerful radiation] therapy. I actually felt lucky to be receiving this cutting-edge treatment, delivered by one of the few proton beam machines in the country.

My radiation treatment ended in 2008, and a follow-up PET-CT scan would tell me if I needed further treatment. I remember when the doctor told me that the scan was all clear, I said, "Great!"—and then went outside and cried on a bench for an hour. More recently, I've been getting follow-up scans every year. Honestly, I'm relieved when the scan is clear, but I am also afraid and aware of the possibility of recurrence and of developing a secondary cancer as a result of the extensive radiation treatment. Since my mother passed away in 2013, I've been getting regular mammograms, and because of the radiation effects on my thyroid gland, I'm taking thyroid hormone to treat hypothyroidism.

I know that my Hodgkin lymphoma experience will always be with me, but I still have an inherently positive attitude, which has enabled and empowered me to start a new, exciting business and think optimistically about the future.

Lenore Estrada is the CEO and Co-Founder of Three Babes Bakeshop, a pie business in San Francisco that works to bring awareness to the economic, social and environmental issues at play in working-class American communities. She is also the President of the Board of Bay Leaf Kitchen, a non-profit that helps children learn through hands-on cooking and farming experiences.

14

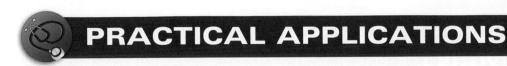

PRACTICAL APPLICATIONS

Answers to the questions are on page 574.

SHORT CLINICAL CASES

Circle the correct answer in **boldface** for the diagnosis.

1. John was a healthy baby until the age of 22 months, when he developed angioedema [swelling induced while eating a cookie containing peanut butter]. The symptoms disappeared in about an hour. A month later, while eating the same type of cookie, he started to vomit, became hoarse, had great difficulty in breathing, started to wheeze, and developed a swollen face. He was taken immediately to the ED of Children's Hospital, where he was given a subcutaneous injection of epinephrine [adrenaline]. Within minutes of the epinephrine injection, John's hoarseness decreased, the wheezing diminished, and his breathing was less labored. His parents were advised to avoid giving him foods containing peanuts in any form.
Diagnosis: **(multiple myeloma, acute systemic anaphylaxis, acquired immunodeficiency syndrome)**

2. Mark Scott is a 48-year-old band leader who has always been in good health. Six months ago he went to the ED at the local hospital complaining of fever and sudden swelling of his right hand from a cat scratch. He was admitted to the hospital for the hand infection. His blood lymphocyte count was very low, so a blood sample was sent to be tested for antibodies against HIV. Both ELISA and a Western blot revealed presence of anti-HIV antibodies. His CD4+ T cell count was very low at 170 [normal is 500 to 1600]. Mr. Scott told his doctor that he had several homosexual encounters before his marriage. His physician prescribed trimethoprim-sulfamethoxazole for prophylaxis against *Pneumocystis* pneumonia, and Mark also was given HAART. After 5 weeks of therapy, his HIV viral load declined to undetectable levels and his CD4+ T cell count rose. He remains well and active and works full time.
Diagnosis: **(T cell lymphoma, severe combined immunodeficiency disease, acquired immunodeficiency syndrome)**

3. Mrs. Archer is a 55-year-old housewife who began to experience excessive fatigue. A blood sample revealed mild anemia and slightly lowered white blood cell count. Her sedimentation rate was elevated, and electrophoresis of serum proteins showed marked elevation of IgG. She returned for regular visits to her physician, and on each occasion serum IgG levels were gradually increasing. After she experienced sudden onset of upper back pain, a thoracic spine MRI study was performed and showed destruction of a portion of a vertebra. A bone marrow biopsy specimen showed a proliferation of plasma cells. She was given chemotherapy (vincristine, Adriamycin, and Decadron), but a year later she developed fever and chest pain. Chest x-ray revealed pneumonia, and antibiotics were given. The outlook for her survival is poor.
Diagnosis: **(Hodgkin lymphoma, hemolytic anemia, multiple myeloma)**

14

IN PERSON: LYMPHOMA TREATMENT

14

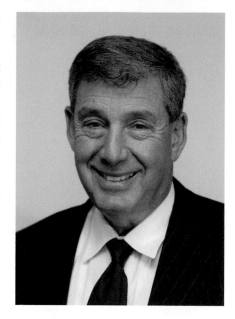

This account was written by a medical oncologist who specializes in the treatment of patients with lymphoma.

Of the many challenges of practicing medical oncology, the treatment of patients with lymphoma is among the most satisfying, and at times the most difficult. Lymphomas were the first common solid tumor to become curable with drugs alone. In 1969, investigators at the National Cancer Institute published their promising results with combination chemotherapy for Hodgkin lymphoma. At that time, this was a tumor that was treatable and curable with radiation therapy in only a small fraction of patients, when disease was limited to involvement of only a few lymph nodes. Very soon thereafter, chemotherapy proved to be curative for almost one half of patients with a more aggressive disease— large B cell lymphocytic lymphoma, a malignancy that affects 20,000 new subjects every year in the United States. In succeeding years, for patients not cured with conventional drugs, bone marrow transplantation following ultra-high-dose chemotherapy salvaged at least half of those patients who experienced a relapse of disease. New drugs, particularly monoclonal antibodies that attack proteins on the surface of tumors and initiate immune destruction of tumors, have added to that success. Thus, at present, with use of chemotherapy, irradiation, and high-dose drug treatment, most patients with lymphoma can be cured.

The experience of treating a patient with lymphoma is not simple. The first step is making the correct diagnosis, which requires obtaining an adequate biopsy specimen from the involved lymph nodes, bone marrow, or other disease sites. Next, the physician in charge of the case must establish the sites and extent of disease, and this requires sophisticated x-ray and even MR imaging of lungs, abdomen, bones, and in some cases the spinal canal. The choice of drug regimens and other treatments depends on making a correct assessment of these factors.

The doctor must explain all of this information to the patient so that he or she has a clear understanding of what lies ahead. The long-term plan of management involves numerous hospital outpatient visits for evaluation and treatment, including possible biopsy and repeat biopsy of sites of disease to establish whether the tumor has been effectively treated. I also spend considerable time with patients explaining the potential side effects of treatments, some of which can affect the lungs, heart, and immune system. In addition, patients need guidance after chemotherapy about susceptibility to serious infections when blood counts are low. Overall, the psychological stress and uncertainty of outcome plus the impact on work and family responsibilities make the need for support from friends and family crucial.

For most patients, all of these issues are successfully managed during treatment, and no experience is more gratifying for me, as an oncologist, than to achieve cure of a potentially lethal disease. All of this is accomplished at a price. For a few patients, the stresses of disease and its impact on family and work prove nearly overwhelming. I call upon the intervention of social workers, nurses, and even psychiatrists to help my patients deal with the difficulty of disease and life-changing experiences. The added rigors of bone marrow transplantation increase the burden on patients who are not cured by conventional treatments. Finally, even more stressful and demanding are the challenges faced by those patients, a minority to be sure, whose disease progresses despite all interventions, and who are destined not to survive. For these patients, experimental treatments at times are the best option and again may reverse the downward course. Through it all, as a physician, I find that we must all work as a team to provide the best medical advice, psychological support, and hope for 60,000 new patients who develop lymphoma each year.

Dr. Bruce A. Chabner is a professor of medicine at Harvard Medical School and the Director of Clinical Research at the Massachusetts General Hospital Cancer Center.

? EXERCISES

Remember to check your answers carefully with the Answers to Exercises, page 573.

A Match the listed terms with the descriptions that follow.

adenoids   lymph node   thoracic duct
interstitial fluid   right lymphatic duct   thymus gland
lymph capillaries   spleen

1. collection of stationary lymphatic tissue along lymph

   vessels _____

2. large lymphatic vessel that drains lymph from the lower and left side of the

   body _____

3. organ in the left upper quadrant of the abdomen that destroys worn-out erythrocytes, activates

   lymphocytes, and stores blood _____

4. mass of lymphatic tissue in the nasopharynx _____

5. lymphoid organ in the mediastinum that conditions T cells to react to foreign cells in the

   immune response _____

6. tiniest lymphatic vessels _____

7. large lymphatic vessel in the chest that drains lymph from the upper right part of the body

   _____

8. fluid in the spaces between cells _____

B Give the locations of the following lymph nodes.

1. inguinal nodes _____

2. axillary nodes _____

3. cervical nodes _____

4. mediastinal nodes _____

5. paraaortic nodes _____

6. mesenteric nodes _____

14

C ● Circle the correct answer in boldface in each sentence.

1. Cytotoxic T cells are (**CD8+ T cells, helper T cells, suppressor T cells**) and directly kill foreign cells.

2. Lymphocytes that directly act on antigens are (**B cells, T cells, macrophages**).

3. CD4+ T cells are (**helper T cells, Tregs, B cells**) and are deficient in people with AIDS.

4. Lymphocytes that mature into plasma cells and secrete antibodies are (**B cells, T cells, macrophages**).

5. The type of immunity in which B cells produce antibodies after exposure to antigens is (**natural immunity, cytotoxic immunity, humoral immunity**).

6. The type of immunity that is the ability to recognize and remember specific antigens and mount an attack on them is (**adaptive immunity, natural immunity**).

D ● Match the following cell names with their meanings as given below.

complement system	helper T cell	plasma cell
dendritic cell	macrophage	suppressor T cell

1. lymphocyte that matures from a B lymphocyte and secretes antibodies _____

2. large phagocyte found in lymph nodes and other tissues of the body _____

3. CD4+ T cell that aids B cells in recognizing antigens _____

4. Treg that inhibits the activity of B and T lymphocytes _____

5. proteins in the blood that help antibodies and T cells kill their target _____

6. antigen-presenting cell; shows B cells and T cells what to attack _____

E ● Match the terms in Column I with their descriptions in Column II. Write your answers in the spaces provided.

COLUMN I

1. immunoglobulins _____

2. toxins _____

3. helper T cells _____

4. suppressor T cells _____

5. cytotoxic T cells _____

6. plasma cells _____

7. interferons and interleukins _____

COLUMN II

A. Antibodies—IgA, IgE, IgG, IgM, IgD

B. Lymphocytes that aids B cells; CD4+ T cell

C. Poisons (antigens)

D. T lymphocytes that inhibit the activity of B and T cells

E. Cytokines secreted by cytotoxic T cells

F. Transformed B cells that secrete antibodies

G. T lymphocytes that directly kill foreign cells (CD8+ T cells)

F **Use the given definitions to build medical terms.**

1. removal of the spleen: _____

2. enlargement of the spleen: _____

3. formation of lymph: _____

4. malignant tumor of the thymus gland: _____

5. inflammation of lymph glands (nodes): _____

6. deficiency of lymph cells: _____

7. pertaining to poison: _____

8. disease of lymph glands (nodes): _____

G **Match the listed terms with the descriptions/definitions that follow.**

AIDS   Hodgkin lymphoma   lymphoid organs
allergen   hypersplenism   thymectomy
anaphylaxis   lymphedema

1. syndrome marked by enlargement of the spleen and associated with anemia, leukopenia, and

   thrombocytopenia _____

2. extraordinary hypersensitivity to a foreign protein; marked by hypotension, shock, and

   respiratory distress _____

3. antigen capable of causing allergy (hypersensitivity) _____

4. disorder in which the immune system is suppressed by exposure to HIV _____

5. removal of a mediastinal organ _____

6. malignant tumor of lymphoid tissue in the lymph nodes and spleen; Reed-Sternberg cells are in

   lymph nodes _____

7. spleen, thymus, and tonsils _____

8. swelling of tissues due to interstitial fluid accumulation _____

H Match the listed terms or abbreviations related to AIDS with the descriptions that follow.

CD4+ T cells   Kaposi sarcoma   viral load test
ELISA   opportunistic infections wasting syndrome
HAART   protease inhibitor
HIV   reverse transcriptase inhibitor

1. malignant condition associated with AIDS (purplish skin nodules appear)

  _____

2. human immunodeficiency virus; the retrovirus that causes AIDS _____

3. white blood cells that are destroyed by the AIDS virus _____

4. group of infectious diseases associated with AIDS _____

5. measures the amount of HIV in blood _____

6. weight loss with decreased muscular strength, appetite, and mental activity

  _____

7. drug used to treat AIDS by blocking an enzyme needed to make copies of HIV

  _____

8. drug used to treat AIDS by blocking the production of an enzyme that creates new viral pieces for HIV _____

9. use of combinations of drugs to treat AIDS _____

10. test to detect anti-HIV antibodies _____

I Complete the following terms according to the definitions provided. Pay close attention to the proper spelling of each term.

1. chronic, disabling diseases caused by abnormal production of antibodies to normal tissue:

  auto _____ diseases

2. a hypersensitivity or allergic state with an inherited predisposition: a _____

3. a malignant tumor of lymph nodes; follicular and large cell are types of this disease:

  non _____

4. fluid that lies between cells throughout the body: inter _____ fluid

5. formation of lymphocytes or lymphoid tissue: lympho _____

6. chronic swelling of a part of the body due to collection of fluid between tissues secondary to obstruction of lymph vessels and nodes: lymph _____

7. an unusual or exaggerated allergic reaction to a foreign protein: ana _____

8. introduction of altered antigens to produce an immune response and protection from disease:

  vac _____

9. test that separates immunoglobulins: immuno _____

10. antibody used in immunotherapy; produced in a laboratory to attack antigens and destroy cells:

  mono _____ antibody

14

J Circle the correct term(s) in boldface to complete each sentence.

1. Mr. Blake had been HIV-positive for 5 years before he developed (*Pneumocystis* pneumonia, thymoma, multiple myeloma) and was diagnosed with (**Hodgkin lymphoma, non-Hodgkin lymphoma, AIDS**).

2. Mary developed rhinitis, rhinorrhea, and red eyes every spring when pollen was prevalent. She consulted her doctor about her severe (**hypersplenism, allergies, lymphadenitis**).

3. Paul felt some marble-sized lumps in his left groin. His doctor told him that he had an infection in his foot and had developed secondary (**axillary, cervical, inguinal**) lymphadenopathy.

4. Mr. Jones was referred to a dermatologist and an oncologist when his primary physician noticed purple spots on his arms and legs. Because he had AIDS, his physician was concerned about the possibility of (**Kaposi sarcoma, splenomegaly, thrombocytopenic purpura**).

5. Fifteen-year-old Peter was allergic to peanuts. His allergy was so severe that he carried epinephrine with him at all times to prevent (**adaptive immunity, anaphylaxis, immunosuppression**) in case he came in contact with peanut butter at school.

6. When she was in her mid-20s, Rona was diagnosed with a lymph node malignancy known as (**sarcoidosis, Kaposi sarcoma, Hodgkin lymphoma**). Because the disease was primarily in her chest, her (**inguinal, mediastinal, axillary**) lymph nodes were irradiated [radiation therapy], and she was cured. When she developed lung cancer in her mid-40s, her oncologist told her she had a/an (**iatrogenic, hereditary, metastatic**) radiation induced secondary tumor.

7. Mary has suffered from hay fever, asthma, and chronic dermatitis ever since she was a young child. She has been particularly bothered by the severely pruritic [itching], erythematous [reddish] patches on her hands. Her dermatologist gave her topical steroids for her (**toxic, atopic, opportunistic**) dermatitis and told her to avoid soaps, cosmetics, and irritating chemicals.

8. Bernie noticed pain in his pelvis, spine, and ribs and was evaluated by his physician. Blood tests showed high levels of plasma cells and abnormal globulins. Increased numbers of plasma cells were revealed on (**chest x-ray, stem cell transplantation, bone marrow biopsy**). Radiologic studies showed bone loss. The physician's diagnosis was multiple (**sclerosis, thymoma, myeloma**).

9. AIDS is caused by (**herpes simplex virus, monoclonal antibodies, human immunodeficiency virus**). Lymphocytes called (**CD4+ cells, suppressor cells, B cells**) are destroyed, leading to (**anaphylaxis, atopy, opportunistic infections**).

10. Drugs used to treat AIDS are (**immunosuppressants, protease inhibitors, interferons**). Other anti-AIDS drugs are (**reverse transcriptase inhibitors, monoclonal antibodies, immunoglobulins**).

ANSWERS TO EXERCISES

A

1. lymph node	4. adenoids	7. right lymphatic duct
2. thoracic duct	5. thymus gland	8. interstitial fluid
3. spleen	6. lymph capillaries	

B

1. groin region	4. space between the lungs in the chest	5 near the aorta in the lumbar area of the body
2. armpit region		
3. neck (of the body) region		6. intestinal region

14

C

1. CD8+ T cells
2. T cells
3. helper T cells
4. B cells
5. humoral immunity
6. adaptive immunity

D

1. plasma cell
2. macrophage
3. helper T cell
4. suppressor T cell
5. complement system
6. dendritic cell

E

1. A
2. C
3. B
4. D
5. G
6. F
7. E

F

1. splenectomy
2. splenomegaly
3. lymphopoiesis
4. thymoma
5. lymphadenitis
6. lymphocytopenia
7. toxic
8. lymphadenopathy

G

1. hypersplenism
2. anaphylaxis
3. allergen
4. AIDS
5. thymectomy
6. Hodgkin lymphoma
7. lymphoid organs
8. lymphedema

H

1. Kaposi sarcoma
2. HIV
3. CD4+ T cells
4. opportunistic infections
5. viral load test
6. wasting syndrome
7. reverse transcriptase inhibitor
8. protease inhibitor
9. HAART (highly active antiretroviral therapy)
10. ELISA (enzyme-linked immunosorbent assay)

I

1. autoimmune
2. atopy
3. non-Hodgkin lymphoma
4. interstitial
5. lymphopoiesis
6. lymphedema
7. anaphylaxis
8. vaccination
9. immunoelectrophoresis
10. monoclonal

J

1. *Pneumocystis* pneumonia; AIDS
2. allergies
3. inguinal
4. Kaposi sarcoma
5. anaphylaxis
6. Hodgkin lymphoma; mediastinal; iatrogenic
7. atopic
8. bone marrow biopsy; myeloma
9. human immunodeficiency virus; CD4+ cells; opportunistic infections
10. protease inhibitors; reverse transcriptase inhibitors

Answers to Practical Applications

Short Clinical Cases

1. acute systemic anaphylaxis—Allergic reactions occur when already sensitized people are reexposed to the same allergen. The first exposure generates allergen-specific antibodies and/or T cells, and reexposure to the same allergen can produce a severe allergic reaction or anaphylaxis.

2. acquired immunodeficiency syndrome
3. multiple myeloma

PRONUNCIATION OF TERMS

To test your understanding of the terminology in this chapter, write the meaning of each term in the space provided. In addition, you may wish to cover the terms and write them by looking at your definitions. Make sure your spelling is correct. The page number after each term indicates where it is defined or used in the book, so you can easily check your responses. You will find complete definitions for all of these terms and their audio pronunciations on the Evolve website.

Pronunciation Guide

ā as in āpe	ă as in ăpple
ē as in ēven	ĕ as in ĕvery
ī as in īce	ĭ as in ĭnterest
ō as in ōpen	ŏ as in pŏt
ū as in ūnit	ŭ as in ŭnder

Vocabulary and Terminology

TERM	PRONUNCIATION	MEANING
adaptive immunity (555)	ă-DĀP-tĭv ĭ-MŪ-nĭ-tē	_____
adenoids (555)	ĂD-ĕ-noydz	_____
anaphylaxis (559)	ăn-ă-fă-LĂK-sĭs	_____
antibody (555)	ĂN-tĭ-bŏ-dē	_____
antigen (555)	ĂN-tĭ-jĕn	_____
asplenia (559)	ā-SPLĒN-ē-ă	_____
autoimmune disease (558)	aw-tō-ĭ-MŪN dĭ-ZĒZ	_____
axillary nodes (556)	AKS-ĭ-lăr-ē nōdz	_____
B cell (556)	B sĕl	_____
cell-mediated immunity (556)	sĕl mē-dē-Ā-tĕd ĭ-MŪN-ĭ-tē	_____
cervical nodes (556)	SĔR-vĭ-kl nōdz	_____
complement system (556)	CŎM-plĕ-mĕnt SĭS-tĕm	_____
cytokines (556)	SĪ-tō-kĭnz	_____
cytotoxic T cell (556)	sī-tō-TŎK-sĭk T sĕl	_____
dendritic cell (556)	dĕn-DRĬ-tĭk sĕl	_____
helper T cell (556)	HĔL-pĕr T sĕl	_____
humoral immunity (556)	HŪ-mĕr-ăl ĭm-MŪN-ĭ-tē	_____
hypersplenism (559)	hī-pĕr-SPLĔN-ĭzm	_____
immunity (556)	ĭm-MŪN-ĭ-tē	_____
immunoglobulins (556)	ĭm-ū-nō-GLŎB-ū-lĭnz	_____
immunosuppression (558)	ĭm-ū-nō-sŭ-PRĔ-shŭn	_____
immunotherapy (556)	ĭ-mū-nō-THĔR-ă-pē	_____

14

TERM	PRONUNCIATION	MEANING
inguinal node (556)	ĬNG-gwĭ-năl nōd	
interferons (556)	ĭn-tĕr-FĒR-ŏnz	
interleukins (556)	ĭn-tĕr-LOO-kĭnz	
interstitial fluid (556)	ĭn-tĕr-STĬSH-ăl FLOO-ĭd	
lymph (556)	lĭmf	
lymphadenitis (559)	lĭm-făh-dĕ-NĪ-tĭs	
lymphadenopathy (559)	lĭm-făd-ĕ-NŎP-ăh-thē	
lymph capillaries (556)	lĭmf KĂP-ĭ-lă-rēz	
lymphedema (558)	lĭmf-ĕ-DĒ-mă	
lymph node (556)	lĭmf nōd	
lymphocytes (548)	LĬM-fō-sītz	
lymphocytosis (558)	lĭm-fō-sī-TŌ-sĭs	
lymphocytopenia (558)	lĭm-fō-sī-tō-PĒ-nē-ă	
lymphoid organs (556)	LĬM-foid ŎR-gănz	
lymphopoiesis (558)	lĭm-fō-poy-Ē-sĭs	
lymph vessel (556)	lĭmf VĚS-ĕl	
macrophage (556)	MĂK-rō-fāj	
mediastinal nodes (556)	mē-dē-ăs-TĪ-năl nōdz	
mesenteric nodes (557)	mĕs-ĕn-TĔR-ĭk nōdz	
monoclonal antibody (557)	mŏn-ō-KLŌ-năl ĂN-tĭ-bŏd-ē	
natural immunity (557)	NĂ-tū-răl ĭm-MŪ-nĭ-tē	
paraaortic nodes (557)	pă-ră-ā-ŎR-tĭk nōdz	
plasma cell (557)	PLĂZ-mă sĕl	
right lymphatic duct (557)	rīt lĭm-FĂ-tĭk dŭkt	
spleen (557)	splēn	
splenectomy (559)	splĕ-NĚK-tō-mē	
splenomegaly (559)	splĕ-nō-MĚG-ă-lē	
suppressor T cell (557)	sŭ-PRĚ-sŏr T sĕl	
T cell (557)	T sĕl	
thoracic duct (557)	thō-RĂ-sĭk dŭkt	
thymectomy (559)	thī-MĚK-tō-mē	
thymus gland (557)	THĪ-mŭs glănd	
tolerance (557)	TŎL-ĕr-ăntz	
tonsils (557)	TŎN-sĭlz	

14

TERM	PRONUNCIATION	MEANING
toxic (559)	TŎK-sĭk	_____
toxin (557)	TŎK-sĭn	_____
vaccination (557)	văk-sĭ-NĀ-shŭn	_____
vaccine (557)	văk-SĒN	_____

Pathology and Laboratory Tests

TERM	PRONUNCIATION	MEANING
acquired immunodeficiency syndrome (559)	ă-KWĪRD ĭm-ū-nō-dĕ-FĬSH-ĕn-sē SĬN-drōm	_____
allergen (564)	ĂL-ĕr-jĕn	_____
allergy (562)	ĂL-ĕr-jē	_____
atopy (564)	ĂT-ō-pē	_____
CD4+ cell (564)	CD4 PŎS-ĭ-tĭv sĕl	_____
ELISA (564)	ĕ-LĪ-ză	_____
Hodgkin lymphoma (564)	HŎJ-kĭn lĭm-FŌ-mă	_____
human immunodeficiency virus (564)	HŪ-măn ĭm-ū-nō-dĕ-FĬSH-ĕn-sē VĪ-rŭs	_____
immunoelectrophoresis (565)	ĭm-ū-nō-ē-lĕk-trō-phŏr-Ē-sĭs	_____
Kaposi sarcoma (564)	KĂ-pō-sē (or kă-PŌS-sē) săr-KŌ-mă	_____
lymphoma (562)	lĭm-FŌ-mă	_____
multiple myeloma (563)	MŬLT-ĭ-pl mī-ĕ-LŌ-mă	_____
non-Hodgkin lymphoma (564)	nŏn-HŎJ-kĭn lĭm-FŌ-ma	_____
opportunistic infections (564)	ŏp-pŏr-tū-NĬS-tĭk ĭn-FĔK-shŭnz	_____
protease inhibitors (564)	PRŌ-tē-ās ĭn-HĬB-ĭ-tŏrz	_____
reverse transcriptase inhibitors (564)	rē-VĔRS trăns-SCRĬPT-āz ĭn-HĬB-ĭ-tŏrz	_____
severe combined immunodeficiency disease (559)	sĕ-VĔR kŏm-BĪND ĭm-ū-nō-dĕ-FĬSH-ĕn-sē dĭ-ZĒZ	_____
thymoma (563)	thī-MŌ-mă	_____
viral load test (565)	vī-răl lōd tĕst	_____
wasting syndrome (564)	WĀST-ĭng SĬN-drōm	_____
Western blot (564)	WĔS-tĕrn blŏt	_____

14

REVIEW SHEET

Write the meaning of the word parts in the spaces provided. Check your answers with the information in the chapter or in the *Glossary (Medical Word Parts—English)* at the end of the book.

Combining Forms

COMBINING FORM	MEANING	COMBINING FORM	MEANING
axill/o	_____	lymphaden/o	_____
cervic/o	_____	splen/o	_____
immun/o	_____	thym/o	_____
inguin/o	_____	tox/o	_____
lymph/o	_____		

Suffixes

SUFFIX	MEANING	SUFFIX	MEANING
-cytosis	_____	-pathy	_____
-edema	_____	-penia	_____
-globulin	_____	-phylaxis	_____
-megaly	_____	-poiesis	_____
-oid	_____	-stitial	_____
-oma	_____	-suppression	_____

Prefixes

PREFIX	MEANING	PREFIX	MEANING
ana-	_____	inter-	_____
auto-	_____	retro-	_____
hyper-	_____		

evolve *Please refer to the Evolve website for additional exercises and images related to this chapter.*

CHAPTER
15

Musculoskeletal System

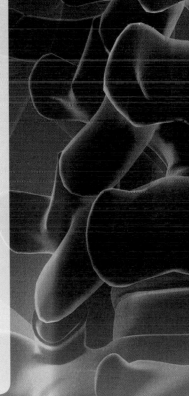

Chapter Sections:

CHAPTER GOALS

- Define terms relating to the structure and function of bones, joints, and muscles.
- Describe the process of bone formation and growth.
- Locate and name the major bones of the body.
- Analyze the combining forms, prefixes, and suffixes used to describe bones, joints, and muscles.
- Explain various musculoskeletal disease conditions and terms related to bone fractures.
- Describe important laboratory tests and clinical procedures relating to the musculoskeletal system, and recognize relevant abbreviations.
- Apply your new knowledge to understanding medical terms in their proper contexts, such as medical reports and records.

INTRODUCTION

The musculoskeletal system includes the bones, muscles, and joints. All have important functions in the body.

Bones provide the framework on which the body is constructed and protect and support internal organs. Bones also assist the body in movement, because they serve as a point of attachment for muscles. The inner core of bones is composed of hematopoietic tissue (red bone marrow, which manufactures blood cells), whereas outer parts of bone are storage areas for minerals necessary for growth, such as calcium and phosphorus.

Joints are the places at which bones come together. Several different types of joints are found within the body. The type of joint found in any specific location is determined by the need for greater or lesser flexibility of movement.

Muscles, whether attached to bones or to internal organs and blood vessels, are responsible for movement. Internal movement involves the contraction and relaxation of muscles found in viscera, and external movement is accomplished by the contraction and relaxation of muscles that are attached to the bones. **Tendons** are connective tissue that bind muscles to bones, while **ligaments** bind bones to other bones.

Orthopedists are physicians who treat (surgically and medically) bone, joint, and muscle conditions. Originally, orthopedics was a branch of medicine correcting deformities in children (**orth/o** means straight, **ped/o** means child). **Rheumatologists** are physicians (nonsurgical) who specialize primarily in joint problems, such as arthritis; in this context, **rheumat/o,** meaning watery flow, refers to joint fluid. **Physiatrists** are medical doctors whose focus is on rehabilitation after injury or illness to muscles, bones, and nerves.

Both a **medical doctor (MD)** and an **osteopathic physician (DO)** can specialize in orthopedics or rheumatology. MD and DO medical education programs are similar, and both kinds of physicians perform surgery as well as prescribe medication. An osteopath has added training in the musculoskeletal system, with an emphasis on body mechanics to promote good health. A **chiropractor** (**chir/o** means hand) is not a physician but has extensive and specialized training in using physical means to manipulate the spinal column, joints, and soft tissues. Chiropractic medicine considers that disease is related to pressure on nerves by spinal misalignment.

A **physical therapist** is a master's or doctoral degree–prepared health care professional who develops a treatment plan based on a physician's diagnosis. The goals of physical therapy (PT) are to restore function, improve mobility, and relieve pain. **Athletic trainers** are health care professionals who, working with a physician, provide therapeutic intervention and rehabilitation of injuries and medical conditions. Training includes a bachelor's or master's degree from an accredited school. Passing a certification examination also is required to work in this field.

BONES

FORMATION AND STRUCTURE

Formation

Bones are complete organs composed chiefly of connective tissue called **osseous** (bony) **tissue,** plus a rich supply of blood vessels and nerves. Osseous tissue consists of a combination of **osteocytes** (bone cells), dense connective tissue strands known as **collagen,** and intercellular **calcium salts.**

During fetal development, the bones of the fetus are composed of **cartilage,** which resembles osseous tissue but is more flexible and less dense because of a lack of calcium salts in its intercellular spaces. As the embryo develops, the process of depositing calcium salts in the soft, cartilaginous tissue occurs and continues throughout the life of the individual after birth. The gradual replacement of cartilage and its intercellular substance by immature bone cells and calcium deposits is **ossification** (bone formation).

Osteoblasts are the immature osteocytes that produce the bony tissue that replaces cartilage during ossification. **Osteoclasts** (**-clast** is from the Greek word meaning to break) are large cells that function to reabsorb, or digest, bony tissue. Osteoclasts (also called **bone phagocytes**) digest bone tissue from the inner sides of bones thus enlarging the inner bone cavity so that the bone does not become overly thick and heavy. When a bone breaks, osteoblasts lay down the mineral bone matter (calcium salts) and osteoclasts remove excess bone debris (smooth out the bone).

Osteoblasts and osteoclasts work together in all bones throughout life, tearing down (osteoclasts) and rebuilding (osteoblasts) bony tissue. This allows bone to respond to mechanical stresses placed on it and thus enables it to be a living tissue, constantly rebuilding and renewing itself.

The formation of bone depends largely on a proper supply of **calcium** and **phosphorus** to the bone tissue. These minerals must be taken into the body along with a sufficient amount of vitamin D. Vitamin D helps calcium to pass through the lining of the small intestine and into the bloodstream. Once calcium and phosphorus are in the bones, osteoblastic activity produces an enzyme that forms calcium phosphate, a substance that gives bone its characteristic hard quality. It is the major calcium salt.

Not only are calcium and phosphorus part of the hard structure of bone tissue, but calcium also is stored elsewhere in bones, and small quantities are present in the blood. If the proper amount of calcium is lacking in the blood, nerve fibers are unable to transmit impulses effectively to muscles, the heart muscle becomes weak, and muscles attached to bones undergo spasms.

The necessary level of calcium in the blood is maintained by the parathyroid gland, which secretes a hormone that signals the release of calcium from bone storage. An excess of the hormone (caused by tumor or another pathologic process) will raise blood calcium at the expense of the bones, which become weakened by the loss of calcium.

Structure

There are 206 bones of various types in the body. **Long bones** are found in the thigh, lower leg, and upper and lower arm. These bones are very strong, are broad at the ends where they join with other bones, and have large surface areas for muscle attachment.

Short bones are found in the wrist and ankle and are small with irregular shapes. **Flat bones** are found covering soft body parts. These bones are the skull, shoulder blades, ribs, and pelvic bones. **Sesamoid bones** are small, rounded bones (resembling a sesame seed in shape). They are found near joints, and they increase the efficiency of muscles near a particular joint. The kneecap is the largest example of a sesamoid bone.

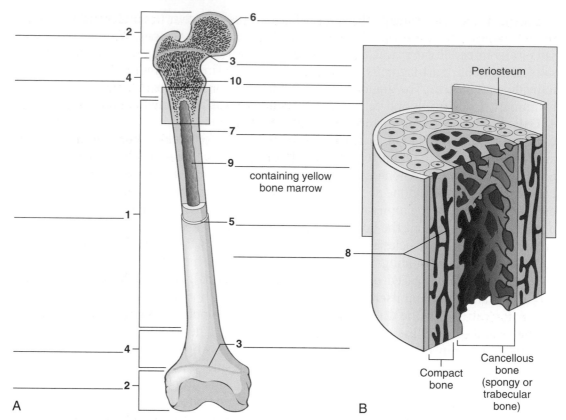

FIGURE 15-1 A, Divisions of a long bone and interior bone structure. B, Composition of compact (cortical) bone.

15

Figure 15-1A shows the anatomic divisions of a long bone such as the thigh bone or upper arm bone. Label the figure as you read the following.

The shaft, or middle region, of a long bone is called the **diaphysis** [1]. Each end of a long bone is called an **epiphysis** [2]. The **epiphyseal line** or **plate** [3] represents an area of cartilage tissue that is constantly being replaced by new bone tissue as the bone grows; it also is commonly known as the growth plate. Cartilage cells at the edges of the epiphyseal plate form new bone, which is responsible for lengthening bones during childhood and adolescence. The plate calcifies and disappears when the bone has achieved its full growth. The **metaphysis** [4] is the flared portion of the bone; it lies between the epiphysis and the diaphysis. It is adjacent to the epiphyseal plate.

The **periosteum** [5] is a strong, fibrous, vascular membrane that covers the surface of long bones, except at the ends of the epiphyses. It has an extensive nerve supply as well. Bones other than long bones are also covered by the periosteum.

The ends of long bones and the surface of any bone that meets another bone to form a joint are covered with **articular cartilage** [6]. When two bones come together to form a joint, the bones themselves do not touch precisely. The articular cartilage that caps the end of one bone comes into contact with that of the other bone. Articular cartilage is a very smooth, strong, and slick tissue. It cushions the joint and allows it to move smoothly and efficiently. Unlike the cartilage of the epiphyseal plate, which disappears when a bone achieves its full growth, articular cartilage is present throughout life.

Compact (cortical) bone [7] is a layer of hard, dense bone that lies under the periosteum in all bones and is located chiefly around the diaphysis of long bones. Within the compact bone is a system of small canals containing blood vessels that bring oxygen and nutrients to the bone and remove waste products such as carbon dioxide. Figure 15-1B shows these channels, called **haversian canals** [8], in the compact bone. Compact bone is tunneled out in the central shaft of the long bones by a **medullary cavity** [9] that contains **yellow bone marrow.** Yellow marrow is composed chiefly of fat cells.

Cancellous bone [10], sometimes called **spongy** or **trabecular bone,** is much more porous and less dense than compact bone. The mineral matter in it is laid down in a series of separated bony fibers that make up a spongy latticework. These interwoven fibers, called **trabeculae,** are found largely in the epiphyses and metaphyses of long bones and in the middle portion of most other bones of the body as well. Spaces in cancellous bone contain **red bone marrow.** The red marrow consists of immature and mature blood cells in various stages of development. **Hematopoiesis** (-poiesis means formation) is the production of all types of blood cells in the bone marrow.

In an adult, the ribs, pelvic bone, sternum (breastbone), and vertebrae, as well as the epiphyses of long bones, contain red bone marrow within cancellous tissue. Red marrow in the medullary cavity of long bones is plentiful in young children but decreases through the years and is replaced by yellow marrow.

PROCESSES AND DEPRESSIONS IN BONES

Bone processes are enlarged areas that extend out from bones to serve as attachments for muscles, tendons, and ligaments. Bone depressions are openings or hollow regions serving as connections between bones, or passageways for blood vessels and nerves. Table 15-1 lists various processes and depressions for your reference.

TABLE 15-1	PROCESSES AND DEPRESSIONS IN BONES

PROCESS (Refer to Figure 15-2)	DESCRIPTION	
1. **Bone head**	Rounded end of a bone	
2. **Condyle**	Rounded knuckle-like process	
3. **Epicondyle**	Small rounded process above the condyle	
4. **Trochanters**	Large and small processes for tendon attachments	
5. **Tuberosity (tubercle)**	Small round elevation where tendons and muscles attach	

DEPRESSION	DESCRIPTION	EXAMPLE
Fissure	Narrow groove or slit-like opening	Orbital (eye socket) fissure (Figure 15-5)
Foramen	Opening for blood vessels and nerves	Foramen magnum of the skull (Figure 15-4)
Fossa	Shallow cavity in or on a bone	Olecranon (elbow) fossa on humerus (Figure 15-2)
Sinus	Hollow cavity within bone	Sinuses of the skull (Figure 15-6)

15

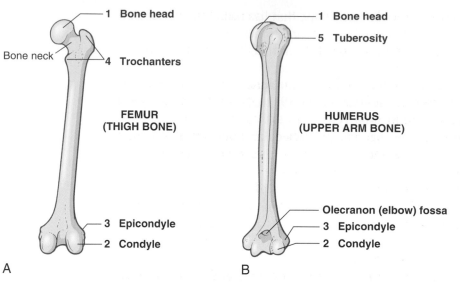

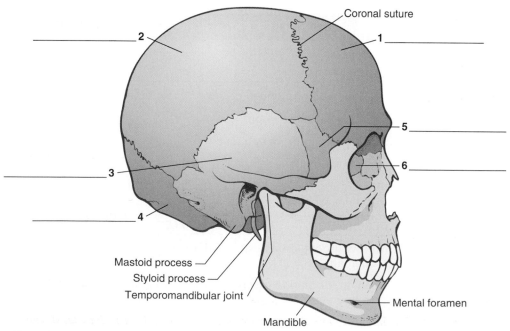

FIGURE 15-2   **Bone processes on the femur** (thigh bone) **(A)** and **humerus** (upper arm bone) **(B)**. The **bone neck** separates the bone head from the rest of the bone. A **fossa** is a shallow depression or cavity in a bone. The fossa on the humerus is a space for the olecranon process on the lower arm bone (ulna) when the elbow is extended.

CRANIAL BONES

The bones of the skull, or cranium, protect the brain and structures related to it, such as the sense organs. Muscles for controlling head movements and chewing motions are connected to the cranial bones. The cranial bones join each other at joints called **sutures.**

The cranial bones of a newborn child are not completely joined. There are gaps of unossified tissue in the skull at birth. These are called soft spots, or **fontanelles** ("little fountains"). The pulse of blood vessels can be felt (palpated) under the skin in those areas.

Figure 15-3 illustrates the bones of the cranium. Label them as you read the following descriptions:

FIGURE 15-3   **Cranial bones,** lateral view. The **mental** (ment/o = chin) **foramen** is the opening in the mandible that allows blood vessels and nerves to enter and leave. The **coronal suture** is the connection across the skull between the two parietal bones and the frontal bone.

Frontal bone [1]—forms the forehead and the roof of the bony sockets that contain the eyes.

Parietal bone [2]—the two bones (one on each side of the skull) that form the roof and upper part of the sides of the cranium.

Temporal bone [3]—the two bones that form the lower sides and base of the cranium. Each bone encloses an ear and contains a fossa for joining with the mandible (lower jawbone). The **temporomandibular joint (TMJ)** is the area of connection between the temporal and mandibular bones. The **mastoid process** is a round (**mast/o** means breast) process of the temporal bone behind the ear. The **styloid process** (**styl/o** means pole or stake) projects downward from the temporal bone.

Occipital bone [4]—forms the back and base of the skull and joins the parietal and temporal bones, forming a suture. The inferior portion of the occipital bone has an opening called the **foramen magnum** through which the spinal cord passes (see Figure 15-4).

Sphenoid bone [5]—the bat-shaped bone that extends behind the eyes and forms part of the base of the skull. Because it joins with the frontal, occipital, and ethmoid bones, it serves as an anchor to hold those skull bones together (**sphen/o** means wedge). The **sella turcica** ("Turkish saddle") is a depression in the sphenoid bone in which the pituitary gland is located (see Figure 15-4).

Ethmoid bone [6]—the thin, delicate bone that supports the nasal cavity and forms part of the sockets of the eyes. It is composed primarily of spongy, cancellous bone, which contains numerous small holes (**ethm/o** means sieve).

Study Figure 15-4, which shows these cranial bones as viewed from above downward, toward the floor of the cranial cavity.

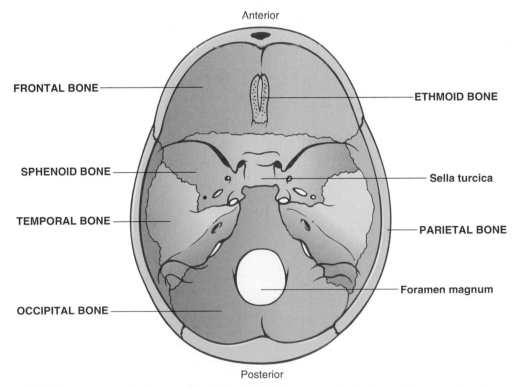

FIGURE 15-4   Cranial bones, viewed from above downward, to the floor of the cranial cavity.

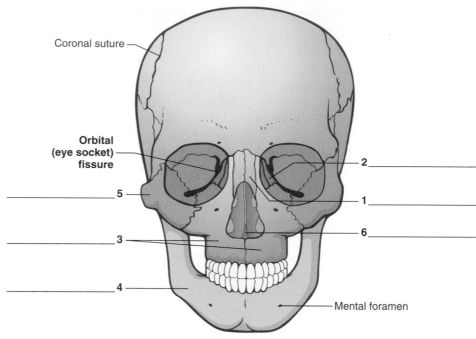

Coronal suture

Orbital
(eye socket)
fissure

5

3

4

2

1

6

Mental foramen

FIGURE 15-5   Facial bones.

FACIAL BONES

All of the facial bones except one are joined together by sutures, so they are immovable. The mandible (lower jawbone) is the only facial bone capable of movement. This ability is necessary for activities such as mastication (chewing) and speaking.

Figure 15-5 shows the facial bones; label it as you read the following descriptions of the facial bones:

Nasal bones [1]—the two slender bones that support the bridge of the nose (**nas/o** means nose). They join with the frontal bone superiorly and form part of the nasal septum.

Lacrimal bones [2]—the two small, thin bones located at the corner of each eye. The lacrimal (**lacrim/o** means tear) bones contain fossae for the lacrimal gland (tear gland) and canals for the passage of the lacrimal duct.

Maxillary bones [3]—the two large bones that compose the massive upper jawbones **(maxillae).** They are joined by a suture in the median plane. If the two bones do not come together normally before birth, the condition known as **cleft palate** results.

Mandibular bone [4]—the lower jawbone **(mandible).** Both the maxilla and the mandible contain the sockets called **alveoli** in which the teeth are embedded. The mandible joins the skull at the region of the temporal bone, forming the TMJ on either side of the skull.

Zygomatic bones [5]—the two bones, one on each side of the face, that form the high portion of the cheek.

Vomer [6]—the thin, single, flat bone that forms the lower portion of the nasal septum.

Sinuses, or air cavities, are located in specific places within the cranial and facial bones to lighten the skull and warm and moisten air as it passes through. Figure 15-6 shows the sinuses of the skull.

Table 15-2 reviews the cranial and facial bones with the location of each bone.

15

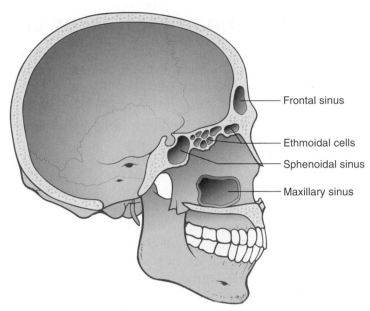

FIGURE 15-6 Sinuses of the skull.

TABLE 15-2	CRANIAL AND FACIAL BONES
CRANIAL BONES	**LOCATION**
Ethmoid bone	Supports nasal cavity and eye sockets
Frontal bone	Forehead; part of eye sockets
Occipital bone	Back and base of skull
Parietal bones	Top and sides of skull
Sphenoid bone	Base of skull and behind eyes (bat-shaped bone)
Temporal bones	Lower sides and back of skull
FACIAL BONES	**LOCATION**
Lacrimal bones	Corners of each eye
Mandible	Lower jawbone
Maxillae	Upper jawbones
Nasal bones	Bridge and septum of nose
Vomer	Nasal septum (thin, flat bone)
Zygomatic bones	Cheek bones

VERTEBRAL COLUMN AND STRUCTURE OF VERTEBRAE

The **vertebral (spinal) column** is composed of 26 bone segments, called **vertebrae,** that are arranged in five divisions from the base of the skull to the tailbone. The bones are separated by pads of cartilage called **intervertebral disks** (discs).

Figure 15-7A illustrates the general structure of a vertebra. Although the individual vertebrae in the separate regions of the spinal column are all slightly different in structure, they do have several parts in common.

A vertebra is composed of an inner, thick, round anterior portion called the **vertebral body** [1]. Between the body of one vertebra and the body of the vertebra lying beneath or above is an **intervertebral disk (disc).** This is a pad of cartilage that provides flexibility and absorbs shocks to the vertebral column (see Figure 15-7B). A spinal disk herniation occurs when a tear in a disk causes a portion of the disk to bulge out into the neural canal.

The posterior portion of a vertebra (vertebral arch) consists of a single **spinous process** [2], a **transverse process** [3], one on each side of the spinous process, and a bar-like **lamina** [4] between each transverse process and the spinous process. The **neural** or **spinal canal** [5] is the space between the vertebral body and the vertebral arch through which the spinal cord passes. Figure 15-7B shows a lateral view of several vertebrae. Note the location of the spinal cord running through the neural canal.

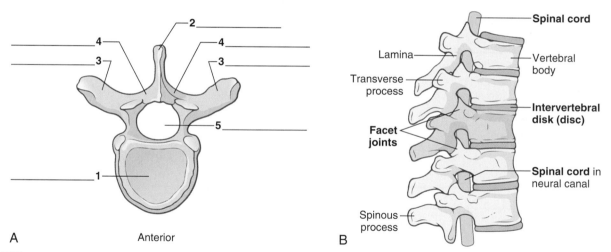

FIGURE 15-7 **A, General structure of a vertebra,** viewed from above. **B, Series of vertebrae,** lateral view, to show the position of the spinal cord running through the spinal canal, behind the vertebral bodies and intervertebral disks. **Facet** (FĂ-set) **joints** connect the vertebrae to each other. They are important in guiding and limiting the movement of the spinal column. When facet joints become inflamed and arthritic, they lead to narrowing of the neural canal and **spinal stenosis**.

Figure 15-8 illustrates the divisions of the vertebral column: cervical, thoracic, lumbar, sacrum, and coccyx.

The first seven bones of the vertebral column, forming the bony aspect of the neck, are the **cervical (C1 to C7) vertebrae.** These vertebrae do not articulate (join) with the ribs.

The second set of 12 vertebrae is known as the **thoracic (T1 to T12) vertebrae.** These vertebrae articulate with the 12 pairs of ribs.

The third set of five vertebral bones is the **lumbar (L1 to L5) vertebrae.** They are the strongest and largest of the vertebrae. Like the cervical vertebrae, these bones do not articulate with the ribs.

The **sacral vertebrae (sacrum)** are five separate bones that fuse in a young child. In an adult, the sacrum is a slightly curved, triangularly shaped bone.

The **coccyx** is the tailbone, and it, too, is a fused bone, having been formed from four small coccygeal bones.

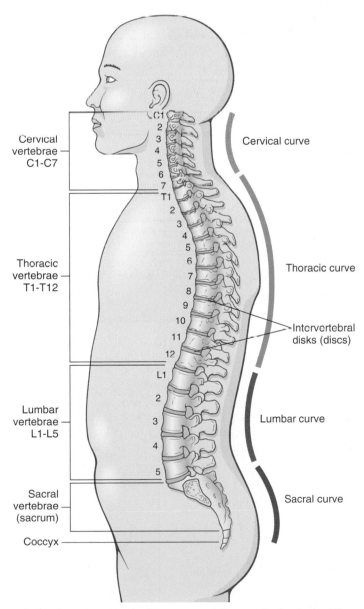

FIGURE 15-8   Vertebral column. Notice the four curves of the vertebral column. The sacral and thoracic curvatures are present at birth. The cervical curvature develops when the infant holds the head erect. The lumbar curvature develops as the infant begins to stand and walk.

BONES OF THE THORAX, PELVIS, AND EXTREMITIES

Label Figure 15-9 as you read the following descriptions of the bones of the thorax (chest cavity), pelvis (hip bone), and extremities (arms, hands, legs, and feet):

Bones of the Thorax

Clavicle [1]—collar bone; a slender bone, positioned ventrally, one on each side, connecting the breastbone (sternum) to each shoulder blade (scapula).

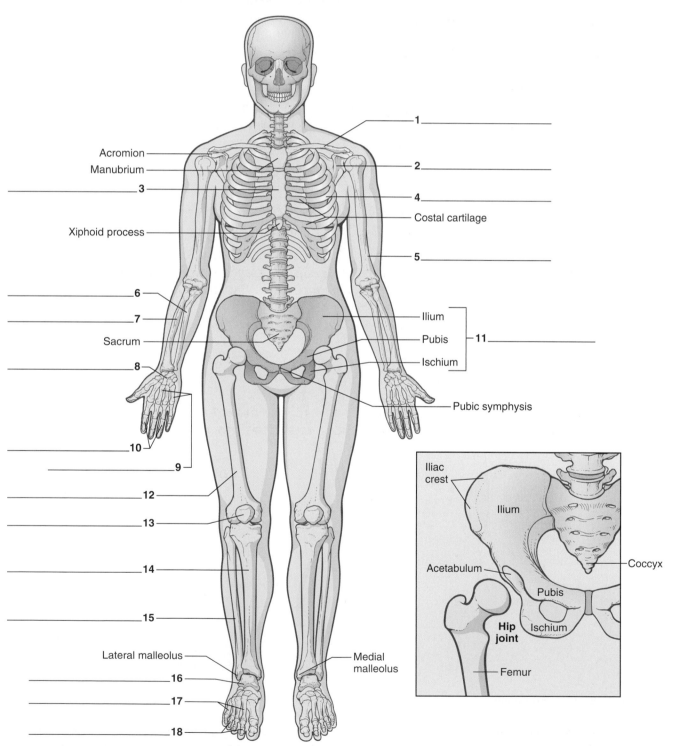

FIGURE 15-9   Bones of the thorax, pelvis, and extremities.

Scapula [2] (*plural*: **scapulae**)—shoulder blade; one of two flat, triangular bones on each dorsal side of the thorax. The extension of the scapula that joins with the clavicle to form a joint above the shoulder is called the **acromion** (**acr/o** means extremity, **om/o** means shoulder). The joint formed by these two bones is known as the **acromioclavicular (AC) joint**. Figure 15-10A shows a posterior view of the scapula. Figure 15-10B shows the anterior acromioclavicular joint.

Sternum [3]—breastbone; a flat bone extending ventrally down the midline of the chest. The upper part of the sternum articulates on the sides with the clavicle and ribs, and the lower, narrower portion is attached to the ribs, diaphragm, and abdominal muscles. The lowest portion of the sternum is the **xiphoid process** (**xiph/o** means sword). The uppermost portion is the **manubrium** (from a Latin term meaning handle).

Ribs [4]—There are 12 pairs of ribs. The first 7 pairs join the sternum anteriorly through cartilaginous attachments called **costal cartilages.** Ribs 1 to 7 are called **true ribs.** They join with the sternum anteriorly and with the vertebral column posteriorly. Ribs 8 to 10 are called **false ribs.** They join with the vertebral column posteriorly but join the 7th rib anteriorly instead of attaching to the sternum. Ribs 11 and 12 are the **floating ribs** because they are completely free at their anterior ends. Figure 15-10A shows a posterior view of the rib cage.

Bones of the Arm and Hand

The bones of the arm and hand are described with the subject in the anatomic position—standing, with the arms held at the sides and the palms forward.

Humerus [5]—upper arm bone; the large head of the humerus is rounded and joins with the glenoid fossa of the scapula to form the shoulder or glenohumeral joint (see Figure 15-10A). A rim of fibrocartilage, called a **labrum,** allows the humerus to move in the glenoid fossa (see Figure 15-10B). The **rotator cuff** is a group of muscles and tendons that surround the shoulder joint. See ***In Person: Rotator Cuff Tear,*** page 624.

Ulna [6]—medial lower arm (forearm) bone; the proximal bony process of the ulna at the elbow is called the **olecranon** (elbow bone). The olecranon is the bony point formed when the elbow is bent. See Figure 15-31 on page 615.

Radius [7]—lateral lower arm (forearm) bone (in line with the thumb).

Carpals [8]—wrist bones; there are two rows of four bones in the wrist.

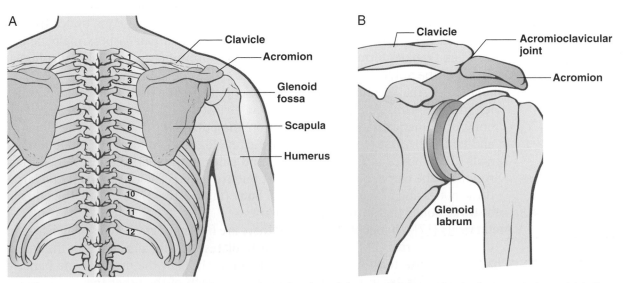

A, Scapulae and rib cage, posterior view. — Clavicle, Acromion, Glenoid fossa, Scapula, Humerus

B — Clavicle, Acromioclavicular joint, Acromion, Glenoid labrum

FIGURE 15-10   A, Scapulae and rib cage, posterior view. The **glenoid fossa** is the depression in the scapula into which the humerus fits. **B,** The **labrum** is a rim of cartilage in the glenoid fossa that forms a suction cup for the end of the humerus to move in. A **labrum tear** can occur with a shoulder injury.

15

Metacarpals [9]—the five bones of the palm of the hand.

Phalanges [10] (*singular:* **phalanx**)—finger bones. Each finger (except the thumb) has three phalanges: a proximal, a middle, and a distal phalanx. The thumb has only two phalanges: a proximal and a distal phalanx.

Bones of the Pelvis

Pelvic girdle [11]—pelvis. This collection of bones supports the trunk of the body and articulates with the femur to form the hip joint. The adult pelvis is composed of three pairs of fused bones: the ilium, ischium, and pubis. The pelvis joins with the single, dorsally located sacrum.

Ilium—uppermost and largest portion of the pelvis. Dorsally, the two parts of the ilium do not meet. Rather, they join the sacrum on either side to form the sacroiliac joints. The connection between the iliac bones and the sacrum is very firm, and very little motion occurs at these joints. The superior part of the ilium is the **iliac crest.** It is filled with red bone marrow and serves as an attachment for abdominal wall muscles as well as strong muscles of the hip and buttocks.

Ischium—inferior or lower part of the pelvis. The ischium and the tendons and muscles attached to it are what you sit on.

Pubis—anterior part of the pelvis. The two pubic bones join by way of a cartilaginous disk. This is the **pubic symphysis.** Like sacroiliac joints, this area is quite rigid.

Pelvic cavity—region within the ring of bone formed by the pelvic girdle. The rectum, sigmoid colon, bladder, and female reproductive organs lie within the pelvic cavity and are protected by the rigid architecture of the pelvic girdle. See Chapter 2, page 57, for comparison of the male pelvis and the female pelvis.

Bones of the Leg and Foot

Femur [12]—thigh bone; this is the longest bone in the body. At its proximal end it has a rounded head that fits into a depression, or socket, in the pelvis. This socket is called the **acetabulum.** The acetabulum was named because of its resemblance to a rounded cup the Romans used for vinegar *(acetum).* The head of the femur and the acetabulum form a ball-and-socket joint otherwise known as the **hip joint.** See inset in Figure 15-9.

Patella [13]—kneecap; this is a small, flat bone that lies in front of the articulation between the femur and one of the lower leg bones called the tibia. It is a sesamoid bone surrounded by protective tendons and held in place by muscle attachments. Together with the femur and the tibia, it forms the knee joint.

Tibia [14]—larger of the two bones of the lower leg; the tibia runs under the skin in the front part of the leg. It joins with the femur and patella proximally, and at its distal end (ankle) forms a flare that is the bony prominence (medial **malleolus**) at the inside of the ankle. The tibia commonly is called the **shin bone.**

Fibula [15]—smaller of the two lower leg bones; this thin bone, well hidden under the leg muscles, runs parallel to the tibia. At its distal part, it forms a flare, which is the bony prominence (lateral **malleolus**) on the outside of the ankle. The tibia, fibula, and **talus** (the first of the tarsal bones) come together to form the **ankle joint.**

Tarsals [16]—bones of the middle and hind parts of the foot; these seven short bones resemble the carpal bones of the wrist but are larger. The **calcaneus** is the largest of these bones and also is called the **heel bone** (Figure 15-11). As noted, the **talus** is one of three bones that form the ankle joint.

Metatarsals [17]—bones of the midfoot; there are five metatarsal bones, which are similar to the metacarpals of the hand. Each articulates with the phalanges of the toes.

Phalanges of the toes [18]—bones of the forefoot; as in the digits of the hand, there are two phalanges in the big toe and three in each of the other toes.

Figure 15-11 illustrates the bones of the foot. Table 15-3 reviews bones and bone processes and their common names.

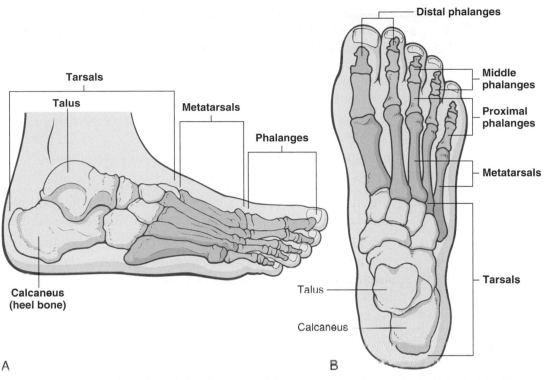

A

B

FIGURE 15-11 **A, Bones of the foot,** lateral view. **B, Bones of the foot,** as viewed from above. Note that the big or great toe has only a distal and proximal phalanx.

TABLE 15-3	BONES OR PROCESSES AND THEIR COMMON NAMES		
BONE OR PROCESS	**COMMON NAME**	**BONE OR PROCESS**	**COMMON NAME**
Acetabulum	Hip socket	Metacarpals	Hand bones
Calcaneus	Heel	Metatarsals	Midfoot bones
Carpals	Wrist bones	Olecranon	Elbow
Clavicle	Collar bone	Patella	Kneecap
Coccyx	Tailbone	Phalanges	Finger and toe bones
Cranium	Skull	Pubis	Anterior part of the pelvic bone
Femur	Thigh bone	Radius	Forearm bone—thumb side
Fibula	Smaller of the two lower leg bones	Scapula	Shoulder blade
Humerus	Upper arm bone	Sternum	Breastbone
Ilium	Upper part of pelvic bone	Tarsals	Hindfoot and midfoot bones
Ischium	Inferior or lower part of the pelvic bone	Tibia	Shin bone—larger of the two lower leg bones
Malleolus	Ankle	Ulna	Forearm bone—little finger side
Mandible	Lower jawbone	Vertebra	Backbone/spine
Maxilla	Upper jawbone		

VOCABULARY—BONES

This list reviews many of the new terms related to bones introduced in the text. Short definitions reinforce your understanding of the terms. Refer to the Pronunciation of Terms on page 643 for help with unfamiliar or difficult terms.

acetabulum	Rounded depression, or socket, in the pelvis that joins the femur (thigh bone), forming the hip joint.
acromion	Outward extension of the shoulder blade forming the point of the shoulder. It overlies the shoulder joint and articulates with the clavicle.
bone	Dense, hard connective tissue composing the skeleton. Examples are long bones (femur), short bones (carpals), flat bones (scapula), and sesamoid bones (patella).
bone depression	Opening or hollow region serving as a connection for bones, or passageways for blood vessels and nerves. Examples are **fissure**, **foramen**, **fossa**, and **sinus**.
bone process	Enlarged area that extends from bones as an attachment for muscles, tendons, and ligaments. Examples are **bone head**, **condyle**, **epicondyle**, **trochanter**, **tubercle**, and **tuberosity**.
calcium	One of the mineral constituents of bone. **Calcium phosphate** is the major calcium salt in bones.
cancellous bone	Spongy, porous, bone tissue in the inner part of a bone.
cartilage	Flexible, connective tissue; found in the immature skeleton, at the epiphyseal growth plate, and on joint surfaces (articular cartilage).
collagen	Dense, connective tissue protein strands found in bone and other tissues.
compact bone	Hard, dense bone tissue, usually found around the outer portion of bones.
cranial bones	Skull bones: **ethmoid, frontal, occipital, parietal, sphenoid,** and **temporal.**
diaphysis	Shaft, or mid-portion, of a long bone.
disk (disc)	Flat, round, plate-like structure. An intervertebral disk is a fibrocartilaginous structure between two vertebrae.
epiphyseal plate	Cartilaginous area at the ends of long bones where lengthwise growth takes place in the immature skeleton.
epiphysis	Each end of a long bone; the area beyond the epiphyseal plate.
facial bones	Bones of the face: **lacrimal, mandibular, maxillary, nasal, vomer,** and **zygomatic.**
fontanelle	Soft spot (incomplete bone formation) between the skull bones of an infant.
foramen magnum	Opening of the occipital bone through which the spinal cord passes.

15

haversian canals	Minute spaces filled with blood vessels; found in compact bone.
ligament	Fibrous connective tissue that binds bones to other bones. Ligaments are bands, or strands, located in and around joints.
malleolus	Round process on both sides of the ankle joint. The lateral malleolus is part of the fibula, and the medial malleolus is part of the tibia.
manubrium	Upper portion of the sternum; joins with the clavicle to form the sternoclavicular joint.
mastoid process	Rounded projection on the temporal bone behind the ear.
medullary cavity	Central, hollowed-out area in the shaft of a long bone.
metaphysis	Flared portion of a long bone, between the diaphysis (shaft) and the epiphyseal plate (in this term, meta- means between).
olecranon	Large process on the proximal end of the ulna at the elbow.
orthopedist	Medical doctor who specializes in bone, joint, and muscle conditions.
osseous tissue	Bone tissue.
ossification	Process of bone formation.
osteoblast	Bone cell that helps form bony tissue.
osteoclast	Bone cell that absorbs and removes unwanted bony tissue.
periosteum	Membrane surrounding bones; rich in blood vessels and nerve tissue.
phosphorus	Mineral substance found in bones in combination with calcium.
physiatrist	Medical doctor specializing in rehabilitation (physi/o means function).
pubic symphysis	Area of confluence (coming together) of the two pubic bones in the pelvis. They are joined (sym- = together, -physis – to grow) by a fibrocartilaginous disk.
red bone marrow	Found in cancellous bone; site of hematopoiesis.
ribs	Twelve pairs of curved bones that form the chest wall. True ribs are the first 7 pairs; false ribs are pairs 8 to 10; floating ribs are pairs 11 and 12.
sella turcica	Depression in the sphenoid bone where the pituitary gland is located.
sinus	Hollow air cavity within a bone.
styloid process	Pole-like process extending downward from the temporal bone on each side of the skull.
suture	Immovable joint between bones, such as the skull (cranium).
temporomandibular joint	Connection on either side of the head between the temporal bone of the skull and mandibular bone of the jaw.
tendon	Fibrous connective tissue that binds muscles to bones.
trabeculae	Supporting bundles of bony fibers in cancellous (spongy) bone.
vertebra	Individual segment of the spine composed of the vertebral body, vertebral arch, spinous process, transverse process, and lamina, enclosing the neural canal and spinal cord.
xiphoid process	Lower, narrow portion of the sternum.
yellow bone marrow	Fatty tissue found in the medullary cavity of most adult long bones.

15

TERMINOLOGY—BONES

The following word parts pertaining to bones are divided into two groups: general terms and terms related to specific bones. Write the meanings of the medical terms in the spaces provided.

General Terms

COMBINING FORMS

COMBINING FORM	MEANING	TERMINOLOGY	MEANING
calc/o, calci/o	calcium	hyper<u>calc</u>emia _____	
		de<u>calci</u>fication _____	
		de- means less or lack of; -fication is the process of making.	
kyph/o	humpback, hunchback (posterior curvature in the thoracic region)	<u>kyph</u>osis _____ *This term (from Greek meaning hill or mountain) indicates a hump on the back. The affected person's height is reduced, and kyphosis may lead to pressure on the spinal cord or peripheral nerves (Figure 15-12).*	
lamin/o	lamina (part of the vertebral arch)	<u>lamin</u>ectomy _____ *An operation often performed to relieve the symptoms of compression of the spinal cord or spinal nerve roots. It involves removal of the lamina and spinous process.*	
lord/o	curve, swayback (anterior curvature in the lumbar region)	<u>lord</u>osis _____ *The normal anterior curvature of the lumbar spine becomes exaggerated (see Figure 15-12). The word lordosis is derived from Greek, describing a person leaning backward in a lordly fashion.*	

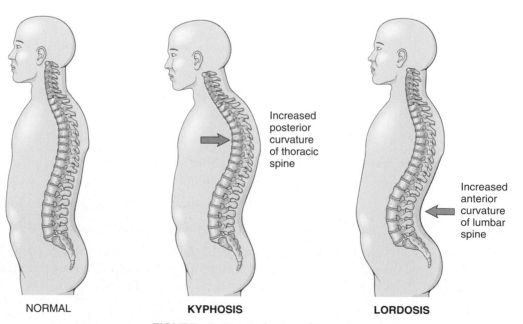

NORMAL   KYPHOSIS   LORDOSIS

Increased posterior curvature of thoracic spine

Increased anterior curvature of lumbar spine

FIGURE 15-12   Kyphosis and lordosis.

COMBINING FORM	MEANING	TERMINOLOGY	MEANING
lumb/o	loins, lower back	lumbar _____	
		Lumbago is a term used to describe low back pain.	
		lumbosacral _____	
myel/o	bone marrow	myelopoiesis _____	
orth/o	straight	orthopedics _____	
		Ped/o means child.	
oste/o	bone	osteitis _____	
		***Osteitis deformans** is better known as **Paget's disease.** Bones become weak and painful, especially in the spine, skull, pelvis, and legs.*	
		osteodystrophy _____	
		osteogenesis _____	
		***Osteogenesis imperfecta** is a genetic disorder involving defective development of bones that are brittle and fragile; fractures occur with the slightest trauma.*	
scoli/o	crooked, bent (lateral curvature)	scoliosis _____	
		The spinal column is bent abnormally to the side. Scoliosis is the most common spinal deformity in adolescent girls (Figure 15-13).	

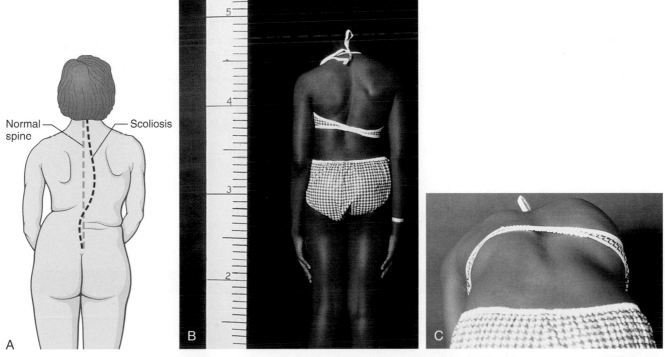

FIGURE 15-13   Moderate thoracic idiopathic adolescent scoliosis. A, Normal spine and **scoliosis. B,** Notice the **scapular asymmetry** in the upright position. This results from rotation of the spine and attached rib cage. **C,** Bending forward reveals a mild rib hump deformity.

COMBINING FORM	MEANING	TERMINOLOGY	MEANING
spondyl/o (used to make words about conditions of the structure)	vertebra	spondylosis ____ *Degeneration of the intervertebral disks in the cervical, thoracic, and lumbar regions. Signs and symptoms include pain and restriction of movement.*	
vertebr/o (used to describe the structure itself)	vertebra	vertebroplasty ____ *Percutaneous vertebroplasty relieves pain caused by compression fractures of the vertebrae. Medical cement is used to fill in the cracks and strengthen bone.*	

SUFFIXES

SUFFIX	MEANING	TERMINOLOGY	MEANING
-blast	embryonic or immature cell	osteoblast ____ *This cell synthesizes collagen and protein to form bone tissue.*	
-clast	to break	osteoclast ____ *This cell breaks down bone to remove bone tissue.*	
-listhesis	slipping	spondylolisthesis ____ *Pronounced* spŏn-dĭ-lō-lĭs-THĒ-sĭs. *The forward slipping (subluxation) of a vertebra over a lower vertebra.*	
-malacia	softening	osteomalacia ____ *A condition in which vitamin D deficiency leads to decalcification of bones; known as rickets in children.*	
-physis	to grow	epiphysis ____	
		pubic symphysis ____	
-porosis	pore, passage	osteoporosis ____ *Loss of bony tissue with decreased mass of bone. See page 602.*	
-tome	instrument to cut	osteotome ____ *This surgical chisel is designed to cut bone.*	

Terms Related to Specific Bones
COMBINING FORMS

COMBINING FORM	MEANING	TERMINOLOGY	MEANING
acetabul/o	acetabulum (hip socket)	acetabular ____	
calcane/o	calcaneus (heel)	calcaneal ____ *The calcaneus is one of the tarsal (hindfoot) bones.*	
carp/o	carpals (wrist bones)	carpal ____	
clavicul/o	clavicle (collar bone)	supraclavicular ____ *Supra- means above.*	

15

COMBINING FORM	MEANING	TERMINOLOGY	MEANING
cost/o	ribs (true ribs, false ribs, and floating ribs)	subcostal _____	
		chondrocostal _____ *Cartilage that is attached to the ribs.*	
crani/o	cranium (skull)	craniotomy _____	
		craniotome _____	
femor/o	femur (thigh bone)	femoral _____	
fibul/o	fibula (smaller lower leg bone)	fibular _____ *See perone/o.*	
humer/o	humerus (upper arm bone)	humeral _____	
ili/o	ilium (upper part of pelvic bone)	iliac _____	
ischi/o	ischium (posterior part of pelvic bone)	ischial _____	
malleol/o	malleolus (process on each side of the ankle)	malleolar _____ *The medial malleolus is at the distal end of the tibia, and the lateral malleolus is at the distal end of the fibula.*	
mandibul/o	mandible (lower jawbone)	mandibular _____	
maxill/o	maxilla (upper jawbone)	maxillary _____	
metacarp/o	metacarpals (hand bones)	metacarpectomy _____	
metatars/o	metatarsals (foot bones)	metatarsalgia _____	
olecran/o	olecranon (elbow)	olecranal _____	
patell/o	patella (kneecap)	patellar _____	
pelv/o	pelvis (hipbone)	pelvimetry _____	
perone/o	fibula	peroneal _____	
phalang/o	phalanges (finger and/or toe bones)	phalangeal _____	

Peroneal/Peritoneal/Perineal

Peroneal means pertaining to the fibula (smaller of two lower leg bones). Don't confuse this term with *peritoneal*, meaning pertaining to the peritoneum (membrane surrounding the abdominal organs), or *perineal*, meaning pertaining to the area between the rectum and the vagina in females, and between the rectum and scrotal sac in males.

15

COMBINING FORM	MEANING	TERMINOLOGY	MEANING
pub/o	pubis (anterior part of the pelvic bone)	<u>pubic</u> _____	
radi/o	radius (forearm bone—thumb side)	<u>radial</u> _____	
scapul/o	scapula (shoulder blade)	<u>scapular</u> _____	
stern/o	sternum (breastbone)	<u>sternal</u> _____	
tars/o	tarsals (bones of the hindfoot)	<u>tarsectomy</u> _____	
tibi/o	tibia (shin bone)	<u>tibial</u> _____	
uln/o	ulna (forearm bone—little finger side)	<u>ulnar</u> _____	

PATHOLOGY—BONES

Ewing sarcoma

Rare malignant tumor arising in bone; most often occurring in children.

Pain and swelling are common, especially if the tumor involves the shaft (medullary cavity) of a long bone. This tumor usually occurs at an early age between 5 and 15 years, and combined treatment with surgery, radiotherapy, and chemotherapy represents the best chance for cure (60% to 70% of patients are cured if metastasis has not occurred).

exostosis

Bony growth (benign) arising from the surface of bone.

Osteochondromas (composed of cartilage and bone) are benign **exostoses** usually found on the metaphyses of long bones near the epiphyseal plates. Ex- means out; -ostosis is condition of bones.

A **bunion** is a swelling of the metatarsophalangeal joint near the base of the big toe and is accompanied by the buildup of soft tissue and underlying bone at the distal medial aspect of the first metatarsal.

fracture

Traumatic breaking of a bone.

In a **simple (closed) fracture,** the bone is broken but there is no open wound in the skin. In a **compound (open) fracture,** the bone is broken and a fragment of bone protrudes through an open wound in the skin. See Figure 15-14A. **Crepitus** is the crackling sound produced when ends of bones rub each other or rub against roughened cartilage. Figure 15-14B illustrates different types of fractures.

Treatment of fractures involves **reduction,** which is restoration of the bone to its normal position. A **closed reduction** is manipulative reduction without a surgical incision; in an **open reduction,** an incision is made for access to the fracture site. A **cast** (solid mold of the body part) is applied to fractures to immobilize the injured bone after a closed reduction. The abbreviation **ORIF** means <u>o</u>pen <u>r</u>eduction/<u>i</u>nternal <u>f</u>ixation. Often this involves insertion of metal plates, screws, rods, or pins to stabilize the bone. See Figure 15-15.

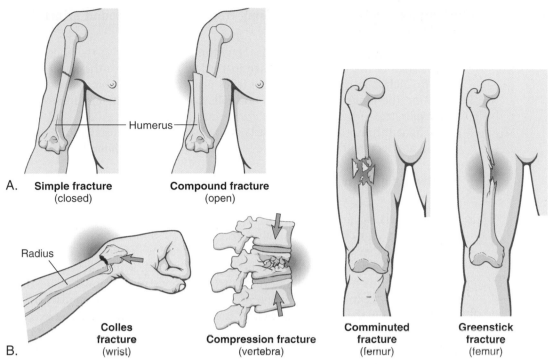

A. **Simple fracture**   **Compound fracture**
    (closed)   (open)

Humerus

Radius

B.   **Colles**   **Compression fracture**   **Comminuted**   **Greenstick**
      fracture   (vertebra)   **fracture**   **fracture**
      (wrist)   (femur)   (femur)

FIGURE 15-14   **A, Simple and compound fractures. B, Types of fractures.** A pathologic fracture (not pictured) is caused by disease of bones (tumor, infection, osteoporosis) that causes them to weaken. Cartilage is found at the site of injury when a bone breaks and is in the process of healing.

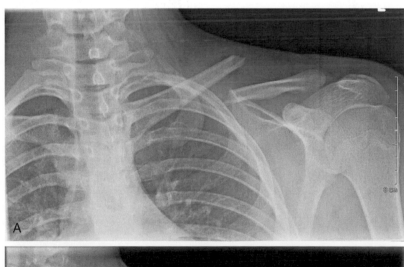

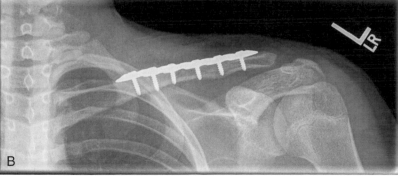

FIGURE 15-15   **Clavicle fracture. A,** This is a clavicle fracture of a 17-year-old rugby player. **B, Open reduction with internal fixation (ORIF)** to align and repair the fracture.

**osteogenic sarcoma
(osteosarcoma)**

Common malignant tumor arising from osteoblasts, found primarily in children and adolescents.

Osteoblasts multiply, forming large, bony tumors, especially at the ends of long bones (half of the lesions are located just below or just above the knee) (Figure 15-16). Metastasis (spread of tumor) takes place through the bloodstream, often affecting the lungs. Surgical resection followed by chemotherapy improves the survival rate.

Malignant tumors from other parts of the body (breast, prostate, lung, thyroid gland, and kidney) that metastasize to bones are **metastatic bone lesions.**

osteomalacia

Softening of bone, with inadequate amounts of mineral (calcium) in the bone.

Osteomalacia occurs primarily as a disease of infancy and childhood and is then known as **rickets.** Bones fail to receive adequate amounts of calcium and phosphorus; they become soft, bend easily, and become deformed.

In affected patients, vitamin D is deficient in the diet, which prevents calcium and phosphorus from being absorbed into the bloodstream from the intestines. Vitamin D is formed by the action of sunlight on certain compounds (such as cholesterol) in the skin; thus, rickets is more common in large, smoky cities during the winter months.

Treatment most often consists of administration of large daily doses of vitamin D and an increase in dietary intake of calcium and phosphorus.

osteomyelitis

Inflammation of the bone and bone marrow secondary to infection.

Bacteria enter the body through a wound and spread to the bone. Children are affected most often, and the infection usually occurs near the ends of long bones of the legs and arms. Adults can be affected too, usually as the result of an open fracture.

The lesion begins as an inflammation with pus collection. Pus tends to spread down the medullary cavity and outward to the periosteum. Antibiotic therapy corrects the condition if the infection is treated quickly. If treatment is delayed, an **abscess** can form. An abscess is a walled-off area of infection that can be difficult or impossible to penetrate with antibiotics. Surgical drainage of an abscess usually is necessary.

osteoporosis

Decrease in bone density (mass); thinning and weakening of bone.

Osteopenia is a condition in which bone mineral density is lower than normal. In some cases, it is a precursor to osteoporosis. In osteoporosis, the interior of bones is diminished in structure, as if the steel skeleton of a building had rusted and deteriorated (Figure 15-17). The condition commonly occurs in older women as a consequence of estrogen deficiency with menopause. Lack of estrogen promotes

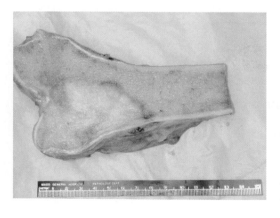

FIGURE 15-16 Osteosarcoma. The tumor has grown through the cortex of the bone and elevated the periosteum. *(Courtesy Dr. Francis Hornicek, Department of Orthopedics, Massachusetts General Hospital, Boston.)*

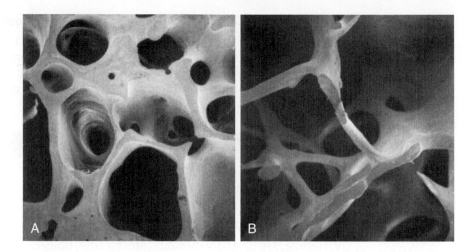

FIGURE 15-17   Scanning electron micrograph of normal bone (A) and bone with osteoporosis (B). Notice the thinning and wide separation of the trabeculae in the osteoporotic bone.

excessive bone resorption (osteoclast activity) and less bone deposition. Weakened bones are subject to fracture (as in the hip); loss of height and kyphosis occur as vertebrae collapse (Figure 15-18).

Osteoporosis can occur with atrophy caused by disuse, as in a limb that is in a cast, in the legs of a person with paraplegia, or in a bedridden patient. It also may occur in men as part of the aging process and in patients who have received corticosteroids (hormones made by the adrenal gland and used to treat inflammatory conditions).

Treatment and prevention of osteoporosis ◣ are critical to maintaining strong bones and avoiding fractures of the spine, hip, or wrist.

15

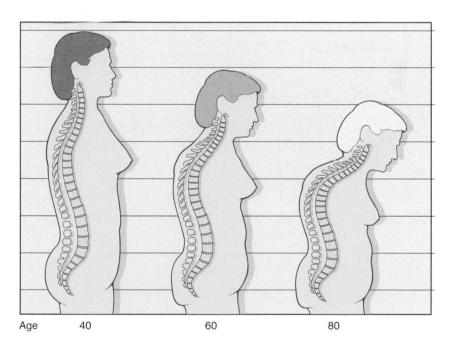

FIGURE 15-18   Kyphosis. Loss of bone mass due to osteoporosis produces posterior curvature of the spine in the thoracic region. A normal spine is shown at the age of 40 years, and osteoporotic changes are illustrated at the ages of 60 and 80 years. The changes in the spine can cause a loss of as much as 6 to 9 inches in height.

Age   40   60   80

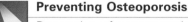

Preventing Osteoporosis

Prevention of osteoporosis includes the following:
- Balanced diet rich in calcium and vitamin D
- Weight-bearing and resistance exercise
- Reduction of smoking and alcohol intake
- Checking bone mineral density (BMD) with a DEXA test (see page 621)
- Medications when appropriate—such as bisphosphonates (Fosamax, Boniva) and selective estrogen receptor modulators (SERMs—Raloxifene, Evista) and hormone replacement therapy (HRT)

talipes

Congenital abnormality of the hindfoot (involving the talus).

Talipes (Latin *talus* = ankle, *pes* = foot) is a congenital anomaly. The most common form is **talipes equinovarus** (**equin/o** = horse), or **clubfoot.** The infant cannot stand with the sole of the foot flat on the ground. The defect can be corrected by applying orthopedic casts in the early months of infancy or, if that fails, by surgery.

JOINTS

TYPES OF JOINTS

A **joint (articulation)** is a coming together of two or more bones. Some joints are immovable, such as the **suture joints** between the skull bones. Other joints, such as those between the vertebrae, are partially movable. Most joints, however, allow considerable movement. These freely movable joints are called **synovial joints.** Examples of synovial joints are the ball-and-socket type (the hip and shoulder joints) and the hinge type (elbow, knee, and ankle joints). Label the structures in Figure 15-19 as you read the following description of a synovial joint.

The bones in a synovial joint are surrounded by a **joint capsule** [1] composed of fibrous tissue. **Ligaments** (thickened fibrous bands of connective tissue) anchor one bone to another and thereby add considerable strength to the joint capsule in critical areas. Bones at the joint are covered with a smooth, glistening white tissue called the **articular cartilage** [2]. The **synovial membrane** [3] lies under the joint capsule and lines the **synovial cavity** [4] between the bones. The synovial cavity is filled with a special lubricating fluid produced by the synovial membrane. This **synovial fluid** contains water and nutrients that nourish as well as lubricate the joints so that friction on the articular cartilage is minimal.

A **meniscus** is a crescent-shaped fibrocartilaginous structure that partly divides a joint cavity and acts as a protective cushion. It is present in the knee (see Figure 15-20).

BURSAE

Bursae (*singular*: **bursa**) are closed sacs of synovial fluid lined with a synovial membrane and are located near but not within a joint. Bursae are present wherever two types of tissue need to slide past one another with as little friction as possible. Bursae serve as layers of lubrication between the tissues. Common sites of bursae are between **tendons** (connective tissue that connects a muscle to bone) and bones, between **ligaments** (connective tissue binding bone to bone) and bones, and between skin and bones in areas where bony anatomy is prominent.

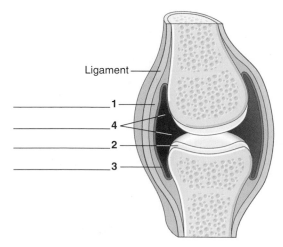

Ligament

1

4

2

3

FIGURE 15-19 **Structure of a synovial joint.**

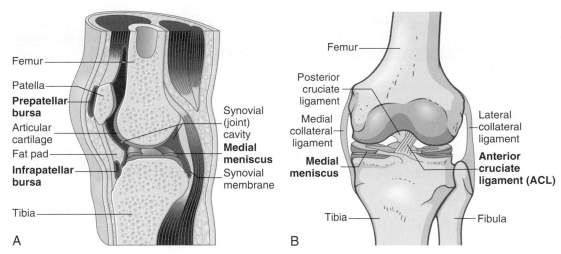

FIGURE 15-20 **A, Sagittal (lateral) section of the knee showing the medial meniscus** (plural menisci), and **bursae.** A "torn cartilage" in the knee is a damaged meniscus and is frequently treated with arthroscopic surgery. **B, Frontal section of the knee.** Notice the **anterior cruciate ligament (ACL),** which may be damaged ("torn ligament") with knee injury. Reconstruction of the ACL can require extensive surgery, and months of physical therapy may be required before return of normal function. See the case study on page 626.

Some common locations of bursae are at the elbow joint (olecranon bursa), knee joint (prepatellar bursa), and shoulder joint (subacromial bursa). Figure 15-20A shows a lateral view of the knee joint with bursae. Figure 15-20B is a frontal (anterior/posterior) view of the knee showing ligaments that provide stability for the joint.

VOCABULARY—JOINTS

This list reviews many new terms related to joints introduced in the text. Short definitions reinforce your understanding of the terms. Refer to the Pronunciation of Terms on page 647 for help with unfamiliar or difficult terms.

articular cartilage	Smooth, glistening white tissue that covers the surface of a joint.
articulation	Any type of joint.
bursa (*plural:* **bursae**)	Sac of fluid near a joint; promotes smooth sliding of one tissue against another.
ligament	Fibrous, connective bands binding bones to other bones; supports, strengthens, and stabilizes the joint.
meniscus	Crescent-shaped fibrocartilaginous structure found in the knee.
suture joint	Immovable joint, such as between the bones of the skull.
synovial cavity	Space between bones at a synovial joint; contains synovial fluid produced by the synovial membrane.
synovial fluid	Viscous (sticky) fluid within the synovial cavity. Synovial fluid is similar in viscosity to egg white; this accounts for the origin of the term (syn- = like, ov/o = egg).
synovial joint	A freely movable joint.
synovial membrane	Tissue lining the synovial cavity; it produces synovial fluid.
tendon	Fibrous, connective tissue muscles to bones.

15

TERMINOLOGY—JOINTS

Write the meanings of the medical terms in the spaces provided.

COMBINING FORMS

COMBINING FORM	MEANING	TERMINOLOGY	MEANING
ankyl/o	stiff	ankylosis	
arthr/o	joint	arthroplasty	

Replacement arthroplasty is replacement of one or both bone ends by a prosthesis (artificial part) of metal or plastic. See page 620. Carpometacarpal arthroplasty is a treatment for arthritis in the thumb (at the basal joint).

arthrotomy

hemarthrosis

hydrarthrosis

Synovial fluid collects abnormally in the joint.

polyarthritis

articul/o	joint	articular cartilage	
burs/o	bursa	bursitis	

Causes of this periarticular condition may be related to stress placed on the bursa or to diseases such as gout or rheumatoid arthritis. The bursa becomes inflamed and movement is limited and painful. Intrabursal injection of corticosteroids and also rest and splinting of the limb are helpful in treatment.

chondr/o	cartilage	achondroplasia	

This is an inherited condition in which the bones of the arms and legs fail to grow to normal size because of a defect in cartilage and bone formation. Dwarfism results, characterized by short limbs and a normal-sized head and trunk. See page 82.

chondrosarcoma

chondromalacia

Chondromalacia patellae *is a softening and roughening of the articular cartilaginous surface of the kneecap, resulting in pain, a grating sensation, and mechanical "catching" behind the patella with joint movement.*

ligament/o	ligament	ligamentous	

Ankylosis/Alkalosis

Ankylosis is a condition of joint stiffening or immobilization. Don't confuse this term with *alkalosis*, meaning increased alkalinity (pH) of blood and tissues.

COMBINING FORM	MEANING	TERMINOLOGY	MEANING
rheumat/o	watery flow	rheumatologist _____ *Various forms of arthritis are marked by collection of fluid in joint spaces.*	
synov/o	synovial membrane	synovitis _____	
ten/o	tendon	tenorrhaphy _____	
		tenosynovitis _____ *Synov/o here refers to the sheath (covering) around the tendon.*	
tendin/o	tendon	tendinitis _____ *Also spelled tendonitis.*	

SUFFIXES

SUFFIX	MEANING	TERMINOLOGY	MEANING
-desis	to bind, tie together	arthrodesis _____ *Bones are fused across the joint space by surgery (artificial ankylosis). This operation is performed when a joint is very painful, unstable, or chronically infected.*	
-stenosis	narrowing	spinal stenosis _____ *Narrowing of the neural (spinal) canal in the lumbar spine. Symptoms (pain, paresthesias, urinary retention, bowel incontinence) come from compression of the cauda equina (nerves that spread out from the lower end of the spinal cord like a horse's tail). See Figure 15-21.*	

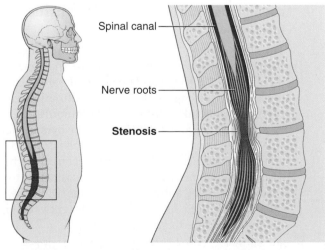

Spinal canal

Nerve roots

Stenosis

FIGURE 15-21   Spinal stenosis. Wear-and-tear effects of aging can lead to narrowing of the spinal (neural) canal.

PATHOLOGY—JOINTS

arthritis

Inflammation of any joint.

Common forms of arthritis are:

1. ankylosing spondylitis

Chronic, progressive arthritis with stiffening of spinal joints, primarily of the spine.

Bilateral sclerosis (hardening) of the sacroiliac joints is a diagnostic sign. Joint changes are similar to those seen in rheumatoid arthritis, and the condition can respond to corticosteroids and anti-inflammatory drugs.

2. gouty arthritis (gout)

Inflammation and painful swelling of joints caused by excessive uric acid in the body.

A congenital defect in the metabolism of uric acid causes too much of it to accumulate in blood (**hyperuricemia**), joints, and soft tissues near joints. The "pointy" uric acid crystals (salts) destroy the articular cartilage and damage the synovial membrane, often resulting in excruciating pain. The joint chiefly affected is the big toe; hence, the condition often is called **podagra** (pod/o = foot, -agra = excessive pain). Treatment consists of drugs to lower uric acid production (allopurinol) and to prevent inflammation (colchicine and indomethacin) and a special diet that avoids foods that are rich in uric acid, such as red meats, red wines, and fermented cheeses.

3. osteoarthritis (OA)

Progressive, degenerative joint disease with loss of articular cartilage and hypertrophy of bone (formation of osteophytes, or bone spurs) at articular surfaces.

This condition, also known as **degenerative joint disease,** can occur in any joint, but occurs mainly in the spine, hips, and knees of older people. It is marked by a narrowing of the joint space (due to loss of cartilage). Treatment consists of aspirin and nonsteroidal anti-inflammatory drugs (NSAIDs) to reduce inflammation and pain and physical therapy to loosen impaired joints. Figure 15-22 compares a normal joint and those with changes characteristic of osteoarthritis and rheumatoid arthritis.

End-stage osteoarthritis is the most common reason for joint replacement surgery (total joint arthroplasty). See the clinical case on page 627.

4. rheumatoid arthritis (RA)

Chronic joint condition with inflammation and pain; caused by an autoimmune reaction against joint tissue, particularly the synovial membrane.

The small joints of the hands and feet are affected first, and larger joints later. Women are more commonly afflicted than men. Synovial membranes become inflamed and thickened, damaging the articular cartilage and preventing easy movement (see Figure 15-22). Sometimes fibrous tissue forms and calcifies, creating a **bony ankylosis** (pathologic union) at the joint and preventing movement. Swollen, painful joints accompanied by **pyrexia** (fever) are symptoms.

Diagnosis is by clinical criteria, blood tests, and x-ray images revealing changes around the affected joints. Treatment consists of heat applications and drugs such as aspirin and other NSAIDs and corticosteroids to reduce inflammation and pain. Disease-modifying antirheumatic drugs (DMARDs) such as methotrexate and gold salts also are used, as well as more recently, biologic medications to change the immune response to synovial tissues.

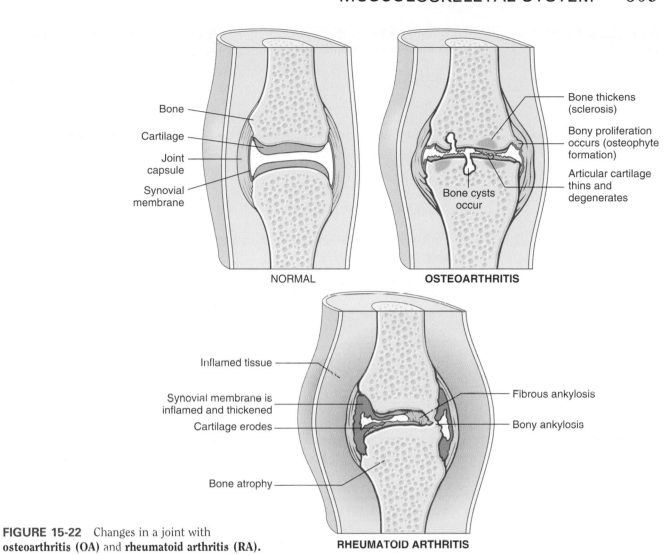

FIGURE 15-22 Changes in a joint with **osteoarthritis (OA)** and **rheumatoid arthritis (RA).**

bunion	**Enlargement of bone or tissue around the joint at the base of the big toe (metatarsophalangeal joint).**
	Chronic irritation from ill-fitting shoes can cause a buildup of soft tissue and underlying bone. Bunionectomy (removal of a bony exostosis and associated soft tissue) is indicated if other measures (changing shoes and use of anti-inflammatory agents) fail. See Figure 15-23. Another name for a bunion is **hallux** (great toe) **valgus** (abnormal angulation of the toe).

FIGURE 15-23 The photograph shows a **bunion** of the left foot. The first x-ray image is before **bunionectomy,** and the second is after surgery to remove tissue and realign the bones.
(Courtesy Dr. Sidra Ezrahi and Dr. Richard de Asia, Massachusetts General Hospital, Boston.)

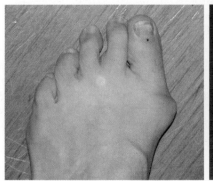
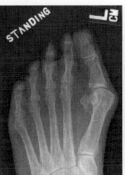
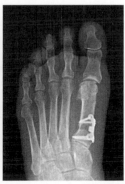

carpal tunnel syndrome (CTS)

Compression of the median nerve as it passes between the transverse ligament, and bones and tendons of the wrist.

CTS is caused by compression of the median nerve (see Figure 15-24) in the carpal tunnel. The compression results from swelling and/or inflammation of the flexor tendons. The thumb, the index and long (middle) fingers, and the radial half of the ring finger become dysesthetic (numb).

Treatment consists of splinting the wrist during sleep to immobilize it, use of anti-inflammatory medications, and injection of corticosteroids such as cortisone into the carpal tunnel. If these measures fail, surgical release of the transverse carpal ligament usually is curative.

dislocation

Displacement of a bone from its joint.

Dislocated bones do not articulate with each other. The most common cause of dislocations is trauma. **Shoulder dislocation** (disruption of articulation between the head of the humerus and the glenoid fossa of the scapula) and **hip dislocation** (disruption of articulation between the head of the femur and the acetabulum of the pelvis) are examples.

Treatment of dislocations involves **reduction,** which is restoration of the bones to their normal positions. A **subluxation** is a partial or incomplete dislocation.

ganglion cyst

Fluid-filled sac arising from joint capsules or tendons.

Most common in the wrist, but can occur in the hand, shoulder, knee, hip, or ankle. See Figure 15-25. Treatment ranges from immobilization and reduced activity to aspiration of fluid, to surgical resection, if necessary.

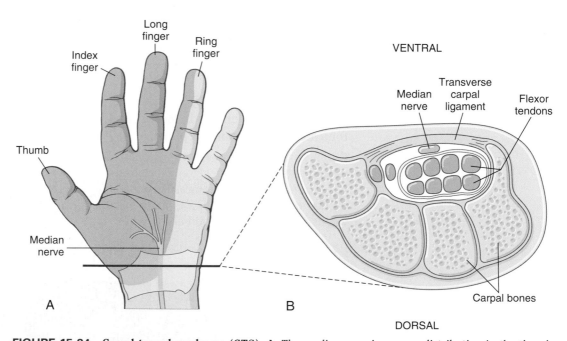

FIGURE 15-24 Carpal tunnel syndrome (CTS). A, The median nerve's sensory distribution in the thumb, first three fingers, and palm. **B,** Cross section of a left hand at the level indicated in **(A)**. Note the position of the median nerve between the carpal ligament and the tendons and carpal bones.

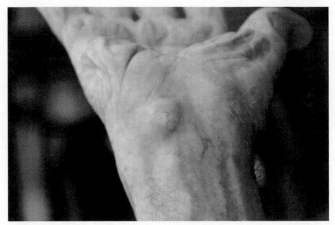

FIGURE 15-25 **Ganglion cyst** on the wrist. This is commonly known as a "Bible cyst" because a frequent treatment in the past was to drop the large family Bible on the cyst to rupture it. Success of such treatment usually was only temporary, with reoccurrence of the cyst over time.

herniation of an intervertebral disk (disc)

Abnormal protrusion of an intervertebral disk into the spinal canal or spinal nerves.

This condition is commonly referred to as a "**slipped disk**." Pain is experienced as the inner portion of the disk (nucleus pulposus) presses on spinal nerves or on the spinal cord. See Figure 15-26A. Low back pain and **sciatica** (pain radiating down the leg) are symptoms when the disk protrudes in the lumbar spine. See Figure 15-26B. Neck pain and burning pain radiating down an arm are characteristic of a herniated disk in the cervical spine. Physical therapy, drugs for pain, and epidural cortisone injections may help initially. In patients with chronic or recurrent disk herniation, **microdiskectomy** (removal of a portion of the protruding disk) may be advised. See Figure 15-27A. In microendoscopic surgery, the disk is removed by inserting a tube through the skin and aspirating the disk through the tube, while the procedure is visualized through a small fiberoptic scope.

15

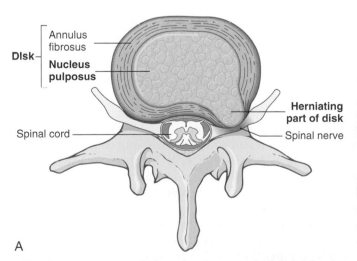

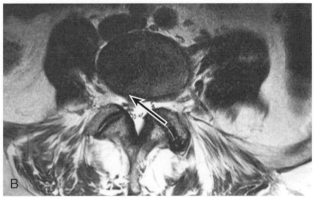

A

B

FIGURE 15-26 **A, Herniation of an intervertebral disk** (view from above the vertebra). The inner portion (nucleus pulposus) of the disk can be seen pressing on the spinal nerve. The condition also is known as **herniated nucleus pulposus (HNP). B, Magnetic resonance image showing a herniated disk impinging on the sciatic nerve root.**

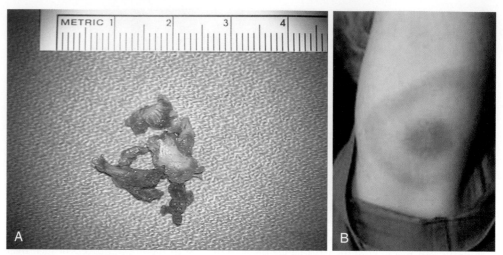

FIGURE 15-27   A, In **microdiskectomy,** fragments of the herniated disk (*shown here*) are removed. **B,** "Bull's eye" rash in Lyme disease. *(A, Courtesy Jean-Valéry Coumans, Massachusetts General Hospital, Boston.)*

Lyme disease (Lyme arthritis)	**Chronic, recurrent disorder marked by severe arthritis, myalgia and malaise; cause is bacterium carried by a tick.** It was first reported in Old Lyme, Connecticut, and is now found throughout the eastern coastal region of the United States. It is often marked by a "bull's eye" rash at the site of the tick bite. See Figure 15-27B. The condition is treated with antibiotics. In some cases, Lyme disease can affect the nervous system. See the ***In Person: Neurologic Lyme,*** page 628.
sprain	**Trauma to a joint with swelling and injury to ligaments.** A **strain** is an injury involving the overstretching of muscle. Application of gentle compressive wraps is an immediate measure to relieve pain and minimize swelling caused by sprains and strains. Application of ice and elevation of the extremity as well as physical therapy are also helpful.
systemic lupus erythematosus (SLE)	**Chronic inflammatory autoimmune disease involving joints, skin, kidneys, central nervous system (CNS), heart, and lungs.** This condition affects connective tissue (specifically a protein component called **collagen**) in tendons, ligaments, bones, and cartilage all over the body. Typically, there is a red, scaly rash over the nose and cheeks ("butterfly" rash) (Figure 15-28). Patients, usually women, experience joint pain in several joints (polyarthralgia), pyrexia (fever), kidney inflammation, and malaise. SLE is an autoimmune disease that is diagnosed by the presence of abnormal antibodies in the blood and characteristic white blood cells called LE cells. Treatment involves giving corticosteroids, hormones made by the adrenal gland that are used to treat inflammatory conditions. New medications that modulate the immune system are being used with increasing success. The name lupus, meaning wolf, has been used since the 13th century, because more severe (erosive) lupus skin lesions were thought to look like the affected person had been attacked by a wolf.

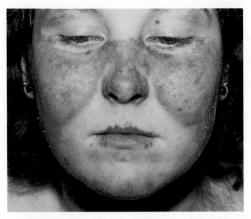

FIGURE 15-28 **Butterfly rash** that may accompany systemic lupus erythematosus.

MUSCLES

TYPES OF MUSCLES

There are three types of muscles in the body. Label Figure 15-29 as you read the following descriptions of the various types of muscles.

Striated muscle [1] makes up the **voluntary** or **skeletal muscles** that move all bones, as well as controlling facial expression and eye movements. Through the central and peripheral nervous systems, we have conscious control over these muscles. Striated muscle fibers (cells) have a pattern of dark and light bands, or fibrils, in their cytoplasm. Fibrous tissue that envelops and separates muscles is called **fascia**.

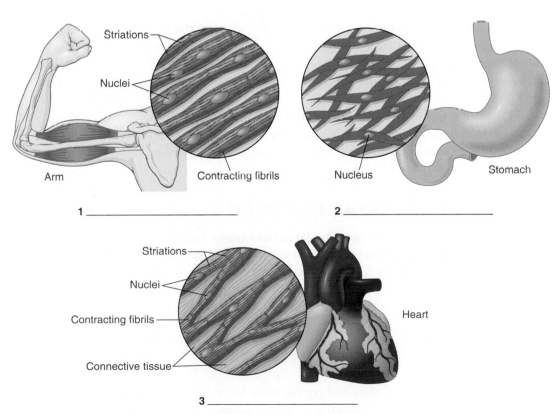

FIGURE 15-29 **Types of muscles.**

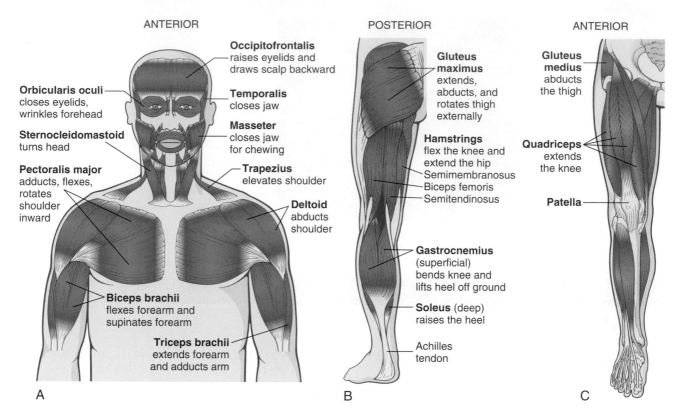

ANTERIOR

Occipitofrontalis
raises eyelids and
draws scalp backward

Orbicularis oculi
closes eyelids,
wrinkles forehead

Temporalis
closes jaw

Sternocleidomastoid
turns head

Masseter
closes jaw
for chewing

Pectoralis major
adducts, flexes,
rotates
shoulder
inward

Trapezius
elevates shoulder

Deltoid
abducts
shoulder

Biceps brachii
flexes forearm and
supinates forearm

Triceps brachii
extends forearm
and adducts arm

A

POSTERIOR

**Gluteus
maximus**
extends,
abducts, and
rotates thigh
externally

Hamstrings
flex the knee and
extend the hip
Semimembranosus
Biceps femoris
Semitendinosus

Gastrocnemius
(superficial)
bends knee and
lifts heel off ground

Soleus (deep)
raises the heel

Achilles
tendon

B

ANTERIOR

**Gluteus
medius**
abducts
the thigh

Quadriceps
extends
the knee

Patella

C

FIGURE 15-30   A, Selected muscles of the head, neck, torso, and arm and their functions. B, Selected muscles of the posterior and anterior aspect of the leg and their functions. The Evolve website contains additional anterior and posterior images of major muscles and their functions.

15

Smooth muscle [2] makes up the **involuntary** or **visceral muscles** that contract to move internal organs such as the digestive tract, the walls of blood vessels, and secretory ducts leading from glands. These muscles are controlled involuntary because they are not controlled by the conscious mind. They are called smooth because they have no dark and light fibrils in their cytoplasm. Smooth muscle forms sheets of fibers that wrap around tubes and vessels while skeletal muscle fibers are arranged in bundles.

Cardiac muscle [3] is striated in appearance but is like smooth muscle in its action. Its movement cannot be consciously controlled. The fibers of cardiac muscle are branching fibers and are found in the heart.

ACTIONS OF SKELETAL MUSCLES

Skeletal (striated) muscles (more than 600 in the human body) are the muscles that move bones. Figure 15-30 shows some skeletal muscles of the head, neck, and torso and muscles of the posterior aspect of the leg. When a muscle contracts, one of the bones to which it is joined remains virtually stationary as a result of other muscles that hold it in place. The point of attachment of the muscle to the stationary bone is called the **origin (beginning)** of that muscle. When the muscle contracts, however, another bone to which it is attached does move. The point of junction of the muscle to the bone that moves is called the **insertion** of the muscle. Most often, the origin of a muscle lies proximal in the skeleton, whereas its insertion lies distal.

Figure 15-31 shows the biceps and triceps muscles in the upper arm. One origin of the biceps is at the scapula, and its insertion is at the radius. Tendons are the connective tissue bands that connect muscles to the bones.

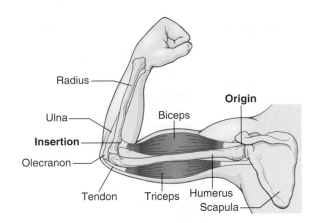

FIGURE 15-31 Origin and insertion of the biceps in the arm. Note also the origin of the triceps at the scapula and the insertion at the olecranon of the ulna.

Muscles can perform a variety of actions. Some of the terms used to describe those actions are listed here, with a short description of the specific type of movement performed (see Figure 15-32 on page 616).

ACTION	MEANING
flexion	Decreasing the angle between two bones; bending a limb.
extension	Increasing the angle between two bones; straightening out a limb.
abduction	Movement away from the midline of the body.
adduction	Movement toward the midline of the body.
rotation	Circular movement around an axis (central point). Internal rotation is toward the center of the body and external rotation is away from the center of the body.
dorsiflexion	Decreasing the angle of the ankle joint so that the foot moves upward, toward the knee or ceiling. This is the opposite movement of stepping on the gas pedal when driving a car.
plantar flexion	Motion that moves the foot downward toward the ground as when pointing the toes or stepping on the gas pedal. Plant/o means sole of the foot.
supination	As applied to the hand and forearm, where the elbow is bent, the act of turning the palm up. As applied to the foot, it is outward roll of the foot/ankle during normal motion.
pronation	As applied to the hand and forearm, where the elbow is bent, the act of turning the palm down. As applied to the foot, it is inward roll of the foot/ankle during normal motion.

15

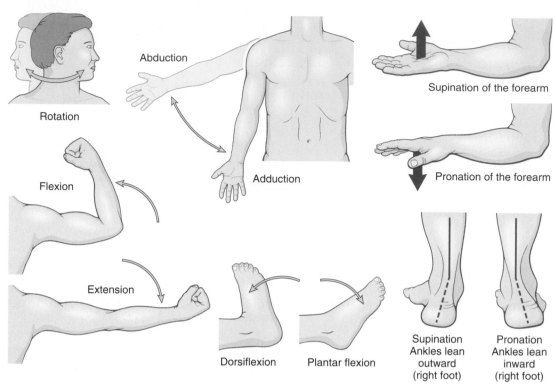

Rotation

Flexion

Extension

Abduction

Adduction

Supination of the forearm

Pronation of the forearm

Dorsiflexion

Plantar flexion

Supination
Ankles lean
outward
(right foot)

Pronation
Ankles lean
inward
(right foot)

FIGURE 15-32   Types of muscular actions.

VOCABULARY—MUSCLES

This list reviews many of the new terms related to muscle introduced in the text. Short definitions reinforce your understanding of the terms. Refer to the Pronunciation of Terms on page 647 for help with unfamiliar or difficult terms.

abduction	Movement away from the midline of the body.
adduction	Movement toward the midline of the body.
dorsiflexion	Upward movement of the foot; achieved through ankle motion.
extension	Straightening of a flexed limb; increasing the angle between the bones of a joint.
fascia	Fibrous membrane separating and enveloping muscles.
flexion	Bending a limb; decreasing the angle between bones.
insertion of a muscle	Connection of the muscle to a bone that moves; usually distal on the skeleton.
origin of a muscle	Connection of the muscle to a stationary bone; usually proximal on the skeleton.
plantar flexion	Downward movement of the foot; achieved through ankle motion.
pronation	Turning the palm downward.
rotation	Circular movement around a central point. Internal rotation is toward the center of the body. External rotation is away from the center of the body.
striated muscle	Muscle connected to bones; voluntary or skeletal muscle.
supination	Turning the palm upward.
visceral muscle	Muscle connected to internal organs; involuntary or smooth muscle.

15

TERMINOLOGY—MUSCLES

Write the meanings of the medical terms in the spaces provided.

COMBINING FORMS

COMBINING FORM	MEANING	TERMINOLOGY	MEANING
fasci/o	fascia (forms sheaths enveloping muscles)	<u>fasciotomy</u> _____ *Fascia is cut to relieve tension or pressure on muscles. See Figure 15-33.*	
fibr/o	fibrous connective tissue	<u>fibromyalgia</u> _____ *Chronic pain and stiffness in muscles, joints, and fibrous tissue, especially of the back, shoulders, neck, hips, and knees. Fatigue is a common complaint. Cause is unknown, and treatment includes physical therapy, stress relief methods, and medications such as Cymbalta (duloxetine) and Lyrica (pregabalin).*	
leiomy/o	smooth (visceral) muscle that lines the walls of internal organs	<u>leiomyoma</u> _____ <u>leiomyosarcoma</u> _____	

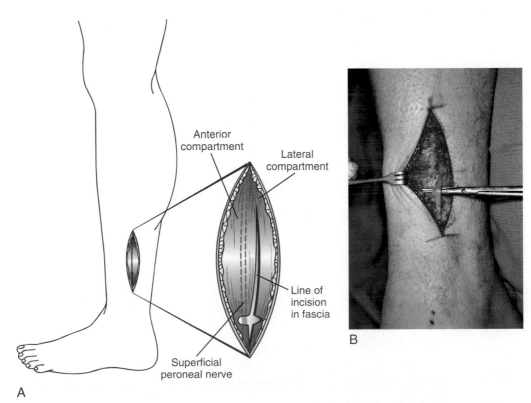

A

B

FIGURE 15-33   A, Fasciotomy as treatment for **compartment syndrome,** which is the compression of muscle, blood vessels, and nerves inside a closed space (compartment) of the body. It most often involves the lower leg. **B, Clinical photograph of fasciotomy procedure and exposed superficial peroneal nerve.**

15

COMBINING FORM	MEANING	TERMINOLOGY	MEANING
my/o	muscle	myalgia _____	
		electromyography _____	
		myopathy _____	
myocardi/o	heart muscle	myocardial _____	
myos/o	muscle	myositis _____	
plant/o	sole of the foot	plantar flexion _____	
rhabdomy/o	skeletal (striated) muscle connected to bones	rhabdomyoma _____	
		rhabdomyosarcoma _____	
sarc/o	muscle and flesh	sarcopenia _____ *Loss of muscle mass and strength associated with aging. Exercise and strength training can help preserve and enhance muscle mass at any age.*	

SUFFIXES

SUFFIX	MEANING	TERMINOLOGY	MEANING
-asthenia	lack of strength	myasthenia gravis _____ *Muscles lose strength because of a failure in transmission of the nervous impulse from the nerve to the muscle cell.*	
-trophy	development, nourishment	atrophy _____ *Decrease in size of an organ or tissue.*	
		hypertrophy _____ *Increase in size of an organ or tissue.*	
		amyotrophic _____ *In **amyotrophic lateral sclerosis (Lou Gehrig disease),** muscles deteriorate (paralysis occurs) as a result of degeneration of nerves in the spinal cord and lower region of the brain.*	

PREFIXES

PREFIX	MEANING	TERMINOLOGY	MEANING
ab-	away from	abduction _____ *Duct/o means to lead.*	
ad-	toward	adduction _____	
dorsi-	back	dorsiflexion _____	

PREFIX	MEANING	TERMINOLOGY	MEANING
poly-	many, much	poly<u>myalgia</u> _____ ***Polymyalgia rheumatica*** *is an autoimmune disorder marked by aching and morning stiffness in the shoulder, hip, or neck for longer than 1 month.*	

PATHOLOGY—MUSCLES

muscular dystrophy	**Group of inherited diseases characterized by progressive weakness and degeneration of muscle fibers without involvement of the nervous system.** **Duchenne muscular dystrophy** is the most common form. Muscles appear to enlarge **(pseudohypertrophy)** as fat replaces functional muscle cells that have degenerated and atrophied. Onset of muscle weakness occurs soon after birth, and diagnosis can be made by muscle biopsy and electromyography. The disease predominantly affects males; muscle weakness produces stumbling, falling, lordosis, winged (prominent) scapulae, and cardiac problems.
polymyositis	**Chronic inflammatory myopathy.** This condition is marked by symmetric muscle weakness and pain, often accompanied by a rash around the eyes and on the face and limbs. Evidence that polymyositis is an autoimmune disorder is growing stronger, and some patients recover completely with immunosuppressive therapy.

LABORATORY TESTS AND CLINICAL PROCEDURES

LABORATORY TESTS

antinuclear antibody test (ANA)	**Detects an antibody often present in serum of patients with systemic lupus erythematosus (SLE) and other autoimmune diseases.**
erythrocyte sedimentation rate (ESR)	**Measures time it takes for erythrocytes to settle to the bottom of a test tube.** Elevated ESR is associated with inflammatory disorders such as rheumatoid arthritis, tumors, and infections, and with chronic infections of bone and soft tissue.
rheumatoid factor test (RF)	**Serum is tested for the presence of an antibody found in many patients with rheumatoid arthritis.**
serum calcium (Ca)	**Measurement of calcium level in serum.** Hypercalcemia may be caused by disorders of the parathyroid gland and malignancy that affects bone metabolism. Hypocalcemia is seen in critically ill patients with burns, sepsis, and acute renal failure.
serum creatine kinase (CK)	**Measurement of the enzyme creatine kinase in serum.** This enzyme normally is present in skeletal and cardiac muscle. Increased levels occur in muscular dystrophy, polymyositis, and with traumatic injuries.

15

uric acid test	**Measurement of uric acid in serum.**
	High levels are associated with gouty arthritis.

CLINICAL PROCEDURES

arthrocentesis	**Surgical puncture to remove fluid from the joint space.**
	Synovial fluid is removed for analysis using a needle and syringe.
arthrography	**Taking x-ray images after injection of contrast material into a joint.**
arthroplasty	**Surgical repair or replacement of a joint.**
	Total hip arthroplasty or **total hip replacement (THR)** is replacement of the femoral head and acetabulum with prostheses that are fastened into the bone (Figure 15-34).
	In a **total knee replacement (TKR)** a metal prosthesis covers the end of the femur, and a tibial component made of metal and plastic covers the tip end of the tibia. See page 627 for a clinical case describing TKR.
	Other examples of arthroplasties are **resection arthroplasty** (small portion of a bone is removed to repair the joint; acromioclavicular joint is a common location), **interposition arthroplasty** (new tissue is placed between damaged surface of a joint such as the elbow), and **revision arthroplasty** (an operation to replace a failing prosthetic joint).

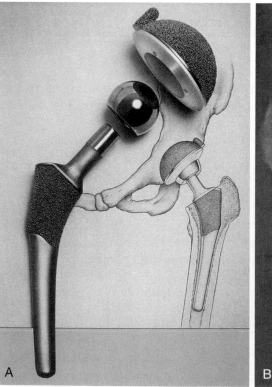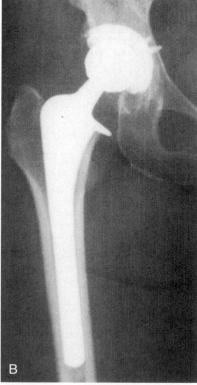

FIGURE 15-34   A, Acetabular and femoral components of a total hip arthroplasty. B, Radiograph showing a hip after placement of a cementless Harris-Galante implant. The bone grows into the porous metal to stabilize it to the skeleton.

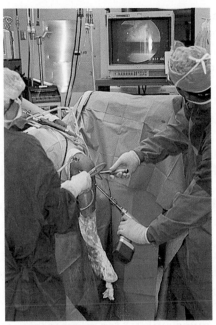

FIGURE 15-35   Knee arthroscopy in progress. Notice the monitor in the background. An arthroscope is used in the diagnosis and treatment of pathologic changes.

arthroscopy	**Visual examination of a joint with an arthroscope, which projects an image on a video monitor.**
	An orthopedist passes small surgical instruments into a joint (knee, shoulder, ankle, wrist, hip) to evaluate and/or remove and repair damaged tissue while viewing the joint simultaneously with a scope. See Figure 15-35.
bone density test (bone densitometry)	**Low-energy x-ray absorption in bones of the spinal column, pelvis, and wrist is used to measure bone mass.**
	An x-ray detector measures how well x-rays penetrate through bones (Figure 15-36). Areas of decreased density indicate osteopenia and osteoporosis. Also called **dual-energy x-ray absorptiometry** (**DEXA** or **DXA**).

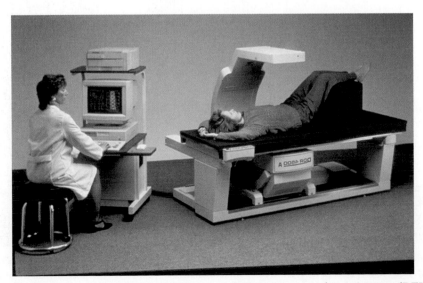

FIGURE 15-36   Patient undergoing **bone density test or dual energy x-ray absorptiometry (DEXA or DXA).**

bone scan	**Uptake of a radioactive substance is measured in bone.**
	After a weak radioactive tracer is injected intravenously into the patient, a nuclear medicine physician uses a special scanning device to detect areas of increased uptake (tumors, infection, inflammation, stress fractures) (Figure 15-37).
computed tomography (CT)	**X-ray beam and computer provide cross-sectional and other images.**
	CT scans identify bone abnormalities, and musculo-skeletal trauma.
diskography	**X-ray examination of cervical or lumbar intervertebral disk after injection of contrast into nucleus pulposus (interior of the disk).**
electromyography (EMG)	**Recording the strength of muscle contraction as a result of electrical stimulation.**
magnetic resonance imaging (MRI)	**A strong magnetic field and advanced computing technology are used to create high-resolution images of soft tissue.**
	MRI shows soft tissue conditions in greater detail than that achieved with CT.
muscle biopsy	**Removal of muscle tissue for microscopic examination.**

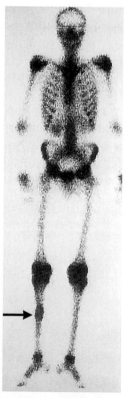

FIGURE 15-37   A technetium-99m bone scan of a skeleton showing an area of increased radioactive uptake on the right tibia (*arrow*) that indicates a bone tumor.

ABBREVIATIONS

AC	acromioclavicular (joint)
ACL	anterior cruciate ligament of the knee
ANA	antinuclear antibody—indicator of systemic lupus erythematosus
BKA	below-knee amputation
BMD	bone mineral density
C1 to C7	cervical vertebrae
Ca	calcium
CK	creatine kinase—enzyme elevated in muscle disease
CMC	carpometacarpal (joint)
CTS	carpal tunnel syndrome
DEXA or DXA	dual-energy x-ray absorptiometry—a test of bone mineral density
DMARD	disease-modifying antirheumatic drug
DO	doctor of osteopathy
DTRs	deep tendon reflexes
EMG	electromyography
ESR (sed rate)	erythrocyte sedimentation rate—indicates inflammation
HNP	herniated nucleus pulposus
IM	intramuscular
L1 to L5	lumbar vertebrae
NSAID	nonsteroidal anti-inflammatory drug—often prescribed to treat musculoskeletal disorders
OA	osteoarthritis
ORIF	open reduction (of fracture)/internal fixation
ortho	orthopedics (or orthopaedics)
OT	occupational therapy—helps patients with impaired musculoskeletal function perform activities of daily living and function in work-related situations
P	phosphorus
PT	physical therapy—helps patients regain use of muscles and joints after injury or surgery
RA	rheumatoid arthritis
RF	rheumatoid factor
ROM	range of motion
SLE	systemic lupus erythematosus
T1 to T12	thoracic vertebrae
TKR	total knee replacement/arthroplasty
THR	total hip replacement/arthroplasty
TMJ	temporomandibular joint

15

IN PERSON: ROTATOR CUFF TEAR

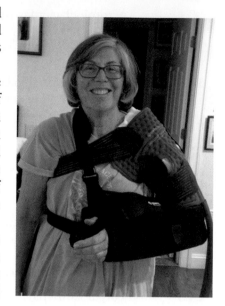

When I took the enormous swing for my drive on the 10th hole and instead of hitting the ball, I hit the ground, I immediately knew that I had done severe damage to my left shoulder. The club flew out of my hands and I felt excruciating pain.

Over the next few weeks, I iced the shoulder and took NSAIDs, but the pain and inability to move my shoulder persisted. After several weeks of physical therapy that didn't improve my mobility or pain, I went to an orthopedic surgeon who specialized in shoulders. He suspected a torn rotator cuff. The rotator cuff is a group of muscles and tendons that hold the bones of the shoulder [humerus, clavicle, and scapula] in place. [See Figure 15-38A for a diagram of the anatomy of shoulder and rotator cuff tendons and muscles.] An MRI of my shoulder made the diagnosis. [See Figure 15-38B for an MRI scan.]

I was told that rotator cuff tears do not repair themselves, but some people gradually get used to the limited mobility and diminished pain. The other alternative is arthroscopic surgery [see Figure 15-38C] to repair the torn tendons and muscles. I decided to have the surgery, which consisted of drilling into the head of the humerus and pulling the tendon (with cords) toward the bone [humerus] to reinsert it in place. [See Figure 15-38D.]

After surgery, I found myself strapped into an elaborate sling to protect my shoulder. I also was given a miraculous ice machine contraption that continuously delivered ice water to my shoulder when I was sleeping (or trying to) sleep!). The sling and ice machine lasted over 6 weeks. Tough going, but now after a year of recovery and physical therapy, I think I can get back on the golf course. It was worth it!

Davi-Ellen Chabner.

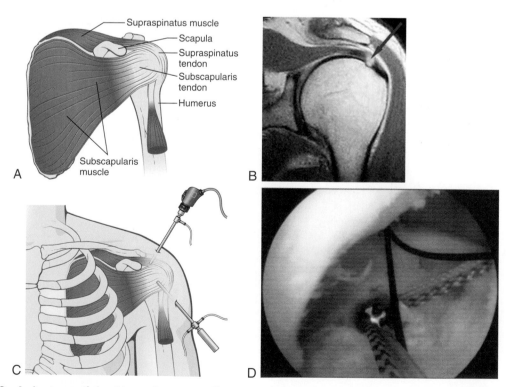

FIGURE 15-38 **A,** Anatomy of shoulder and rotator cuff tendons and muscles. **B,** MRI showing rotator cuff tear. **C,** Arthroscopic surgery to repair torn tendons and muscles. **D,** Arthroscopic view of procedure.

PRACTICAL APPLICATIONS

This section contains an x-ray report, an orthopedic operating room schedule, a case report with findings presented in SOAP format, and a short clinical case. Explanations of more difficult or unfamiliar terms are given in brackets. Answers to the matching questions are found on page 642.

MEDICAL REPORT: RESULTS OF CHEST X-RAY EXAMINATION

PA [posteroanterior] and lateral chest: The heart is enlarged in its transverse diameter. The lungs are fully expanded and free of active disease.

Thoracic spine shows a scoliosis of the upper thoracic spine convex to the left. There is 50% wedge compression fracture of T6 and slight wedge compression fracture of T5. There is also anterior wedge compression fracture of T12.

Lumbar spine shows 90% compression fractures of L1 and L3 with 30% compression fractures of L2 and L5. All bones are markedly osteoporotic. There is calcification within the aortic arch. There are gallstones in the right upper quadrant. The findings in the spine are most compatible with osteoporotic compression fractures. During the procedure, the patient had a sickable [syncopal—this word was incorrectly transcribed!] episode and fell, striking her head. A skull series, done at no cost to the patient, shows no evidence of bony fracture. The pineal gland is calcified and has a midline location. The sella turcica is normal.

OPERATING ROOM SCHEDULE

Match the operation in Column I with an accompanying diagnosis or indication for surgery from Column II.

COLUMN I

1. Excision, osteochondroma, R calcaneus _____

2. TMJ arthroscopy with probable arthrotomy _____

3. L4–5 laminectomy and diskectomy _____

4. Arthroscopy, left knee _____

5. Open reduction, malleolar fracture _____

6. R occipital craniotomy with tumor resection _____

7. Excision, distal end right clavicle, with prob. acromioplasty _____

8. Open reduction and internal fixation of the acetabulum _____

COLUMN II

A. Fracture of the ankle
B. ACL rupture
C. Neoplastic lesion in brain
D. Exostosis on heel bone
E. Pelvic fracture
F. Pain and malocclusion of jawbones
G. Lower back pain radiating down one leg
H. Pain in shoulder joint with bone spur (exostosis) evident on x-ray

15

CASE REPORT—SOAP FORMAT: ACL INJURY

[*Note*: **SOAP** stands for **S**ubjective, **O**bjective, **A**ssessment, and **P**lan.]

S: Patient reports that she fell and twisted her right knee while skiing last month. She notes that she felt a "pop" and experienced immediate pain and swelling of the knee. X-ray was negative for fracture, but MRI revealed a torn ACL [anterior cruciate ligament]. Patient underwent an ACL reconstruction using a patellar tendon autograft 1 week ago. Pain is 3/10 at rest and 6/10 during weight-bearing [on a scale of 0 to 10]. Her goals are to decrease pain, walk normally, and return to prior level of functioning, including skiing and soccer.

O: *Gait*: Ambulates with Bledsoe [hinged] brace and bilateral axillary crutches.

	Left	**Right**
Range of Motion:		
Extension	0°	0°
Flexion	140°	90°
Strength:		
Quadriceps	5/5	3+/5
Hamstrings	5/5	4–/5
Gluteus medius	5/5	4–/5
Gluteus maximus	5/5	4–/5
Gastroc/soleus	5/5	4–/5
Girth:		
Mid-patella	15″	16″

A: Patient is a 20-year-old female presenting with signs and symptoms consistent with status post-ACL reconstruction. Impairments include gait disturbance, decreased range of motion, decreased strength, edema, pain, and decreased functional activities.

P: Treatment will include manual therapy, therapeutic exercise modalities, patient education, and gait training.

15

SHORT CLINICAL CASE: OA OF THE KNEE

A 65-year-old woman has been suffering from right knee joint stiffness, aching pain, and limited movement that is worse when she rises in the morning or after inactivity. She has been taking acetaminophen (Tylenol) and other NSAIDs (Motrin or Advil) to cope with the pain.

An x-ray of her knees (Figure 15-39A) shows deterioration of articular cartilage in the right knee with narrowing of the joint space. See left knee for comparison. Surgery is recommended for TKR and was performed (see Figure 15-39B and C). Follow-up x-ray (Figure 15-39D) shows the prosthesis in place. After successful healing of the incision and removal of surgical clips, the patient had several months of PT and is walking normally without pain.

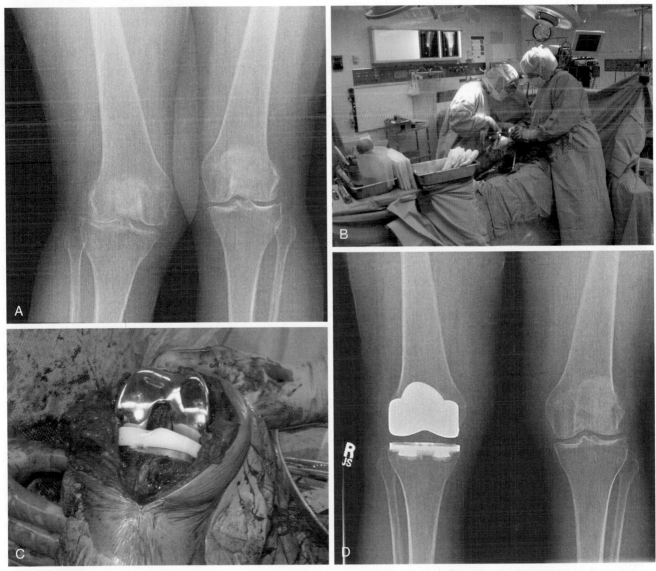

FIGURE 15-39   A, X-ray image of knees showing **osteoarthritis** in right knee. **B,** Patient undergoing **total knee replacement (TKR). C, Prosthetic device** in place. **D,** X-ray image of knees after TKR. *(A to D, Courtesy Dr. Sidra Ezrahi and Dr. Dennis Burke, Massachusetts General Hospital, Boston.)*

IN PERSON: NEUROLOGIC LYME DISEASE

This first-person account was written by a woman diagnosed with neurologic Lyme disease.

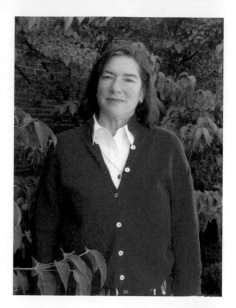

Weeding the garden and pruning the shrubs are chores I have willingly performed many, many times with no ill effects except an occasional backache, some scratches, and the misery of poison ivy. To avoid bending over I would often kneel or sit down in the garden. In late June 2009 I not only got quite dirty, but unknowingly connected with a deer tick and developed acute neurologic Lyme disease. One day shortly after working in the garden, I developed a fever and noticed a rash all over my trunk. I figured I had a summer virus that would go away in a few days. I never suspected Lyme disease. There was no tick and no telltale "bull's eye" pattern in the rash. Indeed, I did feel fine after just a few days—the respite lasted just one day, however. The next day, another rash appeared and I was feeling poorly. My husband Paul drove me to the doctor's office, where a physician's assistant took some blood and gave me a prescription for doxycycline. I had taken just four doses when my condition worsened alarmingly. I lost my balance and could barely lift my head up while lying in bed. My mental processing was slow and I was having difficulty with word finding—more than the usual memory lapses of a healthy 67-year-old. When I called the doctor's office, I was told to stop taking the doxycycline as I could be having an allergic reaction. We went back to the doctor's office, where I was put into an ambulance and sent to the hospital.

Neurologists and infectious disease specialists examined me over the next 5 days and ordered tests, including MRI (to rule out stroke), EMGs (there was delayed nerve conduction in my legs), and a lumbar puncture (spinal tap). The doctors first suspected Guillain-Barré syndrome, a scary paralyzing autoimmune disease, but the blood work indicated that my condition was Lyme disease. I learned that in Lyme disease, the bite of an infected deer tick releases a spirochete (bacterium) into the bloodstream and can affect joints, the nervous system, and other organs.

My treatment was a course of intravenous antibiotics. A PICC [peripherally inserted central catheter] was implanted in my upper arm leading to the superior vena cava to gain access to my bloodstream. I was given a prescription for a powerful antibiotic called ceftriaxone (although I was not allergic to the first antibiotic, doxycycline, after all) and I was allowed to go home. I reclined in a hospital bed in the dining room and received excellent nursing care from my husband, a college professor, who, luckily, could be at home with me 24/7. Paul carefully infused 2000 mg of ceftriaxone daily and kept the PICC sterile. He also held on to me in the bathtub where I sat on a bathtub chair and helped me wash my hair. Now that was an experience!

Physical therapists, occupational therapists, and visiting nurses came to the house over the next 3 weeks. I had to practice writing my name and the numbers 1 to 10. I had to coordinate getting out of bed and standing up—without holding onto the bed. I learned to walk and balance on one foot by holding onto the kitchen counter. I went up stairs slowly holding onto the banister for dear life and went down stairs on my bottom like a crab. Eventually, I had a walker and then a cane, and Paul escorted me on short trips around the top of the driveway. During this time, I also made follow-up visits to doctors. I had strength in my legs and feet but was still wobbly mentally and physically. One day I was able to walk by myself in the neighborhood—this a triumph for a woman who was used to a 3½-mile daily walk and long bike rides. I also exercised in the shallow end of our swimming pool. But I could not drive until the neurologic symptoms resolved. This was the only thing Paul and I fought about! The first time he took me for a "driving test," he flunked me. I was indignant, to say the least. In another few weeks, my timing and coordination had improved, and I was able to drive and begin to take long walks and bike rides once again. I also joined a health club to vary my exercise routine and have kept at it ever since. I no longer get down and dirty when I pull weeds in the garden.

Elizabeth F. Fideler, EdD, is an independent researcher and author of Women Still at Work (2012) and Men Still at Word (2014), Rowman & Littlefield publishing. She ahs two children and five grandchildren.

? EXERCISES

Remember to check your answers carefully with the Answers to Exercises, page 640.

A **Complete the following sentences.**

1. Bones are composed of a type of connective tissue called _____ tissue.

2. Bone cells are called _____.

3. The bones of a fetus are composed mainly of _____.

4. Immature bone cells called _____ produce bony tissue.

5. Large bone cells called _____ digest bone tissue to shape the bone and smooth it out.

6. Mineral substances needed for bone development are _____ and _____.

7. Round, small bone covering the knee joint is a/an _____ bone.

8. Shaft of a long bone is the _____.

9. Ends of a long bone are the _____.

10. Cartilaginous area at the end of a long bone where growth takes place is the _____.

11. Red bone marrow is found in spongy or _____ bone.

12. Yellow bone marrow is composed of _____ tissue.

13. The strong membrane surrounding the surface of a bone is the _____.

14. Hard, dense bone tissue lying under the periosteum is _____.

15. A series of canals containing blood vessels lie within the outer dense tissue of bone and are called the _____ canals.

16. A thin layer of cartilage covering the ends of bones at the joints is _____.

17. The _____ is a central, hollowed-out area in the shaft of long bones.

18. Two physicians who treat bones and bone diseases are a/an _____ and a/an _____.

19. A practitioner who manipulates the patient's spinal column to relieve pressure on nerves is a/an _____.

20. Medical doctor who specializes in restoring patients to functional activity after injuries to bones, nerves, and muscles is a/an _____.

15

B Match the cranial and facial bones with their meanings that follow.

ethmoid bone   maxilla   sphenoid bone
frontal bone   nasal bone   temporal bone
lacrimal bones   occipital bone   vomer
mandible   parietal bone   zygomatic bone

1. forms the roof and upper side parts of the skull _____

2. delicate bone, composed of spongy, cancellous tissue; supports the nasal cavity and orbits of the

   eye _____

3. forms the back and base of the skull _____

4. forms the forehead _____

5. bat-shaped bone extending behind the eyes to form the base of the skull _____

   _____

6. bone near the ear and connecting to the lower jaw _____

7. cheekbone _____

8. bone that supports the bridge of the nose _____

9. thin, flat bone forming the lower portion of the nasal septum _____

10. lower jawbone _____

11. upper jawbone _____

12. two paired bones, one located at the corner of each eye _____

C Identify the following parts associated with a vertebra. See Figure 15-7, page 588.

1. space through which the spinal cord passes: _____

2. piece of cartilage between two vertebrae: _____

3. posterior part of a vertebra: _____

4. anterior part of a vertebra: _____

D Name the five divisions of the spinal column.

1. _____

2. _____

3. _____

4. _____

5. _____

15

E **Give the medical names of the following bones.**

1. shoulder blade _____

2. upper arm bone _____

3. breastbone _____

4. thigh bone _____

5. finger bones _____

6. hand bones _____

7. forearm bone (little finger side) _____

8. forearm bone (thumb side) _____

9. collar bone _____

10. wrist bones _____

11. backbone _____

12. kneecap _____

13. shin bone (larger of two lower leg bones) _____

14. smaller of two lower leg bones _____

15. three parts of the pelvis _____, _____, and

_____

16. midfoot bones _____

F **Give the meanings of the following terms associated with bones.**

1. foramen magnum _____

2. calcaneus _____

3. acromion _____

4. xiphoid process _____

5. lamina _____

6. malleolus _____

7. acetabulum _____

8. pubic symphysis _____

9. olecranon _____

10. fontanelle _____

11. mastoid process _____

12. styloid process _____

15

G **Give the meanings of the following terms.**

1. osteogenesis _____

2. hypercalcemia _____

3. spondylosis _____

4. epiphyseal _____

5. decalcification _____

6. ossification _____

7. osteitis _____

8. costoclavicular _____

H **Build medical terms for the following definitions.**

1. pertaining to the shoulder blade _____

2. instrument to cut the skull _____

3. pertaining to the upper arm bone _____

4. pertaining to below the kneecap _____

5. softening of cartilage _____

6. pertaining to a toe bone _____

7. removal of hand bones _____

8. pertaining to the shin bone _____

9. pertaining to the heel bone _____

10. poor bone development _____

11. removal of the lamina of the vertebral arch _____

12. pertaining to the sacrum and ilium _____

15

I Give medical terms for the following.

1. formation of bone marrow _____

2. clubfoot _____

3. humpback _____

4. high levels of calcium in the blood _____

5. benign tumors arising from the bone surface _____

6. brittle bone disease _____

7. lateral curvature of the spine _____

8. anterior curvature of the spine _____

9. forward slipping (subluxation) of a vertebra over a lower vertebra _____

10. instrument to cut bone _____

J Give the meanings of the following terms.

1. osteoporosis _____

2. osteomyelitis _____

3. osteogenic sarcoma _____

4. crepitus _____

5. osteomalacia _____

6. abscess _____

7. osteopenia _____

8. Ewing sarcoma _____

9. metastatic bone lesion _____

10. compound fracture _____

11. simple fracture _____

12. open reduction _____

15

K **Complete the following sentences.**

1. Immovable joint, as in the skull bones, is called a _____.

2. Connective tissue that binds muscles to bones is a/an _____.

3. Another term for a joint is a/an _____.

4. Connective tissue that binds bones to other bones is a/an _____.

5. Fluid found in a joint is called _____.

6. The membrane that lines the joint cavity is the _____.

7. Sac of fluid near a joint is a/an _____.

8. Smooth cartilage that covers the surface of bones at joints is _____.

9. Surgical repair of a joint is called _____.

10. Inflammation surrounding a joint is known as _____.

L **Complete the following terms based on the definitions provided.**

1. inflammation of a tendon: _____ itis

2. tumor (benign) of cartilage: _____ oma

3. tumor (malignant) of cartilage: _____ oma

4. incision of a joint: arthr _____

5. softening of cartilage: chondro _____

6. abnormal condition of blood in the joint: _____ osis

7. inflammation of a sac of fluid near the joint: _____ itis

8. doctor who specializes in treatment of joint disorders: _____ logist

9. abnormal condition of a stiffened, immobile joint: _____ osis

10. suture of a tendon: ten _____

15

M Select from the list of terms to name the abnormal conditions that follow.

achondroplasia   dislocation   osteoarthritis
ankylosing spondylitis   ganglion cyst   rheumatoid arthritis
bunion   gouty arthritis   systemic lupus erythematosus
carpal tunnel syndrome   Lyme disease   tenosynovitis

1. an inherited condition in which the bones of the arms and the legs fail to grow normally

   because of a defect in cartilage and bone formation; type of dwarfism _____

2. degenerative joint disease; chronic inflammation of bones and joints _____

3. inflammation of joints caused by excessive uric acid in the body (hyperuricemia)

   _____

4. chronic joint disease; inflamed and painful joints owing to autoimmune reaction against normal

   joint tissue, and synovial membranes become swollen and thickened _____

5. tick-borne bacterium causes this condition marked by arthritis, myalgia, malaise, and

   neurologic and cardiac symptoms _____

6. abnormal swelling of a metatarsophalangeal joint _____

7. cystic mass arising from a tendon in the wrist _____

8. chronic, progressive arthritis with stiffening of joints, especially of the spine (vertebrae)

   _____

9. chronic inflammatory disease affecting not only the joints but also the skin (butterfly rash on

   the face), kidneys, heart, and lungs _____

10. inflammation of a tendon sheath _____

11. compression of the median nerve in the wrist as it passes through an area between a ligament,

    tendons, bones, and connective tissue _____

12. displacement of a bone from its joint _____

N Give the meanings of the following terms.

1. subluxation _____

2. arthrodesis _____

3. pyrexia _____

4. podagra _____

5. sciatica _____

15

6. herniation of an intervertebral disk _____

7. laminectomy _____

8. sprain _____

9. strain _____

10. hyperuricemia _____

11. fasciotomy _____

O **Circle the boldface term that best fits the given definition.**

1. fibrous membrane separating and enveloping muscles: **(fascia, flexion)**

2. movement away from the midline of the body: **(abduction, adduction)**

3. connection of the muscle to a stationary bone: **(insertion, origin)** of the muscle

4. connection of the muscle to a bone that moves: **(insertion, origin)** of the muscle

5. muscle that is connected to internal organs; involuntary muscle: **(skeletal, visceral)** muscle

6. muscle that is connected to bones; voluntary muscle: **(skeletal, visceral)** muscle

7. pain of many muscles: **(myositis, polymyalgia)**

8. pertaining to heart muscle: **(myocardial, myasthenia)**

9. process of recording electricity within muscles: **(muscle biopsy, electromyography)**

10. increase in development (size) of an organ or tissue: **(hypertrophy, atrophy)**

P **Match the term for muscle action in Column I with its meaning in Column II. Write the letter of your answer in the space provided.**

COLUMN I

1. extension   _____
2. rotation   _____
3. flexion   _____
4. adduction   _____
5. supination   _____
6. abduction   _____
7. pronation   _____
8. dorsiflexion   _____
9. plantar flexion   _____

COLUMN II

A. movement away from the midline
B. turning the palm downward
C. turning the palm upward
D. straightening of a flexed limb
E. downward movement of the foot
F. circular movement around an axis
G. bending a limb
H. movement toward the midline
I. upward movement of the foot

Q **Give the meanings of the following abnormal conditions affecting muscles.**

1. leiomyosarcoma _____

2. rhabdomyoma _____

3. polymyositis _____

4. fibromyalgia _____

5. muscular dystrophy _____

6. myasthenia gravis _____

7. amyotrophic lateral sclerosis _____

8. sarcopenia _____

R **Match the term in Column I with its meaning in Column II. Write the letter of your answer in the space provided.**

COLUMN I

1. antinuclear antibody test _____

2. serum creatine kinase _____

3. uric acid test _____

4. rheumatoid factor test _____

5. bone scan _____

6. muscle biopsy _____

7. arthroscopy _____

8. acetylcholine _____

9. calcium _____

10. arthrography _____

COLUMN II

A. Radioactive substance is injected and traced in dense, hard connective tissue.

B. Chemical found in myoneural space.

C. Test for presence of an antibody found in the serum of patients with rheumatoid arthritis.

D. Substance necessary for proper bone development.

E. Visual examination of a joint.

F. Test tells if patient has gouty arthritis.

G. Test tells if patient has systemic lupus erythematosus.

H. Removal of soft connective tissue for microscopic examination.

I. Process of taking x-ray pictures of a joint.

J. Elevated blood levels of this enzyme are found in muscular disorders.

15

S **Circle the terms in boldface that best complete the meaning of the sentences.**

1. Selma, a 40-year-old secretary, had been complaining of wrist pain with tingling sensations in her fingers for months. Dr. Ayres diagnosed her condition as (**osteomyelitis, rheumatoid arthritis, carpal tunnel syndrome**).

2. Bill was a marathon runner who developed compartment syndrome in his left lower leg (calf). He had severe pain, and his orthopedist recommended (**tenorrhaphy, arthroplasty, fasciotomy**) to cut through the fibrous connective tissue and relieve pressure. A skin graft was needed later to close the wound.

3. Sally was experiencing chronic muscle pain and stiffness in her shoulder, back, knees, and hips. Most of all, she was very tired all the time. Her doctor diagnosed her condition as (**myasthenia gravis, fibromyalgia, sarcopenia**) and prescribed medication for fatigue and pain plus physical therapy.

4. Paul had a skiing accident and tore ligaments in his knee. Dr. Miller recommended **(electromyography, hypertrophy, arthroscopic surgery)** to repair the ligaments.

5. For several months after her first pregnancy Elsie noticed a red rash on her face and cheeks. Her joints were giving her pain and she had a slight fever. Her ANA was elevated, and her doctor suspected that she had **(SLE, polymyositis, muscular dystrophy)**.

6. David injured his left knee while playing basketball. He was scheduled for arthroscopic repair of his **(ACL, SLE, TMJ)**. However, because of his height (6'7") and the length of the ligament, his **(rheumatologist, orthopedist, chiropractor)** decided to do "open" surgery.

7. James has significant lower back pain radiating down his left leg. This condition is called **(fibromyalgia, sciatica, talipes)**. MRI shows an intervertebral **(disk, bunion, exostosis)** impinging on spinal nerves at the **(L5–S1, C2–C3, T3–T5)** level. Bed rest produced no improvement. His orthopedist decided to perform a **(tenorrhaphy, microdiskectomy, bunionectomy)** to relieve pressure on his nerves.

8. Bruce spent 2 weeks hiking and vacationing on Nantucket Island. A week later he developed a "bull's eye" rash on his chest (from a tick bite), fever, muscle pain, and a swollen, tender right ankle. His physician ordered a blood test that revealed **(antigens, antibodies)** to a spirochete bacterium. The physician told Bruce he had contracted **(ankylosing spondylitis, polymyositis, Lyme disease)**.

9. Scott likes to eat rich food. Lately he has noticed pain and tenderness in his right toe, called **(talipes, podagra, rickets),** and also hard, lumpy deposits over his elbows. His doctor orders a serum uric acid test; the result is abnormally high, revealing **(hemarthrosis, hyperuricemia, hypercalcemia)**, consistent with a diagnosis of **(rheumatoid arthritis, gouty arthritis, osteoarthritis)**.

10. Sara, a 70-year-old widow, has persistent midback pain, and her **(CXR, ESR, EMG)** shows compression fractures of her **(scapula, femur, vertebrae)** and thinning of her bones. A bone density scan confirms the diagnosis of **(osteomyelitis, osteomalacia, osteoporosis)**, and her doctor prescribes calcium, vitamin D, and Fosamax.

T Give meanings for the abbreviations in Column I. Then select the letter in Column II of the best description/definition for each.

COLUMN I

1. ROM _____ _____

2. NSAID _____ _____

3. TMJ _____ _____

4. EMG _____ _____

5. ACL _____ _____

6. SLE _____ _____

7. C1 to C5 _____ _____

8. T1 to T12 _____ _____

9. THR _____ _____

10. ORIF _____ _____

COLUMN II

A. Connection between the lower jawbone and a bone of the skull

B. Band of fibrous tissue connecting bones in the knee

C. Bones of the spinal column in the chest region

D. Test of strength of electrical transmission within muscle

E. Autoimmune disease that affects joints, skin, and other body tissues

F. Measurement in degrees of a circle assesses the extent a joint can be flexed or extended

G. Bones of the spinal column in the neck region

H. Drug used to treat joint diseases

I. Procedure to repair compound fracture

J. Arthroplasty

U **Match images A to F in Figure 15-40 with the following descriptions, and give a medical term for the abnormal condition.**

1. Children who are born with a condition of muscle deterioration and wasting have winged scapulae: _____

2. Children are born with this deformity of the talus: _____

3. This deformity is often the result of a chronic, inflammatory, autoimmune disorder that affects joints, leading to bony ankylosis and inflamed, thickened synovial membranes:

   _____

4. Bleeding disorders can lead to this accumulation of blood in and around a joint:

   _____

5. Inflammation of a bursa causes this abnormality: _____

6. Fluid-filled cyst arising from joint capsules or tendons: _____

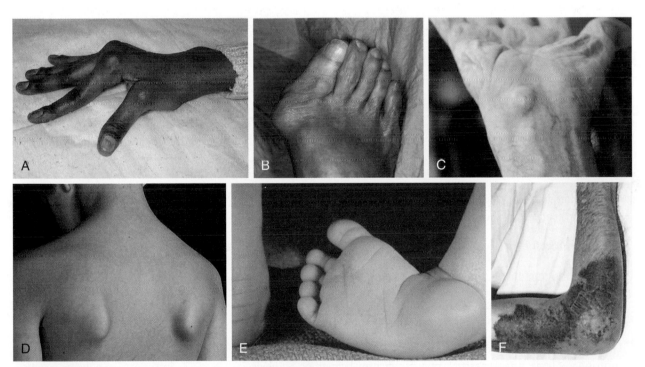

FIGURE 15-40   *A, From Swartz MH: Textbook of Physical Diagnosis, History and Examination, 5th ed., Philadelphia, Saunders, 2006; **B** and **E,** from Canale ST, Beaty JH: Campbell's Operative Orthopaedics, 11th ed., St. Louis, Mosby, 2008; **C,** courtesy Dr. Norman M. Simon; **D,** from Zitelli BJ, Davis HW: Atlas of Pediatric Physical Diagnosis, 5th ed., St. Louis, Mosby, 2007; **F,** from Moll JM: Rheumatology, 2nd ed., London, Churchill Livingstone, 1997.*

15

ANSWERS TO EXERCISES

A

1. osseous
2. osteocytes
3. cartilage
4. osteoblasts
5. osteoclasts
6. calcium, phosphorus
7. sesamoid
8. diaphysis
9. epiphyses
10. epiphyseal plate
11. cancellous or trabecular
12. fat
13. periosteum
14. compact bone
15. haversian
16. articular cartilage
17. medullary cavity
18. orthopedist, osteopath
19. chiropractor
20. physiatrist

B

1. parietal bone
2. ethmoid bone
3. occipital bone
4. frontal bone
5. sphenoid bone
6. temporal bone
7. zygomatic bone
8. nasal bone
9. vomer
10. mandible
11. maxilla
12. lacrimal bones

C

1. neural canal
2. intervertebral disk
3. vertebral arch
4. vertebral body

D

1. cervical
2. thoracic
3. lumbar
4. sacral
5. coccygeal

E

1. scapula
2. humerus
3. sternum
4. femur
5. phalanges
6. metacarpals
7. ulna
8. radius
9. clavicle
10. carpals
11. vertebral column
12. patella
13. tibia
14. fibula
15. ilium, ischium, pubis
16. metatarsals

F

1. opening of the occipital bone through which the spinal cord passes
2. heel bone; largest of the tarsal bones
3. lateral extension of the scapula
4. lower portion of the sternum
5. portion of the vertebral arch
6. the bulge on either side of the ankle joint; the lower end of the fibula is the lateral malleolus, and the lower end of the tibia is the medial malleolus
7. depression in the pelvis into which the femur fits
8. area of convergence of the two pubis bones, at the midline
9. bony process at the proximal end of the ulna; elbow joint
10. soft spot between the bones of the skull in an infant
11. round process on the temporal bone behind the ear
12. pole-like process projecting downward from the temporal bone

G

1. formation of bone; osteogenesis imperfecta is known as brittle bone disease
2. excessive calcium in the blood
3. abnormal condition of the vertebrae; degenerative changes in the spine
4. pertaining to the epiphysis
5. removal of calcium from bones
6. formation of bone
7. inflammation of bone; osteitis deformans (Paget disease) causes deformed bones such as an enlarged skull
8. pertaining to the ribs and clavicle

H

1. scapular
2. craniotome
3. humeral
4. subpatellar
5. chondromalacia
6. phalangeal
7. metacarpectomy
8. tibial
9. calcaneal
10. osteodystrophy
11. laminectomy
12. sacroiliac

15

I

1. myelopoiesis
2. talipes
3. kyphosis
4. hypercalcemia

5. exostoses
6. osteogenesis imperfecta
7. scoliosis

8. lordosis
9. spondylolisthesis
10. osteotome

J

1. increased porosity in bone; decrease in bone density
2. inflammation of bone and bone marrow
3. cancerous tumor of bone; osteoblasts multiply at the ends of long bones
4. crackling sensation as broken bones move against each other

5. softening of bones; rickets in children due to loss of calcium in bones
6. collection of pus
7. deficiency of bone; precursor of osteoporosis
8. malignant tumor of bone in children, often involving the entire shaft of a long bone

9. malignant tumor that has spread to bone from the breast, lung, kidney, or prostate gland
10. break in bone with wound in skin
11. break in bone without wound in skin
12. bone is put in proper place after incision of the skin

K

1. suture joint; a synovial joint is a freely movable joint
2. tendon
3. articulation

4. ligament
5. synovial fluid
6. synovial membrane
7. bursa

8. articular cartilage
9. arthroplasty
10. periarthritis

L

1. tendinitis or tendonitis
2. chondroma
3. chondrosarcoma
4. arthrotomy

5. chondromalacia
6. hemarthrosis
7. bursitis

8. rheumatologist
9. ankylosis
10. tenorrhaphy

M

1. achondroplasia
2. osteoarthritis
3. gouty arthritis
4. rheumatoid arthritis

5. Lyme disease
6. bunion
7. ganglion cyst
8. ankylosing spondylitis

9. systemic lupus erythematosus
10. tenosynovitis
11. carpal tunnel syndrome
12. dislocation

N

1. partial or incomplete displacement of a bone from the joint
2. surgical fixation of a joint (binding it together by fusing the joint surfaces)
3. fever; increase in body temperature
4. pain in a big toe from gouty arthritis

5. pain radiating from the back to the leg (along the sciatic nerve); most commonly caused by a protruding intervertebral disk
6. protrusion of a disk into the neural canal or the spinal nerves
7. removal of a portion of the vertebral arch (lamina) to relieve

pressure from a protruding intervertebral disk
8. trauma to a joint with pain, swelling, and injury to ligaments
9. overstretching of a muscle
10. high levels of uric acid in the bloodstream; present in gouty arthritis
11. incision of fascia

O

1. fascia
2. abduction
3. origin of the muscle
4. insertion of the muscle

5. visceral muscle
6. skeletal muscle
7. polymyalgia

8. myocardial
9. electromyography
10. hypertrophy

P

1. D
2. F
3. G

4. H
5. C
6. A

7. B
8. I
9. E

15

Q

1. malignant tumor of smooth (involuntary, visceral) muscle
2. benign tumor of striated (voluntary, skeletal) muscle
3. inflammation of many muscles; polymyositis rheumatica is a chronic inflammatory condition causing muscle weakness and pain
4. pain of muscle and fibrous tissue (especially of the back); also called fibrositis or rheumatism
5. group of inherited muscular diseases marked by progressive weakness and degeneration of muscles without nerve involvement
6. loss of strength of muscles (often with paralysis) because of a defect at the connection between the nerve and the muscle cell
7. muscles degenerate (paralysis occurs) owing to degeneration of nerves in the spinal cord and lower region of the brain; Lou Gehrig disease
8. deficiency of flesh (muscle mass)

R

1. G
2. J
3. F
4. C
5. A
6. H
7. E
8. B
9. D
10. I

S

1. carpal tunnel syndrome
2. fasciotomy
3. fibromyalgia
4. arthroscopic surgery
5. SLE
6. ACL; orthopedist
7. sciatica; disk; L5–S1; microdiskectomy
8. antibodies; Lyme disease
9. podagra; hyperuricemia; gouty arthritis
10. CXR; vertebrae; osteoporosis

T

1. range of motion: F
2. nonsteroidal anti-inflammatory drug: H
3. temporomandibular joint: A
4. electromyography: D
5. anterior cruciate ligament: B
6. systemic lupus erythematosus: E
7. first cervical vertebra to fifth cervical vertebra: G
8. first thoracic vertebra to twelfth thoracic vertebra: C
9. total hip replacement: J
10. open reduction, internal fixation: I

U

1. D: winged scapulae in muscular dystrophy
2. E: clubfoot—talipes
3. A: rheumatoid arthritis
4. F: hemarthrosis
5. B: bunion
6. C: ganglion cyst

Answers to Practical Applications

Operating Room Schedule
1. D
2. F
3. G
4. B
5. A
6. C
7. H
8. E

15

PRONUNCIATION OF TERMS

To test your understanding of the terminology in this chapter, write the meaning of each term in the space provided. In addition, you may wish to cover the terms and write them by looking at your definitions. Make sure your spelling is correct. The page number after each term indicates where it is defined or used in the book, so you can easily check your responses. You will find complete definitions for all of these terms and their audio pronunciations on the Evolve website.

Pronunciation Guide

ā as in āpe   ă as in ăpple
ē as in ēven   ĕ as in ĕvery
ī as in īce   ĭ as in ĭnterest
ō as in ōpen   ŏ as in pŏt
ū as in ūnit   ŭ as in ŭnder

Terms Related to Bones

TERM	PRONUNCIATION	MEANING
acetabular (598)	ă-cĕ-TĂB-ū-lăr	
acetabulum (594)	ăs-ĕ-TĂB-ū-lŭm	
acromion (594)	ă-KRŌ-mē-ŏn	
articular cartilage (594)	ăr-TĬK-ū-lăr KĂR-tĭ-lăj	
bone (594)	BŌN	
bone depression (594)	BŌN dē-PRĔ-shŭn	
bone process (594)	BŌN PRŎ-sĕs	
calcaneal (598)	kăl-KĀ-nē-ăl	
calcaneus (598)	kăl-KĀ-nē-ŭs	
calcium (594)	KĂL-sē-ŭm	
cancellous bone (594)	KĂN-sĕ-lŭs bōn	
carpals (598)	KĂR-pălz	
cartilage (594)	KĂR-tĭ-lăj	
cervical vertebrae (589)	SĔR-vĭ-kăl VĔR-tĕ-brā	
chondrocostal (599)	kŏn-drō-KŎS-tăl	
clavicle (599)	KLĂV-ĭ-kl	
coccyx (589)	KŎK-sĭks	
collagen (594)	KŎL-ă-jĕn	
compact bone (594)	KŎM-păkt bōn	
cranial bones (594)	KRĀ-nē-ăl bōnz	
craniotome (599)	KRĀ-nē-ō-tōm	
craniotomy (599)	krā-nē-ŎT-ō-mē	

TERM	PRONUNCIATION	MEANING
crepitus (601)	KRĚP-ĭ-tŭs	_____
decalcification (596)	dē-kăl-sĭ-fĭ-KĀ-shŭn	_____
diaphysis (594)	dī-ĂF-ĭ-sĭs	_____
disk (594)	dĭsk	_____
epiphyseal plate (594)	ĕp-ĭ-FĬZ-ē-ăl plāt	_____
epiphysis (594)	ĕ-PĬF-ĭ-sĭs	_____
ethmoid bone (585)	ĔTH-moyd bōn	_____
Ewing sarcoma (600)	Ū-ĭng săr-KŌ-mă	_____
exostosis (600)	ĕk-sŏs-TŌ-sĭs	_____
facial bones (594)	FĀ-shăl bōnz	_____
femoral (599)	FĔM-ŏr-ăl	_____
femur (599)	FĒ-mŭr	_____
fibula (599)	FĬB-ū-lă	_____
fibular (599)	FĬB-ū-lăr	_____
fontanelle (594)	fŏn-tă-NĔL	_____
foramen magnum (594)	fōr-Ā-mĕn MĂG-nŭm	_____
fracture (600)	FRĂK-shur	_____
frontal bone (585)	FRŎN-tăl bōn	_____
haversian canals (595)	hă-VĔR-zhăn kă-NĂLZ	_____
humeral (599)	HŪ-mĕr-ăl	_____
humerus (599)	HŪ-mĕr-ŭs	_____
hypercalcemia (596)	hī-pĕr-kăl-SĒ-mē-ă	_____
iliac (599)	ĬL-ē-ăk	_____
ilium (599)	ĬL-ē-ŭm	_____
ischial (599)	ĬSH-ē-ăl *or* ĬS-kē-ăl	_____
ischium (599)	ĬSH-ē-ŭm *or* ĬS-kē-ŭm	_____
kyphosis (596)	kī-FŌ-sĭs	_____
lacrimal bones (586)	LĂ-krĭ-măl bōnz	_____
lamina (588)	LĂM-ĭ-nă	_____
laminectomy (596)	lăm-ĭ-NĔK-tō-mē	_____
lordosis (596)	lŏr-DŌ-sĭs	_____

15

TERM	PRONUNCIATION	MEANING
lumbar vertebrae (589)	LŬM-băr VĔR-tĕ-brā	
lumbosacral (597)	lŭm-bō-SĀ-krăl	
malleolar (599)	mă-LĒ-ō-lăr	
malleolus (595)	măl-LĒ-ō-lŭs	
mandible (599)	MĂN-dĭ-bl	
mandibular (599)	măn-DĬB-ū-lăr	
manubrium (595)	mă-NOO-brē-ŭm	
mastoid process (595)	MĂS-toyd PRŎS-ĕs	
maxilla (599)	măk-SĬL-ă	
maxillary (599)	măk-sĭ-LĂR-ē	
medullary cavity (595)	MĔD-ū-lăr-ē KĂ-vĭ-tē	
metacarpals (599)	mĕt-ă-KĂR-pălz	
metacarpectomy (599)	mĕt-ă-kăr-PĔK-tō-mē	
metaphysis (595)	mĕ-TĂ-fĭ-sĭs	
metatarsalgia (599)	mĕt-ă-tăr-SĂL-jă	
metatarsals (599)	mĕt ă-TĂR-sălz	
myelopoiesis (597)	mī-ĕ-lō-poy-Ē-sĭs	
nasal bones (586)	NĀ-zăl bōnz	
occipital bone (585)	ŏk-SĬP-ĭ-tăl bōn	
olecranal (599)	ō-LĔK-ră-năl	
olecranon (595)	ō-LĔK-ră-nŏn	
orthopedics (597)	ŏr-thō-PĒ-dĭks	
osseous tissue (595)	ŎS-ē-ŭs TĬSH-ū	
ossification (595)	ŏs-ĭ-fĭ-KĀ-shŭn	
osteitis (597)	ŏs-tē-Ī-tĭs	
osteoblast (595)	ŎS-tē-ō-blăst	
osteoclast (595)	ŎS-tē-ō-klăst	
osteodystrophy (597)	ŏs-tē-ō-DĬS-trō-fē	
osteogenesis imperfecta (597)	ŏs-tē-ō-JĔN-ĕ-sĭs ĭm-pĕr-FĔK-tă	
osteogenic sarcoma (602)	ŏs-tē-ō-JĔN-ĭk săr-KŌ-mă	

TERM	PRONUNCIATION	MEANING
osteomalacia (602)	ŏs-tē-ō-mă-LĀ-shă	
osteomyelitis (602)	ŏs-tē-ō-mī-ĕ-LĪ-tĭs	
osteopenia (602)	ŏs-tē-ō-PĒ-nē-ă	
osteoporosis (602)	ŏs-tē-ō-pŏr-Ō-sĭs	
osteotome (598)	ŎS-tē-ō-tōm	
parietal bone (585)	pă-RĪ-ĕ-tăl bōn	
patella (599)	pă-TĔL-ă	
pelvic (599)	PEL-vic	
periosteum (595)	pĕ-rē-ŎS-tē-ŭm	
peroneal (599)	pĕr-ō-NĒ-ăl	
phalangeal (599)	fă-lăn-JĒ-ăl	
phalanges (600)	fă-LĂN-jēz	
phosphorus (595)	FŎS-fō-rŭs	
physiatrist (595)	fĭ-ZĪ-ă-trĭst	
pubic (600)	PŪ-bĭk	
pubic symphysis (595)	PŪ-bĭk SĬM-fĭ-sĭs	
pubis (600)	PŪ-bĭs	
radial (600)	RĀ-dē-ăl	
radius (600)	RĀ-dē-ŭs	
red bone marrow (595)	rĕd bōn MĂ-rō	
reduction (601)	rĕ-DŬK-shŭn	
ribs (595)	rĭbz	
sacral vertebrae (589)	SĀ-krăl VĔR-tĕ-brā	
scapula (600)	SKĂP-ū-lă	
scapular (600)	SKĂP-ŭ-lăr	
scoliosis (597)	skō-lē-Ō-sĭs	
sella turcica (595)	SĔ-lă TŬR-sĭ-kă	
sinus (595)	SĪ-nŭs	
sphenoid bone (585)	SFĔ-noyd bōn	
spondylolisthesis (598)	spŏn-dĭ-lō-lĭs-THĒ-sĭs	
spondylosis (598)	spŏn-dĭ-LŌ-sĭs	

15

TERM	PRONUNCIATION	MEANING
sternum (600)	STĔR-nŭm	
styloid process (595)	STĪ-loyd PRŎS-ĕs	
subcostal (599)	sŭb-KŎS-tăl	
supraclavicular (598)	soo-pră-klă-VĬK-ū-lăr	
suture (595)	SOO-tŭr	
talipes (604)	TĂL-ĭ-pēz	
tarsals (604)	TĂR-sălz	
tarsectomy (600)	tăr-SĔK-tō-mē	
temporal bone (585)	TĔM-pōr-ăl bōn	
temporomandibular joint (595)	tĕm-pŏr-ō-măn-DĬB-ŭ-lăr joynt	
thoracic vertebrae (589)	thō-RĂS-ĭk VĔR-tĕ-brā	
tibia (600)	TĬB-ē-ă	
tibial (600)	TĬB-ē-ăl	
trabeculae (595)	tră-BĔK-ū-lē	
ulna (600)	ŬL-nă	
ulnar (600)	ŬL-năr	
vertebra; vertebrae (595)	VĔR-tĕ-bră; VĔR-tĕ-brā	
vertebroplasty (598)	vĕr-TĒ-brō-plăs-tē	
vomer (586)	VŌ-mĕr	
xiphoid process (595)	ZĬF-oyd PRŎS-ĕs	
yellow bone marrow (595)	YĔ-lō bōn MĂ-rō	
zygomatic bones (586)	zī-gō-MĂ-tĭk bōnz	

Terms Related to Joints and Muscles

TERM	PRONUNCIATION	MEANING
abduction (616)	ăb-DŬK-shŭn	
achondroplasia (606)	ā-kŏn-drō-PLĀ-zē-ă	
adduction (616)	ă-DŬK-shŭn	
amyotrophic lateral sclerosis (618)	ā-mī-ō-TRŌ-fĭk LĂT-ĕr-ăl sklĕ-RŌ-sĭs	

15

TERM	PRONUNCIATION	MEANING
ankylosing spondylitis (608)	ăng-kĭ-LŌ-sĭng spŏn-dĭ-LĪ-tĭs	
ankylosis (606)	ăng-kĭ-LŌ-sĭs	
arthrodesis (607)	ăr-thrō-DĒ-sĭs	
arthrotomy (606)	ăr-THRŎT-ō-mē	
articular cartilage (605)	ăr-TĬK-ū-lăr KĂR-tĭ-lăj	
articulation (605)	ăr-tĭk-ū-LĀ-shŭn	
atrophy (618)	ĂT-rō-fē	
bunion (609)	BŬN-yŭn	
bursa; bursae (605)	BŬR-să; BŬR-sē	
bursitis (606)	bŭr-SĪ-tis	
carpal tunnel syndrome (610)	KĂR-păl TŬN-nĕl SĬN-drōm	
chondrosarcoma (606)	kŏn-drō-SAR-cōma	
chondromalacia (606)	kŏn-drō-mă-LĀ-shă	
dislocation (610)	dĭs-lō-KĀ-shŭn	
dorsiflexion (616)	dŏr-sē-FLĔK-shŭn	
extension (616)	ĕk-STĔN-shŭn	
fascia (616)	FĂSH-ē-ă	
fasciotomy (617)	făsh-e-ŎT-tō-mē	
fibromyalgia (617)	fī-brō-mī-ĂL-jă	
flexion (616)	FLĔK-shŭn	
ganglion cyst (610)	GĂNG-lē-ŏn sĭst	
gouty arthritis (608)	GŎW-tē ăr-THRĪ-tĭs	
hemarthrosis (606)	hĕm-ăr-THRŌ-sĭs	
herniation of a intervertebral disk (611)	hĕr-nē-Ā-shŭn of a ĭn-tĕr-vĕr-TĒ-brăl dĭsk	
hydrarthrosis (606)	hī-drăr-THRŌ-sĭs	
hypertrophy (618)	hī-PĔR-trō-fē	
hyperuricemia (608)	hī-pĕr-ŭr-ĭ-SĒ-mē-ă	
leiomyoma (617)	lī-ō-mī-Ō-mă	
leiomyosarcoma (617)	lī-ō-mī-ō-săr-KŌ-mă	

TERM	PRONUNCIATION	MEANING
ligament (605)	LĬG-ă-mĕnt	
ligamentous (606)	lĭg-ă-MĔN-tŭs	
Lyme disease (612)	līm dĭ-ZĒZ	
meniscus (605)	mĕ-NĬS-kŭs	
muscular dystrophy (619)	MŬS-kū-lăr DĬS-trŏ-fē	
myalgia (618)	mī-ĂL-jă	
myasthenia gravis (618)	mī-ăs-THĒ-nē-ă GRĂ-vĭs	
myopathy (618)	mī-ŎP-ă-thē	
myositis (618)	mī-ō-SĪ-tĭs	
osteoarthritis (608)	ŏs-tē-ō-ăr-THRĪ-tĭs	
plantar flexion (618)	PLĂN-tăr FLĔK-shun	
podagra (608)	pō-DĂG-ră	
polyarthritis (606)	pŏl-ē-ărth-RĪ-tĭs	
polymyalgia (619)	pŏl-ē-mī-ĂL-jă	
polymyositis (619)	pŏl-ē-mī-ō-SĪ-tĭs	
pronation (616)	prō-NĀ-shŭn	
pyrexia (608)	pī-RĔK-sē-ă	
rhabdomyoma (618)	răb-dō-mī-Ō-mă	
rhabdomyosarcoma (608)	răb-dō-mī-ō-săr-KŌ-mă	
rheumatoid arthritis (608)	ROO-mă-toyd ăr-THRĪ-tĭs	
rheumatologist (607)	roo-mă-TŎL-ō-jĭst	
rotation (616)	rō-TĀ-shŭn	
sarcopenia (618)	săr-kō-PĒ-nē-ă	
spinal stenosis (607)	SPĪ-năl stĕ-NŌ-sĭs	
sprain (612)	sprān	
strain (612)	strān	
striated muscle (616)	STRĪ-ā-tĕd MŬS-l	
subluxation (610)	sŭb-lŭk-SĀ-shŭn	
supination (616)	soo-pĭ-NĀ-shŭn	
suture joint (605)	SOO-chŭr joint	
synovial cavity (605)	sĭ-NŌ-vē-ăl KĂV-ĭ-tē	

15

TERM	PRONUNCIATION	MEANING
synovial fluid (605)	sĭ-NŌ-vē-ăl FLOO-ĭd	_____
synovial joint (605)	sĭ-NŌ-vē-ăl joint	_____
synovial membrane (605)	sĭ-NŌ-vē-ăl MĔM-brān	_____
synovitis (607)	sĭn-ō-VĪ-tĭs	_____
systemic lupus erythematosus (612)	sĭs-TĔM-ĭk LOO-pŭs ĕ-rĭ-thĕ-mă-TŌ-sŭs	_____
tendinitis (607)	tĕn-dĭ-NĪ-tĭs	_____
tendon (605)	TĔN-dŭn	_____
tenorrhaphy (607)	tĕn-ŎR-ă-fē	_____
tenosynovitis (607)	tĕn-ō-sĭ-nō-VĪ-tĭs	_____
visceral muscle (616)	VĬS-ĕr-ăl MŬS-l	_____

Laboratory Tests and Clinical Procedures

TERM	PRONUNCIATION	MEANING
antinuclear antibody test (619)	ăn-tē-NŪ-klē-ăr ĂN-tĭ-bŏd-ē tĕst	_____
arthrocentesis (620)	ăr-thrō-sĕn-TĒ-sĭs	_____
arthrography (620)	ăr-THRŎG-ră-fē	_____
arthroplasty (620)	ăr-thrō-PLĂS-tē	_____
arthroscopy (620)	ăr-THRŎS-kō-pē	_____
bone density test (621)	bōn DĔN-sĭ-tē tĕst	_____
bone scan (622)	bōn skăn	_____
diskography (622)	dĭsk-ŎG-ră-fē	_____
electromyography (622)	ē-lĕk-trō-mī-ŎG-ră-fē	_____
erythrocyte sedimentation rate (619)	ĕ-RĬTH-rō-sīt sĕd-ĭ-mĕn-TĀ-shŭn rāt	_____
muscle biopsy (622)	MŬS-l BĪ-ŏp-sē	_____
rheumatoid factor test (619)	ROO-mă-tŏyd FĂK-tŏr tĕst	_____
serum calcium (619)	SĔR-ŭm KĂL-sē-ŭm tĕst	_____
serum creatine kinase (619)	SĔR-ŭm KRĒ-ă-tĭn KĪ-nās	_____
uric acid test (620)	ŪR-ĭk ĂS-ĭd tĕst	_____

15

REVIEW SHEET

Write the meanings of the word parts in the spaces provided. Check your answers with the information in the chapter or in the *Glossary (Medical Word Parts—English)* at the end of the book.

Combining Forms

COMBINING FORM	MEANING	COMBINING FORM	MEANING
acetabul/o		ligament/o	
ankyl/o		lord/o	
arthr/o		lumb/o	
articul/o		malleol/o	
burs/o		mandibul/o	
calc/o		maxill/o	
calcane/o		metacarp/o	
calci/o		metatars/o	
carp/o		my/o	
cervic/o		myel/o	
chondr/o		myocardi/o	
clavicul/o		myos/o	
coccyg/o		olecran/o	
cost/o		orth/o	
crani/o		oste/o	
fasci/o		patell/o	
femor/o		ped/o	
fibr/o		pelv/o	
fibul/o		perone/o	
humer/o		phalang/o	
ili/o		plant/o	
ischi/o		pub/o	
kyph/o		radi/o	
lamin/o		rhabdomy/o	
leiomy/o		rheumat/o	

15

COMBINING FORM	MEANING	COMBINING FORM	MEANING
sacr/o		tars/o	
sarc/o		ten/o	
scapul/o		tendin/o	
scoli/o		thorac/o	
spondyl/o		tibi/o	
stern/o		uln/o	
synov/o		vertebr/o	

Suffixes

SUFFIX	MEANING	SUFFIX	MEANING
-algia		-penia	
-asthenia		-physis	
-blast		-plasty	
-clast		-porosis	
-desis		-stenosis	
-emia		-tome	
-listhesis		-trophy	
-malacia			

Prefixes

PREFIX	MEANING	PREFIX	MEANING
a-, an-		hyper-	
ab-		meta-	
ad-		peri-	
dia-		poly-	
dorsi-		sub-	
epi-		supra-	
exo-		sym-	

15

16

Skin

Chapter Sections:

CHAPTER GOALS

- Name the layers of the skin and the accessory structures associated with the skin.
- Build medical words using the combining forms that are related to the specialty of dermatology.
- Identify lesions, signs and symptoms, and pathologic conditions that relate to the skin.
- Describe laboratory tests and clinical procedures that pertain to the skin, and recognize relevant abbreviations.
- Apply your new knowledge to understanding medical terms in their proper contexts, such as medical reports and records.

INTRODUCTION

The skin and its accessory structures (hair, nails, and glands) make up the **integumentary system** of the body. Integument means covering, and the skin (weighing 8 to 10 pounds and extending over an area of 22 square feet in an average adult) is the outer covering for the body. It is, however, more than a simple body covering. This complex system of specialized tissues contains glands that secrete several types of fluids, nerves that carry impulses, and blood vessels that aid in the regulation of the body temperature.

The skin has many important functions:

First, as a protective membrane over the entire body, the skin guards the deeper tissues of the body against excessive loss of water, salts, and heat and against invasion of pathogens and their toxins. Specialized cells (Langerhans cells) react to the presence of antigens and have an immune function.

Second, the skin contains two types of glands that produce important secretions. These glands in the skin are the **sebaceous glands** and the **sweat glands.** Sebaceous glands produce **sebum,** an oily secretion, and sweat glands produce **sweat,** a watery secretion. Sebum and sweat pass to the outer edges of the skin through ducts and leave the skin through pores (openings). Sebum lubricates the surface of the skin, and sweat cools the body as it evaporates from the skin surface.

Third, nerve fibers under the skin are receptors for sensations such as pain, temperature, pressure, and touch. Thus, the body's adjustment to the environment depends on sensory messages relayed to the brain and spinal cord by sensitive nerve endings in the skin.

Fourth, different tissues in the skin maintain body temperature (thermoregulation). Nerve fibers coordinate thermoregulation by carrying messages to the skin from heat centers in the brain that are sensitive to increases and decreases in body temperature. Impulses from these fibers cause blood vessels to dilate to bring blood to the surface and cause sweat glands to produce the watery secretion that carries heat away.

ANATOMY OF THE SKIN

Figure 16-1A shows three layers of the skin. Label them from the outer surface inward:

Epidermis [1]—a thin, cellular membrane layer; containing keratin
Dermis [2]—dense, fibrous, connective tissue layer; containing collagen
Subcutaneous layer [3]—thick, fat-containing tissue

EPIDERMIS

The epidermis is the outermost totally cellular layer of the skin. It is composed of **squamous epithelium.** Epithelium is the covering of both the internal and the external surfaces of the body. Squamous epithelial cells are flat and scale-like. In the outer layer of the skin, these cells are arranged in several layers **(strata)** to form **stratified squamous epithelium.**

The epidermis lacks blood vessels, lymphatic vessels, and connective tissue (elastic fibers, cartilage, fat) and is therefore dependent on the deeper dermis layer and its rich network of capillaries for nourishment. In fact, oxygen and nutrients seep out of the capillaries in the dermis, pass through tissue fluid, and supply nourishment to the lower layers of the epidermis.

Figure 16-1B illustrates the multilayered cells of the epidermis. The deepest layer is called the **basal layer** [4]. The cells in the basal layer are constantly growing and multiplying and are the source of all the other cells in the epidermis. As the basal layer cells divide,

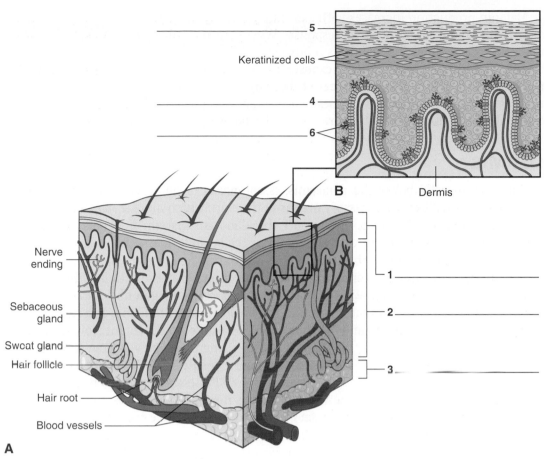

FIGURE 16-1 Skin. A, Three layers of the skin. B, Epidermis.

they are pushed upward and away from the blood supply of the dermal layer by a steady stream of younger cells. In their movement toward the most superficial layer of the epidermis, called the **stratum corneum** [5], the cells flatten, shrink, lose their nuclei, and die, becoming filled with a hard protein material called **keratin.** The cells are then called keratinocytes, reflecting their composition of keratin. Finally, within 3 to 4 weeks after beginning as a basal cell in the deepest part of the epidermis, the keratinized cell is sloughed off from the surface of the skin. The epidermis is thus constantly renewing itself, with cells dying at the same rate at which they are replaced. This process slows with age.

The basal layer of the epidermis contains special cells called **melanocytes** [6]. Melanocytes contain a pigment called **melanin** that is transferred to other epidermal cells and gives color to the skin. ◣ The number of melanocytes in all human races is the same, but the amount of melanin within each cell accounts for the color differences among the races. Individuals with darker skin possess more melanin within the melanocytes, not a greater number of melanocytes. Individuals who are incapable of forming melanin are called **albinos.** Skin and hair are white. In albinos, eye color varies, ranging from red to blue to brown, depending on the amount of melanin present in the iris (pigmented portion of the eye). Occulocutaneous albinism affects eyes, skin, and hair, whereas ocular albinism affects the eyes only.

Types of Melanin: Eumelanin and Pheomelanin

Eumelanin (eu- = true) is more common and is a brown-black pigment. **Pheomelanin** (pheo- = dusky) is a red-yellow pigment. People with darker skin have more eumelanin, whereas people with lighter skin have more pheomelanin. Pheomelanin doesn't protect the skin from damaging ultraviolet rays and makes lighter-skinned people, and especially redheads, more susceptible to skin cancer.

Melanin production increases with exposure to strong ultraviolet light, and this creates a suntan, which is a protective response. When the melanin cannot absorb all of the ultraviolet rays, the skin becomes sunburned and inflamed (redness, swelling, and pain). Over a period of years, excessive exposure to sun tends to cause wrinkles, permanent pigmentary changes, and even cancer of the skin. Because dark-skinned people have more melanin, they acquire fewer wrinkles and they are less likely to develop the types of skin cancer that are associated with ultraviolet light exposure.

DERMIS

The dermis, directly below the epidermis, is composed of blood vessels and lymph and nerve fibers, as well as the accessory organs of the skin, which are the hair follicles, sweat glands, and sebaceous glands. To support the elaborate system of nerves, vessels, and glands, the dermis contains connective tissue cells and fibers that account for the extensibility and elasticity of the skin.

The dermis is composed of interwoven **elastin** (protein that is elastic and helps skin to return to its original position when pinched or poked) and **collagen** fibers. Collagen (**colla** = glue) is a fibrous protein material found in bone, cartilage, tendons, and ligaments, as well as in the skin. It is tough and resistant but also flexible. In the infant, collagen is loose and delicate; it becomes harder as the body ages. During pregnancy, overstretching of the skin with weight gain may break the elastin fibers, resulting in linear markings called **striae** ("stretch marks") on the woman's abdomen and elsewhere. Collagen fibers support and protect the blood and nerve networks that pass through the dermis. Collagen diseases affect connective tissues of the body. An example of a connective tissue collagen disorder is scleroderma.

SUBCUTANEOUS LAYER

The subcutaneous layer (epidermis and dermis are the cutaneous layers) specializes in the formation of fat. **Adipocytes** (fat cells) are predominant in the subcutaneous layer, and they manufacture and store large quantities of fat. Fat deposition varies in different areas of the body and among individual people. Functionally, this layer of the skin is important in protection of the deeper tissues of the body, as a heat insulator, and for energy storage.

ACCESSORY STRUCTURES OF THE SKIN

HAIR

A hair fiber is composed of a tightly fused meshwork of cells filled with the hard protein called **keratin.** Hair growth is similar to the growth of the epidermal layer of the skin. Deep-lying cells in the hair root (Figure 16-2) produce keratinized cells that move upward through **hair follicles** (sacs within which each hair fiber grows). Melanocytes (see Figure 16-2) are located at the root of the hair follicle, and they donate the melanin pigment to the cells of the hair fiber. ◣

Of the 5 million hairs on the body, about 100,000 are on the head. They grow about ½ inch (1.3 cm) per month. Cutting the hair has no effect on its rate of growth.

What causes hair color?

Concentration of eumelanin and pheomelanin cause the variations in hair color. For example:
- Black hair = high levels of black eumelanin
- Brown hair = high levels of brown eumelanin
- Blond hair = low levels of black eumelanin
- Red hair = high levels of pheomelanin
- Gray hair = low concentration of eumelanin and pheomelanin

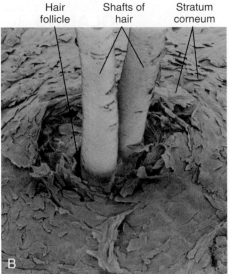

Hair follicle   Shafts of hair   Stratum corneum

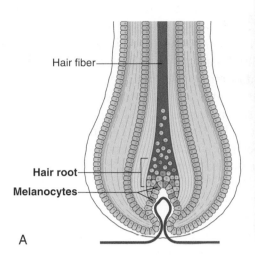

Hair fiber

Hair root

Melanocytes

A

FIGURE 16-2   A, Enlargement of a **hair follicle. B,** Scanning electron micrograph of **hair shafts** (visible parts of hair) extending from their hair follicles.

NAILS

Nails are hard keratin plates covering the dorsal surface of the last bone of each toe and finger. They are composed of keratinocytes that are cemented together tightly and can extend indefinitely unless cut or broken. A nail grows in thickness and length as a result of division of cells in the region of the nail matrix, which is at the base (proximal portion) of the nail plate.

Fingernails grow about 1 mm per week, which means that they can regrow in 3 to 5 months. Toenails grow more slowly than fingernails; it takes approximately 12 months for toenails to be replaced completely.

The **lunula** is a semilunar (half-moon–shaped) whitish region at the base of the nail plate. It generally can be seen in the thumbnail of most people and is evident to varying degrees in other fingernails. Air mixed in with keratin and cells rich in nuclei give the lunula its whitish color. The **cuticle,** a narrow band of epidermis (layer of keratin), is at the base and sides of the nail plate. The **paronychium** is the soft tissue surrounding the nail border. Figure 16-3A illustrates the anatomic structure of a nail.

Nail growth and appearance commonly alter during systemic disease. For example, grooves in nails may occur with high fevers and serious illness, and spoon nails (flattening of the nail plate) develop in iron deficiency anemia. **Onycholysis (onych/o =** nail) is the loosening of the nail plate with separation from the nail bed (Figure 16-3B). It may occur with infection of the nail and is often seen in psoriasis.

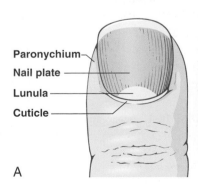

Paronychium

Nail plate

Lunula

Cuticle

A

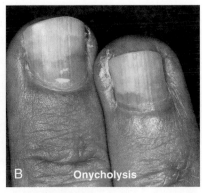

Onycholysis

FIGURE 16-3   A, Anatomic structure of a nail. B, Onycholysis. Infection or trauma to the nail may be the cause of the detachment of the nail plate from the nail bed.

GLANDS

Sebaceous Glands

Sebaceous glands are located in the dermal layer of the skin over the entire body, with the exception of the palms (hands), soles (feet), and lips. They secrete an oily substance called **sebum.** Sebum, containing lipids, lubricates the skin and minimizes water loss. Sebaceous glands are closely associated with hair follicles, and their ducts open into the hair follicle through which the sebum is released. Figure 16-4 shows the relationship of the sebaceous gland to the hair follicle. The sebaceous glands are influenced by sex hormones, which cause them to hypertrophy at puberty and atrophy in old age. Increased production of sebum during puberty contributes to blackhead (comedo) formation and acne in some people.

Sweat Glands

Sweat glands (the most common type are **eccrine sweat glands**) are tiny, coiled glands found on almost all body surfaces (about 2 million in the body). They are most numerous in the palm of the hand (3000 glands per square inch) and in the sole of the foot. As illustrated in Figure 16-4, the coiled eccrine sweat gland originates deep in the dermis and straightens out to extend up through the epidermis. The tiny opening on the surface is a **pore.**

Sweat, or perspiration, is almost pure water, with dissolved materials such as salt making up less than 1% of the total composition. It is colorless and odorless. The odor produced when sweat accumulates on the skin is caused by the action of bacteria on the sweat.

Sweat cools the body as it evaporates into the air. Perspiration is controlled by the sympathetic nervous system, whose nerve fibers are activated by the heart regulatory center in the hypothalamic region of the brain, which stimulates sweating.

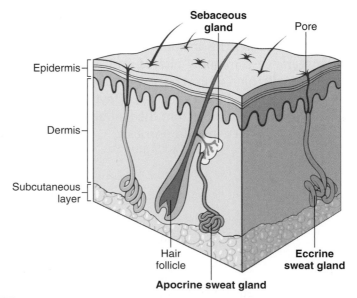

FIGURE 16-4 Sebaceous gland, eccrine sweat gland, and apocrine sweat gland.

A special variety of sweat gland, active only from puberty onward and larger than the ordinary kind, is concentrated in a few areas of the body near the reproductive organs and in the armpits. These glands **(apocrine sweat glands)** secrete an odorless sweat, containing substances easily broken down by bacteria on the skin. The bacterial waste products produce a characteristic human body odor. The milk-producing mammary gland is another type of apocrine gland; it secretes milk after the birth of a child.

 # VOCABULARY

This list reviews many of the new terms introduced in the text. Short definitions reinforce your understanding of the terms. Refer to the Pronunciation of Terms on page 690 for help with unfamiliar or difficult words.

adipocyte	Fat cell.
albino	Person with skin deficient in pigment (melanin).
apocrine sweat gland	One of the large dermal exocrine glands located in the axilla and genital areas. It secretes sweat that, in action with bacteria, is responsible for human body odor.
basal layer	Deepest region of the epidermis; it gives rise to all the epidermal cells.
collagen	Structural protein found in the skin and connective tissue.
cuticle	Band of epidermis at the base and sides of the nail plate.
dermis	Middle layer of the skin.
eccrine sweat gland	Most numerous sweat-producing exocrine gland in the skin.
epidermis	Outermost layer of the skin.
epithelium	Layer of skin cells forming the outer and inner surfaces of the body.
hair follicle	Sac within which each hair grows.
integumentary system	The skin and its accessory structures such as hair and nails.
keratin	Hard protein material found in the epidermis, hair, and nails. Keratin means horn and commonly is found in the horns of animals.
lunula	The half-moon–shaped, whitish area at the base of a nail.
melanin	Skin pigment. It is formed by melanocytes in the epidermis. **Eumelanin** is brown-black pigment, whereas **pheomelanin** is red-yellow.
paronychium	Soft tissue surrounding the nail border.
pore	Tiny opening on the surface of the skin.
sebaceous gland	Oil-secreting gland in the dermis that is associated with hair follicles.
sebum	Oily substance secreted by sebaceous glands.
squamous epithelium	Flat, scale-like cells composing the epidermis.
stratified	Arranged in layers.
stratum (*plural*: strata)	A layer (of cells).
stratum corneum	Outermost layer of the epidermis, which consists of flattened, keratinized cells.
subcutaneous layer	Innermost layer of the skin, containing fat tissue.

TERMINOLOGY

Write the meanings of the medical terms in the spaces provided.

COMBINING FORMS

COMBINING FORM	MEANING	TERMINOLOGY	MEANING
adip/o	fat (*see* **lip/o** and **steat/o**)	adipose _____	
albin/o	white	albinism _____ *Table 16-1 lists combining forms for colors and examples of terms using those combining forms.*	
caus/o	burn, burning	causalgia _____ *Intensely unpleasant burning sensation in skin and muscles when there is damage to nerves.*	
cauter/o	heat, burn	electrocautery _____ *An instrument containing a needle or blade used during surgery to burn through tissue by means of an electrical current. Electrocauterization is very effective in minimizing blood loss.*	
cutane/o	skin (*see* **derm/o**)	subcutaneous _____ *Epidermis and dermis are the cutaneous layers of the skin.*	
derm/o, dermat/o	skin	epidermis _____ dermatitis _____ dermatologist _____ dermabrasion _____ *Abrasion means a scraping away. Dermabrasion using a sandpaper-like material removes acne scars and fine wrinkles.* epidermolysis _____ *Loosening of the epidermis with the development of large blisters; occurs after injury, or with blister-producing diseases.*	
diaphor/o	profuse sweating (*see* **hidr/o**)	diaphoresis _____ *Commonly called sweating.*	
erythem/o, erythemat/o	redness	erythema _____ *Flushing; widespread redness of the skin. Pronunciation is ĕr-ĭ-THĒ-mă.* **Erythematous** *means pertaining to erythema.*	
hidr/o	sweat	anhidrosis _____ *Do not confuse hidr/o with hydr/o (water)!*	
ichthy/o	dry, scaly (fish-like)	ichthyosis _____ *This is usually a hereditary condition in which the skin is dry, rough, and scaly (resembling fish scales) because of a defect in keratinization. Ichthyosis also can be acquired, appearing with malignancies such as lymphomas and multiple myeloma. Greek ichthys means fish (Figure 16-5A).*	

16

TABLE 16-1 | COLORS

COMBINING FORM	MEANING	TERMINOLOGY
albin/o	white	albinism
anthrac/o	black (as coal)	anthracosis
chlor/o	green	chlorophyll
cirrh/o	tawny yellow	cirrhosis
cyan/o	blue	cyanosis
eosin/o	rosy	eosinophil
erythr/o	red	erythrocyte
jaund/o	yellow	jaundice
leuk/o	white	leukoderma
lute/o	yellow	corpus luteum
melan/o	black	melanocyte
poli/o	gray	poliosis (decrease of melanin in hair, eyebrows, and eyelashes)
xanth/o	yellow	xanthoma

COMBINING FORM	MEANING	TERMINOLOGY	MEANING
kerat/o	hard	keratosis *See page 672.*	
leuk/o	white	leukoplakia *The suffix -plakia means plaques (Figure 16-5B).*	
lip/o	fat	lipoma	
		liposuction *Removal of subcutaneous fat tissue through a tube that is introduced into the fatty area via a small incision. The fat is aspirated (suctioned out).*	
melan/o	black	melanocyte	
		melanoma *This is a malignant skin tumor. See page 674.*	

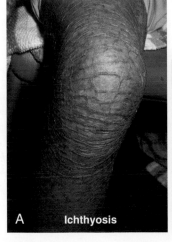
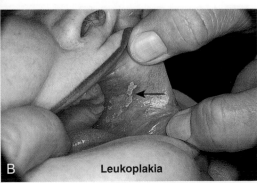

FIGURE 16-5 A, Ichthyosis. B, Leukoplakia.

A Ichthyosis

B Leukoplakia

16

COMBINING FORM	MEANING	TERMINOLOGY	MEANING
myc/o	fungus (fungi include yeasts, molds, and mushrooms)	mycosis ___ *An example of a mycosis (fungal infection) is **tinea pedis**, commonly called **"athlete's foot"** (Figure 16-6A). Another fungal infection is tinea corporis (ringworm). See page 671.*	
onych/o	nail (*see* **ungu/o**)	onycholysis ___ *Separation of the nail plate from the nail bed in fungal infections or after trauma. See Figure 16-3, page 667. Onycholysis is often seen in psoriasis.*	
		onychomycosis ___ *Fungal infection of the nails, which become white, opaque, thick, and brittle.*	
		paronychia ___ *Par- means near or beside. Paronychia is inflammation and swelling of the soft tissue around the nail and is associated with torn cuticles or ingrown nails (Figure 16-6B).*	
phyt/o	plant	dermatophytosis ___ *Examples are fungal infections (mycoses) (see Figure 16-6A).*	
pil/o	hair (*see* trich/o), hair follicle	pilosebaceous ___ *Sebace/o indicates a gland that secretes sebum. The pilosebaceous unit is the combination of the hair follicle and attached sebaceous gland.*	
py/o	pus	pyoderma ___ *Pus within the skin (-derma). **Impetigo** is a purulent (pus-containing) skin disease caused by bacterial infection. See page 669.*	
rhytid/o	wrinkle	rhytidectomy ___ *Cosmetic plastic surgery to remove wrinkles and excess skin; also called rhytidoplasty or face lift. Laser treatments, **Botox Cosmetic** (purified botulinum toxin) injections, and injectable fillers are used to soften facial lines and wrinkles.*	
seb/o	sebum (oily secretion from sebaceous glands)	seborrhea ___ *Excessive secretion from sebaceous glands. **Seborrheic dermatitis** commonly is known as **dandruff.***	
squam/o	scale-like	squamous epithelium ___ *Cells are flat and scale-like; "pavement" epithelium.*	

Is Botox Cosmetic Safe?

Botox Cosmetic (onabotulinumtoxin A) has been FDA approved since 2002, for cosmetic use to the brow and facial frown lines. Over a million patients have been treated with Botox Cosmetic, and there have been no reported fatal or permanent adverse effects related to its use. Botox Cosmetic works by blocking the connection between nerves and muscles. Muscles do not contract, thus preventing lines and wrinkles in the skin. When injected in small doses directly into the muscle, Botox Cosmetic can reduce specific facial lines for several months.

The FDA also has approved injectable dermal fillers for deep facial wrinkles and folds. These include Restylane, Perlane, Juvederm, Radiesse, Belotero Balance, and Voluma. New additional neuromodulators similar to Botox Cosmetic are also available: Xeomin (incobotulinumtoxin A) and Dysport (abobotulinumtoxin A).

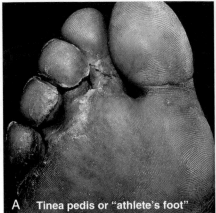
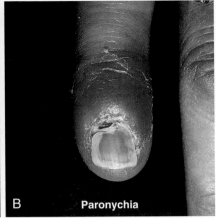

A   Tinea pedis or "athlete's foot"   B   Paronychia

FIGURE 16-6   A, Mycosis. B, Acute paronychia most commonly occurs from nail biting, finger sucking, aggressive manicuring, or penetrating trauma. The most common infecting organism is *Staphylococcus aureus*.

COMBINING FORM	MEANING	TERMINOLOGY	MEANING
steat/o	fat	steatoma *Cystic collection of sebum (fatty material) that forms in a sebaceous gland and can become infected; **sebaceous cyst.** See Figure 16-7A.*	
trich/o	hair	hypertrichosis	
ungu/o	nail	subungual	
xanth/o	yellow	xanthoma *Nodules develop under the skin owing to excess lipid deposits and can be associated with a high cholesterol level. A xanthoma that appears on the eyelids is a **xanthelasma** (-elasma = a flat plate) (Figure 16-7B).*	
xer/o	dry	xerosis *This is very dry skin.*	

16

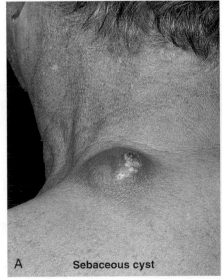
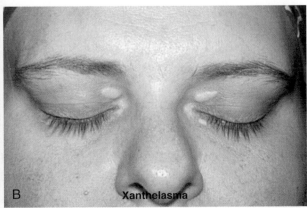

A   Sebaceous cyst   B   Xanthelasma

FIGURE 16-7   A, Sebaceous cyst. B, Xanthelasma.

PATHOLOGY

CUTANEOUS LESIONS

A **lesion** is an area of abnormal tissue anywhere on or in the body. It may be caused by disease or trauma (external forces). The following terms describe common skin lesions, which are illustrated in Figure 16-8A to L.

A. crust

Collection of dried serum and cellular debris.

A scab is a crust. It forms from the drying of a body exudate, as in eczema, impetigo, and seborrhea.

B. cyst

Thick-walled, closed sac or pouch containing fluid or semisolid material.

Examples of cysts are the **pilonidal cyst,** which is found over the sacral area of the back in the midline and contains hairs (**pil/o** = hair, **nid/o** = nest); and a **sebaceous cyst,** a collection of yellowish, cheesy sebum commonly found on the scalp, vulva, and scrotum.

C. erosion

Wearing away or loss of epidermis.

Erosions do not penetrate below the dermoepidermal junction. They occur as a result of inflammation or injury and heal without scarring.

D. fissure

Groove or crack-like sore.

An anal fissure is a break in the skin lining of the anal canal.

E. macule

Flat, pigmented lesion measuring less than 1 cm in diameter.

Freckles, tattoo marks, and flat moles are examples. A **patch** is a large macule, greater than 1 cm in diameter.

F. nodule

Solid, round or oval elevated lesion 1 cm or more in diameter.

An enlarged lymph node and solid growths are examples.

G. papule

Small (less than 1 cm in diameter), solid elevation of the skin.

Pimples are examples of papules. Papules may become confluent (run together) and form **plaques,** which are elevated flat lesions.

H. polyp

Growth extending from the surface of mucous membrane.

Polyps (a type of papule) commonly are found in the nose and sinuses, colon, urinary bladder, and uterus.

I. pustule

Papule containing pus.

A pustule is a small **abscess** (collection of pus) on the skin.

J. ulcer

Open sore on the skin or mucous membranes (deeper than an erosion).

Decubitus ulcers (bedsores) are caused by pressure that results from lying in one position (Latin *decubitus* means lying down). Pressure ulcers usually involve loss of tissue substance and pus or exudate formation.

K. vesicle

Small collection (papule) of clear fluid (serum); blister.

Vesicles form in skin after burns and may be seen with allergies and dermatitis. A **bulla** (*plural*: bullae) is a large vesicle.

L. wheal

Smooth, edematous (swollen) papule or plaque that is centrally redder or paler than the surrounding skin.

Wheals may be papular, as in a mosquito bite, or may involve a wide area, as in some allergic reactions. Wheals often are accompanied by itching and are seen in hives, anaphylaxis, and insect bites.

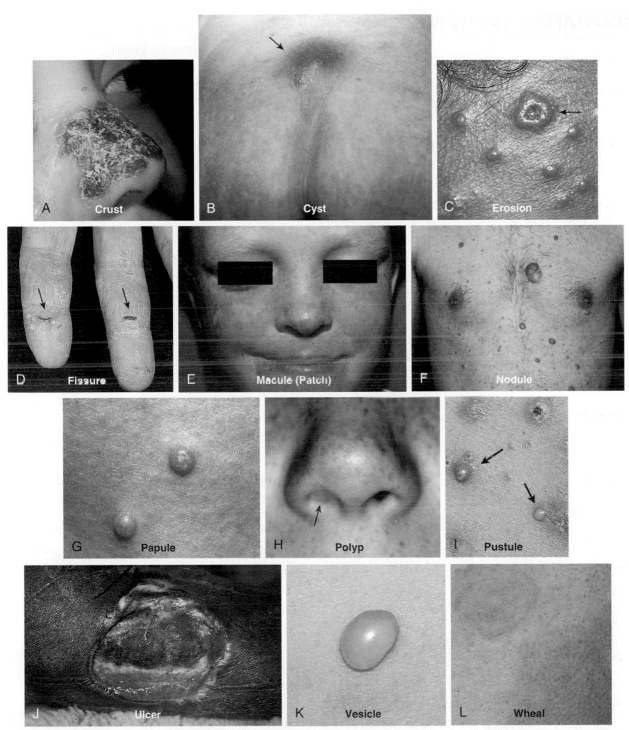

FIGURE 16-8 Cutaneous lesions. **A, Crust**—scab. **B, Cyst**—pilonidal cyst. **C, Erosion**—in varicella (chickenpox after rupture of blister). **D, Fissures. E, Macule**—freckles. **F, Nodules. G, Papules. H, Polyp**—nasal polyp. **I, Pustules**—acne. **J, Ulcer**—decubitus ulcer. **K, Vesicle**—bulla. **L, Wheal**—urticaria.

SIGNS AND SYMPTOMS

alopecia

Absence of hair from areas where it normally grows.

Alopecia, or baldness, may be hereditary (usual progressive loss of scalp hair in men) or it may be caused by disease, injury, or treatment (chemotherapy) or may occur with old age. **Alopecia areata** is an autoimmune disease in which hair falls out in patches without scarring or inflammation (Figure 16-9A).

ecchymosis (*plural: ecchymoses*)

Bluish-purplish mark (bruise) on the skin.

Ecchymoses (**ec-** = out, **chym/o** = pour) are caused by hemorrhages into the skin from injury or spontaneous leaking of blood from vessels (Figure 16-9B).

petechia (*plural: petechiae*)

Small, pinpoint hemorrhage.

Petechiae (pĕ-TĒ-kē-ī) are smaller versions of ecchymoses (Figure 16-9C). Both ecchymoses and petechiae are forms of **purpura** (bleeding into the skin).

pruritus

Itching.

Pruritus is a symptom associated with most forms of dermatitis and with other conditions as well. It arises as a result of stimulation of nerves in the skin by substances released in allergic reactions or by irritation caused by substances in the blood or by foreign bodies.

ABNORMAL CONDITIONS

acne

Chronic papular and pustular eruption of the skin with increased production of sebum.

Acne vulgaris (Latin *vulgaris* means ordinary) is caused by the buildup of sebum and keratin in the pores of the skin. A **blackhead** is called an open **comedo** or **comedone** (plural **comedones**.) It is a sebum plug that partially blocks the pore (Figure 16-10A). If the pore becomes completely blocked, a **whitehead** (closed

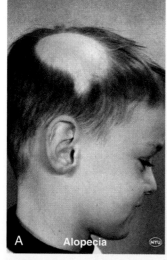
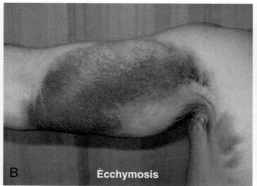
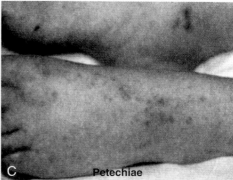

FIGURE 16-9   A, Alopecia areata. B, Ecchymosis. High-grade tear at the myotendinous junction in the right pectoralis major muscle. **C, Petechiae.**

Pruritus

Be sure to spell **pruritus** correctly. It is a condition, not an inflammation (-itis).

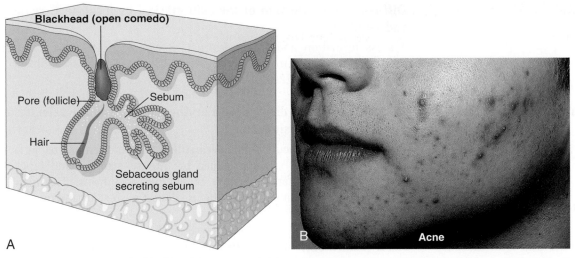

FIGURE 16-10 **A,** Formation of a **blackhead (open comedo)** in a dilated pore filled with oxidized sebum and bacteria. **B, Acne vulgaris** on the face.

comedone) forms. Bacteria in the skin break down the sebum, producing inflammation in the surrounding tissue. Papules, pustules, and cysts can thus form. Treatment can include antibiotic use and medications to decrease inflammation in the skin. Benzoyl peroxide and tretinoin (Retin-A) are topical medications used to prevent comedone formation; isotretinoin (Accutane) is an oral retinoid used in severe cystic or treatment-resistant acne.

burns

Injury to tissues caused by heat contact.

Burns may be caused by dry heat (fire), moist heat (steam or liquid), chemicals, lightning, electricity, or radiation. Burns usually are classified as follows:

  first-degree burns—superficial epidermal lesions, erythema, hyperesthesia, and no blisters.
  second-degree burns (partial-thickness burn injury)—epidermal and dermal lesions, erythema, blisters, and hyperesthesia (Figure 16-11A).
  third-degree burns (full-thickness burn injury)—epidermis and dermis are destroyed (necrosis of skin), and subcutaneous layer is damaged, leaving charred, white tissue (Figure 16-11B).

16

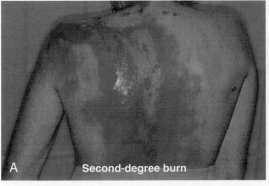

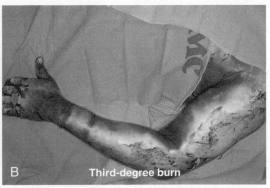

FIGURE 16-11 **Burns. A, Second-degree burn.** Wound is painful and very sensitive to touch and air currents. **B, Third-degree burn** showing variable color (deep-red, white, black, and brown). The wound itself is insensate (patient does not respond to pinprick).

cellulitis	**Diffuse, acute infection of the skin marked by local heat, redness, pain, and swelling.**
	Abscess formation and tissue destruction can occur if appropriate antibiotic therapy is not given. Areas of poor lymphatic drainage are susceptible to this skin infection (Figure 16-12A).
eczema (atopic dermatitis)	**Inflammatory skin disease with erythematous, papulovesicular, or papalosquamous lesions.**
	This is a chronic or acute **atopic dermatitis** ◣ (rash often begins on face, hands, elbows, or knees) It is accompanied by intense pruritus and tends to occur in patients with a family history of allergic conditions. Treatment depends on the cause but usually includes the use of corticosteroids and moisturizers. See Figure 16-12B.
exanthematous viral diseases	**Rash (exanthem) of the skin due to a viral infection.**
	Examples are **rubella** (German measles), **rubeola** (measles), and **varicella** (chickenpox). These conditions are no longer as common in children because of vaccination programs. However, **erythema infectiosum** (fifth disease) is a common exanthematous viral disease. See Figure 16-13A. **Hand-foot-and-mouth disease** is another common viral illness in children. See Figure 16-13B.

16

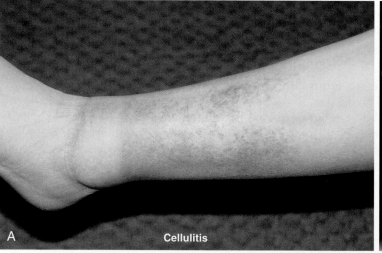
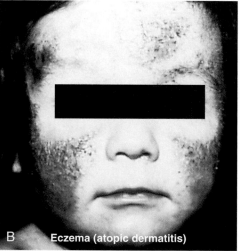

FIGURE 16-12   A, Cellulitis. Traveling on a safari in Botswana, a 63-year-old woman noticed swelling, redness, and pain in her lower leg. After a local physician prescribed oral antibiotics, she was advised to interrupt her trip to get intravenous antibiotics at a major hospital. Her cellulitis cleared in a week. **B, Eczema (atopic dermatitis)** in an infant. More than 70% of affected patients have a family history of other atopic conditions such as allergic rhinitis, hay fever, and asthma.

◣ **Atopic Dermatitis**

Atopic means pertaining to **atopy**, which means out of place or unusual (a = no, top = place). It is a hyperallergic condition that may be hereditary, but contact with an allergen must occur before a hypersensitivity reaction can develop.

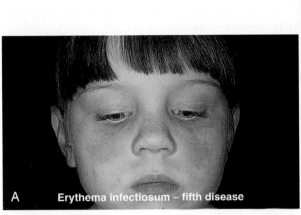

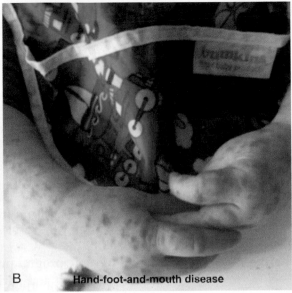

| A   Erythema infectiosum – fifth disease | B   Hand-foot-and-mouth disease |

FIGURE 16-13   A, Erythema infectiosum—fifth disease. It is marked by fever and an erythematous rash that has a "slapped cheek" appearance on the face and later involving the arms, buttocks, and trunk. It is caused by a parvovirus. **B, Hand-foot-and-mouth disease.** It is caused by an enterovirus.

gangrene	**Death of tissue associated with loss of blood supply.**
	In this condition, ischemia resulting from injury, inflammation, frostbite, diseases such as diabetes, or arteriosclerosis can lead to necrosis of tissue followed by bacterial invasion and putrefaction (proteins are decomposed by bacteria). See Figure 16-14A.
impetigo	**Bacterial inflammatory skin disease characterized by vesicles, pustules, and crusted-over lesions.**
	This is a contagious **pyoderma** (**py/o** = pus) and usually is caused by staphylococci or streptococci. Systemic use of antibiotics combined with proper cleansing of lesions is effective treatment. See Figure 16-14B.

16

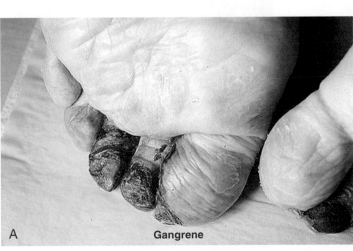

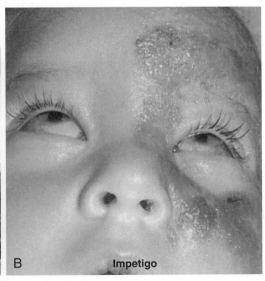

| A   Gangrene | B   Impetigo |

FIGURE 16-14   A, Gangrene. B, Impetigo.

psoriasis

Chronic, recurrent dermatosis marked by itchy, scaly, red plaques covered by silvery gray scales (Figure 16-15A).

Psoriasis commonly involves the forearms, knees, legs, and scalp. It is neither infectious nor contagious but is caused by an increased rate of growth of the basal layer of the epidermis. It is an autoinflammatory disease that can run in families. Treatment is **palliative** (relieving but not curing) and includes topical lubricants, keratolytics, and steroids. Systemic treatments include psoralen–ultraviolet A (PUVA) light therapy and immunomodulators.

scabies

Contagious, parasitic infection of the skin with intense pruritus (Figure 16-15B).

Scabies (from Latin *scabere*, to scratch) commonly affects areas such as the groin, nipples, and skin between the fingers. Treatment is with topical medicated cream to destroy the scabies mites (tiny parasites).

scleroderma

Chronic progressive disease of the skin and internal organs with hardening and shrinking of connective tissue. See Figure 16-16A.

Fibrous scar-like tissue forms in the skin, and the heart, lungs, kidneys, and esophagus may be affected as well. Skin is thick, hard, and rigid, with areas of both depigmentation and hyperpigmentation. It is an autoimmune disease for which palliative treatment consists of immunosuppressive and anti-inflammatory agents, antifibrotics, and physical therapy.

systemic lupus erythematosus (SLE)

Chronic autoimmune inflammatory disease of collagen in skin, joints, and internal organs.

Lupus, meaning wolf-like (the shape and color of the erosive skin lesions and tissue loss resembling a wolf attack), produces a characteristic "butterfly" pattern of redness over the cheeks and nose. See Figure 16-16B. In more severe cases, the extent of erythema increases, and all exposed areas of the skin may be involved. Primarily a disease of females, lupus is an autoimmune disorder. High levels of certain autoantibodies are found in the patient's blood. Corticosteroids and immunosuppressive drugs are used to control symptoms.

SLE should be differentiated from chronic **discoid lupus erythematosus (DLE),** which is a photosensitive, scaling, plaque-like eruption of the skin confined to the face, scalp, ears, chest, arms, and back, which heals with scarring. SLE should also be differentiated from **lupus vulgaris,** which refers to a cutaneous form of tuberculosis.

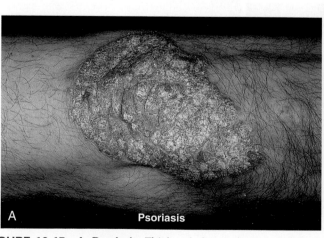
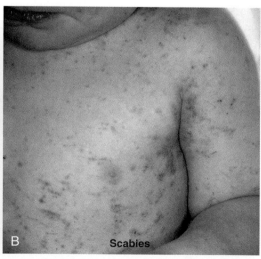

FIGURE 16-15 A, Psoriasis. Thick red plaques have a sharply defined border and an adherent silvery scale. **B, Scabies.**

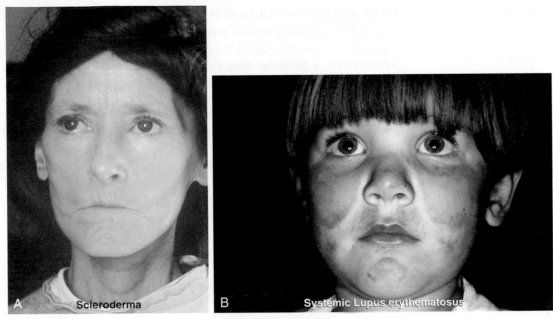

FIGURE 16-16   A, Scleroderma. B, Systemic lupus erythematosus.

tinea

Infection of the skin caused by a fungus.

Tinea corporis, or ringworm, so called because the infection is in a ring-like pattern (Figure 16-17A), is highly contagious and causes severe pruritus. Other examples are **tinea pedis** (athlete's foot, which affects the skin between the toes), **tinea capitis** (on the scalp), **tinea barbae** (affecting the skin under a beard), and **tinea unguium** (affecting the nails) (Figure 16-17B). Treatment is with antifungal agents. (Latin *tinea* means worm or moth—apparently the Romans thought that skin affected with tinea looked "moth-eaten.")

16

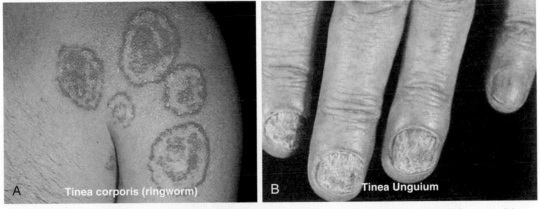

FIGURE 16-17   A, Tinea corporis (ringworm). B, Tinea unguium. Fungal infection of the nail (onychomycosis) causes the distal nail plate to turn yellow or white. Hyperkeratotic debris accumulates, causing the nail to separate from the nail bed (**onycholysis**).

urticaria (hives)	**Acute allergic reaction in which red, round wheals develop on the skin.**

Hives often are a reaction to foods (shellfish, nuts, eggs) or to medication. Histamine is released into the bloodstream, causing **pruritus** and **edema** (swelling). **Angioedema** is swelling around the face. Other substances and events that can trigger hives are animal dander, insect bites and stings, and pollen. See Figure 16-18A.

vitiligo	**Loss of pigment (depigmentation) in areas of the skin (milk-white patches).**

This is a form of **leukoderma** (Figure 16-18B). The skin changes result from an autoimmune process, and there is an increased association of vitiligo with autoimmune disorders such as thyroiditis, hyperthyroidism, and diabetes mellitus.

SKIN NEOPLASMS

Benign Neoplasms

callus	**Increased growth of cells in the keratin layer of the epidermis caused by pressure or friction.**

The feet (Figure 16-19A) and the hands are common sites for callus formation. A **corn** is a type of callus that develops a hard core (a whitish, cone-shaped central kernel).

keloid	**Excess hypertrophied, thickened scar developing after trauma or surgical incision.**

Keloids (Figure 16-19B) result from excessive collagen formation in the skin during connective tissue repair. Keloids extend beyond the boundaries of the original injury. The term comes from the Greek *kelis*, meaning blemish. Surgical excision often is combined with intralesional steroid injections or ablative laser treatments.

A normal scar left by a healed wound is called a **cicatrix** (SĬK-ă-trĭks).

keratosis	**Thickened and rough lesion of the epidermis; associated with aging or skin damage.**

Actinic keratosis is caused by long-term ultraviolet light exposure and is a precancerous lesion that can evolve into squamous cell carcinoma (Figure 16-20A). **Seborrheic keratosis** is a benign lesion that results from overgrowth of the upper epidermis and is dark in color.

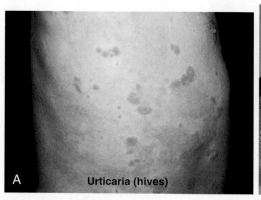 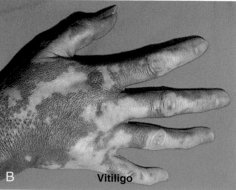

FIGURE 16-18 A, Urticaria (hives). Erythematous, edematous, often circular plaques. **B, Vitiligo** on the hand (from Latin *vitium*, blemish). Epidermal melanocytes are completely lost in depigmented areas through an autoimmune process.

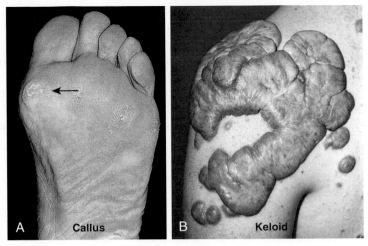

FIGURE 16-19   **A, Callus** on the sole of the foot. **B, Keloid.**

leukoplakia	**White, thickened patches on mucous membrane tissue of the tongue or cheek (evolves to squamous cell carcinoma).** See Figure 16-5B, page 661.
	One type is a precancerous lesion that is common in smokers and may be caused by chronic inflammation.
nevus (*plural:* **nevi**)	**Pigmented lesion of the skin** (see Figure 16-20B).
	Nevi are commonly known as moles. Many are present at birth, but some are acquired.
	Dysplastic nevi are moles that have atypical cells and may progress to form a type of skin cancer called melanoma (see **malignant melanoma**).
verruca (*plural:* **verrucae**)	**Epidermal growth (wart) caused by a virus.**
	Verruca vulgaris (common wart) is the most frequent type of wart (Figure 16-20C). **Plantar warts** occur on the soles of the feet, juvenile warts occur on the hands and face of children, and venereal warts occur on the genitals and around the anus. Warts are removed with acids, or freezing with liquid nitrogen (cryosurgery), or immune therapy. If the virus remains in the skin, the wart frequently regrows.

16

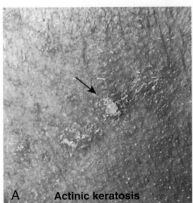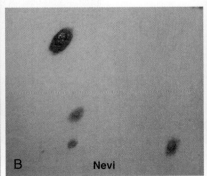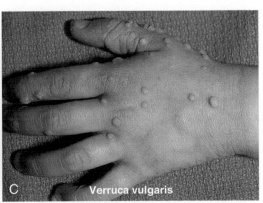

FIGURE 16-20   **A, Actinic (solar) keratosis. B, Nevi. C, Verruca vulgaris.** A wart consists of multiple papules with rough, pebble-like surfaces.

Cancerous Lesions

basal cell carcinoma

Malignant tumor of the basal cell layer of the epidermis.

This is the most common cancer in humans and the most common skin cancer. It is a slow-growing tumor that usually occurs on chronically sun-exposed skin, especially near or on the nose (Figure 16-21A). It almost never metastasizes.

squamous cell carcinoma

Malignant tumor of the squamous epithelial cells in the epidermis.

This tumor may grow in places other than the skin, wherever squamous epithelium is found (mouth, larynx, bladder, esophagus, lungs). **Actinic** (sun-related) **keratoses** are premalignant (precursor) lesions in people with sun-damaged skin. Progression to squamous cell carcinoma (Figure 16-21B) may occur if lesions are not removed. Treatment is removal by surgical excision, cryotherapy, electrodesiccation and curettage, or radiotherapy.

malignant melanoma

Cancerous growth composed of melanocytes.

This malignancy is attributed to a genetic predisposition and to exposure to ultraviolet light. Melanoma usually begins as a mottled, light brown to black macule with irregular borders (Figure 16-22). The lesion may turn shades of red, blue, and white and may crust on the surface and bleed. Melanomas may arise in preexisting moles (dysplastic nevi) and frequently appear on the upper back, lower legs, arms, head, and neck.

Biopsy is required to confirm the diagnosis of melanoma, and prognosis is best determined by measuring tumor thickness in millimeters.

Melanomas often metastasize to the lung, liver, bone, and brain. Treatment may include excision of the tumor, regional lymphadenectomy, chemotherapy/ immunotherapy, or radiotherapy. See ***In Person: Metastatic Melanoma***, page 679.

Kaposi sarcoma

Malignant, vascular, neoplastic growth characterized by cutaneous nodules.

Frequently arising on the lower extremities, nodules range in color from deep pink to dark blue and purple. One form of this condition is associated with acquired immunodeficiency syndrome (AIDS). See Figure 14-11, page 661.

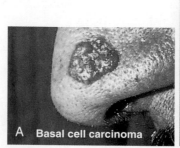
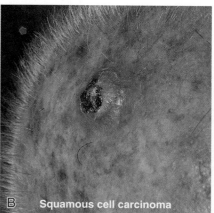

FIGURE 16-21   A, Basal cell carcinoma. B, Squamous cell carcinoma. Advanced lesions often are nodular and ulcerated.

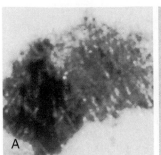 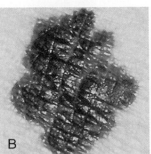 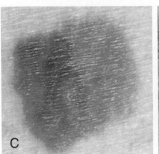 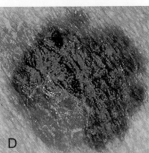

FIGURE 16-22   The ABCDEs of melanoma:
Asymmetry: one half unlike the other half
Border: irregular or poorly circumscribed border
Color: varies from one area to another; shades of tan and brown, black, and sometimes white, red, or blue
Diameter: usually larger than 6 mm (diameter of a pencil eraser)
Evolution: change in the lesion over time

LABORATORY TESTS AND CLINICAL PROCEDURES

LABORATORY TESTS

bacterial analyses	**Samples of skin are examined for presence of microorganisms.**
	Purulent (pus-filled) material or exudate (fluid that accumulates) often is taken for examination.
fungal tests	**Scrapings from skin lesions, hair specimens, or nail clippings are sent to a laboratory for culture and microscopic examination.**
	The specimen also may be treated with a potassium hydroxide (KOH) preparation and examined microscopically. Positive result reveals fungal infection.

CLINICAL PROCEDURES

cryosurgery	**Use of subfreezing temperature achieved with liquid nitrogen application to destroy tissue.**
curettage	**Use of a sharp dermal curette to scrape away a skin lesion.**
	A curette is shaped like a spoon or scoop.
electrodesiccation	**Tissue is destroyed by burning with an electric spark.**
	This procedure is used along with curettage to remove and destroy small cancerous lesions with well-defined borders.
Mohs surgery	**Thin layers of malignant tissue are removed, and each slice is examined microscopically to check for adequate extent of the resection.**
	Mohs surgery (also called Mohs micrographic surgery) is a specialized form of excision to treat basal cell carcinomas, squamous cell carcinomas, and other tumors. It is used in areas in which a wide local excision is not feasible (such as on the face) or tissue sparing is required (as with large skin cancers). See Figure 16-23.

16

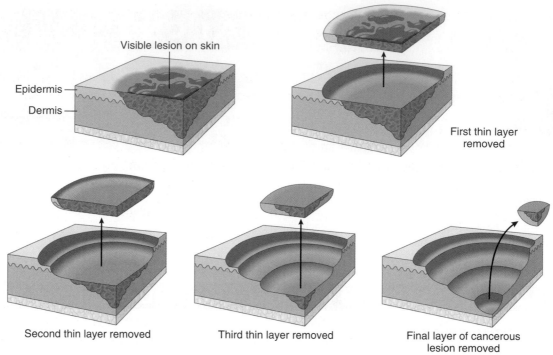

Epidermis —

Dermis —

Visible lesion on skin

First thin layer removed

Second thin layer removed

Third thin layer removed

Final layer of cancerous lesion removed

FIGURE 16-23 Mohs surgery is microscopically controlled excision of skin cancer.

16

skin biopsy	**Suspicious skin lesions are removed or sampled and examined microscopically by a pathologist.**

In a **punch biopsy,** a surgical instrument removes a core of tissue obtained by rotation of its sharp, circular edge. In a shave biopsy, tissue is excised using a cut parallel to the surface of the surrounding skin.

skin test	**Substances are injected intradermally or applied to the skin, and results are observed.**

Skin tests are used to diagnose allergies and disease. In the **patch test,** an allergen-treated piece of gauze or filter paper is applied to the skin. If the skin becomes red or swollen, the result is positive. In the **scratch test,** several scratches are made in the skin, and a very minute amount of test material is inserted into the scratches. The Schick test (for diphtheria) and the Mantoux and purified protein derivative (PPD) tests (for tuberculosis) are other skin tests.

ABBREVIATIONS

ABCDE	asymmetry (of shape), border (irregularity), color (variation within one lesion), diameter (greater than 6 mm), evolution (change)—characteristics associated with melanoma	**PPD**	purified protein derivative—used in skin test for tuberculosis
		PUVA	psoralen–ultraviolet A light therapy; treatment for psoriasis and other skin conditions
Bx	biopsy	**SLE**	systemic lupus erythematosus
Derm	dermatology	**SC**	subcutaneous
DLE	discoid lupus erythematosus		

PRACTICAL APPLICATIONS

This section contains disease descriptions, a medical record, and a case report using terms that you have studied in this and previous chapters. Explanations of more difficult terms are added in brackets.

DISEASE DESCRIPTIONS

1. **Candidiasis** (*Candida* is a yeast-like fungus): This fungus is normally found on mucous membranes, skin, and vaginal mucosa. Under certain circumstances (excessive warmth and moisture; administration of antibiotics and corticosteroids; debilitated states; infancy), it can proliferate and cause localized or generalized mucocutaneous disease. Examples are paronychial lesions, lesions in areas of the body where the rubbing of opposed surfaces is common (groin, perianal, axillary, inframammary, and interdigital), thrush (white plaques attached to oral or vaginal mucous membranes), and vulvovaginitis.

2. **Cellulitis:** This is a common nonsuppurative infection of connective tissue with severe inflammation of the dermal and subcutaneous layers of the skin. Cellulitis appears on an extremity as a warm reddish area of tender edematous skin. A surgical wound, puncture, insect bite, skin ulcer, or patch of dermatitis is the usual means of entry for bacteria (most cases are caused by streptococci or Staphylococcus aureus). Therapy includes rest, elevation, hot wet packs, and antibiotics. Any cellulitis on the face should be given special attention because the infection may extend directly to the brain.

3. **Mycosis fungoides (cutaneous T cell lymphoma):** This rare, chronic skin condition is caused by the infiltration of the skin by atypical lymphocytes. Contrary to its name (myc/o = fungus), it is not caused by a fungus but was formerly thought to be of fungal origin. It can manifest with generalized erythroderma or large, reddish, raised tumors that spread and ulcerate. In some cases, the malignant cells may involve lymph nodes and other organs. Treatment with cortisone ointments, topical nitrogen mustard, psoralen–ultraviolet light A (PUVA), and systemic retinoids or immunomodulators can be effective in controlling the disease.

MEDICAL RECORD: FINDINGS ON DERMATOLOGIC EXAMINATION

A wide variety of lesions are seen on the face, shoulders, and back. The predominant lesions are pustules or papules. Many pustules are confluent [running together] over the chin and forehead. Comedones are present on the face, especially along the midface. Inflammatory papules are present on the lower cheeks and chin. Large abscesses and ulcerated cysts are present over the upper shoulder area. Numerous scars are present over the face and upper back.

Questions about the Medical Record
See page 689 for answers.

1. In this skin condition, the primary lesions are:
   a. Discolored flat lesions
   b. Grooves or crack-like sores
   c. Small elevations containing pus

2. Comedones are:
   a. Sebum plugs partially blocking skin pores
   b. Contagious, infectious plugs of sebum
   c. Small, pinpoint hemorrhages

16

3. The papules described are known as:
   a. Purpura
   b. Pimples
   c. Freckles

4. In the scapular region, lesions are:
   a. Large pigmented areas
   b. Numerous collections of blisters
   c. Large collections of sacs containing pus with erosion of skin

5. What is your diagnosis of this skin condition, based on the physical examination?
   a. Acne vulgaris
   b. Leukoplakia
   c. Scabies

CASE REPORT: SQUAMOUS CELL CARCINOMA

A 76-year-old woman noticed a 1-inch-diameter flaky patch on her scalp. Over a period of months, the lesion increased in size and became ulcerated, with the skull bone visible (Figure 16-24A). A biopsy was performed and pathologic examination revealed squamous cell carcinoma. Mohs micrographic surgery was attempted but a CT study of the head/brain with contrast showed the likelihood of residual tumor extending into the skull (Figure 16-24B).

Major surgery was performed to resect residual malignant tissue. A large portion of skull was removed and replaced with titanium mesh on which muscle from her back and skin from her leg were grafted. The primary surgical area healed well. Pathologic examination confirmed the presence of tumor invading the skull and underlying dura at the surgical margin. The patient is now receiving radiation therapy for 6 weeks to treat the affected area.

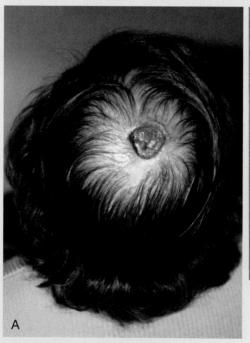
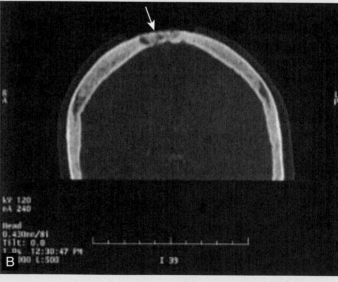

FIGURE 16-24 **A, Squamous cell carcinoma** on scalp. **B,** CT scan showing defect (*arrow*) in skull from tumor invasion.

IN PERSON: METASTATIC MELANOMA

This is a first-person account describing the course of metastatic melanoma. It was written by the husband of a patient.

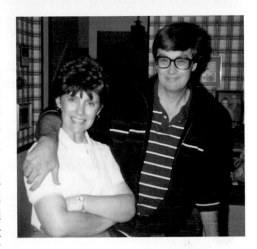

Mary Ann showed me the mole on her arm near her armpit and I knew immediately that this was not going to be a good thing. It was raised, red and black, irregular shape. That was more than 30 years ago, before the Internet, and no way to confirm our fear. Four days later the mole was excised, and within a week, we received confirmation that it was a melanoma.

We had various opinions about the next step, but Mary Ann had always been convinced that you always go to a teaching hospital and find the experts. We selected a surgeon at Georgetown Hospital and she underwent a resection of an area on her arm that was about 3 × 4 inches. The nodes in her armpit also were removed, which I questioned. If the cancer had spread to her nodes, then it was already metastatic, and either way, she risked getting edema in her arm. Fortunately, there was no node involvement and she didn't get edema. Again, with no Internet we had to spend several nights at the Library of Medicine trying to educate ourselves about what we were dealing with. We didn't know about the classifications, and TNM [tumor-node-metastasis] readings weren't mentioned to us. We only knew the depth of the tumor, and relating that to the charts, we found it implied a 30% to 40% 5-year survival rate.

Living in anticipation of recurrence was extremely stressful. Mary Ann dwelled a lot on her demise despite my and her friends' efforts to put on a happy face and trying to fill the days with distractions. Her 6-month chest x-rays and checkups gradually became less stressful, leaving us with the feeling that it was okay to enjoy life again. Two and a half years after her operation, that changed. A tumor showed up in her lung. Again, she found the best thoracic surgeon in the area and had it removed. Six weeks later, two small tumors appeared below her ribcage right where the drain from her operation had been. These were the first of many that appeared just below the dermis, in her abdomen, thigh, and back. This was over a period of about 8 months, and during this time Mary Ann entered her first trial in which she received an injectable, specific antigen that was designed to boost her immune system. Remarkably, Mary Ann the fighter began to emerge. With two pre-teen daughters to nurture, she put tumor removal and weekly injections on her to-do list.

At this time, she was under increased stress dealing with the loss of her mother to a heart attack. During the funeral she complained of severe back pain, and when we returned home tests revealed metastases on her spinal cord. Again, she found the best neurologic surgeon and had them removed. She had to learn how to walk again and had barely begun to recover when her sisters called to tell her that their father had died of a heart attack. She knew even before I told her, and I remember her words: "Bring it on, give me all you've got, I can take it."

Shortly after his funeral she began to have "dancing spots" in her right eye, a sign of a metastatic brain tumor. Her oncologist was adamantly opposed to surgery. His advice was to stick to the protocol, and not put her through an operation because she would be dead in 6 months. Mary Ann and I believed that the drug protocol alone was not going to give her more time. She was determined to have the surgery and subsequent radiation. Recovery was difficult and she lost her hair in the radiation field, but it was a fortunate time in that she met Davi Chabner, who was to be her best friend and catalyst for enjoying life again. A year later there was another brain tumor, which was removed and followed by more radiation. She then took part in a brief trial using monoclonal antibodies. A couple more surface tumors were removed, but then: no more! Remission! Life was good. Vacations, golf with friends, visits to college to see our daughters, trips to see Mary Ann's sisters, all was a pleasant blend of what you do with the time you have. Although she had a multitude of friends whom she saw often, it was Mary Ann's time with Davi and her husband that kept her enthused over every day.

16

Five years later Mary Ann woke up with night sweats and a low-grade fever that wouldn't go away. Our worst fears were realized. A large, inoperable tumor was in her spleen. Less than 4 months later she died. Looking back, it's easy to see she went through a lot during her 9-year ordeal, but she beat the odds and, through sheer willpower, enjoyed her time to the fullest. That was over 20 years ago, and to this day, I still meet people who remember her fondly and remark that she was one of their best friends. That was Mary Ann. No matter what she was going through she was still interested in *your* life.

Bob Rowe is a retired software engineer and avid golfer.

Author's note: In recent years, promising therapies for metastatic melanoma are emerging using a new targeted agent, Vemurafenib, and new monoclonal antibodies that promote an immune response to the tumor.

 EXERCISES

Remember to check your answers carefully with the Answers to Exercises, page 688.

A **Select from the listed terms to complete the sentences that follow.**

adipocyte	dermis	melanin
basal layer	keratin	sebum
collagen	lunula	stratum corneum
cuticle		

1. A fat cell is a/an _____.

2. The half-moon–shaped white area at the base of a nail is the _____.

3. A structural protein found in skin and connective tissue is _____.

4. A pigment found in the epidermis is _____.

5. The deepest region of the epidermis is the _____.

6. The outermost layer of the epidermis, which consists of flattened, keratinized cells, is the

   _____.

7. An oily substance secreted by sebaceous glands is _____.

8. The middle layer of the skin is the _____.

9. A hard, protein material found in epidermis, hair, and nails is _____.

10. A band of epidermis at the base and sides of the nail plate is the _____.

B **Complete the following terms based on their meanings as given.**

1. the outermost layer of skin: epi _____

2. profuse sweating: dia _____

3. excessive secretion from sebaceous glands: sebo _____

4. inflammation and swelling of soft tissue around a nail: par _____

5. fungal infections of hands and feet: dermato _____

6. burning sensation (pain) in skin: caus _____

C Match the terms in Column I with the descriptive meanings in Column II. Write the letter of the answer in the space provided.

COLUMN I

1. squamous epithelium _____

2. sebaceous gland _____

3. albinism _____

4. electrocautery _____

5. subcutaneous tissue _____

6. collagen _____

7. dermis _____

8. melanocyte _____

9. erythema _____

10. dermabrasion _____

COLUMN II

A. Connective tissue layer of skin
B. Surgical procedure to scrape away tissue
C. Flat, scale-like cells
D. Connective tissue protein
E. Pigment deficiency of the skin
F. Contains a dark pigment
G. Redness of skin
H. Contains lipocytes
I. Oil-producing organ
J. Knife used to burn through tissue

D Build medical terms based on the definitions and word parts given.

1. pertaining to under the skin: sub _____

2. abnormal condition of lack of sweat: an

3. abnormal condition of proliferation of horny, keratinized cells: kerat _____

4. abnormal condition of dry, scaly skin: _____ osis

5. loosening of the epidermis: epidermo _____

6. yellow tumor (nodule under the skin): _____ oma

7. pertaining to under the nail: sub _____

8. abnormal condition of excessive hair growth: hyper _____

9. abnormal condition of nail fungus: onycho _____

10. removal of wrinkles: _____ ectomy

16

E **Give the meanings for the following combining forms.**

1. melan/o _____

2. adip/o _____

3. squam/o _____

4. xanth/o _____

5. myc/o _____

6. onych/o _____

7. pil/o _____

8. xer/o _____

9. trich/o _____

10. erythem/o _____

11. albin/o _____

12. ichthy/o _____

13. hidr/o _____

14. ungu/o _____

15. cauter/o _____

16. steat/o _____

17. rhytid/o _____

18. py/o _____

19. hydr/o _____

20. cutane/o _____

16

F **Match each of the following lesions with their illustrations in Figure 16-25.**

crust (scab)   macule   pustule
cyst   nodule   ulcer
erosion   papule   vesicle
fissure   polyp   wheal

1.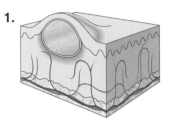

_____
pus-filled

2.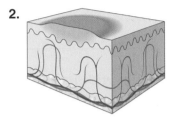

_____
smooth, edematous, reddish
papule or plaque

3.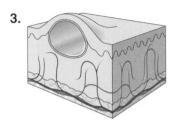

_____
fluid or semisolid thick-walled
filled sac

4.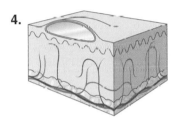

_____
clear fluid, blister

5.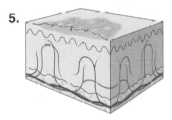

_____
dried serum and cellular debris

6.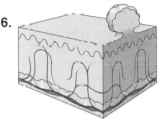

_____
benign growth extending from
mucous membrane surface

7.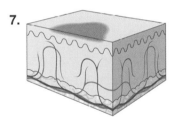

_____
discolored, flat

8.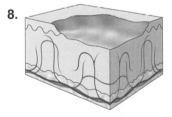

_____
wearing away, loss of epidermis

9.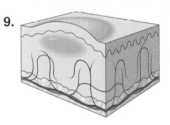

_____
solid, elevated mass,
more than 1 cm

10.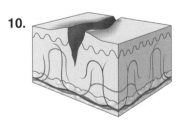

_____
slit, groove

11.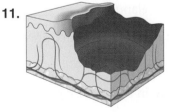

_____
open sore on skin or
mucous membrane

12.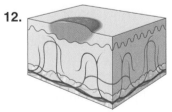

_____
small, solid elevation,
pimple or plaque

FIGURE 16-25 Cutaneous lesions.

16

G Give the medical terms for the following.

1. baldness _____

2. bluish black mark (macule) caused by hemorrhages into the skin _____

3. itching _____

4. acute allergic reaction in which red, round wheals develop on the skin _____

5. blackhead _____

6. small, pinpoint hemorrhages _____

H Match the pathologic skin condition with its description from the numbered list that follows.

acne vulgaris	gangrene	scleroderma
basal cell carcinoma	impetigo	squamous cell carcinoma
decubitus ulcer	malignant melanoma	systemic lupus erythematosus
eczema	psoriasis	tinea

1. malignant neoplasm originating in scale-like cells of the epidermis _____

2. buildup of sebum and keratin in pores of the skin leading to papular and pustular eruptions

_____

3. fungal skin infection _____

4. chronic disease marked by hardening and shrinking of connective tissue in the skin

_____

5. bedsore _____

6. necrosis of skin tissue resulting from ischemia _____

7. chronic or acute inflammatory skin disease with erythematous, pustular, or papular lesions

_____

8. widespread inflammatory disease of the joints and collagen of the skin with "butterfly" rash on

the face _____

9. cancerous tumor composed of melanocytes _____

10. chronic, recurrent dermatosis marked by silvery-gray scales covering red patches on the skin

_____

11. malignant neoplasm originating in the basal layer of the epidermis _____

12. contagious, infectious pyoderma _____

16

I   **Circle the boldface term that best fits the definition given.**

1. contagious parasitic infection with intense pruritus: **(scleroderma, scabies)**

2. measles: **(rubella, rubeola)**

3. chickenpox: **(varicella, eczema)**

4. thickened excess cicatrix (scar): **(tinea, keloid)**

5. white patches on mucous membrane of tongue or inner cheek: **(leukoplakia, albinism)**

6. characterized by a rash: **(gangrene, exanthematous)**

7. thickening of epidermis related to sunlight exposure: **(actinic keratosis, callus)**

8. small, pinpoint hemorrhages: **(psoriasis, petechiae)**

9. large blisters: **(bullae, pustules)**

10. hyperpigmented macule or papule of skin (mole): **(nevus, verruca)**

11. sac of fluid and hair over sacral region: **(ecchymosis, pilonidal cyst)**

12. acute allergic reaction in which hives develop: **(vitiligo, urticaria)**

J   **Describe the following types of burns.**

1. second-degree burn: _____

2. first-degree burn: _____

3. third-degree burn: _____

K   **Match the medical terms with the more common names or descriptions provided.**

alopecia	exanthem	tinea pedis
comedones	nevi	urticaria
decubitus ulcer	pruritus	verrucae
ecchymosis	seborrheic dermatitis	vesicles

1. blackheads _____

2. moles _____

3. baldness _____

4. itching _____

5. hives _____

6. bedsore _____

7. warts _____

8. athlete's foot _____

9. "black-and-blue" mark _____

10. dandruff _____

11. blisters _____

12. rash _____

16

L **Describe how the following conditions affect the skin.**

1. pyoderma: _____

2. xerosis: _____

3. leukoderma: _____

4. erythema: _____

5. callus: _____

6. keloid: _____

7. gangrene: _____

M **Give short answers to complete the following sentences.**

1. Two skin tests for allergy are _____ and _____.

2. The _____ test is an intradermal test for diphtheria.

3. The _____ test and the _____ test are skin tests for tuberculosis.

4. Purulent means _____.

5. A surgical procedure to core out a disk of skin for microscopic analysis is a/an

   _____.

6. The procedure in which thin layers of a malignant growth are removed and each is examined

   under the microscope is _____.

7. A type of skin cancer associated with AIDS and marked by dark blue-purple lesions over the skin

   is _____.

8. Abnormal, premalignant moles are _____.

9. Removal of skin tissue using a cut parallel to the surface of the surrounding skin is called a/an

   _____.

10. Destruction of tissue using intensely cold temperatures is _____.

11. Scraping away skin to remove acne scars and fine wrinkles on the skin is

    _____.

12. Removal of subcutaneous fat tissue by aspiration is _____.

13. Destruction of tissue using an electric spark is _____.

14. Use of a sharp, spoon-like instrument to scrape away tissue is _____.

16

N **Circle the terms in boldface that best complete the meaning of the sentences.**

1. Since he was a teenager, Jim had had red, scaly patches on his elbows and the front of his knees. Dr. Horn diagnosed Jim's dermatologic condition as **(vitiligo, impetigo, psoriasis)** and prescribed a special cream.

2. Clarissa noticed a rash across the bridge of her nose and aching in her joints. She saw a rheumatologist, who did some blood work and diagnosed her condition as **(rheumatoid arthritis, systemic lupus erythematosus, scleroderma)**.

3. Bea had large red plaques develop all over her trunk and neck after eating shrimp. The doctor prescribed hydrocortisone cream to relieve her itching **(seborrhea, acne, urticaria)**.

4. The poison ivy Maggie touched caused very uncomfortable **(pruritus, calluses, keratosis)**, and she was scratching her arms raw.

5. Kelly was fair-skinned with red hair. She had many benign nevi on her arms and legs, but Dr. Keefe was especially worried about one pigmented lesion with an irregular, raised border, which he biopsied and found to be malignant **(melanoma, Kaposi sarcoma, pyoderma)**.

6. After 5 days of high fever, 3-year-old Sadie developed a red rash all over her body. The pediatrician described it as a viral **(eczema, purpura, exanthem)** and told her mother it was a case of **(rubeola, impetigo, scabies)**.

7. Several months after her surgery, Mabel's scar became raised and thickened and grew beyond the boundaries of the incision. It had **(atrophied, stratified, hypertrophied)**, and her physician described it as a **(nevus, verruca, keloid)**.

8. Perry had a bad habit of biting his nails and picking at the **(follicle, cuticle, subcutaneous tissue)** surrounding his nails. Often, he developed inflammation and swelling of the soft tissue around the nail, a condition known as **(onychomycosis, onycholysis, paronychia)**.

9. Brenda noticed a small papillomatous wart on her hand. Her **(oncologist, dermatologist, psychologist)** explained that it was a **(pustule, polyp, verruca)** and was caused by a **(bacterium, virus, toxin)**. The doctor suggested removing it by **(Mohs surgery, cryosurgery, dilation and curettage)**.

10. Sarah, a teenager, was self-conscious about the inflammatory lesions of papules and pustules on her face. She noticed blackheads or **(wheals, bullae, open comedones)** and whiteheads (closed comedones). She was advised to begin taking antibiotics and applying topical medications to treat her **(acne vulgaris, scleroderma, gangrene)**.

16

ANSWERS TO EXERCISES

A

1. adipocyte
2. lunula
3. collagen
4. melanin

5. basal layer
6. stratum corneum
7. sebum

8. dermis
9. keratin
10. cuticle

B

1. epidermis
2. diaphoresis
3. seborrhea
4. paronychia

5. dermatophytosis or dermatomycosis (tinea)
6. causalgia

C

1. C
2. I
3. E
4. J

5. H
6. D
7. A

8. F
9. G
10. B

D

1. subcutaneous
2. anhidrosis
3. keratosis
4. ichthyosis

5. epidermolysis
6. xanthoma
7. subungual

8. hypertrichosis
9. onychomycosis
10. rhytidectomy

E

1. black
2. fat
3. scale-like
4. yellow
5. fungus
6. nail
7. hair

8. dry
9. hair
10. redness
11. white
12. scaly, dry
13. sweat
14. nail

15. heat, burn
16. fat
17. wrinkle
18. pus
19. water
20. skin

F

1. pustule
2. wheal
3. cyst
4. vesicle

5. crust (scab)
6. polyp
7. macule
8. erosion

9. nodule
10. fissure
11. ulcer
12. papule

G

1. alopecia
2. ecchymosis
3. pruritus

4. urticaria
5. comedo
6. petechiae

H

1. squamous cell carcinoma
2. acne vulgaris
3. tinea
4. scleroderma

5. decubitus ulcer
6. gangrene
7. eczema
8. systemic lupus erythematosus

9. malignant melanoma
10. psoriasis
11. basal cell carcinoma
12. impetigo

I

1. scabies
2. rubeola
3. varicella
4. keloid

5. leukoplakia
6. exanthematous
7. actinic keratosis
8. petechiae

9. bullae
10. nevus
11. pilonidal cyst
12. urticaria

J

1. damage to the epidermis and dermis with blisters, erythema, and hyperesthesia
2. damage to the epidermis with erythema and hyperesthesia; no blisters
3. destruction of both epidermis and dermis and damage to subcutaneous layer

K

1. comedones
2. nevi
3. alopecia
4. pruritus
5. urticaria
6. decubitus ulcer
7. verrucae
8. tinea pedis
9. ecchymosis
10. seborrheic dermatitis
11. vesicles
12. exanthem

L

1. collections of pus in the skin
2. dry skin
3. white patches of skin (vitiligo)
4. redness of skin
5. increased growth of epidermal horny-layer cells due to excess pressure or friction
6. thickened, hypertrophied scar tissue
7. necrosis (death) of skin tissue

M

1. scratch test; patch test
2. Schick
3. Mantoux; PPD
4. pus-filled
5. punch biopsy
6. Mohs surgery
7. Kaposi sarcoma
8. dysplastic nevi
9. shave biopsy
10. cryosurgery
11. dermabrasion
12. liposuction
13. electrodesiccation
14. curettage

N

1. psoriasis
2. systemic lupus erythematosus
3. urticaria
4. pruritus
5. melanoma
6. exanthem; rubeola
7. hypertrophied; keloid
8. cuticle; paronychia
9. dermatologist; verruca; virus; cryosurgery
10. open comedones; acne vulgaris

Answers to Practical Applications

1. c
2. a
3. b
4. c
5. a

16

PRONUNCIATION OF TERMS

To test your understanding of the terminology in this chapter, write the meaning of each term in the space provided. In addition, you may wish to cover the terms and write them by looking at your definitions. Make sure your spelling is correct. The page number after each term indicates where it is defined or used in the book, so you can easily check your responses. You will find complete definitions for all of these terms and their audio pronunciations on the Evolve website.

Pronunciation Guide

ā as in āpe   ă as in ăpple

ē as in ēven   ĕ as in ĕvery

ī as in īce   ĭ as in ĭnterest

ō as in ōpen   ŏ as in pŏt

ū as in ūnit   ŭ as in ŭnder

Terminology

TERM	PRONUNCIATION	MEANING
adipocyte (659)	ĂD-ĭ-pō-sīt	_____
adipose (660)	ĂD-ĭ-pōs	_____
albinism (660)	ĂL-bĭ-nĭzm	_____
albino (659)	ăl-BĪ-nō	_____
anhidrosis (660)	ăn-hī-DRŌ-sĭs	_____
apocrine sweat gland (659)	ĂP-ō-krĭn swĕt glănd	_____
basal layer (659)	BĀ-săl LĀ-ĕr	_____
causalgia (660)	kăw-ZĂL-jă	_____
collagen (659)	KŎL-ă-jĕn	_____
cuticle (659)	KŪ-tĭ-kl	_____
dermabrasion (660)	dĕrm-ă-BRĀ-zhŭn	_____
dermatitis (660)	dĕr-mă-TĪ-tŭs	_____
dermatologist (660)	dĕr-mă-TŎL-ō-jĭst	_____
dermatophytosis (662)	dĕr-mă-tō-fī-TŌ-sĭs	_____
dermis (659)	DĔR-mĭs	_____
diaphoresis (660)	dī-ă-fŏr-RĒ-sĭs	_____
eccrine sweat gland (659)	Ĕ-krĭn swĕt glănd	_____
electrocautery (660)	ĕ-lĕk-trō-KĂW-tĕr-ē	_____
epidermis (659)	ĕp-ĭ-DĔR-mĭs	_____
epidermolysis (660)	ĕp-ĭ-dĕr-MŎL-ĭ-sĭs	_____
epithelium (659)	ĕp-ĭ-THĒL-ē-ŭm	_____
erythema (660)	ĕr-ĭ-THĒ-mă	_____
erythematous (660)	ĕr-ĭ-THĒ-mă-tŭs	_____
hair follicle (659)	hār FŎL-ĭ-kl	_____

TERM	PRONUNCIATION	MEANING
hypertrichosis (663)	hī-pĕr-trĭ-KŌ-sĭs	
ichthyosis (660)	ĭk-thē-Ō-sĭs	
integumentary system (659)	ĭn-tĕg-ū-MĔN-tăr-ē SĬS-tĕm	
keratin (659)	KĔR-ă-tĭn	
keratosis (661)	kĕr-ă-TŌ-sĭs	
leukoplakia (661)	loo-kō-PLĀ-kē-ă	
lipoma (661)	lĭ-PŌ-mă *or* lī-PŌ-mă	
liposuction (661)	lī-pō-SŬK-shun	
lunula (659)	LŪ-nū-lă	
melanin (659)	MĔL-ă-nĭn	
melanocyte (661)	mĕ-LĂN-ō-sīt	
mycosis (662)	mī-KŌ-sĭs	
onycholysis (662)	ŏn-ĭ-KŎL-ĭ-sĭs	
onychomycosis (662)	ŏn-ĭ-kō-mī-KŌ-sĭs	
paronychia (662)	păr ō NĬK ē-ă	
paronychium (659)	păr-ŏn-NĬK-ē-um	
pilosebaceous (662)	pī-lō-sĕ-BĀ-shŭs	
pore (659)	PŎR	
pyoderma (662)	pī-ō-DĔR-mă	
rhytidectomy (662)	rĭt-ĭ-DĔK-tō-mē	
sebaceous gland (659)	sĕ-BĀ-shŭs glănd	
seborrhea (662)	sĕb-ō-RĒ-ă	
seborrheic dermatitis (662)	sĕb-ō-RĒ-ĭk dĕr-mă-TĪ-tĭs	
sebum (659)	SĒ-bŭm	
squamous epithelium (659)	SKWĀ-mŭs ĕp-ĭ-THĒ-lē-ŭm	
steatoma (663)	stē-ă-TŌ-mă	
stratified (659)	STRĂT-ĭ-fīd	
stratum; (strata) (659)	STRĂ-tŭm; STRĂ-tă	
stratum corneum (659)	STRĂ-tŭm KŎR-nē-ŭm	
subcutaneous layer (659)	sŭb-kū-TĀ-nē-ŭs LĀ-ĕr	
subungual (663)	sŭb-ŬNG-wăl	
xanthoma (663)	zăn-THŌ-mă	
xerosis (663)	zĕr-Ō-sĭs	

16

Pathology; Laboratory Tests and Clinical Procedures

TERM	PRONUNCIATION	MEANING
abscess (664)	ĂB-sĕs	
acne (666)	ĂK-nē	
alopecia areata (666)	ăl-ō-PĒ-shē-ă ăr-ē-ĂT-ă	
atopic dermatitis (668)	ā-TŎP-ĭk dĕr-mă-TĪ-tĭs	
bacterial analyses (675)	băk-TĒR-ē-ăl ă-NĂL-ĭ-sēz	
basal cell carcinoma (674)	BĀ-săl sĕl kăr-sĭ-NŌ-mă	
bulla; bullae (664)	BŬL-ă; BŬL-ē	
burns (667)	bŭrnz	
callus (672)	KĂL-ŭs	
cellulitis (668)	sĕl-ū-LĪ-tĭs	
cicatrix (672)	SĬK-ă-trĭks	
comedo; comedones (666)	KŎM-ĕ-dō; kŏm-ĕ-DŌNĒZ	
crust (664)	krŭst	
cryosurgery (675)	krī-ō-SŬR-gĕr-ē	
curettage (675)	kū-rĕ-TĂZH	
cyst (664)	sĭst	
decubitus ulcer (664)	dē-KŪ-bĭ-tŭs ŬL-sĕr	
dysplastic nevi (673)	dĭs-PLĂS-tik NĒ-vī	
ecchymosis; ecchymoses (666)	ĕk-ĭ-MŌ-sĭs; ĕk-ĭ-MŌ-sēz	
eczema (668)	ĔK-zĕ-mă	
electrodesiccation (675)	ĕ-lĕk-trō-dĕ-sĭ-KĀ-shun	
erosion (664)	ĕ-RŌ-zhŭn	
exanthematous viral disease (668)	ĕg-zăn-THĔM-ă-tŭs VĪ-răl dĭ-ZĒZ	
fissure (664)	FĬSH-ŭr	
fungal tests (676)	FŬNG-ăl tĕsts	
gangrene (669)	găng-GRĒN	
impetigo (669)	ĭm-pĕ-TĪ-gō	
Kaposi sarcoma (674)	KĂH-pō-sē săr-KŌ-mă	
keloid (672)	KĒ-loyd	
keratosis (672)	kĕr-ă-TŌ-sĭs	

16

TERM	PRONUNCIATION	MEANING
macule (664)	MĂK-ūl	
malignant melanoma (674)	mă-LĬG-nănt mĕ-lă-NŌ-mă	
Mohs surgery (675)	mōz SŬR-jĕ-rē	
nevus; nevi (673)	NĒ-vŭs; NĒ-vī	
nodule (664)	NŎD-ūl	
papule (664)	PĂP-ūl	
petechia; petechiae (666)	pĕ-TĒ-kē-ă; pĕ-TĒ-kē-ī	
pilonidal cyst (664)	pī-lō-NĪ-dăl sĭst	
polyp (664)	PŎL-ĭp	
pruritus (666)	proo-RĪ-tŭs	
psoriasis (670)	sō-RĪ-ă-sĭs	
purpura (666)	PŬR-pŭr-ă	
pustule (664)	PŬS-tūl	
rubella (668)	roo-BĔL-ă	
rubeola (668)	roo-be-Ō-lă	
scabies (670)	SKĀ-bēz	
scleroderma (670)	sklĕr-ō-DĔR-mă	
sebaceous cyst (663)	sĕ-BĀ-shŭs sĭst	
skin biopsy (676)	skĭn BĪ-ŏp-sē	
skin test (676)	skĭn tĕst	
squamous cell carcinoma (674)	SKWĀ-mŭs sĕl kăr-sĭ-NŌ-mă	
systemic lupus erythematosus (670)	sĭs-TĔM-ĭk LOO-pŭs ĕr-ĭ-thē-mă-TŌ-sŭs	
tinea (671)	TĬN-ē-ă	
ulcer (664)	ŬL-sĕr	
urticaria (672)	ŭr-tĭ-KĀ-rē-ă	
varicella (668)	văr-ĭ-SĔL-ă	
verruca; verrucae (673)	vĕ-ROO-kă; vĕ-ROO-kē	
vesicle (664)	VĔS-ĭ-kl	
vitiligo (672)	vĭt-ĭl-Ī-gō	
wheal (664)	wēl	

REVIEW SHEET

Write the meanings of the word parts in the spaces provided, and test yourself. Check your answers with the information in the chapter or in the *Glossary (Medical Word Parts—English)* at the end of the book.

Combining Forms

COMBINING FORM	MEANING	COMBINING FORM	MEANING
adip/o	_____	melan/o	_____
albin/o	_____	myc/o	_____
caus/o	_____	onych/o	_____
cauter/o	_____	phyt/o	_____
cutane/o	_____	pil/o	_____
derm/o	_____	py/o	_____
dermat/o	_____	rhytid/o	_____
diaphor/o	_____	seb/o	_____
erythem/o	_____	sebace/o	_____
erythemat/o	_____	squam/o	_____
hidr/o	_____	steat/o	_____
hydr/o	_____	trich/o	_____
ichthy/o	_____	ungu/o	_____
kerat/o	_____	xanth/o	_____
leuk/o	_____	xer/o	_____
lip/o	_____		

16

Suffixes

SUFFIX	MEANING	SUFFIX	MEANING
-algia	_____	-osis	_____
-derma	_____	-ous	_____
-esis	_____	-plakia	_____
-lysis	_____	-plasty	_____
-ose	_____	-rrhea	_____

Give combining forms for the following (first letters are given).

fat	a _____	sweat	d _____
	l _____		h _____
	s _____	yellow	x _____
white	a _____	dry	x _____
	l _____	dry, scaly (fish-like)	i _____
skin	c _____	redness	e _____
	d _____		e _____
nail	o _____	hard	k _____
	u _____	heat, burn	c _____
hair	p _____	black	m _____
	t _____	fungus	m _____
plant	p _____		

16

Identify the following skin conditions shown in the accompanying figure:

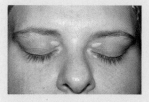

A._____

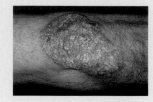

B._____

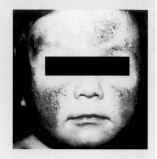

C._____

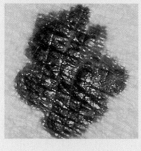

D._____

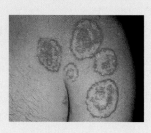

E._____

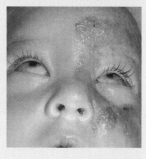

F._____

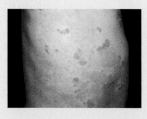

G._____

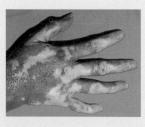

H._____

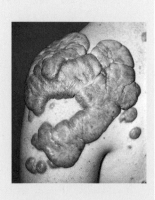

I._____

16

Sense Organs:
The Eye and the Ear

Chapter Sections:

CHAPTER GOALS

- Identify locations and functions of the major parts of the eye and the ear.
- Name the combining forms, prefixes, and suffixes most commonly used to describe these organs and their parts.
- Describe the abnormal conditions that may affect the eye and the ear.
- Identify clinical procedures that pertain to ophthalmology and otology.
- Apply your new knowledge to understanding medical terms in their proper contexts, such as medical reports and records.

INTRODUCTION

The **eye** and the **ear** are sense organs, like the skin, taste buds, and **olfactory** (centers of smell in the nose) regions. As such, they are receptors whose sensitive cells may be activated by a particular form of energy or stimulus in the external or internal environment. The sensitive cells in the eye and ear respond to the stimulus by initiating a series of nerve impulses along sensory nerve fibers that lead to the brain.

No matter what stimulus affects a particular receptor, the resulting sensation is determined by regions in the brain connected to that receptor. Thus, mechanical injury that stimulates receptor cells in the eye and the ear may produce sensations of vision (flashes of light) and sound (ringing in the ears). If a workable connection could be made between the sensitive receptor cells of the ear and the area in the brain associated with sight, it would be possible to "see" sounds.

Figure 17-1 reviews the general pattern of events that occur when such stimuli as light and sound are received by sense organs such as the eye and the ear.

THE EYE

ANATOMY AND PHYSIOLOGY

Label Figure 17-2 as you read the following:

Light rays enter the central dark opening of the eye, the **pupil** [1], which is surrounded by the colored portion of the eye, or **iris** (see the photo inset). The **conjunctiva** [2] is a membrane lining the inner surfaces of the eyelids and anterior portion of the eyeball over the white of the eye. The conjunctiva is clear and almost colorless except when blood vessels are dilated. Dust and smoke may cause the blood vessels to dilate, giving the conjunctiva a reddish appearance—commonly known as bloodshot eyes. Also, the same blood vessels may dilate when the eye is infected or inflamed by allergies. This condition is known as conjunctivitis.

Before entering the eye through the pupil, light passes through the **cornea** [3]. The cornea is a fibrous, transparent tissue that extends like a dome over the pupil and iris. The function of the cornea is to bend, or **refract,** the rays of light so they are focused properly on the sensitive receptor cells in the posterior region of the eye. The normal, healthy cornea is avascular (has no blood vessels) but receives nourishment from blood vessels near its junction with the opaque white of the eye, the **sclera** [4]. Corneal transplants for people with scarred or opaque corneas are often successful because antibodies responsible for rejection of foreign tissue usually do not reach the avascular, transplanted corneal tissue. The sclera is a fibrous layer under the conjunctiva. It extends from the cornea on the anterior surface of the eyeball to the optic nerve in the posterior of the eye.

The **choroid** [5] is a dark brown membrane inside the sclera. It contains many blood vessels that supply nutrients to the eye. The choroid is continuous with the pigment-containing **iris** [6] and the **ciliary body** [7] in the anterior portion of the eye. The choroid, iris, and ciliary body are known as the **uvea** of the eye.

The iris is the colored portion of the eye (it can appear blue, green, hazel, gray, or brown), which has a circular opening in the center that forms the pupil. Muscles of the

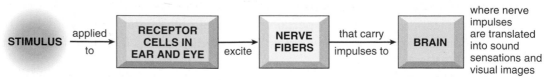

FIGURE 17-1　Pattern of events in the stimulation of a sense organ.

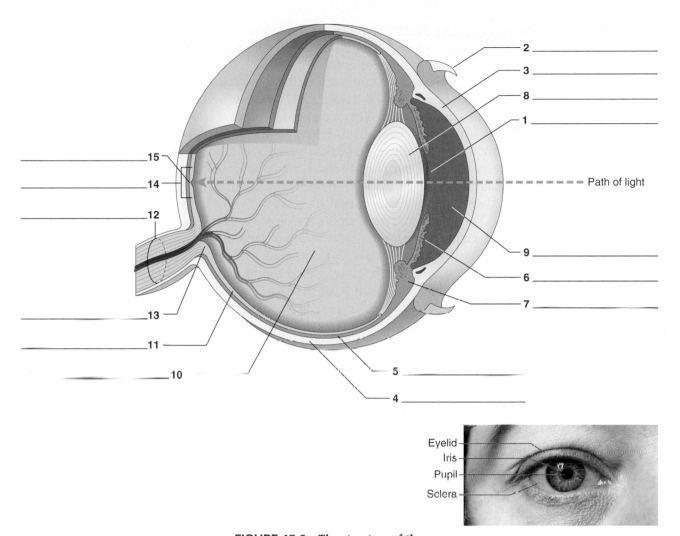

Path of light

Eyelid
Iris
Pupil
Sclera

FIGURE 17-2   The structure of the eye.

17

iris constrict the pupil in bright light and dilate the pupil in dim light, thereby regulating the amount of light entering the eye.

The ciliary body surrounds the outside of the **lens** [8] in circular fashion for a full 360 degrees. There are fine, thread-like attachments (zonules) that connect the ciliary body and the lens, allowing the muscles in the ciliary body to adjust the shape and thickness of the lens. These changes in the shape of the lens cause **refraction** of light rays. Refraction is the bending of rays as they pass through the cornea, lens, and other tissues. Muscles of the ciliary body produce flattening of the lens (for distant vision) and thickening and rounding of the lens (for close vision). This refractory adjustment to focus on an object from far to near is called **accommodation.** When people get older, their eyes' ability to accommodate decreases, so they may need magnifying glasses to see close objects and to read.

Besides regulating the shape of the lens, the ciliary body also secretes a fluid called **aqueous humor,** which is found in the **anterior chamber** [9] of the eye. Aqueous humor maintains the shape of the anterior portion of the eye and nourishes the structures in that region. The fluid is constantly produced and leaves the eye through a canal that carries it into the bloodstream. Another cavity of the eye is the **vitreous chamber,** which is a large region behind the lens filled with a soft, jelly-like material, the **vitreous humor** [10]. Vitreous humor maintains the shape of the eyeball and is not constantly re-formed. Its escape (due to trauma or surgical damage) may result in significant damage to the eye, leading to possible retinal damage and blindness. Both the aqueous and the vitreous humors further refract light rays.

The **retina** [11] is the thin, delicate, and sensitive nerve layer of the eye. As light energy, in the form of waves, travels through the eye, it is refracted (by the cornea, lens, and fluids), so that it focuses on sensitive receptor cells of the retina called the **rods** and **cones.** There are approximately 6.5 million cones and 120 million rods in the retina. The cones function in bright levels of light and are responsible for color and central vision. There are three types of cones, each stimulated by one of the primary colors in light (red, green, or blue). Most cases of color blindness affect either the green or the red receptors, so that the two colors cannot be distinguished from each other. Rods function at reduced levels of light and are responsible for peripheral vision and vision in dim light.

When light rays are focused on the retina, a chemical change occurs in the rods and cones, initiating nerve impulses that then travel from the eye to the brain via the **optic nerve** [12]. The region in the eye where the optic nerve meets the retina is called the **optic disc** [13]. Because there are no light receptor cells in the optic disc, it is known as the blind spot of the eye. The **macula** [14] is a small, oval, yellowish area adjacent to the optic disc. It contains a central depression called the **fovea centralis** [15], which is composed largely of cones and is the location of the sharpest vision in the eye. If a portion of the fovea or macula is damaged, vision is reduced and central-vision blindness occurs. Figure 17-3 shows the retina of a normal eye as seen through an ophthalmoscope. The **fundus** of the eye is this posterior, inner part that is visualized through the ophthalmoscope.

Figure 17-4 illustrates what happens when you look at an object and "see" it. If an object is in your **left visual field** (purple area), sensitive cells—rods and cones—in the **right** half

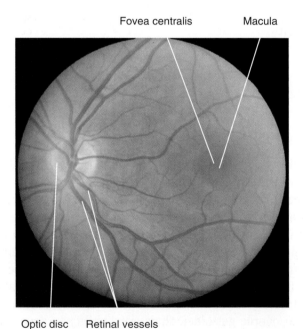

Fovea centralis   Macula

Optic disc   Retinal vessels

FIGURE 17-3 **The posterior, inner part (fundus) of the eye,** showing the retina as seen through an ophthalmoscope.

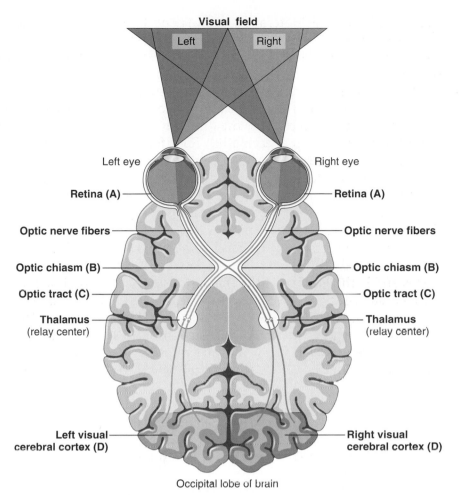

FIGURE 17-4 **Visual pathway from the retina (A) to the visual cerebral cortex (D)** (occipital lobe of the brain). Objects in the left visual field are "seen" by the right side of the brain, whereas objects in the right visual field are projected into the left visual cerebral cortex.

of each **retina** (labeled A in the figure) are stimulated. Similarly, if an object is in your **right visual field** (orange color), rods and cones are stimulated in the left half of each retina. Nervous impulses then travel along optic nerve fibers from each retina and then merge to form the **optic chiasm** (B). Here, medial optic nerve fibers cross and temporal fibers do not. Thus, fibers from the right half of each retina (purple color) form an **optic tract** (C) leading, via the **thalamus** (relay center), to the **right visual cerebral cortex** (D). Similarly, fibers from the left half of each retina (orange color) form an optic tract leading to the **left visual cerebral cortex** (D). Images (one from each eye) are then fused in the occipital lobe of the brain, producing a single visual sensation with the three-dimensional effect. This is **binocular vision.**

Brain damage to nerve cells in the right visual cerebral cortex (such as in a stroke) causes loss of vision in the left visual field (purple), whereas damage in the left cerebral cortex causes loss of vision in the right visual field (gold). This loss of vision, which occurs in both eyes, on the contralateral (opposite side) visual field is called **hemianopsia** (**hemi-** means half, **an-** means without, **-opsia** means vision). In the right eye, the loss is in the left nasal visual field, and in the left eye, the loss is in the left temporal visual field.

Figure 17-5 reviews the pathway of light rays from the cornea to the cerebral cortex of the brain.

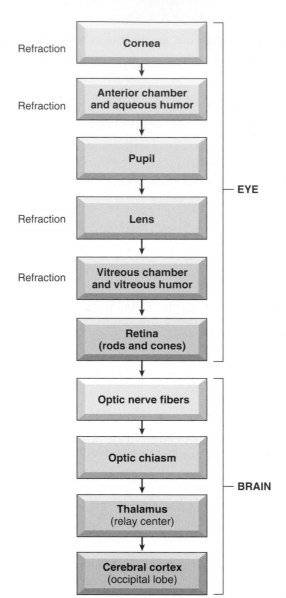

FIGURE 17-5   Pathway of light rays from the cornea of the eye to the cerebral cortex of the brain.

VOCABULARY—THE EYE

This list reviews many new terms relating to the eye introduced in the text. Short definitions reinforce your understanding of the terms. Refer to the Pronunciation of Terms on page 742 for help with unfamiliar or difficult words.

accommodation	Normal adjustment of the eye to focus on objects from far to near. The ciliary body adjusts the lens (rounding it) and the pupil constricts. When the eye focuses from near to far, the ciliary body flattens the lens and the pupil dilates.
anterior chamber	Area behind the cornea and in front of the lens and iris. It contains aqueous humor.
aqueous humor	Fluid produced by the ciliary body and found in the anterior chamber. A humor (Latin *humidus* means moist) is any body fluid, including blood and lymph.

biconvex	Consisting of two surfaces that are rounded, elevated, and curved evenly, like part of a sphere. The lens of the eye is a biconvex body.
choroid	Middle, vascular layer of the eye, between the retina and the sclera.
ciliary body	Structure on each side of the lens that connects the choroid and iris. It contains ciliary muscles, which control the shape of the lens, and it secretes aqueous humor.
cone	Photoreceptor cell in the retina that transforms light energy into a nerve impulse. Cones are responsible for color and central vision.
conjunctiva	Delicate membrane lining the eyelids and covering the eyeball.
cornea	Fibrous transparent layer of clear tissue that extends over the anterior portion of the eyeball. Derived from Latin *corneus*, meaning horny, perhaps because as it protrudes outward, it was thought to resemble a horn.
fovea centralis	Tiny pit or depression in the retina that is the region of clearest vision.
fundus of the eye	Posterior, inner part of the eye; visualized with an ophthalmoscope.
iris	Pigmented (colored) layer that opens and closes to allow more or less light into the eye. The central opening of the iris is the pupil.
lens	Transparent, biconvex body behind the pupil of the eye. It bends (refracts) light rays to bring them into focus on the retina.
macula	Yellowish region on the retina lateral to and slightly below the optic disc; contains the fovea centralis, which is the area of clearest vision.
optic chiasm	Point at which optic nerve fibers cross in the brain (Latin *chiasma* means crossing).
optic disc	Region at the back of the eye where the optic nerve meets the retina. It is the blind spot of the eye because it contains only nerve fibers, no rods or cones, and is thus insensitive to light.
optic nerve	Cranial nerve carrying impulses from the retina to the brain (cerebral cortex).
pupil	Central opening of the eye, surrounded by the iris, through which light rays pass. It appears dark.
refraction	Bending of light rays by the cornea, lens, and fluids of the eye to bring the rays into focus on the retina. Refract means to break (-fract) back (re-).
retina	Light-sensitive nerve cell layer of the eye containing photoreceptor cells (rods and cones).
rod	Photoreceptor cell of the retina essential for vision in low light and for peripheral vision.
sclera	Tough, white outer coat of the eyeball.
thalamus	Relay center of the brain. Optic nerve fibers pass through the thalamus on their way to the cerebral cortex.
vitreous humor	Soft, jelly-like material behind the lens in the vitreous chamber; helps maintain the shape of the eyeball.

17

TERMINOLOGY—THE EYE

Write the meanings of the medical terms relating to the eye in the spaces provided.

COMBINING FORMS: STRUCTURES AND FLUIDS

COMBINING FORM	MEANING	TERMINOLOGY	MEANING
aque/o	water	aqueous humor _____	
blephar/o	eyelid (*see* **palpebr/o**)	blepharitis _____ *See Figure 17-6A.*	
		blepharoptosis _____ *Pronounced blĕf-ă-rŏp-TŌ-sĭs. Also called **ptosis.** This condition may be caused by abnormalities of the eyelid muscle or by nerve damage.*	
conjunctiv/o	conjunctiva	conjunctivitis _____ *Commonly called **pinkeye** (Figure 17-6B). Conjunctivitis occurs when blood vessels dilate from allergens like pollen (allergic conjunctivitis), bacterial infection (bacterial conjunctivitis), or virus (viral conjunctivitis).*	
cor/o	pupil (*see* **pupill/o**)	anisocoria _____ *Anis/o means unequal. Anisocoria may be an indication of neurologic injury or disease (Figure 17-7A).*	

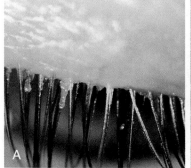
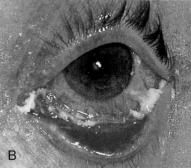

FIGURE 17-6   A, Blepharitis. Notice the crusting on the eyelid and eyelashes. **B, Acute bacterial conjunctivitis.** Notice the discharge of pus characteristic of this highly contagious infection of the conjunctiva.

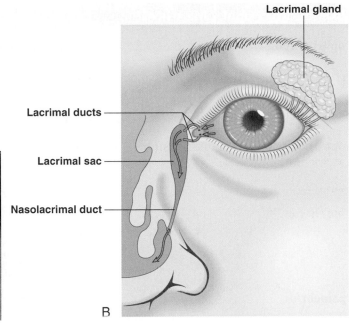

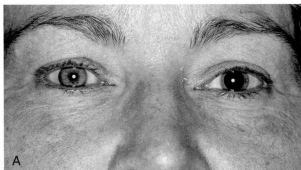

FIGURE 17-7   A, Anisocoria. B, Lacrimal (tear) gland and ducts.

COMBINING FORM	MEANING	TERMINOLOGY	MEANING
corne/o	cornea (*see* **kerat/o**)	corneal abrasion _____	
cycl/o	ciliary body or muscle of the eye	cycloplegic _____	
dacry/o	tears, tear duct (*see* **lacrim/o**)	dacryoadenitis _____ *Figure 17-7B shows the lacrimal gland and lacrimal ducts.*	
ir/o, irid/o	iris (colored portion of the eye around the pupil)	iritis _____ *Characterized by pain, sensitivity to light, and lacrimation. A corticosteroid is prescribed to reduce inflammation.*	
		iridic _____	
		iridectomy _____ *A portion of the iris is removed to improve drainage of aqueous humor or to extract a foreign body.*	
kerat/o	cornea	keratitis _____ *Note that kerat/o here does not refer to keratin (protein in skin tissue).*	
lacrim/o	tears	lacrimal _____	
		lacrimation _____	
ocul/o	eye	intraocular _____	

17

COMBINING FORM	MEANING	TERMINOLOGY	MEANING
ophthalm/o	eye	ophthalmologist _____ *Medical doctor who specializes in treating disorders of the eye.* ophthalmic _____ ophthalmoplegia _____	
opt/o, optic/o	eye, vision	optic _____ optometrist _____ *Nonmedical professional who can examine eyes to determine vision problems and prescribe lenses; a doctor of optometry (O.D.).* optician _____ *Nonmedical professional who grinds lenses and fits glasses but cannot prescribe lenses.*	
palpebr/o	eyelid	palpebral _____	
papill/o	optic disc; nipple-like	papilledema _____ *The suffix -edema means swelling. This condition is associated with increased intracranial pressure and hyperemia (increased blood flow) in the region of the optic disc.*	
phac/o, phak/o	lens of the eye	phacoemulsification _____ *Technique of cataract extraction using ultrasonic vibrations to fragment (emulsify) the lens and aspirate the pieces from the eye.* aphakia _____ *This condition may be congenital, but most often it is the result of extraction of a cataract (clouded lens) without placement of an artificial lens (pseudophakia).*	
pupill/o	pupil	pupillary _____	
retin/o	retina	retinitis _____ ***Retinitis pigmentosa** is a genetic disorder (pigmented scar forms on the retina) that destroys retinal rods. Decreased vision and night blindness (nyctalopia) occur.* hypertensive retinopathy _____ *Lesions such as narrowing of arterioles, microaneurysms, hemorrhages, and **exudates** (fluid leakage) are found on examination of the fundus.*	
scler/o	sclera (white of the eye); hard	corneoscleral _____ scleritis _____	

Palpebral/Palpable

Don't confuse *palpebral* with *palpable*, which means detectable or distinguishable by touch.

scler/o

The combining form scler/o also means hard, as in **scler**oderma (a hardening and thickening of the skin) and arterio**scler**osis (hardening of arteries with collection of plaque).

COMBINING FORM	MEANING	TERMINOLOGY	MEANING
uve/o	uvea; vascular layer of the eye (iris, ciliary body, and choroid)	uveitis _____	
vitre/o	glassy	vitreous humor _____	

COMBINING FORMS: CONDITIONS

COMBINING FORM	MEANING	TERMINOLOGY	MEANING
ambly/o	dull, dim	amblyopia _____ *The suffix -opia means vision. Amblyopia is unilateral or bilateral reduction of visual acuity. Early in life (before age 7 to 10) ocular misalignment, such as with strabismus, uncorrected errors of refraction, or other eye disorders, can lead to amblyopia (also known as lazy eye).*	
dipl/o	double	diplopia _____	
glauc/o	gray	glaucoma _____ *Here, -oma means mass or collection of fluid (aqueous humor). The term comes from the dull gray-green color of the affected eye in advanced cases. See page 711.*	
mi/o	smaller, less	miosis _____ *Contraction of the pupil. A **miotic** is a drug (such as pilocarpine) that causes the pupil to contract.*	
mydr/o	widen, enlarge	mydriasis _____ *Enlargement of pupils. Tropicamide, atropine, and cocaine cause dilation, or enlargement, of pupils.*	
nyct/o	night	nyctalopia _____ *-opia means vision; -al comes from Greek ala, meaning blindness. Night blindness is poor vision at night but good vision on bright days. Deficiency of vitamin A leads to nyctalopia.*	
phot/o	light	photophobia _____ *Sensitivity to light.*	
presby/o	old age	presbyopia _____ *See page 709.*	
scot/o	darkness	scotoma _____ *Area of decreased vision surrounded by an area of normal vision; a blind spot. This can result from damage to the retina or the optic nerve.*	
xer/o	dry	xerophthalmia _____	

17

SUFFIXES

SUFFIX	MEANING	TERMINOLOGY	MEANING
-opia	vision	hyperopia _____ *Hypermetropia (farsightedness).*	
-opsia	vision	hemianopsia _____ *Absence of vision in half of the visual field (space of vision of each eye). Stroke victims frequently have damage to the brain on one side of the visual cortex and experience hemianopsia (the visual loss is in the right or the left visual field of both eyes).*	
-tropia	to turn	esotropia _____ *Inward (eso-) turning of an eye. **Exotropia** is an outward turning of an eye. These conditions are examples of **strabismus** (defect in eye muscles so that both eyes cannot be focused on the same point at the same time).*	

ERRORS OF REFRACTION

astigmatism

Defective curvature of the cornea or lens of the eye.

This problem results from one or more abnormal curvatures of the cornea or lens. This causes light rays to be unevenly and not sharply focused on the retina, so that the image is distorted. A cylindrical lens placed in the proper position in front of the eye can correct this problem (Figure 17-8A).

hyperopia (hypermetropia)

Farsightedness.

As Figure 17-8B illustrates, the eyeball in this condition is too short (front to back) or the refractive power of the lens is too weak. Parallel rays of light tend to focus behind the retina, which results in a blurred image. A convex lens (thicker in the middle than at the sides) bends the rays inward before they reach the cornea, and thus the rays can be focused properly on the retina.

myopia

Nearsightedness.

In myopia the eyeball is too long (front to back) or the refractive power of the lens so strong that light rays do not properly focus on the retina. The image perceived is blurred because the light rays are focused in front of the retina. Concave glasses (thicker at the periphery than in the middle) correct this condition because the lenses spread the rays out before they reach the cornea, so that they can be properly focused directly on the retina (Figure 17-8C).

Myopia/Miotic

In myopia, my- comes from Greek *myein*, meaning to shut, referring to the observation that myopic persons frequently peer through half-closed eyelids. Don't confuse **myopia** with **miotic,** which is a drug that contracts the pupil of the eye.

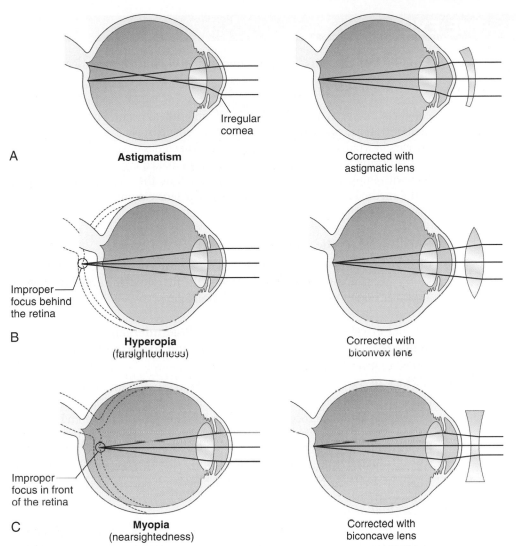

Irregular
cornea

A   **Astigmatism**

Corrected with
astigmatic lens

Improper
focus behind
the retina

B   **Hyperopia**
(farsightedness)

Corrected with
biconvex lens

Improper
focus in front
of the retina

C   **Myopia**
(nearsightedness)

Corrected with
biconcave lens

FIGURE 17-8   Errors of refraction. A, Astigmatism and its correction. **B, Hyperopia** and its correction.
C, Myopia and its correction. *Dashed lines* in **B** and **C** indicate the contour and size of the normal eye.

17

presbyopia

Impairment of vision as a result of old age.

With increasing age, loss of elasticity of the ciliary body impairs its ability to adjust
the lens for accommodation to near vision. The lens of the eye cannot thicken to
bend the rays coming from near objects (less than 20 feet away). The light rays
focus behind the retina, as in hyperopia. Therefore, a convex lens is needed to
refract the rays coming from objects closer than 20 feet.

PATHOLOGY—THE EYE

cataract

Clouding of the lens, causing decreased vision (Figure 17-9A).

A cataract is a type of degenerative eye disease (protein in the lens aggregates and clouds vision) and is linked to the process of aging (senile cataracts). Some cataracts, however, are present at birth, and others occur with diabetes mellitus, ocular trauma, and prolonged high-dose corticosteroid administration. Vision appears blurred as the lens clouds over and becomes opaque. Lens cloudiness can be seen using an ophthalmoscope or with the naked eye. Surgical removal of the lens with implantation of an artificial lens behind the iris (the preferred position) is the method of treatment. If an intraocular lens cannot be inserted, the patient may wear eyeglasses or contact lenses to help refraction.

chalazion

Small, hard, cystic mass (granuloma) on the eyelid.

Chalazions (kă-LĀ-zē-ŏnz) are formed as a result of chronic inflammation of a sebaceous gland (meibomian gland) along the margin of the eyelid (Figure 17-9B). Treatment often requires incision and drainage.

diabetic retinopathy

Retinal effects of diabetes mellitus include microaneurysms, hemorrhages, dilation of retinal veins, and neovascularization (new blood vessels form in the retina).

Macular edema occurs as fluid leaks from blood vessels into the retina and vision is blurred. **Exudates** (fluid leaking from the blood) appear in the retina as yellow-white spots. Laser photocoagulation is helpful for patients in whom hemorrhaging on the retina has been severe. Also, vitrectomy is done to remove nonresolving hemorrhage into the vitreous jelly. The latest treatment for diabetic macular edema involves injecting medications into the vitreous jelly. Corticosteroids, which promote regression of abnormal blood vessels, are used to decrease fluid leakage and neovascularization.

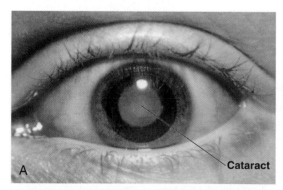 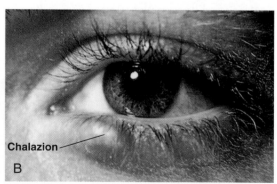

FIGURE 17-9   **A, Cataract.** The lens appears cloudy. **B, Chalazion.** *(A, Courtesy Ophthalmic Photography at the University of Michigan, WK Kellogg Eye Center, Ann Arbor. From Black JM, Hawks JH: Medical-Surgical Nursing: Clinical Management for Positive Outcomes, 7th ed., Philadelphia, Saunders, 2005. B, Courtesy Ophthalmic Photography at the University of Michigan, WK Kellogg Eye Center, Ann Arbor. From Black JM, Hawks JH, Keene AM: Medical-Surgical Nursing, 5th ed., Philadelphia, Saunders, 1997.)*

glaucoma

Increased intraocular pressure results in damage to the retina and optic nerve with loss of vision.

Intraocular pressure is elevated because of the inability of aqueous humor to drain from the eye and enter the bloodstream. Normally, aqueous humor is formed by the ciliary body, flows into the anterior chamber, and leaves the eye at the angle where the cornea and the iris meet. If fluid cannot leave or too much fluid is produced, pressure builds up in the anterior chamber (Figure 17-10).

Glaucoma is diagnosed by means of **tonometry** (see page 715), with an instrument applied externally to the eye after administration of local anesthetic. Acute glaucoma is marked by extreme ocular pain, blurred vision, redness of the eye, and dilation of the pupil. If untreated, it causes blindness. Chronic glaucoma may produce no symptoms initially. A patient with glaucoma may experience a gradual loss of peripheral vision, with headaches, blurred vision, and halos around bright lights, or they may experience no symptoms at all.

Administration of drugs to lower intraocular pressure can control the condition. Sometimes, laser therapy is used to treat narrow-angle glaucoma by creating a hole in the periphery of the iris (iridotomy), which allows aqueous humor to flow more easily out of the anterior chamber and reduces intraocular pressure. **Trabeculoplasty** (laser therapy) for chronic open-angle glaucoma causes scarring in the drainage angle, improving aqueous humor outflow and reducing intraocular pressure. **Argon laser trabeculoplasty (ALT)** and **selective laser trabeculoplasty (SLT)** are used. SLT, which is as effective as ALT, uses a lower power laser and may be repeated, because the lower level of energy should cause less scarring.

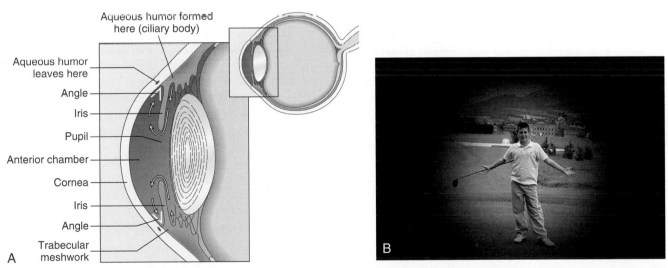

FIGURE 17-10   A, Glaucoma and circulation of aqueous humor. Circulation is impaired in glaucoma, so that aqueous fluid builds up in the anterior chamber, with consequent increase in intraocular pressure. The most common type of glaucoma is **open-angle glaucoma,** in which the chamber angles are open but the underlying problem is resistance to the flow of aqueous humor or too much aqueous production. **B, How a person with glaucoma sees an image.** Damage to the optic nerve usually starts as loss of peripheral vision. (**B,** *Courtesy Solomon J. Thompson.*)

Trabeculoplasty

Trabecul/o means a small beam, rod, or plank of wood.

TABLE 17-1	EYELID ABNORMALITIES

LESION/ ABNORMALITY	DESCRIPTION
Blepharitis	Inflammation of eyelid, causing redness, crusting, and swelling along lid margins
Chalazion	Granuloma formed around an inflamed sebaceous gland
Dacryocystitis	Blockage, inflammation, and infection of a nasolacrimal duct and lacrimal sac, causing redness and swelling in the region between the nose and the lower lid
Ectropion	Outward sagging and eversion of the eyelid, leading to improper lacrimation and corneal drying and ulceration
Entropion	Inversion of the eyelid, causing the lashes to rub against the eye; corneal abrasion may result
Hordeolum (stye)	Small, superficial white nodule along lid margin due to infection of a sebaceous gland
Ptosis	Drooping of upper lid margin from neuromuscular problems or trauma
Xanthelasma	Raised yellowish plaque on eyelid caused by lipid disorder (xanth/o = yellow, -elasma = plate)

hordeolum (stye *or* sty)

Localized, purulent, inflammatory staphylococcal infection of a sebaceous oil-producing gland in the eyelid.

Hot compresses may help localize the infection and promote drainage. In some cases, surgical incision is necessary. In Latin, *hordeolum* (hŏr-DĒ-ō-lŭm) means barley. See Table 17-1 for a list of common eyelid abnormalities.

macular degeneration

Progressive damage to the macula of the retina.

Macular degeneration is one of the leading causes of blindness in the elderly. It causes severe loss of central vision (Figure 17-11). Peripheral vision (using the part of the retina that is outside the macular region) is retained.

Macular degeneration occurs in both a "dry" and a "wet" form. The dry form (affecting about 85% of patients) is marked by atrophy and degeneration of retinal cells and deposits of clumps of extracellular debris, or **drusen.** The wet form results from development of new (neovascular) and leaky (exudative) blood vessels close to the macula.

There is no treatment for the dry form of macular degeneration except attempting to slow the progression of the disease by taking vitamin and mineral supplements, and actions such as smoking cessation. Wet macular degeneration may be treated with laser photocoagulation of the leaking vessels and injection of medication into the vitreous jelly that promotes regression of abnormal blood

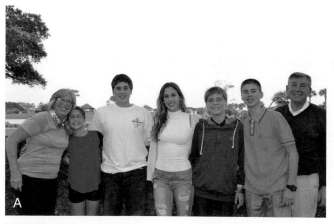

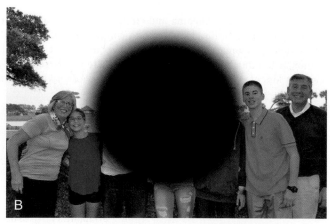

FIGURE 17-11   A, Picture as seen with **normal vision. B,** The same picture as it would appear to a person with **macular degeneration.** *(Photograph shows Louisa, Solomon, Bebe, Ben, and Gus with proud grandparents.)*

vessels. Unfortunately, in many cases, patients with wet macular degeneration have more severe vision loss, and success of treatment is limited.

nystagmus   **Repetitive rhythmic movements of one or both eyes.**

Brain tumors or diseases of the inner ear may cause nystagmus. Nystagmus is normal in newborns.

retinal detachment   **Two layers of the retina separate from each other.**

Trauma to the eye, head injuries, bleeding, scarring from infection, or shrinkage of the vitreous humor can produce holes or tears in the retina and result in the separation of layers. Patients often experience **photopsia** (bright flashes of light) and see **floaters** (black spots or filmy shapes), which are vitreous clumps that detach from the retina. Later, they may notice a shadow or curtain falling across the field of vision. In some cases, floaters may be a sign of a retinal hole, tear, or detachment caused by pigmented cells from the damaged retina or bleeding that has occurred as a result of a detachment. See ***In Person: Retinal Tear*** page 728.

Photocoagulation (making pinpoint burns to form scar tissue and seal holes) and cryotherapy (creating a "freezer burn" that forms a scar and knits a tear together) are used to repair smaller retinal tears. For larger retinal detachments, a **scleral buckle** (see page 717) made of silicone is sutured to the sclera directly over the detached portion of the retina to push the two retinal layers together.

In selected retinal detachments, a procedure called **pneumatic retinopexy** is performed. A gas bubble is injected into the vitreous cavity to put pressure on the area of retinal tear until the retina is reattached.

strabismus   **Abnormal deviation of the eye.**

A failure of the eyes to look in the same direction because of weakness of a muscle controlling the position of one eye (Figure 17-12). Different forms of strabismus include **esotropia** (one eye turns inward; "cross-eyed"), **exotropia** (one eye turns outward; "wall-eye"), **hypertropia** (upward deviation of one eye), and **hypotropia** (downward deviation of one eye). Treatment may include medications in the form of eye drops, corrective lenses, eye exercises with patching of the normal eye, or surgery to restore muscle balance.

In children, strabismus may lead to **amblyopia** (partial loss of vision from "lazy eye"). Amblyopia is reversible until the retina is fully developed, at the age of 7 to 10 years. When strabismus develops in an adult, **diplopia** (double vision) is a common problem.

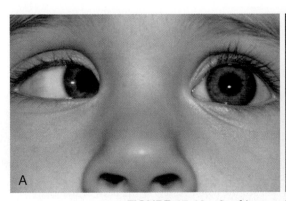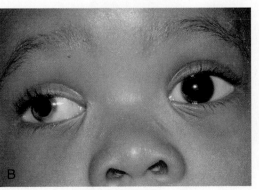

FIGURE 17-12   Strabismus. A, Esotropia. B, Exotropia.

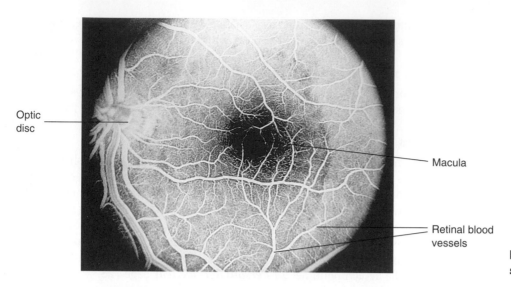

Optic disc

Macula

Retinal blood vessels

FIGURE 17-13 Normal eye seen on fluorescein angiogram.

CLINICAL PROCEDURES—THE EYE

DIAGNOSTIC

fluorescein angiography

Intravenous injection of fluorescein (a dye) followed by serial photographs of the retina through dilated pupils.

This test provides diagnostic information about blood flow in the retina, detects vascular changes in diabetic and hypertensive retinopathy, and identifies lesions in the macular area of the retina (Figure 17-13).

ophthalmoscopy

Visual examination of the interior of the eye.

Ideally, the pupil is dilated and the physician holds the ophthalmoscope close to the patient's eye, shining the light into the back of the eye (Figure 17-14). Ophthalmologists also may use special lenses in conjunction with a head lamp or a slit lamp (Figure 17-15).

slit lamp microscopy

Examination of anterior ocular structures under microscopic magnification.

This procedure provides a magnified view of the conjunctiva, sclera, cornea, anterior chamber, iris, lens, and vitreous. Devices attached to a slit lamp expand

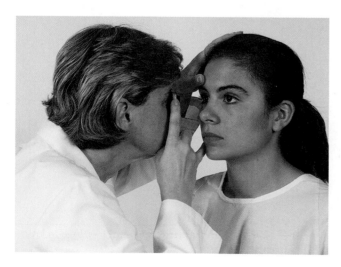

FIGURE 17-14 Ophthalmoscopy. In addition to inspecting the cornea, lens, and vitreous humor for opacities (cloudiness), the examiner can see the blood vessels at the back of the eye (fundus) and note degenerative changes in the retina.

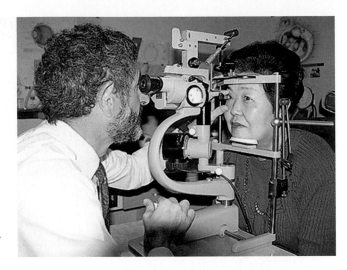

FIGURE 17-15   **Slit lamp examination measuring intraocular pressure by tonometry.**

the scope of the examination. **Tonometry** (ton/o = tension) measures intraocular pressure to detect glaucoma (see Figure 17-15). Special magnifying lenses also permit examination of the fundus, as with a direct ophthalmoscope.

visual acuity test

Clarity of vision is assessed (Figure 17-16A).

A patient reads from a **Snellen chart** at 20 feet (distance vision test). Visual acuity is expressed as a ratio, such as 20/20. The first number is the distance the patient is standing from the chart. The second number is the distance at which a person with normal vision could read the same line of the chart. If the best a patient can see is the 20/200 line on the chart, then at 20 feet the patient can see what a "healthy" eye sees at 200 feet.

Mirrors are used so that measurements can be taken at less than 20 feet and still be equivalent to those for vision measured at 20 feet.

visual field test

Measurement of the entire scope of vision (peripheral and central). See Figure 17-16B.

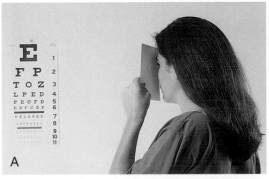
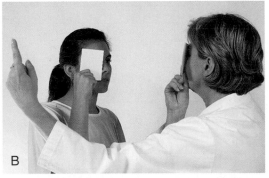

FIGURE 17-16   A, Snellen chart assesses visual acuity. **B, Visual field test** is performed with the eyes fixes, looking straight ahead without movement of the head.

Direct Ophthalmoscopy and Slit Lamp Microscopy

As part of a visual examination, both of these procedures are often used. **Direct ophthalmoscopy** examines the fundus and interior of the eye, whereas **slit lamp microscopy** visualizes the anterior part of the eye.

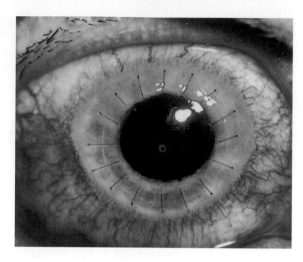

FIGURE 17-17 Clinical appearance of the eye after keratoplasty. *(Courtesy Ophthalmic Photography at the University of Michigan, WK Kellogg Eye Center, Ann Arbor. From Black JM, Hawks JH: Medical-Surgical Nursing: Clinical Management for Positive Outcomes, 7th ed., Philadelphia, Saunders, 2005, p. 1958.)*

TREATMENT

enucleation

Removal of the entire eyeball.

This surgical procedure is necessary to treat tumors such as ocular melanoma (malignant tumor of pigmented cells in the choroid layer) or if an eye has become blind and painful from trauma or disease, such as glaucoma.

keratoplasty

Surgical repair of the cornea.

Also known as a **corneal transplant** procedure (**penetrating keratoplasty**). The ophthalmic surgeon removes the patient's scarred or opaque cornea and replaces it with a donor cornea ("button" or graft), which is sutured into place (Figure 17-17).

17

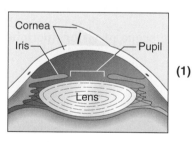

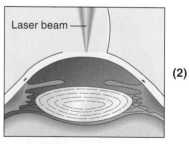

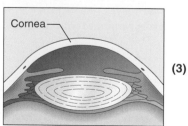

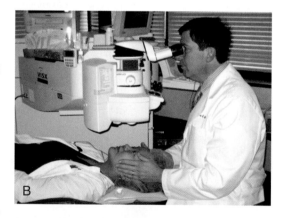

FIGURE 17-18 **A, LASIK refractive surgery:** (1) An instrument to cut the cornea (microkeratome) creates a hinged cap of tissue, which then is lifted off the corneal surface. (2) An excimer laser vaporizes and reshapes the cornea to correct the refraction. (3) The corneal flap is replaced. **B,** Ophthalmologists typically perform LASIK surgery as an office procedure. The patient with corrected vision returns home that day and is visually functioning normally or close to it the next day. *(**B,** Courtesy Eric R. Mandel, MD, Mandel Vision, New York.)*

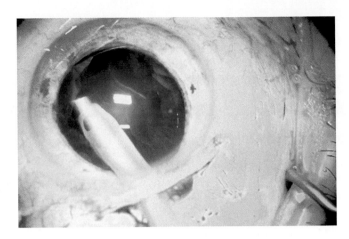

FIGURE 17-19   Phacoemulsification of a cataractous lens through a small scleral tunnel incision.

laser photocoagulation	**Intense, precisely focused light beam (argon laser) creates an inflammatory reaction that seals retinal tears and leaky retinal blood vessels.** This procedure is useful to treat retinal tears, diabetic retinopathy, and wet macular degeneration. ✱ **HINT:** Laser is an acronym for <u>l</u>ight <u>a</u>mplification by <u>s</u>timulated <u>e</u>mission of <u>r</u>adiation.
LASIK	**Use of an excimer laser to correct errors of refraction (myopia, hyperopia, and astigmatism).** Performed as an outpatient procedure with use of local anesthesia. The surgeon lifts the top layer of the cornea (a flap is made) and uses a laser to sculpt the cornea. The corneal flap is then repositioned. LASIK is an acronym for <u>l</u>aser <u>i</u>n situ <u>k</u>eratomileusis (shaping the cornea) (Figure 17-18).
phacoemulsification	**Ultrasonic vibrations break up the lens; the pieces are then aspirated through the ultrasonic probe (Figure 17-19).** This is the typical surgery for **cataract removal**. The ophthalmic surgeon uses a small, scleral tunnel or self-sealing corneal incision. In most patients, a foldable intraocular lens (IOL) is implanted at the time of surgery.
scleral buckle	**Suture of a silicone band to the sclera over a detached portion of the retina.** The band pushes the two parts of the retina against each other to bring together the two layers of the detached retina (Figure 17-20).

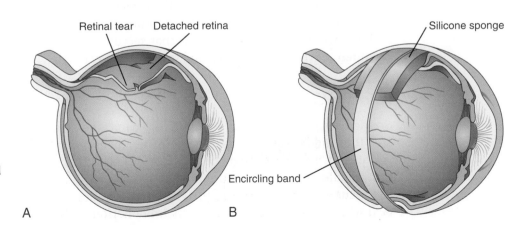

FIGURE 17-20   A, Detached retina. B, Scleral buckling procedure to repair retinal detachment.

vitrectomy   **Removal of the vitreous humor.**

The vitreous is replaced with a clear solution. This is necessary when blood and scar tissue accumulate in the vitreous humor (a complication of diabetic retinopathy).

ABBREVIATIONS—THE EYE

ALT	argon laser trabeculoplasty	**PERRLA**	pupils equal, round, reactive to light and accommodation
AMD	age-related macular degeneration	**POAG**	primary open-angle glaucoma
HEENT	head, eyes, ears, nose, and throat	**PRK**	photorefractive keratectomy—a laser beam flattens the top layer of the cornea to correct myopia
IOL	intraocular lens		
IOP	intraocular pressure		
LASIK	laser in situ keratomileusis	**SLT**	selective laser trabeculoplasty
OD	right eye (Latin, *oculus dexter*)	**VA**	visual acuity
OS	left eye (Latin, *oculus sinister*)	**VF**	visual field
OU	both eyes (Latin, *oculus uterque*, "each eye")		

THE EAR

ANATOMY AND PHYSIOLOGY

Sound waves are received by the outer ear, conducted to special receptor cells within the ear, and transmitted by those cells to nerve fibers that lead to the auditory region of the brain in the cerebral cortex. Sensations of sound are perceived within the nerve fibers of the cerebral cortex.

Label Figure 17-21 as you read the following paragraphs describing the anatomy and physiology of the ear.

The ear can be divided into three separate regions: outer ear, middle ear, and inner ear. The outer and middle ears function in the conduction of sound waves through the ear, and the inner ear contains structures that receive the auditory waves and relay them to the brain.

Outer Ear

Sound waves enter the ear through the **pinna, or auricle** [1], which is the projecting part, or flap, of the ear. The **external auditory meatus (auditory canal)** [2] leads from the pinna and is lined with numerous glands that secrete a yellowish brown, waxy substance called **cerumen.** Cerumen lubricates and protects the ear canal.

Middle Ear

Sound waves travel through the auditory canal and strike a membrane between the outer and the middle ear. This is the **tympanic membrane, or eardrum** [3]. As the eardrum vibrates, it moves three small bones, or **ossicles,** that conduct the sound waves through the middle ear. These bones, in the order of their vibration, are the **malleus** [4], the **incus** [5], and the **stapes** [6]. As the stapes moves, it touches a membrane called the **oval window** [7], which separates the middle from the inner ear.

Before proceeding with the pathway of sound conduction and reception into the inner ear, an additional structure that affects the middle ear should be mentioned. The **auditory** or **eustachian tube** [8] is a canal leading from the middle ear to the pharynx. It normally is closed but opens on swallowing. In an efficient way, this tube can prevent damage to the eardrum and shock to the middle and inner ears. Normally the pressure of air in the middle ear is equal to the pressure of air in the external environment; however, if you ascend in the atmosphere, as in flying in an airplane, climbing a high mountain, or riding a fast elevator, the atmospheric pressure, along with that in the outer ear, drops, while the pressure in the middle ear remains the same—greater than in the outer ear. This inequality of air pressure on the inside and outside of the eardrum forces the eardrum to bulge outward and potentially burst if the difference in pressures increases. Swallowing opens the eustachian tube so that air can leave the middle ear and enter the throat until the atmospheric and middle ear pressures are balanced. The eardrum then relaxes, and the danger of its bursting is averted.

Inner Ear

Sound vibrations, having been transmitted by the movement of the eardrum to the bones of the middle ear, reach the inner ear via the fluctuations of the oval window that separates the middle and inner ears. The inner ear is also called the **labyrinth** because of its circular, maze-like structure. The part of the labyrinth that leads from the oval window is a bony, snail shell–shaped structure called the **cochlea** [9]. The cochlea contains special auditory liquids called **perilymph** and **endolymph** through which the vibrations travel. Also present in the cochlea is a sensitive auditory receptor area called the **organ of Corti.** In the organ of Corti, tiny hair cells receive vibrations from the auditory liquids and relay the sound waves to **auditory nerve fibers** [10], which end in the auditory center of the cerebral cortex, where these impulses are interpreted and "heard."

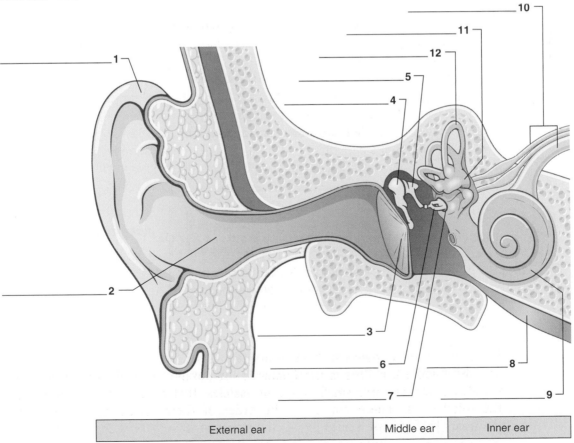

FIGURE 17-21   Anatomy of the ear.

Study Figure 17-22, which is a schematic representation of the pathway of sound vibrations from the outer ear to the brain.

The ear is an important organ of equilibrium (balance), as well as an organ for hearing. Refer back to Figure 17-21. The **vestibule** [11] connects the cochlea (for hearing) to three **semicircular canals** [12] (for balance). The semicircular canals (containing two membranous sacs called the saccule and utricle) contain a fluid, endolymph, as well as sensitive hair cells. In an intricate manner, the fluid and hair cells fluctuate in response to the movement of the head. This sets up impulses in nerve fibers that lead to the brain. Messages are then sent to muscles in all parts of the body to ensure that equilibrium is maintained.

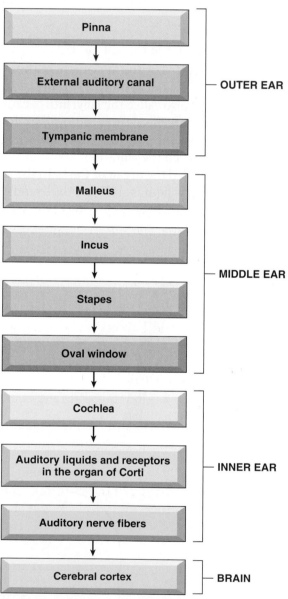

FIGURE 17-22   Pathway of sound vibrations from the outer ear to the brain (cerebral cortex.)

VOCABULARY—THE EAR

This list reviews many new terms related to the ear introduced in the text. Short definitions reinforce your understanding of the terms. Refer to the Pronunciation of Terms on page 745 for help with unfamiliar or difficult words.

auditory canal	Channel that leads from the pinna to the eardrum.
auditory meatus	Auditory canal.
auditory nerve fibers	Carry impulses from the inner ear to the brain (cerebral cortex). These fibers compose the vestibulocochlear nerve (cranial nerve VIII).
auditory tube	Channel between the middle ear and the nasopharynx; **eustachian tube.**
auricle	Flap of the ear; the protruding part of the external ear, or **pinna.**
cerumen	Waxy substance secreted by the external ear; **earwax.**
cochlea	Snail shell–shaped, spirally wound tube in the inner ear; contains hearing-sensitive receptor cells.
endolymph	Fluid within the labyrinth of the inner ear.
eustachian tube	Auditory tube.
incus	Second ossicle (small bone) of the middle ear; incus means **anvil.**
labyrinth	Maze-like series of canals of the inner ear. This includes the cochlea, vestibule, and semicircular canals.
malleus	First ossicle of the middle ear; malleus means **hammer.**
organ of Corti	Sensitive auditory receptor area found in the cochlea of the inner ear.
ossicle	Small bone of the ear; includes the malleus, incus, and stapes.
oval window	Membrane between the middle ear and the inner ear.
perilymph	Fluid contained in the labyrinth of the inner ear.
pinna	Auricle; flap of the ear.
semicircular canals	Passages in the inner ear associated with maintaining equilibrium.
stapes	Third ossicle of the middle ear. Stapes means **stirrup**.
tympanic membrane	Membrane between the outer and the middle ear; also called the **eardrum.**
vestibule	Central cavity of the labyrinth, connecting the semicircular canals and the cochlea. The vestibule contains two structures, the **saccule** and **utricle**, that help to maintain equilibrium.

Cerumen

This normal product of wax glands in the external ear canal protects the ear from dust, water, and infection. However, too much earwax increases the incidence of infection and may lead to hearing loss.

17

TERMINOLOGY—THE EAR

Write the meanings of the medical terms relating to the ear in the spaces provided.

COMBINING FORMS

COMBINING FORM	MEANING	TERMINOLOGY	MEANING
acous/o	hearing	acoustic	
audi/o	hearing; the sense of hearing	audiogram	
		audiologist	
		A health care professional specializing in the evaluation and rehabilitation of people with hearing loss.	
audit/o	hearing	auditory	
aur/o, auricul/o	ear (*see* ot/o)	aural	
		postauricular	
cochle/o	cochlea	cochlear	
mastoid/o	mastoid process	mastoiditis	
		*The **mastoid process** is the posterior portion of the temporal bone extending downward behind the external auditory meatus. Mastoiditis, caused by bacterial infection, spreads from the middle ear.*	
myring/o	eardrum, tympanic membrane (*see* **tympan/o**)	myringotomy	
		myringitis	
ossicul/o	ossicle	ossiculoplasty	
ot/o	ear	otic	
		otomycosis	
		otopyorrhea	
		otolaryngologist	
		An otolaryngologist is a medical doctor specializing in the ear, nose, and throat.	
salping/o	eustachian tube, auditory tube	salpingopharyngeal	
		In the context of female reproductive anatomy, salping/o means the fallopian tubes.	

17

Audiogram/Audiometry

An **audiogram** is the record (chart) produced when a person's hearing is tested by **audiometry** (see page 726).

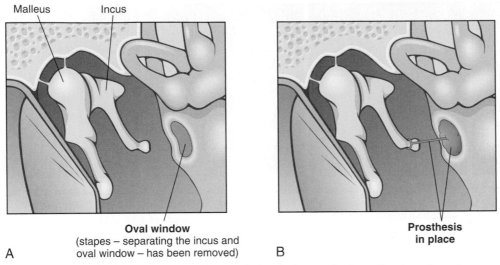

FIGURE 17-23   A, Stapedectomy. Using microsurgical technique and a laser, the stapes bone is removed from the middle ear. **B, A prosthetic device** (wire, Teflon, or metal) is placed into the incus and attached to a hole in the oval window.

COMBINING FORM	MEANING	TERMINOLOGY	MEANING
staped/o	stapes (third bone of the middle ear)	<u>staped</u>ectomy _____ *After stapedectomy a prosthetic device is used to connect the incus and the oval window (Figure 17-23). Also see otosclerosis, page 725.*	
tympan/o	eardrum, tympanic membrane	<u>tympan</u>oplasty _____ *Surgical reconstruction of the bones of the middle ear with reconnection of the eardrum to the oval window. Figure 17-24 shows a normal tympanic membrane (eardrum).*	
vestibul/o	vestibule	<u>vestibul</u>ocochlear _____	

SUFFIXES

SUFFIX	MEANING	TERMINOLOGY	MEANING
-acusis *or* **-cusis**	hearing	hyper<u>acusis</u> _____ *Abnormally acute sensitivity to sounds.* presby<u>cusis</u> _____ *This type of nerve deafness occurs with the process of aging.*	
-meter	instrument to measure	audio<u>meter</u> _____	
-otia	ear condition	macr<u>otia</u> _____ *Abnormally large ears; congenital anomaly.*	

17

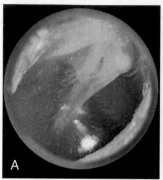
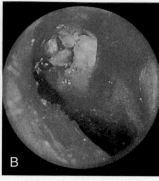
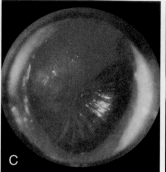
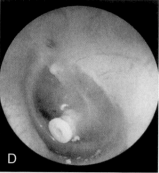

FIGURE 17-24 A, Healthy tympanic membrane. B, Tympanic membrane with cholesteatoma. C, Tympanic membrane with acute otitis media. D, Myringotomy with tympanostomy tube. *(A to C, Courtesy Richard A. Buckingham, Clinical Professor, Otolaryngology, Abraham Lincoln School of Medicine, University of Illinois, Chicago. From Barkauskas VH et al: Health and Physical Assessment, 3rd ed., St. Louis, Mosby, 2002, pp. 278 and 290. D, From Fireman P, Slavin RG: Atlas of Allergies, 2nd ed., London, Glower Medical Publishing, 1996.)*

PATHOLOGY—THE EAR

17

acoustic neuroma	**Benign tumor arising from the acoustic vestibulocochlear nerve (eighth cranial nerve) in the brain.**

Initially, this tumor causes tinnitus (ringing in the ears), vertigo (dizziness), and decreased hearing. Small tumors are resected by microsurgical techniques or ablated (removed) by radiosurgery (using powerful and precise x-ray beams rather than a surgical incision).

cholesteatoma

Collection of skin cells and cholesterol in a sac within the middle ear.

These cyst-like masses produce a foul-smelling discharge and are most often the result of chronic otitis media. They are associated with perforations of the tympanic membrane (Figure 17-24B).

deafness

Loss of the ability to hear.

Nerve deafness (sensorineural hearing loss) results from impairment of the cochlea or auditory (acoustic) nerve. **Conductive deafness** results from impairment of the middle ear ossicles and membranes transmitting sound waves into the cochlea. Hearing aids help people with conductive or sensorineural hearing loss. These devices have a microphone to pick up sounds, an amplifier to increase their volume, and a speaker to transmit amplified sounds. See Figure 17-25.

Meniere disease

Disorder of the labyrinth of the inner ear; elevated endolymph pressure within the cochlea (cochlear hydrops) and semicircular canals (vestibular hydrops).

Signs and symptoms are tinnitus, heightened sensitivity to loud sounds, progressive loss of hearing, headache, nausea, and vertigo. Attacks last minutes or continue for hours. The cause is unknown, and treatment is bed rest, sedation, and drugs to combat nausea and vertigo. Surgery may be necessary to relieve accumulation of fluid from the inner ear.

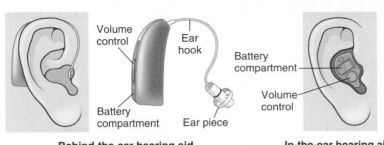

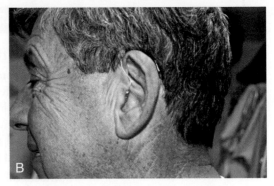

Behind-the-ear hearing aid   **In-the-ear hearing aid**

A

FIGURE 17-25   Hearing aids: A, Two types of hearing aid devices. B, Behind-the-ear hearing aid device in place.

otitis media	**Inflammation of the middle ear.**

Acute otitis media is infection of the middle ear, often following an upper respiratory infection (URI). Pain and fever with redness and loss of mobility of the tympanic membrane occur (Figure 17-24C). As bacteria invade the middle ear, pus formation occurs (**suppurative otitis media**). It is treated with antibiotics, but if the condition becomes chronic, myringotomy may be required to ventilate the middle ear.

Serous otitis media is a noninfectious inflammation with accumulation of serous fluid. It often results from a dysfunctional or obstructed auditory tube. Treatment includes myringotomy to aspirate fluid and placement of tympanostomy tubes in the eardrum to allow ventilation of the middle ear (Figure 17-24D).

otosclerosis	**Hardening of the bony tissue of the middle ear.**

The result of this hereditary condition is that bone forms around the oval window and causes fixation or **ankylosis** (stiffening) of the stapes bone (ossicle). Conduction deafness occurs, as the ossicles cannot pass on vibrations when sound enters the ear. Stapedectomy with replacement by a **prosthesis** (artificial part) is effective in restoring hearing (see Figure 17-23 on page 723). In order to perform this operation, the oval window must be **fenestrated** (opened) using a laser.

tinnitus	**Sensation of noises (ringing, buzzing, whistling, booming) in the ears.**

Caused by irritation of delicate hair cells in the inner ear, this disease symptom may be associated with presbycusis, Meniere disease, otosclerosis, chronic otitis, labyrinthitis, and other disorders. Tinnitus can be persistent and severe and can interfere with the affected person's daily life. Treatment includes medication and biofeedback to manage stress and anxiety if these are contributing factors. Tinnitus, a Latin-derived term, means tinkling.

vertigo	**Sensation of irregular or whirling motion either of oneself or of external objects.**

Vertigo can result from disease in the labyrinth of the inner ear or in the nerve that carries messages from the semicircular canals to the brain. Equilibrium and balance are affected, and nausea may occur as well.

17

Tinnitus

Note the spelling! Tinnitus is a condition (-itus), not an inflammation (-itis).

CLINICAL PROCEDURES—THE EAR

audiometry

Testing the sense of hearing.

An **audiometer** is an electrical device that delivers acoustic stimuli of specific frequencies to determine a patient's hearing loss for each frequency (Figure 17-26A). Results are shown on a chart or **audiogram** (Figure 17-26B).

cochlear implant procedure

Surgical insertion of a device that allows sensorineural hearing–impaired persons to understand speech.

Electrical signals are sent directly into the auditory nerve by means of multiple electrodes inserted into the cochlea. An external microphone and speech processor pick up sound signals and convert them to electrical impulses (Figure 17-27A).

ear thermometry

Measurement of the temperature of the tympanic membrane by detection of infrared radiation from the eardrum.

A device is inserted into the auditory canal, and results, which reflect the body's temperature, are obtained within 2 seconds.

otoscopy

Visual examination of the ear canal with an otoscope (see Figure 17-27B).

tuning fork test

Test of ear conduction using a vibration source (tuning fork).

To perform the **Rinne test,** the examiner places the base of the vibrating fork against the patient's mastoid bone (bone conduction) and in front of the auditory meatus (air conduction). In the **Weber test,** the tuning fork is placed on the center of the forehead. The perceived loudness of sound is the same in both ears if hearing is normal.

17

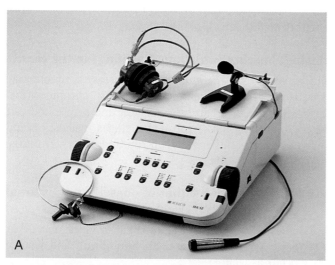

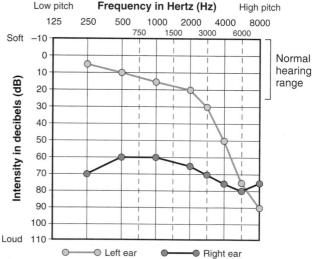

FIGURE 17-26   A, Pure-tone audiometer. B, Audiogram for a person with normal hearing in the left ear only for low frequencies (pitch). Notice the *blue line* sloping downward, showing severe high-frequency hearing loss in the left ear. There is moderate to severe hearing loss in the right ear. The decibel (dB) level of the softest sound you are able to hear is called your threshold. Thresholds of 0 to 25 dB (*yellow area*) are considered normal (for adults). (**A,** *Courtesy Maico, Inc., Minneapolis, Minnesota. In Ignatavicius DD, Workman ML: Medical-Surgical Nursing: Critical Thinking for Collaborative Care, 5th ed., Philadelphia, Saunders, 2005, p. 1120.*)

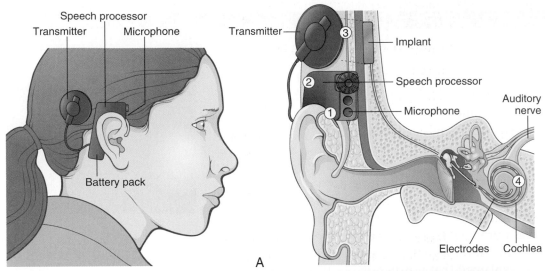

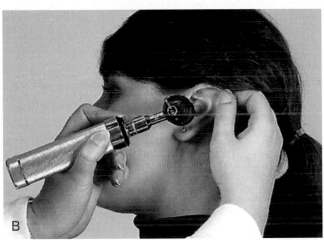

FIGURE 17-27 A, Cochlear implant.
(1). Microphone receives sound. (2). Speech processor converts sounds into digital signals. (3). Signals are sent to a transmitter that relays them to an implant, where they are converted to electrical impulses.
(4). Impulses are sent to electrodes that stimulate nerve cells in the cochlea, which sends them to the auditory nerve and brain.
B, Otoscopic examination. The auricle is pulled up and back. The examiner's hand holding the otoscope is braced against the patient's face for stabilization.

17

ABBREVIATIONS—THE EAR

AD	right ear (Latin, *auris dextra*)	**ENT**	ears, nose, and throat
AOM	acute otitis media	**ETD**	eustachian tube dysfunction
AS	left ear (Latin, *auris sinistra*)	**HEENT**	head, eyes, ears, nose, and throat
EENT	eyes, ears, nose, and throat	**PE tube**	pressure-equalizing tube—a polyethylene ventilating tube placed in the eardrum (to treat recurrent episodes of acute otitis media)
ENG	electronystagmography—a test of the balance mechanism of the inner ear by assessing eye movements (**nystagmus** is rapidly twitching eye movements)		
		SOM	serous otitis media

IN PERSON: RETINAL TEAR

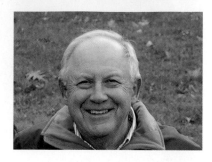

One day, while out for my usual walk, I sneezed on account of the higher seasonal pollen in our area. It was not an easy sneeze, and I was aware of the result immediately: I noticed some new floaters in my left eye. No pain, but a little feeling that something wasn't right. I did not see flashes of bright light (a good thing).

I hoped that the floaters would minimize and when they did not, I called my optometrist for an appointment. My appointment was at 10:30, and by 11:00 he had discovered a possible tear in my left retina. He walked me down the hall to an ophthalmologist, who confirmed the tear and suggested cryopexy, which involves numbing the eye, inserting a probe into the area, and freezing the torn retina to the back of the eye. I was through all of this by 11:30. Timing is everything.

The ophthalmologist explained that waiting two or three days could have allowed the tear to progress to a detachment—which, if not caught, could cause more serious problems.

If you think about a sneeze, it involves the head moving forward and stopping abruptly. As we get older, the clear jell (vitreous) inside the eye may pull away from the retina at the back of the eye. If this pulls away gradually, usually there is no problem. However, if there is a hard pull with a tear, the vitreous can pass through the tear, lifting the retina off the back of the eye, much like the way wallpaper can peel off a wall. There are a number of conditions that may lead to the chance of retinal problems, such as nearsightedness, cataract surgery, glaucoma, or family history.

As explained to me, if you are going to sneeze, grasp your head with both hands (perhaps while holding a tissue to your nose) to prevent the head from moving radically. That may stop a sudden front-to-back movement of your head.

The bad news is that I couldn't play golf for a couple of weeks after the cryopexy. My left eye looked horrible (itching and swollen) and I had a bunch of dark floaters in it. It was like trying to dodge three or four gnats right in front of my face. The good news is that my vision is intact.

My doctor told me that once you have had one episode, there is a 15% chance of developing the same problem in the other eye. Right on schedule, a year later, my right eye had a tear/separation. This time, though, the separation was located on the nasal side of the eye, which precluded using the cryogenic method of sealing the retina. My choice, in his office at least, was for a laser correction. I asked about the particulars, including safety, whether it would correct the problem, and how long the procedure would take. I was given assurances for my first two concerns, and told the procedure might take 5 minutes. I agreed to do it, but had concerns about how I could stay still for 5 minutes while he fired laser shots through my eye to stitch up the tear. After numbing the eye and putting me in the correct position, the doctor proceeded to light up my eye with 30 very bright flashes. He finished in 15 seconds. While I was pulling back from the head rest, I asked why had he told me that it would take 5 minutes. He said, with a little smile, that he didn't want me to starting figuring his fee based on a per second basis while I was undergoing the treatment. Pretty clever, and worth the smile that I gave him.

Needless to say, both eyes are fine. I still have floaters in both eyes and occasionally swipe at nonexistent gnats.

It may have no relation, but my golf handicap has dropped four shots lower since last spring and two below my historical prior low. Isn't technology great or what?!

Mac McGinnis is a retired businessman and dedicated golfer.

PRACTICAL APPLICATIONS

This section contains an operating room schedule and an operative report. Explanations of more difficult terms are added in brackets. Answers to the matching questions are on page 741.

OPERATING ROOM SCHEDULE: EYE AND EAR PROCEDURES

Match the operation in Column I with a diagnosis/surgical indication in Column II.

COLUMN I

1. phacoemulsification with IOL; OS _____

2. blepharoplasty _____

3. scleral buckle _____

4. vitrectomy _____

5. radical mastoidectomy _____

6. keratoplasty _____

7. cochlear implant _____

8. laser photocoagulation of the macula _____

9. incision and drainage of hordeolum _____

COLUMN II

A. scarred and torn cornea
B. ptosis of eyelid skin
C. retinal detachment
D. diabetic retinopathy
E. macular degeneration
F. chronic stye
G. chronic infection of a bone behind the ear
H. severe deafness
I. cataracts

OPERATIVE REPORT

Preoperative Diagnosis: Bilateral chronic serous otitis media; tonsilloadenoiditis.

Operation: Bilateral myringotomies and ventilation tube insertion; T&A.

Procedure: With the patient in the supine position and under general endotracheal anesthesia, inspection of AD was made under the operating microscope. The external canal was clear; tympanic membrane was divided. A purulent discharge appeared to be present. This drainage was suctioned out and the ear thoroughly lavaged [washed out]. A ventilating tube was put in place and otic drops were administered. Same procedure for AS.

The patient was placed in the Rose position [supine with the head over the table edge in full extension] and the adenoids were removed with adenoid curettes and adenoid biopsy forceps. A nasopharyngeal sponge was put in place. The right tonsil was then grasped with tonsil forceps, dissected free, and removed with snare. Bleeding was controlled with suction cautery. The nasopharyngeal sponge was removed and no further bleeding noted. The patient tolerated the procedure well and left the OR in good condition.

17

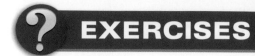

EXERCISES

Remember to check your answers carefully with the Answers to Exercises, page 739.

A Match the structure of the eye in Column I with its description in Column II. Write the letter of your answer in the space provided.

COLUMN I

1. pupil _____
2. conjunctiva _____
3. cornea _____
4. sclera _____
5. choroid _____
6. iris _____
7. ciliary body _____
8. lens _____
9. retina _____
10. vitreous humor _____

COLUMN II

A. Contains sensitive cells called rods and cones that transform light energy into nerve impulses.
B. Contains muscles that control the shape of the lens and secretes aqueous humor.
C. Transparent structure behind the iris and in front of the vitreous humor; it refracts light rays onto the retina.
D. Jelly-like material behind the lens that helps maintain the shape of the eyeball.
E. Open center of the iris through which light rays enter.
F. Vascular layer of the eyeball that is continuous with the iris.
G. Delicate membrane lining the eyelids and covering the anterior sclera of the eyeball.
H. Fibrous layer of clear tissue that extends over the anterior portion of the eyeball.
I. Colored portion of the eye; surrounds the pupil.
J. Tough, white outer layer of the eyeball.

B Supply the terms that complete the following sentences.

1. The region at the back of the eye where the optic nerve meets the retina is the

    _____.

2. The normal adjustment of the lens (becoming fatter) to bring an object into focus for near

    vision on the retina is _____.

3. A yellowish region on the retina lateral to the optic disc is the _____.

4. The tiny pit or depression in the retina that is the region of clearest vision is the

    _____.

5. The bending of light rays by the cornea, lens, and fluids of the eye is _____.

6. The point at which the fibers of the optic nerve cross in the brain is the

    _____.

7. The photoreceptor cells in the retina that make the perception of color possible are the

    _____.

17

8. The photoreceptor cells in the retina that make vision in dim light possible are the

   _____.

9. The _____ is the area behind the cornea and in front of the lens and iris.

   It contains aqueous humor.

10. The posterior, inner part of the eye is the _____.

C **Arrange the following terms in proper sequence to show the pathway of light rays to the visual region of the brain.**

anterior chamber and aqueous humor   optic nerve fibers
cerebral cortex (occipital lobe)   pupil
cornea   retina
lens   thalamus
optic chiasm   vitreous chamber and vitreous humor

1. _____ fibrous transparent layer of clear tissue over the eyeball

2. _____ space and fluid in the front of the eye

3. _____ central opening of the iris

4. _____ transparent, biconvex body that refracts light rays

5. _____ space and soft, jelly-like material in the posterior (back) of eye

6. _____ light-sensitive inner nerve cell layer; rods and cones

7. _____ cranial nerve

8. _____ area of brain where optic nerve fibers cross

9. _____ relay center of the brain

10. _____ visual region of the brain

D **Give the meanings of the following terms.**

1. optic nerve _____

2. biconvex _____

3. anisocoria _____

4. cycloplegic _____

5. palpebral _____

6. mydriasis _____

7. miosis _____

8. papilledema _____

9. photophobia _____

10. scotoma _____

17

E **Complete the medical terms based on their meanings and the word parts given.**

1. inflammation of an eyelid: _____ itis

2. inflammation of the conjunctiva: _____ itis

3. inflammation of a tear gland: _____ itis

4. inflammation of the iris: _____ itis

5. inflammation of the cornea: _____ itis

6. inflammation of the white of the eye: _____ itis

7. inflammation of the retina: _____ itis

8. prolapse of the eyelid: blephar _____

9. pertaining to tears: _____ al

10. pertaining to within the eye: intra _____

F **Select from the list of terms to match the descriptions/definitions that follow.**

aphakia   hemianopsia   optometrist
corneal ulcer   ophthalmologist   uveitis
esotropia   optician   xerophthalmia
exotropia

1. Fibrous layer of clear tissue over the front of the eyeball has a defect resulting from infection:

   _____

2. Inflammation of the vascular layer of the eye (iris, ciliary body, and choroid): _____

3. Condition of dry eyes: _____

4. Absence of vision in half of the visual field: _____

5. Eye abnormally turns outward: _____

6. Medical doctor who treats diseases of the eyes: _____

7. Nonmedical professional who can examine eyes and prescribe glasses: _____

8. Nonmedical professional who grinds lenses and fits glasses: _____

9. Absence of the lens of the eye: _____

10. Eye abnormally turns inward: _____

G **Describe the following visual conditions.**

1. amblyopia: _____

2. hyperopia: _____

3. presbyopia: _____

4. myopia: _____

17

5. nyctalopia: _____

6. diplopia: _____

7. astigmatism: _____

H **Complete the following sentences.**

1. In the myopic eye, light rays do not focus properly on the _____. Either

   the eyeball is too _____ or the refractive power of the lens is too

   _____, so that the image is blurred and comes to a focus in

   _____ of the retina. The type of lens used to correct this refractive error

   is called a/an _____ lens.

2. In the hyperopic eye, the eyeball is too _____ or the refractive power of the

   lens too _____, so that the image is blurred and focused in

   _____ of the retina. The type of lens used to correct this refractive error is

   called a/an _____ lens.

3. A miotic is a drug that _____ the pupil of the eye.

4. A mydriatic is a drug that _____ the pupil of the eye.

I **Match the abnormal conditions of the eye with the descriptions/definitions that follow.**

cataract   hordeolum (stye)   retinal detachment
chalazion   macular degeneration   retinitis pigmentosa
diabetic retinopathy   nystagmus   strabismus
glaucoma

1. Retinal microaneurysms, hemorrhages, dilation of retinal veins, and neovascularization occur

   secondary to an abnormal endocrine condition: _____

2. Two layers of the retina separate from each other: _____

3. Abnormal deviations of the eye occur (esotropia and exotropia): _____

4. Clouding of the lens causes decreased vision: _____

5. Loss of central vision caused by deterioration of the macula of the retina: _____

6. Localized, purulent infection of a sebaceous gland in the eyelid: _____

7. Small, firm, cystic mass on the eyelid; formed as a result of chronic inflammation of a

   sebaceous gland: _____

8. Increased intraocular pressure results in optic nerve damage: _____

9. Pigmented scarring forms throughout the retina: _____

10. Repetitive rhythmic movements of one or both eyes: _____

17

J Label the drawing of the eye using the list of terms provided.

anterior chamber
choroid
ciliary body
conjunctiva
cornea

fovea centralis
iris
lens
macula
optic disc

optic nerve
pupil
retina
sclera
vitreous humor

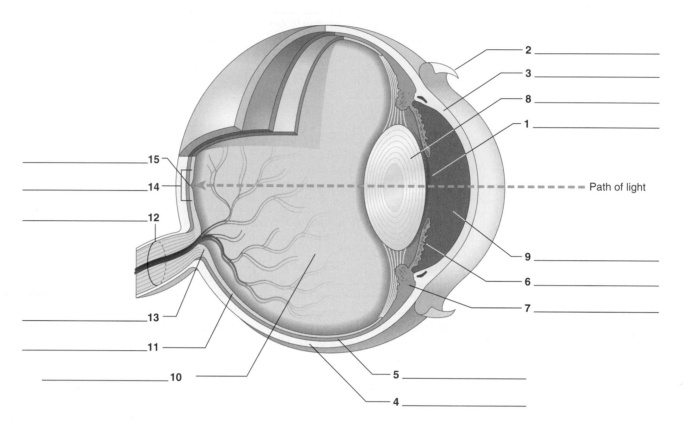

Path of light

K Match the pathologic conditions of the eye with the images that follow. Write the letter of the image in the space provided

1. stroke (hemianopsia) _____   2. glaucoma _____   3. cataract _____

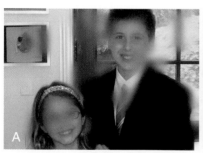

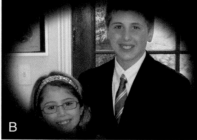

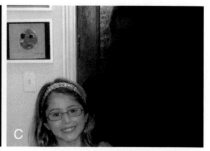

L **Give the meaning of the following combining forms.**

1. lacrim/o _____

2. dacry/o _____

3. kerat/o _____

4. corne/o _____

5. blephar/o _____

6. palpebr/o _____

7. cor/o _____

8. pupill/o _____

9. phac/o _____

10. phak/o _____

11. ocul/o _____

12. ophthalm/o _____

13. opt/o _____

14. scot/o _____

M **Give the meanings of the following abbreviations for terms relating to the eye or ear.**

1. OU _____

2. VA _____

3. OD _____

4. OS _____

5. VF _____

6. IOL _____

7. IOP _____

8. PERRLA _____

N Match the clinical procedures with the descriptions/definitions that follow.

fluorescein angiography | ophthalmoscopy | tonometry
keratoplasty | phacoemulsification | visual acuity test
laser photocoagulation | scleral buckle | visual field test
LASIK | slit lamp microscopy | vitrectomy

1. Ultrasonic vibrations break up the lens, and the fragments are aspirated from the eye: _____

2. Test of clearness of vision: _____

3. Measurement of tension or pressure within the eye; glaucoma test: _____

4. High-energy light radiation beams are used to stop retinal hemorrhaging:

   _____

5. A laser removes corneal tissue (sculpts it) to correct myopia: _____

6. Intravenous injection of dye followed by photographs of the eye through dilated pupils:

   _____

7. Suture of a silicone band to the sclera to correct retinal detachment: _____

8. Test to measure central and peripheral vision (area within which objects are seen) when the

   eyes are looking straight ahead: _____

9. Removal (and replacement) of diseased fluid in the chamber behind the lens of the eye:

   _____

10. Visual examination of the interior of the eye after dilation of the pupil: _____

11. Use of an instrument for microscopic examination of parts of the eye: _____

12. Corneal transplant surgery: _____

O Arrange the following terms in the correct order to indicate their sequence in the transmission of sound waves to the brain from the outer ear. See page 720.

auditory liquids and receptors | external auditory canal | pinna (auricle)
auditory nerve fibers | incus | stapes
cerebral cortex | malleus | tympanic membrane
cochlea | oval window

1. _____

2. _____

3. _____

4. _____

5. _____

6. _____

7. _____

8. _____

9. _____

10. _____

11. _____

P **Give short definitions for the following medical terms.**

1. labyrinth _____

2. semicircular canals _____

3. auditory (eustachian) tube _____

4. stapes _____

5. organ of Corti _____

6. perilymph and endolymph _____

7. cerumen _____

8. vestibule _____

9. oval window _____

10. tympanic membrane _____

Q **Complete the following terms based on their definitions.**

1. instrument to examine the ear: _____ scope

2. removal of the third bone of the middle ear: _____ ectomy

3. pertaining to the auditory tube and throat: _____ pharyngeal

4. flow of pus from the ear: oto _____

5. instrument to measure hearing: _____ meter

6. incision of the eardrum: _____ tomy

7. surgical repair of the eardrum: _____ plasty

8. deafness due to old age: _____ cusis

9. small ear: micr _____

10. inflammation of the middle ear: ot _____

R **Give short definitions for the following medical terms.**

1. vertigo _____

2. Meniere disease _____

3. otosclerosis _____

4. tinnitus _____

5. labyrinthitis _____

6. cholesteatoma _____

7. suppurative otitis media _____

8. acoustic neuroma _____

9. mastoiditis _____

10. myringitis _____

17

S Give the meanings of the following abbreviations of terms relating to otology.

1. ENG _____

2. AS _____

3. AD _____

4. EENT _____

5. ENT _____

6. PE tube _____

T Circle the correct term(s) in boldface to complete each sentence.

1. Dr. Jones specializes in pediatric ophthalmology. His examination of children with poor vision often leads to the diagnosis of **(cataract, amblyopia, glaucoma)**, or lazy eye.

2. Stella's near vision became progressively worse as she aged. Her physician told her that she had a common condition called **(presbyopia, detached retina, anisocoria)**, which often develops beginning in middle age.

3. Matthew rubbed his itchy eyes constantly and thus spread his "pinkeye" or **(conjunctivitis, blepharitis, myringitis)** from one eye to the other. Dr. Chang prescribed antibiotics for this common condition, because Matthew had a purulent discharge suggestive of an infection.

4. As Paul's **(mastoiditis, otitis media, tinnitus)** became progressively worse, his doctor worried that this ringing in his ears might be caused by a benign brain tumor, a/an **(cholesteatoma, acoustic neuroma, glaucoma)**.

5. Before her second birthday, Sally had so many episodes of **(vertigo, otosclerosis, suppurative otitis media)** that Dr. Sills recommended the placement of PE tubes.

6. Sixty-eight-year-old Bob experienced blurred vision in the central portion of his visual field. After careful examination of his **(cornea, sclera, retina)**, his **(ophthalmologist, optician, optometrist)** diagnosed his condition as **(glaucoma, iritis, macular degeneration)**. The doctor explained that the form of this condition was atrophic or **(dry, wet)**, causing photoreceptor rods and cones to die.

7. If Bob's condition had been diagnosed as the **(dry, wet)** form, it might have been treated with **(cryotherapy, intraocular lenses, laser photocoagulation)** to seal leaky blood vessels.

8. Sarah suddenly experienced bright flashes of light in her right eye. She also told her physician that she had a sensation of a curtain being pulled over part of the visual field in that eye. Her doctor examined her eye with **(keratoplasty, ophthalmoscopy, tonometry)** and determined that she had **(retinal refraction, retinal detachment, diabetic retinopathy)**. Corrective surgery, known as **(enucleation, vitrectomy, scleral buckling)**, was recommended.

9. Carol awakened with a sensation of dizziness or **(vertigo, tinnitus, presbycusis)** as she tried to get out of bed. She was totally incapacitated for several days and noticed hearing loss in her left ear. Her physician explained that fluid called **(pus, endolymph, mucus)** had accumulated in her **(auditory tube, middle ear, cochlea)** and her condition was **(otosclerosis, cholesteatoma, Meniere disease)**. He prescribed drugs to control her dizziness and nausea.

10. Patients with conductive hearing loss are helped by reconstruction of the **(labyrinth, tympanic membrane, auditory tube)**, a procedure known as **(myringoplasty, audiometry, otoscopy)**. Patients with sensorineural hearing loss may be helped by a **(hearing aid, cochlear implant, stapedectomy)**.

17

ANSWERS TO EXERCISES

A

1. E
2. G
3. H
4. J

5. F
6. I
7. B

8. C
9. A
10. D

B

1. optic disc
2. accommodation
3. macula
4. fovea centralis

5. refraction
6. optic chiasm
7. cones

8. rods
9. anterior chamber
10. fundus

C

1. cornea
2. anterior chamber and aqueous humor
3. pupil

4. lens
5. vitreous chamber and vitreous humor
6. retina

7. optic nerve fibers
8. optic chiasm
9. thalamus
10. cerebral cortex (occipital lobe)

D

1. cranial nerve that carries impulses from the retina to the brain
2. having two sides that are rounded, elevated, and curved evenly
3. condition of pupils of unequal (anis/o) size
4. pertaining to paralysis of the ciliary muscles, which would

result in dilation or enlargement of the pupil
5. pertaining to the eyelid
6. condition of enlargement of the pupil
7. condition of constriction of the pupil

8. swelling in the region of the optic disc
9. condition of sensitivity to ("fear of") light
10. blind spot; area of darkened (diminished) vision surrounded by clear vision

E

1. blepharitis
2. conjunctivitis
3. dacryoadenitis
4. iritis

5. keratitis
6. scleritis
7. retinitis

8. blepharoptosis
9. lacrimal
10. intraocular

F

1. corneal ulcer
2. uveitis
3. xerophthalmia
4. hemianopsia

5. exotropia
6. ophthalmologist
7. optometrist

8. optician
9. aphakia
10. esotropia

G

1. decreased (dim) vision; lazy eye (resulting from strabismus and uncorrected refractive errors in childhood)
2. farsightedness

3. decreased vision at near, resulting from increasing age
4. nearsightedness
5. night blindness; decreased vision at night

6. double vision
7. defective curvature of the lens and cornea leading to blurred vision

H

1. retina; long; strong; front; concave
2. short; weak; back; convex

3. constricts
4. dilates

17

I

1. diabetic retinopathy
2. retinal detachment
3. strabismus
4. cataract
5. macular degeneration
6. hordeolum (stye)
7. chalazion
8. glaucoma
9. retinitis pigmentosa
10. nystagmus

J

1. pupil
2. conjunctiva
3. cornea
4. sclera
5. choroid
6. iris
7. ciliary body
8. lens
9. anterior chamber
10. vitreous humor
11. retina
12. optic nerve
13. optic disc
14. macula
15. fovea centralis

K

1. C. Stroke (hemianopsia)—loss of half of the visual field caused by a stroke affecting the left visual cortex
2. B. Glaucoma—loss of peripheral vision first (darkness around the edges of the picture)
3. A. Cataract—causes blurred vision

L

1. tears
2. tears
3. cornea
4. cornea
5. eyelid
6. eyelid
7. pupil
8. pupil
9. lens
10. lens
11. eye
12. eye
13. eye
14. darkness

M

1. both eyes
2. visual acuity
3. right eye
4. left eye
5. visual field
6. intraocular lens
7. intraocular pressure
8. pupils equal, round, reactive to light and accommodation

N

1. phacoemulsification
2. visual acuity test
3. tonometry
4. laser photocoagulation
5. LASIK
6. fluorescein angiography
7. scleral buckle
8. visual field test
9. vitrectomy
10. ophthalmoscopy
11. slit lamp microscopy
12. keratoplasty

O

1. pinna (auricle)
2. external auditory canal
3. tympanic membrane
4. malleus
5. incus
6. stapes
7. oval window
8. cochlea
9. auditory liquids and receptors
10. auditory nerve fibers
11. cerebral cortex

P

1. cochlea and organs of equilibrium (semicircular canals and vestibule)
2. organ of equilibrium in the inner ear
3. passageway between the middle ear and the throat
4. third ossicle (little bone) of the middle ear
5. region in the cochlea that contains auditory receptors
6. auditory fluids circulating within the inner ear
7. wax in the external auditory meatus
8. central cavity of the inner ear that connects the semicircular canals and the cochlea
9. delicate membrane between the middle and the inner ears
10. eardrum

Q

1. otoscope
2. stapedectomy
3. salpingopharyngeal
4. otopyorrhea

5. audiometer
6. myringotomy (tympanotomy)
7. tympanoplasty (myringoplasty)

8. presbycusis
9. microtia
10. otitis media

R

1. sensation of irregular or whirling motion either of oneself or of external objects
2. disorder of the labyrinth marked by elevation of ear fluids and pressure within the cochlea (tinnitus, vertigo, and nausea result)

3. hardening in the bony tissue of the ossicles of the middle ear
4. noise (ringing, buzzing) in the ears
5. inflammation of the labyrinth of the inner ear
6. collection of skin cells and cholesterol in a sac within the middle ear

7. inflammation of the middle ear with bacterial infection and pus collection
8. benign tumor arising from the acoustic nerve in the brain
9. inflammation of the mastoid process (behind the ear)
10. inflammation of the eardrum

S

1. electronystagmography; a test of balance
2. left ear

3. right ear
4. eyes, ears, nose, and throat
5. ears, nose, and throat

6. pressure-equalizing tube; ventilating tube placed in the eardrum

T

1. amblyopia
2. presbyopia
3. conjunctivitis
4. tinnitus; acoustic neuroma
5. suppurative otitis media

6. retina; ophthalmologist; macular degeneration; dry
7. wet; laser photocoagulation
8. ophthalmoscopy; retinal detachment; scleral buckling

9. vertigo; endolymph; cochlea; Meniere disease
10. tympanic membrane; myringoplasty; cochlear implant

17

Answers to Practical Applications

Operating Room Schedule: Eye and Ear Procedures

1. I
2. B
3. C
4. D
5. G
6. A
7. H
8. E
9. F

PRONUNCIATION OF TERMS

To test your understanding of the terminology in this chapter, write the meaning of each term in the space provided. In addition, you may wish to cover the terms and write them by looking at your definitions. Make sure your spelling is correct. The page number after each term indicates where it is defined or used in the book, so you can easily check your responses. You will find complete definitions for all of these terms and their audio pronunciations on the Evolve website.

Pronunciation Guide

ā as in āpe	ă as in ăpple
ē as in ēven	ĕ as in ĕvery
ī as in īce	ĭ as in ĭnterest
ō as in ōpen	ŏ as in pŏt
ū as in ūnit	ŭ as in ŭnder

Vocabulary and Terminology: Eye

TERM	PRONUNCIATION	MEANING
accommodation (702)	ă-kŏm-ō-DĀ-shŭn	
amblyopia (707)	ăm-blē-Ō-pē-ă	
anisocoria (704)	ăn-ī-sō-KŌ-rē-ă	
anterior chamber (702)	ăn-TĒ-rē-ŏr CHĀM-bĕr	
aphakia (706)	ă-FĀ-kē-ă	
aqueous humor (702)	ĂK-wē-ŭs *or* Ā-kwē-ŭs HŪ-mŏr	
astigmatism (708)	ă-STĪG-mă-tĭzm	
biconvex (703)	bī-KŎN-vĕks	
blepharitis (704)	blĕf-ă-RĪ-tĭs	
blepharoptosis (704)	blĕf-ă-rŏp-TŌ-sĭs	
cataract (710)	KĂT-ă-răkt	
chalazion (710)	kă-LĀ-zē-ŏn	
choroid (703)	KŎR-oyd	
ciliary body (703)	SĬL-ē-ăr-ē BŎD-ē	
cone (703)	kōn	
conjunctiva (703)	kŏn-jŭnk-TĪ-vă	
conjunctivitis (704)	kŏn-jŭnk-tĭ-VĪ-tĭs	
cornea (703)	KŎR-nē-ă	
corneal abrasion (705)	KŎR-nē-ăl ă-BRĀ-zhŭn	
corneoscleral (706)	kŏr-nē-ō-SKLĔ-răl	
cycloplegic (705)	sī-klō-PLĒ-jĭk	
dacryoadenitis (705)	dăk-rē-ō-ăd-ĕ-NĪ-tĭs	
diabetic retinopathy (710)	dī-ă-BĔT-ĭk rĕ-tĭn-NŎP-ă-thē	

17

TERM	PRONUNCIATION	MEANING
diplopia (707)	dĭp-LŌ-pē-ă	
enucleation (716)	ē-nū-klē-Ā-shun	
esotropia (708)	ĕs-ō-TRŌ-pē-ă	
exotropia (713)	ĕk-sō-TRŌ-pē-ă	
fluorescein angiography (714)	floo-ō-RĔS-ē-ĭn ăn-jē-ŎG-ră-fē	
fovea centralis (703)	FŌ-vē-ă sĕn-TRĂ-lĭs	
fundus of the eye (703)	FŬN-dŭs of the ī	
glaucoma (711)	glaw-KŌ-mă	
hemianopsia (708)	hĕ-mē-ă-NŎP-sē-ă	
hordeolum (712)	hŏr-DĒ-ō-lŭm	
hyperopia (708)	hī-pĕr-Ō-pē-ă	
hypertensive retinopathy (706)	hī-pĕr-TĔN-sĭv rĕ-tĭ-NŎP-ă-thē	
intraocular (705)	ĭn-tră-ŎK-ū-lăr	
iridectomy (705)	ĭr-ĭ-DĔK-tō-mē	
iridic (705)	ĭ RĪD ĭk	
iris (703)	Ī-rĭs	
iritis (705)	ī-RĪ-tĭs	
keratitis (705)	kĕr-ă-TĪ-tĭs	
keratoplasty (716)	kĕr-ă-tō-PLĂS-tē	
lacrimal (705)	LĂK-rĭ-măl	
lacrimation (705)	lă-krĭ-MĀ-shŭn	
laser photocoagulation (717)	LĀ-zĕr fō-tō-kō-ăg-ū-LĀ-shŭn	
lens (703)	lĕnz	
macula (703)	MĂK-ū-lă	
macular degeneration (712)	MĂK-ū-lăr dē-jĕn-ĕ-RĀ-shŭn	
miosis (707)	mī-Ō-sĭs	
miotic (707)	mī-ŎT-ĭk	
mydriasis (707)	mĭ-DRĪ-ă-sĭs	
myopia (708)	mī-Ō-pē-ă	
nyctalopia (707)	nĭk-tă-LŌ-pē-ă	
nystagmus (713)	nĭ-STĂG-mŭs	

TERM	PRONUNCIATION	MEANING
ophthalmic (706)	ŏf-THĂL-mĭk	
ophthalmologist (706)	ŏf-thăl-MŎL-ō-jĭst	
ophthalmoplegia (706)	ŏf-thăl-mō-PLĒ-jă	
ophthalmoscopy (714)	ŏf-thăl-MŎS-kō-pē	
optic chiasm (703)	ŎP-tĭk KĪ-ăzm	
optic disc (703)	ŎP-tĭk dĭsk	
optician (706)	ŏp-TĬSH-ăn	
optic nerve (703)	ŎP-tĭk nĕrv	
optometrist (706)	ŏp-TŎM-ĕ-trĭst	
palpebral (706)	PĂL-pĕ-brăl	
papilledema (706)	păp-ĭ-lĕ-DĒ-mă	
phacoemulsification (717)	făk-ō-ĕ-mŭl-sĭ-fĭ-KĀ-shŭn	
photophobia (707)	fō-tō-FŌ-bē-ă	
presbyopia (709)	prĕz-bē-Ō-pē-ă	
pupil (703)	PŪ-pĭl	
pupillary (706)	PŪ-pĭ-lăr-ē	
refraction (703)	rē-FRĂK-shŭn	
retina (703)	RĔT-ĭ-nă	
retinal detachment (713)	RĔ-tĭ-năl dē-TĂCH-mĕnt	
retinitis pigmentosa (706)	rĕt-ĭ-NĪ-tĭs pĭg-mĕn-TŌ-să	
rod (703)	rŏd	
sclera (703)	SKLĔ-ră	
scleral buckle (717)	SKLĔ-răl BŬ-kl	
scleritis (706)	sklĕ-RĪ-tĭs	
scotoma (707)	skō-TŌ-mă	
slit lamp microscopy (714)	slĭt lămp mī-KRŎS-kō-pē	
strabismus (713)	stră-BĬZ-mŭs	
thalamus (703)	THĂL-ă-mŭs	
tonometry (715)	tō-NŎM-ĕ-trē	
trabeculoplasty (711)	tră-bĕk-ū-lō-PLĂS-tē	
uveitis (707)	ū-vē-Ī-tĭs	
visual acuity test (715)	VĬZ-ū-ăl ă-KŪ-ĭ-tē tĕst	

17

TERM	PRONUNCIATION	MEANING
visual field test (715)	VĬZ-ū-ăl fēld tĕst	_____
vitrectomy (718)	vĭ-TRĔK-tō-mē	_____
vitreous humor (703)	VĬT-rē-ŭs HŪ-mŏr	_____
xerophthalmia (707)	zĕr-ŏf-THĂL-mē-ă	_____

Vocabulary and Terminology: Ear

TERM	PRONUNCIATION	MEANING
acoustic (722)	ă-KOOS-tĭk	_____
acoustic neuroma (724)	ă-KOOS-tĭk nū-RŌ-mă	_____
audiogram (726)	ĂW-dē-ō-grăm	_____
audiologist (722)	ăw-dē-ŎL-ō-gĭst	_____
audiometer (726)	ăw-dē-ŎM-ĕ-tĕr	_____
audiometry (726)	ăw-dē-ŎM-ĕ-trē	_____
auditory canal (721)	ĂW-dĭ-tō-rē kă-NĂL	_____
auditory meatus (721)	ĂW-dĭ-tō-re mē-Ā-tŭs	_____
auditory nerve fibers (721)	ĂW-dĭ-tō-re nĕrv FĪ-bĕrz	_____
auditory tube (721)	ĂW-dĭ-tō-rē toob	_____
aural (722)	ĂW-răl	_____
auricle (721)	ĂW-rĭ-kl	_____
cerumen (721)	sĕ-ROO-mĕn	_____
cholesteatoma (724)	kō-lē-stē-ă-TŌ-mă	_____
cochlea (721)	KŎK-lē-ă	_____
cochlear (722)	KŎK-lē-ăr	_____
deafness (724)	DĔF-nĕs	_____
ear thermometry (726)	ēr thĕr-MŎM-ĕ-trē	_____
endolymph (721)	ĔN-dō-lĭmf	_____
eustachian tube (721)	ū-STĀ-shŭn toob	_____
hyperacusis (723)	hī-pĕr-ă-KŪ-sis	_____
incus (721)	ĬNG-kŭs	_____
labyrinth (721)	LĂB-ĭ-rĭnth	_____
macrotia (723)	măk-RŌ-shē-ă	_____

17

TERM	PRONUNCIATION	MEANING
malleus (721)	MĂL-ē-ŭs	
mastoiditis (722)	măs-toy-DĪ-tĭs	
Meniere disease (724)	měn-ē-ĀR dĭ-ZĒZ	
myringitis (722)	mĭr-ĭn-JĪ-tĭs	
myringotomy (722)	mĭr-ĭn-GŎT-ō-mē	
organ of Corti (721)	ŎR-găn of CŎR-tē	
ossicle (721)	ŎS-ĭ-kl	
ossiculoplasty (722)	ŏs-ĭ-kū-lō-PLĂS-tē	
otic (722)	Ō-tĭk	
otitis media (725)	ō-TĪ-tĭs MĒ-dē-ă	
otolaryngologist (722)	ō-tō-lă-rĭn-GŎL-ō-jĭst	
otomycosis (722)	ō-tō-mī-KŌ-sĭs	
otopyorrhea (722)	ō-tō-pī-ō-RĒ-ă	
otosclerosis (725)	ō-tō-sklĕ-RŌ-sĭs	
otoscopy (726)	ō-TŎS-kō-pē	
oval window (721)	Ō-văl WĬN-dō	
perilymph (721)	PĔR-ĭ-lĭmf	
pinna (721)	PĬN-ă	
postauricular (722)	pōst-aw-RĬK-ū-lăr	
presbycusis (723)	prĕz-bē-KŪ-sĭs	
salpingopharyngeal (722)	săl-pĭng-gō-fă-RĬN-gē-ăl	
semicircular canals (721)	sĕ-mē-SĔR-kū-lăr kă-NĂLZ	
stapedectomy (723)	stā-pĕ-DĔK-tō-mē	
stapes (721)	STĀ-pēz	
tinnitus (725)	TĬN-nĭ-tŭs	
tuning fork test (726)	TOO-nĭng fŏrk tĕst	
tympanic membrane (721)	tĭm-PĂN-ĭk MĔM-brān	
tympanoplasty (723)	tĭm-pă-nō-PLĂS-tē	
vertigo (725)	VĔR-tĭ-gō	
vestibule (721)	VĔS-tĭ-būl	
vestibulocochlear (723)	vĕs-tĭb-ū-lō-KŎK-lē-ăr	

17

REVIEW SHEET

Write the meaning of the word parts in the spaces provided and test yourself. Check your answers with the information in the chapter or in the *Glossary (Medical Word Parts—English)* at the end of the book.

Combining Forms

COMBINING FORM	MEANING	COMBINING FORM	MEANING
acous/o		myring/o	
ambly/o		nyct/o	
anis/o		ocul/o	
aque/o		ophthalm/o	
audi/o		opt/o	
audit/o		optic/o	
aur/o		ossicul/o	
auricul/o		ot/o	
blephar/o		palpebr/o	
cochle/o		papill/o	
conjunctiv/o		phac/o	
cor/o		phak/o	
corne/o		phot/o	
cycl/o		presby/o	
dacry/o		pupill/o	
dipl/o		retin/o	
glauc/o		salping/o	
ir/o		scler/o	
irid/o		scot/o	
kerat/o		staped/o	
lacrim/o		tympan/o	
mastoid/o		uve/o	
mi/o		vestibul/o	
myc/o		vitre/o	
mydr/o		xer/o	

17

Suffixes

SUFFIX	MEANING	SUFFIX	MEANING
-acusis	_____	-opsia	_____
-cusis	_____	-otia	_____
-meter	_____	-phobia	_____
-metry	_____	-plegic	_____
-opia	_____	-tropia	_____

Use the following terms to label the accompanying diagram.

auditory nerve fibers   incus   semicircular canals
cochlea   malleus   stapes
eustachian tube   oval window   tympanic membrane (eardrum)
external auditory meatus   pinna (auricle)   vestibule

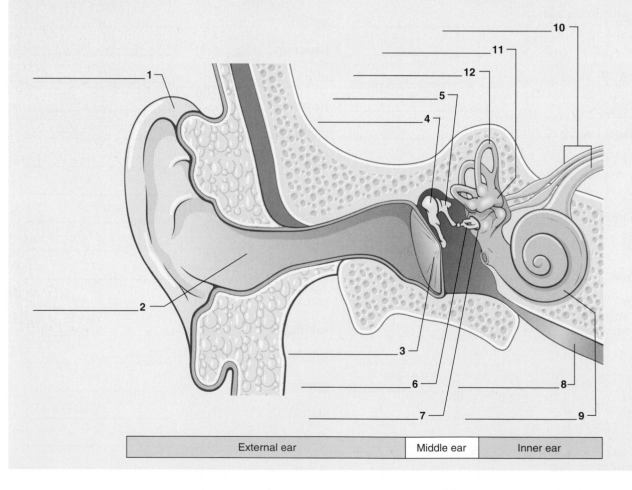

External ear   Middle ear   Inner ear

evolve   *Please refer to the Evolve website for additional exercises and images related to this chapter.*

Endocrine System

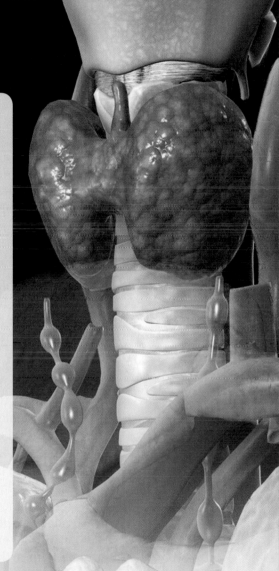

Chapter Sections:

CHAPTER GOALS

- Identify the endocrine glands and their hormones.
- Gain an understanding of the functions of these hormones in the body.
- Analyze medical terms related to the endocrine glands and their hormones.
- Identify the abnormal conditions resulting from excessive and deficient secretions of the endocrine glands.
- Describe laboratory tests and clinical procedures related to endocrinology, and recognize relevant abbreviations.

INTRODUCTION

The endocrine system is an information signaling system much like the nervous system. However, the nervous system uses nerves to conduct information, whereas the endocrine system uses blood vessels as information channels. **Glands** located in many regions of the body release into the bloodstream specific chemical messengers called **hormones** (from the Greek word *hormōn,* meaning urging on) that regulate the many and varied functions of an organism. For example, one hormone stimulates the growth of bones, another causes the maturation of sex organs and reproductive cells, and another controls the metabolic rate (metabolism) within all the individual cells of the body. In addition, one powerful endocrine gland below the brain secretes a wide variety of different hormones that travel through the bloodstream and regulate the activities of other endocrine glands.

Hormones produce their effects by binding to **receptors,** which are recognition sites in the various **target tissues** on which the hormones act. The receptors initiate specific biologic effects when the hormones bind to them. Each hormone has its own receptor, and binding of a receptor by a hormone is much like the interaction of a key and a lock.

Endocrine glands, no matter which hormones they produce, secrete their hormones directly into the bloodstream. **Exocrine glands** send chemical substances (tears, sweat, milk, saliva) via ducts to the outside of the body. Examples of exocrine glands are sweat, mammary, mucous, salivary, and lacrimal (tear) glands.

The ductless, internally secreting **endocrine glands** are listed as follows. Locate these glands on Figure 18-1.

[1] thyroid gland
[2] parathyroid glands (four glands)
[3] adrenal glands (one pair)
[4] pancreas (islets of Langerhans)

[5] pituitary gland
[6] ovaries in female (one pair)
[7] testes in male (one pair)
[8] pineal gland

The last gland on this list, the **pineal gland,** is included as an endocrine gland because it is ductless, although less is known about its endocrine function. Located in the central portion of the brain, the pineal secretes melatonin. **Melatonin** functions to support the body's "biologic clock" and is thought to induce sleep. The pineal gland has been linked to a mental condition, **seasonal affective disorder (SAD),** in which the person suffers from depression in winter months. Melatonin secretion increases with deprivation of light and is inhibited by sunlight. Calcification of the pineal gland can occur and can be an important radiologic landmark when x-rays of the brain are examined.

Hormones are also secreted by endocrine tissue in other organs apart from the major endocrine glands. Examples are **erythropoietin** (kidney), **human chorionic gonadotropin** (placenta), and **cholecystokinin** (gallbladder). **Prostaglandins** are hormone-like substances that affect the body in many ways. First found in semen (produced by the prostate gland) but now recognized in cells throughout the body, prostaglandins have three functions: (1) stimulate the contraction of the uterus; (2) regulate body temperature, platelet aggregation, and acid secretion in the stomach; and (3) have the ability to lower blood pressure.

Endocrine tissue (apart from the major glands) is reviewed in Table 18-1. Use it as a reference.

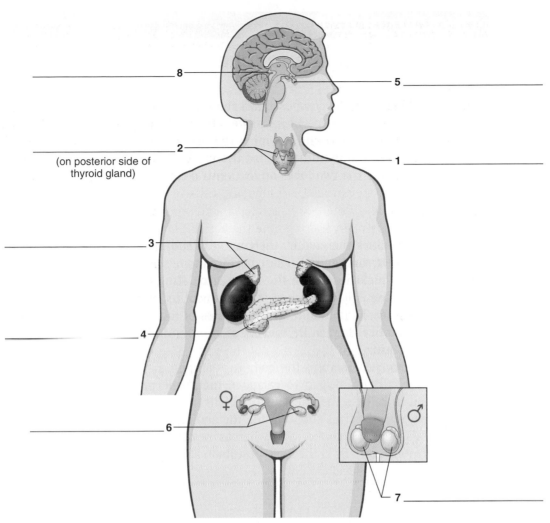

FIGURE 18-1 The endocrine system.

TABLE 18-1	ENDOCRINE TISSUE (APART FROM MAJOR GLANDS): LOCATION, SECRETION, AND ACTION	
LOCATION	**SECRETION**	**ACTION**
Body cells	Prostaglandins	Aggregation of platelets Contract uterus Lower acid secretion in stomach Lower blood pressure
Gastrointestinal tract	Cholecystokinin Gastrin Secretin	Contracts gallbladder Stimulates gastric secretion Stimulates pancreatic enzymes
Kidney	Erythropoietin	Stimulates erythrocyte production
Placenta	Human chorionic gonadotropin	Sustains pregnancy
Skin	Vitamin D	Affects absorption of calcium

(on posterior side of thyroid gland)

18

THYROID GLAND

LOCATION AND STRUCTURE

Label Figure 18-2.

The **thyroid gland** [1] is composed of a right and a left lobe on either side of the **trachea** [2], just below a large piece of cartilage called the **thyroid cartilage** [3]. The thyroid cartilage covers the larynx and produces the prominence on the neck known in men as the "Adam's apple." The **isthmus** [4] of the thyroid gland is a narrow strip of glandular tissue that connects the two lobes on the ventral (anterior) surface of the trachea.

FUNCTION

Two of the hormones secreted by the thyroid gland are **thyroxine** or **tetraiodothyronine (T4)** and **triiodothyronine (T3).** These hormones are synthesized in the thyroid gland from **iodine,** which is picked up from the blood circulating through the gland, and an amino acid called tyrosine. T4 (containing four atoms of iodine) is much more concentrated in the blood, whereas T3 (containing three atoms of iodine) is far more potent in affecting the metabolism of cells. Most thyroid hormone is bound to protein molecules as it travels in the bloodstream.

T4 and T3 are necessary in the body to maintain a normal level of metabolism in all body cells. Cells need oxygen to carry on metabolic processes, one aspect of which is burning food to release the energy stored within it. Thyroid hormone aids cells in their uptake of oxygen and thus supports the metabolic rate in the body. Injections of thyroid hormone raise the metabolic rate, whereas removal of the thyroid gland, diminishing thyroid hormone content in the body, results in a lower metabolic rate, heat loss, and poor physical and mental development.

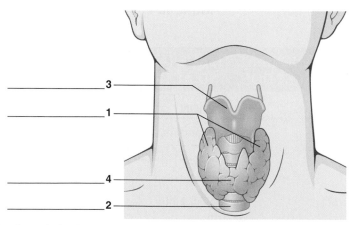

FIGURE 18-2   The thyroid gland, anterior view. Notice how the thyroid gland covers the trachea like a shield (*thyr/o* = shield).

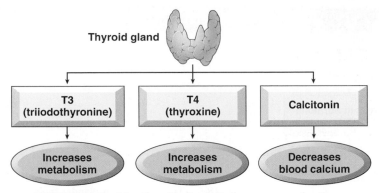

FIGURE 18-3   The thyroid gland: its hormones and actions.

A more recently discovered hormone produced by the thyroid gland is **calcitonin.** Calcitonin is secreted when calcium levels in the blood are high. It stimulates calcium to leave the blood and enter the bones, thereby lowering blood calcium back to normal. Calcitonin contained in a nasal spray may be used for treatment of osteoporosis (loss of bone density). By increasing calcium storage in bone, calcitonin strengthens weakened bone tissue and prevents spontaneous bone fractures. Figure 18-3 summarizes the hormones secreted by the thyroid gland.

PARATHYROID GLANDS

LOCATION AND STRUCTURE

Label Figure 18-4.

The **parathyroid glands** [1] are four small oval bodies located on the dorsal aspect of the **thyroid gland** [2].

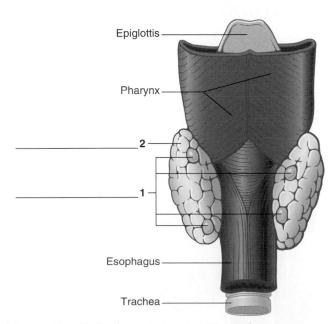

FIGURE 18-4   **The parathyroid glands,** posterior view. The prefix para- means near, or alongside.

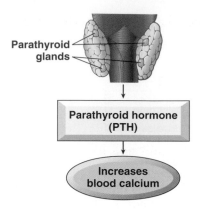

FIGURE 18-5   The parathyroid glands: their hormone and action.

FUNCTION

Parathyroid hormone (PTH) is secreted by the parathyroid glands. This hormone (also known as **parathormone**) mobilizes **calcium** (a mineral substance) from bones into the bloodstream, where calcium is necessary for proper functioning of body tissues, especially muscles. Normally, calcium in the food we eat is absorbed from the intestine and carried by the blood to the bones, where it is stored. The adjustment of the level of calcium in the blood is a good example of the way hormones in general control the **homeostasis** (equilibrium or constancy in the internal environment) of the body. If blood calcium decreases (as in pregnancy or with vitamin D deficiency), parathyroid hormone secretion increases, causing calcium to leave bones and enter the bloodstream. In this way, blood calcium levels are brought back to normal (Figure 18-5).

18

ADRENAL GLANDS

LOCATION AND STRUCTURE

Label Figure 18-6.

The **adrenal glands** are two small glands, one on top of each **kidney** [1]. Each gland consists of two parts: an outer portion, the **adrenal cortex** [2], and an inner portion, the **adrenal medulla** [3]. The adrenal cortex and the adrenal medulla are two glands in one, secreting different hormones. The adrenal cortex secretes **steroids** or **corticosteroids**

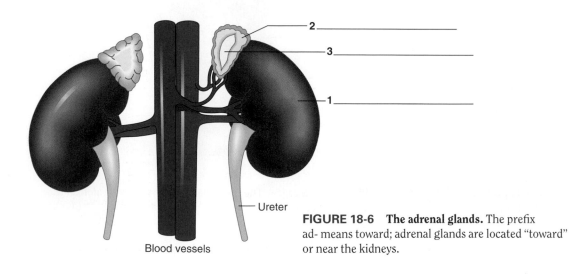

FIGURE 18-6   The adrenal glands. The prefix ad- means toward; adrenal glands are located "toward" or near the kidneys.

(complex chemicals derived from cholesterol); the adrenal medulla secretes **catecholamines** (chemicals derived from amino acids).

FUNCTION

The **adrenal cortex** secretes three types of **corticosteroids.**

1. **Glucocorticoids**—These steroid hormones have an important influence on the metabolism of sugars, fats, and proteins within all body cells and have a powerful anti-inflammatory effect.

    Cortisol helps regulate glucose, fat, and protein metabolism. It raises blood glucose as part of a response to stress. **Cortisone** is a hormone very similar to cortisol and can be prepared synthetically. Cortisone is useful in treating inflammatory conditions such as rheumatoid arthritis.

2. **Mineralocorticoids**—The major mineralocorticoid is **aldosterone.** It regulates the concentration of mineral **salts (electrolytes)** in the body. Aldosterone acts on the kidney to reabsorb **sodium** (an important **electrolyte**) and water and to excrete **potassium** (another major **electrolyte**). Thus, it regulates blood volume and blood pressure and electrolyte concentration.

3. **Sex hormones**—**Androgens** (testosterone) and **estrogens** are secreted in small amounts and influence secondary sex characteristics, such as pubic and axillary hair in boys and girls. In females, the masculinizing effects of adrenal androgens (such as increased body hair) may appear when levels of ovarian estrogen decrease after menopause.

Think of the "three S's" to recall the main adrenal cortex hormones, which influence <u>s</u>ugar (cortisol), <u>s</u>alt (aldosterone), and <u>s</u>ex (androgens and estrogens).

The **adrenal medulla** secretes two types of **catecholamine** hormones:

1. **Epinephrine (adrenaline)**—Increases heart rate and blood pressure, dilates bronchial tubes, and releases glucose (sugars) from glycogen (storage substance) when the body needs it for more energy.

2. **Norepinephrine (noradrenaline)**—Constricts blood vessels to raise blood pressure.

Both epinephrine and norepinephrine are **sympathomimetic** agents because they mimic, or copy, the actions of the sympathetic nervous system. They are released to help the body meet the challenges of stress in response to stimulation by the sympathetic nervous system.

Figure 18-7 summarizes hormones secreted by the adrenal glands and their actions.

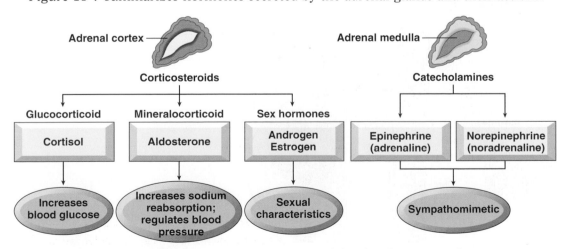

FIGURE 18-7 **The adrenal cortex and adrenal medulla: their hormones and actions.**

PANCREAS

LOCATION AND STRUCTURES

Label Figure 18-8.

The **pancreas** [1] is located near and partly behind the **stomach** [2] at the level of the first and second lumbar vertebrae. The endocrine tissue of the pancreas consists of specialized hormone-producing cells called the **islets of Langerhans** [3] or **islet cells.** More than 98% of the pancreas consists of exocrine cells (glands and ducts). These cells secrete digestive enzymes into the gastrointestinal tract.

FUNCTION

The islets of Langerhans produce **insulin** (produced by beta cells) and **glucagon** (produced by alpha cells). Both play a role regulating blood **glucose** (sugar) levels. When blood glucose rises, insulin lowers blood sugar by helping it enter body cells. Insulin also lowers blood sugar by causing conversion of **glucose** to **glycogen** (a starch storage form of sugar) in the liver. If blood glucose levels fall too low, glucagon raises blood sugar by acting on liver cells to promote conversion of glycogen back to glucose. Thus, the endocrine function of the pancreas is another example of **homeostasis,** the body's ability to regulate its inner environment to maintain stability.

Figure 18-9 reviews the secretions of the islet cells and their actions.

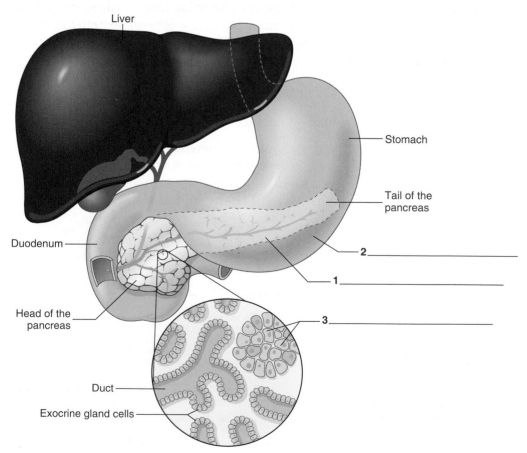

FIGURE 18-8   The **pancreas** and surrounding organs.

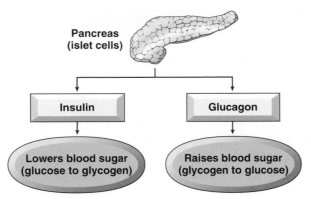

FIGURE 18-9 The pancreas (islet cells): its hormones and actions. Insulin is the only hormone that lowers blood sugar levels.

PITUITARY GLAND

LOCATION AND STRUCTURE

Label Figure 18-10.

The **pituitary gland,** also called the **hypophysis,** is a small pea-sized gland located at the base of the brain in a small pocket-like depression of the skull called the **sella turcica.** It is a well-protected gland, with the entire mass of the brain above it and the nasal cavity below. The ancient Greeks incorrectly imagined that its function was to produce *pituita,* or nasal secretion.

The pituitary consists of two distinct parts: an **anterior lobe** or **adenohypophysis** [1], composed of glandular epithelial tissue, and a **posterior lobe** or **neurohypophysis** [2], composed of nervous tissue. The **hypothalamus** [3] is a region of the brain under the thalamus and above the pituitary gland. Signals transmitted from the hypothalamus control secretions by the pituitary gland. Special secretory neurons in the hypothalamus send releasing and inhibiting factors (hormones) via capillaries to the anterior pituitary gland.

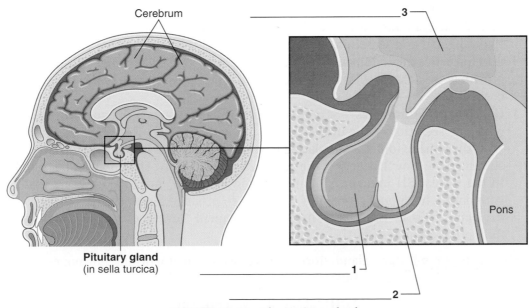

FIGURE 18-10 The pituitary gland.

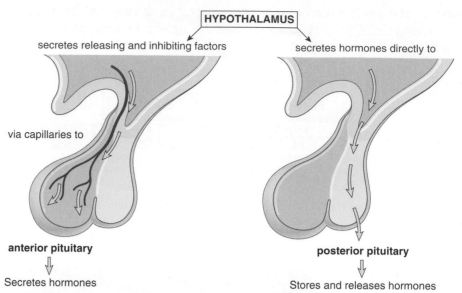

FIGURE 18-11 The relationship of the hypothalamus to the anterior and posterior lobes of the pituitary gland.

These factors stimulate or inhibit secretion of hormones from the anterior lobe of the pituitary gland. The hypothalamus also produces and secretes hormones directly to the posterior lobe of the pituitary gland, where the hormones are stored and then released (Figure 18-11).

FUNCTION

Although no bigger than a pea, the **pituitary gland** is often called the **"master gland"** because it makes hormones that control several other endocrine glands.

The major hormones of the **anterior pituitary gland** are:

1. **Growth hormone (GH),** or **somatotropin (STH)**—Promotes protein synthesis that results in the growth of bones, muscles, and other tissues. GH also stimulates the liver to make insulin-like growth factor (also called IGF), which stimulates the growth of bones. It increases blood glucose levels and is secreted during exercise, sleep, and hypoglycemia.
2. **Thyroid-stimulating hormone (TSH),** or **thyrotropin**—Stimulates the growth of the thyroid gland and secretion of thyroxine (T4) and triiodothyronine (T3).
3. **Adrenocorticotropic hormone (ACTH),** or **adrenocorticotropin**—Stimulates the growth of the adrenal cortex and increases its secretion of steroid hormones (primarily cortisol).
4. **Gonadotropic hormones**—Several gonadotropic hormones influence the growth and hormone secretion of the ovaries in females and the testes in males.
    In the female, **follicle-stimulating hormone (FSH)** and **luteinizing hormone (LH)** stimulate the growth of eggs in the ovaries, the production of hormones, and ovulation. In the male, FSH influences the production of sperm, and LH (an interstitial cell–stimulating hormone) stimulates the testes to produce testosterone.
5. **Prolactin (PRL)**—Stimulates breast development during pregnancy and sustains milk production after birth.

The **posterior pituitary gland** stores and releases two important hormones that are synthesized in the hypothalamus:

1. **Antidiuretic hormone (ADH),** also called **vasopressin**—Stimulates the reabsorption of water by the kidney tubules. In addition, ADH also increases blood pressure by constricting arterioles.

2. **Oxytocin (OT)**—Stimulates the uterus to contract during childbirth and maintains labor during childbirth. OT also is secreted during suckling and causes the production of milk from the mammary glands.

Figure 18-12 summarizes hormones secreted by the pituitary gland and their functions.

OVARIES

LOCATION AND STRUCTURE

The **ovaries** are two small glands located in the lower abdominal region of the female. The ovaries produce the female gamete, the ovum, as well as hormones that are responsible for female sex characteristics and regulation of the menstrual cycle.

FUNCTION

The ovarian hormones are **estrogens** (**estradiol** and estrone) and **progesterone.** Estrogens stimulate development of ova (eggs) and development of female secondary sex characteristics. Progesterone is responsible for the preparation and maintenance of the uterus in pregnancy.

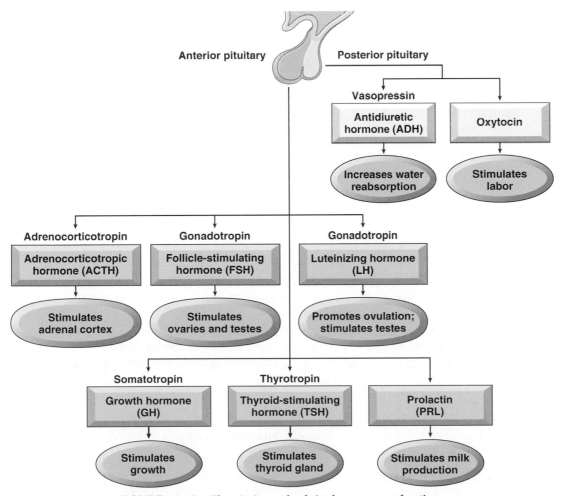

FIGURE 18-12   The pituitary gland: its hormones and actions.

18

TESTES

LOCATION AND STRUCTURE

The **testes** are two small ovoid glands suspended from the inguinal region of the male by the spermatic cord and surrounded by the scrotal sac. The testes produce the male gametes, spermatozoa, as well as the male hormone called **testosterone.**

FUNCTION

Testosterone is an **androgen** (male steroid hormone) that stimulates development of sperm and secondary sex characteristics in the male (deepening of voice and development of beard and pubic hair).

Figure 18-13 reviews the hormones secreted by the ovaries and testes.

Table 18-2 lists the major endocrine glands, their hormones, and the actions they produce.

TABLE 18-2	MAJOR ENDOCRINE GLANDS: THE HORMONES THEY PRODUCE AND THEIR ACTIONS	
ENDOCRINE GLAND	**HORMONE**	**ACTION**
Thyroid	• Thyroxine (T4); triiodothyronine (T3) • Calcitonin	• Increases metabolism in body cells • Decreases blood calcium
Parathyroids	• Parathyroid hormone	• Increases blood calcium
Adrenals		
Cortex	• Cortisol (glucocorticoid) • Aldosterone (mineralocorticoid) • Androgens, estrogens (sex hormones)	• Increases blood sugar • Increases reabsorption of sodium • Secondary sex characteristics
Medulla	• Epinephrine (adrenaline) • Norepinephrine (noradrenaline)	• Sympathomimetic • Sympathomimetic
Pancreas		
Islet cells	• Insulin • Glucagon	• Decreases blood sugar (glucose to glycogen) • Increases blood sugar (glycogen to glucose)
Pituitary		

Anterior lobe	• Growth hormone (GH) (somatotropin)
	 • Thyroid-stimulating hormone (TSH)
	
	 • Adrenocorticotropic hormone (ACTH)
	
	 • Gonadotropins
	   • Follicle-stimulating hormone (FSH)
	   • Luteinizing hormone (LH)
	 • Prolactin (PRL)
		• Increases bone and tissue growth
		 • Stimulates thyroid gland and thyroxine secretion
		 • Stimulates adrenal cortex, especially cortisol secretion
		
		 • Oogenesis and spermatogenesis
		 • Promotes ovulation; testosterone secretion
		 • Promotes growth of breast tissue and milk secretion

Posterior lobe	• Antidiuretic hormone (ADH) (vasopressin) • Oxytocin	• Stimulates reabsorption of water by kidney tubules • Stimulates contraction of the uterus during labor and childbirth
Ovaries	• Estrogens • Progesterone	• Promote development of ova and female secondary sex characteristics • Prepares and maintains the uterus in pregnancy
Testes	• Testosterone	• Promotes development of sperm and male secondary sex characteristics

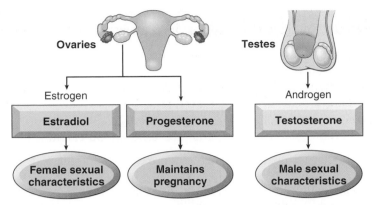

FIGURE 18-13   The ovaries and testes: their hormones and actions.

VOCABULARY

This list reviews many new terms introduced in the text. Short definitions reinforce your understanding of the terms. Refer to the Pronunciation of Terms on page 792 for help with unfamiliar or difficult words.

MAJOR ENDOCRINE GLANDS

adrenal cortex	Outer section (cortex) of each adrenal gland; secretes cortisol, aldosterone, and sex hormones.
adrenal medulla	Inner section (medulla) of each adrenal gland; secretes epinephrine and norepinephrine.
ovaries	Located in the lower abdomen of a female; responsible for egg production and estrogen and progesterone secretion.
pancreas	Located behind the stomach. Islet (alpha and beta) cells (islets of Langerhans) secrete hormones from the pancreas. The pancreas also contains cells that are exocrine in function. They secrete enzymes, via a duct, into the small intestine to aid digestion.
parathyroid glands	Four small glands on the posterior of the thyroid gland. Some people may have three or five parathyroid glands.
pituitary gland (hypophysis)	Located at the base of the brain in the sella turcica; composed of an **anterior lobe (adenohypophysis)** and a **posterior lobe (neurohypophysis).** It weighs only $\frac{1}{16}$ of an ounce and is a half-inch across.
testes	Two glands enclosed in the scrotal sac of a male; responsible for sperm production and testosterone secretion.
thyroid gland	Located in the neck on either side of the trachea; secretes thyroxine, triiodothyronine, and calcitonin.

HORMONES

adrenaline (epinephrine)	Secreted by the adrenal medulla; increases heart rate and blood pressure.
adrenocorticotropic hormone (ACTH)	Secreted by the anterior lobe of the pituitary gland; also called **adrenocorticotropin.** ACTH stimulates the adrenal cortex.

18

aldosterone	Secreted by the adrenal cortex; increases salt (sodium) reabsorption.
androgen	Male hormone secreted by the testes and to a lesser extent by the adrenal cortex; testosterone is an example.
antidiuretic hormone (ADH)	Secreted by the posterior lobe of the pituitary gland. **ADH (vasopressin)** increases reabsorption of water by the kidney.
calcitonin	Secreted by the thyroid gland; decreases blood calcium levels.
cortisol	Secreted by the adrenal cortex; increases blood sugar. It is secreted in times of stress and has an anti-inflammatory effect.
epinephrine (adrenaline)	Secreted by the adrenal medulla; increases heart rate and blood pressure and dilates airways (sympathomimetic). It is part of the body's "fight or flight" reaction.
estradiol	Estrogen (female hormone) secreted by the ovaries.
estrogen	Female hormone secreted by the ovaries and to a lesser extent by the adrenal cortex. Examples are estradiol and estrone.
follicle-stimulating hormone (FSH)	Secreted by the anterior lobe of the pituitary gland. **FSH** stimulates hormone secretion and egg production by the ovaries and sperm production by the testes.
glucagon	Secreted by alpha islet cells of the pancreas; increases blood sugar by conversion of glycogen (starch) to glucose.
growth hormone (GH); somatotropin	Secreted by the anterior lobe of the pituitary gland; stimulates growth of bones and soft tissues.
insulin	Secreted by beta islet cells (Latin *insula* means island) of the pancreas. Insulin helps glucose (sugar) to pass into cells, and it promotes the conversion of glucose to glycogen.
luteinizing hormone (LH)	Secreted by the anterior lobe of the pituitary gland; stimulates ovulation in females and testosterone secretion in males.
norepinephrine	Secreted by the adrenal medulla; increases heart rate and blood pressure (sympathomimetic). Nor- in chemistry means a parent compound from which another is derived. Also called noradrenaline.
oxytocin (OT)	Secreted by the posterior lobe of the pituitary gland; stimulates contraction of the uterus during childbirth.
parathormone (PTH)	Secreted by the parathyroid glands; increases blood calcium.
progesterone	Secreted by the ovaries; prepares the uterus for pregnancy.
prolactin (PRL)	Secreted by the anterior lobe of the pituitary gland; promotes milk secretion.
somatotropin (STH)	Secreted by the anterior lobe of the pituitary gland; **growth hormone.**
testosterone	Male hormone secreted by the testes.
thyroid-stimulating hormone (TSH); thyrotropin	Secreted by the anterior lobe of the pituitary gland. TSH acts on the thyroid gland to promote its functioning. ✹ **HINT**: TSH is not secreted by the thyroid gland.

18

thyroxine (T4)	Secreted by the thyroid gland; also called **tetraiodothyronine.** T4 increases metabolism in cells.
triiodothyronine (T3)	Secreted by the thyroid gland; T3 increases metabolism in cells ✱ **HINT**: The extra n in -thyronine (pronounced THĪ-rō-nēn) avoids the combination of two vowels (o and i).
vasopressin	Secreted by the posterior lobe of the pituitary gland; **antidiuretic hormone (ADH).** Vasopressin increases water reabsorption and raises blood pressure.

RELATED TERMS

catecholamines	Hormones derived from an amino acid and secreted by the adrenal medulla. Epinephrine is a catecholamine.
corticosteroids	Hormones (steroids) produced by the adrenal cortex. Examples are cortisol (raises sugar levels), aldosterone (raises salt reabsorption by kidneys), and androgens and estrogens (sex hormones).
electrolyte	Mineral salt found in the blood and tissues and necessary for proper functioning of cells; potassium, sodium, and calcium are electrolytes.
glucocorticoid	Steroid hormone secreted by the adrenal cortex; regulates glucose, fat, and protein metabolism. Cortisol raises blood sugar and is part of the stress response.
homeostasis	Tendency of an organism to maintain a constant internal environment.
hormone	Chemical, secreted by an endocrine gland, that travels through the blood to a distant organ or gland where it influences the structure or function of that organ or gland.
hypothalamus	Region of the brain lying below the thalamus and above the pituitary gland. It secretes releasing factors and hormones that affect the pituitary gland.
mineralocorticoid	Steroid hormone secreted by the adrenal cortex to regulate mineral salts (electrolytes) and water balance in the body. Aldosterone is an example.
receptor	Cellular or nuclear protein that binds to a hormone so that a response can be elicited.
sella turcica	Cavity at the base of the skull; contains the pituitary gland.
sex hormones	Steroids (androgens and estrogens) produced by the adrenal cortex to influence male and female sexual characteristics.
steroid	Complex substance related to fats (derived from a sterol, such as cholesterol), and of which many hormones are made. Examples of steroids are estrogens, androgens, glucocorticoids, and mineralocorticoids. **Ster/o** means solid; **-ol** means oil.
sympathomimetic	Pertaining to mimicking or copying the effect of the sympathetic nervous system. Adrenaline (epinephrine) is a sympathomimetic hormone (it raises blood pressure and heart rate and dilates airways).
target tissue	Cells of an organ that are affected or stimulated by specific hormones.

18

TERMINOLOGY

Write the meanings of the medical terms in the spaces provided.

COMBINING FORMS: GLANDS

COMBINING FORM	MEANING	TERMINOLOGY	MEANING
aden/o	gland	adenitis _____	
adrenal/o	adrenal gland	adrenalectomy _____	
gonad/o	sex glands (ovaries and testes)	gonadotropin _____ *Here, -tropin means to act on. Gonadotropins act on (stimulate) gonads. Examples of gonadotropins are FSH and LH, secreted by the pituitary gland.*	
		hypogonadism _____ *Deficiency of gonadotropins can produce hypogonadism.*	
pancreat/o	pancreas	pancreatectomy _____	
parathyroid/o	parathyroid gland	parathyroidectomy _____	
pituitar/o	pituitary gland; hypophysis	hypopituitarism _____ *Pituitary dwarfism (see page 776) is caused by hypopituitarism.*	
thyr/o, thyroid/o	thyroid gland	thyrotropic hormone _____ *Thyroid-stimulating hormone (TSH) is a thyrotropic hormone secreted by the pituitary gland.*	
		thyroiditis _____ *May result from bacterial or viral infection, or an autoimmune reaction. Symptoms are throat pain, swelling, tenderness, and signs of hyperthyroidism. The condition may progress to destruction of the thyroid gland and hypothyroidism. In* **Hashimoto disease,** *or* **autoimmune thyroiditis,** *antibodies trigger lymphocytes to destroy follicular cells in the thyroid gland, producing hypothyroidism.*	

COMBINING FORMS: RELATED TERMS

COMBINING FORM	MEANING	TERMINOLOGY	MEANING
andr/o	male	androgen _____ *Androgens are produced by the testes in males and by the adrenal cortex in males and females.*	
calc/o, calci/o	calcium	hypercalcemia _____	
		hypocalcemia _____	
		hypercalciuria _____	

18

COMBINING FORM	MEANING	TERMINOLOGY	MEANING
cortic/o	cortex, outer region	corticosteroid _____	
crin/o	secrete	endocrinologist _____	
dips/o	thirst	polydipsia _____ *Poly- means many or increased. Uncontrolled diabetes (mellitus or insipidus) causes increased thirst. See page 773.*	
estr/o	female	estrogenic _____	
gluc/o	sugar	glucagon _____ *In this term, -agon means to assemble or gather together. Glucagon raises blood sugar by stimulating its release from glycogen into the bloodstream.*	
glyc/o	sugar	hyperglycemia _____	
		glycemic _____ *A patient with diabetes mellitus requires glycemic control.*	
		glycogen _____ *Glycogen is animal starch that can be converted to glucose by the liver. Glucagon promotes glycogenolysis.*	
home/o	sameness	homeostasis _____ *The suffix -stasis means controlling.*	
hormon/o	hormone	hormonal _____	
kal/i	potassium	hypokalemia _____ *This condition can occur in dehydration and with excessive vomiting and diarrhea. The heart is particularly sensitive to potassium loss.*	
lact/o	milk	prolactin _____ *The suffix -in means a substance.*	
myx/o	mucus	myxedema _____ *Mucus-like material accumulates under the skin. See page 769.*	
natr/o	sodium	hyponatremia _____ *Occurs with hyposecretion of the adrenal cortex as salts and water leave the body.*	

18

Potassium and Sodium

In patients' medical charts, potassium is abbreviated as **K** and sodium is abbreviated as **Na**. As electrolytes, they are written as **K⁺** and **Na⁺**.

COMBINING FORM	MEANING	TERMINOLOGY	MEANING
phys/o	growing	hypophysectomy _____ *The hypophysis is the pituitary gland, which is so named because it grows from the undersurface (hypo-) of the brain (Figure 18-14).*	
somat/o	body	somatotropin _____ *Growth hormone.*	
ster/o	solid structure	steroid _____ *This complex, solid, ring-shaped molecule resembles a sterol (such as cholesterol); many hormones (androgens, estrogens, glucocorticoids, and mineralocorticoids) are steroids.*	
toc/o	childbirth	oxytocin _____ *Oxy- means rapid, sharp, or acute.*	
toxic/o	poison	thyrotoxicosis _____ *Condition caused by excessive thyroid gland activity and oversecretion of thyroid hormone. Signs and symptoms are sweating, weight loss, tachycardia, and nervousness.*	
ur/o	urine	antidiuretic hormone _____ *Posterior pituitary hormone that affects the kidneys and reduces water loss.*	

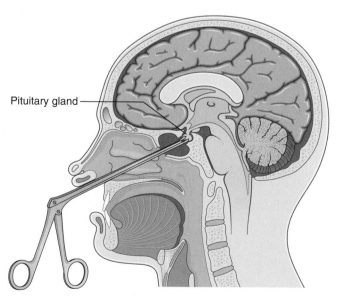

Pituitary gland

FIGURE 18-14   Hypophysectomy. Abnormal pituitary gland tissue is removed with instruments passed through the nasal passages and an opening created in the sphenoid bone (transsphenoidal hypophysectomy). The gland is removed to slow the growth of endocrine-dependent malignant tumors or to excise a pituitary tumor. Other treatments to destroy pituitary tissue include radiation therapy, radioactive implants, and cryosurgery.

18

SUFFIXES

SUFFIX	MEANING	TERMINOLOGY	MEANING
-agon	assemble, gather together	gluc<u>agon</u> _____	
-emia	blood condition	hypoglyc<u>emia</u> _____	
-in, -ine	substance	epinephr<u>ine</u> _____	
-tropin	stimulating the function of (to turn or act on)	adrenocortico<u>tropin</u> _____ *The ending -tropic is the adjective form (adrenocorticotropic hormone).*	
-uria	urine condition	glycos<u>uria</u> _____ *Sign of diabetes mellitus.*	

PREFIXES

PREFIX	MEANING	TERMINOLOGY	MEANING
eu-	good, normal	<u>eu</u>thyroid _____	
hyper-	excessive; above	<u>hyper</u>kalemia _____ *Seen in acute renal failure, massive trauma, and major burns.*	
hypo-	deficient; below; under; less than normal	<u>hypo</u>insulinism _____ *Deficient secretion of insulin by the pancreas.*	
oxy-	rapid, sharp, acid	<u>oxy</u>tocin _____	
pan-	all	<u>pan</u>hypopituitarism _____	
poly-	many or increased	<u>poly</u>uria _____ *This is a sign of uncontrolled diabetes (mellitus and insipidus).*	
tetra-	four	<u>tetra</u>iodothyronine _____ *Iod/o means iodine.*	
tri-	three	<u>tri</u>iodothyronine _____	

Oxy- Meaning Acid

In 1774, the French scientist Antoine Lavoisier named a new gas **oxygen** because he incorrectly believed that the gas was an essential part of all **acids.**

18

PATHOLOGY

THYROID GLAND

Enlargement of the thyroid gland is **goiter** (Figure 18-15A). **Endemic** (**en-** = in; **dem/o** = people) **goiter** occurs in certain regions where there is a lack of **iodine** in the diet. Goiter develops when low iodine levels lead to low T3 and T4 levels. This causes feedback to the hypothalamus and adenohypophysis, stimulating them to secrete releasing factors and TSH. TSH then promotes the thyroid gland to secrete T3 and T4, but because there is no iodine available, the only effect is to increase the size of the gland (goiter). Prevention includes increasing the supply of iodine (as iodized salt) in the diet.

Another type of goiter is **nodular** or **adenomatous goiter,** in which hyperplasia occurs as well as formation of nodules and adenomas. Some patients with nodular goiter develop hyperthyroidism with clinical signs and symptoms such as rapid pulse, tremors, nervousness, and excessive sweating. Treatment is with thyroid-blocking drugs or radioactive iodine to suppress thyroid functioning.

Hypersecretion

hyperthyroidism

Overactivity of the thyroid gland; thyrotoxicosis.

The most common form of this condition is **Graves disease** (resulting from autoimmune processes). Because metabolism is faster, the condition is marked by an increase in heart rate (with irregular beats), higher body temperature, hyperactivity, weight loss, and increased peristalsis (diarrhea occurs). In addition, **exophthalmos** (protrusion of the eyeballs, or **proptosis**) occurs as a result of swelling of tissue behind the eyeball, pushing it forward. Treatment of Graves disease includes management with antithyroid drugs to reduce the amount of thyroid hormone produced by the gland and administration of radioactive iodine, which destroys the overactive glandular tissue. Figure 18-15B shows a patient with Graves disease.

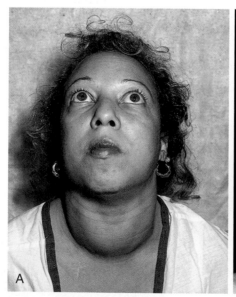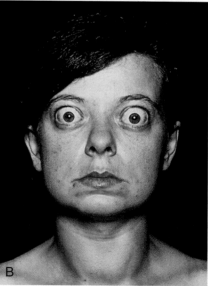

FIGURE 18-15   A, Goiter. Notice the wide neck, indicating enlargement of the thyroid gland. Goiter comes from the Latin *guttur,* meaning throat. **B, Exophthalmos in Graves disease.** Note the staring or startled expression resulting from periorbital edema (swelling of tissue around the eyeball or orbit of the eye). Exophthalmos usually persists despite treatment of Graves disease.

Hyposecretion

hypothyroidism

Underactivity of the thyroid gland.

Any of several conditions can produce hypothyroidism (thyroidectomy, thyroiditis, endemic goiter, destruction of the gland by irradiation), but all have similar physiologic effects. These include fatigue, muscular and mental sluggishness, weight gain, fluid retention, slow heart rate, low body temperature, and constipation. Two examples of hypothyroid disorders are myxedema and cretinism.

Myxedema is advanced hypothyroidism in adulthood. Atrophy of the thyroid gland occurs, and practically no hormone is produced. The skin becomes dry and puffy (edema) because of the collection of mucus-like (myx/o = mucus) material under the skin. Many patients also develop atherosclerosis because lack of thyroid hormone increases the quantity of blood lipids (fats). Recovery may be complete if thyroid hormone is given soon after symptoms appear. Figure 18-16A on page 770 shows a patient with myxedema.

In **cretinism,** extreme hypothyroidism during infancy and childhood leads to a lack of normal physical and mental growth. Skeletal growth is more inhibited than soft tissue growth, so the affected person has the appearance of an obese, short, and stocky child. Treatment consists of administration of thyroid hormone, which may be able to reverse some of the hypothyroid effects.

Neoplasms

thyroid carcinoma

Cancer of the thyroid gland.

More than one half of thyroid malignancies are slow-growing papillary carcinomas, and about one third are slow-growing follicular carcinomas. Others include rapidly growing anaplastic (widely metastatic) tumors. Radioactive iodine scans distinguish hyperfunctioning areas from hypofunctioning areas. "Hot" tumor areas (those collecting more radioactivity than surrounding tissues) usually indicate hyperthyroidism and benign growth; "cold," nonfunctional nodules can be either benign or malignant. Ultimately, fine needle aspiration, surgical biopsy, or excision is required to make the diagnosis. Total or subtotal thyroidectomy with lymph node removal is indicated for most thyroid carcinomas. Postsurgical treatment with radioactive iodine destroys remaining tissue, and high doses of exogenous thyroid hormone are given to suppress TSH, in an effort to cause regression of residual tumor dependent on TSH.

PARATHYROID GLANDS

Hypersecretion

hyperparathyroidism

Excessive production of parathormone.

Hypercalcemia occurs as calcium leaves the bones and enters the bloodstream, where it can produce damage to the kidneys and heart. Bones become decalcified with generalized loss of bone density (osteoporosis) and susceptibility to fractures and formation of cysts. Kidney stones can occur as a result of hypercalcemia and hypercalciuria. The cause is parathyroid hyperplasia or a parathyroid tumor. Treatment is resection of the overactive tissue. Medical therapy is another option for the patient who is not a surgical candidate. Bisphosphonates, such as alendronate (Fosamax), decrease bone turnover and decrease hypercalcemia.

18

Hyposecretion

hypoparathyroidism

Deficient production of parathyroid hormone.

Hypocalcemia results as calcium remains in bones and is unable to enter the bloodstream. This leads to muscle and nerve weakness with spasms of muscles, a condition called **tetany** (constant muscle contraction). Administration of calcium plus large quantities of vitamin D (to promote absorption of calcium) can control the calcium level in the bloodstream.

ADRENAL CORTEX

Hypersecretion

adrenal virilism

Excessive secretion of adrenal androgens.

Adrenal hyperplasia or more commonly adrenal adenomas or carcinomas can cause **virilization** in adult women. Signs and symptoms include amenorrhea, **hirsutism** (excessive hair on the face and body), acne, and deepening of the voice. Drug therapy to suppress androgen production and adrenalectomy are possible treatments.

Cushing syndrome

Group of signs and symptoms produced by excess cortisol from the adrenal cortex.

A number of signs and symptoms occur as a result of increased cortisol secretion, including obesity, moon-like fullness of the face, excess deposition of fat in the thoracic region of the back (so-called buffalo hump), hyperglycemia, hypernatremia, hypokalemia, osteoporosis, virilization, and hypertension. The cause may be excess ACTH secretion or tumor of the adrenal cortex. Tumors and disseminated cancers can be associated with ectopic secretion of hormone, such as ectopic ACTH produced by nonendocrine neoplasms (lung and thyroid tumors). Figure 18-16B shows a woman with Cushing syndrome. See **In Person: My Cushing's Journey**, page 783.

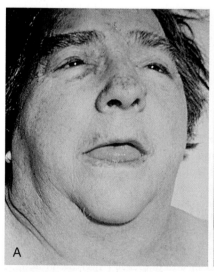
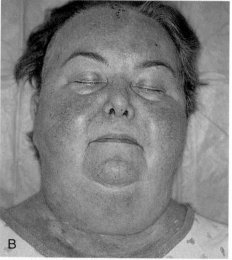

FIGURE 18-16   A, Myxedema. Note the dull, puffy, yellowed skin; coarse, sparse hair; prominent tongue. **B, Cushing syndrome.** Elevated plasma levels of cortisol (steroids) produce obesity, rounded facial appearance (moon-face), thin skin that bruises easily, and muscle weakness. *(A, Courtesy Paul W. Ladenson, MD, Johns Hopkins University and Hospital, Baltimore, Maryland.)*

Cushing Disease

Cushing disease is one cause of Cushing syndrome. In Cushing disease, a benign tumor of the pituitary gland (pituitary adenoma) increases ACTH secretion, stimulating the adrenal cortex to produce excess cortisol. The cure for Cushing disease is removal of the pituitary adenoma. Dr. Harvey Cushing described the condition in 1932.

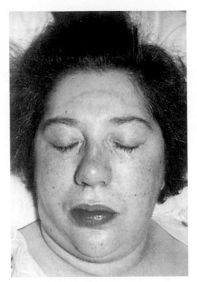

FIGURE 18-17   Addison disease. Notice the darker skin discoloration, especially evident on the face.

In clinical practice, most cases of Cushing syndrome result from chronic use of cortisone-like drugs, such as steroids. Examples are the cases in young athletes seeking to improve their performance and in patients treated for autoimmune disorders, asthma, kidney, and skin conditions. Steroids (prednisone is an example) are never discontinued abruptly because the adrenal cortex and pituitary gland (ACTH producer) need time to "restart" after long periods of prescribed cortisol use (the adrenal gland stops producing cortisol when cortisol is given as therapy).

Hyposecretion

Addison disease

Hypofunctioning of the adrenal cortex.

The adrenal cortex is essential to life. When aldosterone and cortisol blood levels are low, the patient experiences generalized malaise, weakness, muscle atrophy, and severe loss of fluids and electrolytes (with hypoglycemia, low blood pressure, and hyponatremia). An insufficient supply of cortisol signals the pituitary to secrete more ACTH, which increases pigmentation of scars, skin folds, and breast nipples (hyperpigmentation) (Figure 18-17).

Primary insufficiency is believed to be due to autoimmune adrenalitis. Treatment consists of daily cortisone administration and intake of salts or administration of a synthetic form of aldosterone.

ADRENAL MEDULLA

Hypersecretion

pheochromocytoma

Benign tumor of the adrenal medulla; tumor cells stain a dark or dusky (phe/o) color (chrom/o).

The tumor cells produce excess secretion of epinephrine and norepinephrine. Signs and symptoms are hypertension, tachycardia, palpitations, severe headaches, sweating, flushing of the face, and muscle spasms. Surgery to remove the tumor and administration of antihypertensive drugs are possible treatments.

PANCREAS

Hypersecretion

hyperinsulinism

Excess secretion of insulin causing hypoglycemia.

The cause is an overdose of insulin. Hypoglycemia occurs as insulin draws sugar out of the bloodstream. Fainting spells, convulsions, and loss of consciousness are common because a minimal level of blood sugar is necessary for proper mental functioning.

Hyposecretion

diabetes mellitus (DM)

Lack of insulin secretion or resistance of insulin in promoting sugar, starch, and fat metabolism in cells.

In diabetes mellitus (mellitus means sweet or sugary), insulin insufficiency or ineffectiveness prevents sugar from leaving the blood and entering the body cells, where it is used to produce energy. There are two types of diabetes mellitus.

Type 1 diabetes is an **autoimmune disease.** Autoantibodies against normal pancreatic islet cells are present. Onset is usually in early childhood but can occur in adulthood, and the etiology involves des truction of the beta islet cells, producing complete deficiency of insulin in the body. Patients usually are thin and require frequent injections of insulin to maintain a normal level of glucose in the blood. Type 1 requires patients to monitor their blood glucose levels several times a day using a glucometer. To test sugar levels with this device, the user pricks a finger to draw blood. At a minimum, patients test before each meal and at bedtime, but many test up to 12 times a day. Patients must continually (every day) balance insulin levels with food and exercise (see *In Person: Living with Diabetes*, pages 781-782). In addition to injecting insulin into the body (buttocks, thighs, abdomen and arms), it also is possible to administer insulin through a portable pump, which infuses the drug continuously through a indwelling needle under the skin (Figure 18-18).

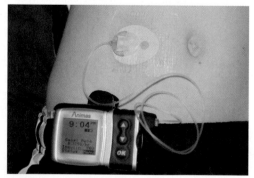

FIGURE 18-18   Insulin pump. This device can be programmed to deliver doses of insulin according to varying body needs. **Basal insulin** is delivered continuously over 24 hours and mimics the normal secretion by the pancreas. **Bolus insulin** is delivered or injected at mealtimes to "cover" a specific amount of sugar or starch ingested. *(Courtesy Ruthellen Sheldon.)*

Insulin

There are many different types of insulin. Insulins can be **rapid-acting** (peak at 30 to 60 minutes and last 3 to 5 hours), **short-acting** (peak at 1½ to 2 hours and last 6 to 8 hours), **intermediate-acting** (peak at 4 to 12 hours and last 14 to 24 hours), or **long-acting** (peak at 1 to 2 hours and last up to 24 hours). The rapid- and short-acting insulins are taken before a meal to reduce the blood sugar spike that normally occurs after eating. Intermediate- and long-acting insulins mimic the natural production of insulin by the pancreas.

Type 2 diabetes is a separate disease from type 1. Patients often are older, usually with a family history of type 2 diabetes. Obesity is very common. The islet cells are not initially destroyed, and there is a relative deficiency of insulin secretion with a resistance by target tissues to insulin. **Insulin resistance** usually develops 5 to 10 years before type 2 diabetes is diagnosed, and is associated with an increased risk of cardiovascular disease. Often, high blood pressure, high cholesterol, and central abdominal obesity are seen in people who have insulin resistance. Treatment of type 2 diabetes is with diet, weight reduction, exercise, and, if necessary, insulin or oral hypoglycemic agents. Oral hypoglycemic agents stimulate the release of insulin from the pancreas and improve the body's sensitivity to insulin.

Table 18-3 compares the clinical features, symptoms, and treatment of type 1 and type 2 diabetes.

Both type 1 and type 2 diabetes are associated with primary and secondary complications. The **primary complication** of type 1 is **hyperglycemia.** Hyperglycemia can lead to **ketoacidosis** (fats are improperly burned, leading to an accumulation of ketones and acids in the body). Ketoacidosis also can result from illness or infection, and initial symptoms may be upset stomach and vomiting. **Hypoglycemia** occurs when too much insulin is taken. **Insulin shock** is severe hypoglycemia caused by an overdose of insulin, decreased intake of food, or excessive exercise. Signs and symptoms are sweating, hunger, confusion, trembling, nervousness, and numbness. Treatment of severe hypoglycemia is with either a shot of glucagon or intravenous glucose to restore normal blood glucose levels. Convulsions, coma, and loss of consciousness can result if treatment is not given.

TABLE 18-3	COMPARISON OF TYPE 1 AND TYPE 2 DIABETES MELLITUS	
CATEGORY	**TYPE 1***	**TYPE 2†**
Clinical features	Usually occurs before age 30 Abrupt, rapid onset of symptoms Little or no insulin production Thin or normal body weight at onset Ketoacidosis often occurs	Usually occurs after age 30 Gradual onset; asymptomatic Insulin usually present Obesity in 85% of affected persons Ketoacidosis seldom occurs
Symptoms	Polyuria (glycosuria promotes loss of water) Polydipsia (dehydration causes thirst) Polyphagia (tissue breakdown causes hunger)	Polyuria sometimes seen Polydipsia sometimes seen Polyphagia sometimes seen
Treatment	Insulin	Diet (weight loss); oral hypoglycemics or insulin

*Type 1 formerly was called juvenile (juvenile-onset) diabetes.
†Type 2 formerly was called adult-onset diabetes.

18

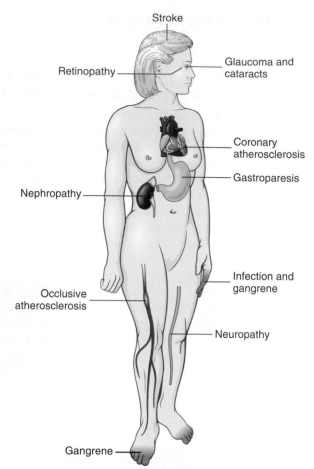

FIGURE 18-19   Secondary complications of diabetes mellitus. Complications can be avoided or minimized with optimal glycemic control.

Secondary (long-term) **complications** may appear many years after the patient develops diabetes. These include destruction of retinal blood vessels **(diabetic retinopathy)**, causing visual loss and blindness; destruction of the kidneys **(diabetic nephropathy)**, causing renal insufficiency and often requiring hemodialysis or renal transplantation; destruction of blood vessels, with **atherosclerosis** leading to stroke, heart disease, and peripherovascular ischemia (gangrene, infection, and loss of limbs); and destruction of nerves **(diabetic neuropathy)** involving pain or loss of sensation, most commonly in the extremities. Loss of gastric motility **(gastroparesis)** also occurs. Figure 18-19 reviews the secondary complications of diabetes mellitus.

As a result of hormonal changes during pregnancy, **gestational diabetes** can occur in women with a predisposition to diabetes during the second or third trimester of pregnancy. After delivery, blood glucose usually returns to normal. Type 2 diabetes may develop in these women later in life.

PITUITARY GLAND: ANTERIOR LOBE

Hypersecretion

acromegaly

Hypersecretion of growth hormone from the anterior pituitary after puberty, leading to enlargement of extremities.

An excess of growth hormone (GH) is produced by adenomas of the pituitary gland that occur during adulthood. This excess GH stimulates the liver to secrete a hormone (somatomedin C, or insulin-like growth factor [IGF]) that causes the clinical manifestations of acromegaly (acr/o in this term means extremities). Bones in the hands, feet, face, and jaw grow abnormally large, producing a characteristic "coarsened" facial appearance. The pituitary adenoma can be irradiated or surgically removed. Figure 18-20 shows the features of a woman with acromegaly. Measurement of blood levels of somatomedin C as GH fluctuates is a test for acromegaly.

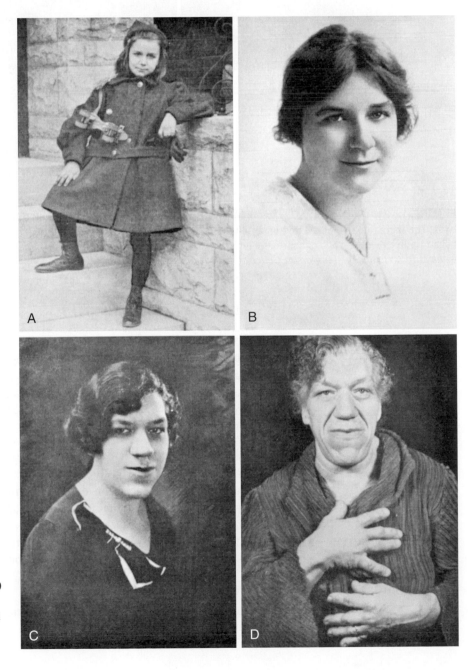

FIGURE 18-20   Progression of acromegaly. A, The patient at the age of 9 years; **B,** at age 16, with possible early features of acromegaly; **C,** at age 33, with well-established acromegaly; **D,** at age 52, with end-stage acromegaly.

18

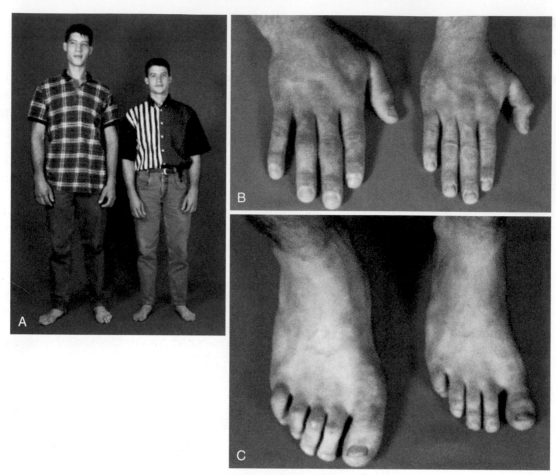

FIGURE 18-21 **Gigantism.** A 22-year-old man with gigantism due to excess growth hormone is standing next to his identical twin. The increased height (**A**) and enlarged hand (**B**) and foot (**C**) of the affected twin are apparent. Their height and features began to diverge at the age of approximately 13 years. (*A to C, Courtesy Robert F. Gagel, MD, and Ian E. McCutcheon, MD, University of Texas M.D. Anderson Cancer Center, Houston, Texas.*)

gigantism	**Hypersecretion of growth hormone from the anterior pituitary before puberty, leading to abnormal overgrowth of body tissues.**

Benign adenomas of the pituitary gland that occur before a child reaches puberty produce an excess of growth hormone. See Figure 18-21. The underlying hormonal problem caused by gigantism can be corrected by early diagnosis in childhood.

Hyposecretion

dwarfism	**Congenital hyposecretion of growth hormone; hypopituitary dwarfism.**

Children who are affected are normal mentally, but their bones remain small. Treatment consists of administration of growth hormone. Achondroplastic dwarfs differ from hypopituitary dwarfs in that they have a genetic defect in cartilage formation that limits the growth of long bones.

panhypopituitarism	**Deficiency of all pituitary hormones.**

Tumors of the sella turcica as well as arterial aneurysms may be etiologic factors, causing a failure of the pituitary to secrete hormones that stimulate major glands in the body.

PITUITARY GLAND: POSTERIOR LOBE

Hypersecretion

syndrome of inappropriate ADH (SIADH)   **Excessive secretion of antidiuretic hormone.**

Hypersecretion of ADH produces excess water retention in the body. Treatment consists of dietary water restriction. Tumor, drug reactions, and head injury are some of the possible causes.

Hyposecretion

diabetes insipidus (DI)   **Insufficient secretion of antidiuretic hormone (vasopressin).**

Deficiency of antidiuretic hormone causes the kidney tubules to fail to hold back (reabsorb) needed water and salts. Clinical manifestations include polyuria and polydipsia. Synthetic preparations of ADH are administered with nasal sprays or intramuscularly as treatment. **Insipidus** means tasteless, reflecting the condition of dilute urine, as opposed to **mellitus,** meaning sweet or like honey, reflecting the sugar content of urine in diabetes mellitus. The term diabetes comes from the Greek *diabainein*, meaning to pass through. Both diabetes insipidus and diabetes mellitus are characterized by polyuria.

Table 18-4 reviews the abnormal conditions associated with hypersecretions and hyposecretions of the endocrine glands.

TABLE 18-4	ABNORMAL CONDITIONS OF ENDOCRINE GLANDS	
ENDOCRINE GLAND	**HYPERSECRETION**	**HYPOSECRETION**
Adrenal cortex	• Adrenal virilism • Cushing syndrome	• Addison disease
Adrenal medulla	• Pheochromocytoma	
Pancreas	• Hyperinsulinism	• Diabetes mellitus
Parathyroid glands	• Hyperparathyroidism (hypercalcemia, osteoporosis, kidney stones)	• Hypoparathyroidism (tetany, hypocalcemia)
Pituitary—anterior lobe	• Acromegaly • Gigantism	• Dwarfism • Panhypopituitarism
Pituitary—posterior lobe	• Syndrome of inappropriate antidiuretic hormone	• Diabetes insipidus
Thyroid gland	• Exophthalmic goiter (Graves disease, thyrotoxicosis) • Nodular (adenomatous) goiter	• Cretinism (children) • Endemic goiter • Myxedema (adults)

18

LABORATORY TESTS

fasting plasma glucose (FPG)	**Also known as fasting blood sugar test. Measures circulating glucose level in a patient who has fasted at least 8 hours.**

This test can diagnose **diabetes** and **prediabetes** (blood glucose is higher than normal but not high enough for diagnosis of diabetes). A normal result is 99 mg/dL or belower. Prediabetes levels are 100 to 125 mg/dL, and diabetes is diagnosed with levels of 126 mg/dL and above. A casual non-fasting plasma glucose level of 200 mg/dL plus the presence of signs and symptoms such as increased urination, increased thirst, and unexplained weight loss also can diagnose diabetes. An oral **glucose tolerance test** is used to diagnose prediabetes and gestational diabetes.

The **glycosylated hemoglobin (HbA1C) test (A1C** for short), performed by measuring the percentage of red blood cells with glucose attached, monitors long-term glucose control. A high level indicates poor glucose control in diabetic patients.

serum and urine tests	**Measurement of hormones, electrolytes, glucose, and other substances in serum (blood) and urine as indicators of endocrine function.**

Serum studies include assays for growth hormone, somatomedin C (insulin-like growth factor), prolactin level, gonadotropin levels, parathyroid hormone, calcium, and cortisol. A high reading on blood glucose testing by **glucometer** in a doctor's office may be the first indication of a diabetes diagnosis (levels may be as high as 750 mg/dL, whereas normal is about 100 mg/dL).

Urine studies include dipstick testing for glucose (Clinistix, Labstix) and ketones (Acetest, Ketostix) and measurement of 17-ketosteroids (to check adrenal and gonadal function). A **urinary microalbumin assay** may detect small quantities of albumin in urine as a marker or harbinger of diabetic nephropathy.

thyroid function tests	**Measurement of T3, T4, and TSH in the bloodstream.**

CLINICAL PROCEDURES

exophthalmometry	**Measurement of eyeball protrusion (as in Graves disease) with an exophthalmometer.**
computed tomography (CT) scan	**X-ray imaging of endocrine glands in cross section and other views, to assess size and infiltration by tumor.**
magnetic resonance imaging (MRI)	**Magnetic waves produce images of the hypothalamus and pituitary gland to locate abnormalities.**
thyroid scan	**Scanner detects radioactivity and visualizes the thyroid gland.**

Administration of radioactivity is either intravenous (with radioactive technetium) or oral (with radioactive iodine). The latter is called **RAIU (radioactive iodine uptake scan)**. Thyroid function is assessed; nodules and tumors can be evaluated.

ultrasound examination	**Sound waves show images of endocrine organs.**

Thyroid ultrasound is the best method to evaluate thyroid structures and abnormalities (nodules).

18

ABBREVIATIONS

A1C	blood test that measures glycosylated hemoglobin (HbA1C) to assess glucose control
ACTH	adrenocorticotropic hormone
ADH	antidiuretic hormone— vasopressin
Ca^{++}	calcium, an important electrolyte
CGMS	continuous glucose monitoring system—senses and records blood glucose levels continuously
DI	diabetes insipidus
DKA	diabetic ketoacidosis
DM	diabetes mellitus
FBG	fasting blood glucose
FBS	fasting blood sugar
FSH	follicle-stimulating hormone
GH	growth hormone
GTT	glucose tolerance test—measures ability to respond to a glucose load; a test for diabetes
HbA1C (test)	test for the presence of glucose attached to hemoglobin (glycosylated hemoglobin)—a high level indicates poor glucose control in diabetic patients; also called A1C
hCG or HCG	human chorionic gonadotropin

IGF	insulin-like growth factor
K$^+$	potassium—an important electrolyte
LH	luteinizing hormone
MDI	multiple daily injection—for delivery of either basal or bolus insulin; a diabetes management regimen
Na$^+$	sodium—an important electrolyte
OT, OXT	oxytocin
PRL	prolactin
PTH	parathyroid hormone (parathormone)
RAI	radioactive iodine—treatment for Graves disease
RIA	radioimmunoassay—measures hormone levels in plasma
RAIU	radioactive iodine uptake (imaging test or scan)
SIADH	syndrome of inappropriate antidiuretic hormone (secretion)
SMBG	self-monitoring of blood glucose
STH	somatotropin—growth hormone
T3	triiodothyronine
T4	thyroxine—tetraiodothyronine
TFT	thyroid function test
TSH	thyroid-stimulating hormone— secreted by the anterior pituitary gland

18

PRACTICAL APPLICATIONS

The following table lists endocrine medicines and how they are used. Answers are found on page 791.

ENDOCRINE MEDICINES (brand names are in parentheses)

Antidiabetic Medicines

• insulin	Injected synthetic hormone; lowers blood sugar; comes in short-acting and long-acting forms; used in type 1 and type 2 diabetes
• metformin (Glucophage)	Oral hypoglycemic medication that reduces glucose production by the liver and increases the body's sensitivity to insulin; used in type 2 diabetes

• sulfonylureas
  glipizide (Glucotrol)
  glyburide (Diabeta or Micronase)
	Oral hypoglycemic medications that stimulate pancreatic beta cells to produce insulin; used in type 2 diabetes

Thyroid Medicines

• levothyroxine (Synthroid, Levoxyl)	Oral synthetic thyroid hormone (T4); used in hypothyroidism
• liothyronine (Cytomel)	Oral synthetic thyroid hormone (T3); used in hypothyroidism
• thyroid ISP (Armour thyroid)	Desiccated thyroid extract (combination of T3 and T4); used in hypothyroidism
• methimazole (Tapazole)	Inhibits thyroid hormone production; used in Graves hyperthyroidism
• prophylthiouracil (PTU)	Inhibits thyroid hormone production; used in Graves hyperthyroidism
• beta blockers (atenolol, propranolol)	Reduce the symptoms of hyperthyroidism (palpitations, tachycardia, tremors)

Corticosteroids

• prednisone • hydrocortisone	Used in the treatment of hypoadrenalism

Bisphosphonates

• alendronate (Fosamax) • ibandronate (Boniva)	Used to build bone strength in osteoporosis and to treat hyperparathyroidism

Diabetes Insipidus Medicine

• desmopressin (DDAVP, Stimate)	Intranasal or oral synthetic form of vasopressin (antidiuretic hormone); used to treat diabetes insipidus

QUESTIONS:

1. Which endocrine medicine treats hypothyroidism?
   a. Prednisone
   b. Prophylthiouracil
   c. Liothyronine

2. Which endocrine medicine treats type 2 diabetes?
   a. Desmopressin
   b. Metformin
   c. Hydrocortisone

3. Which endocrine medicine treats osteoporosis?
   a. Alendronate
   b. Beta blockers
   c. Insulin

18

IN PERSON: LIVING WITH DIABETES

This first-person account was written by the mother of a 12-year-old boy who was diagnosed with diabetes at age 8.

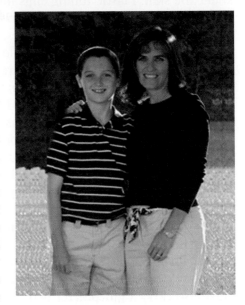

On school days, I wake up Jake at 6:30 AM. He tests his blood sugar by pricking his finger until it bleeds and sticking a test strip into the drop of blood. Then he inserts the strip into a small handheld glucometer and waits 3 to 5 seconds for a reading of his blood sugar. If this is 120 mg/dL or higher, he gives himself insulin 10 to 15 minutes before breakfast. I calculate how many carbohydrates (by reading labels and measuring food quantities precisely) he will have in his breakfast so that he can bolus [give himself enough insulin to cover the food he will eat] correctly. He has an insulin pump, so he types in the amount of carbohydrates he will eat plus his current blood sugar reading. The pump calculates how much insulin he needs to cover the carbs and any extra insulin he may need to bring down a high blood sugar. After he boluses he waits 15 minutes to eat breakfast. If his blood sugar is less than 120 mg/dL he will not bolus until he starts eating, because if the insulin acts too rapidly his blood sugar can drop too low.

As I cook his breakfast, I count carbs exactly—3 eggs (he needs protein to keep his blood sugar stable throughout the morning), 15 carbs of fruit (15 grapes, ½ banana, ½ small apple, or 1½ clementines), one 8-oz cup of low-carb juice, and 3 waffles.

I then count carbs for his lunch and place an index card in his lunch bag to show the nurse before his lunchtime bolus. At school, he visits the nurse if he feels high or low, and at lunch as well . . ... I worry about his exposure to all the sick kids at school when he visits the nurse. At school, if his blood sugar is high, he drinks water and tests his urine for ketones to make sure he does not have ketonuria, which may indicate ketoacidosis. If it is positive for ketones, he is sent home from school (fortunately, this has never happened).

At lunch, he leaves class early to test his blood sugar and does the same calculations as at breakfast. He waits for the nurse to manually compute the amount of insulin he needs to make sure that it matches the calculation of the pump. Then he boluses and goes to lunch. If his blood sugar is less than 70, he can't go to lunch with his friends. He eats or drinks some fast-acting sugar (Skittles, Smarties, or Sprite) and waits for his blood sugar to rise to an acceptable range.

We plan ahead for all field trips and food snacks that are brought into the classroom. If Jake is playing sports, he times his meals with the start of the activity so his blood sugar is around 150. He disconnects his pump during sports. Jake is an avid soccer player. At halftime he tests his blood sugar. If it is low, he needs to eat. If it is high, he needs to reconnect his pump and get more insulin. After sports, his blood sugar usually spikes because of an adrenaline [epinephrine] rush and then crashes down 3 to 10 hours later. This is unpredictable and never consistent, so it takes guesswork to keep him in range after a sports game or practice.

During the night, his dad and I set alarms to wake up every few hours to test him. If his blood sugar is high while he sleeps, we use his pump to give him a correction. If it is low, we wake him and have him drink Sprite or eat Smarties. Sometimes we check him four or five times during the night. Even if his numbers are stable, it's not a guarantee that he won't drop suddenly and have a seizure (this happened once after we had tested him at 11 PM and 2 AM and he was steady). He never complains about all the interruptions to his sleep and does a great job of falling right back to sleep when awakened.

18

Every 2 days he changes his insertion site for the insulin pump. He can't do this alone. The pump is connected to his body with a small cannula [tube]. It is inserted manually via a needle into his hip region. The needle is then removed and the tiny Teflon cannula remains in his body, delivering fast-acting insulin under the skin. Plastic tubing clips into the cannula and then attaches to the side of his pump. He clips his pump to his waistband or places it in his pocket. When he bathes, he disconnects from his pump, and when he sleeps, he places it on the mattress next to his body.

His body naturally rejects the Teflon cannula, so after 2 days his pump site must be changed. We realize this because his blood sugar numbers start rising for no apparent reason. Typically, we will change out the pump site and notice that it is red and sometimes the cannula tip is bent. Although changing the pump site is time-consuming and expensive, a bad site means that not enough insulin is getting into his body, which can quickly spiral into stomach pains, ketonuria, and ketoacidosis (DKA [diabetic ketoacidosis]).

Jake has just started to wear a continuous glucose monitoring system (CGMS). This has a small sensor that is inserted into his arm to measure blood sugar in his interstitial fluid every minute. It is new technology that will actually beep at night if his blood sugar is dropping. Jake doesn't like the system because it is painful to insert and is cumbersome to carry. Plus, it doesn't replace fingersticks for blood sugar readings. It is also difficult to calibrate his CGMS, so the readings are not 100% reliable. This is still very new technology; we are very hopeful that future generations will be more reliable!

In general, Jake's diabetes doesn't disrupt his life other than the nighttime checks, wearing an insulin pump, and paying attention to how many carbs he eats. We encourage him to make good nutritional choices (not always easy for a kid) and to limit certain foods (doughnuts, Slurpees, candy) for special occasions. He must also carry a glucometer with him at all times and a sugar to take when his blood glucose is low.

Having a child with diabetes forces me to carefully plan the preparation and timing of meals. I always have certain foods and medical supplies in the house and I carry snacks and sugar sources wherever I go. I am

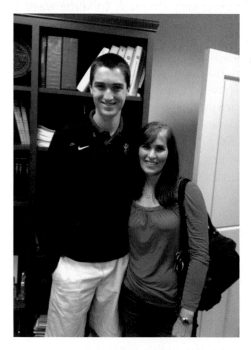

18

always available to Jake and to the school nurse. I don't always have a good night's sleep. I think I would sleep better if I were not so driven to keep his blood sugar in a healthy range. Right now, my body has adjusted to this new sleep pattern and I'm happy to wake up for him. I try to be at all his sports events to help him manage his blood sugars properly before, during, and after games. He can't go to a friend's house for a sleepover and he cannot attend overnight camp. His dad or I must always be in town. Keeping Jake's blood sugar in tight control hopefully means that he will avoid many of the complications frequently encountered later in life by people with type 1 diabetes.

Update 2015: Jake is now 18 and attending college. Throughout high school, Jake took over all diabetes management tasks and managed his diabetes 100 percent independently before his graduation. Moving out of state to college, Jake has had to learn how cafeteria foods, late nights, and new social situations affect his blood sugars. Jake is also learning how to manage ordering and maintaining a vast number of diabetes supplies and prescriptions in his dorm room. Jake will also be transitioning from his pediatric endocrinologist to an adult endocrinologist this year.

Ruthellen Sheldon and her son, Jake, now 18 years old.

IN PERSON: MY CUSHING'S JOURNEY

This first-person account was written by a young woman about her experience with Cushing syndrome.

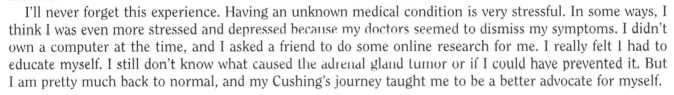

I've always been a bit of a "skinny-Minnie" and had no major health issues. But in 1997 I started having irregular periods. Not only that, but I started gaining weight—6 to 9 pounds every month. I knew something was wrong.

This began my year-long journey with Cushing syndrome. Initially, I saw two general practitioners, had blood work done, and was told I was fine. As I gained more weight, Cushing's symptoms became more apparent. I developed striae (purplish marks on my thighs*), a big round "moon face," and a humpback.[†] I also became extremely fatigued when performing simple tasks. At the time, however, I had no idea or clue of what was happening.

Next, I saw my gynecologist. Again, more blood work, and I was told I'm fine. This process continued on with three other doctors. I pressed on from feeling misunderstood, depressed, and utterly tired and found an endocrinologist. After 3 months of testing, he located the problem: a tumor on my right adrenal gland. A month later I had a right adrenalectomy. Thankfully, my left adrenal works great, and I don't have to take any hormone pills. I was also thrilled that the 72 pounds I gained over the year melted away in a few months.

I'll never forget this experience. Having an unknown medical condition is very stressful. In some ways, I think I was even more stressed and depressed because my doctors seemed to dismiss my symptoms. I didn't own a computer at the time, and I asked a friend to do some online research for me. I really felt I had to educate myself. I still don't know what caused the adrenal gland tumor or if I could have prevented it. But I am pretty much back to normal, and my Cushing's journey taught me to be a better advocate for myself.

Tanzie Johnson is a professional photographer living in New York City.

---

*The weight gain in Cushing syndrome stretches the skin, which becomes thin and weakened, allowing small hemorrhages to occur in the thinned-out tissue.

[†]Fat pads accumulate along the collarbone and on the back of the neck ("buffalo hump").

Note: The diagnosis of Cushing syndrome can take months to years, because its symptoms can be confused with those of many other conditions.

18

? EXERCISES

Remember to check your answers carefully with the Answers to Exercises, page 790.

A **Match the endocrine gland with its location.**

adrenal cortex   pancreas   testis
adrenal medulla   parathyroid   thyroid
ovary   pituitary (hypophysis)

1. behind the stomach _____

2. posterior side of the thyroid gland _____

3. inner section of glands above each kidney _____

4. in the scrotal sac _____

5. on either side of the trachea _____

6. outer section of gland above each kidney _____

7. lower abdomen of a female _____

8. below the brain in the sella turcica _____

B **Name the endocrine organs (including the appropriate lobe or region) that produce the following hormones.**

1. follicle-stimulating hormone _____

2. vasopressin _____

3. aldosterone _____

4. insulin _____

5. thyroxine _____

6. cortisol _____

7. gonadotropic hormones _____

8. epinephrine _____

9. oxytocin _____

10. prolactin _____

11. growth hormone _____

12. glucagon _____

13. adrenocorticotropic hormone _____

14. estradiol _____

15. progesterone _____

16. testosterone _____

17. thyroid-stimulating hormone _____

18

C Spell out the following abbreviations for hormones.

1. ADH _____

2. ACTH _____

3. LH _____

4. FSH _____

5. TSH _____

6. PTH _____

7. GH _____

8. PRL _____

9. T4 _____

10. T3 _____

11. OT _____

12. STH _____

D Match the hormones with their actions.

ACTH	epinephrine	parathyroid hormone
ADH	estradiol	testosterone
aldosterone	insulin	thyroxine
cortisol		

1. sympathomimetic; raises heart rate and blood pressure _____

2. promotes growth and maintenance of male sex characteristics _____

3. stimulates water reabsorption by kidney tubules; decreases urine output

   _____

4. increases metabolism in body cells _____

5. raises blood calcium _____

6. increases reabsorption of sodium by kidney tubules _____

7. stimulates secretion of hormones from the adrenal cortex _____

8. increases blood sugar _____

9. helps transport glucose to cells; decreases blood sugar _____

10. develops and maintains female sex characteristics _____

18

E Indicate whether the following conditions are related to hypersecretion or hyposecretion. Also, select from the following the endocrine glands and hormones involved in each disease.

Glands		Hormones	
adenohypophysis	pancreas	ADH	GH
adrenal cortex	parathyroid gland	aldosterone	insulin
adrenal medulla	testes	cortisol	parathyroid hormone
neurohypophysis	thyroid	epinephrine	thyroxine
ovaries			

Condition	Hypo or Hyper	Gland and Hormone
1. Cushing syndrome	_____	_____
2. tetany	_____	_____
3. Graves disease	_____	_____
4. diabetes insipidus	_____	_____
5. acromegaly	_____	_____
6. myxedema	_____	_____
7. diabetes mellitus	_____	_____
8. Addison disease	_____	_____
9. gigantism	_____	_____
10. endemic goiter	_____	_____
11. cretinism	_____	_____
12. pheochromocytoma	_____	_____

F Build medical terms based on the definitions and word parts given.

1. removal of the pancreas: _____ectomy

2. condition of deficiency or underdevelopment of the sex organs: hypo _____

3. pertaining to producing female (characteristics): _____genic

4. removal of the pituitary gland: _____ectomy

5. deficiency of calcium in the blood: hypo _____

6. excessive sugar in the blood: _____emia

7. inflammation of the thyroid gland: _____itis

8. specialist in the study of hormone disorders: _____ist

G Give the meanings of the following conditions.

1. hyponatremia _____

2. polydipsia _____

3. hyperkalemia _____

4. hypercalcemia _____

5. hypoglycemia _____

6. glycosuria _____

7. euthyroid _____

8. hyperthyroidism _____

9. tetany _____

10. ketoacidosis _____

H The following hormones are all produced by the anterior lobe of the pituitary gland (note that they all have the same suffix, -tropin). Name the target tissue they act on or stimulate in the body.

1. gonadotropins: _____

2. somatotropin: _____

3. thyrotropin: _____

4. adrenocorticotropin: _____

I Give the meanings of the following medical terms.

1. steroids _____

2. catecholamines _____

3. adenohypophysis _____

4. tetany _____

5. exophthalmos _____

6. mineralocorticoids _____

7. homeostasis _____

8. sympathomimetic _____

9. glucocorticoids _____

10. epinephrine _____

18

11. glycogen _____

12. androgen _____

13. corticosteroid _____

14. oxytocin _____

15. tetraiodothyronine _____

16. adrenal virilism _____

17. thyroid carcinoma _____

18. hirsutism _____

19. acromegaly _____

20. estradiol _____

J Give the meanings of the following terms related to diabetes mellitus.

1. type 1 _____

2. diabetic neuropathy _____

3. ketoacidosis _____

4. hypoglycemia _____

5. type 2 _____

6. diabetic retinopathy _____

7. diabetic coma _____

8. diabetic nephropathy _____

9. atherosclerosis _____

10. hyperglycemia _____

11. gastroparesis _____

12. insulin shock _____

K Explain the following laboratory tests or clinical procedures related to the endocrine system.

1. thyroid scan _____

2. fasting plasma glucose _____

3. exophthalmometry _____

4. thyroid function test _____

L **Circle the boldface terms that best complete the meaning of the sentences.**

1. Phyllis was diagnosed with Graves disease when her husband noticed her (**panhypopituitarism, hirsutism, exophthalmos**). Her eyes seemed to be bulging out of their sockets.

2. Helen had a primary brain tumor called a (**pituitary, thyroid, adrenal**) adenoma. Her entire endocrine system was disrupted, and her physician recommended surgery and radiation therapy to help relieve her symptoms.

3. Bessie's facial features gradually became "rough" in her late thirties and forties. By the time she was 50, her adult children noticed her very large hands and recommended that she see an endocrinologist, who diagnosed her chronically progressive condition as (**hyperinsulism, gigantism, acromegaly**).

4. Bobby was brought into the emergency department because he was found passed out in the kitchen. He had not taken his usual dose of insulin and had developed (**Cushing disease, hyperparathyroidism, diabetic ketoacidosis**).

5. Because her 1-hour test of blood sugar was slightly abnormal, Selma's obstetrician ordered a (**glucose tolerance test, thyroid function test, Pap smear**) to rule out gestational (**hyperthyroidism, chlamydial infection, diabetes**).

6. Bill noticed that he was passing his urine more frequently, a condition known as (**polyphagia, polyuria, hyperglycemia**), and was experiencing increased thirst, manifested as (**polydipsia, hypernatremia, polyphagia**). His wife urged him to see a physician, who performed a (**serum calcium test, urinalysis, serum sodium test**) that revealed inappropriately dilute (**blood, sweat, urine**). Measurement of the hormone (**PTH, ADH, STH**) in his blood showed low levels. His diagnosis was (**DI, DM, SIADH**). Treatment with (**oxytocin, cortisol, vasopressin**) delivered by nasal spray was prescribed, and his condition improved.

7. Mary noticed that she had gained weight recently and that her face had a moon-like fullness with new heavy hair growth. Her blood pressure was high at her doctor's appointment. Blood and urine tests showed high levels of blood sugar and (**cortisol, vasopressin, thyroid hormone**). Her diagnostic workup included a/an (**CT scan of the abdomen, thyroid ultrasound, thyroid scan**), which revealed a tumor in the (**pancreas, thyroid gland, adrenal gland**). Her doctor made the diagnosis of (**hyperthyroidism, Cushing syndrome, Addison disease**).

8. Jack had several fractures of ribs and vertebrae in a skiing accident. X-ray images of his bones revealed a generalized decrease in bone density, a condition known as (**osteoporosis, tetany, acromegaly**). A blood test showed high serum (**sodium, calcium, growth hormone**) and high levels of (**mineralocorticoids, somatotropin, parathyroid hormone**). An ultrasound scan of the neck revealed a (**thymus, parathyroid, thyroid**) adenoma, which was removed surgically. His bone disease and other abnormalities were all related to (**hypoparathyroidism, hyperparathyroidism, hypothyroidism**).

18

ANSWERS TO EXERCISES

A

1. pancreas
2. parathyroid
3. adrenal medulla
4. testis
5. thyroid gland
6. adrenal cortex
7. ovary
8. pituitary (hypophysis)

B

1. anterior pituitary gland (adenohypophysis)
2. posterior pituitary gland (neurohypophysis)
3. adrenal cortex
4. beta islet cells of the pancreas
5. thyroid gland
6. adrenal cortex
7. anterior pituitary gland; these hormones are FSH and LH
8. adrenal medulla
9. posterior pituitary gland
10. anterior pituitary gland
11. anterior pituitary gland
12. alpha islet cells of the pancreas
13. anterior pituitary gland
14. ovaries
15. ovaries
16. testes
17. anterior pituitary gland

C

1. antidiuretic hormone
2. adrenocorticotropic hormone
3. luteinizing hormone
4. follicle-stimulating hormone
5. thyroid-stimulating hormone
6. parathyroid hormone
7. growth hormone
8. prolactin
9. thyroxine; tetraiodothyronine
10. triiodothyronine
11. oxytocin
12. somatotropin (growth hormone)

D

1. epinephrine
2. testosterone
3. ADH
4. thyroxine
5. parathyroid hormone
6. aldosterone
7. ACTH
8. cortisol
9. insulin
10. estradiol

E

1. hypersecretion; adrenal cortex; cortisol
2. hyposecretion; parathyroid gland; parathyroid hormone
3. hypersecretion; thyroid gland; thyroxine
4. hyposecretion; neurohypophysis; ADH
5. hypersecretion; adenohypophysis; GH
6. hyposecretion; thyroid gland; thyroxine
7. hyposecretion; pancreas; insulin
8. hyposecretion; adrenal cortex; aldosterone and cortisol
9. hypersecretion; adenohypophysis; GH
10. hyposecretion; thyroid gland; thyroxine
11. hyposecretion; thyroid gland; thyroxine
12. hypersecretion; adrenal medulla; epinephrine

F

1. pancreatectomy
2. hypogonadism
3. estrogenic
4. hypophysectomy
5. hypocalcemia
6. hyperglycemia
7. thyroiditis
8. endocrinologist

G

1. deficient sodium in the blood
2. condition of excessive thirst
3. excessive potassium in the blood
4. excessive calcium in the blood
5. deficient sugar in the blood
6. condition of sugar in the urine
7. normal thyroid function
8. condition of increased secretion from the thyroid gland
9. constant muscle contraction (result of hypoparathyroidism)
10. condition of excessive ketones (acids) in the blood as a result of diabetes mellitus

H

1. the male and female sex organs (ovaries and testes); examples of gonadotropins are FSH and LH
2. bones; another name for somatotropin is growth hormone
3. thyroid gland; another name for thyrotropin is thyroid-stimulating hormone (TSH)
4. adrenal cortex; another name for adrenocorticotropin is adrenocorticotropic hormone (ACTH)

18

I

1. complex substances derived from cholesterol; hormones from the adrenal cortex and sex hormonesare steroids
2. complex substances derived from an amino acid; epinephrine (adrenaline) and norepinephrine (noradrenaline) are examples
3. anterior lobe of the pituitary gland
4. continuous contractions of muscles associated with low levels of parathyroid hormone
5. eyeballs that bulge outward; associated with hyperthyroidism
6. steroid hormones from the adrenal cortex (outer region of the adrenal gland) that influence salt (minerals such as sodium and potassium) metabolism

7. tendency of an organism to maintain a constant internal environment
8. substance that mimics the action of the sympathetic nerves; epinephrine (adrenaline) is an example
9. steroid hormones from the adrenal cortex that influence sugar metabolism in the body
10. catecholamine hormone from the adrenal medulla; adrenaline
11. animal starch; storage form of glucose
12. male hormone; testosterone is an example
13. hormone secreted by the adrenal cortex; cortisol is an example

14. hormone from the posterior lobe of the pituitary that stimulates contraction of the uterus during labor
15. major hormone from the thyroid gland; thyroxine (contains four iodine atoms)
16. abnormal secretion of androgens from the adrenal cortex produces masculine characteristics in a female
17. cancerous tumor of the thyroid gland
18. excessive hair on the body (result of excessive secretion of androgens)
19. enlargement of extremities (excessive secretion of growth hormone after puberty)
20. female hormone; an estrogen

J

1. destruction of the beta cells (islets of Langerhans); insulin is not produced
2. destruction of nerves as a secondary complication of diabetes mellitus
3. abnormal condition of high levels of ketones (acids) in the blood as a result of improper burning of fats; fats are burned because the cells do not have sugar available as a result of lack of insulin or inability of insulin to act

4. too little sugar in the blood; this can occur if too much insulin is taken by a diabetic patient
5. insulin deficiency and resistance by target tissue to the action of insulin
6. destruction of blood vessels in the retina as a secondary complication of diabetes mellitus
7. unconsciousness caused by high levels of sugar in the blood; water leaves cells to balance the large amounts of sugar in the blood, leading to cellular dehydration

8. destruction of the kidneys as a secondary complication of diabetes mellitus
9. collection of fatty plaque in arteries
10. high level of sugar in the blood; insulin is unavailable or unable to transport sugar from the blood into cells
11. decreased gastric motility (-paresis means slight paralysis); secondary complication of diabetes
12. hypoglycemic shock caused by an overdose of insulin, decreased intake of food, or excessive exercise

K

1. Radioactive compound is given, and the thyroid gland is imaged using a scanning device.

2. Measurement of blood sugar levels in a fasting patient (at least 4 hours) and after intervals of 30 minutes and 1, 2, and 3 hours after ingestion of glucose.

3. Measurement of eyeball protrusion (symptom of Graves disease)
4. Measurement of T3, T4, and TSH in the bloodstream

L

1. exophthalmos
2. pituitary
3. acromegaly
4. diabetic ketoacidosis
5. glucose tolerance test; diabetes

6. polyuria; polydipsia; urinalysis; urine; ADH; DI; vasopressin
7. cortisol; CT scan of the abdomen; adrenal glands; Cushing syndrome

8. osteoporosis; calcium; parathyroid hormone; parathyroid; hyperparathyroidism

Answers to Practical Applications

Endocrine Medicines
1. c
2. b
3. a

18

PRONUNCIATION OF TERMS

To test your understanding of the terminology in this chapter, write the meaning of each term in the space provided. In addition, you may wish to cover the terms and write them by looking at your definitions. Make sure your spelling is correct. The page number after each term indicates where it is defined or used in the book, so you can easily check your responses. You will find complete definitions for all of these terms and their audio pronunciations on the Evolve website.

Pronunciation Guide

ā as in āpe	ă as in ăpple
ē as in ēven	ĕ as in ĕvery
ī as in īce	ĭ as in ĭnterest
ō as in ōpen	ŏ as in pŏt
ū as in ūnit	ŭ as in ŭnder

Vocabulary and Terminology

TERM	PRONUNCIATION	MEANING
adenitis (764)	ăd-ĕ-NĪ-tĭs	
adenohypophysis (761)	ăd-ĕ-nō-hī-PŎF-ĭ-sĭs	
adrenal cortex (761)	ă-DRĒ-năl KŎR-tĕks	
adrenalectomy (764)	ă-drē-năl-ĔK-tō-mē	
adrenaline (761)	ă-DRĔN-ă-lĭn	
adrenal medulla (761)	ă-DRĒ-năl mĕ-DŪ-lăh	
adrenocorticotropic hormone (761)	ă-drē-nō-kŏr-tĭ-kō-TRŌP-ĭk HŎR-mōn	
adrenocorticotropin (767)	ă-drē-nō-kŏr-tĭ-kō-TRŌ-pĭn	
aldosterone (762)	ăl-DŎS-tĕ-rōn	
androgen (762)	ĂN-drō-jĕn	
antidiuretic hormone (762)	ăn-tĭ-dī-ū-RĔT-ĭk HŎR-mōn	
calcitonin (762)	kăl-sĭ-TŌ-nĭn	
catecholamines (763)	kăt-ĕ-KŌL-ă-mēnz	
corticosteroids (763)	kŏr-tĭ-kō-STĔ-roydz	
cortisol (762)	KŎR-tĭ-sōl	
electrolyte (763)	ĕ-LĔK-trō-līt	
endocrinologist (765)	ĕn-dō-krĭ-NŎL-ō-jĭst	
epinephrine (762)	ĕp-ĭ-NĔF-rĭn	
estradiol (762)	ĕs-tră-DĪ-ŏl	
estrogen (762)	ĔS-trō-jĕn	
estrogenic (765)	ĕs-trō-JĔN-ĭk	
euthyroid (767)	ū-THĪ-royd	

18

TERM	PRONUNCIATION	MEANING
follicle-stimulating hormone (762)	FŎL-ĭ-kl STĬM-ū-lā-tĭng HŎR-mōn	
glucagon (762)	GLOO-kă-gŏn	
glucocorticoid (763)	gloo-kō-KŎR-tĭ-koyd	
glycemic (765)	glī-SĒ-mĭk	
glycogen (765)	GLĪ-kō-jĕn	
glycosuria (767)	glī-kōs-Ū-rē-ă	
gonadotropin (764)	gō-năd-ō-TRŌ-pĭn	
growth hormone (762)	grōth HŎR-mōn	
homeostasis (763)	hō-mē-ō-STĀ-sĭs	
hormonal (765)	hŏr-MO-năl	
hormone (763)	HŎR-mon	
hypercalcemia (764)	hī-pĕr-kăl-SĒ-mē-ă	
hypercalciuria (764)	hī-pĕr-kăl-sē-ŪR-ē-ă	
hyperglycemia (765)	hī-pĕr-glī-SĒ-mē-ă	
hyperkalemia (767)	hī-pĕr-kā-LĒ-mē-ă	
hypocalcemia (764)	hī-pō-kăl-SĒ-mē-ă	
hypoglycemia (767)	hī-pō-glī-SĒ-mē-ă	
hypogonadism (764)	hī-pō-GŌ-năd-ĭzm	
hypoinsulinism (767)	hī-pō-ĬN-sū-lĭn-ĭzm	
hypokalemia (765)	hī-pō-kā-LĒ-mē-ă	
hyponatremia (765)	hī-pō-nā-TRĒ-mē-ă	
hypophysectomy (766)	hī-pō-fĭ-ZĔK-tō-mē	
hypophysis (761)	hī-PŎF-ĭ-sĭs	
hypopituitarism (764)	hī-pō-pĭ-TOO-ĭ-tă-rĭzm	
hypothalamus (763)	hī-pō-THĂL-ă-mŭs	
insulin (762)	ĬN-sū-lĭn	
luteinizing hormone (762)	LOO-tē-ĭn-īz-ĭng HŎR-mōn	
mineralocorticoid (763)	mĭn-ĕr-ăl-ō-KŎR-tĭ-koyd	
neurohypophysis (761)	noo-rō-hī-PŎF-ĭ-sĭs	
norepinephrine (762)	nŏr-ĕp-ĭ-NĔF-rĭn	

18

TERM	PRONUNCIATION	MEANING
ovaries (761)	ō-vă-rēz	_____
oxytocin (762)	ŏk-sĭ-TŌ-sĭn	_____
pancreas (761)	PĂN-krē-ăs	_____
pancreatectomy (764)	păn-krē-ă-TĔK-tō-mē	_____
parathormone (762)	păr-ă-THŎR-mōn	_____
parathyroidectomy (764)	păr-ă-thī-roy-DĔK-tō-mē	_____
parathyroid glands (761)	păr-ă-THĪ-royd glănz	_____
pineal gland (750)	pī-NĒ-ăl glănd	_____
pituitary gland (761)	pĭ-TOO-ĭ-tĕr-ē glănd	_____
polydipsia (765)	pŏl-ē-DĬP-sē-ă	_____
polyuria (767)	pŏl-ē-Ū-rē-ă	_____
progesterone (762)	prō-JĔS-tĕ-rōn	_____
prolactin (762)	prō-LĂK-tĭn	_____
receptor (763)	rē-SĔP-tŏr	_____
sella turcica (763)	SĔL-ă TŬR-sĭ-kă	_____
sex hormones (763)	sĕx HŎR-monz	_____
somatotropin (762)	sō-mă-tō-TRŌ-pĭn	_____
steroid (763)	STĔR-oyd	_____
sympathomimetic (763)	sĭm-pă-thō-mĭ-MĔT-ĭk	_____
target tissue (763)	TĂR-gĕt TĬS-ū	_____
testes (761)	TĔS-tēz	_____
testosterone (762)	tĕs-TŎS-tĕ-rōn	_____
tetraiodothyronine (767)	tĕ-tră-ī-ō-dō-THĪ-rō-nēn	_____
thyroid gland (761)	THĪ-royd glănd	_____
thyroiditis (764)	thī-royd-Ī-tĭs	_____
thyrotropin (762)	thī-rō-TRŌ-pĭn	_____
thyroxine (763)	thī-RŎK-sĭn	_____
triiodothyronine (763)	trī-ī-ō-dō-THĪ-rō-nēn	_____
vasopressin (763)	văz-ō-PRĔS-ĭn	_____

18

Pathology, Laboratory Tests, and Clinical Procedures

TERM	PRONUNCIATION	MEANING
acromegaly (775)	ăk-rō-MĚG-ă-lē	_____
Addison disease (771)	ĂD-ĭ-sŏn dĭ-ZĒZ	_____
adrenal virilism (770)	ă-DRĒ-năl VĬR-ĭ-lĭzm	_____
cretinism (769)	KRĒ-tĭn-ĭzm	_____
Cushing syndrome (770)	KŬSH-ĭng SĬN-drōm	_____
diabetes insipidus (777)	dī-ă-BĒ-tēz ĭn-SĬP-ĭ-dŭs	_____
diabetes mellitus (772)	dī-ă-BĒ-tēz MĚL-ĭ-tŭs	_____
dwarfism (776)	DWĂRF-ĭzm	_____
endemic goiter (768)	ĕn-DĚM-ĭk GOY-tĕr	_____
exophthalmometry (778)	ĕk-sŏf-thăl-MŎM-ĕ-trē	_____
exophthalmos (768)	ĕk-sŏf-THĂL-mōs	_____
fasting plasma glucose (778)	FĂS-tĭng PLĂS-măh GLŪ-kōs	_____
gastroparesis (774)	găs-trō-păr-Ē-sĭs	_____
gigantism (776)	JĪ-găn-tĭzm	_____
glucose tolerance test (778)	GLOO-kōs TŎL-ĕr-ăns tĕst	_____
goiter (768)	GOY-tĕr	_____
Graves disease (768)	GRĀVZ dĭ-ZĒZ	_____
hirsutism (770)	HĚR-soot-ĭzm	_____
hyperinsulinism (772)	hī-pĕr-ĬN-sū-lĭn-ĭzm	_____
hyperparathyroidism (769)	hī-pĕr-pă-ră-THĪ-royd-ĭzm	_____
hyperthyroidism (768)	hī-pĕr-THĪ-royd-ĭsm	_____
hypoparathyroidism (770)	hī-pō-pă-ră-THĪ-royd-ĭzm	_____
hypothyroidism (769)	hī-pō-THĪ-royd-ĭzm	_____
ketoacidosis (773)	kē-tō-ă-sĭ-DŌ-sĭs	_____
myxedema (769)	mĭk-sĕ-DĒ-mă	_____
nodular goiter (768)	NŎD-ū-lăr GOY-tĕr	_____
panhypopituitarism (776)	păn-hī-pō-pĭ-TOO-ĭ-tăr-ĭzm	_____
pheochromocytoma (771)	fē-ō-krō-mō-sī-TŌ-mă	_____

18

TERM	PRONUNCIATION	MEANING
syndrome of inappropriate ADH (777)	SĬN-drōm of ĭn-ă-PRŌ-prē-ĭt ADH	_____
tetany (770)	TĔT-ă-nē	_____
thyroid carcinoma (769)	THĪ-royd kăr-sĭ-NŌ-mă	_____
thyroid function tests (778)	THĪ-royd FŬNK-shŭn tests	_____
thyroid scan (778)	THĪ-royd skăn	_____
thyrotoxicosis (768)	thī-rō-tŏk-sĭ-KŌ-sĭs	_____

18

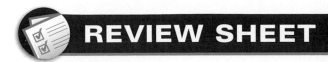

REVIEW SHEET

Write the meanings of the word parts in the spaces provided and test yourself. Check your answers with the information in the chapter or in the **Glossary (Medical Word Parts—English)** at the end of the book.

Combining Forms

COMBINING FORM	MEANING	COMBINING FORM	MEANING
aden/o		lact/o	
adrenal/o		myx/o	
andr/o		natr/o	
calc/o, calci/o		pancreat/o	
cortic/o		parathyroid/o	
crin/o		phys/o	
dips/o		pituitar/o	
estr/o		somat/o	
gluc/o		ster/o	
glyc/o		thyr/o	
gonad/o		thyroid/o	
home/o		toc/o	
hormon/o		toxic/o	
insulin/o		ur/o	
kal/i			

Suffixes

SUFFIX	MEANING	SUFFIX	MEANING
-agon		-osis	
-ectomy		-physis	
-emia		-stasis	
-genic		-tocin	
-in, -ine		-tropin	
-megaly		-uria	
-oid			

18

Prefixes

PREFIX	MEANING	PREFIX	MEANING
eu-	_____	pan-	_____
hyper-	_____	poly-	_____
hypo-	_____	tetra-	_____
oxy-	_____	tri-	_____

Fill in the following chart of pathologic conditions of endocrine glands and check your answers with Table 18-4 on p. 777.

ENDOCRINE GLAND	HYPERSECRETION	HYPOSECRETION
Adrenal cortex	_____	_____
	_____	
Adrenal medulla	_____	
Pancreas	_____	_____
Parathyroid glands	_____	_____
Pituitary—anterior lobe	_____	_____
	_____	_____
Pituitary—posterior lobe	_____	_____
Thyroid gland	_____	_____
	_____	_____
		_____

Give the abbreviations for the following.

1. test to assess glucose control _____
2. sodium; and its electrolyte _____
3. thyroxine _____
4. pregnancy hormone _____
5. potassium; and its electrolyte _____

Cancer Medicine (Oncology)

CHAPTER GOALS

- Identify medical terms that describe the growth and spread of tumors.
- Recognize terms related to the causes, diagnosis, and treatment of cancer.
- Review how tumors are classified and described by pathologists.
- Describe x-ray studies, laboratory tests, and other procedures used by physicians for determining the presence and extent of spread (staging) of tumors.
- Apply your new knowledge to understanding medical terms in their proper contexts, such as medical reports and records.

INTRODUCTION

Cancer is a disease caused by abnormal and excessive growth of cells in the body. It may arise in any tissue and appear at any time of life, although cancer occurs most frequently in older people. Cancer cells accumulate as growths called malignant tumors that compress, invade, and ultimately destroy the surrounding normal tissue. In addition to their local growth, cancerous cells spread throughout the body by way of the bloodstream or lymphatic vessels. In some patients, the spread of cancers from their site of origin to distant organs occurs early in the course of tumor growth and ultimately results in death.

Although more than one half of all patients who develop cancer are cured of their disease, about 550,000 people die of cancer each year. Lung cancers, followed by breast and colorectal cancers, are the most common causes of cancer death for women, whereas lung, colorectal, and prostate cancers are the leading causes of death due to cancer in men. This chapter explores the terminology related to this common and often fatal group of diseases.

CHARACTERISTICS OF TUMORS

Tumors (neoplasms) are new growths that arise from normal tissue. They may be either **malignant** (capable of invasion and spread to surrounding or more distant sites) or **benign** (noninvasive and not spreading to other sites). There are several differences between benign and malignant tumors. Some of these differences are:

1. Benign tumors **grow slowly,** and malignant tumor cells **multiply rapidly.**
2. Benign tumors are often **encapsulated** (contained within a fibrous capsule or cover), so that the tumor cells do not invade the surrounding tissue. Malignant tumors characteristically are **invasive** and **infiltrative,** extending into neighboring normal tissue.
3. Benign tumors are composed of organized and specialized **(differentiated)** cells that closely resemble the normal, mature tissue from which they are derived. For example,

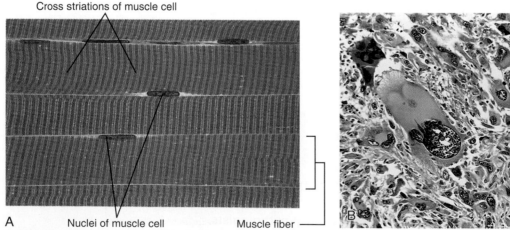
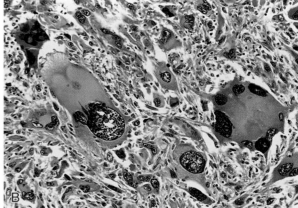

Cross striations of muscle cell

A Nuclei of muscle cell   Muscle fiber

FIGURE 19-1   A, Photomicrograph of normal skeletal muscle cells (fibers). Note the orderly arrangement and the long, narrow, threadlike shape of the cells. There are many nuclei per cell and many cross striations. **B, Anaplastic tumor cells of the skeletal muscle (rhabdomyosarcoma).** Note the variation in size and shape of the nuclei (pleomorphism; pleo = many, morph/o = shape), hyperchromatic (intensely staining) nuclei, and large tumor cells (which may possess more than one nucleus). **(B, Courtesy Trace Worrell, MD, Department of Pathology, University of Texas Southwestern Medical School, Dallas.)**

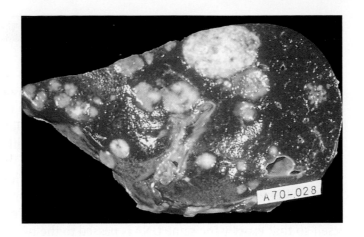

FIGURE 19-2   A liver studded with metastatic cancer.

benign tumors derived from epithelial cells that line the wall of the gastrointestinal tract look very much like their normal counterparts. Malignant tumors are composed of cancerous cells that resemble primitive cells and lack the capacity to perform mature cell functions. This characteristic of malignant tumors is called **anaplasia.** Anaplasia (ana- means backward and -plasia means growth) indicates that the cancerous cells are **dedifferentiated,** or **undifferentiated** (reverting to a less specialized state), in contrast with the normal, differentiated tissue of their origin. Anaplastic cells lack an orderly arrangement. Thus, tumor cells vary in size and shape and are piled one on top of the other in a disorganized fashion. The nuclei in these cells are large and **hyperchromatic** (stain excessively with dyes that recognize genetic material, DNA). Figure 19-1A and B shows normal skeletal muscle and anaplastic malignant muscle tumor cells.

4. Cells from benign tumors do not spread or **metastasize** to form secondary tumor masses in distant places in the body. Cells from malignant tumors, however, can detach themselves from the primary tumor site, penetrate a blood vessel or lymphatic vessel, travel through the bloodstream or lymphatic system, and establish a new tumor site at a distant tissue, such as the lung, liver, or bone marrow. The secondary growth is called a **metastasis.** Figure 19-2 shows metastatic tumors within the liver.

Figure 19-3 reviews the differences between benign and malignant tumors.

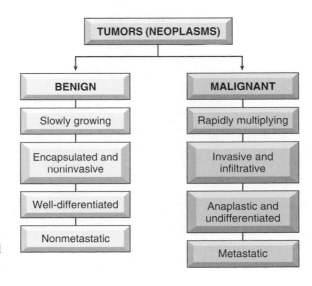

FIGURE 19-3   Differences between benign and malignant tumors.

19

CARCINOGENESIS

WHAT CAUSES CANCER?

The causes of transformation from a normal cell to a cancerous one **(carcinogenesis)** are only partly understood. What is clear is that malignant transformation results from damage to the genetic material, or **DNA (deoxyribonucleic acid),** of the cell. Strands of DNA in the cell nucleus form **chromosomes,** which become readily visible under a microscope when a cell is preparing to divide into two (daughter) cells. In order to understand what causes cancer, it is necessary to learn more about DNA and its functions in a normal cell.

DNA has two main functions in a normal cell. First, DNA controls the production of new cells (cell division). When a cell divides, the DNA material in each chromosome copies itself so that exactly the same DNA is passed to the two new daughter cells that are formed. This process of cell division is called **mitosis** (Figure 19-4A).

Second, DNA controls the production of new proteins **(protein synthesis)** in the cell. Each DNA piece, or **gene,** contains the code for making a single protein. That protein carries out an important specific function in the cell. There are 20,000 to 25,000 human protein-coding genes. Genes are composed of an arrangement of units called **nucleotides** (containing a sugar, phosphate, and a base, such as adenine, guanine, thymine, or cytosine). DNA (as a string of coded nucleotides) sends a molecular message outside the nucleus to the cytoplasm of the cell, directing the synthesis of specific proteins (such as hormones and enzymes) essential for normal cell function and growth. This message is transmitted in the following way: In the nucleus, the coded message with instructions for making a specific protein is copied from DNA onto another molecule called **RNA (ribonucleic acid).** Then RNA travels from the nucleus to the cytoplasm of the cell, carrying the coded message that directs the formation of specific proteins (Figure 19-4B).

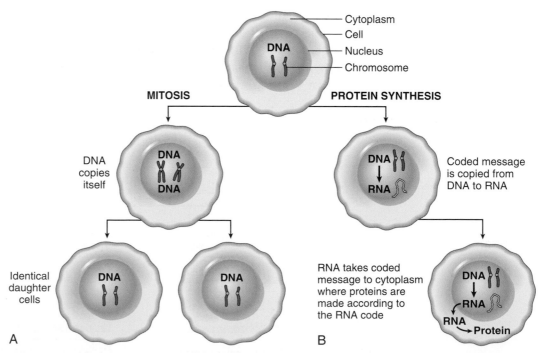

FIGURE 19-4   Two functions controlled by DNA. A, Mitosis (the process of cell division). **B, Protein synthesis** (creating new proteins for cellular growth).

When a cell becomes malignant, however, the processes of mitosis and protein synthesis are disturbed. Cancer cells reproduce almost continuously, and abnormal proteins are made. Malignant cells are **anaplastic**; that is, their DNA stops making normal codes that allow the cells to carry on the function of differentiating mature cells. Instead, new signals lead to malignant growth and spread of tumor cells.

Various kinds of damage to DNA result in malignancy. DNA damage may be caused by toxic chemicals, sunlight, tobacco smoke, and viruses. The specific damage usually involves changes in the cell's DNA codes, creating abnormal genes with changes called **mutations**. Mutations interfere with the accurate synthesis of new proteins and can be passed on to new cells during cell division.

Although most DNA changes, or mutations, lead to higher-than-normal rates of growth, some mutations found in cancer cells actually prevent the cells from dying. In recent years, scientists have recognized that in some types of cancers, the normal blueprints that direct aging or damaged cells to die are missing. Normal cells undergo spontaneous disintegration by a process known as **apoptosis,** or programmed cell death. Some cancer cells have lost elements of this program and thus can live indefinitely.

ENVIRONMENTAL AGENTS

Agents from the environment, such as chemicals, drugs, tobacco smoke, radiation, and viruses, can cause damage to DNA and thus produce cancer. These environmental agents are called **carcinogens.**

Chemical carcinogens are found in a variety of products and drugs, including **hydrocarbons**—in cigarette, cigar, and pipe smoke and automobile exhaust—insecticides, dyes, industrial chemicals, asbestos as in insulation, and hormones. Hormones such as estrogens can cause cancer by stimulating growth of cells in the lining of the uterus or in milk glands of the breast.

Radiation, whatever its source—sunlight, x-rays, radioactive substances—consists of waves of energy. This energy causes DNA damage and mutations that lead to cancer. Leukemia used to be an occupational hazard of radiologists, who were routinely exposed to x-rays. There is a high incidence of leukemia and other cancers among survivors of atomic bomb explosions, as at Hiroshima and Nagasaki. Ultraviolet radiation in sunlight can cause skin cancer, especially in persons with lightly pigmented, or fair, skin.

Some **viruses** are carcinogenic. For example, the human T cell leukemia virus (HTLV1) causes a form of leukemia in adults. Kaposi sarcoma is caused by another virus, herpesvirus type 8. Other viruses are known to cause cervical cancer (human papillomavirus or HPV) and liver cancer (hepatitis B and C viruses). See Table 19-1.

TABLE 19-1	ENVIRONMENTAL CARCINOGENS
Chemicals	• asbestos in insulation • dyes and industrial chemicals • hormones • hydrocarbons • insecticides
Radiation	• sunlight (ultraviolet rays) • x-rays • radioactive substances
Viruses	• human T cell leukemia virus (HTLV1) • human papillomavirus (HPV) • hepatitis B and C viruses

ONCOGENES

Oncogenes are pieces of normal DNA that when activated by a mutation, can convert a normal cell to a cancerous cell. Some examples of oncogenes are **ras** (colon cancer), **myc** (lymphoma), and **abl** (chronic myeloid leukemia or CML).

In chronic myeloid leukemia, the oncogene *abl* is activated when pieces from two different chromosomes switch locations. This mutation is called a **translocation.** What happens is that the oncogene *abl* on chromosome 9 moves to a new location next to a gene called *bcr* on chromosome 22, (see Figure 19-5). When **bcr** (**b**reakpoint **c**luster **r**egion) and **abl** are near each other, they cause the production of an abnormal protein that makes the leukocyte divide and causes a malignancy (chronic myeloid leukemia). The new chromosome formed from the translocation is called the **Philadelphia chromosome** (it was discovered in 1970 in Philadelphia).

HEREDITY

Cancer also may be caused by transmission from parents to offspring through defects in the DNA of the egg or sperm cells. Although most cancers result from chance mutations in body cells during a lifetime, examples of known inherited cancers are **retinoblastoma** (tumor of the retina of the eye), **adenomatous polyposis coli syndrome** (premalignant

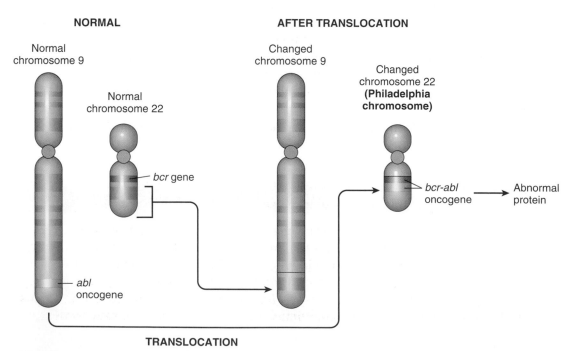

FIGURE 19-5 Oncogene translocation resulting in the Philadelphia chromosome. Notice the translocation of the *abl* oncogene from the long arm of chromosome 9 to the long arm of chromosome 22 (next to the *bcr* gene). This results in a combination *bcr-abl* oncogene, which produces an abnormal protein leading to chronic myeloid leukemia.

| TABLE 19-2 | EXAMPLES OF GENES IMPLICATED IN HEREDITARY CANCERS |

CANCER	GENE	CHROMOSOMAL LOCATION*
Breast; ovarian	BRCA1	17q21
Breast; ovarian	BRCA2	3q12-13
Li-Fraumeni syndrome (multiple cancers)	TP53	17p13
Polyposis coli syndrome	APC	5q21
Renal cell carcinoma	VHL	3p21-26
Retinoblastoma	RB1	13q14
Wilms tumor	WT1	11p13

*The first number is the chromosome; p is the short arm of the chromosome, and q is the long arm of the chromosome. The second number is the region (band) of the chromosome.

polyps that grow in the colon and rectum), and certain forms of colon, breast, and kidney cancer.

In many cases, it is believed that these tumors arise because of inherited or acquired abnormalities in certain genes called **suppressor genes.** In normal persons, these suppressor genes regulate growth, promote differentiation, and suppress oncogenes from causing cancer. Loss of a normal suppressor gene takes the brake off the process of cell division and leads to cancer. Examples of suppressor genes are the **retinoblastoma (Rb) type 1 gene (RB1)** and the **TP53** gene, which leads to brain tumors or breast cancer.

Because inherited changes can be detected by analyzing DNA in any tissue of the body, not simply cancerous cells, blood cells from family members may be tested to determine whether a person has inherited the cancer-causing gene. This is known as **genetic screening.** Affected patients may be watched carefully to detect tumors at an early stage or elect to have prophylactic removal of organs or tissue that may become cancerous. Table 19-2 lists several hereditary cancers and the name of the responsible gene. For a review of the role of environment, oncogenes and heredity in carcinogenesis, see the Evolve site for this chapter.

CLASSIFICATION OF CANCEROUS TUMORS

Almost one half of all cancer deaths are caused by malignancies that originate in lung, breast, or colon; however, in all there are more than 100 distinct types of cancer, each having a unique set of symptoms and requiring a specific type of therapy. It is possible to divide these types of cancer into three broad groups on the basis of **histogenesis**—that is, by identifying the particular type of tissue **(hist/o)** from which the tumor cells arise (**-genesis**). These major groups are **carcinomas, sarcomas,** and **mixed-tissue tumors.**

CARCINOMAS

Carcinomas, the largest group, are solid tumors that are derived from epithelial tissue that lines external and internal body surfaces, including skin, glands, and digestive, urinary, and reproductive organs. Approximately 90% of all malignancies are carcinomas.

Table 19-3 gives examples of specific carcinomas and the epithelial tissue from which they derive. Benign tumors of epithelial origin are usually designated by the term **adenoma,** which indicates that the tumor is of epithelial or glandular (**aden/o**) origin. For example, a gastric adenoma is a benign tumor of the glandular epithelial cells lining the stomach. Malignant tumors of epithelial origin are named by using the term **carcinoma** and adding the type of tissue in which the tumor occurs. Thus, a **gastric adenocarcinoma** is a cancerous tumor arising from glandular cells lining the stomach.

TABLE 19-3	CARCINOMAS AND THE EPITHELIAL TISSUES FROM WHICH THEY DERIVE
TYPE OF EPITHELIAL TISSUE	**MALIGNANT TUMOR (CARCINOMAS)**
Gastrointestinal tract	
Colon	Adeno**carcinoma** of the colon
Esophagus	Esophageal **carcinoma**
Liver	Hepatocellular **carcinoma** (hepatoma)
Stomach	Gastric adeno**carcinoma**
Glandular tissue	
Adrenal glands	**Carcinoma** of the adrenals (adrenocortical **carcinoma**)
Breast	**Carcinoma** of the breast
Pancreas	**Carcinoma** of the pancreas (pancreatic adeno**carcinoma**)
Prostate	**Carcinoma** of the prostate
Salivary glands	Adenoid cystic **carcinoma**
Thyroid	**Carcinoma** of the thyroid
Kidney and bladder	
	Renal cell **carcinoma** (hypernephroma)
	Transitional cell **carcinoma** of the bladder
Lung	
	Adeno**carcinoma** (bronchioloalveolar)
	Large cell **carcinoma**
	Small cell **carcinoma**
	Squamous cell **carcinoma** (epidermoid)
Reproductive organs	
	Adeno**carcinoma** of the uterus
	Squamous cell **carcinoma** of the penis
	Chorio**carcinoma** of the uterus or testes
	Cystadeno**carcinoma** (mucinous or serous) of the ovaries
	Seminoma and embryonal cell **carcinoma** (testes)
	Squamous cell (epidermoid) **carcinoma** of the vagina or cervix
Skin	
Basal cell layer	Basal cell **carcinoma**
Melanocyte	Malignant melanoma
Squamous cell layer	Squamous cell **carcinoma**

SARCOMAS

Sarcomas also are malignant tumors but are less common than carcinomas. They derive from connective tissues in the body, such as bone, fat, muscle, cartilage, and bone marrow and from cells of the lymphatic system. Often, the term **mesenchymal tissue** is used to describe embryonic connective tissue from which sarcomas are derived. The middle, or mesodermal, layer of the embryo gives rise to the connective tissues of the body as well as to blood and lymphatic vessels.

Table 19-4 gives examples of specific types of sarcomas and the connective tissues from which they derive. Benign tumors of connective tissue origin are named by adding the suffix **-oma** to the type of tissue in which the tumor occurs. For example, a benign tumor of bone is called an **osteoma.** Malignant tumors of connective tissue origin are frequently named using the term **sarcoma** (**sarc/o** = flesh). For example, an **osteosarcoma** is a malignant tumor of bone.

TABLE 19-4	SARCOMAS AND THE CONNECTIVE TISSUES FROM WHICH THEY DERIVE
TYPE OF CONNECTIVE TISSUE	**MALIGNANT TUMOR (SARCOMA)**
Bone	Osteosarcoma (osteogenic sarcoma) Ewing **sarcoma**
Muscle	
Smooth (visceral) muscle	Leiomyo**sarcoma**
Striated (skeletal) muscle	Rhabdomyo**sarcoma**
Cartilage	Chondro**sarcoma**
Fat	Lipo**sarcoma**
Fibrous tissue	Fibro**sarcoma**
Blood vessel tissue	Angio**sarcoma**
Blood-forming tissue	
All leukocytes	Leukemias

Lymphocytes	Lymphomas
	    Hodgkin Lymphoma
	    Non-Hodgkin lymphomas
	    1. follicular
	    2. diffuse large cell
	    3. Burkitt
	    4. anaplastic large cell

Plasma cells (bone marrow)	Multiple myeloma
Nerve tissue	
Embryonic nerve tissue	Neuroblastoma
Glial tissue	Astrocytoma (tumor of glial cells called astrocytes) Glioblastoma multiforme
Nerve cells of the gastrointestinal tract	Gastrointestinal stromal tumor (GIST)

19

TABLE 19-5	MIXED-TISSUE TUMORS
TYPE OF TISSUE	**MALIGNANT TUMOR**
Kidney	Wilms tumor (embryonal adenosarcoma)
Ovaries and testes	Teratoma (tumor composed of bone, muscle, skin, gland cells, cartilage, etc.) Germ cell tumor

In addition to the solid tumors of connective tissue origin, sarcomas include tumors arising from blood-forming tissue. **Leukemias** and **multiple myeloma** are tumors derived from bone marrow. **Lymphomas**, such as Hodgkin, Burkitt, and follicular types, are derived from immune cells of the lymphatic system. Glial cells within the brain and other cells of the nervous system give rise to malignancies such as **gliomas** and **neuroblastomas**.

MIXED-TISSUE TUMORS

Mixed-tissue tumors are derived from tissue that is capable of differentiating into both epithelial and connective tissue. These uncommon tumors are thus composed of several different types of cells. Examples of mixed-tissue tumors (Table 19-5) are found in the kidney, ovaries, and testes.

PATHOLOGIC DESCRIPTIONS

The following terms are used to describe the appearance of a malignant tumor, on either gross (visual) or microscopic examination.

GROSS DESCRIPTIONS

cystic

Forming large open spaces filled with fluid.

Mucinous tumors are filled with mucus (thick, sticky fluid), and **serous** tumors are filled with a thin, watery fluid resembling serum. The most common site of cystic tumors is in ovaries (Figure 19-6A).

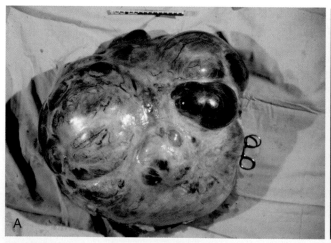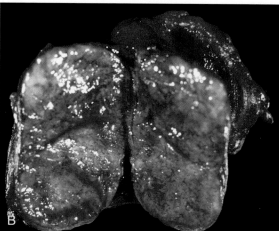

FIGURE 19-6 A, Cystic ovarian adenocarcinoma. Note that the tumor has formed fluid-filled cysts and blood-filled sacs. **B, Medullary carcinoma** of the thyroid. Tumor shows a solid pattern of growth. (*A, Courtesy Dr. Annekathryn Goodman, Massachusetts General Hospital, Boston.*)

fungating	**Mushrooming pattern of growth in which tumor cells pile one on top of another and project from a tissue surface.** Tumors found in the colon are often of this type.
inflammatory	**Having the features of inflammation—that is, redness, swelling, and heat.** Inflammatory changes result from tumor blockage of the lymphatic drainage of the skin, as in breast cancer.
medullary	**Large, soft, fleshy tumors.** Thyroid and breast tumors may be medullary (Figure 19-6B).
necrotic	**Containing dead tissue.** Any type of tumor can outgrow its blood supply with resulting cell death and necrosis of part or all of the tumor.
polypoid	**Growths that form projections extending outward from a base.** **Sessile** polypoid tumors extend from a broad base, and **pedunculated** polypoid tumors extend from a stem or stalk. Both benign and malignant tumors of the colon may grow as polyps. Benign polyps of the colon have a significant risk of becoming malignant over time and should be removed to prevent cancer (Figure 19-7A).
ulcerating	**Characterized by an open, exposed surface resulting from the death of overlying tissue.** Ulcerating tumors often are found in the stomach, breast, colon, and skin (Figure 19-7B).
verrucous	**Resembling a wart-like growth.** Tumors of the gingiva (gum) frequently are verrucous.

MICROSCOPIC DESCRIPTIONS

alveolar	**Tumor cells form patterns resembling small sacs;** commonly found in tumors of muscle, bone, fat, and cartilage.
carcinoma in situ	**Referring to localized tumor cells that have not invaded adjacent structures.** (Latin *in situ* means in place.) Cancer of the cervix may begin as carcinoma in situ.

19

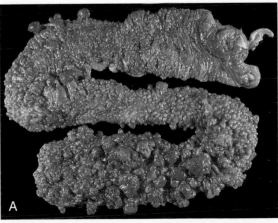
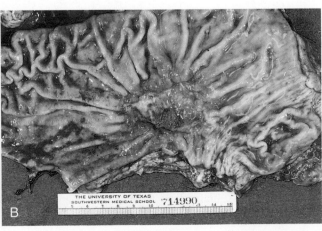

FIGURE 19-7   A, Adenomatous polyposis of the colon. These innumerable polypoid adenomas have a strong tendency for progression to colon adenocarcinoma. **B, Gastric (stomach) carcinoma with a large irregular ulcer.**

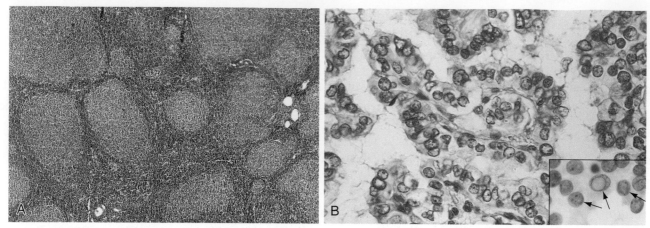

FIGURE 19-8   A, Follicular non-Hodgkin lymphoma involving a lymph node. B, Papillary carcinoma of the thyroid.

diffuse	**Spreading evenly throughout the affected tissue.** Malignant lymphomas may display diffuse involvement of lymph nodes.
dysplastic	**Containing abnormal-appearing cells that are not clearly cancerous.** Dysplastic nevi (moles on skin) are an example. They are often forerunners of skin cancers.
epidermoid	**Resembling squamous epithelial cells (thin, plate-like);** often occurring in the respiratory tract.
follicular	**Forming small glandular sacs.** Thyroid gland cancer and lymphomas are examples (Figure 19-8A).
papillary	**Forming small, finger-like or nipple-like projections of cells.** Bladder and thyroid cancers are examples (Figure 19-8B).
pleomorphic	**Composed of a variety of types of cells.** Mixed-cell tumors are examples.
scirrhous	**Densely packed** (scirrhous means hard) **tumors, due to dense bands of fibrous tissue;** commonly found in breast or stomach cancers.
undifferentiated	**Lacking microscopic structures typical of normal mature cells.**

19

GRADING AND STAGING SYSTEMS

In grading and staging systems, doctors classify tumors on the basis of **microscopic appearance (grade)** and the **extent of spread (stage).** These two properties influence the diagnosis, treatment, and prognosis for cancer patients.

GRADING

When **grading** a tumor, the pathologist is concerned with the microscopic appearance of the tumor cells, specifically with their degree of maturity and differentiation. Often, three or four grades are used. **Grade I** tumors are very well differentiated, so that they closely resemble normal cells. **Grade IV** tumors are so undifferentiated or anaplastic that even recognition of the tumor's tissue of origin may be difficult. **Grades II** and **III** are intermediate in appearance, moderately or poorly differentiated, as opposed to well differentiated (grade I) and undifferentiated (grade IV).

Grading often is of value in determining the prognosis for certain types of cancers, such as cancer of the urinary bladder, prostate gland, and ovary and brain tumors. Patients with grade I tumors have a high survival rate, and patients with grade II, III, and IV tumors have an increasingly poorer survival rate. Grading also is used in evaluating cells obtained from body fluids in preventive screening tests, such as **Papanicolaou (Pap) smears** of the uterine cervix.

STAGING

The **staging** of cancerous tumors is based on the extent of spread of the tumor. It relies on careful definition of the size and possible metastatic spread of the tumor, using computed tomography (CT), combination positron emission tomography (PET-CT), and magnetic resonance imaging (MRI) scans and radionuclide (radioactive) bone scans. See Figure 19-14, page 828, for a PET-CT scan showing lymph node metastases. An example of a staging system is the **tumor-node-metastasis (TNM) International Staging System.** It has been applied to malignancies such as lung and breast cancer, as well as to many other tumors.

Notations in a staging system are:

T = tumor (size and degree of local extension)

N = nodes (number of regional lymph nodes invaded by tumor cells)

M = metastases (spread of tumor cells to distant sites)

Stage groupings I-IV indicate tumor progression. Thus a stage II group may be designated as T2, N1, M0. Stage IV group indicates any T, any N, and distant metastases.

19

CANCER TREATMENT

Major approaches to cancer treatment are **surgery, radiation therapy, chemotherapy, molecularly targeted therapy,** and **immunotherapy.** Each **modality** (method) may be used alone, but often they are used together in combined-modality regimens to improve the overall diagnosis and treatment result.

SURGERY

In many patients with cancer, the tumor is discovered before it has spread, and it may be cured by surgical excision. Some common cancers in which surgery may be curative are those of the stomach, breast, colon, lung, and uterus (endometrium). In other patients who have metastases, surgical removal of the primary tumor prevents local spread or complications, even in the presence of distant disease. A **debulking procedure** may be used to remove as much of the primary tumor mass as possible, even if the tumor is attached to a vital organ and cannot be completely removed. After removal of the primary tumor, the patient often receives **adjuvant** (assisting) radiation therapy and/or chemotherapy to prevent recurrence at local and distant sites.

The following is a list of terms that describe surgical procedures used in diagnosing and treating cancer.

cauterization	Destruction of tissue by burning. Examples are electrocauterization (using a needle or snare heated by electric current), laser, dry ice, and chemicals.
core needle biopsy	Placement of a large-bore needle that extracts a thin core of tissue.
cryosurgery	Use of subfreezing temperature to destroy tissue.
en bloc resection	Tumor is removed along with a large area of surrounding tissue containing lymph nodes. Modified radical mastectomy, colectomy, and gastrectomy are examples.
excisional biopsy	Removal of tumor and a margin of normal tissue. This procedure provides a specimen for diagnosis and may be curative for small noninvasive tumors.
exenteration	Wide resection involving removal of the tumor, its organ of origin, and all surrounding tissue in the body space. Pelvic exenteration with removal of the uterus, ovaries, bladder, and segments of the large bowel may be performed to treat large primary tumors of the uterus.
fine needle aspiration	Placement of a very thin needle inside the tumor mass and extracting cells for microscopic evaluation.
fulguration	Destruction of tissue by electric sparks generated by a high-frequency current.
incisional biopsy	Piece of tumor is removed for examination to establish a diagnosis. More extensive surgical procedure or other forms of treatment, such as chemotherapy or radiation therapy, are then used to treat the bulk of the tumor.

RADIATION THERAPY (RADIATION ONCOLOGY)

The **goal of radiation therapy (RT)** is to deliver a maximal dose of ionizing radiation to the tumor tissue and a minimal dose to the surrounding normal tissue. High-dose **irradiation** (exposure of tissue to radiation) destroys tumor cells and produces damage to DNA. Newer techniques of irradiation use high-energy beams of **protons** (subatomic particles) to improve the uniformity (conformality) of dose and to limit damage to normal tissues.

Terms used in the field of radiation therapy for cancer are as follows:

brachytherapy	Implantation of small, sealed containers or seeds of radioactive material directly into the tumor (interstitial therapy); or in a cavity of the tumor (intracavitary therapy, as in endometrial cancer). An implant may be temporary (as in treatment for tumors of the head and neck or gynecologic malignancies) or permanent (as with prostatic implants, or "seeds," placed into the affected area of the gland).
electron beams	Low-energy beams for treatment of skin or surface tumors.
external beam irradiation (teletherapy)	Radiation therapy applied to a tumor from a distant source (linear accelerator).
fields	Dimensions of the size of radiation area used to treat a tumor from a specific angle. See Figure 19-9.
fractionation	A method of dividing radiation into small, repeated doses rather than fewer large doses. Fractionation allows larger total doses to be given while causing less damage to normal tissue.
gray (Gy)	Unit of absorbed radiation dose. Historically, the unit in use was **rad** (100 rad equal 1 Gy).
linear accelerator	Large electronic device that produces high-energy x-ray (or photon) beams for the treatment of deep-seated tumors (Figure 19-10). Intraoperative radiation therapy (IORT) is direct application of radiation during surgery using a linear accelerator in the operating room.
photon therapy	Radiation therapy using x-rays or gamma rays. A linear accelerator produces photon beams to treat tumors. See ***In Person: Radiotherapy,*** page 830.

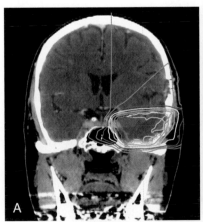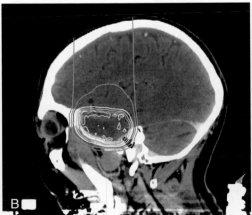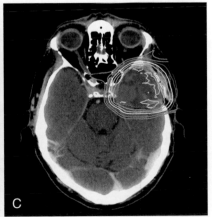

FIGURE 19-9   Radiation fields. Three-color radiation dose distribution image showing radiation fields used to treat a brain tumor. *(Courtesy of Jay Loeffler, MD, Chief, Radiation Oncology Department, Massachusetts General Hospital, Boston.)*

proton therapy   Small subatomic positively charged particles (protons) produced by a cyclotron deposit all the energy at a focused finite point. This reduces the dose affecting normal surrounding tissues by at least 50% (Figure 19-11A).

radiocurable tumor   Tumor that can be completely eradicated by radiation therapy. Usually, this is a localized tumor with no evidence of metastasis. Lymphomas, Hodgkin lymphoma, and seminomas of the testes are examples.

radioresistant tumor   Tumor that requires large doses of radiation to produce death of the cells. Melanoma and renal carcinoma are among the most radioresistant tumors.

radiosensitive tumor   Tumor in which irradiation can cause the death of cells without serious damage to surrounding tissue (morbidity). Tumors of hematopoietic (blood-forming) and lymphatic origins are radiosensitive.

radiosensitizers   Drugs that increase the sensitivity of tumors to x-rays. Many cancer chemotherapy drugs, especially 5-fluorouracil and cisplatin, sensitize tumors and normal tissue to radiation, thereby improving the outcome of treatment.

simulation   An imaging study performed before radiation therapy using CT scan and/ or MRI to map the area to receive treatment. Simulation is required for all patients undergoing radiotherapy.

stereotactic radiosurgery   Single large dose of radiation is delivered under precise three-dimensional (3D) guidance (stereotactic) from multiple angles to destroy vascular abnormalities and small brain tumors (see Figure 19-11B).

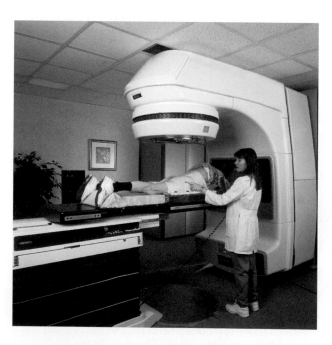

FIGURE 19-10   Linear accelerator. Radiation therapy (photon therapy) delivered to a patient positioned under a linear accelerator. **Intensity-modulated radiation therapy (IMRT)** is an advanced mode of high-precision radiotherapy that uses computer-controlled linear accelerators to deliver precise radiation doses to a malignant tumor. This is a type of **conformal radiation therapy** that uses computer technology to create a three-dimensional image of a tumor so that rotating beams can shape exactly to the contour of the tumor. *(Courtesy Arthur Brimberg, MD, Riverhill Radiation Oncology, Yonkers, New York.)*

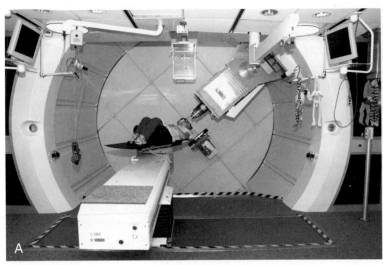 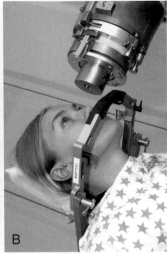

FIGURE 19-11   A, Proton therapy machine. Proton beam radiation therapy is useful in treating a variety of cancers including tumors of the head and neck, brain, eye, and prostate. **B, Proton stereotactic radiosurgery.** A model poses to show how a proton beam device is brought near a patient in preparation for stereotactic radiosurgery. *(Courtesy Jay Loeffler, MD, Chief, Radiation Oncology Department, Massachusetts General Hospital, Boston.)*

Radiotherapy, although it may be either **palliative** (relieving symptoms) or curative, can produce undesirable side effects to any normal body tissues that are caught in the field of irradiation. Some complications due to irradiation of normal tissue surrounding the tumor and in the path of the beam of photons may be reversible with time, and recovery takes place soon after radiotherapy is completed. Side effects may be acute (days to weeks after first dose), subacute (several weeks or months later), or late (months to years later). Radiation side effects are listed in Table 19-6.

TABLE 19-6	RADIOTHERAPY SIDE EFFECTS
Acute	
• **mucositis**	inflammation and ulceration of mucous membranes (mouth, pharynx, vagina, bladder, large or small intestine)
• **myelosuppression**	bone marrow depression (anemia, leukopenia, and thrombocytopenia)
• **nausea and vomiting**	uneasiness of the stomach and emptying of its contents—more common with irradiation of the brain and gastrointestinal tract
• **xerostomia**	dryness of the mouth—with salivary gland irradiation
Subacute	
• **alopecia**	baldness (permanent or temporary)
• **cystitis**	inflammation of the urinary bladder
• **pneumonitis**	inflammation of the lungs
• **proctitis**	inflammation of the rectum and anus
Late	
• **fibrosis**	increase of connective tissue (scarring of skin, lungs, kidneys)
• **secondary tumors**	new types of tumors in separate sites (leukemias and solid tumors such as carcinomas and sarcomas)
• **infertility**	loss of reproductive function

19

CHEMOTHERAPY

Cancer chemotherapy is the treatment of cancer using chemicals (drugs). It is the standard treatment for many types of cancer, and is curative in a number of them, such as testicular cancer, acute lymphocytic leukemia (children), and Hodgkin lymphoma, and large cell lymphomas. Chemotherapy may be used alone or in combination with surgery and irradiation to improve cure rates.

Drugs cause tumor cells to die by damaging their DNA. Tumor cells with damaged DNA undergo apoptosis (self-destruction). This means that they have less capacity to repair their DNA and, in general, are less able to survive DNA damage caused by drugs and radiation.

The ideal is to administer drugs that kill large numbers of tumor cells without harming normal cells. However, rapidly dividing normal cells, such as in the bone marrow and gastrointestinal lining, can suffer considerable damage from chemotherapeutic drugs. Research physicians measure drug levels and disappearance from the bloodstream and tissues. They use information from animal experiments and **clinical trials** to design better routes and schedules of administration to achieve the greatest tumor kill with the least toxicity (harm) to normal cells.

Combination chemotherapy is the use of two or more drugs together to kill tumors. Drugs are given according to a written **protocol,** or plan, that details the route, schedule, and frequency of doses. Usually, drug therapy is continued until the patient achieves a complete **remission** (absence of all signs of disease). **Adjuvant chemotherapy** is the administration of drug treatment after surgery to kill any residual cancer cells. **Neoadjuvant chemotherapy** is administrated before surgery to reduce the size of a tumor, such as breast or head and neck cancer. Neoadjuvant drug treatment allows for a lesser surgery and improvement of outcome.

Clinical Trials

Clinical trials are research studies designed to find treatments that work better than the standard therapies for patients. The studies follow a predefined protocol and are divided into four phases:

Phase I: The experimental drug or treatment is tested in a small group of people (20 to 80) for the first time to evaluate its safety. Phase I trials also determine a safe dosage range and schedule of administration (daily, weekly, or every 3 weeks, oral or intravenous, and so on).

Phase II: Experimental treatment is given to a larger group of subjects (200 to 300) with a specific type of cancer to identify tumor response rate and define safety risks.

Phase III: A larger and more definitive trial is conducted in which hundreds or thousands of subjects take part. Patients are randomly assigned to the new treatment or to a standard, established treatment. The effectiveness and overall risk-versus-benefit ratio for the experimental treatment are compared with those for standard treatment. A new drug may be approved by the FDA (U.S. Food and Drug Administration) based on these results.

Phase IV: Large studies are conducted after the FDA has granted its initial approval of a new treatment for marketing. These trials are designed to monitor safety in large populations and identify new indications and new drug combinations beyond those already approved.

The following are categories of cancer chemotherapeutic agents. Each works by disrupting cell function so that cancer cells die. At the same time, normal cells may be damaged as well. In each category, side effects such as alopecia, nausea and vomiting, and myelosuppression can occur.

1. **Alkylating agents.** These drugs cause crosslinks and breaks in DNA that interfere with cell division. **Cisplatin (Platinol)** and **cyclophosphamide (Cytoxan)** are examples.

2. **Antibiotics.** These drugs are produced by bacteria or fungi and inhibit cell division by causing breaks in DNA strands. **Doxorubicin (Adriamycin)** is an example.

3. **Antimetabolites.** These drugs block synthesis of DNA components (nucleotides) and prevent cells from dividing. **Methotrexate** and **5-fluorouracil (5FU)** are examples.

4. **Antimitotics.** These chemicals block the function of a protein that is necessary for mitosis (cell division). They come from bacteria, fungi, or plants or from animals found on coral reefs in the ocean. **Paclitaxel (Taxol)** is an example.

5. **Hormonal agents.** These drugs block hormone receptors on cells so that growth is inhibited. An example is **tamoxifen (Novadex)**, which blocks an **estrogen receptor** on breast cancer cells. **Flutamide (Eulexin)** blocks androgen receptors in prostate cancer. Aromatase inhibitors, such as **anastrozole (Arimidex)** prevent the conversion of androgen to estrogen and starve breast tumors of their estrogen supply in postmenopausal women.

Figure 19-12 illustrates the mechanisms of action for various types of cancer chemotherapeutic agents. Often, drugs are administered in combination, according to carefully planned **protocols** (regimens). For your reference, see Table 19-7 which lists specific chemotherapeutic drugs in each category and the type of cancer they treat.

19

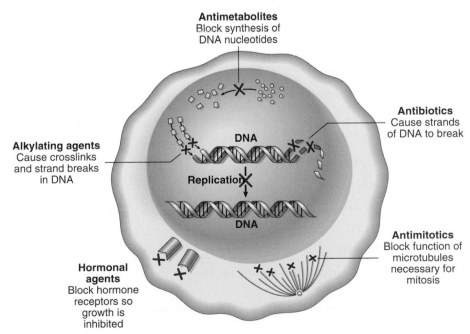

FIGURE 19-12   Mechanisms of action of cancer chemotherapeutic agents.

TABLE 19-7	SELECTED CANCER CHEMOTHERAPEUTIC AGENTS AND THE CANCERS THEY TREAT

CHEMOTHERAPEUTIC AGENT	TYPE OF CANCER
Alkylating Agents	
Bendamustine (Ribomustine)	Non-Hodgkin lymphoma
Carmustine (BCNU)	Brain
Carboplatin (Paraplatin)	Ovarian
Cisplatin (Platinol)	Testicular; ovarian
Cyclophosphamide (Cytoxan)	Lymphoma
Dacarbazine (DTIC-Dome)	Hodgkin lymphoma
Temozolomide (Temodar)	Brain (glioma)
Antibiotics	
Bleomycin (Blenoxane)	Testicular
Daunorubicin (Cerubidine)	Acute myeloid leukemia (AML)
Doxorubicin (Adriamycin, Doxil)	Breast
Antimetabolites	
Capecitabine (Xeloda)	Breast and colon
Cladribine (Leustatin)	Hairy cell leukemia
Cytarabine (ara-C, Cytosar-U)	AML
Fludarabine (Fludara)	Chronic lymphoid leukemia (CLL)
5-Fluorouracil (5-FU) (various)	Colon
Gemcitabine (Gemzar)	Pancreatic cancer
Methotrexate, MTX (Folex, Mexate)	Acute lymphoid leukemia (ALL)
Pemetrexed (Alimta)	Lung cancer
Antimitotics	
Docetaxel (Taxotere)	Breast
Paclitaxel (Taxol)	Breast, ovary
Vinblastine (Velban)	Lymphoma
Vincristine (Oncovin)	Lymphoma
Vinorelbine (Navelbine)	Breast
Hormones and Hormone Antagonists	
Abiraterone (Zyliga)	Prostate cancer
Dexamethasone (Decadron)	Lymphoma
Flutamide (Eulexin)	Prostate
Letrozole (Femara)	Breast
Leuprolide (Lupron)	Prostate
Prednisone (various)	Acute lymphoid leukemia (ALL)
Tamoxifen (Nolvadex)	Breast

Note: Brand names are in parentheses. Often drugs are given in combinations according to carefully planned regimens called **protocols.**

MOLECULARLY TARGETED THERAPY

Molecularly targeted cancer therapy uses drugs to attack specific mutations (targets) that drive cancer cell growth. When these targets are blocked by drugs, the cancer cell dies. Some of the targets are absolutely unique to tumor cells and not found in normal tissues. Thus, in contrast with chemotherapy, blocking these targets will have little or no effect on normal cells. Chemotherapeutic drugs normally are delivered by intravenous infusion, whereas molecularly targeted drugs often are given orally, in pill form.

IMMUNOTHERAPY

Immunotherapy is the use of immune cells (lymphocytes) or antibodies, to kill tumors. An example is the use of **T cells** that have been modified in a laboratory to recognize and destroy a patient's own tumor. This therapy is effective against acute lymphoid leukemia (ALL) and chronic lymphoid leukemia (CLL).

Another example involves making an antibody (monoclomal antibody) that will attack a target on the tumor cell surface. One of the most effective therapeutic antibodies is **Herceptin**, which blocks a receptor and destroys a growth factor on the surface of breast cancer cells. Another antibody called **nivolumab (Opdivo)**, works by blocking a protein (PD-1) on tumor cells. It is effective against melanoma, lung cancer, bladder cancer, kidney cancer, and Hodgkin lymphoma. See Table 19-8 for examples of immunotherapy agents and their modes of action.

TABLE 19-8	IMMUNOTHERAPY AGENTS AND THEIR MODES OF ACTION
AGENT	**MODE OF ACTION**
Bevacizumab (Avastin)	Monoclonal antibody that binds to VEGF
Cetuximab (Erbitux)	Monoclonal antibody that binds to EGFR
Interferons (Roferon, Intron)	Promote broad immune response
Interleukin 2 (IL-2)	Promotes immune response of T lymphocytes Long-acting filgrastim
Rituximab (Rituxan)	Monoclonal antibody binding to cell surface receptor; induces apoptosis
Nivolumab (Opdivo)	Antibody that stimulates immune cells (T cells) to target cancer cells
Trastuzumab (Herceptin)	Monoclonal antibody binding to *HER2* receptor on cell surface; blocks growth-signaling pathways within cell; induces apoptosis

Molecularly Targeted Drugs

Examples are:

Gleevec (imatinib mesylate)—blocks bcr-abl tyrosine kinase in chronic myeloid leukemia cells

Tarceva (erlotinib)—blocks epidermal growth factor (EGFR) in lung cancer cells

Zelboraf (vemurafenib)—blocks mutated BRAF enzyme in 50% of melanoma patients

VOCABULARY

This list reviews many of the new terms introduced in the text. Short definitions reinforce your understanding of the terms. Refer to the Pronunciation of Terms section, page 842, for help with unfamiliar or difficult words.

adjuvant chemotherapy	Drugs are given after primary therapy (surgery or radiation). Adjuvant means to assist.
alkylating agents	Chemotherapeutic synthetic drugs that cause crosslinks and breaks in DNA to stop cells from dividing.
anaplasia	Loss of differentiation of cells; reversion to a more primitive cell type.
antibiotics	Chemotherapeutic drugs found in bacteria and fungi, which cause breaks in DNA strands to inhibit cell division.
antimetabolites	Chemotherapeutic agents that block the synthesis of DNA components (nucleotides) and prevent cells from dividing.
antimitotics	Chemotherapeutic chemicals that block the function of a protein necessary for mitosis.
apoptosis	Programmed cell death. (Apo- means off, away; -ptosis means to fall.) Normal cells undergo apoptosis when damaged or aging. Some cancer cells have lost the ability to undergo apoptosis, and they live forever.
benign tumor	Noncancerous growth (neoplasm).
brachytherapy	Radiotherapy that uses insertion of sealed containers into body cavities or radioactive seeds directly into the tumor.
carcinogens	Agents that cause cancer: chemicals and drugs, radiation, and viruses.
carcinoma	Cancerous tumor made up of cells of epithelial origin.
chemotherapy	Treatment with drugs.
combination chemotherapy	Use of several chemotherapeutic agents together for the treatment of tumors.
dedifferentiation	Loss of differentiation of cells; reversion to a more primitive, embryonic cell type; anaplasia or undifferentiation.
deoxyribonucleic acid (DNA)	Genetic material within the nucleus of a cell; controls cell division and protein synthesis.
differentiation	Specialization of cells.
electron beams	Low-energy beams of radiation for treatment of skin or surface tumors.
encapsulated	Surrounded by a capsule; benign tumors are encapsulated.
external beam irradiation	Radiation is applied to a tumor from a source outside the body.
fields	Dimensions of the area of the body undergoing irradiation.
fractionation	Giving radiation in small, repeated doses.
genetic screening	Patients and family members are tested to determine whether they have inherited a cancer-causing gene.

19

grading of tumors	Evaluating the degree of maturity of tumor cells or degree of differentiation.
gray (Gy)	Unit of absorbed radiation dose.
gross description of tumors	Visual appearance of tumors to the naked eye: cystic, fungating, inflammatory, medullary, necrotic, polypoid, ulcerating, or verrucous.
immunotherapy	Cancer treatment using immune cells and antibodies to kill tumor cells.
infiltrative	Extending beyond normal tissue boundaries into adjacent tissues.
invasive	Having the ability to enter and destroy surrounding tissue.
irradiation	Exposure to any form of radiant energy such as light, heat, or x-rays.
linear accelerator	Large electronic device that produces high-energy x-ray beams for treatment of deep-seated tumors.
malignant tumor	Tumor having the characteristics of continuous growth, invasiveness, and metastasis.
mesenchymal	Embryonic connective tissue (mes = middle, enchym/o = to pour). This is the tissue from which connective tissues (bone, muscle, fat, cartilage, and blood cells) arise.
metastasis	Spread of a malignant tumor to a secondary site; literally, beyond (meta-) control (-stasis).
microscopic description of tumors	Appearance of tumors when viewed under a microscope: alveolar, carcinoma in situ, diffuse, dysplastic, epidermoid, follicular, papillary, pleomorphic, scirrhous, or undifferentiated.
mitosis	Replication of cells; a stage in a cell's life cycle involving the production of two identical cells from a parent cell.
mixed-tissue tumors	Tumors composed of different types of tissue (epithelial as well as connective tissue).
modality	Method of treatment, such as surgery, chemotherapy, or irradiation.
molecularly targeted therapy	Use of drugs to attack specific targets (mutations) that drive cancer cell growth.
morbidity	Condition of being unwell or deficient in normal function.
mucinous	Containing mucus (a thick whitish secretion).
mutation	Change in the genetic material (DNA) of a cell; may be caused by chemicals, radiation, or viruses or may occur spontaneously.
neoadjuvant chemotherapy	Drugs are given before primary therapy (surgery or radiation) to reduce the size of a tumor.
neoplasm	New growth; benign or malignant tumor.
nucleotide	Unit of DNA (gene) composed of a sugar, phosphate, and a base. The sequence or arrangement of nucleotides on a gene is the genetic code.
oncogene	Region of DNA in tumor cells (cellular oncogene) or in viruses that cause cancer (viral oncogene). Oncogenes are designated by a three-letter name, such as *abl*, *erb*, *jun*, *myc*, *ras*, and *src*.

19

palliative	Relieving but not curing symptoms.
pedunculated	Possessing a stem or stalk (peduncle); characteristic of some polypoid tumors.
photon therapy	Radiation therapy using energy in the form of x-rays or gamma rays.
protocol	Detailed plan for treatment of an illness.
proton therapy	Subatomic positively charged particles (protons) produced by a cyclotron deposit a dose of radiation at a tightly focused point in the body.
radiation	Energy carried by a stream of particles.
radiocurable tumor	Tumor that is completely destroyed by radiation therapy. Early Hodgkin lymphoma is an example.
radioresistant tumor	Tumor that surivives large doses of radiation.
radiosensitive tumor	Tumor in which radiation can cause the death of cells without serious damage to surrounding tissue.
radiosensitizers	Drugs that increase the sensitivity of tumors to x-rays.
radiotherapy	Treatment of tumors using doses of radiation; radiation oncology.
relapse	Recurrence of tumor after treatment.
remission	Partial or complete disappearance of symptoms of disease.
ribonucleic acid (RNA)	Cellular substance that represents a copy of DNA and directs the formation of new protein inside cells.
sarcoma	Cancerous tumor derived from connective or flesh tissue.
serous	Having the appearance of a thin, watery fluid (serum).
sessile	Having no stem; characteristic of some polypoid tumors.
simulation	Study using CT scan or MRI to map the area to receive treatment before radiotherapy is given.
solid tumor	Tumor composed of a mass of cells.
staging of tumors	System of evaluating the extent of spread of tumors. An example is the TNM (tumor-node-metastasis) system.
stereotactic radiosurgery	Technique in which a single large dose of radiation is delivered under precise 3D guidance to destroy vascular abnormalities and small brain tumors.
surgical procedures to treat cancer	Methods of removing cancerous tissue: cryosurgery, cauterization, en bloc resection, excisional biopsy, exenteration, fulguration, incisional biopsy.
viral oncogenes	Pieces of DNA from viruses that infect a normal cell and cause it to become malignant.
virus	Infectious agent that reproduces by entering a host cell and using the host's genetic material to make copies of itself.

19

TERMINOLOGY

Write the meanings of the medical terms in the spaces provided.

COMBINING FORMS

COMBINING FORM	MEANING	TERMINOLOGY	MEANING
alveol/o	small sac	alveolar _____ *Microscopic description of tumor cell arrangement (found in connective tissue tumors).*	
cac/o	bad	cachexia _____ *General ill health and malnutrition (wasting of muscle and emaciation) associated with chronic, severe disease (-hexia means state or condition).*	
carcin/o	cancer, cancerous	carcinoma in situ _____ *Localized cancer; confined to the site of origin.*	
cauter/o	burn, heat	electrocauterization _____	
chem/o	chemical, drug	chemotherapy _____	
cry/o	cold	cryosurgery _____	
cyst/o	sac of fluid	cystic tumor _____	
fibr/o	fibers	fibrosarcoma _____	
follicul/o	small glandular sacs	follicular _____ *A microscopic description of cellular arrangement in glandular tumors.*	
fung/i	fungus, mushroom	fungating tumor _____	
medull/o	soft, inner part	medullary tumor _____	
mucos/o	mucous membrane	mucositis _____	
mut/a	genetic change	mutation _____ *-tion means process.*	
mutagen/o	causing genetic change	mutagenic _____	
necr/o	death	necrotic tumor _____	

19

COMBINING FORM	MEANING	TERMINOLOGY	MEANING
neur/o	nerve	neurofibromatosis _____ *Fibromas are tumors of fibrous connective tissue. Tumors begin in supporting cells of nerves and the myelin sheath around nerve cells. Most tumors are benign but some may become cancerous. It is a genetic disorder occurring in 1 in 3000 births, but some cases arise via spontaneous mutation.*	
onc/o	tumor	oncology _____	
papill/o	nipple-like	papillary _____ *A microscopic description of tumor cell growth.*	
plas/o	formation	dysplastic _____ *Microscopic description of cells that are highly abnormal but not clearly cancerous. The suffix -tic means pertaining to.*	
ple/o	many, more	pleomorphic _____ *Microscopic description of tumors that are composed of a variety of cells.*	
polyp/o	polyp	polypoid tumor _____ *The suffix -oid means resembling.*	
prot/o	first	protocol _____ *The ending -col, from Latin* kolla, *means glued page. A protocol is a written plan detailing the procedures to be followed in research or treatment.*	
radi/o	rays	radiation _____ *Use of radioactive substances in the diagnosis and treatment of disease.* **Irradiation** *is exposure to any form of radiation (ionizing, heat, light, or x-rays).*	
sarc/o	flesh, connective tissue	osteosarcoma _____	
scirrh/o	hard	scirrhous _____ *Microscopic description of densely packed, fibrous tumor cell composition.*	
xer/o	dry	xerostomia _____	

SUFFIXES

SUFFIX	MEANING	TERMINOLOGY	MEANING
-blastoma	immature tumor	retino<u>blastoma</u> _____ _Childhood cancer arising from immature cells in the retina (posterior, light-sensitive area of the eye)._ neuro<u>blastoma</u> _____ _This sarcoma of nervous system origin affects infants and children up to the age of 10 years, usually arising in immature tissues of the autonomic nervous system or adrenal medulla._	
-genesis	formation	carcino<u>genesis</u> _____	
-oma	mass, tumor	adenocarcin<u>oma</u> _____	
-plasia	formation, growth	hyper<u>plasia</u> _____	
-plasm	formation, growth	neo<u>plasm</u> _____	
-suppression	to stop	myelo<u>suppression</u> _____	
-therapy	treatment	radio<u>therapy</u> _____ _Ionizing radiation is used to treat malignancies._	

PREFIXES

PREFIX	MEANING	TERMINOLOGY	MEANING
ana-	backward	<u>ana</u>plasia _____	
apo-	off, away	<u>apo</u>ptosis _____	
brachy-	short (distance)	<u>brachy</u>therapy _____ _Radiation delivered in close range to tumor site._	
epi-	upon	<u>epi</u>dermoid _____ _Microscopic description of tumor cells that resemble epidermal tissue._	
meta-	beyond; change	<u>meta</u>stasis _____	
neo-	new	<u>neo</u>adjuvant _____ _Adjuvant means to assist or aid._	
tele-	far	<u>tele</u>therapy _____ _Also called **external beam radiotherapy**._	

Neoadjuvant and Adjuvant

Don't' confuse these terms. **Neoadjuvant drug therapy** is delivered **before** primary treatment, as a first step to shrink a tumor. **Adjuvant drug therapy** is given **after** primary treatment to kill possible hidden tumor cells.

19

LABORATORY TESTS

cytogenetic analysis	**Chromosomes of normal or tumor cells are examined for breaks, translocations, or deletions of DNA.**
	The results of cytogenetic analysis can help confirm the diagnosis of a particular form of leukemia or other cancer.
immunohistochemistry	**Localization of antigens or proteins in tissues using labeled (colored or fluorescent) antibodies.**
	This technique allows for evaluation of the presence and amount of specific molecules in normal and tumor cells.
protein marker tests	**Measure the level of proteins in the blood or on the surface of tumor cells.**
	These tests diagnose cancer or detect its recurrence after treatment. Examples are:

PROTEIN	WHERE MEASURED	TYPE OF CANCER
acid phosphatase	blood	prostate
alpha-fetoprotein (AFP)	blood	liver, testicular
beta-hCG (human chorionic gonadotropin)	blood	choriocarcinoma, testicular
CA-125	blood	ovarian
CEA (carcinoembryonic antigen)	blood	colorectal, GI
estrogen receptor	tumor cells	breast
PSA (prostate-specific antigen)	blood	prostate
15.3 and 29.7	blood	breast
19.9	blood	pancreatic

CLINICAL PROCEDURES

The following specialized procedures are used to detect or treat malignancies. X-rays, CT scans, MRI, and ultrasound imaging (described throughout the text and specifically in Chapter 20) also are important diagnostic procedures in oncology.

bone marrow biopsy	**Aspiration of bone marrow tissue and examination under a microscope for evidence of malignant cells.**
bone marrow or stem cell transplantation	**Bone marrow or stem cells are infused intravenously into a patient.**
	In **autologous marrow transplantation,** marrow previously obtained from the patient and stored is reinfused when needed. In **allogeneic marrow transplantation** (all/o = other), marrow is obtained from a living donor other than the recipient. In **peripheral blood stem cell transplantation,** immature blood cells called stem cells are selected and harvested from the blood of a patient instead of from the bone marrow. After undergoing chemotherapy, the patient gets a reinfusion of the stem cells to repopulate the bone marrow with blood cells.

19

core needle biopsy	**Insertion of a large-bore needle into tissue to remove a core of cells for microscopic examination.** A needle (aspiration) biopsy is the insertion of a fine needle and aspiration (extraction) of a sample from a fluid-filled cavity or solid mass of tumor.
exfoliative cytology	**Cells are scraped from the region of suspected disease and examined under a microscope.** The Pap test (smear) to detect carcinoma of the cervix and vagina is an example (Figure 19-13).
fiberoptic colonoscopy	**Visual examination of the colon using a fiberoptic instrument.** This is an important screening procedure using an endoscope to detect cancer and remove premalignant polyps.
laparoscopy	**Visual examination of the abdominal cavity using small incisions and a laparoscope.** Also known as peritoneoscopy.
mammography	**X-ray examination of the breast to detect breast cancer.**

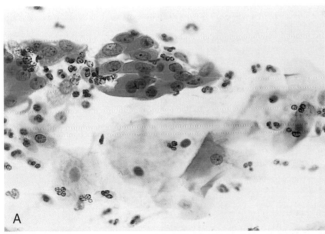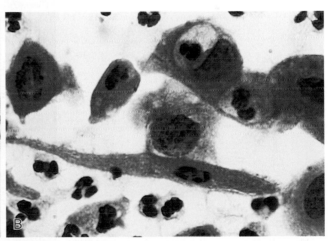

FIGURE 19-13 **A, Normal exfoliative cytologic smear (Pap smear) from the cervicovaginal region.** It shows flattened squamous cells and some neutrophils as well. **B, Abnormal cervicovaginal smear** shows numerous malignant cells that have pleomorphic (irregularly shaped) and hyperchromatic (stained) nuclei. *(A and B, Courtesy Dr. P.K. Gupta, Department of Pathology and Laboratory Medicine, University of Pennsylvania Medical Center, Philadelphia.)*

PET-CT scan	**Diagnostic procedure combining CT (computed tomography) and PET (positron emission tomography).**
	The combination provides a more complete picture of a tumor's location and growth or spread than either done independently. See Figure 19-14. PET-CT uses a combination of two machines: one to examine chemical reactions (PET scan) and the other to examine physical structures (CT scan).
radionuclide scans	**Radioactive substances (radionuclides) are injected intravenously, and scans (images) of organs are obtained.**
	These tests detect tumor and metastases. Examples of radionuclides are gallium-67 (whole-body scan), rose Bengal (liver), and technetium-99m (liver and spleen).

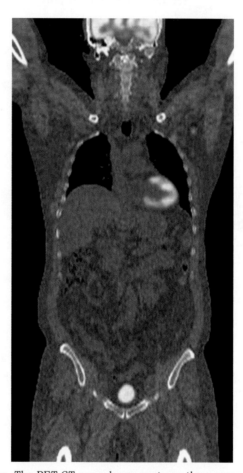

FIGURE 19-14   PET-CT scan. The PET-CT scan shown captures three areas of increased radioactivity, seen in the lymph nodes of the left axilla (armpit). By overlaying PET and CT images, physicians can identify spread of malignancy or metastasis. Brain and heart activity are normal. *(Courtesy Massachusetts General Hospital, Boston, Massachusetts.)*

19

ABBREVIATIONS

AFP	alpha-fetoprotein
bcr	breakpoint cluster region (*bcr-abl* oncogene is a part of the Philadelphia chromosome associated with chronic myeloid leukemia)
BMT	bone marrow transplantation
bx	biopsy
CA	cancer
CEA	carcinoembryonic antigen
cGy	centigray (one hundredth of a gray) or rad
chemo	chemotherapy
CR	complete response—disappearance of all tumor
CSF	colony-stimulating factor—examples: G-CSF (granulocyte colony-stimulating factor) and GM-CSF (granulocyte-macrophage colony-stimulating factor)
DNA	deoxyribonucleic acid
EGFR	epidermal growth factor receptor
ER	estrogen receptor
EPO	erythropoietin; promotes growth of red blood cells
FNA	fine needle aspiration
5-FU	5-fluorouracil
Ga	gallium
GIST	gastrointestinal stromal tumor
Gy	gray—unit of absorbed radiation dose
H&E	hematoxylin and eosin—a dye combination used to stain pathology specimens
HER2	growth factor gene highly activated in cells of certain types of breast cancer
IGRT	intensity-modulated gated radiation therapy—use of imaging mechanism attached to linear accelerator is added to IMRT to gate (track) a tumor moving during respiration
IHC	immunohistochemistry
IMRT	intensity-modulated radiation therapy—high doses of radiation are delivered directly to cancer cells in a targeted way, more precisely than in conventional radiotherapy
IORT	intraoperative radiation therapy
Mets	metastases
MoAb	monoclonal antibody
NED	no evidence of disease
NF	neurofibromatosis
NHL	non-Hodgkin lymphoma
NSCLC	non–small cell lung cancer
Pap smear	Papanicolaou smear
PD	progressive disease—tumor increases in size
PR	partial response—tumor is one-half its original size
prot.	protocol
PSA	prostate-specific antigen
PSCT	peripheral stem cell transplantation
PSRS	proton stereotactic radiosurgery
RNA	ribonucleic acid
RT	radiation therapy
SD	stable disease—tumor does not shrink but does not grow
TNM	tumor-node-metastasis
VEGF	vascular endothelial growth factor
RT, XRT	radiation therapy

19

IN PERSON: RADIOTHERAPY

This first-person narrative is by a woman who experienced radiation therapy for breast cancer.

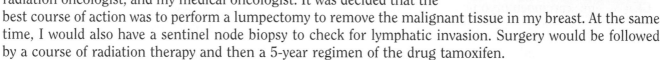

My life changed forever when I got that phone call that no one wants to hear: "Your biopsy is malignant." So after they tell you that you have cancer, you are scared to death, begin to contemplate your mortality, and wonder how to break the news to your husband, children, loved ones, and friends. You settle down, and marshal up your strength to fight this beast that attacks too many of us.

After my biopsy, I met with a team that included my surgeon, my radiation oncologist, and my medical oncologist. It was decided that the best course of action was to perform a lumpectomy to remove the malignant tissue in my breast. At the same time, I would also have a sentinel node biopsy to check for lymphatic invasion. Surgery would be followed by a course of radiation therapy and then a 5-year regimen of the drug tamoxifen.

Approximately 3 weeks after the surgery, I met with my radiation oncologist. She explained all the benefits and risks associated with radiation. At my first radiotherapy appointment, technicians created a mold to hold my breast in the exact position for treatment. I was marked on both sides of my body with indelible ink to place the mold correctly each visit. I also received a small permanent tattoo on the middle of my breastbone that enabled the machine to correctly target the beams.

On my first day of treatment, as I walked into the radiation room, I noticed hundreds of molds for other patients stacked up against the wall. The technicians positioned me into my mold and calibrated the machine against the markings on my body. When all the bodily GPS settings were in sync, they scurried out of the room to stand behind the giant lead walls (the cowards). A giant circular radiation machine began to move closer, gyrating slowly back and forth until it was properly fixed. A pulse of light shot out and a humming sound began. The machine gradually rotated, sending radiation to my breast. The entire treatment session lasted less than 10 minutes.

My side effects of radiation included fatigue and skin irritation from folliculitis (inflammation of hair follicles). Even after my treatments ended, side effects (blisters and even bleeding) continued. Time, however, brought healing.

I am amazed at what my journey revealed. Most of all, it taught me about how wonderful friends can be, how much of a difference support groups can make, and why dedicated medical professionals deserve so much thanks and praise. A very lovely woman I met along the way shared some wisdom that I will pass along to all of you reading my story. She said, "At first cancer is your whole world, then it becomes a room, then it becomes a drawer in that room, and then it becomes a box in the drawer." I still take that box out once in a while, but not as often.

Mary Braun is Vice President, Investments at Chapin Davis, Baltimore, Maryland.

PRACTICAL APPLICATIONS

Answers to questions are on page 841.

FYI: OTHER MALIGNANT TUMORS

A number of malignant tumors do not contain the combining form carcin/o or sarc/o in their names:

MALIGNANT TUMOR	DESCRIPTION
glioma	primary brain tumor
hepatoma	liver tumor (hepatocellular carcinoma)
hypernephroma	kidney tumor
lymphoma	lymph node tumor
melanoma	tumor of pigmented skin cells
mesothelioma	tumor of cells within the pleura
multiple myeloma	bone marrow cell tumor
thymoma	thymus gland tumor

Questions about FYI: Other Malignant Tumors

1. Which tumor develops from a dysplastic nevus? _____

2. Which tumor arises from an organ located within the mediastinum? _____

3. Which tumor arises from an organ in the RUQ of the abdomen? _____

4. Which tumor has types called astrocytoma, ependymoma, glioblastoma multiforme?

   _____

5. Which tumor is also known as a renal cell carcinoma? _____

6. Which tumor is characterized by large numbers of plasma cells (bone marrow antibody-producing

   cells)? _____

7. Which tumor arises from membrane cells surrounding the lungs? _____

8. Which tumor has a type known as Hodgkin disease? _____

CASE STUDY: SUSPECTED BREAST CANCER

A 52-year-old married woman presented to her physician with a painless mass in her left breast. During breast examination a 1.0-cm, firm, nontender mass was palpated in the upper outer quadrant located at the 2 o'clock position, 3 cm from the areola. The mass was not fixed to the skin, and there was no cutaneous erythema or edema. No axillary or supraclavicular lymphadenopathy was noted.

19

An excisional biopsy of the mass was performed. The pathology report described a gross specimen of fatty breast tissue. Microscopic evaluation of the nodule revealed an invasive ductal carcinoma. The margins of the lumpectomy specimen were free of tumor. Sentinel node [first lymph node where cancer cells are likely to spread] biopsy revealed no tumor involvement.

A portion of the specimen was sent for estrogen receptor assay and proved to be positive. The patient was informed of the diagnosis and underwent additional studies, including chest x-ray, liver chemistries, CBC, and bone scan; all results were negative.

The patient's tumor was staged as a T1N0M0, stage I carcinoma of the left breast. She was referred to a radiation oncologist for primary radiation therapy. After completion of radiotherapy, she was treated with tamoxifen. Prognosis is excellent for cure.

Questions about the Case Study

1. Where was the primary breast lesion located?
   a. Under the pigmented area of the breast
   b. About an inch and a half above and to the left of the nipple and pigmented area
   c. Near the axilla and under the shoulder blade

2. Other associated findings were
   a. Redness and swelling
   b. Enlarged lymph nodes under the armpit
   c. None of the above

3. The tumor was composed of
   a. Dense connective tissue surrounding the tumor cells, giving it a hard structure
   b. Glandular tumor with invasion of surrounding tissue
   c. Cells that had extended into the skin overlying the tumor

4. What procedure gave evidence that the tumor had not yet metastasized?
   a. Estrogen receptor assay
   b. Excisional biopsy of the mass
   c. Sentinel node biopsy

5. What additional therapy was undertaken?
   a. Bone scan, liver chemistries, CBC, and chest x-ray
   b. Radiation to the breast
   c. Radiation to the breast and then treatment with an estrogen blocker

6. Tamoxifen was prescribed because
   a. The tumor was found to be nonresponsive to estrogen
   b. The tumor had an estrogen receptor, and tamoxifen is an antiestrogen
   c. The tumor was at an advanced stage

CHART ROUNDS REVIEW: CENTER FOR RADIATION ONCOLOGY

Patient A has metastatic melanoma, with severe chest pain on deep breathing (with one metastasis involving a rib). He is being treated palliatively with 3000 cGy to the painful area.

Patient B is being treated for esophageal carcinoma. Because of previous treatment for breast cancer, the radiation dose to the recurrent field is limited to 3000 cGy.

Patient C is being treated for a pathologic stage I Hodgkin lymphoma with a radiation field to the mediastinum and adjacent lymph nodes.

Patient D is being treated for a GBM [glioblastoma multiforme]. The plan for appropriate fields of irradiation needs to be signed.

19

Questions about the Chart Rounds Review

1. Which patient is being treated for a brain tumor? _____

2. Which patient is being treated for lesions in the ribs? _____

3. Which patient has disease in cervical and thoracic lymph nodes? _____

4. Which patient is being treated for gastrointestinal cancer? _____

PATHOLOGY REPORT: RESECTED SPLEEN, GROSS DESCRIPTION

The spleen weighs 127 grams and measures 13.0 × 9.2 cm. External surface is smooth, leathery, homogeneous, and dark purplish brown. There are no defects in the capsule. The blood vessels of the hilum of the spleen are patent [open], with no thrombi or other abnormalities. On section of the spleen at 2- to 3-mm intervals, there are three well-defined, pale gray nodules on the cut surface, ranging from 3.0 to 4.0 cm in greatest dimension. The remainder of the cut surface is homogeneous and dark purple, and the tissue consistency is firm. *Possible diagnosis*: Hodgkin lymphoma.

Question about the Pathology Report

1. Which information leads the pathologist to the diagnosis of possible Hodgkin lymphoma?
    a. Blood clots in patent blood vessels
    b. Capsular defects
    c. Uniform, smooth surface
    d. Large, pale nodules in spleen

SHORT HISTORIES

As you read these actual patient histories, congratulate yourself on your understanding of medical terms!

1. A 28-year-old man feels a hard, nontender mass in his right testicle. He goes to his doctor, who checks his serum human chorionic gonadotropin and alpha-fetoprotein levels and finds both to be quite elevated. The tentative diagnosis is a germ cell tumor of the testis. A CT scan of the abdomen reveals extensive lymphadenopathy. A chest CT shows nodes in both lungs suggestive of tumor. An orchiectomy confirms the diagnosis of testicular cancer. He is given four cycles of chemotherapy with vinblastine, cisplatin, and bleomycin, and his serum AFP and HCG markers return to normal. His CT scans reveal no evidence of residual tumor.

2. A 42-year-old woman notices repeated episodes of red blood in her stool with each bowel movement. A colonoscopy reveals a 4-cm mass arising from the epithelium of the rectum. A biopsy demonstrates a rectal adenocarcinoma. An abdominal CT shows two large metastases in the liver and enlarged lymph nodes. She first receives four cycles of chemotherapy, which cause the liver lesions to shrink significantly and the lymph nodes to regress. The remaining liver lesions are surgically resected. Radiation therapy with chemotherapy (5-fluorouracil) is then administered to shrink the rectal tumor and lymph nodes, after which the rectal mass shrinks to a small 1-cm nodule. This is resected surgically. The lymph nodes are removed and contain no tumor.

3. A 62-year-old man has a routine PSA blood sample drawn. PSA is elevated at 5.8 (normal is less than 4.0). A transrectal biopsy of the prostate reveals a Gleason grade 6 adenocarcinoma in 4 of 12 biopsy pieces. He chooses to be treated with brachytherapy. Treatment causes dysuria, cystitis, and proctitis, but these symptoms disappear 3 weeks after therapy ends, and his PSA is now undetectable.

? EXERCISES

Remember to check your answers carefully with those given in the Answers to Exercises, page 840.

A Identify the following characteristics of malignant tumors based on their definitions as given below. Word parts are given as clues.

1. loss of differentiation of cells and reversion to a more primitive cell type:

    ana _____

2. extending beyond the normal tissue boundaries: in _____

3. having the ability to enter and destroy surrounding tissue: in _____

4. spreading to a secondary site: meta _____

B Match the terms or abbreviations with the definitions/descriptions that follow.

chemical carcinogen   mitosis   RNA
DNA   mutation   virus
radiation   oncogene

1. replication of cells; two identical cells are produced from a parent cell

    _____

2. change in the genetic material of a cell _____

3. genetic material within the nucleus that controls replication and protein synthesis

    _____

4. cellular substance (ribonucleic acid) that is important in protein synthesis

    _____

5. energy carried by a stream of particles _____

6. infectious agent that reproduces by entering a host cell and using the host's genetic material to

    make copies of itself _____

7. region of genetic material found in tumor cells and in viruses that causes cancer

    _____

8. an agent (hydrocarbon, insecticide, hormone) that causes cancer _____

C Give the meanings of the following terms.

1. solid tumor _____

2. adenoma _____

3. adenocarcinoma _____

4. osteoma _____

5. osteosarcoma _____

6. mixed-tissue tumor _____

7. neoplasm _____

8. neurofibromatosis _____

9. benign _____

10. differentiation _____

D **Name the terms that describe tumor growth as seen through a microscope. Definitions and word parts are given.**

1. small nipple-like projections: pap _____

2. abnormal formation of cells: dys _____

3. localized growth of cells: carcin _____

4. densely packed; containing fibrous tissue: _____ous

5. pattern resembling small, microscopic sacs: alv _____

6. small, round, gland-type clusters: foll _____

7. variety of cell types: pleo _____

8. lacking structures typical of mature cells: un _____

9. spreading evenly throughout the tissue: di _____

10. resembling epithelial cells: epiderm _____

E **Match the gross descriptions of tumors with the descriptions/definitions that follow.**

cystic   medullary   ulcerating
fungating   necrotic   verrucous
inflammatory   polypoid

1. Containing dead tissue: _____

2. Mushrooming pattern of growth: tumor cells pile on top of each other:

   _____

3. Characterized by large, open, exposed surfaces: _____

4. Characterized by redness, swelling, and heat: _____

5. Growths are projections from a base; sessile and pedunculated tumors are examples:

   _____

6. Tumors form large, open spaces filled with fluid; serous and mucinous tumors are examples:

   _____

7. Tumors resemble wart-like growths: _____

8. Tumors are large, soft, and fleshy: _____

19

F **Circle or supply the appropriate medical terms.**

1. A (**carcinoma/sarcoma**) is a cancerous tumor composed of cells of epithelial tissue. An example of such a cancerous tumor is a/an _____.

2. A (**carcinoma/sarcoma**) is a cancerous tumor composed of connective tissue. An example of such a cancerous tumor is a/an _____.

3. Retinoblastoma and adenomatous polyposis coli syndrome are examples of (**chemical carcinogens/inherited cancers**).

4. The assessment of a tumor's degree of maturity or microscopic differentiation is (**grading/ staging**) of the tumor.

5. The assessment of a tumor's extent of spread within the body is known as (**grading/staging**).

6. In the TNM staging system, T stands for (**tissue/tumor**), N stands for (**node/necrotic**), and M stands for (**mitotic/metastasis**).

7. Loss of differentiation of cells is called (**hyperplasia/anaplasia**).

8. Programmed call death is known as (**apoptosis/carcinogenesis**).

G **Match the surgical procedure in Column I with its meaning in Column II. Write the letter of the meaning in the space provided.**

COLUMN I

1. fulguration   _____

2. en bloc resection   _____

3. incisional biopsy   _____

4. excisional biopsy   _____

5. cryosurgery   _____

6. cauterization   _____

7. exenteration   _____

COLUMN II

A. Removal of tumor and a margin of normal tissue for diagnosis and possible cure of small tumors
B. Burning a lesion to destroy tumor cells
C. Wide resection involving removal of tumor, its organ of origin, and surrounding tissue in the body space
D. Destruction of tissue by electric sparks generated by a high-frequency current
E. Removal of entire tumor and regional lymph nodes
F. Freezing a lesion to kill tumor cells
G. Cutting into a tumor and removing a piece to establish a diagnosis

H **Supply medical terms to complete the following sentences.**

1. The method of treating cancer using high-energy radiation is _____.

2. If tumor tissue survives large doses of radiation, it is a/an _____ tumor.

3. If radiation can cause loss of tumor cells without serious damage to surrounding regions, the tumor is _____.

4. A tumor that is completely destroyed by RT is a/an _____ tumor.

5. The method of giving radiation in small, repeated doses is _____.

6. Drugs that increase the sensitivity of tumors to x-rays are _____.

7. Treatment of cancerous tumors with drugs is _____.

19

8. A condition of tumors of fibrous supportive nerve cells is _____.

9. The use of two or more drugs to kill tumor cells is _____.

10. A large electronic device that produces high-energy x-ray or photon beams for treatment of deep-seated tumors is a/an _____.

11. Alkylating agents, antimetabolites, hormones, antibiotics, and antimitotics all are types of _____ agents.

12. Implantation of seeds of radioactive material directly into a tumor is _____.

13. The unit of absorbed radiation dose is _____.

14. Radiation applied to a tumor from a distant source is _____.

15. Technique in which subatomic positively charged particles produced by a cyclotron deposit a dose of radiation at a tightly focused point is _____.

16. The dimension of the area of the body that receives radiation is a/an _____.

17. Study performed using CT or MRI to map the area to receive treatment before radiotherapy is given is _____.

18. Technique in which a single large dose of radiation is delivered under precise 3D guidance to destroy vascular abnormalities and small brain tumors is _____.

❚ **Match the side effects of radiotherapy and chemotherapy with the descriptions/ treatments that follow.**

alopecia	myelosuppression	pneumonitis
cystitis and proctitis	nausea	secondary tumors
fibrosis	oral mucositis	xerostomia
infertility		

1. Inflammation and ulceration of lining cells in the mouth caused by radiation to the jaw:

   _____

2. Radiation to the lungs causes inflammation of the lungs: _____

3. Chemotherapy for ovarian cancer causes loss of hair on the head: _____

4. Bone marrow depression with leukopenia, anemia, and thrombocytopenia:

   _____

5. Radiation to the lungs causes increase in connective tissue: _____

6. Radiation of salivary glands causes dryness of the mouth: _____

7. Chemotherapy may cause this sensation leading to vomiting: _____

8. New type of growths in separate sites from the primary tumor: _____

9. Loss of reproductive function: _____

10. Radiation effects on the urinary bladder and rectum: _____

19

J Give the meanings of the following medical terms.

1. modality _____

2. adjuvant chemotherapy _____

3. protocol _____

4. remission _____

5. relapse _____

6. morbidity _____

7. neoadjuvant chemotherapy _____

8. genetic screening _____

9. external beam irradiation _____

10. immunotherapy _____

11. apoptosis _____

12. cachexia _____

13. palliative _____

14. molecularly targeted therapy _____

15. nucleotide _____

K Match the test or procedure with its description/definition.

beta-hCG test   core needle biopsy   laparoscopy
bone marrow biopsy   estrogen receptor assay   PSA test
CA-125   exfoliative cytology   stem cell transplant
CEA test

1. test for the presence of a portion of human chorionic gonadotropin hormone (a marker for testicular cancer) _____

2. protein marker for ovarian cancer detected in the blood _____

3. visual examination of the abdominal cavity; peritoneoscopy _____

4. test for the presence of a hormone receptor on breast cancer cells _____

5. removal of bone marrow tissue for microscopic examination _____

6. obtaining a plug of tissue for microscopic examination _____

7. blood test for the presence of an antigen related to prostate cancer _____

8. blood test for carcinoembryonic antigen (marker for GI cancer) _____

9. cells are scraped off tissue and microscopically examined _____

10. an intravenous infusion of blood-forming cells _____

L **Circle the correct boldface terms to complete the sentences.**

1. Pauline was diagnosed with a meningioma, which usually is a/an **(benign, anaplastic, necrotic)** tumor. The doctor told her that it was not malignant, but that it should be removed because of the pressure it was causing on the surrounding tissues.

2. Marlene underwent surgical resection of her breast mass. After surgery, Dr. Mendez recommended **(dedifferentiated, modality, adjuvant)** chemotherapy because her tumor was large and she had one positive lymph node.

3. Unfortunately, at the time of diagnosis, the tumor had spread to distant sites because it was **(pleomorphic, metastatic, mutagenic)**. The oncologist recommended beginning chemotherapy as soon as possible.

4. The polyp in Lisa's colon was *not* pedunculated, and Dr. Sidney described it as flat and **(fungating, scirrhous, sessile)**.

5. Mr. Elder had difficulty urinating and had an elevated PSA blood level. Dr. Jones examined him and found a hard prostate gland. **(Laparoscopy, Electrocauterization, Biopsy)** demonstrated adenocarcinoma.

6. During the days following her chemotherapy for breast cancer, Mrs. Yang experienced loss of appetite and **(fibrosis, nausea, xerostomia)**. Blood tests revealed low levels of blood cells, indicating **(hematopoiesis, myeloma, myelosuppression)**.

7. One year after Mr. Smith's diagnosis and treatment for lung cancer, he underwent follow-up **(bone marrow biopsy, PET-CT scan, exfoliative cytology)**, which enabled his doctors to **(restage, regrade)** his disease using the **(ABCD, 1234, TNM)** system.

8. Mrs. Broom's doctor told her she needed **(CA-125, RT, PSA)** because her tumor was nonoperable and could not be **(resected, irradiated, electrocauterized)**.

19

ANSWERS TO EXERCISES

A

1. anaplasia
2. infiltrative
3. invasive
4. metastasis

B

1. mitosis
2. mutation
3. DNA
4. RNA
5. radiation
6. virus
7. oncogene
8. chemical carcinogen

C

1. tumor composed of a mass of cells
2. tumor of glandular tissue (benign)
3. cancerous (malignant) tumor of glandular tissue
4. tumor of bone (benign)
5. flesh (connective tissue) tumor of bone (malignant)
6. tumor composed of different types of tissue (both epithelial and connective tissues)
7. new formation (tumor)
8. tumors of fibrous supportive nerve tissue; often benign but may become malignant
9. noncancerous
10. specialization of cells

D

1. papillary
2. dysplastic
3. carcinoma in situ
4. scirrhous
5. alveolar
6. follicular
7. pleomorphic
8. undifferentiated
9. diffuse
10. epidermoid

E

1. necrotic
2. fungating
3. ulcerating
4. inflammatory
5. polypoid
6. cystic
7. verrucous
8. medullary

F

1. carcinoma; thyroid adenocarcinoma, squamous cell carcinoma
2. sarcoma; liposarcoma, chondrosarcoma, osteogenic sarcoma
3. inherited cancers
4. grading
5. staging
6. tumor; node; metastasis
7. anaplasia
8. apoptosis

G

1. D
2. E
3. G
4. A
5. F
6. B
7. C

H

1. radiation therapy
2. radioresistant
3. radiosensitive
4. radiocurable
5. fractionation
6. radiosensitizers
7. chemotherapy
8. neurofibromatosis
9. combination chemotherapy
10. linear accelerator
11. chemotherapeutic agents
12. brachytherapy
13. gray
14. external beam radiation (teletherapy)
15. proton therapy
16. field
17. simulation
18. stereotactic radiosurgery

I

1. oral mucositis
2. pneumonitis
3. alopecia
4. myelosuppression
5. fibrosis
6. xerostomia
7. nausea
8. secondary tumors
9. infertility
10. cystitis and proctitis

19

J

1. method of treatment
2. assisting primary treatment with drugs. This is given after surgery or radiation to attack small deposits of cancer cells undetected by diagnostic techniques.
3. report or plan of steps taken in an experiment or disease case
4. absence of all signs of disease
5. symptoms of disease return
6. conditions of damage to normal tissue; disease
7. use of drugs to reduce the size of a tumor before surgery. This lessens the extent of suregy and improves outcome.
8. patients and family members are tested to determine whether they have inherited a cancer causing gene
9. radiation applied to a tumor from a source outside the body
10. cancer treatment using immune cells and antibodies to kill tumor cells
11. programmed cell death
12. malnutrition marked by weakness and emaciation; usually associated with later stages of cancer
13. relieving but not curing symptoms of disease
14. use of drugs to attack specific targets (mutations) that drive cancer cell growth
15. unit of DNA composed of a sugar, phosphate, and base (adenine, cytosine, guanine, or thymine)

K

1. beta-hCG test
2. CA-125
3. laparoscopy
4. estrogen receptor assay
5. bone marrow biopsy
6. core needle biopsy
7. PSA test
8. CEA test
9. exfoliative cytology
10. stem cell transplant

L

1. benign
2. adjuvant
3. metastatic
4. sessile
5. biopsy
6. nausea; myelosuppression
7. PET-CT scan; restage; TNM
8. RT; resected

Answers to Practical Applications

FYI: Other Malignant Tumors
1. melanoma (a nevus is a benign pigmented lesion or mole)
2. thymoma
3. hepatoma
4. glioma
5. hypernephroma
6. multiple myeloma
7. mesothelioma
8. lymphoma (previously known as lymphosarcoma)

Case Study
1. b
2. c
3. b
4. c
5. c
6. b

Chart Rounds Review
1. patient D
2. patient A
3. patient C
4. patient B

Pathology Report
1. d

19

PRONUNCIATION OF TERMS

To test your understanding of the terminology in this chapter, write the meaning of each term in the space provided. In addition, you may wish to cover the terms and write them by looking at your definitions. Make sure your spelling is correct. The page number after each term indicates where it is defined or used in the book, so you can easily check your responses. You will find complete definitions for all of these terms and their audio pronunciations on the Evolve website.

Pronunciation Guide

ā as in āpe	ă as in ăpple
ē as in ēven	ĕ as in ĕvery
ī as in īce	ĭ as in ĭnterest
ō as in ōpen	ŏ as in pŏt
ū as in ūnit	ŭ as in ŭnder

TERM	PRONUNCIATION	MEANING
adenocarcinoma (825)	ăd-ĕ-nō-kăr-sĭ-NŌ-mă	_____
adjuvant chemotherapy (820)	ĂD-jū-vănt kē-mō-THĔR-ă-pē	_____
alkylating agents (820)	ĂL-kĭ-lā-tĭng Ā-jents	_____
alopecia (815)	ăl-ō-PĒ-shē-ă	_____
alveolar (823)	ăl-vē-Ō-lăr _or_ ăl-VĒ-ō-lăr	_____
anaplasia (820)	ăn-ă-PLĀ-zē-ă	_____
antibiotics (820)	ăn-tĭ-bī-ŎT-ĭks	_____
antimetabolites (820)	ăn-tē-mĕ-TĂB-ō-līts	_____
antimitotics (820)	ăn-tĭ-mī-TŎT-ĭks	_____
apoptosis (820)	ăp-ō-TŌ-sĭs _or_ ā-pŏp-TŌ-sĭs	_____
benign tumor (820)	bē-NĪN TOO-mŏr	_____
bone marrow biopsy (826)	bōn MĂ-rō BĪ-ŏp-sē	_____
bone marrow transplantation (826)	bōn MĂ-rō trănz-plănt-Ā-shŭn	_____
brachytherapy (820)	brā-kē-THĔ-ră-pē	_____
cachexia (823)	kă-KĔK-sē-ă	_____
carcinogens (820)	kăr-SĬN-ō-jĕnz	_____
carcinoma (820)	kăr-sĭ-NŌ-mă	_____
carcinoma in situ (823)	kăr-sĭ-NŌ-ma ĭn SĪ-too	_____

TERM	PRONUNCIATION	MEANING
cauterization (812)	kăw-tĕr-ĭ-ZĀ-shŭn	_____
chemotherapy (820)	kē-mō-THĔR-ă-pē	_____
combination chemotherapy (820)	KŎM-bĭ-NĀ-shŭn kē-mō-THĔR-ă-pē	_____
core needle biopsy (827)	kŏr NĒ-dl BĪ-ŏp-sē	_____
cryosurgery (823)	krī-ō-SŬR-jĕr-ē	_____
cystic tumor (823)	SĬS-tĭk TOO-mŏr	_____
cytogenetic analysis (826)	sī-tō-jĕ-NĔT-ĭk ă-NĂL-ĕ-sĭs	_____
dedifferentiation (820)	dē-dĭf-ĕr-ĕn-shē-Ā-shŭn	_____
deoxyribonucleic acid (820)	dē-ŏx-ē-rī-bō-noo-KLĒ-ĭk ĂS-ĭd	_____
differentiation (820)	dĭf-ĕr-ĕn-shē-Ā-shŭn	_____
diffuse (810)	dĭ-FŪS	_____
dysplastic (824)	dĭs-PLĂS-tĭk	_____
electrocauterization (812)	ē-lĕk-trō-kaw-tĕr-ĕ-ZĀ-shun	_____
electron beams (820)	ē-LĔK-trŏn bēmz	_____
en bloc resection (812)	ĕn blŏk rē-SĔK-shŭn	_____
encapsulated (820)	ĕn-KĂP-sū-lāt-ĕd	_____
epidermoid (825)	ĕp-ĭ-DĔR-moyd	_____
excisional biopsy (812)	ek-SIZH-ŭn-ăl BĪ-ŏp-sē	_____
exenteration (812)	ĕks-ĕn-tĕ-RĀ-shŭn	_____
exfoliative cytology (827)	ĕks-FŌ-lē-ā-tĭv sī-TŎL-ō-jē	_____
external beam radiation (820)	ĕks-TĔR-năl bēm rā-dē-Ā-shŭn	_____
fiberoptic colonoscopy (827)	fī-bĕr-ŎP-tĭk kō-lōn-ŎS-kō-pē	_____
fibrosarcoma (823)	fī-brō-săr-KŌ-mă	_____
fibrosis (815)	fī-BRŌ-sĭs	_____
fields (820)	fēldz	_____
fine needle aspiration (812)	FĪN NĒ-dl ăs-pĕ-RĀ-shŭn	_____
follicular (823)	fō-LĬK-ū-lăr	_____
fractionation (820)	frăk-shă-NĀ-shŭn	_____

19

TERM	PRONUNCIATION	MEANING
fulguration (812)	fŭl-gū-RĀ-shŭn	_____
fungating tumor (823)	fŭng-GĀ-tĭng *or* FŬNG-gă-tĭng TOO-mŏr	_____
genetic screening (820)	jĕ-NĔT-ĭk SCRĒ-nĭng	_____
grading of tumors (821)	GRĀ-dĭng of TOO-mŏrz	_____
gray (Gy) (821)	grā	_____
hyperplasia (825)	hī-pĕr-PLĀ-zē-ă	_____
immunohistochemistry (836)	ĭm-ū-nō-hĭs-tō-KĔM-ĭs-trē	_____
immunotherapy (821)	ĭm-ū-nō-THĔ-ră-pē	_____
incisional biopsy (812)	ĭn-SĬZH-ŭn-ăl BĪ-ŏp-sē	_____
infertility (815)	ĭn-fĕr-TĬL-ĭ-tē	_____
infiltrative (821)	ĬN-fĭl-trā-tĭv	_____
invasive (821)	ĭn-VĀ-sĭv	_____
irradiation (821)	ĭr-rā-dē-Ā-shŭn	_____
laparoscopy (827)	lă-păr-ŎS-kō-pē	_____
linear accelerator (821)	LĬN-ē-ăr ăk-sĕl-ĕ-RĀ-tŏr	_____
malignant tumor (821)	mă-LĬG-nănt TOO-mŏr	_____
mammography (827)	mă-MŎG-ră-fē	_____
medullary tumor (823)	MĔD-ū-lār-ē TOO-mŏr	_____
mesenchymal (821)	mĕs-ĕn-KĪ-măl	_____
metastasis (821)	mĕ-TĂS-tă-sĭs	_____
mitosis (821)	mī-TŌ-sĭs	_____
mixed-tissue tumors (821)	MĬKSD TĬ-shū TOO-mŏrz	_____
modality (821)	mō-DĀL-ĭ-tē	_____
molecularly targeted therapy (821)	mō-LĔK-ū-lăr-lē TĂR-gĕt-ĕd THĔR-ā-pē	_____
morbidity (821)	mŏr-BĬD-ĭ-tē	_____
mucinous (821)	MŪ-sĭ-nŭs	_____

19

TERM	PRONUNCIATION	MEANING
mucositis (821)	mū-kō-SĪ-tĭs	
mutagenic (823)	mū-tă-JĔN-ĭk	
mutation (823)	mū-TĀ-shŭn	
myelosuppression (825)	mī-ĕ-lō-sū-PRĔ-shŭn	
necrotic tumor (823)	nĕ-KRŎT-ĭk TOO-mŏr	
neoadjuvant chemotherapy (821)	nē-ō-ĂD ū-vănt kē-mō-THĔR-ă-pē	
neoplasm (821)	NĒ-ō-plăzm	
neuroblastoma (825)	noo-rō-blăs-TŌ-mă	
neurofibromatosis (824)	noo-rō-fī-brō-mă-TŌ-sĭs	
nucleotide (821)	NOO-klē-ō-tīd	
oncogene (821)	ŎNGK-ō-jēn	
oncology (824)	ŏn-KŎL-ō-jē	
osteosarcoma (824)	ŏs-tē-ō-săr-KŌ-mă	
palliative (822)	PĂL-ē-ă-tĭv	
papillary (824)	PĂP-ĭ-lăr-ē	
pedunculated (822)	pĕ-DŬNG-kū-lāt-ĕd	
PET-CT scan (828)	PĔT-CT skăn	
photon therapy (822)	FŌ-tŏn THĔR-ă-pē	
pleomorphic (824)	plē-ō-MŎR-fĭk	
pneumonitis (815)	noo-mō-NĪ-tĭs	
polypoid tumor (824)	PŎL-ĭ-poyd TOO-mŏr	
protein marker tests (826)	PRŌ-tēn MĂRK-ĕr tĕsts	
protocol (824)	PRŌ-tō-kŏl	
proton therapy (822)	PRŌ-tŏn THĔR-ă-pē	
radiation (822)	rā-dē-Ā-shŭn	
radiocurable tumor (822)	rā-dē-ō-KŪR-ă-bl TOO-mŏr	
radionuclide scans (828)	rā-dē-ō-NOO-klīd skănz	
radioresistant tumor (822)	rā-dē-ō-rĕ-ZĬS-tănt TOO-mŏr	
radiosensitive tumor (822)	rā-dē-ō-SĔN-sĭ-tĭv TOO-mŏr	
radiosensitizers (822)	rā-dē-ō-SĔN-sĭ-tī-zĕrz	
radiotherapy (822)	rā-dē-ō-THĔR-ă-pē	

19

TERM	PRONUNCIATION	MEANING
relapse (822)	rē-LĂPS	
remission (822)	rē-MĬSH-ŭn	
retinoblastoma (825)	rĕt-ĭ-nō-blăs-TŌ-mă	
ribonucleic acid (RNA) (822)	rī-bō-noo-KLĒ-ik ĂS-ĭd	
sarcoma (822)	săr-KŌ-mă	
scirrhous (824)	SKĬR-ŭs	
secondary tumors (815)	SĔ-kŏn-dă-rē TOO-mŏrz	
serous (822)	SĒ-rŭs	
sessile (822)	SĔS-ĭl	
simulation (822)	sĭm-ū-LĀ-shŭn	
solid tumor (822)	SŎL-ĭd TOO-mŏr	
staging of tumors (822)	STĀ-jĭng of TOO-mŏrz	
stem cell transplantation (826)	stĕm sĕl trănz-plăn-TĀ-shŭn	
stereotactic radiosurgery (822)	stĕ-rē-ō-TĂK-tĭc rā-dē-ō-SŬR-jĕr-ē	
teletherapy (825)	tĕl-ē-THĔ-ră-pē	
ulcerating tumor (809)	ŬL-sĕ-rā-tĭng TOO-mŏr	
undifferentiated (810)	ŭn-dĭf-ĕr-ĔN-shē-ā-ĕd	
verrucous tumor (809)	vĕ-ROO-kŭs TOO-mŏr	
viral oncogenes (822)	VĪ-răl ŎNGK-ō-jēnz	
virus (822)	VĪ-rŭs	
xerostomia (824)	zĕr-ō-STŌ-mē-ă	

19

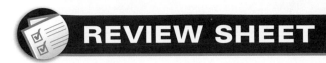

REVIEW SHEET

Write the meanings of the combining forms in the spaces provided and test yourself. Check your answers with the information in the chapter or in the *Glossary (Medical Word Parts—English)* at the end of the book.

Combining Forms

COMBINING FORM	MEANING	COMBINING FORM	MEANING
aden/o		mutagen/o	
alveol/o		necr/o	
cac/o		neur/o	
carcin/o		onc/o	
cauter/o		papill/o	
chem/o		pharmac/o	
cry/o		plas/o	
cyst/o		ple/o	
fibr/o		polyp/o	
follicul/o		radi/o	
fung/i		sarc/o	
medull/o		scirrh/o	
mucos/o		xer/o	
mut/a			

Suffixes

SUFFIX	MEANING	SUFFIX	MEANING
-ary		-ptosis	
-blastoma		-stasis	
-oid		-stomia	
-oma		-suppression	
-plasia		-therapy	
-plasm		-tion	

19

Prefixes

PREFIX	MEANING	PREFIX	MEANING
ana-	_____	epi-	_____
anti-	_____	hyper-	_____
apo-	_____	meta-	_____
brachy-	_____	tele-	_____
dys-	_____		

Write the terms used in cancer medicine next to their meanings below.

adjuvant chemotherapy   exenteration   protein markers
brachytherapy   external beam radiotherapy   protocol
cachexia   fine needle aspiration   sarcoma
carcinoma   metastasis   simulation
carcinoma in situ   myelosuppression

1. Cancerous tumor composed of cells of epithelial origin _____

2. Drug treatment given after primary treatment _____

3. Detailed plan of treatment _____

4. Study using CT scan or MRI to map the area to receive treatment before radiation therapy

   _____

5. Wide and complete resection of tumor in a cavity of the body _____

6. Cancerous tumor derived from connective (flesh) tissue _____

7. Chemicals in the blood that measure the presence of tumor in the body _____

8. General ill health and malnutrition associated with disease _____

9. Teletherapy _____

10. Insertion of radioactive seeds or sealed containers into tumor _____

11. Malignancy that is localized and not invasive _____

12. Cancerous tumor that has spread to lymph nodes and other organs _____

13. Stopping the growth of cells in the bone marrow _____

14. Extraction of cells for microscopic (biopsy) evaluation _____

19

Radiology and Nuclear Medicine

CHAPTER GOALS

- List the physical properties of x-rays.
- Identify diagnostic techniques used by radiologists and nuclear physicians.
- Name the x-ray views and patient positions used in x-ray examinations.
- Describe the role of radioactivity in the diagnosis of disease.
- Recognize medical terms used in the specialties of radiology and nuclear medicine.
- Apply your new knowledge to understanding medical terms in their proper contexts, such as medical reports and records.

INTRODUCTION

Radiology is the medical specialty concerned with the study and application of x-rays and other technologies (such as ultrasound and magnetic resonance) to produce and interpret images of the human body for the diagnosis of disease. **X-rays** are invisible waves of energy that are produced by an energy source (such as an x-ray machine or cathode ray tube) and are useful in the diagnosis and treatment of disease.

Nuclear medicine is the medical specialty that uses **radioactive substances** in the diagnosis and treatment of disease. These radioactive substances **(radionuclides)** are materials that emit high-speed particles and energy-containing rays from the interior of their matter. The emitted particles and rays are called **radioactivity** and can be of three types: **alpha particles, beta particles,** and **gamma rays. Gamma rays** are used effectively as a diagnostic label to trace the path and uptake of chemical substances in the body.

The professionals involved in these medical fields differ in practice and level of education or training. A **radiologist** is a physician who specializes in the practice of diagnostic radiology. A **nuclear medicine physician** specializes in diagnostic radionuclide scanning procedures.

Allied health care professionals who work with physicians in the fields of radiology and nuclear medicine are **radiologic technologists.** Different types of radiologic technologists are **radiographers,** who aid physicians in administering diagnostic x-ray procedures; **nuclear medicine technologists,** who attend to patients undergoing nuclear medicine procedures and operate devices under the direction of a nuclear physician; and **sonographers,** who aid physicians in performing ultrasound procedures.

RADIOLOGY

CHARACTERISTICS OF X-RAYS

Several characteristics of x-rays are useful to physicians in the diagnosis and treatment of disease. Some of these characteristics are the following:

1. **Ability to cause exposure of a photographic plate.** If a photographic plate is placed in front of a beam of x-rays, the x-rays, traveling unimpeded through the air, will expose the silver coating of the plate and cause it to blacken.
2. **Ability to penetrate different substances to varying degrees.** X-rays pass through the different types of substances in the human body (air in the lungs, water in blood vessels and lymph, fat around muscles, and metal such as calcium in bones) with varying ease. Air is the least dense substance and allows the greatest transmission. Fat is denser, water is next, followed by hard materials, such as calcium in bone, which is the densest and transmits least. If the x-rays are absorbed (stopped) by the denser body substance (e.g., calcium in bones), they do not reach the photographic plate held behind the patient, and white areas are left in the x-ray detector (plate). Figure 20-1 is an example of an x-ray photograph.

   A substance is said to be **radiolucent** if it permits passage of most of the x-rays. Lung tissue (containing air) is an example of a radiolucent substance, and it appears dark on an x-ray image. **Radiopaque** substances (bones) are those that absorb most of the x-rays they are exposed to, allowing only a small fraction of the x-rays to reach the x-ray plate. Thus, normally radiopaque, calcium-containing bone appears white on an x-ray image.
3. **Invisibility.** X-rays cannot be detected by sight, hearing, or touch. Workers exposed to x-rays must wear a **film badge** to detect and record the amount of radiation to which they have been exposed. The film badge contains a special film that reacts when

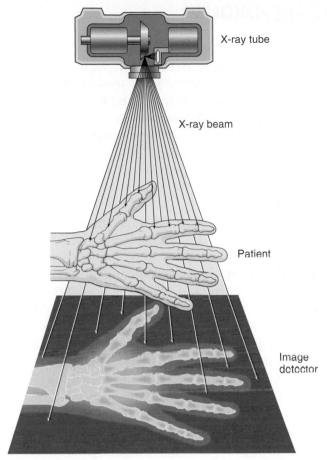

FIGURE 20-1   X-ray photograph (radiograph) of the hand. Relative positions of x ray tube, patient (hand), and image detector necessary to make the x-ray photograph are shown. Bones tend to stop (absorb) diagnostic x-rays, but absorption of the x-ray energy occurs to a lesser degree with soft tissue. This results in the light and dark regions that form the image.

exposed to x-rays. The amount of blackness on the film is an indication of the amount of x-rays or gamma rays received by the wearer.

4. **Travel in straight lines.** This property allows the formation of precise shadow images on the x-ray plate and also permits x-ray beams to be directed accurately at a tissue site during radiotherapy.

5. **Scattering of x-rays.** Scattering occurs when x-rays come into contact with any material. Greater scatter occurs with dense objects and less scatter with those substances that are radiolucent. In addition, because scatter can cause blurring (radiographic density that serves no useful purpose) on images, a grid (containing thin lead strips arranged parallel to the x-ray beams) is placed in front of the image detector to absorb scattered radiation before it strikes the x-ray film. In digital imaging, an image receptor replaces film.

6. **Ionization.** X-rays have the ability to ionize substances through which they pass. Ionization is a chemical process in which the energy of an x-ray beam causes rearrangement and disruption within a substance, so that previously neutral particles are changed to charged particles called **ions**. This strongly ionizing ability of x-rays is a double-edged sword. In x-ray or radiation therapy, the ionizing effect of high-energy x-ray beams can help kill cancerous cells and stop tumor growth; however, ionizing x-rays in even small doses can affect normal body cells, leading to tissue damage and malignant changes. Thus, persons exposed to high doses of x-rays are at risk for the development of leukemia, thyroid tumors, breast cancer, or other malignancies.

20

DIAGNOSTIC TECHNIQUES

X-Ray Studies

X-ray imaging is used in a variety of ways to detect pathologic conditions. **Digital radiography** is a form of x-ray imaging in which digital x-ray sensors are used instead of traditional photographic film. Thus images can be enhanced and transferred easily, and less radiation can be used than in conventional radiography. The chest x-ray is the most commonly performed diagnostic x-ray examination. Another common use of x-rays is in dental practice to locate caries in teeth. **Mammography** uses low-dose x-rays to visualize breast tissue. Some special diagnostic x-ray techniques are described next.

Computed Tomography (CT)

The CT scan, sometimes called "CAT scan" (because the technique originally was known as "computerized axial tomography"), is made by beaming x-rays at multiple angles through a section of the patient's body. The absorption of all of these x-rays, after they pass through the body, is recorded and used by a computer to create multiple cross-sectional images (Figure 20-2). The ability of a CT scanner to detect abnormalities is increased with the use of iodine-containing contrast agents, which outline blood vessels and confer additional density to soft tissues.

CT scanners are highly sensitive in detecting disease in bones and can actually provide images of internal organs that are impossible to visualize with ordinary x-ray technique. Figure 20-3 shows a series of CT scans through various regions of the body. New ultrafast CT scanners can produce a three-dimensional (3D) image of a beating heart and surrounding blood vessels. State-of-the-art scanners produce 64, 128, 256, and 320 images per rotation and are called **multidetector CT** or **MDCT scanners.**

Contrast Studies

In radiography, the natural differences in the density of body tissues (e.g., from air in lung or from calcium in bone) produce contrasting shadows on the radiographic image. However, when x-rays pass through two adjacent body parts composed of substances of the same density (e.g., different digestive organs in the abdomen), their shadows cannot be distinguished from one another on the film or on the screen. It is necessary, then, to place a **contrast medium** into the structure or fluid to be visualized so that a specific part, organ, tube, or liquid can be seen as a negative imprint on the dense contrast agent.

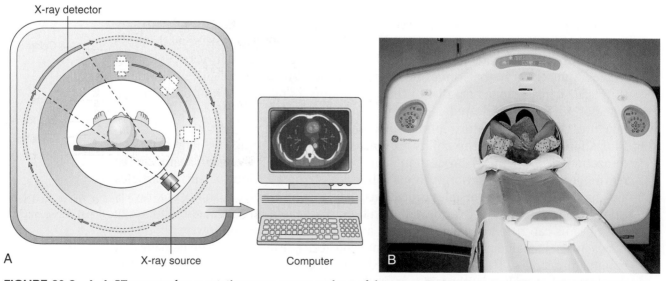

FIGURE 20-2   A, A CT scanner has a rotating x-ray source and set of detectors. B, A patient in a CT scanner. This patient has her arms above her head during a chest CT examination.

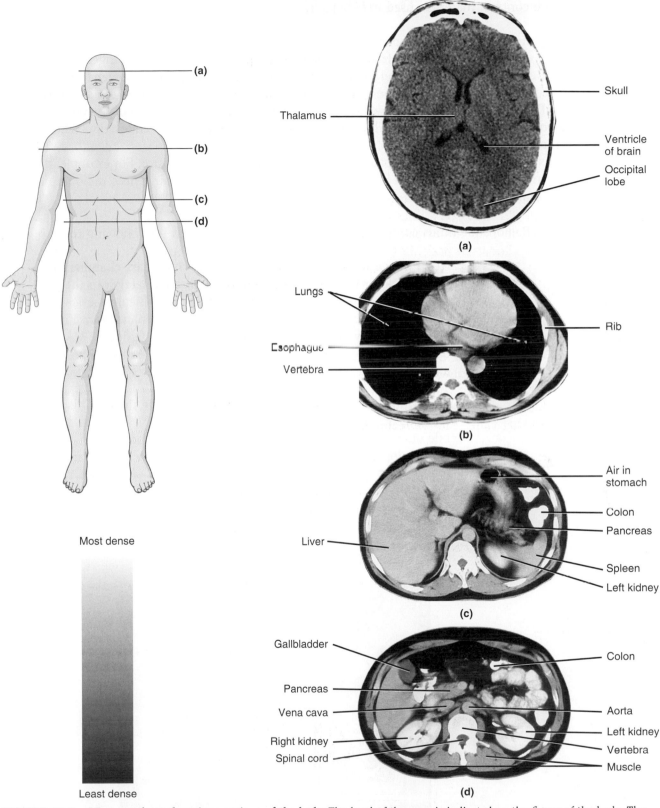

FIGURE 20-3 CT scans through various regions of the body. The level of the scan is indicated on the figure of the body. The *bar* below the figure indicates the gray scale of structure density from black (least dense, such as air) to white (most dense, such as bone).

The following are contrast materials used in diagnostic radiologic studies:

Barium Sulfate. Barium sulfate is a radiopaque substance that is mixed in water and used for examination of the upper and lower GI (gastrointestinal) tract. An **upper GI series (UGI)** involves oral ingestion of barium sulfate so that the esophagus, stomach, and duodenum can be visualized. A **small bowel follow-through (SBFT)** series traces the passage of barium in a sequential manner as it moves through the small intestine. A **barium enema (BE)** study is a lower GI series that opacifies the lumen (passageway) of the large intestine using an enema containing barium sulfate. This test has largely been replaced by endoscopy, which allows visualization of the inside of the bowel.

A **double-contrast study** uses both a radiopaque and a radiolucent contrast medium. For example, the walls of the stomach or intestine are coated with barium and the lumen is filled with air. These radiographs show the pattern of mucosal ridges.

Iodine Compounds. Radiopaque fluids containing up to 50% iodine are used in the following tests:

angiography	**X-ray image (angiogram) of blood vessels and heart chambers is obtained after contrast is injected through a catheter into the appropriate blood vessel or heart chamber.** In clinical practice, the terms angiogram and arteriogram are used interchangeably. Figure 20-4 shows **coronary angiography,** which determines the degree of obstruction of the arteries that supply blood to the heart. Figure 20-5A and B shows coronary angiograms before and after stenting of the artery.
cholangiography	**X-ray imaging after injection of contrast into bile ducts.** This is typically accomplished by injecting contrast directly into the common bile duct in a procedure called **endoscopic retrograde cholangiopancreatography (ERCP)** or after surgery of the gallbladder or biliary tract **(intraoperative cholangiography).** An alternative route for injection of contrast is via a needle through the skin and into the liver. This is **percutaneous transhepatic cholangiography** (Figure 20-6).

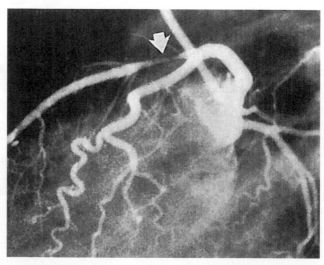

FIGURE 20-4 Coronary angiography shows stenosis (*arrow*) of the left anterior descending coronary artery.

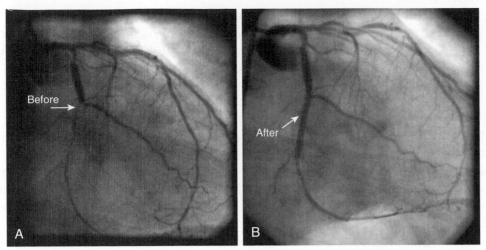

FIGURE 20-5   Coronary angiograms before and after stenting. A, Coronary angiogram before stenting shows narrowed coronary artery (*arrow*) preventing blood flow to the heart muscle. **B,** Coronary angiogram after stenting shows opening of coronary artery (*arrow*). (*Courtesy Dr. Daniel Simon and Mr. Paul Zampino.*)

digital subtraction angiography (DSA)	**X-ray image of contrast-injected blood vessels is produced by taking two x-ray pictures (the first without contrast) and using a computer to subtract obscuring shadows from the second image.**
hysterosalpingography	**X-ray record of the endometrial cavity and fallopian tubes is obtained after injection of contrast material through the vagina and into the endocervical canal.** This procedure determines the patency of the fallopian tubes.
myelography	**X-ray imaging of the spinal cord (myel/o) after injection of contrast agent into the subarachnoid space surrounding the spinal cord.** It usually is performed in patients who cannot undergo MRI (magnetic resonance imaging). After injection of contrast, x-ray films and a CT scan are obtained. This procedure is **CT myelography.**

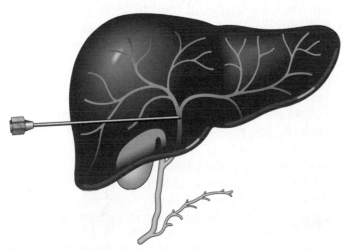

FIGURE 20-6   Percutaneous transhepatic cholangiography. The needle is passed through the abdominal wall into liver tissue until the tip penetrates the hepatic duct. Contrast medium is introduced, and x-ray pictures are taken to visualize the biliary tree.

pyelography

X-ray imaging of the renal pelvis and urinary tract. In **retrograde pyelography,** a catheter is placed through the urethra, bladder, or ureter and into the renal pelvis to inject contrast. **Urography** also describes the process of recording x-ray images of the urinary tract after the introduction of contrast.

Patients may experience side effects caused by iodine-containing contrast substances. These effects can range from mild reactions such as flushing, nausea, warmth, tingling sensations, or hives to severe, life-threatening reactions characterized by airway spasm, laryngeal edema (swelling of the larynx), vasodilation, and tachycardia. Treatment of severe reactions involves immediate establishment of an airway and ventilation followed by injections of epinephrine (adrenaline), corticosteroids, or antihistamines.

Digital imaging techniques can be used to enhance conventional and fluoroscopic x-ray images. A lower dose of x-rays is used to achieve higher-quality images, and digital images can be sent by way of networks to other locations and computer monitors so that many people can share information and assist in the diagnostic process.

Interventional Radiology. Interventional radiologists perform invasive procedures (therapeutic or diagnostic) usually under CT or ultrasound guidance or with fluoroscopic imaging. **Fluoroscopy** is the use of x-rays and a fluorescent screen to produce real-time video images. Procedures include percutaneous biopsy, placement of drainage catheters, drainage of abscesses, occlusion of bleeding vessels, and catheter instillation of antibiotics or chemotherapy agents. In addition, interventional radiologists perform **radiofrequency ablation** (destruction) of tumors and tissues (liver, kidney, lungs, and adrenals). Neurointerventional radiologists perform endovascular procedures including intracranial thrombolysis; head, neck, and intracranial tumor embolizations; extracranial angioplasty; and stenting. They also perform nonvascular procedures, such as intervertebral facet injections, nerve root blocks, and vertebroplasties. Vascular interventional radiologists perform laser treatments for varicose veins and uterine fibroid embolization.

Ultrasound Imaging

Ultrasound imaging, or **ultrasonography,** uses high-frequency inaudible sound waves that bounce off body tissues and are then recorded to give information about the anatomy of an internal organ. An instrument called a **transducer** or **probe** is placed near or on the skin, which is covered with a thin coating of gel to ensure good transmission of sound waves. The transducer emits sound waves in short, repetitive pulses. The ultrasound waves move through body tissues and detect interfaces between tissues of different densities. An echo reflection of the sound waves is formed as they hit the various body tissues and bounce back to the transducer.

These ultrasonic echoes are then recorded as a composite picture of the area of the body over which the instrument has passed. The record produced by ultrasound imaging is called a **sonogram.**

Ultrasound imaging is used as a diagnostic tool not only by radiologists but also by neurosurgeons and ophthalmologists to detect intracranial and ophthalmic lesions. Cardiologists use ultrasound techniques to detect heart valve and blood vessel disorders **(echocardiography),** and gastroenterologists use it to locate abdominal masses outside the digestive organs. Similarly, pulmonologists use ultrasound procedures for locating and sampling lesions outside the bronchial tubes. Obstetricians and gynecologists use ultrasound imaging to differentiate single from multiple pregnancies, as well as to help in performing amniocentesis. Other uses are to image benign and malignant tumors and

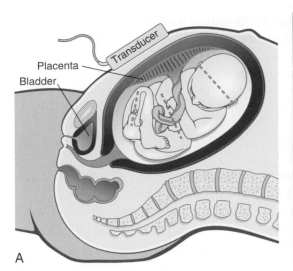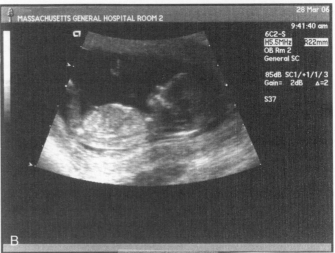

FIGURE 20-7   **A, Fetal measurements taken with ultrasound imaging.** Dashed lines indicate the image planes for measurements of the fetal head, abdomen, and femur. **B, Fetal ultrasound scan** at 13 weeks gestation. (**B,** *Courtesy Joelle Reidy.*)

to determine the size and development of the fetus. Measurements of the head, abdomen, and femur are made from ultrasound images obtained in various fetal planes (Figure 20-7).

Ultrasound imaging has several advantages in that the sound waves are not ionizing and do not injure tissues at the energy ranges used for diagnostic purposes. Because water is an excellent conductor of the ultrasound beams, patients are requested to drink large quantities of water before examination so that the urinary bladder will be distended, allowing better viewing of pelvic and abdominal organs.

Two ultrasound techniques, **Doppler ultrasound** and **color flow imaging,** make it possible to record blood flow velocity (speed). These techniques are used to image major blood vessels to detect obstructions caused by atherosclerotic plaques in patients at risk for stroke. Figure 20-8A and B shows Doppler ultrasound scanning and color flow imaging.

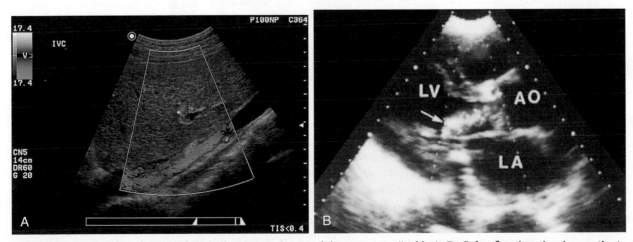

FIGURE 20-8   **A, Doppler ultrasound scan** showing an image of the vena cava (in *blue*). **B, Color flow imaging in a patient with aortic regurgitation.** The brightly colored, high-velocity jet (*arrow*) can be seen passing from the aorta (AO) to the left ventricle (LV). The center of the jet is *white*, and the edges are shades of *blue*.

Ultrasonography is used in interventional radiology to guide needle biopsy for the puncture of cysts, for placing needles during amniocentesis, and for inserting radioactive seeds into the prostate (brachytherapy). In **endoscopic ultrasonography,** a small ultrasound transducer is attached to the tip of an endoscope that is inserted into the body. This technique is used by gastroenterologists and pulmonologists to obtain high-quality and accurate detailed images of the digestive and respiratory systems.

Magnetic Resonance Imaging

Magnetic resonance imaging (MRI) uses magnetic fields and radiowaves rather than x-rays. Hydrogen protons are aligned and synchronized by placing the body in a strong magnetic field and exposing it to radiowaves. The rates of alignment and relaxation vary from one tissue to the next, producing a sharply defined picture. Because bone is virtually devoid of water, it is not well visualized on MRI. This technique produces sagittal (lateral), frontal (coronal), and axial (cross-sectional) images (Figure 20-9), as well as images in oblique (slanted) planes.

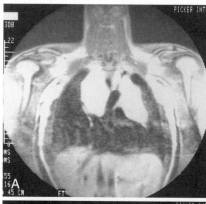
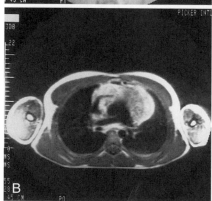
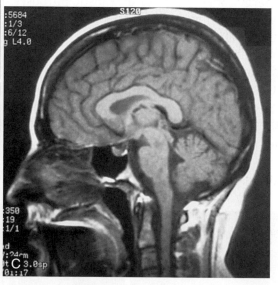

FIGURE 20-9 Magnetic resonance images. A, Frontal (coronal) view of the upper body. *White* masses in the chest are Hodgkin lymphoma lesions. **B, Axial (cross-sectional) view** of the upper body in the same patient, who had a chest mass. **C, Sagittal (lateral) view** of the head showing cerebrum, ventricles, cerebellum, and medulla oblongata.

MRI versus CT Scanning

Why do doctors choose MRI or CT scanning? Differences in use depend on the part of the body viewed. In general, CT is useful for visualizing bones, lungs, and solid masses of the chest and abdomen, whereas MRI is better at giving detail in soft tissues that have more water molecules.

CT
1. bones
2. chest lesions and pneumonia
3. bleeding in the brain from head trauma and ruptured arteries

MRI
1. spinal cord and brain tumors
2. joints, tendons, and ligaments
3. liver masses
4. head and neck lesions

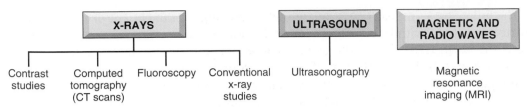

FIGURE 20-10 Summary of radiologic diagnostic techniques.

MRI examinations are performed with and without contrast. The contrast agent most commonly used is **gadolinium (Gd).** As iodine contrast does with CT, gadolinium enhances vessels and tissues, increases the sensitivity for lesion detection, and helps differentiate between normal and abnormal tissues and structures. MRI provides excellent soft tissue images, detecting edema in the brain, providing direct imaging of the spinal cord, detecting tumors in the chest and abdomen, and visualizing the cardiovascular system.

MRI is contraindicated for patients with pacemakers or metallic implants because the powerful magnet can alter position and functioning of such devices. However, the U.S. Food and Drug Administration (FDA) has recently approved new pacemakers that can be safely used with MRI. The sounds (loud tapping) heard during the test are caused by the pulsing of the magnetic field components as the device scans the body. See ***In Person: CT and MRI,*** page 868.

Figure 20-10 summarizes radiologic diagnostic techniques.

X-RAY POSITIONING

In order to take the best picture of the part of the body being radiographed, the patient, detector, and x-ray tube must be positioned in the most favorable alignment possible. Radiologists use special terms to refer to the direction of travel of the x-rays through the patient's body. Listed next are terms for radiographic views that are defined by the direction of the x-ray beam relative to the patient, who is positioned between the source and the detector; the relevant orientations are illustrated in Figure 20-11.

1. **Posteroanterior (PA) view.** In this most commonly requested chest x-ray view, x-rays travel from a posteriorly placed source to an anteriorly placed detector.
2. **Anteroposterior (AP) view.** X-rays travel from an anteriorly placed source to a posteriorly placed detector.
3. **Lateral view.** In a left lateral view, x-rays travel from a source located to the right of the patient to a detector placed to the left of the patient.
4. **Oblique view.** X-rays travel in a slanting direction at an angle from the perpendicular plane. Oblique views show regions or structures ordinarily hidden or superimposed in routine PA and AP views.

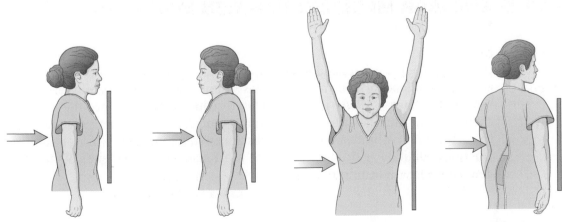

1. Posteroanterior (PA) view   2. Anteroposterior (AP) view   3. Left lateral view   4. Oblique view

FIGURE 20-11 **Positions for x-ray views.** The *arrow* denotes the direction of the x-ray beam through the patient's body.

The following terms are used to describe the position of the patient or part of the body in the x-ray examination:

abduction	Movement away from the midline of the body.
adduction	Movement toward the midline of the body.
decubitus	Lying down. A **lateral decubitus** position is lying down on the side.
eversion	Turning outward.
extension	Lengthening or straightening a flexed limb.
flexion	Bending a part of the body.
inversion	Turning inward.
pr<u>one</u>	Lying <u>on</u> the belly (face down).
recumbent	Lying down (may be prone or supine).
su<u>pine</u>	Lying on the back (face <u>up</u>).

NUCLEAR MEDICINE

RADIOACTIVITY AND RADIONUCLIDES

The spontaneous emission of energy in the form of particles or rays coming from the interior of a substance is called **radioactivity.** A **radionuclide** (or **radioisotope**) is a substance that gives off high-energy particles or rays as it disintegrates. Radionuclides are produced in either a nuclear reactor or a charged-particle accelerator (cyclotron) or by irradiating stable substances, causing disruption and instability. **Half-life** is the time required for a radioactive substance (radionuclide) to lose half of its radioactivity by disintegration. Knowledge of a radionuclide's half-life is important in determining how long the radioactive substance will emit radioactivity when in the body. The half-life must be long enough to allow for diagnostic imaging but as short as possible to minimize patient exposure to radiation.

Radionuclides emit three types of radioactivity: **alpha particles, beta particles,** and **gamma rays.** Gamma rays, which have greater penetrating ability than alpha and beta particles, and more ionizing power, are especially useful to physicians in both the diagnosis and the treatment of disease. **Technetium-99m** (^{99m}Tc) is essentially a pure gamma emitter with a half-life of 6 hours. Its properties make it the most frequently used radionuclide in diagnostic imaging.

NUCLEAR MEDICINE TESTS: IN VITRO AND IN VIVO PROCEDURES

Nuclear medicine physicians use two types of tests in the diagnosis of disease: **in vitro** (in the test tube) procedures and **in vivo** (in the body) procedures. **In vitro** procedures involve analysis of blood and urine specimens using radioactive chemicals. For example, a **radioimmunoassay (RIA)** is an in vitro procedure that combines the use of radioactive chemicals and antibodies to detect hormones and drugs in a patient's blood. The test allows the detection of minute amounts of substances or compounds. RIA is used to monitor the amount of digitalis, a drug used to treat heart disease, in a patient's bloodstream and can detect hypothyroidism in newborn infants.

In vivo tests trace the amounts of radioactive substances within the body. They are given directly to the patient to evaluate the function of an organ or to image it. For example, in **tracer studies,** a specific radionuclide is incorporated into a chemical substance and administered to a patient. The combination of the radionuclide and a drug or chemical is called a **radiopharmaceutical** (or **radiolabeled compound**). Each radiopharmaceutical is designed to concentrate in a certain organ. The organ can then be imaged using the radiation given off by the radionuclide.

A sensitive, external detection instrument called a **gamma camera** is used to determine the distribution and localization of the radiopharmaceutical in various organs, tissues, and fluids (Figure 20-12). The amount of radiopharmaceutical at a given location is proportional to the rate at which the gamma rays are emitted. Nuclear medicine studies depict the physiologic behavior (how the organ works) rather than the specific anatomy of an organ.

The procedure of making an image by tracking the distribution of radioactive substance in the body is **radionuclide scanning. Uptake** refers to the rate of absorption of the radiopharmaceutical into an organ or tissue.

Radiopharmaceuticals are administered by different routes to obtain a scan of a specific organ in the body. For example, during a **lung scan,** a radiopharmaceutical is given intravenously (**perfusion study)** so that the radioactive compound travels through the capillaries of the lungs, where it can be imaged. In a **ventilation study**, a radiolabeled gas or aerosol is inhaled to fill the air sacs (alveoli) before imaging. The combination of these tests, a **ventilation-perfusion study,** permits sensitive and specific diagnosis of clots in the lung arteries (pulmonary emboli).

Other diagnostic procedures that use radionuclides include the following:

1. **Bone scan.** Technetium-99m (Tc-99m) is used to label a phosphate-containing substance, which then is injected intravenously. The radioactive phosphate compound is taken up preferentially by bone, and the skeleton is imaged in 2 or 3 hours. Waiting 2 to 3 hours allows much of the radiopharmaceutical to be excreted in urine and allows for better visualization of the radioactive material remaining in the skeleton. The scan detects infection, inflammation, or tumors involving the skeleton, which appear as areas of high uptake ("hot spots") on the scan. See Figure 15-36 on page 622.

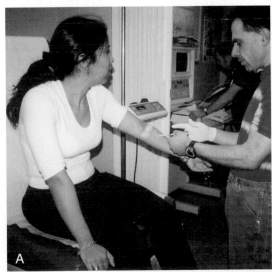
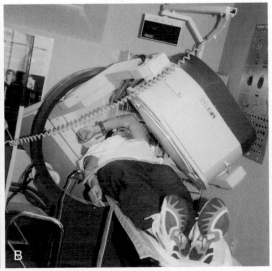

FIGURE 20-12   A, Patient receiving intravenous injection of radionuclide for detection of heart function. B, Gamma camera moves around the patient, detecting radioactivity in heart muscle.

2. **Lymphoscintigraphy.** ◤ This type of nuclear medicine imaging provides pictures (scintigrams) of the lymphatic system. A **radiotracer** (radioactive isotope) is injected under the skin, or deeper, using a small needle. A gamma camera then takes a series of images of an area of the body. Physicians perform lymphoscintigraphy to identify a **sentinel lymph node** (the first lymph node to receive lymph drainage from a tumor), identify areas of lymph node blockage, or evaluate lymphedema (accumulation of fluid in soft tissues leading to swelling).

3. **Positron emission tomography (PET or PET scan).** This radionuclide technique produces images of the distribution of radioactivity in the body through emission of positrons. It is similar to the CT scan, but radioisotopes are used instead of contrast and x-rays. After intravenous injection, the radionuclides are incorporated into the tissues and an image is made showing where the radionuclide is or is not being metabolized. The most common radionuclide is radiolabeled fluorodeoxyglucose (18F-FDG), but others are in use. PET scanning has determined that schizophrenics do not metabolize glucose equally in all parts of the brain and that drug treatment can bring improvement to these regions. Areas of metabolic deficiency can be pinpointed by PET, making it helpful in diagnosing and treating other neurologic disorders such as stroke, epilepsy, and Alzheimer disease. Areas of infection, inflammation, and tumor demonstrate increased metabolic activity, highlighted as hot spots on the PET scan (Figure 20-13).

4. **PET-CT scan.** This scan combines PET and CT techniques to produce a more accurate image than PET or CT alone. See Figure 20-14. It is often used to detect cancer and metastases, especially to determine if the cancer is responding to treatment.

5. **Single photon emission computed tomography (SPECT).** This technique involves an intravenous injection of radioactive tracer (such as Tc-99m) and the computer reconstruction of a 3D image based on a composite of many views. Clinical applications include detecting liver tumors, detecting cardiac ischemia, and evaluating bone disease of the spine.

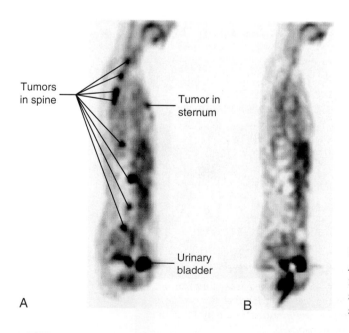

Tumors in spine

Tumor in sternum

Urinary bladder

A   B

FIGURE 20-13   Whole-body sagittal PET images.
A, 18F-FDG image obtained in a patient with breast cancer metastases. Numerous tumors (*dark spots*) are seen along the spine and sternum. **B, Image obtained after chemotherapy** shows regression of the cancer.

◤ **Scintigraphy**

Scintigraphy is the process of obtaining an image using a radioisotope. The term is derived from Latin *scintilla,* meaning spark. Bone scintigraphy is commonly called a bone scan, and lung scintigraphy is commonly called a lung scan.

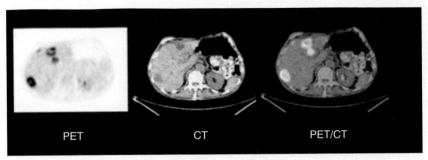

FIGURE 20-14   PET scan, CT scan, and PET-CT scan. *(Courtesy UPMC, University of Pittsburgh.)*

6. **Technetium Tc99m sestamibi (Cardiolite) scan.** For this scan, the technetium radiopharmaceutical is injected intravenously and traced to heart muscle. An exercise tolerance test (ETT) is used with it for an ETT-MIBI scan. In a **mu**ltiple **g**ated **acquisition (MUGA)** scan, Tc-99m is injected intravenously to study the motion of the heart wall muscle and the ventricle's ability to eject blood (ejection fraction).

7. **Thallium scan.** Thallium-201 (Tl-201) is injected intravenously to evaluate myocardial perfusion. A high concentration of Tl-201 is present in well-perfused heart muscle cells, but infarcted or scarred myocardium does not take up any thallium, showing up as "cold spots." If the defective area is ischemic, the cold spots fill in (become "warm") on delayed images (obtained later).

8. **Thyroid scan.** In a thyroid scan, an iodine radionuclide, usually iodine-123 (I-123), is administered orally, and the scan reveals the size, shape, and position of the thyroid gland. Alternatively, radioactive technetium can be administered intravenously. Hyperfunctioning thyroid nodules (adenomas) accumulate higher amounts of radioactivity and are termed "hot." Thyroid carcinoma does not concentrate radioiodine well and is seen as a "cold" spot on the scan. Figure 20-15 shows thyroid scans.

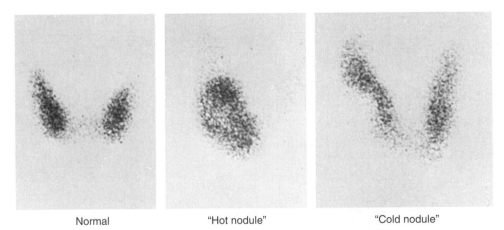

Normal   "Hot nodule"   "Cold nodule"

FIGURE 20-15   I-123 thyroid scans. The scan of a "hot nodule" shows a darkened area of increased uptake of radioactive iodine, which indicates an active nodule. Chances are very good that the nodule is benign. The scan of a "cold nodule" shows an area of decreased uptake, which indicates a nonfunctioning region, a common occurrence when normal tissue is replaced by malignancy.

20

NUCLEAR MEDICINE TESTS

IN VITRO	Radioimmunoassay

IN VIVO	**Tracer Studies:**
	Bone scan
	Lung scan (ventilation-perfusion)
	Lymphoscintigraphy
	PET/CT scan
	Positron emission tomography (PET)
	Radioactive iodine uptake (RAIU)
	Single photon emission computed tomography (SPECT)
	Technetium Tc 99m-sestamibi scan
	Thallium-201 scan
	Thyroid scan

FIGURE 20-16   In vitro and in vivo nuclear medicine diagnostic tests.

A **radioactive iodine uptake (RAIU)** study is performed to assess the function of the thyroid gland (such as hyperthyroidism). The patient is given radioactive iodine (in this case, I-131), also called radioiodine, in liquid or capsule form, and then a sensor is placed over the thyroid gland. It detects gamma rays emitted from the radioactive tracer, which is taken up by the thyroid more readily than by other tissues. Radioiodine also is used in larger doses to treat hyperthyroidism, thyroid nodules, or thyroid cancer. After the patient swallows the I-131, it is absorbed into the bloodstream and then travels to the thyroid gland, where it destroys overactive thyroid tissue.

Figure 20-16 reviews in vitro and in vivo nuclear medicine diagnostic tests.

20

 # VOCABULARY

This list reviews many of the new terms introduced in the text. Short definitions reinforce your understanding of the terms. Refer to the Pronunciation of Terms on page 876 for help with unfamiliar or difficult words.

computed tomography (CT)	Diagnostic x-ray procedure whereby a cross-sectional image of a specific body segment is produced. Newer CT scanners can create 3D images as well.
contrast studies	Radiopaque materials (contrast media) are injected to obtain contrast between tissues that would be indistinguishable from one another.
gamma camera	Machine to detect gamma rays emitted from radiopharmaceuticals during scanning for diagnostic purposes.
gamma rays	High-energy rays emitted by radioactive substances used in tracer studies.
half-life	Time required for a radioactive substance to lose half its radioactivity by disintegration.
interventional radiology	Therapeutic or diagnostic procedures performed by a radiologist. Examples are needle biopsy of a mass and drainage of an abscess, typically under the guidance of CT, ultrasound, or fluoroscopy.
in vitro	Process, test, or procedure is performed, measured, or observed outside a living organism, often in a test tube.
in vivo	Process, test, or procedure is performed, measured, or observed within a living organism.

ionization	Transformation of electrically neutral substances into electrically charged particles. X-rays cause ionization of particles within tissues.
magnetic resonance imaging (MRI)	Magnetic field and radio waves produce sagittal, coronal, and axial images of the body.
nuclear medicine	Medical specialty that uses radioactive substances (radionuclides) in the diagnosis and treatment of disease.
positron emission tomography (PET)	Positron-emitting radioactive substances given intravenously create a cross-sectional image of cellular metabolism based on local concentration of the radioactive substance. PET scans give information about metabolic activity.
radioimmunoassay	Test combines radioactive chemicals and antibodies to detect minute quantities of substances in a patient's blood.
radioisotope	Radioactive form of an element substance; radionuclide.
radiolabeled compound	Radiopharmaceutical; used in nuclear medicine studies.
radiology	Medical specialty concerned with the study of x-rays and their use in the diagnosis of disease. It includes other forms of energy, such as ultrasound and magnetic waves. Also called **diagnostic radiology.**
radiolucent	Permitting the passage of x-rays. Radiolucent structures appear black on x-ray images.
radionuclide	Radioactive form of an element that gives off energy in the form of radiation; radioisotope.
radiopaque	Obstructing the passage of x-rays. Radiopaque structures appear white on the x-ray images.
radiopharmaceutical	Radioactive drug (radionuclide plus chemical) that is administered safely for diagnostic and therapeutic purposes; a radiotracer. An example is technetium-99m, which combines with albumin (for lung perfusion) and DTPA (for renal imaging).
scan	Image of an area, organ or tissue of the body obtained from ultrasonography, radioactive tracer studies, computed tomography, or magnetic resonance imaging.
scintigraphy	Diagnostic nuclear medicine test using radiopharmaceuticals and gamma cameras to create images.
single photon emission computed tomography (SPECT)	Radioactive tracer is injected intravenously and a computer reconstructs a 3D image based on a composite of many views.
tagging	Attaching a radionuclide to a chemical and following its path in the body.
tracer studies	Radionuclides are used as tags, or labels, attached to chemicals and followed as they travel through the body.
ultrasonography (US, U/S)	Diagnostic technique that projects and retrieves high-frequency sound waves as they echo off parts of the body.
ultrasound transducer	Handheld device that sends and receives ultrasound signals.
uptake	Rate of absorption of a radionuclide into an organ or tissue.
ventilation-perfusion study (V/Q scan)	Consists of two scans: a ventilation scan performed using an inhaled radiopharmaceutical and a perfusion scan using an intravenously injected radiopharmaceutical. Used to evaluate for pulmonary embolism.

TERMINOLOGY

Write the meanings of the medical terms in the spaces provided.

COMBINING FORMS

COMBINING FORM	MEANING	TERMINOLOGY	MEANING
is/o	same	radioisotope _____ *Top/o means place; isotopes of an element have similar structures but different weights and stability. A radioisotope (radionuclide) is an unstable form of an element that emits radioactivity.*	
pharmaceut/o	drug	radiopharmaceutical _____ *In this term, radi/o stands for radioactive.*	
radi/o	x-rays	radiographer _____	
		radiology _____	
son/o	sound	hysterosonogram _____ *Saline solution is injected through a catheter inserted into the vagina and cervical canal to the uterus, which is then examined by ultrasound imaging.*	
therapeut/o	treatment	therapeutic _____	
vitr/o	glass	in vitro _____	
viv/o	life	in vivo _____	

SUFFIXES

SUFFIX	MEANING	TERMINOLOGY	MEANING
-gram	record	angiogram _____	
		hysterosalpingogram _____	
		pyelogram _____	
-graphy	process of recording	computed tomography _____ *Tom/o means to cut, as in viewing in slices.*	
-lucent	to shine	radiolucent _____ *Radiolucent (indicating that x-rays pass through easily) areas on x-ray images appear dark.*	
-opaque	obscure	radiopaque _____ *Radiopaque (indicating that x-rays do not penetrate) areas on x-ray images appear white/light.*	

20

PREFIXES

PREFIX	MEANING	TERMINOLOGY	MEANING
echo-	a repeated sound	echocardiography	_____
ultra-	beyond	ultrasonography	_____
		Sound waves are beyond the normal range of those that a human can hear.	

ABBREVIATIONS

Angio	angiography
AP	anteroposterior
Ba	barium
BE	barium enema
C-spine	cervical spine
CT	computed tomography
CXR	chest x-ray
Decub	decubitus—lying down
DICOM	digital image communication in medicine—standard protocol for storage and transmission of images between imaging devices (e.g., CT scans and PACS workstations)
DI	diagnostic imaging
DSA	digital subtraction angiography
ECHO	echocardiography
EUS	endoscopic ultrasonography
18F-FDG	fluorodeoxyglucose—radiopharmaceutical used in PET scanning; ^{18}F-FDG
Gd	gadolinium—MRI contrast agent
I-123	isotope of radioactive iodine—used in thyroid scans
I-131	isotope of radioactive iodine—used in diagnosis (thyroid scan) and treatment for thyroid cancer
IVP	intravenous pyelogram
KUB	kidneys-ureters-bladder (series)—x-ray imaging of these organs without contrast medium
LAT	lateral
LS films	lumbosacral (spine) films
L-spine	lumbar spine
MDCT	multidetector CT scanner

MR, MRI	magnetic resonance, magnetic resonance imaging
MRA	magnetic resonance angiography
MRV	magnetic resonance venography
MUGA	multiple-gated acquisition (scan)—radioactive test to show heart function
PA	posteroanterior
PACS	picture archival and communications system—replacement of traditional films with digital equivalents that can be accessed from several places and retrieved more rapidly
PET	positron emission tomography
PET-CT	positron emission tomography–computed tomography—both studies are performed using a single machine
RAIU	radioactive iodine uptake (test)—evaluates the function of the thyroid gland
RFA	radiofrequency ablation
SBFT	small bowel follow-through
SPECT	single photon emission computed tomography—radioactive substances and a computer are used to create 3D images
Tc-99m	radioactive technetium—used in heart, brain, thyroid, liver, bone, and lung scans
Tl-201	thallium-201—radioisotope used in scanning heart muscle
T-spine	thoracic spine
UGI	upper gastrointestinal (series)
US, U/S	ultrasound; ultrasonography
V/Q scan	ventilation-perfusion scan of the lungs (Q stands for rate of blood flow or blood volume)

IN PERSON: CT AND MRI

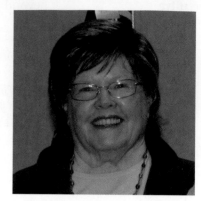

The following first-person narrative provides a detailed look at two common diagnostic procedures—CT and MRI—from the perspective of the patient. It was written by a 77-year-old woman with head and neck cancer.

CT—COMPUTED TOMOGRAPHY

Before an upcoming surgical procedure, I was told that I would need to have a CT scan. The doctors wanted to see if the cancer on my scalp had spread into the bones in my skull. They explained that these images of my head would be in thin "slices," taken as the CT camera rotated around me.

When I arrived in the room, I saw the CT machine. It was a large, circular hollow tube about 18 inches wide. There was a narrow table through the center. It was clear to me immediately that I would not have to worry about feeling "closed in." I lay down on the table, and the technician explained he would add contrast through an intravenous (IV) line halfway through the procedure.

The table was rolled into the machine to a specific spot where a series of pictures were taken. There were several short periods when I was asked to stay as still as possible and hold my breath. The noise was minimal, just soft whirring and clicking. Halfway through the procedure, I was slid out of the machine on the table so that the contrast could be added to the IV line. Once I was back in the machine, more pictures were taken and the test was completed with a minimum of discomfort, much to my grateful surprise.

MRI—MAGNETIC RESONANCE IMAGING

Before yet another surgery procedure, my doctors requested an MRI exam. This time, they wanted to get the best possible image of my malignant tumor and the surrounding area. They explained that the MRI and CT procedures are similar in that they both produce images in thin slices, but that MRI shows more detail, especially of soft tissue.

The technician confirmed I had nothing metal (such as a pacemaker or surgical screws) inside or on my body. The magnet that is used in the MRI machine is so strong that it could cause any metal objects to shift. This movement could disrupt the imaging process or cause damage to tissue in my body.

The MRI machine is a 6-foot-long round tube, open on both ends. Because the body part to be examined was my head, a rubber shield was placed over and very close to my face to hold me in the correct position. I was then rolled inside to the middle of the tube. This was really uncomfortable for me because I have mild claustrophobia. I took deep breaths to relax myself.

Although the technicians had told me the procedure would be loud, I was still taken aback by just how loud it was inside the tube. Even though I was wearing earplugs, the sound was like the pounding of huge hammers held by giant arms, or of heavy-duty jackhammers. At the same time, there was an abrupt shaking of the entire machine from side to side. I knew immediately that this could be an overwhelming experience, so I used the "relax-substitution" method to replace these violent sounds with more familiar ones. I remembered a very loud time as my family and I made our way to Nantucket Island on a ferry for a brief vacation. Now the previously strident and threatening sound was replaced by the welcoming sound of the ferry horn bellowing a happy welcome to the visitors' smiling faces as they came onto the ferry with straw hats, sunscreen, backpacks, and duffel bags. This relaxation method was extremely effective for me. I was then rolled out of the machine for addition of the IV contrast, and the process was repeated.

I am still amazed that the doctors could get such detailed information on what was going on inside my body using these two tests.

PRACTICAL APPLICATIONS

Answers to the questions are found on page 876.

CASE STUDY: MELANOMA FOLLOW-UP

Bill Smith, a 51-year-old sales representative, was initially diagnosed with stage III melanoma 4 years ago. He underwent surgery and received interferon treatment at that time. At his 3-month follow-up CT evaluation last year, Mr. Smith received bad news. The CT scan indicated a small 1-cm nodule that could be a melanoma metastasis. To confirm the diagnosis, Mr. Smith underwent a PET scan.

He was admitted to the nuclear medicine unit of the hospital on the morning of the scan. He had been instructed to fast (no food or beverage 12 hours before the scan). The nuclear medicine physician had told him especially not to eat any type of sugar, which would compete with the radiopharmaceutical 18F-FDG (radiolabeled fluorodeoxyglucose, ^{18}F-FDG), a radioactive glucose molecule that travels to every cell in the body.

The PET scan began with an injection of a trace amount of 18F-FDG by the physician. Bill was asked to lie still for about an hour in a dark, quiet room and to avoid talking to prevent the compound from concentrating in the tongue and vocal cords. The waiting time allowed the 18F-FDG to be absorbed and released from normal tissue. After emptying his bladder, Bill reclined on a bed that moved slowly and quietly through a PET scanner, a large tube similar to a CT scanner. The radioactive glucose emits charged particles called positrons, which interact with electrons, producing gamma rays that are in turn detected by the scanner. Color-coded images indicate the intensity of metabolic activity throughout the body. Cancerous cells absorb more radioactive glucose than noncancerous cells. The malignant cells show up brighter on the PET scan.

Bill's PET scan proved the CT wrong: His melanoma had not metastasized. He returned home quite relieved.

Questions about the Case Study: Melanoma Follow-up

1. In CT scanning:
   a. A radioactive tracer is used
   b. Magnetic images reveal images in all three planes of the body
   c. A nuclear physician performs the ultrasound procedure
   d. X-rays and a computer produce images in the axial plane

2. In PET scanning:
   a. A radioactive tracer is used
   b. X-ray images reveal images in all three planes of the body
   c. A nuclear physician performs the ultrasound procedure
   d. Doppler ultrasound is used

3. Bill's case showed that:
   a. CT scanning and PET scanning are equally effective in diagnosis of metastases
   b. PET scanning is useful in cancer diagnosis and staging
   c. Melanoma never progresses to stage IV
   d. A diet high in glucose helps concentrate the radioactive 18F-FDG before the PET scan

20

GENERAL HOSPITAL: NUCLEAR MEDICINE DEPARTMENT

Available Radionuclides

Radionuclide	Radiopharmaceutical	Administration Route	Target Organ
Xe-133	xenon gas	inhaled	lungs
Tc-99m	albumin microspheres	IV	lungs
Sr-87m (strontium)	solution	IV	bone
Tc-99m	diphosphonate	IV	bone
Tc-99m	pertechnetate	IV	brain
Tc-99m	sulfur colloid	IV	liver/spleen
Tc-99m	HIDA	IV	gallbladder
Tc-99m	DTPA	IV	kidney
Tc-99m	DMSA	IV	kidney
I-123	sodium iodide	PO	thyroid
I-131	sodium iodide	PO	thyroid
TI-201 (thallium)	thallium chloride	IV	heart
Tc-99m	sestamibi	IV	heart
Ga-67 (gallium)	gallium citrate	IV	tumors and abscesses

DMSA, dimercaptosuccinic acid; DTPA, diethylenetriaminepentaacetic acid; HIDA, N-(2,6-dimethyl)iminodiacetic acid; IV, intravenous; PO, oral (Latin per os, by mouth).

Questions about the General Hospital: Nuclear Medicine Department

1. Which radionuclide is used with sestamibi in an ETT of heart function?
   a. Thallium-201
   b. Iodine-131
   c. Gallium-67
   d. Technetium-99m

2. Which radionuclide would be used to diagnose disease in an endocrine gland?
   a. Ga-67
   b. I-123
   c. Xe-123
   d. Sr-87m

? EXERCISES

Remember to check your answers carefully with the Answers to Exercises, page 875.

A **Complete the medical terms based on the definitions and word parts given.**

1. Obstructing the passage of x-rays: radio _____

2. Permitting the passage of x-rays: radio _____

3. Aids physicians in performing ultrasound procedures: _____grapher

4. Transformation of stable substances into charged particles: _____ization

5. Radioactive drug administered for diagnostic purposes: radio _____

6. Radioactive chemical that gives off energy in the form of radiation: radio _____

7. A physician who specializes in diagnostic radiology: radi _____

8. Study of the uses of radioactive substances in the diagnosis of disease: _____ medicine

B **Match the special diagnostic techniques below with their definitions.**

computed tomography   magnetic resonance imaging
contrast studies   ultrasonography
interventional radiology

1. Radiopaque substances are given and conventional x-rays taken _____.

2. Use of echoes of high-frequency sound waves to diagnose disease _____.

3. A magnetic field and radio waves are used to form images of the body _____.

4. X-ray pictures are taken circularly around an area of the body, and a computer synthesizes the

   information into composite images _____.

5. Therapeutic procedures are performed by a radiologist under the guidance of CT, MRI, or

   ultrasonography _____.

C **Match the diagnostic x-ray test in Column I with the part of the body that is imaged in Column II.**

COLUMN I		COLUMN II
1. myelography	_____	A. spinal cord
2. retrograde pyelography	_____	B. uterus and fallopian tubes
3. angiography	_____	C. blood vessels
4. upper GI series	_____	D. esophagus, stomach, and small intestine
5. cholangiography	_____	E. lower gastrointestinal tract
6. barium enema	_____	F. urinary tract
7. hysterosalpingography	_____	G. bile vessels (ducts)

20

D Match the x-ray views or positions in Column I with their meanings in Column II. Write the letter of the answer in the space provided.

COLUMN I

1. PA _____

2. supine _____

3. prone _____

4. AP _____

5. lateral _____

6. oblique _____

7. lateral decubitus _____

8. adduction _____

9. inversion _____

10. abduction _____

11. recumbent _____

12. eversion _____

13. flexion _____

14. extension _____

COLUMN II

A. on the side
B. turned inward
C. movement away from the midline
D. lying on the belly
E. x-ray tube positioned on an angle
F. bending a part
G. straightening a limb
H. lying on the back
I. lying down on the side
J. lying down; prone or supine
K. anteroposterior view (front to back)
L. turning outward
M. posteroanterior view (back to front)
N. movement toward the midline

E Give the meanings of the following medical terms.

1. in vitro _____

2. in vivo _____

3. radiopharmaceutical _____

4. tracer studies _____

5. uptake _____

6. perfusion lung scan _____

7. ventilation lung scan _____

8. bone scan _____

9. thyroid scan _____

10. technetium Tc99m sestamibi scan _____

20

F **Give the meanings of the following terms.**

1. gamma camera _____

2. positron emission tomography (PET) _____

3. radioisotope _____

4. transducer _____

5. echocardiography _____

6. lymphoscintigraphy _____

7. radioactive iodine uptake test _____

8. PET-CT scan _____

G **Give the meanings of the following word parts.**

1. -gram _____   5. pharmaceut/o _____

2. ultra- _____   6. son/o _____

3. vitr/o _____   7. therapeut/o _____

4. viv/o _____

H **Give the meanings of the abbreviations in Column I, and then select the best association for each from Column II.**

COLUMN I	COLUMN II
1. MRI _____ ____	A. X-ray examination of the kidney after injection of contrast
2. SPECT _____ ____	B. Diagnostic procedure frequently used to assess fetal size and development
3. PACS _____ ____	C. X-ray examination of the esophagus, stomach, and intestines
4. UGI _____ ____	D. X-ray of blood vessels made by taking two images (with and without contrast) and subtracting the digitized data for one from the data for the other
5. CXR _____ ____	E. Radioisotope used in nuclear medicine (tracer studies)
6. DSA _____ ____	F. Radioactive substances and a computer used to create 3D images
7. RP _____ ____	G. Diagnostic procedure produces magnetic resonance images of all three planes of the body and visualizes soft tissue in the nervous and musculoskeletal systems
8. LAT _____ ____	H. Replacement of traditional films with digital equivalents
9. U/S _____ ____	I. X-ray view from the side
10. Tc-99m _____ ____	J. Diagnostic procedure (x-rays are used) necessary to investigate thoracic disease

Ⅰ Circle the correct boldface **terms to complete the sentences.**

1. Mr. Jones was scheduled for ultrasound-guided thoracentesis. He was sent to the **(interventional radiology, radiation oncology, nuclear medicine)** department for the procedure.

2. In order to better visualize Mr. Smith's small intestine, Dr. Wong ordered a **(perfusion study, SBFT, hysterosalpingography).** She hoped to determine why he was having abdominal pain and diarrhea.

3. After a head-on automobile collision, Sam was taken to the emergency department in an unconscious state. The paramedics suspected head trauma, and the doctors ordered an emergency **(PET scan, U/S, CT scan)** of his head.

4. In light of Sue's symptoms of fever, cough, and malaise, the doctors thought that the consolidated, hazy **(radioisotope, radiolucent, radiopaque)** area on the chest x-ray represented a pneumonia.

5. Fred, a lung cancer patient, experienced a seizure recently. His oncologist ordered a brain **(ultrasound, pulmonary angiogram, MRI),** which showed a tumor involving the left frontal lobe of the brain. Fred was treated with Gamma Knife irradiation, and the tumor decreased in size. He has had no further seizures.

6. Tom recently developed a cough and fever. A chest x-ray and **(CT, myelogram, IVP)** of the chest show that a **(pelvic, spinal, mediastinal)** mass is present. **(Mediastinoscopy, Cystoscopy, Lumbar puncture)** and biopsy of the mass reveal Hodgkin disease on histopathologic examination. He is treated with chemotherapy, and his symptoms disappear. A repeat x-ray shows that the mass has decreased remarkably, and a **(SPECT, MRI, PET)** scan shows no uptake of ^{18}F-FDG in the chest, indicating that the mass is fibrosis and not tumor.

7. Paola, a 50-year-old woman with diabetes, experiences chest pain during a stress test, and her **(U/S, ECG, EEG)** shows evidence of ischemia. A **(contrast agent, transducer, radiopharmaceutical)** called technetium Tc99m sestamibi (Cardiolite) is injected intravenously, and uptake is assessed with a **(probe, CT scanner, gamma camera)**, which shows an area of poor perfusion in the left ventricle.

8. Sally has a routine pelvic examination, and her **(neurologist, gynecologist, urologist)** detects an irregular area of enlargement in the anterior wall of the uterus. A pelvic **(angiogram, U/S study, PET scan)** is performed, which demonstrates the presence of fibroids in the uterine wall. The examination involves placing a gel over her abdominopelvic area and applying a **(ultrasound transducer, radionuclide, MRI scanner)** to send/receive sound vibrations to/from the pelvic region.

9. Sally was having palpitations in the early evening. An ECG revealed possible left ventricular hypertrophy. Her physician ordered an **(ECHO, EUS, UGI)** to rule out valvular heart disease.

10. Joe, a 75-year-old man with a long smoking history, noticed blood in his sputum. His primary care physician ordered a/an **(abdominal CT, chest CT, ultrasound of his heart)** for further evaluation.

20

ANSWERS TO EXERCISES

A

1. radiopaque
2. radiolucent
3. sonographer
4. ionization
5. radiopharmaceutical
6. radioisotope or radionuclide
7. radiologist
8. nuclear

B

1. contrast studies
2. ultrasonography
3. magnetic resonance imaging
4. computed tomography
5. interventional radiology

C

1. A
2. F
3. C
4. D
5. G
6. E
7. B

D

1. M
2. H
3. D
4. K
5. A
6. E
7. I
8. N
9. B
10. C
11. J
12. L
13. F
14. G

E

1. process, test, or procedure in which something is measured or observed outside a living organism
2. process, test, or procedure in which something is measured or observed in a living organism
3. radioactive drug (radionuclide plus chemical) that is given for diagnostic or therapeutic purposes
4. tests in which radioactive substance (radioisotopes) are administered with chemicals and followed as they travel throughout the body
5. the rate of absorption of a radionuclide into an organ or tissue
6. imaging technique in which a radiopharmaceutical is injected intravenously and traced within the blood vessels of the lung scanned
7. imaging technique in which a radiopharmaceutical is inhaled and its passage through the respiratory tract is traced on a scan
8. imaging technique in which a radiopharmaceutical is given intravenously and taken up by bone tissue, followed by scanning to detect the amount of the radioactive substance in the bone
9. imaging technique in which a radioactive substance is given orally and a scan (image) is made to assess its uptake in the thyroid gland
10. test of heart muscle function

F

1. machine that detects rays emitted by radioactive substances
2. radioactive glucose is injected and traced to body cells
3. a radioactive form (radionuclide) of a substance; gives off radiation
4. handheld device that sends and receives ultrasound signals
5. ultrasound is used to create an image of the heart
6. nuclear medicine imaging of the lymphatic system
7. nuclear medicine test to evaluate the function of the thyroid gland
8. combination of a PET scan and a CT scan to show both structure and function of the body

G

1. record
2. beyond
3. glass
4. life
5. drug
6. sound
7. treatment

20

H

1. magnetic resonance imaging: G
2. single photon emission computed tomography: F
3. picture archival and communications system: H

4. upper gastrointestinal (series): C
5. chest x-ray: J
6. digital subtraction angiography: D
7. retrograde pyelogram: A

8. lateral: I
9. ultrasound: B
10. radioactive technetium: E

I

1. interventional radiology
2. SBFT (small bowel follow-through)
3. CT scan
4. radiopaque
5. MRI

6. CT, mediastinal, mediastinoscopy, PET
7. ECG, radiopharmaceutical, gamma camera

8. gynecologist, U/S, transducer
9. ECHO
10. chest CT

Answers to Practical Applications

Case Study: Melanoma Follow-up
1. d
2. a
3. b

General Hospital: Nuclear Medicine Department
1. d
2. b

PRONUNCIATION OF TERMS

To test your understanding of the terminology in this chapter, write the meaning of each term in the space provided. In addition, you may wish to cover the terms and write them by looking at your definitions. Make sure your spelling is correct. The page number after each term indicates where it is defined or used in the book, so you can easily check your responses. You will find complete definitions for all of these terms and their audio pronunciations on the Evolve website.

Pronunciation Guide

ā as in āpe   ă as in ăpple
ē as in ēven   ĕ as in ĕvery
ī as in īce   ĭ as in ĭnterest
ō as in ōpen   ŏ as in pŏt
ū as in ūnit   ŭ as in ŭnder

TERM	PRONUNCIATION	MEANING
abduction (860)	ăb-DŬK-shŭn	
adduction (860)	ă-DŬK-shŭn	
angiogram (866)	ĂN-jē-ō-grăm	
anteroposterior (859)	ăn-tĕr-ō-pōs-TĒ-rē-ŏr	
bone scan (861)	bōn skăn	
cholangiography (854)	kō-lăn-jē-ŎG-ră-fē	
computed tomography (864)	kŏm-PŪ-tĕd tō-MŎG-ră-fē	
contrast studies (864)	KŎN-trăst STŬD-ēz	
decubitus (860)	dĕ-KŪ-bĭ-tŭs	
echocardiography (867)	ĕk-ō-kăr-dē-ŎG-ră-fē	
eversion (860)	ē-VĔR-zhŭn	
extension (860)	ĕk-STĔN-shŭn	
flexion (860)	FLĔK-shŭn	

TERM	PRONUNCIATION	MEANING
fluoroscopy (856)	floo-RŎS-kō-pē	
gamma camera (864)	GĂ-mă KĂM-ĕr-ă	
gamma rays (864)	GĂ-mă rāz	
half-life (860)	HĂF-līf	
hysterosalpingogram (866)	hĭs-tĕr-ō-săl-PĬNG-gō-grăm	
hysterosonogram (866)	hĭs-tĕr-ō-SŎN-ō-grăm	
interventional radiology (864)	ĭn-tĕr-VĔN-shŭn-ăl rā-dē-ŎL-ō-jē	
inversion (860)	ĭn-VĔR-zhŭn	
in vitro (864)	ĭn VĒ-trō	
in vivo (864)	ĭn VĒ-vō	
ionization (865)	ī ŏn ĭ-ZĀ-shŭn	
lymphoscintigraphy (862)	lĭm-fō-sĭn-TĬG-ră-fē	
magnetic resonance imaging (865)	măg-NĔT-ĭk RĔZ-ō-năns ĬM-ă-jĭng	
myelography (855)	mī-ĕ-LŎG-ră-fē	
nuclear medicine (865)	NOO-klē-ăr MĔD-ĭ-sĭn	
oblique (859)	ŏ-BLĒK	
PET-CT scan (862)	PĔT-CT scăn	
positron emission tomography (865)	PŎS-ĭ-trŏn ē-MĬSH-ŭn tō-MŎG-ră-fē	
posteroanterior (859)	pōs-tĕr-ō-ăn-TĒ-rē-ŏr	
prone (860)	prōn	
pyelogram (866)	PĪ-ē-lō-grăm	
radiographer (866)	rā-dē-ŎG-ră-fĕr	
radioimmunoassay (865)	rā-dē-ō-ĭ-mū-nō-ĂS-ā	
radioisotope (865)	rā-dē-ō-Ī-sō-tōp	
radiolabeled compound (865)	rā-dē-ō-LĀ-bĕld KŎM-pownd	
radiology (865)	rā-dē-ŎL-ō-gē	
radiolucent (865)	rā-dē-ō-LOO-sĕnt	
radionuclide (865)	rā-dē-ō-NOO-klīd	

20

TERM	PRONUNCIATION	MEANING
radiopaque (865)	rā-dē-ō-PĀK	
radiopharmaceutical (865)	rā-dē-ō-făr-mă-SOO-tĭ-kăl	
recumbent (860)	rē-KŬM-bĕnt	
scan (865)	scăn	
scintigraphy (865)	SĬN-tĕ- gră-fē	
single photon emission computed tomography (865)	SĬNG-l PHŌ-tŏn ē-MĬ-shŭn kŏm-PŪ-tĕd tō-MŎG-ră-fē	
sonogram (856)	SŎN-ō-grăm	
supine (860)	SOO-pīn	
tagging (865)	TĂG-ĭng	
technetium Tc99m sestamibi scan (863)	tĕk-NĒ-shē-ŭm Tc99m sĕs-tă-MĬ-bē skăn	
thallium scan (863)	THĂL-ē-ŭm skăn	
therapeutic (866)	thĕr-ă-PŪ-tik	
thyroid scan (863)	THĪ-rŏyd skăn	
tracer studies (865)	TRĀ-sĕr STŬ-dēz	
ultrasonography (865)	ŭl-tră-sō-NŎG-ră-fē	
ultrasound transducer (865)	ŭl-tră-SOWND trănz-DOO-sĕr	
uptake (865)	ŬP-tāk	
urography (856)	ū-RŎG-ră-fē	
ventilation-perfusion study (865)	vĕn-tĭ-LĀ-shŭn-pĕr-FŪ-zhŭn STŬ-dē	

20

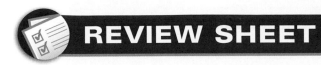

REVIEW SHEET

Write the meanings of the combining forms in the spaces provided, and test yourself. Check your answers with the information in the text or in the **Glossary (Medical Word Parts—English)** at the end of the book.

Combining Forms

COMBINING FORM	MEANING	COMBINING FORM	MEANING
ion/o		son/o	
is/o		therapeut/o	
myel/o		vitr/o	
pharmaceut/o		viv/o	
radi/o			

Suffixes

SUFFIX	MEANING	SUFFIX	MEANING
-gram		-lucent	
-graphy		-opaque	

Prefixes

PREFIX	MEANING	PREFIX	MEANING
echo-		ultra-	

20

Give meanings for the following patient positions or movements:

1. abduction _____

2. adduction _____

3. decubitus _____

4. eversion _____

5. extension _____

6. flexion _____

7. inversion _____

8. prone _____

9. recumbent _____

10. supine _____

20

Match the following abbreviations used in nuclear medicine with their diagnostic uses. Write each abbreviation on the line provided. Check your answers on pg 867.

18F-FDG   Tl-201   V/Q scan
Tc-99m   MUGA   RAIU

_____ Lung study to diagnose a pulmonary embolus

_____ Radiopharmaceutical used in a PET scan

_____ Radioisotope used in scanning heart muscle

_____ Study to evaluate the function of the thyroid gland

_____ Study to evaluate the function of the heart muscle

_____ Radioisotope used in multiple organ scans

evolve *Please refer to the Evolve website for additional exercises, games, and images related to this chapter.*

Pharmacology

Chapter Sections:

CHAPTER GOALS

- Describe the various subspecialty areas of pharmacology.
- Identify the various routes and schedule of drug administration.
- Differentiate among the various classes of drugs and name their primary actions and side effects.
- Define medical terms using combining forms and prefixes that relate to pharmacology.
- Apply your new knowledge to understanding medical terms in their proper contexts, such as medical reports and records.

INTRODUCTION

Drugs (medicines) are substances used to prevent or treat a disease or condition. Some drugs are obtained from **plants** such as the roots, leaves, and fruit. An example of a plant-derived drug is a cardiac medicine, digitalis (from the foxglove plant). Other drugs (antibiotics such as penicillin) are derived from molds. Drugs also are obtained from **animals.** For example, some pharmaceutical hormones are secretions from the glands of animals, and antivenoms are prepared from the venom of snakes, spiders, or other species with poisonous bites or stings. Virtually all drugs are **synthesized** for commercial purposes in a laboratory. **Vitamins** are drugs that are isolated from plant or animal sources and are contained in foods.

A **pharmacist** prepares and dispenses drugs through a **pharmacy** (drugstore) on a written order from a physician. The order is called a **prescription**. Currently, most schools or colleges of pharmacy offer a PharmD (doctor of pharmacy) degree after 6 years of study. As a health care professional, a pharmacist cooperates with, consults with, and sometimes advises licensed practitioners concerning drugs. In addition, the pharmacist answers patients' questions about their prescription. A **pharmacy technician** helps licensed pharmacists provide medication and other health care products to patients.

Pharmacology is the study of the discovery, properties, and uses of drugs. A **pharmacologist** is either an MD (doctor of medicine) or a PhD (doctor of philosophy) who specializes in the study of medicines. Pharmacology contains many subdivisions of study: **medicinal chemistry, pharmacodynamics, pharmacokinetics, molecular pharmacology, chemotherapy,** and **toxicology.**

Medicinal chemistry is the study of new drug synthesis and the relationship between chemical structure and biologic effects. **Pharmacodynamics** involves the study of a drug's effects in the body. **Pharmacokinetics** is the study of a drug's absorption (how drugs pass into the bloodstream), distribution into body compartments, metabolism (changes that drugs undergo within the body), and excretion (removal of the drug from the body) over a period of time.

Molecular pharmacology involves the interaction of drugs and subcellular entities, such as DNA, RNA, and enzymes. It provides important information about the mechanism of action of drugs.

Chemotherapy is the study of drugs that destroy microorganisms, parasites, or malignant cells within the body. Chemotherapy includes treatment of infectious diseases and cancer.

Toxicology is the study of the harmful effects of drugs and chemicals on the body. Toxicologic studies are conducted in animals, as required by law, before new drugs can be tested in humans. A toxicologist also is interested in finding proper **antidotes** to any harmful effects of drugs. Antidotes are substances given to neutralize unwanted effects of drugs.

Figure 21-1 reviews the subspecialty areas of pharmacology.

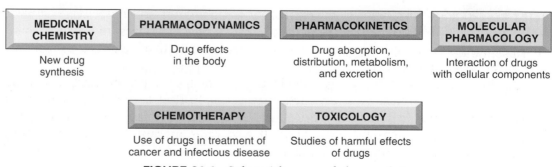

FIGURE 21-1 Subspecialty areas of pharmacology.

DRUG NAMES, STANDARDS, AND REFERENCES

NAMES

A drug can have three different names. The **chemical name** specifies the exact chemical makeup of the drug. This name often is long and complicated.

The **generic name,** typically shorter and less complicated, identifies the drug legally and scientifically. The generic name becomes public property after 17 years of use by the original manufacturer, and any drug manufacturer may use it thereafter. There is only one generic name for each drug.

The **brand name** or trademark is the private property of the individual drug manufacturer, and no competitor may use it. A brand name (also called trade name) often has the superscript ® after or before the name, indicating that it is a registered brand name. Drugs can have several brand names, because each manufacturer producing the drug gives it a different name. When a specific brand name is ordered on a prescription by a physician, it must be dispensed by the pharmacist; no other brand name may be substituted. It is usual practice to capitalize the first letter of a brand name.

The following example shows the chemical, generic, and brand names for the antibiotic drug amoxicillin; note that the drug has several brand names but only one generic, or official, name:

CHEMICAL NAME	GENERIC NAME	BRAND NAMES
[2S,5R,6R]-6-[(R)-(–)-2-amino-2-(p-hydroxyphenyl) acetamido]-3,3-dimethyl-7-oxo-4-thia-1-azabicyclo[3.2.0] heptane-2-carboxylic acid	amoxicillin	Amoxil Polymox Trimox

STANDARDS

The U.S. **Food and Drug Administration (FDA)** has the legal responsibility for deciding whether a drug may be distributed and sold. It sets strict standards for efficacy (effectiveness), safety, and purity. The FDA requires extensive experimental testing in animals and people before it approves a new drug for sale for a specific medical use. An independent committee of physicians, pharmacologists, pharmacists, and manufacturers, called the **United States Pharmacopeia (USP),** reviews the available commercial drugs and continually reappraises their effectiveness in specific medical conditions.

REFERENCES

Two large reference listings of drugs are available at libraries and hospitals. The most complete and up-to-date listing is the **hospital formulary,** which gives information about the characteristics of drugs and their clinical usage (application to patient care) as approved by that particular hospital.

The *Physicians' Desk Reference* **(PDR)** is published by a private firm, and drug manufacturers pay to have their products listed. The PDR is a useful reference with several different indices to identify drugs, along with a complete description of the drug's properties and approved indications. It also gives precautions, warnings about side effects, and information about the recommended dosage and administration of each drug.

21

ADMINISTRATION OF DRUGS

The route of administration of a drug (how it is taken into the body) determines how well it is absorbed into the blood, and its speed and duration of action.

Various methosds of administering drgus are:

Oral administration. Drugs given by mouth are slowly absorbed into the bloodstream through the stomach or intestinal wall. This method, although convenient for the patient, has several disadvantages. If the drug is destroyed in the digestive tract by digestive juices, or if the drug is unable to pass through the intestinal wall, it will be ineffective. Oral administration is also a disadvantage if a rapid onset of action is desired. It takes several hours for oral medication to be fully absorbed into the bloodstream.

Sublingual administration. Drugs placed under the tongue dissolve in the saliva. For some agents, absorption may be rapid. Nitroglycerin tablets are administered in this way to treat attacks of angina (chest pain).

Rectal administration. Suppositories (cone-shaped objects containing drugs) and aqueous solutions are inserted into the rectum. Drugs are given by rectum when oral administration presents difficulties, as when the patient is nauseated and vomiting.

Parenteral administration. Injection of drug from a **syringe** (tube) through a hollow needle placed under the skin, into a muscle, vein, or body cavity. There are several types of parenteral injections and instillations:

1. **Intracavitary instillation.** This injection is made into a body cavity, such as the peritoneal or pleural cavity. For example, drugs may be introduced into the pleural cavity in people who have pleural effusions due to malignant disease. The drug causes the pleural surfaces to adhere, thereby obliterating the pleural space and preventing the accumulation of fluid. This procedures is known as **pleurodesis.**
2. **Intradermal injection.** This shallow injection is made into the upper layers of the skin and is used chiefly in skin testing for allergic reactions.
3. **Subcutaneous (hypodermic) injection (subQ).** A small hypodermic needle is introduced into the subcutaneous tissue under the skin, usually on the upper arm, thigh, or abdomen. Insulin is injected daily via this route.
4. **Intramuscular injection (IM).** The buttock or upper arm is the usual site for this injection into muscle. When drugs are irritating to the skin or when a large volume of solution must be administered, IM injections are used.
5. **Intrathecal instillation.** This instillation is into the space under the membranes (meninges) surrounding the spinal cord and brain. Methotrexate (a cancer chemotherapeutic drug) is introduced intrathecally for treatment of leukemia involving the spinal canal.
6. **Intravenous injection (IV).** This injection is given directly into a vein. It is used when an immediate effect from the drug is desired or when the drug is poorly absorbed into the bloodstream after oral administration. Good technical skill is needed with intravenous injections because leakage of a drug into surrounding tissues may result in irritation and inflammation. Some medicines, such as anticancer drugs, are dissolved in a large volume of fluid and given by a several-hour-long intravenous infusion.

Inhalation. Vapors, or gases, taken into the nose or mouth are absorbed into the bloodstream through the thin walls of air sacs in the lungs. **Aerosols** (particles of drug suspended in air) are administered by inhalation, as are many anesthetics. Aerosolized medicines are used to treat asthma (spasm of the lung airways).

TABLE 21-1	ROUTES OF DRUG ADMINISTRATION					
ORAL	**SUBLINGUAL**	**RECTAL**	**PARENTERAL**		**INHALATION**	**TOPICAL**

Caplets
Capsules
Tablets
	Tablets	Suppositories	Injections and instillations
			   Intracavitary
			   Intradermal
			   Intramuscular (IM)
			   Intrathecal
			   Intravenous (IV)
			   Subcutaneous (subQ)
					Aerosols	Lotions
						Creams
						Ointments
						Transdermal
						   patches

Topical application. Drugs are applied locally on the skin or mucous membranes of the body. **Antiseptics** (against infection) and **antipruritics** (against itching) commonly are used as ointments, creams, and lotions. **Transdermal patches** are used to deliver drugs (such as estrogen for hormone replacement therapy, slow-release pain medications, and nicotine for smoking cessation programs) continuously through the skin.

Table 21-1 summarizes the various routes of drug administration. Figure 21-2 illustrates examples of vehicles for drug administration.

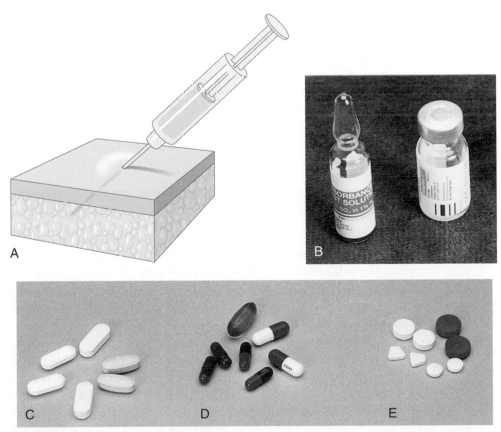

FIGURE 21-2   Examples of vehicles for drug administration. A, Hypodermic syringe. B, Ampule (small, sterile glass or plastic container containing a single dose of drug) and **vial** (glass container with a metal-enclosed rubber seal). **C, Caplets** (coated like a capsule, but solid like a tablet). **D, Capsules** (small soluble containers, usually made of gelatin, with a dose of medication). **E, Tablets** (small solid pills containing a dose of medication).

DRUG ACTIONS AND INTERACTIONS

When a drug enters the body, it produces its effect by interacting with a specific target, or **receptor**. A drug may cross the cell membrane to reach its intracellular receptor or may react with a receptor on the cell's surface. The **dose** of a drug is the amount of drug administered, usually measured in milligrams or grams. **Schedule** is the exact timing and frequency of drug administration.

Various actions and interactions of drugs in the body can occur after they have been absorbed into the bloodstream.

Additive action. If the combination of two similar drugs is equal to the **sum** of the effects of each, then the drugs are called additive. For example, if drug A gives 10% tumor kill as a chemotherapeutic agent and drug B gives 20% tumor kill, using A and B together would give 30% tumor kill.

If two drugs give less than an additive effect, they are called **antagonistic.** If they produce greater than additive effects, they are **synergistic** (as described next).

Synergism. A combination of two drugs sometimes can cause an effect that is **greater** than the sum of the individual effects of each drug given alone. For example, INH (isoniazid) and rifampin, two antibiotic drugs, are given together in the treatment of tuberculosis because of their synergistic action to cure the disease. Individually, the drugs are not as effective.

Response. This is a desired and beneficial effect of a drug. Lowering blood pressure by antihypertensive drugs is an example.

Tolerance. For some drugs, the effects of a given dose diminish as treatment continues, and increasing amounts are needed to produce the same effect. Tolerance is a feature of addiction to drugs such as morphine and meperidine hydrochloride (Demerol). **Addiction** is the physical and psychological **dependence** on and craving for a drug and the presence of clearly unpleasant effects when that drug or other agent such as a narcotic is stopped. **Controlled substances** are drugs such as opioids or narcotics that produce dependence and have potential for abuse or addiction. See pages 906-907 in the Practical Applications section for information about these drugs.

DRUG TOXICITY

Drug toxicity is an unpleasant and potentially dangerous effect of a drug. **Idiosyncrasy** is an example of an unpredictable type of drug toxicity. This is any unexpected and uncommon side effect that develops after administration of a drug. For example, in some people, penicillin causes an **idiosyncratic reaction,** such as **anaphylaxis** (acute hypersensitivity with asthma and shock). Anaphylaxis occurs as a result of exposure to a previously encountered drug or foreign substance (antigen).

Other types of drug toxicity are more predictable and expected, such as stomach upset after aspirin use. Physicians are trained to be aware of the potential toxic effects of all drugs that they prescribe. **Iatrogenic** (produced by treatment) disorders can occur, however, as a result of mistakes in drug use or because of individual sensitivity to a given agent.

Side effects are unpleasant effects that routinely result from the use of a drug. They often occur with the usual therapeutic dosage of a drug and generally are tolerable and reversible when the drug is discontinued. For example, nausea, vomiting, and alopecia are common side effects of the chemotherapeutic drugs used to treat cancer. Other, rare side effects may be life-threatening, such as severe allergic reactions.

Contraindications are factors in a patient's condition that make the use of a particular drug dangerous and ill-advised. For example, in the presence of kidney failure, it is unwise to administer a drug, such as methotrexate, that is normally eliminated by the kidneys because excess drug will accumulate in the body and cause adverse effects.

Drug resistance is the reduction in effectiveness of a drug. It is seen when drugs are unable to control the disease process in a particular patient. Resistance results from an important mutation (genetic change) in the disease (bacterial, viral, or cancer.)

CLASSES OF DRUGS

The following are major classes of drugs with indications for their uses. Specific drugs in each class are included in tables for your reference (note that the brand names are capitalized). Appendix IV presents a complete list of these drugs and their class or type. Notice that many drug types end with the adjectival suffix -ic, meaning pertaining to, although they are used as nouns.

The class of anticancer drugs (chemotherapeutic, molecularly targeted, and immunotherapeutic drugs) is discussed in Chapter 19, pages 816–819.

ANALGESICS

An **analgesic** (alges/o = sensitivity to pain) is a drug that lessens pain. Mild analgesics relieve mild to moderate pain, such as myalgias, headaches, and toothaches. More potent analgesics are **narcotics** or **opioids,** which are derived from opium. These drugs may induce stupor (a condition of near-unconsciousness and reduced mental and physical activity). They are used only to relieve severe pain because they may produce dependence.

Some non-narcotic analgesics reduce fever, pain, and inflammation and are used for joint disorders (osteoarthritis and rheumatoid arthritis), painful menstruation, and acute pain due to minor injuries or infection. These agents are not steroid hormones (such as cortisone) and are known as **nonsteroidal anti-inflammatory drugs (NSAIDs).** NSAIDs act on tissues to inhibit prostaglandins (hormone-like substances that sensitize peripheral pain receptors). A newer class of stronger NSAIDs is the COX-2 (cyclooxygenase-2) inhibitors. These agents block prostaglandin production. They relieve pain and inflammation as do traditional NSAIDs but produce fewer gastrointestinal side effects than with NSAIDs. However, they may increase the risk of clot formation and heart attacks (myocardial infarctions). Examples of COX-2 inhibitors are Celebrex and Bextra, which are listed in Table 21-2 with other analgesics.

TABLE 21-2	ANALGESICS AND ANESTHETICS

ANALGESICS	Nonsteroidal Anti-inflammatory Drugs (NSAIDs)
Mild	aspirin (Anacin, Ascriptin, Excedrin)
	celecoxib (Celebrex)
acetaminophen (Tylenol)	diclofenac sodium (Voltaren)
aspirin	ibuprofen (Motrin, Advil)
	ketorolac (Toradol)
Narcotic (Opioid)	naproxen (Aleve)
	valdecoxib (Bextra)
codeine	
fentanyl patch (Duragesic)	**ANESTHETICS**
hydrocodone w/APAP* (Lortab, Vicodin)	**General**
hydromorphone (Dilaudid)	
meperidine (Demerol)	ketamine (Ketalar)
morphine	nitrous oxide
oxycodone (OxyContin, Roxicodone)	propofol (Diprivan)
oxycodone with APAP* (Percocet, Roxicet, Endocet)	thiopental (Pentothal)
tramadol (Ultram)	
	Local
	lidocaine (Xylocaine)
	lidocaine-prilocaine (EMLA—eutectic mixture of local anesthetics)
	procaine (Novocain)

Note: Brand names are in parentheses.
*APAP, acetyl-*p*-aminophenol—acetaminophen (Tylenol, others).

21

ANESTHETICS

An **anesthetic** is an agent that reduces or eliminates sensation. This effect may occur in all tissues of the body **(general anesthetic)** and puts a patient asleep, or may be limited to a particular region **(local anesthetic).** General anesthetics are used for surgical procedures. They depress the activity of the central nervous system, producing loss of consciousness, and block the perception of pain. Local anesthetics inhibit the conduction of pain impulses in sensory nerves in the region in which they are injected or applied. An example is dental anesthesia with a local Novocain injection.

Table 21-2 gives examples of specific anesthetics.

ANTIBIOTICS AND ANTIVIRALS

An **antibiotic** is a chemical substance produced by a microorganism (bacterium, yeast, or mold) that inhibits **(bacteriostatic)** or kills **(bactericidal)** bacteria, fungi, or parasites. The use of antibiotics (penicillin was first in general use in the 1940s) has made it possible to cure many conditions such as pneumonia, urinary tract infection, and streptococcal pharyngitis ("strep throat"). Caution about the use of antibiotics is warranted because they are powerful agents. Like all drugs, they have side effects. Also, with indiscriminate use of antibiotics, bacteria and fungi can develop resistance to a particular agent. Infections caused by these resistant bacteria can spread and may be difficult or impossible to cure.

Antifungal drugs treat fungal infections. These infections commonly occur in the skin (ringworm), vagina (moniliasis or candidiasis), mouth, bloodstream, or lungs. **Antitubercular drugs** treat tuberculosis, a chronic and often drug-resistant infection.

Antiviral drugs are used against infections due to viruses, such as herpesviruses, Epstein-Barr virus, cytomegalovirus (CMV), human immunodeficiency virus (HIV), and hepatitis C virus.

Table 21-3 lists types of antibiotics (such as antifungal and antitubercular drugs) and antiviral drugs and gives specific examples of each.

ANTICOAGULANTS AND ANTIPLATELET DRUGS

Anticoagulants prevent clotting (coagulation) of blood. They prevent formation of clots or break up clots in blood vessels in conditions such as thrombosis and embolism. They also are used to prevent coagulation in preserved blood used for transfusions. **Heparin** is a natural anticoagulant purified from pig intestine or bovine (cow) lung. It is found in the granules of certain white blood cells. A more easily administered form of heparin called low-molecular-weight heparin (Fragmin, Lovenox) is self-injected on a daily basis and requires no monitoring of blood clotting ability, as is done with regular heparin. Other anticoagulants, including **warfarin (Coumadin),** are chemically synthesized. Coumadin blocks the formation of a number of clot-forming factors in the blood. Its action is reversed by vitamin K. **Tissue-type plasminogen activator (tPA)** dissolves clots and is used to open vessels after myocardial infarction.

New anticoagulant drugs that greatly reduce the risk of stroke are called **NOACs** (new oral anticoagulants). Examples are apixaban (Eliquis), dabigatran (Pradaxa), and rivaroxaban (Xarelto).

TABLE 21-3 | ANTIBIOTICS AND ANTIVIRALS

ANTIBIOTICS

Antifungal Drugs

amphotericin B (Fungilin)
clotrimazole (Lotrimin, Mycelex)
econazole topical (Spectazole)
fluconazole (Diflucan)
itraconazole (Sporanox)
miconazole (Monistat)
nystatin (Nilstat)
terbinafine (Lamisil)

Antiturburcular Drugs

ethambutol (Myambutol)
isoniazid [INH] (Nydrazid)
p-aminosalicylic acid granules (PASER)
rifampin (Rifadin)

Cephalosporins—*bactericidal and similar to penicillins*

ceftazidime (Fortaz)
cefuroxime axetil (Ceftin)

Macrolides—*bacteriostatic*

azithromycin (Zithromax)
clarithromycin (Biaxin)
erythromycin (Ery-Tab)

Penicillins—*bactericidal*

amoxicillin trihydrate (Amoxil, Trimox)
amoxicillin with clavulanate (Augmentin)
oxacillin (Bactocill)

Quinolones—*bactericidal and wide-spectrum*

ciprofloxacin (Cipro)
levofloxacin (Levaquin)
ofloxacin (Floxin)

Sulfonamides *or Sulfa Drugs*—*bactericidal*

sulfamethoxazole with trimethoprim (Bactrim)

Tetracyclines—*bacteriostatic*

doxycycline
tetracycline

ANTIVIRAL DRUGS

acyclovir (Zovirax)
efavirenz + tenofovir + emtricitabine (Atripla)*
entecavir (Baraclude)**
indinavir (Crixivan)[†]
lamivudine (Epivir)[‡]
ribavirin (Copegus, Rebetol)
simeprevir (Olysio)
sofosbuvir (Sovaldi)

Note: Brand names are in parentheses.
*Anti-HIV combination drug—all in one combination tablet.
[†]Anti-HIV drug—protease inhibitor.
[‡]Anti-HIV drug—nucleoside reverse transcriptase inhibitor (NRTI).
**Anti-hepatitis B drug.

21

Antiplatelet drugs reduce the tendency of platelets to stick together. Aspirin is an example of an antiplatelet drug; daily aspirin prophylaxis is recommended for patients with coronary artery disease and for those who have had heart attacks. Clopidogrel (Plavix) inhibits clumping of platelets and is used to prevent clotting after heart attacks and blood vessel procedures, such as angioplasty.

Table 21-4 lists anticoagulants and antiplatelet drugs.

ANTICONVULSANTS

An **anticonvulsant** prevents or reduces the frequency of convulsions in various types of seizure disorders or epilepsy. Ideally, anticonvulsants depress abnormal spontaneous activity of the brain arising from areas of scar or tumor, without affecting normal brain function. Table 21-4 lists examples of anticonvulsants.

TABLE 21-4 | ANTICOAGULANTS AND ANTIPLATELET DRUGS, ANTICONVULSANTS, ANTIDEPRESSANTS, ANTI-ALZHEIMER DRUGS, AND ANTIDIABETICS

ANTICOAGULANTS AND ANTIPLATELET DRUGS

apixaban (Eliquis)
aspirin
clopidogrel (Plavix)
dabigatran (Pradaxa)
dalteparin (Fragmin)*
enoxaparin sodium (Lovenox)*
lepirudin (Refludan)†
prasugrel (Effient)
rivaroxaban (Xarelto)
ticagrelor (Brilinta)
tissue plasminogen activator [tPA]
warfarin (Coumadin)

ANTICONVULSANTS

carbamazepine (Tegretol)
felbamate (Felbatol)
gabapentin (Neurontin)
levetiracetam (Keppra)
phenytoin sodium (Dilantin)
pregabalin (Lyrica)
valproic acid (Depakote)

ANTIDEPRESSANTS

amitriptyline (Elavil)‡
bupropion (Wellbutrin SR)
citalopram hydrobromide (Celexa)§
duloxetine (Cymbalta)
escitalopram (Lexapro)§
fluoxetine (Prozac)§
paroxetine (Paxil)§
sertraline (Zoloft)§
trazodone (Desyrel)§

ANTI-ALZHEIMER DRUGS

donepezil (Aricept)
memantine (Namenda)

ANTIDIABETICS

Insulins

Rapid-acting

insulin aspart (NovoLog)
insulin glulisine (Apidra)
insulin lispro (Humalog)

Short-acting

insulin regulator (Humulin R)

Intermediate-acting

insulin NPH (Humulin N)

Long-acting

insulin detemir (Levemir)
insulin glargine (Lantus)
insulin zinc suspension (Ultralente)

Other Diabetes Drugs—Oral

acarbose (Precose)—alpha-glucosidase inhibitor
glipizide (Glucotrol XL)—sulfonylurea
glyburide (Diabeta, Micronase)—sulfonylurea
metformin (Glucophage)—biguanide
pioglitazone (Actos)—thiazolidinedione
repaglinide (Prandin)—meglitinide
rosiglitazone (Avandia)—thiazolidinedione

Note: Brand names are in parentheses.
*Low-molecular-weight heparin.
†Derived from the saliva of the medicinal leech.
‡Tricyclic antidepressant drug.
§Selective serotonin reuptake inhibitor (SSRI).

ANTIDEPRESSANTS AND ANTI-ALZHEIMER DRUGS

Antidepressants treat symptoms of depression. They can elevate mood, increase physical activity and mental alertness, and improve appetite and sleep patterns. Many antidepressants also are mild sedatives and treat mild forms of depression associated with anxiety.

The largest class of antidepressants increases the action of neurotransmitters by blocking their removal (reuptake) from the synapses (spaces between nerve cells). These drugs include **tricyclic antidepressants (TCAs)** and **selective serotonin reuptake inhibitors (SSRIs).** Other antidepressants are **monoamine oxidase inhibitors (MAOIs),** which increase the length of time neurotransmitters work by blocking monoamine oxidase, an enzyme that normally inactivates neurotransmitters.

Lithium is a drug that is used to stabilize the mood swings and unpredictable behavior of people with bipolar disorder (manic-depressive illness).

Anti-Alzheimer drugs, used to treat symptoms of Alzheimer disease, act by aiding brain neurotransmitters (acetylcholine) or shielding brain cells from glutamate, a neurotransmitter that at high levels contributes to death of brain cells. Table 21-4 lists examples of antidepressants and anti-Alzheimer drugs.

ANTIDIABETICS

Antidiabetics are used to treat diabetes mellitus (condition in which either the hormone insulin is not produced, or the body's tissues have developed insensitivity to insulin). Patients with type 1 diabetes have lost the ability to produce insulin as children or young adults and must receive daily injections of **insulin.** Human insulin and synthetic derivations produced by recombinant DNA research have largely replaced animal-derived insulin in the management of diabetes. Rapid-acting insulins start working in 15 to 30 minutes and last 3 to 5 hours. Short-acting insulin begins working within 30 minutes to an hour and lasts 5 to 8 hours. Long-acting insulins have a time to onset of 1 to 3 hours and last between 24 and 36 hours.

Patients with type 2 diabetes usually develop the disease later in life and have insensitivity to insulin. Their diabetes may be well controlled by limiting sugars in their diet and by taking **oral antidiabetic drugs.** These include **sulfonylureas** (lower the levels of glucose in the blood by stimulating the production of insulin), **biguanides** (increase the body's sensitivity to insulin and reduce the production of glucose by the liver), **alpha-glucosidase inhibitors** (temporarily block enzymes that digest sugars), **thiazolidinediones** (enhance glucose uptake into tissues), and **meglitinides** (stimulate the beta cells in the pancreas to produce insulin).

An **insulin pump** is a device strapped to the patient's waist that periodically delivers (through a subcutaneous needle inserted in the abdomen) the desired amount of insulin.

Table 21-4 lists antidiabetic drugs.

ANTIHISTAMINES

Antihistamines block the action of histamine, which normally is released in the body in allergic reactions. Histamine causes allergic symptoms such as hives, bronchial asthma, hay fever, and in severe cases, **anaphylactic shock** (dyspnea, hypotension, and loss of consciousness). Antihistamines cannot cure the allergic reaction, but they relieve its symptoms. Many antihistamines have strong **antiemetic** (prevention of nausea) activity and are used to prevent motion sickness. The most common side effects of antihistamines are drowsiness, blurred vision, tremors, digestive upset, and lack of motor coordination.

Table 21-5 lists common antihistamines.

21

TABLE 21-5	ANTIHISTAMINES AND ANTIOSTEOPOROSIS DRUGS
ANTIHISTAMINES	**ANTIOSTEOPOROSIS DRUGS**
cetirizine (Zyrtec)	**Bisphosphonates—prevent bone loss**
chlorpheniramine maleate (Chlor-Trimeton)	
diphenhydramine (Benadryl)	alendronate (Fosamax)
fexofenadine (Allegra)	ibandronate sodium (Boniva)
loratadine (Claritin)	zoledronic acid (Zometa)
meclizine (Antivert)	**Selective Estrogen Receptor Modulators (SERMs)**
promethazine (Phenergan)	
	raloxifene (Evista)
	tamoxifen (Nolvadex)
	Other Antiosteoporosis Drugs
	denosumab (Prolia)*
	teriparatide (Forteo)†

Note: Brand names are in parentheses.
*Monoclonal antibody against a protein that signals bone removal.
†Hormone that stimulates bone formation.

ANTIOSTEOPOROSIS DRUGS

Osteoporosis is a disorder marked by loss of bone density. Calcium, vitamin D, and estrogen may increase calcium deposition in bone. Several different drugs are used to treat osteoporosis. **Bisphosphonates** prevent bone loss, and hormone-like drugs called **selective estrogen receptor modulators (SERMs)** increase bone formation. See Table 21-5.

CARDIOVASCULAR DRUGS

Cardiovascular drugs act on the heart or the blood vessels to treat hypertension, angina (pain due to decreased oxygen delivery to heart muscle), myocardial infarction (heart attack), congestive heart failure, and arrhythmias. Often, before other drugs are used, daily aspirin therapy (to prevent clots in blood vessels) and sublingual **nitroglycerin** (to dilate coronary blood vessels) are prescribed. **Digoxin (Lanoxin)** helps the heart pump more forcefully in heart failure. Other cardiovascular drugs include:

Angiotensin-converting enzyme (ACE) inhibitors—dilate blood vessels to lower blood pressure, improve the performance of the heart, and reduce its workload. They prevent the conversion of angiotensin I into angiotensin II, which is a powerful vasopressor (vasoconstrictor). ACE inhibitors reduce the risk of heart attack, stroke, heart failure and death even if a patient is not hypertensive.

Angiotensin II receptor blockers (ARBs)—lower blood pressure by preventing angiotensin from acting on receptors in blood vessels. They are used in patients who do not tolerate ACE inhibitors. An exciting new combination antihypertensive drug to treat heart failure is Entresto, formerly known as LCZ696. It combines two agents: valsartan and sacubitril.

Antiarrhythmics—reverse abnormal heart rhythms. They slow the response of heart muscle to nervous system stimulation or slow the rate at which nervous system impulses are carried through the heart.

Beta blockers—decrease muscular tone in blood vessels (leading to vasodilation), slow heart rate, decrease output of the heart, and reduce blood pressure by blocking the action of epinephrine at receptor sites in the heart muscle and in blood vessels. Beta blockers are prescribed for angina, hypertension, arrhythmias (such as fibrillation), and prevention of a second heart attack.

Calcium channel blockers—dilate blood vessels and lower blood pressure and are used to treat arrhythmias. They inhibit the entry of calcium (necessary for blood vessel contraction) into the muscles of the heart and blood vessels.

Cardiac glycosides—made from digitalis (foxglove plant). These drugs increase the force of contraction of the heart and are used to treat heart failure and atrial fibrillation.

Cholesterol-binding drugs—bind to dietary cholesterol and prevent its uptake from the gastrointestinal tract.

Cholesterol-lowering drugs (statins)—control hypercholesterolemia (high levels of cholesterol in the blood), which is a major factor in the development of heart disease. These drugs lower cholesterol by reducing its production in the liver.

Diuretics—reduce the volume of blood in the body by promoting the kidney to remove water and salt through urine. They treat hypertension (high blood pressure) and congestive heart failure.

Table 21-6 gives examples of cardiovascular drugs.

TABLE 21-6 | CARDIOVASCULAR DRUGS

ANGIOTENSIN-CONVERTING ENZYME (ACE) INHIBITORS

enalapril maleate (Vasotec)
lisinopril (Prinivil, Zestril)
quinapril (Accupril)
ramipril (Altace)

ANGIOTENSIN II RECEPTOR BLOCKERS

irbesartan (Avapro)
losartan (Cozaar)
valsartan (Diovan)
(Entresto; formerly LCZ696)

ANTIARRHYTHMICS

amiodarone (Cordarone)
ibutilide (Corvert)
sotalol (Betapace)

BETA BLOCKERS

atenolol (Tenormin)
carvedilol (Coreg)
metoprolol (Lopressor, Toprol-XL)
propranolol (Inderal)

CALCIUM CHANNEL BLOCKERS

amlodipine
amlodipine besylate (Norvasc)
diltiazem (Cardizem CD)
nifedipine (Adalat CC, Procardia)

CARDIAC GLYCOSIDES

digoxin (Lanoxin)

CHOLESTEROL-BINDING DRUGS (RESINS)

cholestyramine (Questran)
colestipol (Colestid)

CHOLESTEROL-LOWERING DRUGS (STATINS)

atorvastatin (Lipitor)
pravastatin (Pravachol)
rosuvastatin (Crestor)
simvastatin (Zocor)

DIURETICS

bumetanide (Bumex)
furosemide (Lasix)
hydrochlorothiazide (HydroDiuril)
spironolactone (Aldactone)
triamterene (Dyazide)

Note: Brand names are in parentheses.

21

ENDOCRINE DRUGS

Endocrine preparations act in much the same manner as the naturally occurring (endogenous) hormones discussed in Chapter 18. **Androgens,** normally made by the testes and adrenal glands, are used for male hormone replacement and to treat endometriosis and anemia. **Antiandrogens** interfere with the production of androgens or with their binding in tissues. They are prescribed for prostate cancer. **Estrogens** are female hormones, normally produced by the ovaries, that are used for symptoms associated with menopause (estrogen replacement therapy) and to prevent postmenopausal osteoporosis. **Aromatase inhibitors** also reduce the amount of estrogen (estradiol) in the blood and are effective against breast cancer.

Selective estrogen receptor modulators (SERMs) have estrogen-like effects on bone (increase in bone density) and on lipid metabolism (decrease in cholesterol levels). However, they lack estrogenic effects on uterus and breast tissue. SERMs are used to treat postmenopausal osteoporosis and breast cancer. Tamoxifen and raloxifene are SERMs. **Progestins** are prescribed for abnormal uterine bleeding caused by hormonal imbalance and, together with estrogen, in hormone replacement therapy and oral contraceptives.

Thyroid hormone is administered when there is a low output of hormone from the thyroid gland. **Calcitonin** (a thyroid hormone) is used to treat osteoporosis. It increases calcium in the blood and promotes bone deposition. **Glucocorticoids** (adrenal corticosteroids) are prescribed for reduction of inflammation and a wide range of other disorders, including arthritis, severe skin and allergic conditions, respiratory and blood disorders, gastrointestinal ailments, and malignant conditions.

A fragment of human **parathyroid hormone (PTH)** has been approved for osteoporosis treatment. This agent stimulates new bone formation. **Growth hormone release–inhibiting factor (somatostatin)** can be manufactured and given to treat gastrointestinal symptoms associated with acromegaly and other tumors.

Table 21-7 gives examples of endocrine drugs.

TABLE 21-7	ENDOCRINE DRUGS	

ANDROGENS

fluoxymesterone (Halotestin)
methyltestosterone (Virilon)

ANTIANDROGENS

abiraterone (Zytiga)
enzalutamide (XTANDI)
flutamide (Eulexin)
goserelin (Zoladex)
leuprolide (Lupron)
nilutamide (Casodex)

AROMATASE INHIBITORS

anastrozole (Arimidex)
exemestane (Aromasin)
fulvestrant (Faslodex)
letrozole (Femara)

ESTROGENS

estrogens (Premarin, Prempro)

GLUCOCORTICOIDS

dexamethasone (Decadron)
hydrocortisone
prednisone (Deltasone)
triamcinolone (Aristocort)

GROWTH HORMONE–RELEASE INHIBITING FACTOR

octreotide (Sandostatin)

PARATHYROID HORMONE FRAGMENT

teriparatide (Forteo)

PROGESTINS

medroxyprogesterone acetate (Cycrin, Provera)
megestrol (Megace)

SELECTIVE ESTROGEN RECEPTOR MODULATORS (SERMS)

raloxifene (Evista)
tamoxifen (Nolvadex)

THYROID HORMONES

calcitonin (Cibacalcin)
levothyroxine (Levoxyl, Synthroid)
liothyronine (Cytomel)
thyroid ISP (Armour Thyroid)

Note: Brand names are in parentheses.

GASTROINTESTINAL DRUGS

Gastrointestinal drugs often are used to relieve uncomfortable and potentially dangerous symptoms, rather than as cures for specific diseases. **Antacids** neutralize the hydrochloric acid in the stomach to relieve symptoms of peptic ulcer, esophagitis, and reflux. **Antiulcer** drugs block secretion of acid by cells in the lining of the stomach and are prescribed for patients with gastric and duodenal ulcers and **gastroesophageal reflux disease (GERD).** Histamine H₂ receptor antagonists such as **ranitidine (Zantac)** and **cimetidine (Tagamet)** turn off histamine, which promotes secretion of stomach acid. Another drug, **omeprazole (Prilosec),** works by stopping acid production by a different method (proton pump inhibition).

Antidiarrheal drugs relieve diarrhea and decrease the rapid movement (peristalsis) in the muscular walls of the colon. **Cathartics** relieve constipation and promote defecation for diagnostic and operative procedures and are used to treat disorders of the gastrointestinal tract. Some cathartics increase the intestinal salt content to cause fluid to fill the intestines; others increase the bulk of the feces to promote peristalsis. Another type of cathartic lubricates the intestinal tract to produce soft stools. **Laxatives** are mild cathartics, and **purgatives** are strong cathartics.

Antinauseants (antiemetics) relieve nausea and vomiting and overcome vertigo, dizziness, motion sickness, and similar symptoms due to labyrinthitis (inflammation of the inner ear).

Anti-TNF (tumor necrosis factor) drugs are used to treat **autoimmune diseases** such as **Crohn's.** These drugs also are used against rheumatoid arthritis.

Table 21-8 lists the various types of gastrointestinal drugs and examples of each.

TABLE 21-8 | GASTROINTESTINAL DRUGS

ANTACIDS

aluminum and magnesium antacid
    (Gaviscon)
magnesium antacid (milk of magnesia)
aluminum antacid (Rolaids)

ANTIDIARRHEALS

diphenoxylate + atropine (Lomotil)
loperamide (Imodium)
paregoric

ANTINAUSEANTS (ANTIEMETICS)

metoclopramide (Reglan)
ondansetron (Zofran)
promethazine (Phenergan)
prochlorperazine maleate (Compazine)

ANTI–TUMOR NECROSIS FACTOR (TNF) DRUGS

adalimumab (Humira)
certolizumab pegol (Cimzia)
etanercept (Enbrel)
golimumab (Simponi)
infliximab (Remicade)

ANTIULCER AND ANTI–GASTROINTESTINAL REFLUX DISEASE (GERD) DRUGS

cimetidine (Tagamet)
esomeprazole (Nexium)
famotidine (Pepcid)
lansoprazole (Prevacid)
omeprazole (Prilosec)
ranitidine (Zantac)

CATHARTICS

casanthranol + docusate sodium (Peri-
    Colace)

Note: Brand names are in parentheses.

RESPIRATORY DRUGS

Respiratory drugs are prescribed for the treatment of asthma and COPD (chronic obstructive pulmonary diseases such as emphysema and chronic bronchitis.) **Bronchodilators** open bronchial tubes and are administered by injection or aerosol inhalers. **Steroid drugs** are inhaled or given intravenously and orally to reduce chronic inflammation in respiratory passageways. **Leukotriene modifiers** are recent additions to the anti-inflammatory therapy of asthma. They prevent asthma attacks and bronchospasms by blocking leukotriene (bronchoconstrictor) from binding to receptors in respiratory tissues. Table 21-9 gives examples of respiratory drugs.

TABLE 21-9 | RESPIRATORY DRUGS

BRONCHODILATORS

albuterol (Proventil, Ventolin HFA)*
formoterol + budesonide (Symbicort)†
ipratropium + albuterol (Combivent)*
salmeterol + fluticasone (Advair Diskus)†
tiotropium bromide (Spiriva)‡

LEUKOTRIENE MODIFIERS

montelukast (Singulair)
zafirlukast (Accolate)
zileuton (Zyflo)

STEROIDS: INHALERS

fluticasone (Flovent)
mometasone (Asmanex)
triamcinolone (Azmacort)

STEROIDS: INTRAVENOUS OR ORAL

dexamethasone (Decadron)
methylprednisolone (Medrol)
prednisone

Note: Brand names are in parentheses.
*Short-acting; inhaled.
†Long-acting.
‡Anticholinergic; bronchodilator enhancers.

SEDATIVE-HYPNOTICS

Sedative-hypnotics are medications that depress the central nervous system and promote drowsiness (sedatives) and sleep (hypnotics). They are prescribed for insomnia and sleep disorders. These products have a very high abuse potential and should be used only for short periods of time and under close supervision. **Barbiturates** and **benzodiazepines** are the two major categories of sedative-hypnotics.

Low doses of **benzodiazepines** (which influence the part of the brain responsible for emotions) may act as sedatives. In higher doses, benzodiazepines may act as hypnotics (to promote sleep).

Table 21-10 gives examples of sedative-hypnotics.

STIMULANTS

Stimulants are drugs that act on the brain to speed up vital processes (heart and respiration) in cases of shock and collapse. They also increase alertness and inhibit hyperactive behavior in children. High doses can produce restlessness, insomnia, and hypertension. Examples of stimulants are **amphetamines**—used to prevent narcolepsy (seizures of sleep), to suppress appetite, and to calm hyperkinetic children. **Caffeine** also is a cerebral stimulant. It is used in drugs to relieve certain types of headache by constricting cerebral blood vessels. Table 21-10 lists examples of stimulants.

TRANQUILIZERS

Tranquilizers are useful for controlling anxiety. Minor tranquilizers **(benzodiazepines)** control minor symptoms of anxiety. Major tranquilizers **(phenothiazines)** control more severe disturbances of behavior. Table 21-10 lists examples of minor and major tranquilizers.

21

TABLE 21-10	SEDATIVE-HYPNOTICS, STIMULANTS, AND TRANQUILIZERS
SEDATIVE-HYPNOTICS	**TRANQUILIZERS**
methaqualone (Quaalude)	**Minor**
temazepam (Restoril)*	
triazolam (Halcion)*	alprazolam (Xanax)*
zolpidem tartrate (Ambien)	buspirone (BuSpar)
	diazepam (Valium)*
STIMULANTS	lorazepam (Ativan)*
caffeine	**Major**
dextroamphetamine sulfate (Dexedrine)	
dextroamphetamine and amphetamine (Adderall)	aripiprazole (Abilify)
lisdexamfetamine (Vyvanse)	chlorpromazine (Thorazine)†
methylphenidate (Ritalin)	haloperidol (Haldol)
modafinil (Provigil)	lithium carbonate (Eskalith)
	olanzapine (Zyprexa)
	risperidone (Risperdal)
	thioridazine (Mellaril)†
	trifluoperazine (Stelazine)†

Note: Brand names are in parentheses.
*Benzodiazepine.
†Phenothiazine.

VOCABULARY

This list reviews many of the new terms introduced in the text. Short definitions reinforce your understanding of the terms. Refer to the Pronunciation of Terms on page 916 for help with unfamiliar or difficult words.

GENERAL TERMS

addiction	Physical and psychological dependence on and craving for a drug.
additive action	Drug action in which the combination of two similar drugs is equal to the sum of the effects of each.
aerosol	Particles of drug suspended in air and inhaled.
anaphylaxis	Exaggerated hypersensitivity reaction to a previously encountered drug or foreign protein.
antagonistic action	Combination of two drugs gives less than an additive effect (action).
antidote	Agent given to counteract an unwanted effect of a drug.
brand name	Commercial name for a drug; trademark or trade name.
chemical name	Chemical formula for a drug.
contraindications	Factors that prevent the use of a drug or treatment.
controlled substances	Drugs that produce tolerance and dependence and have potential for abuse or addiction. See page 906.
dependence	Physiologic need for a drug with prolonged use.
dose	Amount of drug administered, usually measured in milligrams.
Food and Drug Administration (FDA)	Government agency having the legal responsibility for enforcing proper drug manufacture and clinical use.
generic name	Legal noncommercial name for a drug.
iatrogenic	Condition caused by treatment (drugs or procedures) given by physicians or medical personnel.
idiosyncratic reaction	Unexpected effect produced in a particularly sensitive patient but not seen in most people.
inhalation	Administration of drugs in gaseous or vapor form through the nose or mouth.
medicinal chemistry	Study of new drug synthesis; relationship between chemical structure and biological effects.
molecular pharmacology	Study of interaction of drugs and their target molecules such as enzymes, or cell surface receptors.
oral administration	Drugs are given by mouth.
parenteral administration	Drugs are given by injection into the skin, muscles, or veins (any route other than through the digestive tract). Examples are subcutaneous, intradermal, intramuscular, intravenous, intrathecal, and intracavitary injections and instillations.

21

pharmacist	Specialist in preparing and dispensing drugs.
pharmacy	Location for preparing and dispensing drugs; also the study of preparing and dispensing drugs.
pharmacodynamics	Study of drug effects within the body.
pharmacokinetics	Study of drug absorption, distribution, metabolism, and excretion over a period of time.
pharmacologist	Specialist in the study of the properties, uses, and side effects of drugs.
pharmacology	Study of the preparation, properties, uses, and side effects of drugs.
***Physicians' Desk Reference* (PDR)**	Reference book that lists drug products.
receptor	Target substance with which a drug interacts in the body.
rectal administration	Drugs are inserted through the anus into the rectum.
resistance	Lack of beneficial response; seen when drugs are unable to control the disease process.
response	Desired and beneficial effect of a drug.
schedule	Exact timing and frequency of drug administration.
side effect	Adverse reaction, usually minor, that routinely results from the use of a drug.
sublingual administration	Drugs are given by placement under the tongue.
synergism	Combination of two drugs causes an effect that is greater than the sum of the individual effects of each drug alone.
syringe	Instrument (tube) for introducing or withdrawing fluids from the body.
tolerance	Larger and larger drug doses must be given to achieve the desired effect. The patient becomes resistant to the action of a drug as treatment progresses.
topical application	Drugs are applied locally on the skin or mucous membranes of the body; ointments, creams, and lotions are applied topically.
toxicity	Harmful effects of a drug.
toxicology	Study of harmful chemicals and their effects on the body.
transport	Movement of a drug across a cell membrane into body cells.
United States Pharmacopeia (USP)	Authoritative list of drugs, formulas, and preparations that sets a standard for drug manufacturing and dispensing.
vitamin	Substance found in foods and essential in small quantities for growth and good health.

21

CLASSES OF DRUGS AND RELATED TERMS

ACE inhibitor	Lowers blood pressure by dilating blood vessels. Angiotensin-converting enzyme (ACE) inhibitors block the conversion of angiotensin I to angiotensin II (a powerful vasoconstrictor).
amphetamine	Central nervous system stimulant.
analgesic	Relieves pain.
androgen	Male hormone.
anesthetic	Reduces or eliminates sensation; general and local.
angiotensin II receptor blocker	Lowers blood pressure by preventing angiotensin from acting on receptors in blood vessels.
antacid	Neutralizes acid in the stomach.
antiandrogen	Blocks the formation of androgens or interferes with their effect in tissues.
antiarrhythmic	Treats abnormal heart rhythms.
antibiotic	Chemical substance, produced by a plant or microorganism, that has the ability to inhibit or destroy foreign organisms in the body. Examples are antifungals, antiviral agents, cephalosporins, macrolides, tetracyclines, antituberculosis drugs, penicillins, quinolones, and sulfonamides.
anticoagulant	Prevents blood clotting.
anticonvulsant	Prevents convulsions (abnormal brain activity).
antidepressant	Relieves symptoms of depression.
antidiabetic	Drug given to prevent or treat diabetes mellitus.
antidiarrheal	Prevents diarrhea.
antiemetic	Prevents nausea and vomiting.
antihistamine	Blocks the action of histamine and helps prevent symptoms of allergy.
antinauseant	Relieves nausea and vomiting; antiemetic.
antiplatelet	Reduces the tendency of platelets to stick together and form a clot.
antiulcer	Inhibits the secretion of acid by cells lining the stomach.
antiviral	Acts against viruses such as herpesviruses and HIV.
aromatase inhibitor	Reduces estrogen in the blood by blocking the enzyme aromatase.
bactericidal	Kills bacteria (-cidal means able to kill).
bacteriostatic	Inhibits bacterial growth (-static means stopping or controlling).
beta blocker	Blocks the action of epinephrine at sites on receptors of heart muscle cells, the muscle lining of blood vessels, and bronchial tubes; antiarrhythmic, antianginal, and antihypertensive. Can also be written as beta-blocker.
bisphosphonate	Prevents bone loss in osteoporosis.
caffeine	Central nervous system stimulant (found in coffee and tea).

21

calcium channel blocker	Blocks the entrance of calcium into heart muscle and muscle lining of blood vessels; used as an antiarrhythmic, antianginal, and antihypertensive; also called calcium antagonist.
cardiac glycoside	Increases the force of contraction of the heart.
cardiovascular drug	Acts on the heart and blood vessels. This category of drug includes ACE inhibitors, beta blockers, calcium channel blockers, cholesterol-lowering drugs or statins, and diuretics.
cathartic	Relieves constipation.
cholesterol-binding drug	Binds to dietary cholesterol and prevents its uptake from the gastrointestinal tract.
cholesterol-lowering drug	Lowers cholesterol by preventing its production by the liver; statin.
diuretic	Increases the production of urine and thus reduces the volume of fluid in the body; antihypertensive.
emetic	Promotes vomiting.
endocrine drug	Hormone or hormone-like drug. Examples are androgens, estrogens, progestins, SERMs, thyroid hormones, and glucocorticoids.
estrogen	Female hormone that promotes development of secondary sex characteristics and supports reproductive tissues.
gastrointestinal drug	Relieves symptoms of diseases in the gastrointestinal tract. Examples are antacids, antiulcer drugs, antidiarrheal drugs, cathartics, laxatives, purgatives, and antinauseants (antiemetics).
glucocorticoid	Hormone from the adrenal cortex that raises blood sugar and reduces inflammation.
hypnotic	Produces sleep or a trance-like state.
laxative	Weak cathartic.
narcotic	Habit-forming drug (potent analgesic) that relieves pain by producing stupor or insensibility; morphine and opium are examples.
progestin	Female hormone that stimulates the uterine lining during pregnancy and is also used in treatment of abnormal uterine bleeding and for hormone replacement therapy.
purgative	Relieves constipation; strong cathartic.
respiratory drug	Treats asthma, emphysema, and infections of the respiratory system. Bronchodilators are examples.
sedative	Mildly hypnotic drug that relaxes without necessarily producing sleep. **Benzodiazepines** are examples.
stimulant	Excites and promotes activity. Caffeine and amphetamines are examples.
thyroid hormone	Stimulates cellular metabolism.
tranquilizer	Controls anxiety and severe disturbances of behavior.

21

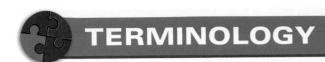

TERMINOLOGY

Write the meaning of the medical term in the space provided.

COMBINING FORMS

COMBINING FORM	MEANING	TERMINOLOGY	MEANING
aer/o	air	aerosol _____ *The suffix -sol means solution.*	
alges/o	sensitivity to pain	analgesic _____	
bronch/o	bronchial tube	bronchodilator _____ *Theophylline is a smooth muscle relaxant used to treat asthma, emphysema, and chronic bronchitis.*	
chem/o	drug	chemotherapy _____	
cras/o	mixture	idiosyncrasy _____ *Idi/o means individual, peculiar; syn- means together. An idiosyncrasy is an abnormal, unexpected effect of a drug that is peculiar to an individual patient.*	
cutane/o	skin	subcutaneous _____	
derm/o	skin	hypodermic _____	
erg/o	work	synergism _____	
esthes/o	feeling, sensation	anesthesia _____	
hist/o	tissue	antihistamine _____ *The suffix -amine indicates a nitrogen-containing compound.* **Histamine** *is a substance found in all body tissues (it causes capillary dilation and gastric acid secretion and constricts bronchial tube smooth muscle); an excess of histamine is released when the body comes into contact with substances to which it is sensitive.*	
hypn/o	sleep	hypnotic _____	
iatr/o	treatment	iatrogenic _____	
lingu/o	tongue	sublingual _____	
myc/o	mold, fungus	erythromycin _____	
narc/o	stupor	narcotic _____	
or/o	mouth	oral _____	
pharmac/o	drug	pharmacology _____	
prurit/o	itching	antipruritic _____	
pyret/o	fever	antipyretic _____	
thec/o	sheath (of brain and spinal cord)	intrathecal _____	

21

COMBINING FORM	MEANING	TERMINOLOGY	MEANING
tox/o	poison	toxic _____	
toxic/o	poison	toxicology _____	
vas/o	vessel	vasodilator _____	
ven/o	vein	intravenous _____	
vit/o	life	vitamin _____	

The term comes from the original thought that vitamins contained amino acids. The first vitamins discovered were nitrogen-containing substances called amines. Table 21-11 lists vitamins, their medical names, and foods that are a major source of each.

PREFIXES

PREFIX	MEANING	TERMINOLOGY	MEANING
ana-	upward, excessive, again	anaphylaxis _____ The suffix -phylaxis means protection.	
anti-	against	antidote _____ The suffix -dote comes from Greek, meaning what is given.	
		antibiotic _____	
contra-	against, opposite	contraindication _____ Alternatively, **drug indications** are reasons to prescribe a medication; a bacterial infection may be an indication to prescribe a specific antibiotic.	
par-	other than, apart from	parenteral _____ Enter/o means intestine.	
syn-	together, with	synergistic _____	

TABLE 21-11	VITAMINS

VITAMIN	CHEMICAL NAME(S)	FOOD SOURCES
vitamin A	retinol; dehydroretinol	leafy, green and yellow vegetables; liver, eggs, cod liver oil
vitamin B_1	thiamine	yeast, ham, liver, peanuts, milk
vitamin B_2	riboflavin	milk, liver, green vegetables
vitamin B_3	niacin (nicotinic acid)	yeast, liver, peanuts, fish, poultry
vitamin B_6	pyridoxine	liver, fish, yeast
vitamin B_9	folic acid	vegetables, liver, yeast, sunflower seeds, cereals
vitamin B_{12}	cyanocobalamin	milk, eggs, liver
vitamin C	ascorbic acid	citrus fruits, vegetables
vitamin D	calciferol	cod liver oil, milk, egg yolk
vitamin E	alpha-glucosidase	wheat germ oil, cereals, egg yolk
vitamin K	phytonadione; menaquinone; menadione	kale, spinach, collards, mustard greens

21

ABBREVIATIONS

Many of the notations used by physicians in writing prescriptions are abbreviations for Latin phrases, which appear in *italics* within parentheses. An Official "Do Not Use" list of abbreviations is on the next page.

a.c., ac	before meals (*ante cibum*)
ACE	angiotensin-converting enzyme
ad lib	freely, as desired (*ad libitum*)
APAP	acetaminophen (Tylenol)
ARB	angiotensin II receptor blocker
b.i.d., bid	two times a day (*bis in die*)
c̄	with
Caps	capsules
cc	cubic centimeter
FDA	U.S. Food and Drug Administration
gm, g	gram
gtt	drops (*guttae*)
h	hour (*hora*)
h.s., hs	at bedtime (*hora somni*)
H2 blocker	histamine H_2 receptor antagonist
HRT	hormone replacement therapy
IM	intramuscular
INH	isoniazid—antituberculosis agent
IV	intravenous
MAOI	monoamine oxidase inhibitor
mg	milligram
ml, mL	milliliter
NPO	nothing by mouth (*nil per os*)
NSAID	nonsteroidal anti-inflammatory drug
p̄	after (*post*)
p.c., pc	after meals (*post cibum*)

PCA	patient-controlled analgesia
PDR	*Physicians' Desk Reference*
PO, p.o., po	by mouth (*per os*)
p.r.n., prn	as needed (*pro re nata*)
Pt	patient
q	every (*quaque*)
q.h., qh	every hour (*quaque hora*)
q2h	every 2 hours
q.i.d., qid	four times a day (*quater in die*)
q.s., qs	sufficient quantity (*quantum satis*)
qAM	every morning
qPM	every evening
Rx	prescription
s̄	without (*sine*)
SERM	selective estrogen receptor modulator
Sig.	directions—how to take medication
SL	sublingual
s.o.s.	if it is necessary (*si opus sit*)
SSRI	selective serotonin reuptake inhibitor
subQ	subcutaneous
tab	tablet
TCA	tricyclic antidepressant
t.i.d., tid	three times daily (*ter in die*)

21

Official "Do Not Use" List

Do Not Use	Potential Problem	Use Instead
U, u (unit)	Mistaken for "0" (zero), the number "4" (four), or "cc"	Write "unit"
IU (International Unit)	Mistaken for "IV" (intravenous) or the number "10" (ten)	Write "International Unit"
Q.D., QD, q.d., qd (daily) Q.O.D., QOD, q.o.d., qod (every other day)	Mistaken for each other Period after Q mistaken for "I" and "O" mistaken for "I"	Write "daily" Write "every other day"
Trailing zero (X.0 mg)[†] Lack of leading zero (.X mg)	Decimal point is missed	Write X mg Write 0.X mg
MS MSO$_4$ and MgSO$_4$	Can mean morphine sulfate or magnesium sulfate Confused for one another	Write "morphine sulfate" Write "magnesium sulfate"

*Applies to all orders and all medication-related documentation that is handwritten (including free-text computer entry) or on pre-printed forms. See the Evolve website for additional abbreviations and symbols that may be included in the future "Do Not Use" list.
[†]**Exception:** A "trailing zero" may be used only when required to demonstrate the level of precision of the value being reported, such as for laboratory results, imaging studies that report size of lesions, or catheter/tube sizes. It may not be used in medication orders or other medication-related documentation.

PRACTICAL APPLICATIONS

21

DOS AND DON'TS OF TAKING MEDICINES

Check the DO or DON'T box for the following scenarios.

1. If your medicine prescription label says: 1 tab PO a.c., you take it before meals.   DO ☐   DON'T ☐

   Answer: DO (a.c. means *ante cibum* "before meals". Some medications are better absorbed on an empty stomach, such as 1 hour before eating or 2 hours after eating. READ labels carefully!)

2. If your medicine prescription label says: 1 PO qPM prn pain, you take it every morning.   DO ☐   DON'T ☐

   Answer: DON'T (qPM means "every evening" and PRN means "when needed.")

3. If you feel 100% better, skip the last few doses of antibiotic medication.   DO ☐   DON'T ☐

   Answer: DON'T (Antibiotics work best when an optimal blood level of the drug is reached and then maintained for a period of time. If you stop your course of treatment early, you may prevent complete eradication of infection. Finish your entire course of medication and call your doctor if you are not feeling better.)

4. Lend a friend your pills if she has the same condition or is taking the same medication.   DO ☐   DON'T ☐

   Answer: DON'T (People take different doses of medications and for different reasons. NEVER SHARE. Any mistake could have serious side effects.)

5. You may take your cholesterol-lowering statin pill with grapefruit juice.   DO □   DON'T □

   Answer: DON'T (Grapefruit juice alters the absorption of statins, such as Lipitor, into the bloodstream.)

6. It's a good idea to take your ACE inhibitor (blood pressure medication) with bananas.   DO □   DON'T □

   Answer: DON'T (Bananas contain potassium, and ACE inhibitors cause the body to retain potassium. If you combine the two, you may end up with a dangerously high level of potassium in the blood.)

7. Add vegetables like kale, mustard greens, and spinach to your diet when you are taking the anticoagulant warfarin (Coumadin).   DO □   DON'T □

   Answer: DON'T (Kale and similar vegetables are rich in vitamin K. Warfarin works as an anticoagulant by decreasing the activity of vitamin K, which is necessary for clotting. Therefore, kale and other vegetables can counteract the anti-clotting benefits of warfarin.)

8. After taking your heart medicine digoxin, you may enjoy a treat of black licorice.   DO □   DON'T □

   Answer: DON'T (Black licorice, or glycyrrhiza glabra, decreases potassium levels in the body. Low potassium levels can increase the side effects that may occur with digoxin usage. These side effects are nausea, vomiting, headache, loss of appetite and diarrhea.)

9. Enjoy a glass or two of wine when you are taking the antibiotic Flagyl (metronidazole).   DO □   DON'T □

   Answer: DON'T (Flagyl interferes with how alcohol is processed in the body and results in gastrointestinal symptoms like nausea and vomiting.)

10. Eat walnuts, Brazil nuts, soybean flour, or foods with high fiber content when you are taking thyroid medication (levothyroxine).   DO □   DON'T □

   Answer: DON'T (Walnuts, Brazil nuts, soybean flour, and high-fiber foods can prevent your body from absorbing thyroid medication.)

PRESCRIPTIONS

The usual order of drug prescription information is as follows: name of the drug, dosage, route of administration, timing of administration. Frequently, the physician will include a qualifying phrase to indicate why the prescription is being written. Not all information is listed with every prescription.

Exercise: Answers are found page 915.

Match the prescriptions as written with the explanations that follow.
   a. Fluoxetine (Prozac) 20 mg PO b.i.d.
   b. Lisinopril (Zestril) 20 mg 1 cap qAM
   c. Ondansetron (Zofran) 4 mg 1 tab/cap t.i.d. p.r.n. for nausea
   d. Ranitidine (Zantac) 300 mg 1 tab p.c. t.i.d.
   e. Olanzapine (Zyprexa) 5 mg 1 tab qPM
   f. Acetaminophen (300 mg) & codeine (30 mg) 1 tab q.i.d. p.r.n. for pain

1. anti-GERD drug taken after meals 3 times a day   _____
2. Tylenol with a narcotic taken 4 times a day as needed   _____
3. antidepressant taken by mouth twice a day   _____
4. antiemetic taken 3 times a day as needed   _____
5. antihypertensive taken every morning   _____
6. antipsychotic, one tablet every evening   _____

21

CONTROLLED SUBSTANCES

Controlled substances are drugs regulated under existing federal law. The substances are divided into five classes (schedules) based on the substance's medicinal value, harmfulness, and potential for abuse or addiction. Schedule I includes the most dangerous drugs that have no recognized medicinal use, and Schedule V includes the least dangerous drugs. The following table lists examples of drugs in each class with their type, trade and/or "street" names, and medical uses.

DRUG	TYPE	TRADE OR OTHER NAME(S)	MEDICAL USE(S)
Class (Schedule) I			
heroin	narcotic	diacetylmorphine, horse, smack	None
LSD (lysergic acid diethylamide)	hallucinogen	acid, microdot	None
mescaline, peyote	hallucinogen	mesc, buttons, cactus	None
methaqualone	depressant	Quaalude,* Parest	sedative-hypnotic

*Quaaludes have been discontinued in the United States, but methaqualone (ab)use continues owing to Internet availability.

Class (Schedule) II

Dangerous substances with general medical indications and high potential for abuse and addiction.

hydromorphone	narcotic	Dilaudid	analgesic
marijuana	cannabis	pot, Acapulco, grass, reefer	under investigation
meperidine	narcotic	Demerol	analgesic
cocaine	stimulant	coke, flake, snow	local anesthetic
methylphenidate	stimulant	Ritalin	hyperkinesis
oxycodone	narcotic	Tylox, Percodan, OxyContin, OC, OX, Oxy	analgesic, pain management
crystal methamphetamine	stimulant	crystal meth, ice	weight control
phencyclidine	hallucinogen	PCP, angel dust, hog	veterinary anesthetic
opium	narcotic	Dover's powder, paregoric	analgesic, antidiarrheal
morphine	narcotic	morphine, pectoral syrup	analgesic, antitussive
barbiturates	depressant	amobarbital (Amytal), pentobarbital (Nembutal), secobarbital (Seconal)	anesthetic, anticonvulsant, sedative-hypnotic
amphetamines	stimulant	Dexedrine, Desoxyn	weight control, narcolepsy

21

DRUG	TYPE	TRADE OR OTHER NAME(S)	MEDICAL USE(S)
Class (Schedule) III			
Carries less potential for abuse, but casual use can lead to psychological addiction and dependence.			
anabolic steroids	male sex hormones	testosterone, Anavar, Winstrol, Dianabol	hormone deficiency, increasing muscle mass
barbiturates	depressant	aprobarbital (Alurate), butalbital (Fiorinal), butabarbital (Butisol)	anesthetic, anticonvulsant, sedative-hypnotic
codeine	narcotic	codeine	analgesic, antitussive
Class (Schedule) IV			
Carries low potential for abuse but a risk of psychological or limited physical dependence.			
barbiturates	depressant	phenobarbital	anesthetic, anticonvulsant, sedative-hypnotic
benzodiazepines	minor tranquilizer	lorazepam (Ativan), diazepam (Valium), chlordiazepoxide (Librium), clonazepam (Klonopin), triazolam (Halcion), alprazolam (Xanax)	antianxiety, sedative-hypnotic, anticonvulsant
nonbenzodiazepine agent	hypnotic	eszopiclone (Lunesta)	insomnia
Class (Schedule) V			
This class includes codeine preparations (Robitussin A-C) and opium/opioid preparations (Kapectolin PG—antidiarrheal, Lomotil—antidiarrheal, Motofen—antidiarrheal).			

21

? EXERCISES

Remember to check your answers carefully with the Answers to Exercises, page 914.

A **Name the pharmacologic specialty based on its description as given.**

1. use of drugs in the treatment of disease _____

2. study of new drug synthesis _____

3. study of how drugs interact with their target molecules _____

4. study of the harmful effects of drugs _____

5. study of drug effects in the body _____

6. measurement of drug absorption, distribution, metabolism, and excretion over a period of time

    _____

B **Match the general pharmacology terms with the definitions/descriptions that follow.**

antidote   generic name   toxicologist
chemical name   pharmacist   trade (brand) name
Food and Drug   pharmacologist   United States
  Administration   *Physicians' Desk Reference*   Pharmacopeia

1. Specialist in the study of the harmful effects of drugs on the body is a/an

    _____.

2. Agent given to counteract harmful effects of a drug is a/an _____.

3. Government agency with legal responsibility for enforcing proper drug manufacture and clinical

    use is _____.

4. The _____ is the commercial name for a drug.

5. The _____ is the complete chemical formula for a drug.

6. The _____ is the legal noncommercial name for a drug.

7. Professional who prepares and dispenses drugs is a/an _____.

8. Specialist (MD or PhD) who studies the properties, uses, and side effects of drugs is a/an

    _____.

9. Reference book listing drug products is _____.

10. Authoritative listing of drugs, formulas, and preparations that sets a standard for drug

    manufacturing and dispensing is _____.

21

C Name the route of drug administration based on its description as given.

1. administered via suppository or fluid into the anus _____

2. administered via vapor or gas into the nose or mouth _____

3. administered under the tongue _____

4. applied locally on skin or mucous membrane _____

5. injected via syringe under the skin or into a vein, muscle, or body cavity _____

6. given by mouth and absorbed through the stomach or intestinal wall _____

D Give the meanings of the following terms.

1. intravenous _____

2. intrathecal _____

3. antiseptic _____

4. antipruritic _____

5. aerosol _____

6. intramuscular _____

7. subcutaneous _____

8. intracavitary _____

9. addiction _____

10. dose _____

11. drug resistance _____

12. response _____

13. schedule _____

14. dependence _____

E Match the routes of drug administration in Column I with the medications or procedures in Column II. Write the letter of the answer in the space provided.

COLUMN I

1. intravenous _____

2. rectal _____

3. oral _____

4. topical _____

5. inhalation _____

6. intrathecal _____

7. intramuscular _____

8. intradermal _____

COLUMN II

A. lotions, creams, ointments
B. tablets and capsules
C. skin testing for allergy
D. lumbar puncture
E. deep injection, usually in buttock
F. suppositories
G. blood transfusions
H. aerosol medications

21

F **For the following descriptions of drug actions, supply the word that fits the description.**

1. Combination of two drugs is greater than the total effects of each drug by itself:

   _____

2. Combination of two drugs that is equal to the sum of the effects of each: _____

3. Effects of a given drug dose become less as treatment continues, and larger and larger doses

   must be given to achieve the desired effect: _____

4. An unexpected effect that may appear in a patient after administration of a drug:

   _____

5. Two drugs give less than an additive effect (action): _____

G **Give the meanings of the following terms that describe classes of drugs.**

1. antibiotic _____

2. antidepressant _____

3. antihistamine _____

4. analgesic _____

5. anticoagulant _____

6. anesthetic _____

7. antidiabetic _____

8. sedative _____

9. stimulant _____

10. tranquilizer _____

H **Match the term in Column I with the associated term in Column II. Write the letter of the answer in the space provided.**

COLUMN I

1. antihistamine   _____

2. analgesic   _____

3. antidiabetic   _____

4. anticoagulant   _____

5. antibiotic   _____

6. stimulant   _____

7. sedative-hypnotic   _____

8. tranquilizer   _____

COLUMN II

A. caffeine or amphetamines
B. penicillin or erythromycin
C. insulin
D. benzodiazepine
E. heparin
F. nonsteroidal anti-inflammatory drug
G. phenothiazine
H. anaphylactic shock

I **Give the meanings of the following terms.**

1. beta blocker _____

2. androgen _____

3. glucocorticoid _____

4. calcium channel blocker _____

5. estrogen _____

6. antacid _____

7. cathartic _____

8. antiemetic _____

9. bronchodilator _____

10. hypnotic _____

11. diuretic _____

12. cholesterol-lowering drug _____

J **Match the type of drug in Column I with the condition it treats in Column II. Write the letter of the answer in the space provided.**

COLUMN I

1. anticonvulsant _____

2. anticoagulant _____

3. antacid _____

4. progestins _____

5. antibiotic _____

6. ACE inhibitor _____

7. bronchodilator _____

8. antihistamine _____

9. tranquilizer _____

10. analgesic _____

COLUMN II

A. abnormal uterine bleeding caused by hormonal imbalance

B. severe behavior disturbances and anxiety

C. epilepsy

D. congestive heart failure and hypertension

E. epigastric discomfort

F. myalgia and neuralgia

G. anaphylactic shock

H. thrombosis and embolism

I. streptococcal pharyngitis

J. asthma

21

K Complete the following terms based on definitions given.

1. agent that reduces fever: anti _____

2. agent that reduces itching: anti _____

3. habit-forming analgesic: _____ tic

4. two drugs cause an effect greater than the sum of each alone: syn _____

5. antibiotic derived from a red mold: _____ mycin

6. legal nonproprietary name of a drug: _____ name

7. factor in a patient's condition that prevents the use of a particular drug:

   contra _____

8. drug that produces an absence of sensation or feeling: an _____

L Select from the list of drug terms to complete the following sentences.
Consult Appendix IV (Drugs), pages 998–1002, for help with this exercise.

ACE inhibitor	antidepressant	diuretic
anesthetic	antiestrogen	NSAID
antibiotic	antihistamine	oral antidiabetic
anticonvulsant	antiviral	SERM

1. Cephalosporins (such as cefuroxime and cefprozil) and penicillins are examples of

   _____ drugs.

2. Advil (ibuprofen) is an example of a/an _____.

3. Tegretol (carbamazepine) and Dilantin (phenytoin) are examples of a/an _____
   drug.

4. Zovirax (acyclovir) and Crixivan (indinavir) are both types of a/an _____
   drug.

5. Nolvadex (tamoxifen), used to treat estrogen receptor–positive breast cancer in women, is an

   example of a/an _____ drug.

6. Patients with high blood pressure may need Vasotec (enalapril) or Zestril (lisinopril). Both of

   these are examples of a/an _____.

7. Glucophage (metformin) and Avandia (rosiglitazone) are two types of _____
   drugs.

8. Evista (raloxifene), used to treat osteoporosis in postmenopausal women, is an example of a

   selective estrogen receptor modulator, or _____.

9. Elavil (amitriptyline) and Prozac (fluoxetine) are two types of a/an _____
   drug.

10. If you have an allergy, your doctor may prescribe Allegra (fexofenadine), which is a/an

    _____ drug.

11. Two agents that reduce the amount of fluid in the blood and thus lower blood pressure are

    Lasix (furosemide) and Aldactone (spironolactone). These are _____ drugs.

12. Xylocaine (lidocaine) and Pentothal (thiopental) are examples of a/an _____ drug.

21

M **Give the meanings of the following abbreviations.**

1. NSAID _____

2. p.r.n. _____

3. q.i.d. _____

4. ad lib _____

5. t.i.d. _____

6. mg _____

7. c̄ _____

8. s̄ _____

9. NPO _____

10. p.c. _____

11. b.i.d. _____

12. q.h. _____

13. PO _____

14. q _____

N **Translate the following prescription orders.**

1. 1 tab PO q.i.d. p.c. and h.s. _____

2. 15-60 mg IM q4-6h _____

3. 2 caps p.o. h.s. _____

4. 1 tab SL p.r.n. _____

5. Apply topically qhs prn _____

O **Circle the boldface terms that best complete the meaning of the sentences.**

1. After his heart attack, Bernie was supposed to take many drugs, including diuretics and a/an **(progestin, laxative, anticoagulant)** to prevent blood clots.

2. Estelle was always anxious and had a hard time sleeping. Dr. Max suggested that a mild **(antacid, anticonvulsant, tranquilizer)** would help her relax and concentrate on her work.

3. During chemotherapy Helen was very nauseated. Dr. Cohen prescribed an **(antihypertensive, antiemetic, antianginal)** to relieve her symptoms of queasy stomach.

4. The two antibiotics worked together and were therefore **(idiosyncratic, generic, synergistic)** in killing the bacteria in Susan's bloodstream.

5. The label warned that the drug might impair fine motor skills. It listed the **(side effects, antidote, pharmacodynamics)** of the sedative.

6. After receiving the results of Judy's sputum culture, her physician, an expert in **(endocrinology, cardiology, infectious disease)**, recommended Biaxin and other **(antihistamines, antibiotics, antidepressants)** to combat the *Mycobacterium avium* complex disease in her **(heart, thyroid gland, lungs)**.

21

7. Our dog, Eli, has had seizures since he was hit by a car last year. The veterinarian currently prescribes phenobarbital, an **(anticoagulant, antinauseant, anticonvulsant)**, 45 mg b.i.d. **(every other day, twice a day, every evening)**.

8. To control his type 1 **(heart disease, asthma, diabetes)**, David gives himself daily injections of **(oral drugs, insulin, aromatase inhibitors)**.

9. Many students who want to stay awake to study are taking **(stimulants, sedatives, tranquilizers)** containing **(lithium, caffeine, butabarbital)**.

10. Shelly's wheezing, coughing, and shortness of breath when she is stressed and exposed to animal dander all pointed to a diagnosis of **(pneumonia, asthma, heart disease)**, which required treatment with steroids and **(antivirals, diuretics, bronchodilators)**.

ANSWERS TO EXERCISES

A

1. chemotherapy
2. medicinal chemistry
3. molecular pharmacology
4. toxicology
5. pharmacodynamics
6. pharmacokinetics

B

1. toxicologist
2. antidote
3. (U.S.) Food and Drug Administration
4. trade (brand) name
5. chemical name
6. generic name
7. pharmacist
8. pharmacologist
9. *Physicians' Desk Reference*
10. United States Pharmacopeia

C

1. rectal
2. inhalation
3. sublingual
4. topical
5. parenteral
6. oral

D

1. within a vein
2. within a sheath (membranes around the spinal cord or brain)
3. an agent that works against infection
4. an agent that works against itching
5. particles of drug suspended in air and inhaled
6. within a muscle
7. under the skin
8. within a cavity
9. physical and psychological dependence on a drug
10. amount of drug administered
11. lack of beneficial response
12. desired and beneficial effect of a drug
13. exact timing and frequency of drug administration
14. prolonged use of a drug that may lead to physiologic need for its actions in the body

E

1. G
2. F
3. B
4. A
5. H
6. D
7. E
8. C

F

1. synergism (potentiation)
2. additive action
3. tolerance
4. idiosyncrasy
5. antagonistic

G

1. an agent that inhibits or kills germ life (microorganisms)
2. an agent that relieves the symptoms of depression
3. an agent that blocks the action of histamine and relieves allergic symptoms
4. an agent that relieves pain
5. an agent that prevents blood clotting
6. an agent that reduces or eliminates sensation
7. an agent used to prevent diabetes mellitus
8. an agent (mildly hypnotic) that relaxes and calms nervousness
9. an agent that excites and promotes activity
10. a drug used to control anxiety and severe disturbances of behavior

H

1. H
2. F
3. C
4. E
5. B
6. A
7. D
8. G

I

1. drug that blocks the action of epinephrine at sites of receptors of heart muscles, blood vessels, and bronchial tubes (antihypertensive, antianginal, and antiarrhythmic)
2. a drug that produces male sexual characteristics
3. a hormone from the adrenal glands that reduces inflammation and raises blood sugar
4. a drug that blocks the entrance of calcium into heart muscle and blood vessel walls (antianginal, antiarrhythmic, and antihypertensive)
5. a hormone that produces female sexual characteristics
6. a drug that neutralizes acid in the stomach
7. a drug that relieves constipation
8. a drug that prevents nausea and vomiting
9. a drug that opens air passages
10. an agent that produces sleep
11. a drug that reduces the volume of blood and lowers blood pressure
12. a drug that reduces cholesterol levels (treats hypercholesterolemia)

J

1. C
2. H
3. E
4. A
5. I
6. D
7. J
8. G
9. B
10. F

K

1. antipyretic
2. antipruritic
3. narcotic
4. synergism
5. erythromycin
6. generic
7. contraindication
8. anesthetic

L

1. antibiotic
2. NSAID
3. anticonvulsant
4. antiviral
5. antiestrogen
6. ACE inhibitor
7. oral antidiabetic for type 2 diabetes
8. SERM
9. antidepressant
10. antihistamine
11. diuretic
12. anesthetic

M

1. nonsteroidal anti-inflammatory drug
2. as needed
3. four times a day
4. freely as desired
5. three times a day
6. milligram
7. with
8. without
9. nothing by mouth
10. after meals
11. twice a day
12. every hour
13. by mouth
14. every

N

1. take one tablet by mouth, four times a day, after meals and at bedtime
2. administer 15 to 60 milligrams intramuscularly, every 4-6 hours
3. take two capsules by mouth at bedtime
4. place one tablet under the tongue, as needed
5. apply to the skin, at bedtime as needed

O

1. anticoagulant
2. tranquilizer
3. antiemetic
4. synergistic
5. side effects
6. infectious disease, antibiotics, lungs
7. anticonvulsant, twice a day
8. diabetes, insulin
9. stimulants, caffeine
10. asthma, bronchodilators

Answers to Practical Applications—Prescriptions

1. d
2. f
3. a
4. c
5. b
6. e

PRONUNCIATION OF TERMS

To test your understanding of the terminology in this chapter, write the meaning of each term in the space provided. In addition, you may wish to cover the terms and write them by looking at your definitions. Make sure your spelling is correct. The page number after each term indicates where it is defined or used in the book, so you can easily check your responses. You will find complete definitions for all of these terms and their audio pronunciations on the Evolve website.

Pronunciation Guide

ā as in āpe   ă as in ăpple
ē as in ēven   ĕ as in ĕvery
ī as in īce   ĭ as in ĭnterest
ō as in ōpen   ŏ as in pŏt
ū as in ūnit   ŭ as in ŭnder

21

TERM	PRONUNCIATION	MEANING
ACE inhibitor (899)	ĀCE ĭn-HĬB-ĭ-tŏr	
addiction (897)	ă-DĬK-shŭn	
additive action (897)	ĂD-ĭ-tĭv ĂK-shŭn	
aerosol (897)	ĀR-ō-sōl	
amphetamine (899)	ăm-FĔT-ă-mēn	
analgesic (899)	ăn-ăl-JĒ-zĭk	
anaphylaxis (897)	ăn-ă-fĭ-LĂK-sĭs	
androgen (899)	ĂN-drō-jĕn	
anesthesia (901)	ăn-ĕs-THĒ-zē-ă	
anesthetic (899)	ăn-ĕs-THĔ-tĭk	
angiotensin II receptor blocker (899)	ăn-jē-ō-TĔN-sĭn II rē-CĔP-tŏr BLŎK-ĕr	
antacid (899)	ănt-ĂS-ĭd	
antagonistic action (897)	ăn-tă-gŏn-NĬS-tĭk ĂK-shŭn	
antiandrogen (899)	ăn-tē-ĂN-drō-jĕn	
antiarrhythmic (899)	ăn-tē-ā-RĬTH-mĭk	
antibiotic (899)	ăn-tĭ-bī-ŎT-ĭk	
anticoagulant (899)	ăn-tĭ-kō-ĂG-ū-lănt	
anticonvulsant (899)	ăn-tĭ-kŏn-VŬL-sănt	
antidepressant (899)	ăn-tĭ-dĕ-PRĔS-ănt	
antidiabetic (899)	ăn-tĭ-dī-ă-BĔT-ĭk	
antidiarrheal (899)	ăn-tĭ-dī-ă-RĒ-ăl	
antidote (897)	ĂN-tĭ-dōt	

TERM	PRONUNCIATION	MEANING
antiemetic (899)	ăn-tē-ĕ-MĔ-tĭk	
antihistamine (899)	ăn-tĭ-HĬS-tă-mēn	
antinauseant (899)	ăn-tĭ-NAW-zē-ănt	
antiplatelet (899)	ăn-tĭ-PLĀT-lĕt	
antipruritic (901)	ăn-tĭ-proo-RĬT-ĭk	
antipyretic (901)	ăn-tĭ-pĭ-RĔT-ĭk	
antiulcer (899)	ăn-tē-ŬL-sĕr	
antiviral (899)	ăn-tē-VĪ-răl	
aromatase inhibitor (899)	ă-RŌ-mă-tās ĭn-HĬB-ĭ-tŏr	
bactericidal (899)	băk-tĕ-rĭ-SĪ-dăl	
bacteriostatic (899)	băk-tĕ-rē-ō-STĂ-tĭk	
beta blocker (899)	BĀ-lă BLŎK-ĕr	
bronchodilator (901)	brŏng-kō-DĪ-lā-tŏr	
bisphosphonate (899)	bĭs-FŎS-fō-nāt	
brand name (897)	brănd nām	
caffeine (899)	kăf-EN	
calcium channel blocker (899)	KĂL-sē-ŭm CHĂN-ĕl BLŎK-ĕr	
cardiac glycoside (900)	KĂR-dē-ăk GLĪ-kō-sīd	
cardiovascular drug (900)	kăr-dē-ō-VĂS-kū-lăr drŭg	
cathartic (900)	kă-THĂR-tĭk	
chemical name (897)	KĔM-ĭ-kal nām	
chemotherapy (901)	kē-mō-THĔR-ă-pē	
cholesterol-binding drug (900)	kō-LĔS-tĕr-ŏl BĪN-dĭng drŭg	
cholesterol-lowering drug (900)	kō-LĔS-tĕr-ŏl LŌ-wĕr-ĭng drŭg	
contraindications (897)	kŏn-tră-ĭn-dĭ-KĀ-shŭnz	
controlled substances (897)	kŏn-TRŌLD SŬB-stăn-sĕz	
dependence (897)	dē-PEN-dents	
diuretic (900)	dī-ū-RĔT-ĭk	
dose (897)	dōs	

21

TERM	PRONUNCIATION	MEANING
emetic (900)	ĕ-MĔT-ĭk	
erythromycin (901)	ĕ-rīth-rō-MĪ-sĭn	
endocrine drug (900)	ĔN-dō-krĭn drŭg	
estrogen (900)	ĔS-trō-jĕn	
gastrointestinal drug (900)	găs-trō-ĭn-TĔS-tĭ-năl drŭg	
generic name (897)	jĕ-NĔR-ĭk nām	
glucocorticoid (900)	gloo-kō-KŎR-tĭ-koyd	
hypnotic (900)	hĭp-NŎT-ĭk	
hypodermic (901)	hī-pō-DĔR-mĭk	
iatrogenic (897)	ī-ăt-rō-JĔN-ĭk	
idiosyncrasy (901)	ĭd-ē-ō-SĬN-kră-sē	
idiosyncratic reaction (897)	ĭd-ē-ō-sĭn-KRĂ-tĭk rē-ĂK-shŭn	
inhalation (897)	ĭn-hă-LĀ-shŭn	
intrathecal (901)	ĭn-tră-THĒ-kăl	
intravenous (902)	ĭn-tră-VĒ-nŭs	
laxative (900)	LĂK-să-tĭv	
medicinal chemistry (897)	mĕ-DĬ-sĭ-năl KĔM-ĭs-trē	
molecular pharmacology (897)	mō-LĔK-ū-lăr făr-mă-KŎL-ō-jē	
narcotic (900)	năr-KŎT-ĭk	
oral administration (897)	ŎR-ăl ăd-mĭn-ĭs-TRĀ-shŭn	
parenteral administration (897)	pă-RĔN-tĕr-ăl ăd-mĭn-ĭs-TRĀ-shŭn	
pharmacist (898)	FĂR-mă-sĭst	
pharmacy (898)	FĂR-mă-sē	
pharmacodynamics (898)	făr-mă-kō-dī-NĂM-ĭks	
pharmacokinetics (898)	făr-mă-kō-kī-NĔT-ĭks	
pharmacologist (898)	făr-mă-KŎL-ō-gĭst	
pharmacology (898)	făr-mă-KŎL-ō-gē	
progestin (900)	prō-JĔS-tĭn	
purgative (900)	PŬR-gă-tĭv	

21

TERM	PRONUNCIATION	MEANING
receptor (898)	rē-SĔP-tŏr	
rectal administration (898)	RĔK-tăl ăd-mĭn-ĭs-TRĀ-shŭn	
resistance (898)	rē-SĬS-tăns	
respiratory drug (900)	rĕs-pĭr-ă-TŎR-ē drŭg	
response (898)	rĕ-SPŌNS	
schedule (898)	SKĔD-ūl	
sedative (900)	SĔD-ă-tĭv	
side effect (898)	sīd ĕ-FĔKT	
stimulant (900)	STĬM-ū-lănt	
subcutaneous (901)	sŭb-kū-TA-nē-ŭs	
sublingual administration (898)	sŭb-LĬNG-wăl ăd-mĭn-ĭs-TRĀ-shŭn	
synergism (898)	SĬN-ĕr-jĭzm	
synergistic (902)	sĭn-ĕr-JĬS-tĭk	
syringe (898)	sĭ-RĬNJ	
thyroid hormone (900)	THĪ-royd HŎR-mon	
tolerance (898)	TŎL-ĕr-ănz	
topical application (898)	TŎP-ĭ-kl ăp-lĭ-KĀ-shŭn	
toxic (902)	TŎK-sĭk	
toxicity (898)	tŏk-SĬS-ĭ-tē	
toxicology (898)	tŏk-sĭ-KŎL-ō-jē	
tranquilizer (900)	TRĂN-kwĭ-lī-zĕr	
transport (898)	TRĂNS-pŏrt	
vasodilator (902)	văz-ō-DĪ-lā-tŏr	
vitamin (898)	VĪ-tă-mĭn	

21

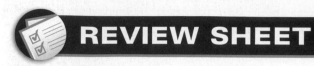

REVIEW SHEET

Write the meanings of the word parts in the spaces provided, and test yourself. Check your answers with the information in the chapter or in the *Glossary (Medical Word Parts—English)* at the end of the book.

Combining Forms

COMBINING FORM	MEANING	COMBINING FORM	MEANING
aer/o	_____	lingu/o	_____
alges/o	_____	myc/o	_____
bronch/o	_____	narc/o	_____
chem/o	_____	or/o	_____
cras/o	_____	pharmac/o	_____
cutane/o	_____	prurit/o	_____
derm/o	_____	pyret/o	_____
enter/o	_____	thec/o	_____
erg/o	_____	tox/o	_____
esthes/o	_____	toxic/o	_____
hist/o	_____	vas/o	_____
hypn/o	_____	ven/o	_____
iatr/o	_____	vit/o	_____

Suffixes

SUFFIX	MEANING	SUFFIX	MEANING
-amine	_____	-in	_____
-dote	_____	-phylaxis	_____
-genic	_____	-sol	_____

Prefixes

PREFIX	MEANING	PREFIX	MEANING
ana-	_____	par-	_____
anti-	_____	syn-	_____
contra-	_____		

evolve *Please refer to the Evolve website for additional exercises, games, and images related to this chapter.*

Psychiatry

Chapter Sections:

CHAPTER GOALS

- Differentiate among psychiatrist, a psychologist, and other mental health specialists.
- Describe tests used by clinical psychologists to evaluate a patient's mental health and intelligence.
- Define terms that describe major psychiatric disorders.
- Identify terms that describe psychiatric symptoms.
- Compare different types of therapy for psychiatric disorders.
- Identify the categories of psychiatric drugs, and name commonly used drugs in each category.
- Define combining forms, suffixes, prefixes, and abbreviations related to psychiatry.
- Apply your new knowledge to understanding medical terms in their proper contexts, such as medical reports and records.

INTRODUCTION

You will find this chapter different from others in the book. Some, but not all, psychiatric disorders are not readily explainable in terms of abnormalities in the structure or chemistry of an organ or tissue, as are other illnesses. In addition, the causes of mental disorders are complex and include significant psychological and social as well as chemical and structural elements. This chapter provides a simple outline of psychiatric disorders and definitions of major psychiatric terms. For more extensive and detailed information, you may wish to consult the *Diagnostic and Statistical Manual of Mental Disorders,* **fifth edition, (DSM-5),** published by the American Psychiatric Association.

Psychiatry (psych/o = mind, **iatr/o** = treatment) is the branch of medicine that deals with the diagnosis, treatment, and prevention of mental illness. It is a specialty of clinical medicine like surgery, internal medicine, pediatrics, and obstetrics.

Psychiatrists complete the same medical training (4 years of medical school) as for other physicians and receive an MD (doctor of medicine) or OD (doctor of osteopathy) degree. Then they spend a variable number of years training in the methods and practice of **psychotherapy** (psychological techniques for treating mental disorders) and **psychopharmacology** (drug therapy). Psychiatrists complete 3 years of residency training and then extra years of fellowship training to specialize in various aspects of psychiatry. **Child psychiatrists** specialize in the treatment of children; **forensic psychiatrists** specialize in the legal aspects of psychiatry, such as the determination of mental competence in criminal cases. **Psychoanalysts** complete 3 to 5 additional years of training in a special psychotherapeutic technique called **psychoanalysis** in which the patient freely relates her or his thoughts and associations to the analyst, who does not interfere with the process. Interpretations are offered at appropriate times.

A **psychologist** is a nonmedical professional who is trained in methods of psychological testing, psychotherapy, analysis, and research and completes a doctor of philosophy (PhD) or doctor of education (EdD) degree program in a specific field of interest, such as **clinical** (patient-oriented) **psychology, experimental research,** or **social psychology** (focusing on social interaction and the ways the actions of others influence the behavior of the individual). A **clinical psychologist,** like a psychiatrist, can use various methods of psychotherapy to treat patients but, unlike a psychiatrist, cannot prescribe drugs or electroconvulsive therapy (ECT). Other nonphysicians trained in the treatment of mental illness include licensed clinical social workers, psychiatric nurses, and licensed mental health clinicians (LMHCs).

Clinical psychologists are trained in the use of tests to evaluate various aspects of a patient's mental health and intelligence. Examples are **intelligence (IQ) tests** such as the **Wechsler Adult Intelligence Scale (WAIS)** and the **Stanford-Binet Intelligence Scale.** Two projective **(personality) tests** are the use of **Rorschach technique,** in which inkblots, as shown in Figure 22-1, are used to bring out associations, and the **Thematic Apperception Test (TAT),** in which pictures are used as stimuli for making up stories (Figure 22-2). Both tests are revealing of personality structure. Examples of **graphomotor projection tests** are the **Draw a Person Test,** in which the patient is asked to copy a body, and the **Bender-Gestalt Test,** in which the patient is asked to draw certain geometric designs. The Bender-Gestalt Test picks up deficits in mental processing and memory caused by brain damage and is used to screen children for developmental delays. The **Minnesota Multiphasic Personality Inventory (MMPI)** contains true-false questions that reveal aspects of personality, such as sense of duty or responsibility, ability to relate to others, and dominance (assertiveness, resourcefulness). This test is widely used as a measure of psychological health in adolescents and adults. The patient's responses to questions are compared with responses made by patients with diagnoses of schizophrenia, depression, and so on.

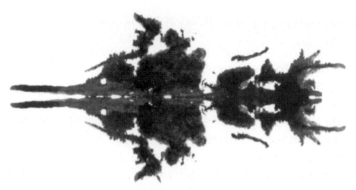

FIGURE 22-1   **Inkblots like this one are presented on 10 cards in the Rorschach test.** The patient describes images that he or she sees in the blot.

PSYCHIATRIC CLINICAL SYMPTOMS

The following terms describe abnormalities that are evident to an examining mental health professional. Familiarity with these terms will help you understand the next section, Psychiatric Disorders.

amnesia	Loss of memory.
anxiety	Varying degrees of uneasiness, apprehension, or dread often accompanied by palpitations, tightness in the chest, breathlessness, and choking sensations.
apathy	Absence of emotions; lack of interest, emotional involvement, or motivation.
compulsion	Uncontrollable urge to perform an act repeatedly in an attempt to reduce anxiety.
conversion	Anxiety becomes a bodily symptom, such as blindness, deafness, or paralysis, that does not have a physical basis.

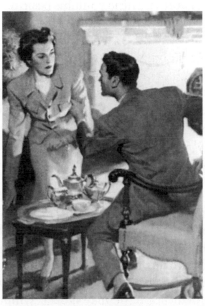

FIGURE 22-2   A sample picture from the **Thematic Apperception Test.** The patient is asked to tell the story that the picture illustrates.

delusion	Fixed, false belief that cannot be changed by logical reasoning or evidence.
dissociation	Uncomfortable thoughts are split off from the person's conscious awareness to avoid mental distress. In extreme cases, dissociation can lead to multiple personalities.
dysphoria	Intense feelings of depression, discontent, and generalized dissatisfaction with life.
euphoria	Intense feelings of well-being, elation, happiness, excitement, and joy.
hallucination	False or unreal sensory perception as, for example, hearing voices when none are present. An **illusion** is a misperception of an actual sensory stimulus, such as hearing voices in the sound of rustling leaves.
labile	Variable; undergoing rapid emotional change.
mania	Elevated, expansive state with talkativeness, hyperactivity, and racing thoughts.
mutism	No, or very little, ability to speak.
obsession	Involuntary, persistent idea or emotion; the suffix -mania indicates a strong obsession with something (e.g., pyromania is an obsession with fire).
paranoia	Overly suspicious system of thinking; fixed delusion that one is being harassed, persecuted, or unfairly treated.

PSYCHIATRIC DISORDERS

Sigmund Freud's ideas of personality structure play an important role in the understanding of many types of psychiatric disorders. Freud believed that personality is made up of three major parts: the **id**, the **ego**, and the **superego**. The **id** represents the unconscious instincts and psychic energy present from birth. The id contains basic drives that, operating according to the pleasure principle, seek immediate gratification regardless of the reality of the situation.

The **ego** is the central coordinating branch of the personality. It is the mediator between the id and the outside world. It is the part of the personality that evaluates and assesses the reality of a situation **(reality testing)** and, if necessary, postpones the gratification of a need or drive (id) until a satisfactory object or situation arises. The ego is perceived as being "self" by the individual.

The **superego** is the internalized conscience and moral part of the personality. It encompasses the sense of discipline derived from parental authority and society. Guilt feelings, for example, arise from behavior and thoughts that do not conform to the standards of the superego.

Freud believed that certain psychological disorders occur when conflicts arise between two or more of these aspects of the personality. **Defense mechanisms,** such as denial, are techniques people use to ward off the anxiety produced by these conflicts. For example, a person afflicted with a serious illness may avoid confronting his or her present or future problems by denial. Thus, he or she may refuse to believe the diagnosis, may miss appointments, may neglect medication, or may ignore symptoms. All people use defense mechanisms to cope with difficult problems. The use of these mechanisms may be regarded as abnormal or normal according to whether that use makes a constructive or destructive contribution to the individual's personality.

22

The term **psychosis** frequently is used to describe mental illness. A **psychosis** involves significant impairment of reality testing, with symptoms such as **delusions** (false beliefs), **hallucinations** (false sensory perceptions), and bizarre behavior. Schizophrenic disorders are examples of psychoses. Patients exhibit a disturbed sense of self, inappropriate affect (emotional reactions), and withdrawal from the external world.

Psychiatric disorders that are discussed in this section are **anxiety disorders, bipolar disorders, depressive disorders, dissociative disorders, eating disorders, neurocognitive disorders, neurodevelopmental disorders, schizophrenia spectrum disorders, sexual dysfunctions and gender dysphoria, somatic symptom disorders,** and **substance-related and addictive disorders.**

ANXIETY DISORDERS

Anxiety disorders are characterized by the experience of unpleasant tension, distress, troubled feelings, and avoidance behavior. A **panic attack** is an abrupt surge of intense fear or discomfort that reaches a peak within minutes. Symptoms and clinical signs may include the following:

- Palpitations
- Sweating
- Trembling
- Sensations of shortness of breath
- Feeling of choking
- Chest pain or discomfort
- Nausea or abdominal distress
- Feeling dizzy or faint
- Feelings of unreality or being detached from oneself
- Fear of losing control or "going crazy"
- Fear of dying
- Numbness or tingling

Panic disorder is recurrent, unexpected panic attacks and persistent concern about having another panic attack in between episodes. A panic attack can occur in the context of other anxiety disorders, such as phobic, obsessive-compulsive, post-traumatic stress, and generalized anxiety disorders.

Phobic disorders are characterized by irrational or debilitating fears associated with a specific object or situation. The patient with a phobic disorder goes to extreme lengths to avoid the object of her or his fear. The object that is feared often is symbolic of an unconscious conflict that is the cause of the phobia and thus diverts the patient's attention from the conflict, keeping it unconscious. Panic attacks can occur in anticipation of the phobic situation.

Agoraphobia (**agora-** = marketplace) is the fear of being in open, crowded, public places from which escape would be difficult or in which help might not be available, or of going out alone in "unsafe" places. Persons with agoraphobia limit their normal activities to avoid situations that trigger their anxiety. Thus, they may feel comfortable only when at home or in the company of a friend or relative.

A **social phobia (social anxiety disorder)** is the fear of situations in which the affected person is open to public scrutiny, which could result in possible embarrassment and humiliation. For example, the fear may focus on speaking in public, using public lavatories, or eating in public.

Other specific phobias are **claustrophobia** (fear of closed-in places; **claustr/o** = barrier), **acrophobia** (fear of heights; in this term, **acr/o** = a high point), and **zoophobia** (fear of animals; **zo/o** = animals).

Obsessive-compulsive disorder (OCD) involves recurrent thoughts **(obsessions)** and repetitive acts **(compulsions)** that dominate the patient's life. The patient experiences anxiety if he or she is prevented from performing special rituals. Often the OCD consumes time and interferes with the person's social or occupational functioning. Several antidepressant drugs, including clomipramine, have been used to treat OCD, with considerable success, particularly when combined with cognitive-behavioral therapy.

22

Post-traumatic stress disorder (PTSD) is the development of symptoms (intense fear, helplessness, insomnia, nightmares, and diminished responsiveness to the external world) following exposure to a traumatic event. Flashbacks, bothersome thoughts, and anxiety often triggered by reminders occur in episodes long after a life-threatening or major emotional event. People avoid situations with reminders. Many survivors of the September 11, 2001, attack on the World Trade Center towers and the Pentagon experienced PTSD.

Generalized anxiety disorder (GAD) is characterized by chronic anxiety and exaggerated worry and tension even when there is little or nothing to provoke such feelings.

BIPOLAR DISORDERS

Bipolar disorders (bi- = two; **pol/o** = extreme) are characterized by one or more **manic episodes** alternating with **depressive episodes.** A manic episode is a period during which the predominant mood is excessively elevated (euphoria), expansive, or irritable. Associated symptoms include inflated self-esteem, or grandiosity, decreased need for sleep, a nearly continuous flow of rapid speech with quick changes of topic, distractibility, an increase in goal-directed activity, and excessive involvement in pleasurable activities that have a high potential for painful consequences. Often there are increased sociability and participation in multiple activities marked by intrusive, domineering, and demanding behavior. **Hypomania** (in this term, **hypo-** = decrease) describes a mood resembling mania, but of lesser intensity. **Bipolar disorder I** is characterized by one or more manic episodes, often alternating with major depressive episodes. **Bipolar disorder II** is characterized by recurrent major depressive episodes alternating with hypomanic episodes.

Cyclothymic disorder (**cycl/o** = cycle, **thym/o** = mind) is a mild form of bipolar disorder characterized by at least 2 years of numerous periods with hypomanic symptoms that do not meet the criteria for mania and depressive symptoms that do not meet the criteria for a major depressive disorder.

DEPRESSIVE DISORDERS

Depressive disorders are marked by the occurrence of one or more major depressive episodes without a history of mania or hypomania. **Major depressive disorder** involves episodes of severe **dysphoria** (sadness, hopelessness, worry, discouragement). Other signs and symptoms are appetite disturbances (increase or decrease) and changes in weight; sleep disorders such as insomnia or hypersomnia; fatigue or low energy; feelings of worthlessness, hopelessness, or excessive or inappropriate guilt; difficulty thinking or concentrating; and recurrent thoughts of death or suicide. **Persistent depressive disorder (dysthymia)** is a depressive disorder involving depressed mood (feeling sad or "down in the dumps") that persists over a 2-year period but is not as severe as major depression. Also, there are no psychotic features (delusions, hallucinations, incoherent thinking) as are sometimes found in major depressive disorder.

Researchers have noted a relationship between the onset of an episode of depressive disorder and a particular period of the year. A regular appearance of depression may occur within a period of approximately 60 days, between the beginning of October and the end of November, every year. This is referred to as **seasonal affective** (mood) **disorder (SAD).** A change from depression to mania or hypomania also may occur within a subsequent 60-day period from mid-February to mid-April.

DISSOCIATIVE DISORDERS

A **dissociative disorder** is a condition involving breakdown in memory, identity, or perception. People with dissociative disorder escape reality through amnesia, **fugue** (sudden travel away from home or work), or alternate identities. Examples of dissociative disorders are:

- **Identity disorder**—The presence of two or more distinct personality states.
- **Dissociative amnesia**—Inability to recall autobiographical information.
- **Depersonalization / derealization disorder**—Experiences of unreality, detachment, or being an outside observer with respect to one's thought and surroundings.

EATING DISORDERS

Eating disorders are severe disturbances in eating behavior. Examples are **anorexia nervosa** and **bulimia nervosa.** Anorexia nervosa is characterized by refusal to maintain a minimal normal body weight. The affected person is intensely afraid of gaining weight and has a disturbance in perception of the shape or size of her or his body. (The term **anorexia,** meaning "lack of appetite," is a misnomer because lack of appetite is rare.) The condition predominantly affects adolescent females, and its principal symptom is a conscious, relentless attempt to diet along with excessive, compulsive overactivity, such as exercise, running, or gymnastics. Most postmenarchal females with this disorder are amenorrheic.

Bulimia nervosa (**bulimia** means abnormal increase in hunger) is characterized by binge eating (uncontrolled indulgence in food) followed by purging (eliminating food from the body). Persons with bulimia maintain normal or nearly normal weight because after bingeing they engage in inappropriate purging. Examples of purging are self-induced vomiting and the misuse of laxatives or enemas.

NEUROCOGNITIVE DISORDERS

Neurocognitive disorders marked by disturbances in **cognition** (thinking, perception, reasoning, and judgment). **Delirium** and **dementia** are their primary features.

Delirium is marked by acute episodes of confused thinking, disorientation, and behavioral changes, such as agitation and fear. It is caused by a variety of conditions, including drug intoxication or withdrawal, seizures or head trauma, and metabolic disturbances such as hypoxia, hypoglycemia, electrolyte imbalances, or hepatic or renal failure. **Delirium tremens** is brought on by stopping alcohol consumption suddenly after prolonged periods of heavy alcohol ingestion.

Dementia is marked by progressive loss of intellectual abilities such as judgment, memory, and reasoning as well as changes in personality. It also includes difficulty with language and with simple acts like dressing or brushing the teeth. Dementia may be caused by conditions, some reversible and some progressive, involving damage to the brain. The most common cause is **Alzheimer disease,** but other causes are cerebrovascular disease (stroke), central nervous system (CNS) infection, certain medications and drugs, brain trauma, tumors, and Parkinson and Huntington diseases. It is important to identify treatable causes of dementia.

NEURODEVELOPMENTAL DISORDERS

Neurodevelopmental disorders are a group of childhood disorders characterized by delays in the development of socialization and communication skills. The following are examples of neurodevelopmental disorders:

- **Intellectual disability disorders**—Previously called mental retardation, these disorders include deficits in intellectual functions (reasoning, problem solving, planning and abstract thinking) and inability to adapt and interact in activities of daily life.
- **Communication disorders**—Persistent difficulties in the acquisition and use of language (spoken or written). This includes reduced vocabulary, limited sentence structure, and impairments in speaking, such as stuttering.

- **Autistic spectrum disorders—Autism,** commonly becoming evident during the first 3 years of life, is marked by difficulties in verbal and nonverbal communication and social and play interactions. The following are examples of autistic symptoms and signs:

> Resistance to change; insistence on sameness
> Using gestures or pointing instead of words to communicate needs
> Repeating words or phrases
> Preference for being alone; aloofness of manner
> Tantrums
> Difficulty in interacting with others
> Not wanting to be touched
> Little or no eye contact
> Uneven gross/fine motor skills
> Sensitivity to sound
> Obsessive attachment to objects

Symptoms of autism may lessen as the child develops and receives treatment. See the *In Person: Living with Autism* story on page 943.

Asperger syndrome often is referred to as a less severe type of autism. Children with Asperger syndrome frequently have normal language skills and normal intelligence. They usually want to interact with others but don't know how to do it. They may have fine rote memory skills but have difficulty with abstract concepts. Repetitive and restricted patterns of behavior also may be part of the picture.

- **Attention-deficit/hyperactivity disorder ADHD—**This is a persistent pattern of inattention and/or hyperactivity-impulsivity that interferes with functioning or development.
- **Specific learning disorders—**This category includes difficulties in learning and using academic skills.
- **Motor disorders—**Children with these disorders display lack of coordination (such as clumsiness and poor handwriting), movement disorders, and tics (involuntary, sudden, recurrent motor movement or vocalization).

PERSONALITY DISORDERS

A **personality disorder** is an enduring pattern of thinking and behavior contrary to what is culturally acceptable. Pervasive and inflexible, it typically first becomes evident in early adulthood and leads to distress or conflict with others.

Personality disorders are divided into three clusters or categories:

Cluster A
- **Paranoid—**Pattern of distrust and suspiciousness so that motives of others are interpreted as malicious; quick to take offense.
- **Schizoid—**Pattern of detachment from social relationships with restricted range of emotions; cold, aloof, and indifferent to the feelings of others.
- **Schizotypal—**Pattern of acute discomfort in close relationships, accompanied by odd beliefs or magical thinking, clairvoyance, bizarre fantasies or preoccupations.

Cluster B
- **Antisocial—**Pattern of disregard for, and violation of, the rights of others. Affected persons have no loyality or concern for others and act only in response to their own desires and impulses.
- **Borderline—**Pattern of instability in interpersonal relationships and sense of self. Affected persons alternate between intense, impulsive involvement and rejection of other people.
- **Histrionic—**Pattern of excessive emotionality and attention seeking. Affected persons are immature, dependent, flamboyant and theatrical. They often have irrational outbursts and tantrums with general angry feelings about themselves and the world.

- **Narcissistic**—Pattern of grandiosity, need for admiration, and lack of empathy. Affected persons have a preoccupation with their own self importance and fantasies of success and power.

Cluster C
- **Avoidance**—Pattern of social inhibition, feelings of inadequacy, and hypersensitivity to negative evaluation. Affected persons are unwilling to get involved with others for fear of being criticized or rejected.
- **Dependent**—Pattern of submissive and clinging behaviour related to an excessive need to be taken care of. Affected persons have a lack of self-confidence and difficulty making everyday decisions without advice or reassurance from others.
- **Obsessive-compulsive**—Pattern of orderliness, perfectionism, and control. At the expense of flexibility and openness, affected persons are preoccupied with details, rules, lists, organization, and schedules. As compared to patients with obsessive compulsive anxiety disorder (OCD), individuals with obsessive-compulsive personality disorder are not aware that their thoughts and behaviors are unreasonable.

SCHIZOPHRENIA SPECTRUM AND OTHER PSYCHOTIC DISORDERS

Schizophrenia spectrum and other psychotic disorders are chronic psychoses marked by disturbed thinking and disorganized speech. Key features that define these disorders are:

Delusions. Fixed beliefs that are not easy to change in light of conflicting evidence. Examples are persecutory delusions ("people are out to get me") or grandiose delusions ("I am the wealthiest, most famous, and important person in the world").

Hallucinations. Hearing voices or sounds that do not exist but seem real.

Disorganized thinking (speech). The person may switch from one topic to another, resulting in incoherent, incomprehensible speech.

Abnormal motor behavior. This disorganized behavior includes involuntary movements and mannerisms from childlike "silliness" to unpredictable agitation. **Catatonic behavior** is marked by decrease in reactivity to the environment, such as maintaining a rigid, inappropriate, or bizarre posture.

Negative symptoms. Two negative symptoms that are prominent in schizophrenia are flatness of affect (diminished emotional expression) and unwillingness to initiate purposeful activities.

SEXUAL DYSFUNCTIONS, PARAPHILIAS, AND GENDER DYSPHORIA

Sexual dysfunctions are disturbances in a person's ability to respond sexually or to experience sexual pleasure. Examples of sexual dysfunctions are delayed or premature ejaculation, orgasmic disorders, sexual interest/arousal disorders, and pelvic pain disorders.

Paraphilias (para- = abnormal, -philia = attraction to or love of) are characterized by recurrent, intense, sexual urges, fantasies, or behaviors that involve sexual objects, activities, or situations. Examples of paraphilias are:

- **Exhibitionism**—compulsive need to expose one's body, particularly the genitals, to an unsuspecting stranger.
- **Fetishism**—use of nonliving objects (articles of clothing) as substitutes for a human sexual love object.
- **Pedophilia**—sexual urges and fantasies involving sexual activity with a prepubescent child (age 13 or younger).
- **Sexual masochism**—sexual gratification is gained by being humiliated, beaten, bound, or otherwise made to suffer.

- **Sexual sadism**—sexual gratification is gained by inflicting physical or psychological pain or humiliation on others.
- **Transvestic fetishism**—cross-dressing; wearing clothing of the opposite sex accompanied by recurrent and intense sexual arousal.
- **Voyeurism**—sexual excitement is achieved by observing unsuspecting people who are naked, undressing, or engaging in sexual activity.

Gender dysphoria is a strong and persistent cross-gender identification manifested in preference for dressing and gender roles typical for the opposite sex. There must also be evidence of distress about this difference in gender identification.

SOMATIC SYMPTOM DISORDERS

In somatic sympton disorders, the patient's psychic (mental) conflicts are expressed as physical symptoms. Abdominal or chest pain, nausea, vomiting, diarrhea, palpitations, deafness, blindness, and paralysis, are not explained by a physical or other mental disorder or by injury and are not side effects of medication, drugs, or alcohol. Examples are:

- **Somatic symptom disorder.** This is classified as the presence of one or more somatic symptoms that are distressing or result in significant disruption of daily life. Typically patients have persistent thoughts and a high level of anxiety about their symptoms.
- **Illness anxiety disorder.** This is marked by preoccupation with having or acquiring a severe illness. Somatic symptoms are not present or if present, only mild in intensity. There is a high level of anxiety about health, and affected people engage in excessive health-related behaviors such as checks on their body for signs of illness. Ruling out a physical abnormality does not reassure the person with an illness anxiety disorder.
- **Conversion disorder.** This is marked by specific neurologic signs or symptoms (such as numbness, paralysis, or blindness) with no actual, organic basis. These symptoms are the result of anxiety and unconscious inner conflict. In a conversion disorder, an unconscious conflict threatens to escape from **repression** (a defense mechanism in which a person removes unacceptable ideas or impulses from consciousness), and is experienced as a physical symptom. The conversion symptom (paralysis, blindness, seizures, and paresthesias) enables the affected person to avoid the conflict and get support from the surrounding environment. For example, a person with repressed anger and desire to physically harm a family member may suddenly develop paralysis of the arm (conversion symptom). Another example of a conversion symptom might be paralysis of the finger used to pull the trigger of a gun if there was internal conflict about firing the weapon.

SUBSTANCE-RELATED AND ADDICTIVE DISORDERS

Substance-related and addictive disorders are characterized by symptoms and behavioral changes associated with regular use or discontinuation of substances that affect the central nervous system (CNS). Continued or periodic use of certain drugs produces a state of dependence. **Psychological dependence** is a compulsion to continue taking a drug despite adverse consequences, and **physiologic dependence** is characterized by the onset of withdrawal symptoms when the drug is discontinued abruptly. A significant feature of physiologic dependence is **tolerance.** Tolerance is the declining effect of the drug so that the dose must be increased to give the same effect.

Examples of substances that are associated with drug abuse (use of a drug for purposes other than those for which it is prescribed) and dependence are:

Alcohol. Alcohol's effects vary from person to person depending on how much is consumed and how often drinking occurs, and on the drinker's age, health status, and family history. Signs of alcohol dependence and intoxication include slurred speech, incoordination, unsteady gait, nystagmus (rapid, rhythmic movement of the eyeball), impairment in attention or memory, stupor, or coma. Alcohol dependence often is associated with the use and abuse of other psychoactive drugs (cannabis, cocaine, heroin, amphetamines). It also is associated with depression, as either a cause or a consequence of the drinking.

Amphetamines. These CNS stimulants are taken orally or administered intravenously. Examples are amphetamine (Benzedrine), dextroamphetamine (Dexedrine), methamphetamine (Desoxyn, or "speed"), and methylphenidate (Ritalin). Some appetite suppressants (diet pills) are amphetamine-like drugs. Psychological and behavioral changes associated with amphetamine dependence include anger, tension or anxiety, impaired judgment, inability to enjoy what was previously pleasurable, and social isolation. Physical signs and symptoms include tachycardia or bradycardia, dilated pupils, nausea, elevated or low blood pressure, and muscular weakness. Serious depression can occur during withdrawal.

Cannabis. This class of drugs includes all substances with psychoactive properties derived from the cannabis plant plus chemically similar synthetic substances. Examples are **marijuana,** hashish, and purified delta-9-tetrahydrocannabinol (THC), the major psychoactive ingredient in these substances. Psychological and physical signs and symptoms after the smoking of cannabis include euphoria, impaired motor coordination, anxiety, sensation of slowed time, social withdrawal, and impaired memory and judgment. Other signs of cannabis intoxication are increased appetite, dry mouth, tachycardia, and paranoia.

Cocaine. Cocaine is a powerfully addictive stimulant drug made from the leaves of the coca plant native to South America. It commonly is inhaled through nostrils or injected intravenously. Short-term effects are euphoria, erratic and violent behavior, vasoconstriction, tachycardia, hypertension, and enlarged pupils. Possible long-term effects are loss of sense of smell, nasal damage and nosebleeds, infection, and bowel necrosis from decreased blood flow. Often, the user of cocaine also is dependent on alcohol or sedatives, which are taken in an attempt to alleviate the unpleasant aftereffects (anxiety, depression, and fatigue) of cocaine intoxication or withdrawal.

Hallucinogens. These drugs produce a state of CNS excitement, hyperactivity, hallucinations, delusions, hypertension, and mood changes. Examples of hallucinogens are **lysergic acid diethylamide (LSD), mescaline (peyote),** and **phencyclidine (PCP).** Other hallucinogens are ayahuasca (hallucinogenic tea) and DMT (*N,N*-dimethyltryptamine, a synthetic drug producing a short-lived hallucinogenic experience). These drugs can disrupt the user's ability to think and communicate rationally. They cause an inability to recognize reality, sometimes resulting in bizarre or dangerous behavior.

Opioids. This group of drugs includes **heroin** and **morphine** and synthetic drugs with morphine-like action, such as **codeine,** meperidine (Demerol), and oxycodone (OxyContin is sustained-release oxycodone). These compounds are prescribed as analgesics (painkillers), anesthetics, or cough suppressants. Typical signs and symptoms of opioid intoxication are pupillary constriction, euphoria, slowness in movement, drowsiness, and slurred speech. Effects of overdose are slow and shallow breathing, convulsions, coma, and possible death.

Sedatives, hypnotics, or anxiolytics. These drugs have a soothing, relaxing, euphoric effect and also can produce sleep (hypnotics). Sleeping pills include **barbiturates** such as phenobarbital and secobarbital. Other drugs that produce a barbiturate-like effect are **benzodiazepines,** including temazepam (Restoril), clonazepam (Klonopin), alprazolam (Xanax), and diazepam (Valium). Intoxication is characterized by slurred speech and disorientation.

Figure 22-3 reviews the types of psychoactive substances that lead to drug dependence and abuse.

Table 22-1 reviews psychiatric disorders and gives examples of each type.

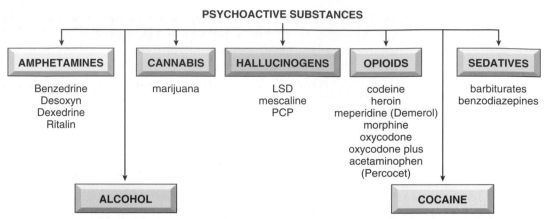

FIGURE 22-3　**Psychoactive substances** that if abused can lead to drug dependence.

TABLE 22-1	PSYCHIATRIC DISORDERS	
CATEGORY	**EXAMPLE(S)**	
Anxiety disorders	• Panic disorder • Phobic disorders • Obsessive-compulsive disorder	• Post-traumatic stress disorder • Generalized anxiety disorder
Bipolar disorders	• Bipolar I • Bipolar II • Cyclothymic disorder	
Depressive disorders	• Major depressive disorder • Persistent depressive disorder (dysthymia) • Seasonal affective disorder (SAD)	
Dissociative disorders	• Identity disorder • Dissociative amnesia • Depersonalization/Derealization disorder	
Eating disorders	• Anorexia nervosa • Bulimia nervosa	
Neurocognitive disorders	• Delirium • Dementia	
Neurodevelopmental disorders	• Intellectual disability disorders • Communication disorders	• Autistic spectrum disorder • Attention-deficit/hyperactivity disorder
Personality disorders	Cluster A: • paranoid • schizoid • schizotypal	Cluster B: • antisocial • borderline • histrionic • narcissistic　　Cluster C: • avoidant • dependent • obsessive-compulsive
Schizophrenia spectrum and other psychotic disorders	Key features: • Delusions • Hallucinations	• Disorganized thinking (speech) • Abnormal motor behavior • Negative symptoms
Sexual dysfunctions, paraphilias, and gender dysphoria disorders	• Delayed or premature ejaculation/orgasmic disorders • Exhibitionism • Voyeurism	
Somatic symptom disorders	• Conversion disorder • Illness anxiety disorder	
Substance-related and addictive disorders	Use/Abuse of: • Alcohol • Cannabis • Hallucinogens • Sedatives	• Amphetamines • Cocaine • Opioids

THERAPEUTIC MODALITIES

Some major therapeutic techniques that are used to treat psychiatric disorders are **psychotherapy, electroconvulsive therapy (ECT),** and **drug therapy (psychopharmacology).**

PSYCHOTHERAPY

Psychotherapy is the treatment of emotional problems and disorders using psychological techniques. The following are psychotherapeutic techniques used by psychiatrists, psychologists, and other mental health professionals.

Cognitive-Behavioral Therapy (CBT). This is a relatively short-term, focused psychotherapy for a wide range of psychological problems, including depression, anxiety, anger, marital conflict, fears, and substance abuse. The focus is on how the person who is experiencing difficulty is thinking, behaving, and communicating today, rather than on early childhood experiences. Because CBT is based on the idea that thoughts cause feelings and behaviors (not people, situations, or events), if the person can change established ways of thinking, then he or she can feel better even if the situation does not change. CBT techniques often are used to reduce anxiety.

Family Therapy. Treatment of an entire family can help the individual members resolve and understand their conflicts and problems.

Group Therapy. In a group with a mental health professional leader as a neutral moderator, patients with similar problems gain insight into their own personalities through discussions and interaction with each other. In **psychodrama,** patients express their feelings by acting out family and social roles along with other patient-actors on a stage. After a scene has been presented, the audience (composed of other patients) is asked to make comments and offer interpretations about what they have observed.

Hypnosis. A **trance** (state of altered consciousness) is created to help in recovery of deeply repressed memories. Hypnotic techniques also are used for anxiety reduction, for creating a sense of psychological safety, and for problem solving.

Insight-Oriented Psychotherapy. This type of psychotherapy uses face-to-face discussion of life problems and associated feelings. The aim is to increase understanding of underlying conflicts, themes, thoughts, and behavior patterns to improve mood (depressive feelings).

Play Therapy. In this form of therapy, the child uses play with toys to express conflicts and feelings that he or she is unable to communicate in a direct manner.

Psychoanalysis. This long-term and intense form of psychotherapy seeks to influence behavior and resolve internal conflicts by allowing patients to bring their unconscious emotions to the surface. Through techniques such as **free association** (the patient speaks his or her thoughts one after another without censorship), **transference** (the patient relates to the therapist as to a person who figured prominently in early childhood, such as a parent or sibling), and **dream interpretation,** the patient is able to bring unconscious emotional conflicts to awareness and thus can overcome these problems.

Sex Therapy. This form of therapy can help people overcome sexual dysfunctions such as **frigidity** (inhibited sexual response in women), **impotence** (inability of a man to achieve and/or maintain an erection), and **premature ejaculation** (release of semen before coitus can be achieved).

Supportive Psychotherapy. The therapist offers encouragement, support, and hope to patients facing difficult life transitions and events.

22

ELECTROCONVULSIVE THERAPY

In **electroconvulsive therapy (ECT),** an electrical current is applied to the brain (usually to one hemisphere) after the patient is anesthetized, with assisted ventilation, and given a very short-acting muscle paralytic agent. Actual physical convulsions are therefore imperceptible. This therapy is used chiefly for serious depression and the depressive phase of bipolar (manic-depressive) disorder. ECT is a particularly effective treatment for psychotic depression and can be life-saving when a rapid response is needed.

DRUG THERAPY

The following are categories of drugs used to treat psychiatric disorders. Figure 22-4 reviews these groups and lists specific drugs in each category.

- **Antianxiety and antipanic agents.** These drugs lessen anxiety, tension, and agitation, especially when they are associated with panic attacks. Examples are **benzodiazepines (BZDs),** which act rapidly as antianxiety angents, sedatives, or anticonvulsants (clonazepam). Benzodiazepines directly affect the brain to stabilize the transmission of excitatory nerve impulses. Other antianxiety and antipanic agents are **selective serotonin reuptake inhibitors (SSRIs).** These agents prevent the reuptake of serotonin (a neurotransmitter) into nerve endings, allowing it to linger in the space between it and the next nerve cell.
- **Antidepressants.** These drugs gradually reverse depressive symptoms and return the patient to a more even state, with less persistent and less severe depressive symptoms. The basic cause of depression is thought to be related to neurotransmitters in the brain. Several groups of drugs are used as antidepressants. These include:
  1. **SSRIs (selective serotonin reuptake inhibitors)** such as fluoxetine (Prozac), paroxetine (Paxil), and sertraline (Zoloft). They improve mood, mental concentration, physical activity, and sleep patterns.
  2. **Atypical antidepressants.** These are antidepressants that do not fit in defined categories. **Serotonin-norepinephrine reuptake inhibitors (SNRIs)** are antidepressant drugs that modulate the two neurotransmitters serotonin and norepinephrine in the brain. Examples are venlafaxine (Effexor), desvenlafaxine (Pristiq), and duloxetine (Cymbalta).
  3. **Tricyclic antidepressants.** These drugs contain three fused rings in their chemical structure (that is, hence the designation *tricyclic*). They disrupt neurotransmission at nerve endings. **Tetracyclic antidepressants** such as mirtazapine (Remeron) also are used to treat depression symptoms. Mirtazapine helps with insomnia, but patients can gain weight.
  4. **Monoamine oxidase (MAO) inhibitors.** These drugs suppress an enzyme, monoamine oxidase, that normally breaks down neurotransmitters. MAO inhibitors are not as widely prescribed as other antidepressants because serious cardiovascular and liver complications can occur with their use. Significant dietary restrictions also are necessary to avoid adverse reactions.
- **Anti–obsessive-compulsive disorder (OCD) agents.** These drugs are prescribed to relieve the symptoms of OCD. Tricyclic antidepressants and SSRIs are examples of these agents.
- **Antipsychotics (neuroleptics).** These drugs suppress psychotic symptoms and behavior (Greek *lepsis* means a taking hold). **Atypical antipsychotics** are the major examples. They are used to treat schizophrenia, bipolar disorder, and other mental illnesses. They reduce anxiety, tension, agitation, and aggressiveness and modify psychotic symptoms such as delusions and hallucinations. Other drugs, such as **first-generation** (early) **antipsychotics,** such as **phenothiazines,** are still used as well. An important potential adverse effect of older neuroleptic drugs taken over long periods is **tardive dyskinesia (TD);** tardive means late, and dyskinesias are abnormal movements. This is a potentially irreversible condition marked by involuntary movements. Early detection is important.

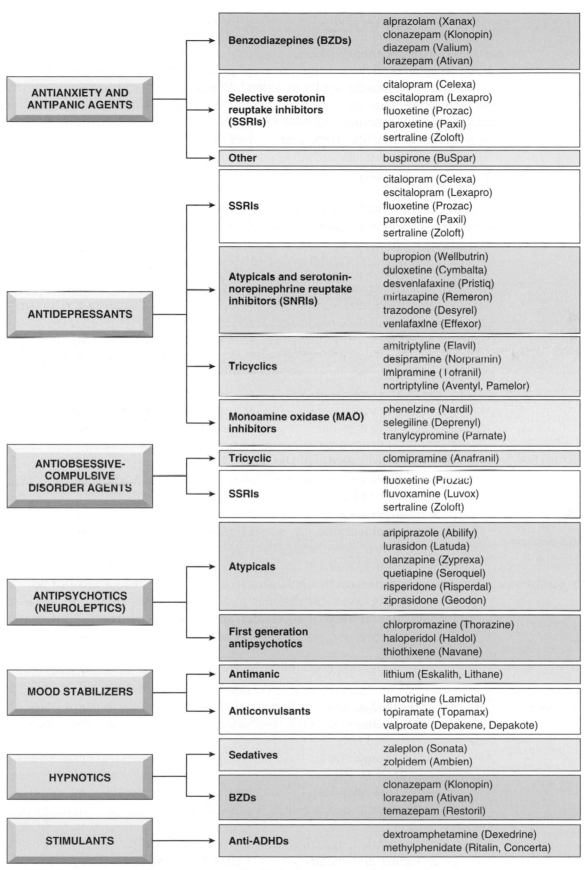

FIGURE 22-4 Psychiatric drug categories and specific drugs.

22

The AIMS (abnormal involuntary movement scale) is used to monitor patients for signs of TD. Weight gain and increased risk for developing diabetes also are important side effects of atypical antipsychotics.

- **Mood stabilizers.** These drugs are used primarily to treat patients with the mood changes associated with bipolar disorder. **Lithium** (Eskalith, Lithane) is commonly used to reduce the frequency and severity of manic symptoms, such as rapid speech, hyperactive movements, grandiose ideas, agitation and irritability, and impaired sleep patterns (decreased need for sleep is typical). It also is used as an adjunct in the treatment of depression. Lithium is a simple salt that is thought to stabilize nerve membranes. **Anticonvulsant drugs** (valproate and lamotrigine) also are used as mood stabilizers.
- **Hypnotics.** These drugs are used to produce sleep (hypn/o = sleep) and relieve insomnia. Examples are sedatives and benzodiazepines.
- **Stimulants.** These drugs **(amphetamines)** are prescribed for **attention-deficit/hyperactivity disorder** in children and, to a lesser extent, adults. Common manifestations of ADHD are a short attention span and easy distractibility, emotional unstability, impulsivity, and moderate to severe hyperactivity.

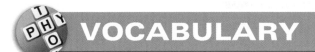

VOCABULARY

This list reviews many of the new terms introduced in the text. Short definitions reinforce your understanding of the terms. Refer to the Pronunciation of Terms on page 954 for help with unfamiliar or difficult words.

GENERAL TERMINOLOGY, SYMPTOMS, AND DISORDERS

affect	External expression of emotion, or emotional response.
amnesia	Loss of memory.
anorexia nervosa	Eating disorder with excessive dieting and refusal to maintain a normal body weight.
anxiety disorders	Characterized by unpleasant tension, distress, and avoidance behavior; examples are panic disorder, phobias, obsessive-compulsive disorder, post-traumatic stress disorder, and generalized anxiety disorder.
apathy	Absence of emotions; lack of interest or emotional involvement.
autism	Neurodevelopmental disorder characterized by inhibited social interaction and communication and by restricted, repetitive behavior.
bipolar disorders	These disorders are marked by alternating periods of mania and depression.
bulimia nervosa	Eating disorder with binge eating followed by vomiting, purging, and depression.
cannabis	Plant substance from which marijuana is obtained.
compulsion	Uncontrollable urge to perform an act repeatedly in an attempt to reduce anxiety.
conversion disorder	Condition marked by neurologic symptoms with no organic (physical) basis, appearing as a result of anxiety and unconscious inner conflict.
defense mechanism	Unconscious technique (coping mechanism) used to resolve or conceal conflicts and anxiety. It protects the person against anxiety and stress; examples are acting out, denial, and repression.

22

delirium	Acute episodes of confused thinking, disorientation, agitation, and fearfulness. This usually is a reversible impairment. **Delirium tremens** is associated with alcohol withdrawal.
delusion	Fixed, false belief that cannot be changed by logical reasoning or evidence.
dementia	Progressive loss of intellectual abilities such as memory, judgment, and reasoning as well as changes in personality.
depressive disorders	Major psychiatric disorders with chronic sadness, loss of energy, hopelessness, worry, discouragement, and, commonly, suicidal impulses and thoughts.
dissociative disorders	Conditions involving breakdown in memory, identity, or perception; examples are identity disorder, dissociative amnesia, and depersonalization/derealization disorder.
ego	Central coordinating branch of the personality or mind.
fugue	Unconscious flight from customary surroundings; a sign of dissociative disorder.
gender dysphoria	Strong and persistent cross-gender identification with the opposite sex that causes clinically significant distress.
hallucination	False sensory perception (hearing voices and seeing things).
id	Major unconscious part of the personality; energy from instinctual drives and desires.
labile	Unstable; undergoing rapid emotional change.
mania	Elevated expansive state (euphoria) with hyperactivity, talkativeness, and racing thought. ✳ **HINT:** Don't confuse with the suffix -mania (see page 940), meaning obsession.
mutism	No, or very little, ability to speak.
neurodevelopmental disorders	Group of childhood disorders characterized by delays in socialization and communication skills; **autism spectrum disorder** is an example.
obsession	Involuntary, persistent idea, urge or emotion.
obsessive-compulsive disorder	Anxiety disorder in which recurrent thoughts and repetitive acts dominate behavior.
paranoia	Overly suspicious system of thinking with fixed delusions of being harassed, persecuted, or unfairly treated.
paraphilia	Recurrent intense sexual urge, fantasy, or behavior that involves unusual objects, activities, or situations.
personality disorders	Lifelong personality patterns marked by inflexibility and impairment of social functioning.
phobia	Irrational or disabling fear (avoidance) of an object or situation.
post-traumatic stress disorder	Anxiety-related symptoms appear after personal experience of a traumatic event.
projective (personality) test	Diagnostic personality test using stimuli (inkblots, pictures, abstract patterns, incomplete sentences) to evoke responses that reflect aspects of an individual's personality.
psychiatrist	Physician (MD degree) or osteopath (DO degree) with medical training in the diagnosis, prevention, and treatment of mental disorders. Examples are a **child psychiatrist** (diagnosing and treating children) and a **forensic psychiatrist** (specializing in legal considerations such as criminal responsibility, guardianship, and competence to stand trial). Forensic comes from the Latin *forum*, meaning public place.

22

psychologist	Nonmedical professional (often with a PhD or an EdD degree) specializing in mental processes and how the brain functions in health and disease. Areas of interest are **clinical psychology** (providing testing and counseling services to patients with mental and emotional disorders), **experimental psychology** (performing laboratory tests and experiments in a controlled environment to study mental processes), and **social psychology** (study of the effects of group membership on behavior and attitudes of individuals).
psychosis	Disorder marked by loss of contact with reality, often associated with delusions and hallucinations.
reality testing	Psychological process that distinguishes fact from fantasy; severely impaired in psychosis.
repression	Defense mechanism by which unacceptable thoughts, feelings, and impulses are automatically pushed into the unconscious, out of awareness.
schizophrenia spectrum disorders	Group of chronic psychotic disorders that may include hallucinations, disorganized speech and behavior, flat affect, and lack of initiative.
sexual dysfunctions	Disturbances in a person's ability to respond sexually or to experience sexual pleasure.
somatic symptom disorders	Presence of physical symptoms that cannot be explained by an actual physical disorder or mental disorder such as depression.
substance-related and addictive disorders	A group of disorders marked by regular overuse of or dependence on psychoactive substances (alcohol, amphetamines, cannabis, cocaine, hallucinogens, opioids, and sedatives) that affect the central nervous system.
superego	Internalized conscience and moral aspect of the personality.

THERAPY

amphetamines	Central nervous system stimulants that may be used to treat attention deficit–hyperactivity disorder and depression.
atypical antipsychotics	Drugs that treat psychotic symptoms and behavior (schizophrenia, bipolar disease, and other mental illness).
benzodiazepines	Drugs that lessen anxiety, tension, agitation, and panic attacks.
cognitive behavioral therapy	Focuses on the connection between behavior and thoughts. Conditioning (changing behavior patterns by training and repetition) is used to relieve anxiety and improve symptoms of illness.
electroconvulsive therapy	Electrical current is used to produce convulsions and loss of consciousness; effective in the treatment of major depression. Modern techniques use anesthesia, so the convulsion is not observable.
family therapy	Treatment of an entire family to resolve and shed light on conflicts.
first-generation antipsychotic drugs	Early neuroleptic medications that reduce psychotic symptoms.
free association	Psychoanalytic technique in which the patient verbalizes, without censorship, the passing contents of his or her mind.
group therapy	Group of patients with similar problems gain insight into their personalities through discussion and interaction with each other.
hypnosis	Induced trance (state of altered consciousness).

insight-oriented therapy	Face-to-face discussion of life problems and associated feelings. The patient tells his or her story and has the opportunity to connect emotional patterns in his or her life history with present concerns. Also called psychodynamic therapy.
lithium	Medication used to treat bipolar illness.
neuroleptic drug	Any drug that favorably modifies psychotic symptoms; antipsychotic drug.
play therapy	Treatment in which a child, through use of toys in a playroom setting, expresses conflicts and feelings that cannot be communicated in a direct manner.
psychoanalysis	Treatment that allows the patient to explore inner emotions and conflicts so as to understand and change current behavior.
psychodrama	Group therapy in which a patient expresses feelings by acting out family and social roles with other patients.
psychopharmacology	Treatment of psychiatric disorders with drugs.
sedatives	Drugs that induce calmness, promote sleep, and help lessen anxiety.
supportive psychotherapy	Offering encouragement, support, and hope to patients facing difficult life transitions and events.
transference	Psychoanalytic process in which the patient relates to the therapist as though the therapist were a prominent childhood figure.
tricyclic antidepressants	Drugs used to treat severe depression (characterized by a three-ringed fused molecular structure).

22

 # TERMINOLOGY

Write the meanings of the medical terms in the spaces provided.

COMBINING FORMS

COMBINING FORM	MEANING	TERMINOLOGY	MEANING
anxi/o	uneasy, anxious, distressed	anxiolytic _____ *This type of drug relieves anxiety.* **Benzodiazopines** *are anxiolytics (Valium and Xanax are examples).*	
aut/o	self	autism _____	
hallucin/o	hallucination, to wander in the mind	hallucinogen _____ *A* **hallucination** *is a sensory perception in the absence of any external stimuli, and an* **illusion** *is an error in perception in which sensory stimuli are present but incorrectly interpreted.*	
hypn/o	sleep	hypnosis _____ *The Greek god of sleep (Hypnos) put people to sleep by touching them with his magic wand or by fanning them with his dark wings.*	

COMBINING FORM	MEANING	TERMINOLOGY	MEANING
iatr/o	treatment	psychiatrist _____	
		iatrogenic _____	
ment/o	mind	mental _____	
neur/o	nerve	neurotransmitter _____ *Examples of neurotransmitters are serotonin and norepinephrine.*	
phil/o	attraction to, love	paraphilia _____ *Para- means abnormal.*	
phren/o	mind	schizophrenia _____ *Schiz/o means split.*	
psych/o	mind	psychosis _____ *Loss of contact with reality associated with symptoms such as delusions, hallucinations, and bizarre behavior.*	
		psychopharmacology _____	
		psychotherapy _____	
schiz/o	split	schizoid _____ *A type of personality disorder; emotionally cold, withdrawn and aloof.*	
somat/o	body	psychosomatic _____	

22

SUFFIXES

SUFFIX	MEANING	TERMINOLOGY	MEANING
-genic	produced by	psychogenic _____	
-leptic	to seize hold of	neuroleptic drug _____	
-mania	obsessive preoccupation	kleptomania _____ *Klept/o means to steal.*	
		pyromania _____ *Pyr/o means fire, heat.*	
-phobia	fear (irrational and often disabling)	agoraphobia _____ *Agora- means marketplace. Agoraphobics fear leaving home or a safe place.*	
		xenophobia _____ *Xen/o means stranger. Table 22-2 lists other phobias.*	
-phoria	feeling, bearing	euphoria _____ *The prefix eu- means good. An excited state of joy; a good feeling.*	
		dysphoria _____ *The prefix dys- means bad or unpleasant.*	

TABLE 22-2 | PHOBIAS

SOURCE OF FEAR/ ANXIETY	MEDICAL TERM	SOURCE OF FEAR/ ANXIETY	MEDICAL TERM
air	aerophobia	heights	acrophobia
animals	zoophobia	insects	entomophobia
bees	apiphobia, melissophobia	light	photophobia
blood or bleeding	hematophobia, hemophobia	marriage	gamophobia
		men	androphobia
books	bibliophobia	needles	belonephobia
cats	ailurophobia	pain	algophobia
corpses	necrophobia	sexual intercourse	coitophobia, cypridophobia
crossing a bridge	gephyrophobia	sleep	hypnophobia
darkness	nyctophobia, scotophobia	snakes	ophidiophobia
death	thanatophobia	spiders	arachnophobia
dogs	cynophobia	traveling	hodophobia
drugs	pharmacophobia	vomiting	emetophobia
eating	phagophobia	women	gynephobia, gynophobia
enclosed places	claustrophobia	worms	helminthophobia
hair	trichophobia, trichopathophobia	writing	graphophobia

22

SUFFIX	MEANING	TERMINOLOGY	MEANING
-thymia	mind	cyclothymia _____ *Cycl/o means circle or recurring. Alternating periods of hypomania and depression; lesser intensity than in bipolar disorder.*	
		dysthymia _____ *Depressed mood that is not as severe as in major depression.*	
		euthymia _____ *Normal, non-depressed, positive mood.*	

PREFIXES

PREFIX	MEANING	TERMINOLOGY	MEANING
a-, an-	no, not	anorexia nervosa _____ *-orexia means appetite.*	
cata-	down	catatonia _____ *Ton/o means tension. A state of psychologically induced immobility with muscular rigidity.*	

PREFIX	MEANING	TERMINOLOGY	MEANING
hypo-	deficient, less than, below	<u>hypo</u>mania _____	
para-	abnormal	<u>para</u>noia _____	

The no- in this term comes from the Greek word nous, _meaning mind._

ABBREVIATIONS

AD	Alzheimer disease—a form of dementia
ADHD	attention-deficit/hyperactivity disorder
ADLs	activities of daily living
AIMS	abnormal involuntary movement scale—used to monitor signs of tardive dyskinesia
ASD	autism spectrum disorder
BZD	benzodiazepine
CA	chronologic age
CBT	cognitive-behavioral therapy
CNS	central nervous system
DSM-5	_Diagnostic and Statistical Manual of Mental Disorders, Fifth Edition_
DT	delirium tremens
ECT	electroconvulsive therapy
GAD	generalized anxiety disorder
ID	intellectual disability
IQ	intelligence quotient — An IQ test is a standardized test to determine mental age of an individual. The average person is considered to have an IQ of between 90 and 110. Those who score below 70 are considered to have an intellectual disability.
LSD	lysergic acid diethylamide—a hallucinogen
MA	mental age—as determined by psychological tests

MAOI	monoamine oxidase inhibitor; an example is phenelzine (Nardil)
MDD	major depressive disorder
MMPI	Minnesota Multiphasic Personality Inventory
NCD	neurocognitive disorder
OCD	obsessive-compulsive disorder (anxiety disorder)
OCPD	obsessive-compulsive personality disorder
PTSD	post-traumatic stress disorder
Rx	therapy
SAD	seasonal affective disorder
SNRI	serotonin-norepinephrine reuptake inhibitor; an example is duloxetine (Cymbalta)
SSRI	selective serotonin reuptake inhibitor; an example is fluoxetine (Prozac)
TAT	Thematic Apperception Test
TCA	tricyclic antidepressant
TD	tardive dyskinesia
THC	delta-9-tetrahydrocannabinol—active ingredient in marijuana
WAIS	Wechsler Adult Intelligence Scale
WISC	Wechsler Intelligence Scale for Children
Ψ	symbol for psych- (the uppercase Greek letter psi)
ΨRx	psychotherapy

22

IN PERSON: LIVING WITH AUTISM

This first-person account was written by the mother of a young boy diagnosed with autism.

"What you do from now on will determine whether your son will be able to live on his own as an adult or whether he will have to live in a facility."

I was told this by a physician when my son, Jeff, was diagnosed with autism.

It began early on. For the first year of his life, Jeff had difficulty tolerating many situations and often cried. Loud noises such as barking dogs, motorcycles, and the trash truck sent him into a crying frenzy. If he was in a quiet room, in a swing, or being held, he was comfortable. Most other situations he could tolerate for only 60 to 90 minutes, after which he would cry for 20 to 30 minutes as if relieving stress. As Jeff aged, his tolerance slowly increased, but even at the age of 4, overstimulation caused him to cry daily.

Jeff experienced numerous other challenges as well. His ability to play was impaired. If a toy did not light up or play music he was not interested in it. The exception was Matchbox cars, which he did enjoy. However, he did not play with them appropriately. He merely lined them up. Jeff never engaged in imaginative play, nor could he carry on a back-and-forth conversation. His speech was rote, and he had extreme difficulty communicating and relating to peers.

After visiting several doctors in search of a diagnosis, we were told Jeff was autistic. We also learned that his discomfort and crying were a result of sensory integration challenges that children on the autism spectrum experience. Sensory integration is the process of organizing useful perceptions, emotions and thoughts. When sensory integration is whole and balanced, body movements are highly adaptive and good behavior is a natural outcome. This was not the case with Jeff.

It was difficult to accept the diagnosis, but we had to move on. The next step was finding proper treatment for Jeff. After much consideration, we decided on DIR/Floortime [Developmental, Individual Difference, Relationship-Based–Floortime] Therapy ("Floortime"), supplemented with occupational therapy (OT), to address Jeff's sensory integration needs.

Floortime is a play-based treatment, focusing on helping children master the building blocks of relating, communicating, and thinking. Guided interactions between the child and parent, sibling, grandparent, or caregiver move the child through six Floortime developmental stages, which are:

1. Self-Regulation and Shared Attention
2. Engagement and Relating
3. Two-way Intentional Communication
4. Purposeful Complex Problem Solving/Communication
5. Creating Ideas
6. Logical Reasoning, Thinking Logically

I was taught Floortime by a professional and spent nights watching instructional videos and reading Floortime books. I worked with Jeff each day, including Saturday and Sunday. We did Floortime constantly even during meals, riding in the car, and during bath time. I was working for my son's future. The more therapy he received, the better his chances of "recovery." No opportunity was missed.

Each week, over the course of several years, our program leader would assess Jeff's development and determine when he had mastered a skill and when further interventions were needed.

Over several years, Floortime was resolving Jeff's developmental issues, and OT was helping his sensory integration issues, but another problem was becoming more extreme. By first grade, Jeff had developed anxiety that was so irrational and overwhelming that it impaired his school, social and family life. He was very fearful and always thinking about the worst things that could happen. Conversations often would "spin out of control" as Jeff worried irrationally about things that might happen to him. During these times, I would attempt to distract him, only to have the anxiety recur.

As time went on, Jeff not only was verbalizing his anxiety, but manifested other unconscious behaviors such as eye and verbal tics, chewing on his shirt, and pulling on his hair.

Our team of doctors did not have a specific answer for Jeff's anxiety. We tried numerous treatments including psychotherapy, desensitization therapy, applied behavioral therapy, occupational body-regulating therapy, and cognitive-behavioral therapy. None had much effect on reducing anxiety.

Finally, one of our doctors suggested a study at a nearby university, which was funded by the National Institute of Mental Health. The program was specifically designed for children on the autism spectrum suffering from very high levels of anxiety. It was a treatment protocol based on a collaborative, family-based intervention approach using targeted cognitive-behavioral therapy techniques. It took into consideration Jeff's spectrum-based deficits and taught him how his anxiety could be managed by using a coping plan and actively facing his fears. The program lasted nearly a year. But we used it regularly for months after it ended. It had a noticeable positive impact on Jeff's anxiety.

By his fourth-grade year, Jeff's physical size of 5'0" and 80 pounds allowed his child psychiatrist to prescribe antianxiety medication. This has made a real difference in his functioning and well-being.

Today Jeff is is a mainstreamed student at a public middle school. He is able to relate to others with real warmth. He has a core group of good friends, a love of learning, and a mischievous sense of humor. His anxiety remains his biggest challenge but is under control with medication and psychotherapy.

Through it all, my family and I have learned that with the proper therapies and treatments, we can define an autistic child's potential not by assumed limitations, but by that child's own growth.

PRACTICAL APPLICATIONS

CASE REPORTS

22

Case Report 1: Major Depression

Mrs. Carr, a 58-year-old widow, was brought to the emergency department by her daughter, who found her at home in bed in the middle of the day. For a period of months, Mrs. Carr had become increasingly withdrawn and dysphoric, without any precipitating events. She had become progressively less active and even required encouragement to eat and perform her daily tasks. Her daughter and son-in-law became alarmed but did not know what to do. Mrs. Carr's medical history was unremarkable, but her psychiatric history revealed an episode of postpartum depression after the birth of one of her children.

On examination, the ER [emergency room] physician noted that Mrs. Carr was withdrawn and negativistic, refusing to cooperate with the examination, and even refusing to open her mouth. There were signs of acute dehydration and decline in personal hygiene and grooming.

Further questioning of her daughter revealed that Mrs. Carr had become increasingly paranoid and had delusions of sinfulness and guilt. Recently, she had shown signs of increasing mutism.

The physician recognized signs of major depression and arranged for immediate hospitalization. Mrs. Carr responded favorably to combined use of an antipsychotic and an antidepressant drug. An alternative treatment would have been a course of electroconvulsive therapy, which also produces favorable results.

Case Report 2: Somatic Symptom Disorder

A 35-year-old man presented with a 6-year history of abdominal pain that he was convinced was cancer. For most of his life, the patient evidently had been dominated by a tyrannical father who never gave him the love he craved. When the patient was 29, his father died of carcinoma of the colon, and soon afterward, the patient developed abdominal pain. His complaints gradually increased as his identification with his father, as well as his unconscious hostility toward him, increased. The patient came to the clinic almost daily with complaints of bloody stools (the feces were found to be free of blood) and the belief that he had cancer. He felt that none of the clinic doctors listened to him, just as his father had not.

Treatment included development of a longstanding, trusting, positive relationship with one of the clinic physicians, who allowed the patient time to talk about the illness. His symptoms gradually subsided during a 12-month period of a supportive physician-patient relationship.

Case Report 3: Bipolar Disorder

A 30-year-old woman first presented with depression at age 26. Her depression was characterized by sadness lasting most of the day, crying spells, severe irritability, hypersomnia with some periods of insomnia, anergia (low energy), severe inappropriate guilt feelings, and absence of libido (sex drive). The patient also described periods of high energy when her "mind ran away," and her mood was irritable, with a decreased need for sleep. She stated that initially, these times would last 1 or 2 days at the most. Her family would avoid confrontations with her during those periods of energy and activity. The patient had previously been diagnosed as suffering from dysthymic disorder with major depression. A bipolar illness was suspected based on her 1- or 2-day bursts of energy and activity. History from family members confirmed that she had experienced expansive mood states lasting at least 4 consecutive days and present most of the day that met the DSM-5 criteria for hypomanic episodes. Her diagnosis was changed to bipolar II disorder. She was placed on a regimen of bupropion (Wellbutrin), and the dose was increased to 300 mg/day. Her mood improved in a general way, with less irritability, more energy, and less sadness. She continued to have rather pronounced premenstrual worsening of her mood, however, that did not respond to an increase in the dose of bupropion. In the meantime, her physician added lithium to her medical regimen of fluoxetine (Prozac).

Case Report 4: Schizophrenia

Mike is a 33-year-old divorced man with two children, ages 8 and 10, whom he rarely ever sees. He has never been evaluated by a psychiatrist. His family physician has tried to get him to see a local psychiatrist, but Mike refuses to go. Mike says he knows someone has removed his brain and replaced it with someone else's. He believes that this brain is controlling him and that he is not responsible for his actions. He works every day and has been on his current job for 15 years. He says he has lots of friends, but sometimes he thinks it's one of them who did this to him. He reports incidents in which he has been injected with something while shopping and speaks of a government conspiracy to kill him. He has a college education and has a degree in computer science. His family physician ordered an MRI study, which showed negative findings, and he also had an EEG. The EEG results came back normal.

22

? EXERCISES

Remember to check your answers carefully with the Answers to Exercises, page 952.

A **Give the terms for the following definitions.**

1. physician specializing in treating mental illness _____

2. nonphysician professionals trained in the treatment of mental illness _____

3. therapist who practices psychoanalysis _____

4. branch of psychiatry dealing with legal matters _____

5. unconscious part of the personality _____

6. conscious, coordinating part of the personality _____

7. conscience or moral part of the personality _____

8. psychological process used to distinguish fact from fantasy _____

9. unconscious technique used to resolve or conceal conflicts and anxiety

   _____ mechanism.

10. branch of psychology dealing with patient care _____

B **Match the psychiatric symptoms with their definitions/descriptions that follow.**

amnesia	conversion	mania
anxiety	delusion	mutism
apathy	dissociation	obsession
compulsion	hallucination	

1. nonreactive state marked by inability to speak _____

2. state of excessive excitability; agitation _____

3. loss of memory _____

4. uncontrollable urge to perform an act repeatedly _____

5. persistent idea, emotion, or urge _____

6. feelings of apprehension, uneasiness, dread _____

7. uncomfortable feelings are separated from their real object and redirected toward a second

   object or behavior pattern _____

8. anxiety becomes a bodily symptom that has no organic basis _____

9. absence of emotions; lack of motivation or emotional involvement _____

10. fixed false belief that cannot be changed by logical reasoning or evidence _____

11. false or unreal sensory perception _____

22

C Give the meanings of the following terms.

1. dysphoria _____

2. euphoria _____

3. amnesia _____

4. paranoia _____

5. psychosis _____

6. iatrogenic _____

7. phobia _____

8. agoraphobia _____

9. labile _____

10. affect _____

D Select from the list of pychiatric conditions to complete the sentences that follow.

anxiety disorders   eating disorders   somatic symptom disorders
delirium   bipolar disorders   substance-related and addictive
dementia   personality disorders   disorders
dissociative disorders   sexual dysfunctions

1. Disturbances of memory and identity that hide the anxiety of unconscious conflicts are

   _____.

2. Troubled feelings, unpleasant tension, distress, and avoidance behavior describe a/an

   _____.

3. Conditions related to regular use of drugs and alcohol are _____.

4. Bulimia and anorexia nervosa are examples of _____.

5. A disorder involving paraphilias is a/an _____.

6. Disorders marked by alternating periods of mania and depression are

   _____.

7. Mental conditions in which physical symptoms cannot be explained by an actual physical

   disorder or injury are _____.

8. Lifelong patterns of thought and behavior that are inflexible and causes distress, conflict, and

   impairment of social functioning are _____.

9. Loss of intellectual abilities with impairment of memory, judgment, and reasoning is

   _____.

10. Confusion in thinking with faulty perceptions and irrational behavior is

    _____.

22

E **Provide meanings of the following terms.**

1. obsessive-compulsive disorder _____

2. post-traumatic stress disorder _____

3. bipolar disorder _____

4. fugue _____

5. paranoia _____

6. amphetamines _____

7. cannabis _____

8. schizophrenia _____

9. sexual sadism _____

10. somatic symptom disorder _____

F **Match the general psychiatric disorder in Column I with an association in Column II. Write the letter of the answer in the space provided.**

COLUMN I

1. somatic symptom disorder

2. sexual dysfunction

3. anxiety disorder

4. bipolar disorder

5. substance-related and addictive disorder

6. schizophrenia spectrum

7. dissociative disorder

8. neurocognitive disorder

9. neurodevelopmental disorder

COLUMN II

A. conversion disorder
B. cocaine abuse
C. phobia
D. negative symptoms such as flat affect and lack of initiative
E. pedophilia
F. autism
G. alternating mania and depression
H. delirium and dementia
I. fugue and identity disorder

G **Provide meanings of the following terms.**

1. anorexia nervosa _____

2. bulimia nervosa _____

3. repression _____

4. dementia _____

5. hypomania _____

6. hallucinogen _____

7. opioids _____

8. cocaine _____

9. cyclothymic disorder _____

10. dysthymia _____

H **Match the personality disorder with its description.**

Cluster A	Cluster B	Cluster C
Paranoid	Antisocial	Avoidant
Schizoid	Borderline	Dependent
Schizotypal	Histrionic	Obsessive-compulsive
	Narcissistic	

1. flamboyant, theatrical, emotionally immature _____

2. no loyalty or concern for others; does not tolerate frustration and blames others when he or she

    is at fault _____

3. fantasies of success and power and a grandiose sense of self-importance _____

4. pervasive, unwarranted suspiciousness and mistrust of people _____

5. emotionally cold, aloof, indifferent to praise or criticism or to the feelings of others

    _____

6. instability in personal relationships and sense of self; alternating overinvolvement with and

    rejection of people _____

7. pattern of social inhibition, feelings of inadequacy, and hypersensitivity to negative evaluations

    _____

8. acute discomfort in close relationships with odd beliefs and bizarre fantasies _____

9. needing orderliness, perfectionism and control; preoccupied with details, rules, lists, and

    schedules _____

10. submissive and clinging behavior related to an excessive need to be taken care of _____

I **Identify the psychotherapeutic technique based on its description provided.**

1. Patients express feelings by acting out roles with other patients: _____

2. A trance helps patients recover deeply repressed feelings: _____

3. Long-term and intense exploration of unconscious feelings uses techniques such as transference

    and free association: _____

4. Toys help a child express conflicts and feelings: _____

5. Conditioning changes actual behavior patterns rather than focusing on subconscious thoughts

    and feelings: _____

6. Techniques help patients overcome sexual dysfunctions: _____

7. Electrical current is applied to the brain to reverse major depression: _____

8. Agents (chemicals) relieve symptoms of psychiatric disorders: _____

9. Face-to-face discussion of life's problems and associated feelings: _____

10. Offering encouragement, support, and hope to patients facing difficult life transitions and

    events: _____

22

J **Select from the listed terms relating to psychiatric disorders and their treatment to complete the sentences that follow.**

agoraphobia   first-generation antipsychotics   pyromania
amphetamines   kleptomania   tricyclic and tetracyclic
benzodiazepines   lithium   antidepressants
cyclothymia   MAO inhibitors   xenophobia
dysthymia

1. Fear of strangers is _____.

2. Obsessive preoccupation with stealing is _____.

3. Antidepressant agents that work by blocking the action of a specific enzyme are

   _____.

4. Depression disorder that is milder than major depression is _____.

5. Neuroleptic drugs such as Thorazine and Haldol are _____.

6. Fear of being left alone in unfamiliar surroundings is _____.

7. Stimulants used for treatment of children with attention deficit–hyperactivity disorder are

   _____.

8. Mild form of bipolar disorder in which hypomanic episodes alternate with depression is

   _____.

9. Obsessive preoccupation with fire is _____.

10. Drugs (with molecular structure containing three fused rings) used to elevate mood and

    increase physical activity and mental alertness are _____.

11. Anxiolytic agents that lessen the anxiety associated with panic attacks are

    _____.

12. Drug that is used to treat bipolar illness is _____.

K **Give the meanings of the following word parts.**

1. phren/o _____
2. hypn/o _____
3. somat/o _____
4. phil/o _____
5. iatr/o _____
6. schiz/o _____
7. -mania _____

8. -phobia _____
9. -thymia _____
10. -tropic _____
11. -genic _____
12. para- _____
13. hypo- _____
14. cata- _____

22

L   **Match the psychiatric drugs with their type and the condition(s) they treat (consult Figure 22-5 on page 935).**

alprazolam (Xanax)   lamotrigine (Lamictal)   thiothixene (Navane)
amitriptyline (Elavil)   methylphenidate (Ritalin,   zolpidem (Ambien)
aripiprazole (Abilify)   Concerta)
escitalopram (Lexapro)

1. SSRI; treats anxiety and depression _____

2. atypical antipsychotic; treats schizophrenia and bipolar disorder _____

3. stimulant; treats attention deficit–hyperactivity disorder _____

4. tricyclic antidepressant; treats depression _____

5. benzodiazepine; treats anxiety and panic attacks _____

6. sedative; treats insomnia _____

7. anticonvulsant that also isused to treat bipolar disorders _____

8. first-generation antipsychotic that treats schizophrenia _____

M   **Circle the boldface terms that best complete the meaning of the sentences.**

1. Robin fluctuated between bouts of depression and mania and finally was diagnosed as having a **(xenophobic, histrionic, bipolar)** disorder.

2. Although the root of Jon's problems could hardly be addressed simply with medication, his personality disorder and his depression were treated with a selective serotonin reuptake inhibitor (SSRI) called **(lithium, Prozac, Valium)**.

3. Hillary had an enormous fear of open-air markets, shopping malls, and stadiums. She was diagnosed as having **(agoraphobia, xenophobia, pyromania)**.

4. When Sam was admitted to the hospital after his automobile accident, his physicians were told of his alcoholism. They needed to know Sam's history so that they could prevent **(dementia, dysthymia, delirium tremens)**.

5. Hanna was afraid of everyone she met. She had the **(paranoid, narcissistic, schizoid)** delusion that everyone was out to get her.

6. Bill was told that an important potential side effect of taking neuroleptic drugs such as atypical and first-generation antipsychotics was **(amnesia, gender dysphoria, tardive dyskinesia)**.

7. Ever since she was trapped in an elevator for 3 hours, Lil experienced a **(social phobia, panic attack, somatic symptom disorder)** marked by palpitations, sweating, and trembling when she was unable to get out of an enclosed space.

8. The few survivors of the nightclub fire were diagnosed with **(OCD, dissociative fugue, post-traumatic stress disorder)**. They regularly experienced insomnia, nightmares, and feelings of helplessness.

22

9. Sarah couldn't stop herself from eating a half-gallon of ice cream and a box of cookies every evening. She would then feel very anxious and guilty about overeating and induce vomiting. Her mother took her to a/an (**endocrinologist, psychiatrist, gastroenterologist**), who diagnosed her condition as (**anorexia nervosa, somatic symptom disorder, bulimia nervosa**) and prescribed (**sex therapy, ECT, psychotherapy**).

10. Bill felt depressed during the months of November through February. In March his (**OCD, ADHD, SAD**) changed and his mood was characterized by (**hypomania, dysphoria, paranoia**).

ANSWERS TO EXERCISES

A

1. psychiatrist
2. psychologist, psychiatric nurse, licensed clinical social worker
3. psychoanalyst
4. forensic psychiatry
5. id
6. ego
7. superego
8. reality testing
9. defense
10. clinical

B

1. mutism
2. mania
3. amnesia
4. compulsion
5. obsession
6. anxiety
7. dissociation
8. conversion
9. apathy
10. delusion
11. hallucination

C

1. sadness, hopelessness, unpleasant feeling
2. exaggerated feeling of well-being ("high")
3. loss of memory
4. suspicious system of thinking; fixed delusion that one is being treated unfairly or harassed
5. loss of contact with reality; often delusions and hallucinations
6. pertaining to a disorder caused by a treatment
7. irrational fear (avoidance) of an object or a situation
8. fear of leaving one's home or a safe place
9. unstable; undergoing rapid emotional change; fluctuating
10. expression of emotion

D

1. dissociative disorder
2. anxiety disorder
3. substance-related/addictive disorder
4. eating disorder
5. sexual dysfunction
6. bipolar disorder
7. somatic symptom disorder
8. personality disorder
9. dementia
10. delirium

E

1. recurrent thoughts and repetitive acts that dominate a person's behavior
2. anxiety-related symptoms appear after exposure to personal experience of a traumatic event
3. alternating periods of mania and depression
4. amnesia with flight from customary surroundings
5. delusions of persecution or grandeur
6. CNS stimulants
7. marijuana, hashish; active substance in marijuana; THC
8. psychosis marked by a split from reality; disorganized thinking and behavior
9. achievement of sexual gratification by inflicting physical or psychological pain
10. presence of physical symptoms that cannot be explained by an actual medical disorder or injury

F

1. A
2. E
3. C
4. G
5. B
6. D
7. I
8. H
9. F

22

G

1. eating disorder marked by excessive dieting related to emotional factors
2. eating disorder characterized by binge eating followed by vomiting, purging, and depression
3. a defense mechanism by which unacceptable thoughts, feelings, and impulses are pushed into the unconscious
4. loss of higher mental functioning, memory, judgment, and reasoning
5. mood disorder resembling mania (exaggerated excitement, hyperactivity) but of lesser intensity
6. drug that produces hallucinations (false sensory perceptions)
7. drugs that are derived from opium (morphine and heroin)
8. stimulant drug that causes euphoria and hallucinations
9. alternating periods of hypomania and depressive episodes of lesser intensity than with bipolar illness
10. depressed mood persisting over a 2-year period but not as severe as a major depression

H

1. histrionic
2. antisocial
3. narcissistic
4. paranoid
5. schizoid
6. borderline
7. avoidant
8. schizotypal
9. obsessive-compulsive
10. dependent

I

1. psychodrama
2. hypnosis
3. psychoanalysis
4. play therapy
5. behavioral therapy
6. sexual therapy
7. electroconvulsive therapy
8. psychopharmacology, or drug therapy
9. insight-oriented psychotherapy
10. supportive psychotherapy

J

1. xenophobia
2. kleptomania
3. MAO inhibitors
4. dysthymia
5. first-generation antipsychotics
6. agoraphobia
7. amphetamines
8. cyclothymia
9. pyromania
10. tricyclic and tetracyclic antidepressants
11. benzodiazepines
12. lithium

K

1. mind
2. sleep
3. body
4. love, attraction to
5. treatment
6. split
7. obsessive preoccupation
8. fear
9. mind; mood
10. to influence, turn
11. produced by
12. abnormal
13. deficient, less than, below
14. down

L

1. escitalopram (Lexapro)
2. aripiprazole (Abilify)
3. methylphenidate (Ritalin, Concerta)
4. amitriptyline (Elavil)
5. alprazolam (Xanax)
6. zolpidem (Ambien)
7. lamotrigine (Lamictal)
8. thiothixene (Navane)

M

1. bipolar
2. Prozac
3. agoraphobia
4. delirium tremens
5. paranoid
6. tardive dyskinesia
7. panic attack
8. post-traumatic stress disorder
9. psychiatrist; bulimia nervosa; psychotherapy
10. SAD; dysphoria

22

PRONUNCIATION OF TERMS

To test your understanding of the terminology in this chapter, write the meaning of each term in the space provided. In addition, you may wish to cover the terms and write them by looking at your definitions. Make sure your spelling is correct. The page number after each term indicates where it is defined or used in the book, so you can easily check your responses. You will find complete definitions for all of these terms and their audio pronunciations on the Evolve website.

Pronunciation Guide

ā as in āpe	ă as in ăpple
ē as in ēven	ĕ as in ĕvery
ī as in īce	ĭ as in ĭnterest
ō as in ōpen	ŏ as in pŏt
ū as in ūnit	ŭ as in ŭnder

TERM	PRONUNCIATION	MEANING
affect (936)	ĂF-fĕkt	
agoraphobia (925)	ăg-ŏ-ră-FŌ-bē-ă	
amnesia (936)	ăm-NĒ-zē-ă	
amphetamines (938)	ăm-FĔT-ă-mēnz	
anorexia nervosa (936)	ăn-ō-RĔK-sē-ă nĕr-VŌ-să	
antisocial personality (928)	ăn-tē-SŌ-shăl pĕr-sŏ-NĂL-ĭ-tē	
anxiety disorders (936)	ăng-ZĪ-ĕ-tē dĭs-ŎR-dĕrz	
anxiolytic (939)	ăng-zī-ō-LĬT-ik	
apathy (936)	ĂP-ă-thē	
atypical antipsychotics (938)	ā-TĬP-ĭ-kăl ăn-tĭ-sī-KŎT-ĭks	
autism (936)	AW-tĭzm	
avoidant personality (929)	ă-VŎY-dănt pĕr-sŏ-NĂL-ĭ-tē	
benzodiazepines (938)	bĕn-zō-dī-ĂZ-ĕ-pēnz	
bipolar disorder (936)	bī-PŌ-lăr dĭs-ŎR-dĕr	
borderline personality (928)	BŎR-dĕr-līn pĕr-sŏ-NĂL-ĭ-tē	
bulimia nervosa (936)	bū-LĒ-mē-ă nĕr-VŌ-să	
cannabis (936)	KĂ-nă-bis	
catatonia (941)	kăt-ă-TŌN-ē-ă	
claustrophobia (925)	klaws-trō-FŌ-bē-ă	
cognitive-behavioral therapy (938)	KŎG-nĭ-tĭv bē-HĀV-yŏr-ăl THĔR-ă-pē	
compulsion (936)	kŏm-PŬL-shŭn	
conversion disorder (936)	kŏn-VĔR-zhŭn dĭs-ŎR-dĕr	

TERM	PRONUNCIATION	MEANING
cyclothymia (941)	sī-klō-THĪ-mē-ă	_____
defense mechanism (936)	dē-FĔNS mĕ-kăn-NĬZM	_____
delirium (937)	dĕ-LĒR-ē-ŭm	_____
delirium tremens (937)	dĕ-LĒR-ē-ŭm TRĔ-mĕnz	_____
delusion (937)	dĕ-LOO-zhŭn	_____
dementia (937)	dē-MĔN-shē-ă	_____
dependent personality (929)	dē-PĔN-dănt pĕr-sŏ-NĂL-ĭ-tē	_____
depressive disorders (937)	dē-PRĔ-sĭv dĭs-ŎR-dĕrz	_____
dissociative disorder (937)	dĭs-SŌ-shē-ă-tĭv dĭs-ŎR-der	_____
dysphoria (940)	dĭs-FŎR-ē-ă	_____
dysthymia (941)	dĭs-THĪ-mē-ă	_____
ego (937)	Ē-gō	_____
electroconvulsive therapy (938)	ē-lĕk-trō-kŏn-VŬL-sĭv THĔR-ă-pē	_____
euphoria (940)	ū-FŎR-ē-ă	_____
euthymia (941)	ū-THĪ-ē-ă	_____
exhibitionism (929)	ĕk-sĭ-BĬSH-ŭ-nĭzm	_____
family therapy (938)	FĂM-ĭ-lē THĔR-ă-pē	_____
fetishism (929)	FĔT-ĭsh-ĭzm	_____
free association (938)	frē ă-sō-shē-Ā-shŭn	_____
fugue (937)	fūg	_____
gender dysphoria (937)	GĔN-dĕr dĭs-FŎR-ē-ă	_____
group therapy (938)	groop THĔR-ă-pē	_____
hallucination (937)	hă-loo-sĭ-NĀ-shŭn	_____
hallucinogen (937)	hă-LOO-sĭ-nō-jĕn	_____
histrionic personality (928)	hĭs-trē-ŎN-ĭk pĕr-sŏn-ĂL-ĭ-tē	_____
hypnosis (938)	hĭp-NŌ-sĭs	_____
hypomania (926)	hī-pō-MĀ-nē-ă	_____
iatrogenic (940)	ī-ă-trō-JĔN-ĭk	_____
id (937)	ĭd	_____

22

TERM	PRONUNCIATION	MEANING
insight-oriented therapy (939)	ĬN-sīt ŎR-ē-ĕn-tĕd THĔR-ă-pē	_____
kleptomania (940)	klĕp-tō-MĀ-nē-ă	_____
labile (937)	LĀ-bĭl	_____
lithium (939)	LĬTH-ē-ŭm	_____
mania (937)	MĀ-nē-ă	_____
mental (940)	MĔN-tăl	_____
mutism (937)	MŪ-tĭzm	_____
narcissistic personality (929)	năr-sĭ-SĬS-tĭk pĕr-sŏ-NĂL-ĭ-tē	_____
neurocognitive disorders (927)	noo-rō-KŎG-nă-tĭv dĭs-ŎR-dĕrz	_____
neurodevelopmental disorders (937)	noo-rō-dĕ-VĔL-ōp-mĕn-tăl dĭs-ŎR-dĕrz	_____
neuroleptic drug (939)	noo-rō-LĔP-tĭk drŭg	_____
neurotransmitter (940)	noo-rō-TRĂNZ-mĭt-ĕr	_____
obsession (937)	ŏb-SĔSH-ŭn	_____
obsessive-compulsive personality (929)	ŏb-SĔS-ĭv cŏm-PŬL-sĭv pĕr-sŏn-NĂL-ĭ-tē	_____
opioids (931)	Ō-pē-ŏydz	_____
paranoia (937)	păr-ă-NŎY-ă	_____
paranoid personality (928)	PĂR-ă-nŏyd pĕr-sŏ-NĂL-ĭ-tē	_____
paraphilia (937)	păr-ă-FĬL-ē-ă	_____
pedophilia (929)	pē-dō-FĬL-ē-ă	_____
personality disorders (937)	pĕr-sŏ-NĂL-ĭ-tē dĭs-ŎR-dĕrz	_____
phenothiazines (934)	fē-nō-THĬ-ă-zēnz	_____
phobia (937)	FŌ-bē-ă	_____
play therapy (939)	plā THĔR-ă-pē	_____
post-traumatic stress disorder (937)	pōst-traw-MĂT-ĭk strĕs dĭs-ŎR-dĕr	_____
projective test (937)	prō-JĔK-tĭv tĕst	_____
psychiatrist (937)	sī-KĪ-ă-trĭst	_____
psychiatry (922)	sī-KĪ-ă-trē	_____
psychoanalysis (939)	sī-kō-ă-NĂL-ĭ-sĭs	_____
psychodrama (939)	sī-kō-DRĂ-mă	_____

22

TERM	PRONUNCIATION	MEANING
psychogenic (940)	sī-kō-JĔN-ĭk	
psychologist (938)	sī-KŎL-ō-jĭst	
psychopharmacology (939)	sī-kō-făr-mă-KŎL-ō-jē	
psychosis (938)	sī-KŌ-sĭs	
psychosomatic (940)	sī-kō-sō-MĂT-ĭk	
psychotherapy (933)	sī-kō-THĔR-ă-pē	
pyromania (940)	pī-rō-MĀ-nē-ă	
reality testing (938)	rē-ĂL-ĭ-tē TĔS-tĭng	
repression (938)	rē-PRĔ-shŭn	
schizoid personality (928)	SKĬZ-ŏyd or SKĬT-sŏyd pĕr-sŏ-NĂL-ĭ-tē	
schizophrenia (940)	skĭz-ō-FRĔ-nē-ă	
sedatives (939)	SĔD-ă-tĭvz	
sexual dysfunctions (938)	SĔX-ū-ăl dĭs-FŬNK-shŭnz	
sexual masochism (929)	SĔX-ū-ăl MĂS-ō-kĭzm	
sexual sadism (930)	SĔX-ŭ-ăl SA-dĭzm	
somatic symptom disorders (938)	sō-MĂT-tĭk SĬM-tŏm dĭs-ŎR-dĕrz	
substance-related and addictive disorders (938)	SŬB-stăns rē-LĀ-tĕd and ă-DĬK-tĭv dĭs-ŎR-dĕrz	
superego (938)	sū-pĕr-Ē-gō	
supportive psychotherapy (939)	sū-PŎR-tĭv sī-kō-THĔR-ă-pē	
tolerance (930)	TŎL-ĕr-ăns	
transference (939)	trăns-FŬR-ĕns	
transvestic fetishism (930)	trăns-VĔS-tĭk FĔT-ĭsh-ĭzm	
tricyclic antidepressants (939)	trī-SĬK-lĭk ăn-tĭ-dĕ-PRĔ-săntz	
voyeurism (930)	VŎY-yĕr-ĭzm	
xenophobia (940)	zĕn-ō-FŌ-bē-ă	

22

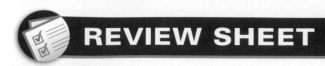

REVIEW SHEET

Write the meanings of the word parts in the spaces provided, and test yourself. Check your answers with the information in the chapter or in the **Glossary (Medical Word Parts—English)** at the end of the book.

Combining Forms

COMBINING FORM	MEANING	COMBINING FORM	MEANING
anxi/o	_____	phil/o	_____
aut/o	_____	phren/o	_____
cycl/o	_____	psych/o	_____
hallucin/o	_____	pyr/o	_____
hypn/o	_____	schiz/o	_____
iatr/o	_____	somat/o	_____
klept/o	_____	ton/o	_____
ment/o	_____	xen/o	_____
neur/o	_____		

Suffixes

SUFFIX	MEANING	SUFFIX	MEANING
-form	_____	-pathy	_____
-genic	_____	-phobia	_____
-kinesia	_____	-phoria	_____
-leptic	_____	-somnia	_____
-mania	_____	-thymia	_____
-oid	_____	-tropic	_____

Prefixes

PREFIX	MEANING	PREFIX	MEANING
a-, an-	_____	eu-	_____
agora-	_____	hypo-	_____
cata-	_____	para-	_____
dys-	_____		

evolve   *Please refer to the Evolve website for additional exercises, games, and images related to this chapter.*

GLOSSARY

MEDICAL WORD PARTS—ENGLISH*

Combining Form, Suffix, or Prefix	Meaning
a-, an-	no; not; without
ab-	away from
abdomin/o	abdomen
-ac	pertaining to
acanth/o	spiny; thorny
acetabul/o	acetabulum (hip socket)
acous/o	hearing
acr/o	extremities; top; extreme point
acromi/o	acromion (extension of shoulder bone)
actin/o	light
acu/o	sharp; severe; sudden
-acusis	hearing
ad-	toward
-ad	toward
aden/o	gland
adenoid/o	adenoids
adip/o	fat
adren/o	adrenal gland
adrenal/o	adrenal gland
aer/o	air
af-	toward
agglutin/o	clumping; sticking together
-agon	assemble, gather
agora-	marketplace
-agra	excessive pain
-al	pertaining to
alb/o	white
albin/o	white
albumin/o	albumin (protein)
alges/o	sensitivity to pain
-algesia	sensitivity to pain
-algia	pain
all/o	other
alveol/o	alveolus; air sac; small sac

Combining Form, Suffix, or Prefix	Meaning
ambly/o	dim; dull
-amine	nitrogen compound
amni/o	amnion (sac surrounding the embryo)
amyl/o	starch
an/o	anus
-an	pertaining to
ana-	up; apart; backward; again, anew
andr/o	male
aneurysm/o	aneurysm (widened blood vessel)
angi/o	vessel (blood)
anis/o	unequal
ankyl/o	stiff
ante-	before; forward
anter/o	front
anthrac/o	coal
anthr/o	antrum of the stomach
anti-	against
anxi/o	uneasy; anxious
aort/o	aorta (largest artery)
-apheresis	removal
aphth/o	ulcer
apo-	off, away
aponeur/o	aponeurosis (type of tendon)
append/o	appendix
appendic/o	appendix
aque/o	water
-ar	pertaining to
-arche	beginning
arter/o	artery
arteri/o	artery
arteriol/o	arteriole (small artery)
arthr/o	joint
-arthria	articulate (speak distinctly)
articul/o	joint

*Page references for all word parts are listed in the Index.

Combining Form, Suffix, or Prefix	Meaning
-ary	pertaining to
asbest/o	asbestos
-ase	enzyme
-asthenia	lack of strength
atel/o	incomplete
ather/o	plaque (fatty substance)
-ation	process; condition
atri/o	atrium (upper heart chamber)
audi/o	hearing
audit/o	hearing
aur/o	ear
auricul/o	ear
aut/o	self, own
aut-, auto-	self, own
axill/o	armpit
azot/o	urea; nitrogen
bacill/o	bacilli (bacteria)
bacteri/o	bacteria
balan/o	glans penis
bar/o	pressure; weight
bartholin/o	Bartholin glands
bas/o	base; opposite of acid
bi-	two
bi/o	life
bil/i	bile; gall
bilirubin/o	bilirubin
-blast	embryonic; immature cell
-blastoma	immature tumor (cells)
blephar/o	eyelid
bol/o	cast; throw
brachi/o	arm
brachy-	short
brady-	slow
bronch/o	bronchial tube
bronchi/o	bronchial tube
bronchiol/o	bronchiole
bucc/o	cheek
bunion/o	bunion
burs/o	bursa (sac of fluid near joints)
byssin/o	cotton dust
cac/o	bad
calc/o	calcium
calcane/o	calcaneus (heel bone)
calci/o	calcium
cali/o, calic/o	calyx (cup-shaped)
capillar/o	capillary (tiniest blood vessel)
capn/o	carbon dioxide
-capnia	carbon dioxide
carcin/o	cancerous; cancer
cardi/o	heart
carp/o	wrist bones (carpals)
cata-	down
caud/o	tail; lower part of body

Combining Form, Suffix, or Prefix	Meaning
caus/o	burn; burning
cauter/o	heat; burn
cec/o	cecum (first part of the colon)
-cele	hernia
celi/o	belly; abdomen
-centesis	surgical puncture to remove fluid
cephal/o	head
cerebell/o	cerebellum (posterior part of the brain)
cerebr/o	cerebrum (largest part of the brain)
cerumin/o	cerumen
cervic/o	neck; cervix (neck of uterus)
-chalasia	relaxation
-chalasis	relaxation
cheil/o	lip
chem/o	drug; chemical
-chezia	defecation; elimination of wastes
chir/o	hand
chlor/o	green
chlorhydr/o	hydrochloric acid
chol/e	bile; gall
cholangi/o	bile vessel
cholecyst/o	gallbladder
choledoch/o	common bile duct
cholesterol/o	cholesterol
chondr/o	cartilage
chore/o	dance
chori/o	chorion (outermost membrane of the fetus)
chorion/o	chorion
choroid/o	choroid layer of eye
chrom/o	color
chron/o	time
chym/o	to pour
cib/o	meal
-cide	killing
-cidal	pertaining to killing
cine/o	movement
cirrh/o	orange-yellow
cis/o	to cut
-clasis	to break
-clast	to break
claustr/o	enclosed space
clavicul/o	clavicle (collar bone)
-clysis	irrigation; washing
coagul/o	coagulation (clotting)
-coccus (-cocci, *pl.*)	berry-shaped bacterium
coccyg/o	coccyx (tailbone)
cochle/o	cochlea (inner part of ear)
col/o	colon
coll/a	glue
colon/o	colon (large intestine)

Combining Form, Suffix, or Prefix	Meaning	Combining Form, Suffix, or Prefix	Meaning
colp/o	vagina	-dote	to give
comat/o	deep sleep	-drome	to run
comi/o	to care for	duct/o	to lead, carry
con-	together, with	duoden/o	duodenum
coni/o	dust	dur/o	dura mater
conjunctiv/o	conjunctiva (lines the eyelids)	-dynia	pain
-constriction	narrowing	dys-	bad; painful; difficult; abnormal
contra-	against; opposite	-eal	pertaining to
cor/o	pupil	ec-	out; outside
core/o	pupil	echo-	reflected sound
corne/o	cornea	-ectasia	dilation; dilatation; widening
coron/o	heart (crown or circle)	-ectasis	dilation; dilatation; widening
corpor/o	body	ecto-	out; outside
cortic/o	cortex, outer region	-ectomy	removal; excision; resection
cost/o	rib	-edema	swelling
crani/o	skull	-elasma	flat plate
cras/o	mixture; temperament	electr/o	electricity
crin/o	secrete	em-	in
-crine	secrete; separate	-ema	condition
-crit	separate	-emesis	vomiting
cry/o	cold	-emia	blood condition
crypt/o	hidden	-emic	pertaining to blood condition
culd/o	cul-de-sac	emmetr/o	in due measure
-cusis	hearing	en-	in; within
cutane/o	skin	encephal/o	brain
cyan/o	blue	end-	in; within
cycl/o	ciliary body of eye; cycle; circle	endo-	in; within
-cyesis	pregnancy	enter/o	intestines (usually small intestine)
cyst/o	urinary bladder; cyst; sac of fluid	eosin/o	red; rosy; dawn-colored
cyt/o	cell	epi-	above; upon; on
-cyte	cell	epididym/o	epididymis
-cytosis	abnormal condition of cells; slight increase in numbers	epiglott/o	epiglottis
		episi/o	vulva (external female genitalia)
dacry/o	tear	epitheli/o	skin; epithelium
dacryoaden/o	tear gland	equin/o	horse
dacryocyst/o	tear sac; lacrimal sac	-er	one who
dactyl/o	fingers; toes	erg/o	work
de-	lack of; down; less; removal of	erythem/o	flushed; redness
dem/o	people	erythr/o	red
dent/i	tooth; teeth	-esis	action; condition; state of
derm/o	skin	eso-	inward
-derma	skin	esophag/o	esophagus
dermat/o	skin	esthes/o	feeling (nervous sensation)
desicc/o	drying	esthesi/o	feeling (nervous sensation)
-desis	bind, tie together	-esthesia	feeling (nervous sensation)
dia-	complete; through	estr/o	female
diaphor/o	sweat	ethm/o	sieve
-dilation	widening; stretching; expanding	eti/o	cause
dipl/o	double	eu-	good; normal; true
dips/o	thirst	-eurysm	widening
dist/o	far; distant	ex-	out; away from
dors/o	back (of body)	exanthemat/o	rash
dorsi-	back	exo-	out; away from

Combining Form, Suffix, or Prefix	Meaning	Combining Form, Suffix, or Prefix	Meaning
extra-	outside	-gravida	pregnant woman
faci/o	face	gynec/o	woman; female
fasci/o	fascia (membrane supporting muscles)	hallucin/o	hallucination
		hem/o	blood
femor/o	femur (thigh bone)	hemat/o	blood
-ferent	to carry	hemi-	half
fibrin/o	fiber	hemoglobin/o	hemoglobin
fibr/o, fibromat/o	fiber	hepat/o	liver
fibros/o	fibrous connective tissue	herni/o	hernia
fibul/o	fibula	-hexia	state of
-fication	process of making	hidr/o	sweat
-fida	split	hist/o, histi/o	tissue
flex/o	bend	home/o	sameness; unchanging; constant
fluor/o	luminous	hormon/o	hormone
follicul/o	follicle; small sac	humer/o	humerus (upper arm bone)
-form	resembling; in the shape of	hydr/o	water
fung/i	fungus; mushroom (lower organism lacking chlorophyll)	hyper-	above; excessive
		hypn/o	sleep
furc/o	forking; branching	hypo-	deficient; below; under; less than normal
-fusion	to pour; to come together		
galact/o	milk	hypophys/o	pituitary gland
ganglion/o	ganglion; collection of nerve cell bodies	hyster/o	uterus; womb
		-ia	condition
gastr/o	stomach	-iac	pertaining to
-gen	substance that produces	-iasis	abnormal condition
-genesis	producing; forming	iatr/o	physician; treatment
-genic	produced by or in	-ic	pertaining to
ger/o	old age	-ical	pertaining to
geront/o	old age	ichthy/o	dry; scaly
gest/o	pregnancy	-icle	small
gester/o	pregnancy	idi/o	unknown; individual; distinct
gingiv/o	gum	-ile	pertaining to
glauc/o	gray	ile/o	ileum
gli/o	glial cells; neuroglial cells (supportive tissue of nervous system)	ili/o	ilium
		immun/o	immune; protection; safe
-globin	protein	in-	in; into; not
-globulin	protein	-in, -ine	substance
glomerul/o	glomerulus	-ine	pertaining to
gloss/o	tongue	infra-	below; inferior to; beneath
gluc/o	glucose; sugar	inguin/o	groin
glyc/o	glucose; sugar	insulin/o	insulin (pancreatic hormone)
glycogen/o	glycogen; animal starch	inter-	between
glycos/o	glucose; sugar	intra-	within; into
gnos/o	knowledge	iod/o	iodine
gon/o	seed	ion/o	ion; to wander
gonad/o	sex glands	-ion	process
goni/o	angle	-ior	pertaining to
-grade	to go	ipsi-	same
-gram	record	ir-	in
granul/o	granule(s)	ir/o	iris (colored portion of eye)
-graph	instrument for recording	irid/o	iris (colored portion of eye)
-graphy	process of recording	is/o	same; equal
gravid/o	pregnancy	isch/o	hold back; back

Combining Form, Suffix, or Prefix	Meaning	Combining Form, Suffix, or Prefix	Meaning
ischi/o	ischium (part of hip bone)	lux/o	slide
-ism	process; condition	lymph/o	lymph
-ist	specialist	lymphaden/o	lymph gland (node)
-itis	inflammation	lymphangi/o	lymph vessel
-itus	condition	-lysis	breakdown; separation; destruction; loosening
-ium	structure; tissue		
jaund/o	yellow	-lytic	reducing, destroying; separating; breakdown
jejun/o	jejunum		
kal/i	potassium	macro-	large
kary/o	nucleus	mal-	bad
kerat/o	cornea; hard, horny tissue	-malacia	softening
kern-	nucleus (collection of nerve cells in the brain)	malleol/o	malleolus
		mamm/o	breast
ket/o	ketones; acetones	mandibul/o	mandible (lower jaw bone)
keton/o	ketones; acetones	-mania	obsessive preoccupation
kines/o	movement	mast/o	breast
kinesi/o	movement	mastoid/o	mastoid process (behind the ear)
-kinesia	movement	maxill/o	maxilla (upper jaw bone)
-kinesis	movement	meat/o	meatus (opening)
klept/o	to steal	medi/o	middle
kyph/o	humpback	mediastin/o	mediastinum
labi/o	lip	medull/o	medulla (inner section); middle; soft, marrow
lacrim/o	tear; tear duct; lacrimal duct		
lact/o	milk	mega-	large
lamin/o	lamina (part of vertebral arch)	-megaly	enlargement
lapar/o	abdominal wall; abdomen	melan/o	black
-lapse	slide, fall, sag	men/o	menses; menstruation
laryng/o	larynx (voice box)	mening/o	meninges (membranes covering the spinal cord and brain)
later/o	side		
leiomy/o	smooth (visceral) muscle	meningi/o	meninges
-lemma	sheath, covering	ment/o	mind; chin
-lepsy	seizure	meso-	middle
lept/o	thin, slender	meta-	change; beyond
-leptic	pertaining to seizing, taking hold of	metacarp/o	metacarpals (hand bones)
leth/o	death	metatars/o	metatarsals (foot bones)
leuk/o	white	-meter	measure
lex/o	word; phrase	metr/o	uterus (womb); measure
-lexia	word; phrase	metri/o	uterus (womb)
ligament/o	ligament	mi/o	smaller; less
lingu/o	tongue	micro-	small
lip/o	fat (a type of lipid)	-mimetic	mimic; copy
lipid/o	lipid	-mission	send
-listhesis	slipping	mon/o	one; single
lith/o	stone; calculus	morph/o	shape; form
-lithiasis	condition of stones	mort/o	death
-lithotomy	incision (for removal) of a stone	-mortem	death
lob/o	lobe	-motor	movement
log/o	study	muc/o	mucus
-logy	study (process of)	mucos/o	mucous membrane (mucosa)
lord/o	curve; swayback	multi-	many
-lucent	to shine	mut/a	genetic change
lumb/o	lower back; loin	mutagen/o	causing genetic change
lute/o	yellow	my/o	muscle

Combining Form, Suffix, or Prefix	Meaning	Combining Form, Suffix, or Prefix	Meaning
myc/o	fungus	-orexia	appetite
mydr/o	wide	orth/o	straight
myel/o	spinal cord; bone marrow	-ose	full of; pertaining to; sugar
myocardi/o	myocardium (heart muscle)	-osis	condition, usually abnormal
myom/o	muscle tumor	-osmia	smell
myos/o	muscle	ossicul/o	ossicle (small bone)
myring/o	tympanic membrane (eardrum)	oste/o	bone
myx/o	mucus	-ostosis	condition of bone
narc/o	numbness; stupor; sleep	ot/o	ear
nas/o	nose	-otia	ear condition
nat/i	birth	-ous	pertaining to
natr/o	sodium	ov/o	egg
necr/o	death	ovari/o	ovary
nect/o	bind, tie, connect	ovul/o	egg
neo-	new	ox/o	oxygen
nephr/o	kidney	-oxia	oxygen
neur/o	nerve	oxy-	rapid; sharp; acid
neutr/o	neither; neutral; neutrophil	oxysm/o	sudden
nid/o	nest	pachy-	heavy; thick
noct/o	night	palat/o	palate (roof of the mouth)
norm/o	rule; order	palpebr/o	eyelid
nos/o	disease	pan-	all
nucle/o	nucleus	pancreat/o	pancreas
nulli-	none	papill/o	nipple-like; optic disc (disk)
nyct/o	night	par-	other than; abnormal
obstetr/o	pregnancy; childbirth	para-	near; beside; abnormal; apart from; along the side of
ocul/o	eye	-para	to bear, bring forth (live births)
odont/o	tooth	-parous	to bear, bring forth
odyn/o	pain	parathyroid/o	parathyroid glands
-oid	resembling; originating from	-paresis	weakness
-ole	little; small	-pareunia	sexual intercourse
olecran/o	olecranon (elbow)	-partum	birth; labor
olig/o	scanty	patell/a	patella
om/o	shoulder	patell/o	patella
-oma	tumor; mass; fluid collection	path/o	disease
omphal/o	umbilicus (navel)	-pathy	disease; emotion
onc/o	tumor	pector/o	chest
-one	hormone	ped/o	child; foot
onych/o	nail (of fingers or toes)	pelv/i	pelvis; hip region
o/o	egg	pelv/o	pelvis; hip region
oophor/o	ovary	pend/o	hang
-opaque	obscure	-penia	deficiency
ophthalm/o	eye	pen/o	penis
-opia	vision condition	-pepsia	digestion
-opsia	vision condition	per-	through
-opsy	view of	peri-	surrounding
opt/o	eye; vision	perine/o	perineum
optic/o	eye; vision	peritone/o	peritoneum
-or	one who	perone/o	fibula
or/o	mouth	-pexy	fixation; to put in place
orch/o	testis	phac/o	lens of eye
orchi/o	testis	phag/o	eat; swallow
orchid/o	testis		

Combining Form, Suffix, or Prefix	Meaning	Combining Form, Suffix, or Prefix	Meaning
-phage	eat; swallow	-poietin	substance that forms
-phagia	condition of eating; swallowing	poikil/o	varied; irregular
phak/o	lens of eye	pol/o	extreme
phalang/o	phalanges (of fingers and toes)	polio-	gray matter (of brain or spinal cord)
phall/o	penis	poly-	many; much; increased
pharmac/o	drug	polyp/o	polyp; small growth
pharmaceut/o	drug	pont/o	pons (a part of the brain)
pharyng/o	throat (pharynx)	-porosis	condition of pores (spaces)
phas/o	speech	post-	after; behind
-phasia	speech	poster/o	back (of body); behind
phe/o	dusky; dark	-prandial	pertaining to eating or mealtime
-pheresis	removal	-praxia	action
phil/o	like; love; attraction to	pre-	before; in front of
-phil	attraction for	presby/o	old age
-philia	attraction for	primi-	first
phim/o	muzzle	pro-	before; forward
phleb/o	vein	proct/o	anus and rectum
phob/o	fear	pros-	before; forward
-phobia	fear	prostat/o	prostate gland
phon/o	voice; sound	prot/o	first
-phonia	voice; sound	prote/o	protein
phor/o	to bear	proxim/o	near
-phoresis	carrying; transmission	prurit/o	itching
-phoria	to bear, carry; feeling (mental state)	pseudo-	false
phot/o	light	psych/o	mind
phren/o	diaphragm; mind	-ptosis	falling; drooping; prolapse
-phthisis	wasting away	-ptysis	spitting
-phylaxis	protection	pub/o	pubis (anterior part of hip bone)
physi/o	nature; function	pulmon/o	lung
phys/o	growing	pupill/o	pupil (dark center of the eye)
-physis	to grow	purul/o	pus
phyt/o	plant	py/o	pus
-phyte	plant	pyel/o	renal pelvis
pil/o	hair	pylor/o	pylorus; pyloric sphincter
pineal/o	pineal gland	pyr/o	fever; fire
pituitar/o	pituitary gland	pyret/o	fever
-plakia	plaque	pyrex/o	fever
plant/o	sole of the foot	quadri-	four
plas/o	development; formation; growth	rachi/o	spinal column; vertebrae
-plasia	development; formation; growth	radi/o	x-rays; radioactivity; radius (lateral lower arm bone)
-plasm	formation; structure		
-plastic	pertaining to formation	radicul/o	nerve root
-plasty	surgical repair	re-	back; again; backward
ple/o	more; many; varied	rect/o	rectum
-plegia	paralysis; palsy	ren/o	kidney
-plegic	pertaining to paralysis; palsy	reticul/o	network
pleur/o	pleura	retin/o	retina
plex/o	plexus; network (of nerves)	retro-	behind; back; backward
-pnea	breathing	rhabdomy/o	striated (skeletal) muscle
pneum/o	lung; air; gas	rheumat/o	watery flow
pneumon/o	lung; air; gas	rhin/o	nose
pod/o	foot	rhytid/o	wrinkle
-poiesis	formation	roentgen/o	x-rays

Combining Form, Suffix, or Prefix	Meaning	Combining Form, Suffix, or Prefix	Meaning
-rrhage	bursting forth (of blood)	spondyl/o	vertebra (backbone)
-rrhagia	bursting forth (of blood)	squam/o	scale
-rrhaphy	suture	-stalsis	contraction
-rrhea	flow; discharge	staped/o	stapes (middle ear bone)
-rrhexis	rupture	staphyl/o	clusters; uvula
rrhythm/o	rhythm	-stasis	stopping; controlling; placing
sacr/o	sacrum	-static	pertaining to stopping or controlling
salpinx	fallopian tube (oviduct); auditory (eustachian) tube	steat/o	fat, sebum
-salpinx	fallopian tube; oviduct	sten/o	narrowing
sarc/o	flesh (connective tissue)	-stenosis	tightening; stricture
scapul/o	scapula; shoulder blade	ster/o	solid structure; steroid
-schisis	split	stere/o	solid; three-dimensional
schiz/o	split	stern/o	sternum (breastbone)
scint/i	spark	steth/o	chest
scirrh/o	hard	-sthenia	strength
scler/o	sclera (white of eye); hard	-stitial	pertaining to standing or positioned
-sclerosis	hardening	stomat/o	mouth
scoli/o	crooked; bent	-stomia	condition of the mouth
-scope	instrument for visual examination	-stomy	new opening (to form a mouth)
-scopy	visual examination	strept/o	twisted chains
scot/o	darkness	styl/o	pole or stake
seb/o	sebum	sub-	under; below
sebace/o	sebum	submaxill/o	mandible (lower jaw bone)
sect/o	to cut	-suppression	stopping
semi-	half	supra-	above, upper
semin/i	semen; seed	sym-	together; with
seps/o	infection	syn-	together; with
sial/o	saliva; salivary	syncop/o	to cut off, cut short; faint
sialaden/o	salivary gland	syndesm/o	ligament
sider/o	iron	synov/o	synovia; synovial membrane; sheath around a tendon
sigmoid/o	sigmoid colon	syring/o	tube
silic/o	glass	tachy-	fast
sinus/o	sinus	tars/o	tarsus; hindfoot or ankle (7 bones between the foot and the leg)
-sis	state of; condition		
-sol	solution	tax/o	order; coordination
somat/o	body	tel/o	complete
-some	body	tele/o	distant
somn/o	sleep	ten/o	tendon
-somnia	sleep	tendin/o	tendon
son/o	sound	-tension	pressure
-spadia	to tear, cut	terat/o	monster; malformed fetus
-spasm	sudden contraction of muscles	test/o	testis (testicle)
sperm/o	spermatozoa; sperm cells	tetra-	four
spermat/o	spermatozoa; sperm cells	thalam/o	thalamus
sphen/o	wedge; sphenoid bone	thalass/o	sea
spher/o	globe-shaped; round	the/o	put; place
sphygm/o	pulse	thec/o	sheath
-sphyxia	pulse	thel/o, theli/o	nipple
splanchn/o	viscera (internal organs)	therapeut/o	treatment
spin/o	spine (backbone)	-therapy	treatment
spir/o	to breathe	therm/o	heat
splen/o	spleen	thorac/o	chest

Combining Form, Suffix, or Prefix	Meaning	Combining Form, Suffix, or Prefix	Meaning
-thorax	chest; pleural cavity	ungu/o	nail
thromb/o	clot	uni-	one
thym/o	thymus gland	ur/o	urine; urinary tract
-thymia	mind (condition of)	ureter/o	ureter
-thymic	pertaining to mind	urethr/o	urethra
thyr/o	thyroid gland; shield	-uria	urination; condition of urine
thyroid/o	thyroid gland	urin/o	urine
tibi/o	tibia (shin bone)	-us	structure; thing
-tic	pertaining to	uter/o	uterus (womb)
toc/o	labor; birth	uve/o	uvea, vascular layer of eye (iris, choroid, ciliary body)
-tocia	labor; birth (condition of)		
-tocin	labor; birth (a substance for)	uvul/o	uvula
tom/o	to cut	vag/o	vagus nerve
-tome	instrument to cut	vagin/o	vagina
-tomy	process of cutting	valv/o	valve
ton/o	tension	valvul/o	valve
tone/o	to stretch	varic/o	varicose veins
tonsill/o	tonsil	vas/o	vessel; duct; vas deferens
top/o	place; position; location	vascul/o	vessel (blood)
-tory	pertaining to	ven/o, ven/i	vein
tox/o	poison	vener/o	venereal (sexual contact)
toxic/o	poison	ventr/o	belly side of body
trache/o	trachea (windpipe)	ventricul/o	ventricle (of heart or brain)
trans-	across; through	venul/o	venule (small vein)
-tresia	opening	-verse	to turn
tri-	three	-version	turning (condition of)
trich/o	hair	vertebr/o	vertebra (backbone)
trigon/o	trigone (area within the bladder)	vesic/o	urinary bladder
-tripsy	crushing	vesicul/o	seminal vesicle
troph/o	nourishment; development	vestibul/o	vestibule of the inner ear
-trophy	nourishment; development (condition of)	viscer/o	internal organs
		vit/o	life
-tropia	to turn	vitr/o	vitreous body (of the eye)
-tropic	pertaining to stimulating	vitre/o	glass
-tropin	stimulate; act on	viv/o	life
tympan/o	tympanic membrane (eardrum); middle ear	vol/o	to roll
		vulv/o	vulva (female external genitalia)
-type	classification; picture	xanth/o	yellow
-ule	little; small	xen/o	stranger
uln/o	ulna (medial lower arm bone)	xer/o	dry
ultra-	beyond; excess	xiph/o	sword
-um	structure; tissue; thing	-y	condition; process
umbilic/o	umbilicus (navel)	zo/o	animal life

ENGLISH—MEDICAL WORD PARTS

Meaning	Combining Form, Suffix, or Prefix	Meaning	Combining Form, Suffix, or Prefix
abdomen	abdomin/o (*use with* -al, -centesis)	apart	ana-
		apart from	para-
	celi/o (*use with* -ac)	aponeurosis	aponeur/o
	lapar/o (*use with* -scope, -scopy, -tomy)	appendix	append/o (*use with* -ectomy)
			appendic/o (*use with* -itis)
abdominal wall	lapar/o	appetite	-orexia
abnormal	dys-	arm	brachi/o
	par-	arm bone, lower lateral	radi/o
	para-		
abnormal condition	-iasis	arm bone, lower, medial	uln/o
	-osis		
above	epi-	arm bone, upper	humer/o
	hyper-	armpit	axill/o
	supra-	arteriole	arteriol/o
acetabulum	acetabul/o	artery	arter/o
acetones	ket/o		arteri/o
	keton/o	articulate (speak distinctly)	-arthria
acid	oxy-		
acromion	acromi/o	asbestos	asbest/o
across	trans-	assemble	-agon
action	-praxia	atrium	atri/o
action	-esis	attraction for	-phil
act on	-tropin		-philia
adenoids	adenoid/o	attraction to	phil/o
adrenal glands	adren/o	auditory tube	salping/o
	adrenal/o		-salpinx
after	post-	away from	ab-
again	ana-, re-		apo-
against	anti-		ex-
	contra-		exo-
air	aer/o	bacilli (rod-shaped bacteria)	bacill/o
	pneum/o		
	pneumon/o	back	re-
air sac	alveol/o		retro-
albumin	albumin/o	back, lower	lumb/o
all	pan-	back portion of body	dorsi-
along side of	para-		dors/o
alveolus	alveol/o		poster/o
anew	ana-	backbone	spin/o (*use with* -al)
amnion	amni/o		spondyl/o (*use with* -itis, -lithesis, -osis, -pathy)
aneurysm	aneurysm/o		
angle	goni/o		vertebr/o (*use with* -al)
animal life	zo/o	backward	ana-
animal starch	glycogen/o		retro-
ankle	tars/o	bacteria	bacteri/o
antrum (of stomach)	anthr/o	bacterium (berry-shaped)	-coccus (-cocci, *pl.*)
anus	an/o	bad	cac/o
anus and rectum	proct/o		dys-
anxiety	anxi/o		mal-
aorta	aort/o	barrier	claustr/o

Meaning	Combining Form, Suffix, or Prefix	Meaning	Combining Form, Suffix, or Prefix
base (not acidic)	bas/o	blood vessel	angi/o (*use with* -ectomy, -genesis, -gram, -graphy, -oma, -plasty, -spasm)
Bartholin glands	bartholin/o		
bear, to	para-		
	-parous		vas/o (*use with* -constriction, -dilation, -motor)
	-phobia		
	phor/o		vascul/o (*use with* -ar, -itis)
before	ante-	blue	cyan/o
	pre-	body	corpor/o
	pro-		somat/o
	pros-		-some
beginning	-arche	bone	oste/o
behind	post-	bone condition	-ostosis
	poster/o	bone marrow	myel/o
	retro-	brain	encephal/o
belly	celi/o	branching	furc/o
belly side of body	ventr/o	break	-clasis
below, beneath	hypo-		-clast
	infra-	breakdown	-lysis
	sub-	breast	mamm/o (*use with* -ary, -gram, -graphy, -plasty)
bend, to	flex/o		
bent	scoli/o		mast/o (*use with* -algia, -dynia, -ectomy, -itis)
beside	para-		
between	inter-	breastbone	stern/o
beyond	hyper-	breathe	spir/o
	meta-	breathing	-pnea
	ultra-	bring forth	-para
bile	bil/i		-parous
	chol/e	bronchial tube	bronch/o
bile vessel	cholangi/o	(bronchus)	bronchi/o
bilirubin	bilirubin/o	bronchiole	bronchiol/o
bind	-desis	bunion	bunion/o
	nect/o	burn	caus/o
birth	nat/i		cauter/o
	-partum	bursa	burs/o
	toc/o	bursting forth	-rrhage
	-tocia		-rrhagia
birth, substance for	-tocin	calcaneus	calcane/o
births, live	-para	calcium	calc/o
black	anthrac/o		calci/o
	melan/o	calyx	cali/o
bladder (urinary)	cyst/o (*use with* -ic, -itis, -cele, -gram, -scopy, -stomy, -tomy)		calic/o
		cancerous	carcin/o
	vesic/o (*use with* -al)	capillary	capillar/o
blood	hem/o (*use with* -dialysis, -globin, lysis, -philia, -ptysis, -rrhage, -stasis, -stat)	carbon dioxide	capn/o
			-capnia
		care for, to	comi/o
	hemat/o (*use with* -crit, -emesis, -logist, -logy, -oma, -poiesis, -uria)	carry	duct/o
			-phoresis
			-phoria
blood condition	-emia	carrying	-ferent
	-emic	cartilage	chondr/o

Meaning	Combining Form, Suffix, or Prefix	Meaning	Combining Form, Suffix, or Prefix
cast; throw	bol/o	condition	-ation
cause	eti/o		-ema
causing genetic change	mutagen/o		-esis
			-ia
cecum	cec/o		-ism
cell	cyt/o		-itus
	-cyte		-sis
cells, condition of	-cytosis		-y
cerebellum	cerebell/o	condition, abnormal	-iasis
cerebrum	cerebr/o		-osis
cerumen	cerumin/o	conjunctiva	conjunctiv/o
cervix	cervic/o	connect	nect/o
change	meta-	connective tissue	sarc/o
cheek	bucc/o	constant	home/o
chemical	chem/o	control	-stasis, -stat
chest	pector/o	contraction	-stalsis
	steth/o	contraction of muscles, sudden	-spasm
	thorac/o		
child	ped/o	coordination	tax/o
childbirth	obstetr/o	copy	-mimetic
chin	ment/o	cornea (of the eye)	corne/o
cholesterol	cholesterol/o		kerat/o
chorion	chori/o	cortex	cortic/o
	chorion/o	cotton dust	byssin/o
choroid layer (of the eye)	choroid/o	crooked	scoli/o
		crushing	-tripsy
ciliary body (of the eye)	cycl/o	cul-de-sac	culd/o
		curve	lord/o
circle or cycle	cycl/o	cut	cis/o
classification	-type		sect/o, -section
clavicle	clavicul/o		tom/o
clot	thromb/o	cut off	syncop/o
clumping	agglutin/o	cutting, process of	-tomy
clusters	staphyl/o	cycle	cycl/o
coagulation	coagul/o	cyst (sac of fluid)	cyst/o
coal dust	anthrac/o	dance	chore/o
coccyx	coccyg/o	dark	phe/o
cochlea	cochle/o	darkness	scot/o
cold	cry/o	dawn-colored	eosin/o
collar bone	clavicul/o	death	leth/o
colon	col/o (*use with* -ectomy, -itis, -pexy, -stomy)		mort/o, -mortem
			necr/o
	colon/o (*use with* -ic, -pathy, -scope, scopy)	deep sleep	comat/o
		defecation (elimination of wastes)	-chezia
color	chrom/o		
come together	-fusion		
common bile duct	choledoch/o	deficiency	-penia
complete	dia-	deficient	hypo-
	tel/o	destroying	-lytic

Meaning	Combining Form, Suffix, or Prefix	Meaning	Combining Form, Suffix, or Prefix
destruction	-lysis	electricity	electr/o
development	plas/o	elimination of wastes	-chezia
	-plasia	embryonic	-blast
	troph/o	enclosed space	claustr/o
	-trophy	enlargement	-megaly
diaphragm	phren/o	enzyme	-ase
difficult	dys-	epididymis	epididym/o
digestion	-pepsia	epiglottis	epiglott/o
dilation	-ectasia	equal	is/o
	-ectasis	esophagus	esophag/o
dim	ambly/o	eustachian tube	salping/o
discharge	-rrhea	excess	-ultra
disease	nos/o	excessive	hyper-
	path/o	excessive pain	-agra
	-pathy	excision	-ectomy
distant	dist/o	expansion	-ectasia
	tele/o		-ectasis
distinct	idi/o	extreme	pol/o
double	dipl/o	extreme point	acr/o
down	cata-	extremities	acr/o
	de-	eye	ocul/o (*use with* -ar, -facial, -motor)
drooping	-ptosis		ophthalm/o (*use with* -ia, -ic, -logist, -logy, -pathy, -plasty, -plegia, -scope, -scopy)
drug	chem/o		
	pharmac/o		opt/o (*use with* -ic, -metrist)
	pharmaceut/o		optic/o (*use with* -al, -ian)
dry	ichthy/o		
	xer/o	eyelid	blephar/o (*use with* -chalasis, -itis, -plasty, -plegia, -ptosis, -tomy)
drying	desicc/o		
duct	vas/o		palpebr/o (*use with* -al)
dull	ambly/o	face	faci/o
duodenum	duoden/o	faint	syncop/o
dura mater	dur/o	falling	-ptosis
dusky	phe/o	fallopian tube	salping/o
dust	coni/o		-salpinx
ear	aur/o (*use with* -al, -icle)	false	pseudo-
	auricul/o (*use with* -ar)	far	dist/o
	ot/o (*use with* -algia, -ic, -itis, -logy, -mycosis, -rrhea, -sclerosis, -scope, -scopy)	fascia	fasci/o
		fast	tachy-
ear condition	-otia	fat	adip/o (*use with* -ose, -osis)
eardrum	myring/o (*use with* -ectomy, -itis, -tomy)		lip/o (*use with* -ase, -cyte, -genesis, -oid, -oma)
	tympan/o (*use with* -ic, -metry, -plasty)		steat/o (*use with* -oma, -rrhea)
eat	phag/o	fear	phob/o
	-phage		-phobia
eating	-phagia	feeling	esthesi/o
egg cell	o/o		-phoria
	ov/o	female	estr/o (*use with* -gen, -genic)
	ovul/o		gynec/o (*use with* -logist, -logy, -mastia)
elbow	olecran/o		

Meaning	Combining Form, Suffix, or Prefix	Meaning	Combining Form, Suffix, or Prefix
femur	femor/o	glass	silic/o
fever	pyr/o		vitre/o
	pyret/o	glial cells	gli/o
	pyrex/o	globe-shaped	spher/o
fiber	fibr/o, fibromat/o, fibrin/o	glomerulus	glomerul/o
fibrous connective tissue	fibros/o	glucose	gluc/o
			glyc/o
fibula	fibul/o (*use with* -ar)		glycos/o
	perone/o (*use with* -al)	glue	coll/a
finger and toe bones	phalang/o		gli/o
		glycogen	glycogen/o
fingers	dactyl/o	go, to	-grade
fire	pyr/o	good	eu-
first	primi-	granule(s)	granul/o
	prot/o	gray	glauc/o
fixation	-pexy	gray matter	polio-
flat plate	-elasma	green	chlor/o
flesh	sarc/o	groin	inguin/o
flow	-rrhea	grow	-physis
fluid collection	-oma	growing	phys/o
flushed	erythem/o	growth	-plasia
follicle	follicul/o	gum	gingiv/o
foot	pod/o	habit	-hexia
foot bones	metatars/o	hair	pil/o
forking	furc/o		trich/o
form	morph/o	half	hemi-
formation	plas/o		semi-
	-plasia	hallucination	hallucin/o
	-plasm	hand	chir/o
	-poiesis	hang	pend/o
forming	-genesis	hard	scirrh/o
forward	ante-, pro-, pros-	hand bones	metacarp/o
four	quadri-	hang, to	pend/o
	tetra-	hard	kerat/o
front	anter/o		scirrh/o
full of	-ose	hardening	-sclerosis
fungus	fung/i (*use with* -cide, -oid, -ous, -stasis)		scler/o
		head	cephal/o
	myc/o (*use with* -logist, -logy, -osis, -tic)	hearing	acous/o
			audi/o
gall	bil/i (*use with* -ary)		audit/o
	chol/e (*use with* -lithiasis)		-acusis
gallbladder	cholecyst/o		-cusis
ganglion	gangli/o	heart	cardi/o (*use with* -ac, -graphy, -logy, -logist, -megaly, -pathy, -vascular)
	ganglion/o		
gas	pneum/o		coron/o (*use with* -ary)
	pneumon/o		
gather	-agon	heart muscle	myocardi/o
genetic change	mut/a	heat	cauter/o
	mutagen/o		therm/o
give, to	-dote	heavy	pachy-
gland	aden/o	heel bone	calcane/o
glans penis	balan/o	hemoglobin	hemoglobin/o

Meaning	Combining Form, Suffix, or Prefix	Meaning	Combining Form, Suffix, or Prefix
hernia	-cele	itching	prurit/o
	herni/o	jaw, lower	mandibul/o
hidden	crypt/o		submaxill/o
hip region	pelv/i, pelv/o	jaw, upper	maxill/o
holding back	isch/o	jejunum	jejun/o
hormone	hormon/o	joint	arthr/o
	-one		articul/o
horn-like	kerat/o	ketones	ket/o
horse	equin/o		keton/o
humerus	humer/o	kidney	nephr/o (*use with* -algia, -ectomy,
humpback	kyph/o		-ic, -itis, -lith, -megaly, -oma,
hydrochloric acid	chlorhydr/o		-osis, -pathy, -ptosis, -sclerosis,
ileum	ile/o		-stomy, -tomy)
ilium	ili/o		ren/o (*use with* -al, -gram,
immature cells	-blast		-vascular)
immature tumor (cells)	-blastoma	killing	-cidal
			-cide
immune	immun/o	knowledge	gnos/o, gno/o
in, into, within	em-	labor	-partum
	en-		toc/o
	endo-		-tocia
	in-	labor, substance for	-tocin
	intra-		
	ir-	lack of	de-
in due measure	emmetr/o	lack of strength	-asthenia
in front of	pre-	lacrimal duct	dacry/o
incomplete	atel/o		lacrim/o
increased	poly-	lacrimal sac	dacryocyst/o
increase in cell numbers (blood cells)	-cytosis	lamina	lamin/o
		large	macro-
			mega-
individual	idi/o	larynx	laryng/o
infection	seps/o	lead	duct/o
inferior to	infra-	lens of eye	phac/o
inflammation	-itis		phak/o
instrument for recording	-graph	less	de-
			mi/o
instrument for visual examination	-scope	less than normal	hypo-
		life	bi/o
			vit/o
instrument to cut	-tome		viv/o
insulin	insulin/o	ligament	ligament/o
internal organs	spanchn/o		syndesm/o
	viscer/o	light	actin/o
intestine, small	enter/o		phot/o
inward	eso-	like	phil/o
iodine	iod/o	lip	cheil/o
ion	ion/o		labi/o
iris	ir/o	lipid	lipid/o
	irid/o	little	-ole
iron	sider/o		-ule
irregular	poikil/o	liver	hepat/o
irrigation	-clysis	lobe	lob/o
ischium	ischi/o	location	top/o

Meaning	Combining Form, Suffix, or Prefix	Meaning	Combining Form, Suffix, or Prefix
loin	lumb/o	**monster**	terat/o
loosening	-lysis	**mood**	-thymia
love	phil/o		-thymic
luminous	fluor/o	**more**	ple/o
lung	pulmon/o	**mouth**	or/o (*use with* -al)
lung	pneum/o (*use with* -coccus, -coniosis, -thorax)		stomat/o (*use with* -itis)
			-stomia
	pneumon/o (*use with* -ectomy, -ia, -ic, -itis, -lysis)	**movement**	cine/o
			kines/o
	pulmon/o (*use with* -ary)		kinesi/o
lymph	lymph/o		-kinesia
lymph gland	lymphaden/o		-kinesis
lymph vessel	lymphangi/o		-motor
make, to	-fication	**much**	poly-
male	andr/o	**mucous membrane**	mucos/o
malformed fetus	terat/o	**mucus**	muc/o
malleolus	malleol/o		myx/o
mandible (lower jaw bone)	mandibul/o	**muscle**	muscul/o (*use with* -ar, -skeletal)
	submaxill/o		my/o (*use with* -algia, -ectomy, -oma, -neutral, -pathy, -rrhaphy, -therapy)
many	multi-		
	ple/o		
	poly-		myos/o (*use with* -in, -itis)
marketplace	agora-	**muscle, smooth (visceral)**	leiomy/o
marrow	medull/o		
mass	-oma	**muscle, striated (skeletal)**	rhabdomy/o
mastoid process	mastoid/o		
maxilla	maxill/o	**muscle tumor**	myom/o
meal	cib/o	**muzzle**	phim/o
	-prandial	**myocardium**	myocardi/o
measure	-meter	**nail**	onych/o
	metr/o		ungu/o
meatus	meat/o	**narrowing**	-constriction
mediastinum	mediastin/o		sten/o
medulla oblongata	medull/o		-stenosis
meninges	mening/o	**nature**	physi/o
	meningi/o	**navel**	omphal/o
menstruation; menses	men/o		umbilic/o
		near	para-
metacarpals	metacarp/o		proxim/o
metatarsals (foot bones)	metatars/o	**neck**	cervic/o
		neither	neutr/o
middle	medi/o	**nerve**	neur/o
	medull/o	**nerve root**	radicul/o
	meso-	**nervous sensation**	esthes/o
middle ear	tympan/o		esthesi/o
milk	galact/o		-esthesia
	lact/o	**nest**	nid/o
mimic	-mimetic	**network**	reticul/o
mind	ment/o	**network of nerves**	plex/o
	phren/o	**neutral**	neutr/o
	psych/o	**neutrophil**	neutr/o
	-thymia	**new**	neo-
	-thymic	**night**	noct/o
mixture	cras/o		nyct/o

Meaning	Combining Form, Suffix, or Prefix	Meaning	Combining Form, Suffix, or Prefix
nipple	thel/o, theli/o	**own**	aut-
nipple-like	papill/o	**oxygen**	ox/o
nitrogen	azot/o		-oxia
nitrogen compound	-amine	**pain**	-algia (*use with* arthr/o, cephal/o, gastr/o, mast/o, my/o, neur/o, ot/o)
no, not	a-, an-		
none	nulli-		
normal	eu-		-dynia (*use with* coccyg/o, pleur/o)
nose	nas/o (*use with* -al)		odyn/o
	rhin/o (*use with* -itis, -rrhea, -plasty)	**pain, excessive**	-agra
		pain, sensitivity to	-algesia
nourishment	troph/o		algesi/o
	-trophy	**painful**	dys-
nucleus	kary/o	**palate**	palat/o
	nucle/o	**palsy**	-plegia
nucleus (collection of nerve cells in the brain)	kern-		-plegic
		pancreas	pancreat/o
		paralysis	-plegia
numbness	narc/o		-plegic
obscure	-opaque	**paralysis, slight**	-paresis
obsessive preoccupation	-mania	**parathyroid glands**	parathyroid/o
		patella	patell/a (*use with* -pexy)
off	apo-		patell/o (*use with* -ar, -ectomy, -femoral)
old age	ger/o		
	geront/o	**pelvis**	pelv/i
	presby/o		pelv/o
olecranon (elbow)	olecran/o	**penis**	pen/o
on	epi-		phall/o
one	mon/o	**people**	dem/o
	mono-	**perineum**	perine/o
	uni-	**peritoneum**	peritone/o
one's own	aut/o	**pertaining to**	-ac (*as in* cardiac)
	auto-		-al (*as in* inguinal)
one who	-er		-an (*as in* ovarian)
	-or		-ar (*as in* palmar)
opening	-tresia		-ary (*as in* papillary)
opening, new	-stomy		-eal (*as in* pharyngeal)
opposite	contra-		-iac (*as in* hypochondriac)
optic disc (disk)	papill/o		-ic (*as in* nucleic)
orange-yellow	cirrh/o		-ical (*as in* psychological)
order	norm/o		-ile (*as in* penile)
	tax/o		-ine (*as in* equine)
organs, internal	viscer/o		-ior (*as in* superior)
originating from	-oid		-ose (*as in* adipose)
ossicle	ossicul/o		-ous (*as in* mucous)
other	all/o		-tic (*as in* necrotic)
other than	par-		-tory (*as in* secretory)
out, outside	ec-	**phalanges**	phalang/o
	ex-	**pharynx (throat)**	pharyng/o
	exo-	**phrase**	-lexia
	extra-	**physician**	iatr/o
outer region	cortic/o	**pineal gland**	pineal/o
ovary	oophor/o (*use with* -itis, -ectomy, -pexy)	**pituitary gland**	hypophys/o
			pituit/o
	ovari/o (*use with* -an)		pituitar/o

Meaning	Combining Form, Suffix, or Prefix	Meaning	Combining Form, Suffix, or Prefix
place	-stasis	put in place	-pexy
	the/o	pyloric sphincter,	pylor/o
	top/o	pylorus	
plant	phyt/o	radioactivity	radi/o
	-phyte	radius (lower arm	radi/o
plaque	ather/o	bone)	
	-plakia	rapid	oxy-
pleura	pleur/o	rash	exanthemat/o
pleural cavity	-thorax	record	-gram
plexus	plex/o	recording, process	-graphy
poison	tox/o	of	
	toxic/o	rectum	rect/o
pole	styl/o	recurring	cycl/o
polyp	polyp/o	red	eosin/o
pons	pont/o		erythr/o
pores, condition of	-porosis	redness	erythem/o
position	top/o		erythemat/o
potassium	kal/i	reduce	-lytic
pour	chyme/o	reflected sound	echo-
	-fusion	relaxation	-chalasia
pregnancy	-cyesis		-chalasis
	gest/o	removal	-apheresis
	gester/o		-ectomy
	gravid/o		-pheresis
	-gravida	renal pelvis	pyel/o
	obstetr/o	repair	-plasty
pressure	bar/o	resembling	-form
	-tension		-oid
process	-ation	retina	retin/o
	-ion	rhythm	rrhythm/o
	-ism	rib	cost/o
	-y	roll, to	vol/o
produced by *or* in	-genic	rosy	eosin/o
producing	-gen	round	spher/o
	-genesis	rule	norm/o
prolapse	-ptosis	run	-drome
prostate gland	prostat/o	rupture	-rrhexis
protection	immun/o	sac, small	alveol/o
	-phylaxis		follicul/o
protein	albumin/o	sac of fluid	cyst/o
	-globin	sacrum	sacr/o
	-globulin	safe	immun/o
	prote/o	sag, to	-ptosis
pubis	pub/o	saliva	sial/o
pulse	sphygm/o	salivary gland	sialaden/o
	-sphyxia	same	ipsi-
puncture to remove	-centesis		is/o
fluid		sameness;	home/o
pupil	cor/o	unchanging;	
	core/o	constant	
	pupill/o	scaly	ichthy/o
pus	purul/o		squam/o
	py/o	scanty	olig/o
put	the/o	scapula	scapul/o

Meaning	Combining Form, Suffix, or Prefix	Meaning	Combining Form, Suffix, or Prefix
sclera	scler/o	sleep	hypn/o
scrotum	scrot/o		somn/o
sea	thalass/o		-somnia
sebum	seb/o	sleep, deep	comat/o
	sebace/o	slender	lept/o
	steat/o	slide, to	lux/o
secrete	crin/o	sliding, condition of	-lapse
	-crine		
seed	gon/o	slipping	-listhesis
	semin/i	slow	brady-
seizure	-lepsy	small	-icle
seizing, taking hold of (pertaining to)	-leptic		micro-
			-ole
self	aut-		-ule
	auto-	small intestine	enter/o
semen	semin/i	smaller	mi/o
seminal vesicle	vesicul/o	smell	-osmia
send, sending	-mission	smooth (visceral) muscle	leiomy/o
sensation (nervous)	-esthesia		
sensitivity to pain	alges/o	sodium	natr/o
	-algesia	soft	medull/o
separate	-crine	softening	-malacia
	-crit	sole (of the foot)	plant/o
	-lytic	solid	ster/o
separation	-lysis		stere/o
set, to	-stitial	solution	-sol
severe	acu/o	sound	echo-
sex glands	gonad/o		phon/o
sexual intercourse	-pareunia		-phonia
shape	-form		son/o
	morph/o	spark	scint/i
sharp	acu/o	specialist	-ist
	oxy-	speech	phas/o
sheath	-lemma		-phasia
	thec/o	sperm cells (spermatozoa)	sperm/o
shield	thyr/o		spermat/o
shin bone	tibi/o	spinal column (spine)	rachi/o
shine	-lucent		spin/o
short	brachy-		vertebr/o
shoulder	om/o	spinal cord	myel/o
side	later/o	spiny	acanth/o
sieve	ethm/o	spitting	-ptysis
sigmoid colon	sigmoid/o	spleen	splen/o
single	mon/o	split	-fida
sinus	sinus/o		-schisis
skin	cutane/o (*use with* -ous)		schiz/o
	derm/o (*use with* -al)	stake (pole)	styl/o
	-derma (*use with* erythr/o, leuk/o)	stapes	staped/o
		starch	amyl/o
	dermat/o (*use with* -itis, -logist, -logy, -osis)	state of	-hexia
			-sis
	epitheli/o (*use with* -al, -lysis, -oid, -oma, -um)	steal	klept/o
		sternum	stern/o
skull	crani/o	steroid	ster/o

Meaning	Combining Form, Suffix, or Prefix	Meaning	Combining Form, Suffix, or Prefix
sticking together	agglutin/o	tearing (cutting)	-spadia
stiff	ankyl/o	tear gland	dacryoaden/o
stimulate	-tropic	tear sac	dacryocyst/o
	-tropin	temperament	cras/o
stomach	gastr/o	tendon	ten/o
stone	lith/o		tend/o
stones, condition of	-lithiasis		tendin/o
stop	-suppression	tension	ton/o
stopping	-stasis	testis	orch/o (*use with* -itis)
	-static		orchi/o (*use with* -algia, -dynia,
straight	orth/o		-ectomy, -pathy, -pexy, -tomy)
stranger	xen/o		orchid/o (*use with* -ectomy, -pexy,
strength	-sthenia		-plasty, -ptosis, -tomy)
stretch	tone/o		test/o (*use with* -sterone)
stretching	-ectasia	thick	pachy-
	-ectasis	thigh bone	femor/o
striated muscle	rhabdomy/o	thalamus	thalam/o
stricture	-stenosis	thin	lept/o
structure	-ium	thing	-um
	-plasm		-us
	-um	thing that produces	-gen
	-us	thirst	dips/o
structure, solid	ster/o	thorny	acanth/o
study of	log/o	three	tri-
	-logy	throat (pharynx)	pharyng/o
stupor	narc/o	through	dia-
substance	-in		per-
	-ine		trans-
substance that forms	-poietin	throw, to	bol/o
substance that produces	-gen	thymus gland	thym/o
		thyroid gland	thyr/o
sudden	acu/o		thyroid/o
	oxysm/o	tibia (shin bone)	tibi/o
sugar	gluc/o	tie	nect/o
	glyc/o	tie together	-desis
	glycos/o	tightening	-stenosis
	-ose	time	chron/o
surgical repair	-plasty	tissue	hist/o
surrounding	peri-		histi/o
suture	-rrhaphy		-ium
swallow	phag/o		-um
swallowing	-phagia	together	con-
swayback	lord/o		sym-
sweat	diaphor/o (*use with* -esis)		syn-
	hidr/o (*use with* -osis)	tongue	gloss/o (*use with* -al, -dynia,
swelling	-edema		-plasty, plegia, -rrhaphy,
sword	xiph/o		-spasm, -tomy)
synovial (fluid)	synov/o		lingu/o (*use with* -al)
synovial membrane	synov/o	tonsil	tonsill/o
tail	caud/o	tooth	dent/i
tailbone	coccyg/o		odont/o
tarsus (ankle)	tars/o	top	acr/o
tear	dacry/o (*use with* -genic, -rrhea)	toward	ad-
	lacrim/o (*use with* -al, -ation)		af-
			-ad

Meaning	Combining Form, Suffix, or Prefix	Meaning	Combining Form, Suffix, or Prefix
trachea (windpipe)	trache/o	vas deferens	vas/o
transmission	-phoresis	vagina	colp/o (*use with* -pexy, -plasty, -scope, -scopy, -tomy)
treatment	iatr/o		
	therapeut/o		vagin/o (*use with* -al, -itis)
	-therapy	vagus nerve	vag/o
trigone	trigon/o	valve	valv/o
true	eu-		valvul/o
tube	syring/o	varicose veins	varic/o
tumor	-oma	varied	ple/o
	onc/o		poikil/o
turn	-tropia	vein	phleb/o (*use with* -ectomy, -itis, -tomy)
	-verse		
	-version		ven/o (*use with* -ous, -gram)
twisted chains	strept/o		ven/i (*use with* -puncture)
two	bi-	vein, small	venul/o
tympanic	myring/o	venereal (sexual	vener/o
membrane	tympan/o	contact)	
(eardrum)		ventricle	ventricul/o
ulcer	aphth/o	vertebra (backbone)	rachi/o (*use with* -itis, -tomy)
ulna	uln/o		spondyl/o (*use with* -itis, -listhesis, -osis, -pathy)
umbilicus (navel)	omphal/o (*use with* -cele, -ectomy, -rrhagia, -rrhexis)		
			vertebr/o (*use with* -al)
	umbilic/o (*use with* -al)	vessel (blood)	angi/o (*use with* -ectomy, genesis, -gram, -graphy, -oma, -plasty, -spasm)
unchanging	home/o		
under	hypo-		
	sub-		vas/o (*use with* -constriction, -dilation, -motor)
uneasy	anxi/o		
unequal	anis/o		vascul/o (*use with* -ar, -itis)
unknown	idi/o	vestibule of the	vestibul/o
up	ana-	inner ear	
upon	epi-	view of	-opsy
urea	azot/o	viscera	splanchn/o
ureter	ureter/o	vision condition	-opia
urethra	urethr/o		-opsia
urinary bladder	cyst/o (*use with* -cele, -ectomy, -itis, -pexy, -plasty, -plegia, -scope, -scopy, -stomy, -tomy)		opt/o
			optic/o
		visual examination	-scopy
	vesic/o (*use with* -al)	vitreous body	vitr/o
urinary tract	ur/o	voice	phon/o
urination	-uria		-phonia
urine	ur/o	voice box (larynx)	laryng/o
	-uria	vomiting	-emesis
	urin/o	vulva	episi/o (*use with* -tomy)
uterus (womb)	hyster/o (*use with* -ectomy, -gram, -graphy, -tomy)		vulv/o (*use with* -ar)
		wander	ion/o
	metr/o (*use with* -rrhagia, -rrhea, -rrhexis)	washing	-clysis
		wasting away	-phthisis
	metri/o (*use with* -osis)	water	aque/o
	uter/o (*use with* -ine)		hydr/o
uvea	uve/o	watery flow	rheumat/o
uvula	staphyl/o (*use with* -ectomy, -plasty, -tomy)	weakness	-paresis
		wedge	sphen/o
	uvul/o (*use with* -ar, -itis, -ptosis)	weight	bar/o

Meaning	Combining Form, Suffix, or Prefix	Meaning	Combining Form, Suffix, or Prefix
white	alb/o	woman	gynec/o
	albin/o	womb	hyster/o
	leuk/o		metr/o
wide	mydr/o		metri/o
widening	-dilation		uter/o
	-ectasia	word	lex/o
	-ectasis		-lexia
	-eurysm	work	erg/o
windpipe (trachea)	trache/o	wrinkle	rhytid/o
with	con-	wrist bones (carpals)	carp/o
	sym-		
	syn-	x-rays	radi/o
within	en-		roentgen/o
	end-	yellow	lute/o
	endo-		jaund/o
	intra-		xanth/o

Plurals

The rules commonly used to form plurals of medical terms are as follows:

1. For words ending in **a**, retain the **a** and add **e**.
   Examples:

Singular	Plural
bulla	bullae
bursa	bursae
vertebra	vertebrae

2. For words ending in **is**, drop the **is** and add **es**.
   Examples:

Singular	Plural
anastomosis	anastomoses
epiphysis	epiphyses
metastasis	metastases
prosthesis	prostheses
pubis	pubes

3. For words ending in **ex** and **ix**, drop the **ex** or **ix** and add **ices**.
   Examples:

Singular	Plural
apex	apices
varix	varices

4. For words ending in **on**, drop the **on** and add **a**.
   Examples:

Singular	Plural
ganglion	ganglia
spermatozoon	spermatozoa

5. For words ending in **um**, drop the **um** and add **a**.
   Examples:

Singular	Plural
bacterium	bacteria
diverticulum	diverticula
ovum	ova

6. For words ending in **us**, drop the **us** and add **i**.
   Examples:

Singular	Plural
bronchus	bronchi
calculus	calculi
nucleus	nuclei

   Two exceptions to this rule are vir*uses* and sin*uses*.

7. Additional rules are used to form plurals in other word families.
   Examples:

Singular	Plural
anomal*y*	anomal*ies*
biops*y*	biops*ies*
fem*ur*	fem*ora*
foram*en*	foram*ina*
ir*is*	ir*ides*
phala*nx*	phala*nges*
thora*x*	thora*ces*

Abbreviations, Acronyms, Eponyms, and Symbols

ABBREVIATIONS

Many of these abbreviations may appear with or without periods and with either a capital or a lowercase first letter. (Latin abbreviations are spelled out in *italics* in parentheses.)

A, B, AB, O	blood types; may have subscript numbers
A1C	blood test that measures glycosylated hemoglobin (HbA1C) to assess glucose control
A2, A$_2$	aortic valve closure (a heart sound)
@	at
ā	before
AAA	abdominal aortic aneurysm
AAL	anterior axillary line
AB, ab	abortion
Ab	antibody
ABCDE	asymmetry (of shape), border (irregularity), color (variation with one lesion), diameter (greater than 6 mm), evolution (change)—characteristics associated with melanoma
abd	abdomen; abduction
ABGs	arterial blood gases
AC	acromioclavicular (joint)
ac, a.c.	before meals (*ante cibum*)
ACE	angiotensin-converting enzyme (ACE inhibitors treat hypertension)
ACh	acetylcholine (a neurotransmitter)
ACL	anterior cruciate ligament (of knee)
ACLS	advanced cardiac life support
ACS	acute coronary syndrome(s)
ACTH	adrenocorticotropic hormone (secreted by the anterior pituitary gland)
AD	Alzheimer disease
AD	right ear (*auris dextra*); better to specify "right ear" rather than abbreviating
ad lib.	as desired (*ad libitum,* "freely")
ADD	attention deficit disorder
add	adduction
ADH	antidiuretic hormone; vasopressin (secreted by posterior pituitary gland)
ADHD	attention deficit–hyperactivity disorder
ADL	activities of daily living
ADT	admission, discharge, transfer
AED	automated external defibrillator
AF	atrial fibrillation
AFB	acid-fast bacillus/bacilli—the TB organism
AFO	ankle-foot orthosis (device for stabilization)
AFP	alpha-fetoprotein
Ag	silver (*argentum*)
AGC	absolute granulocyte count; atypical glandular cells (on Pap smear)
AHF	antihemophilic factor (same as coagulation factor XIII)
AICD	automated implantable cardioverter-defibrillator
AIDS	acquired immunodeficiency syndrome
AIHA	autoimmune hemolytic anemia
AIS	adenocarcinoma in situ (precancerous cells are seen on Pap smear)
AKA	above-knee amputation
alb	albumin (protein)

alk phos	alkaline phosphatase (elevated in liver disease)
ALL	acute lymphoid leukemia
ALS	amyotrophic lateral sclerosis (Lou Gehrig disease)
ALT	alanine aminotransferase (elevated in liver and heart disease); formerly called serum glutamic-pyruvic transaminase (SGPT)
ALT	argon laser trabeculoplasty
AM, a.m., AM	in the morning *or* before noon (*ante meridiem*)
AMA	against medical advice; American Medical Association
amb	ambulate, ambulatory (walking)
AMD	age-related macular degeneration
AMI	acute myocardial infarction
AML	acute myeloid leukemia
ANA	antinuclear antibody
ANC	absolute neutrophil count
AP, A/P	anteroposterior
A&P	auscultation and percussion
APAP	acetyl-*para*-aminophenol
APC	acetylsalicylic acid/aspirin, phenacetin, caffeine
aq.	water (*aqua*); aqueous
ARB	angiotensin II receptor blocker
ARDS	acute respiratory distress syndrome
AROM	active range of motion
AS	aortic stenosis
AS	left ear (*auris sinistra*); better to specify "left ear," rather than abbreviating
ASA	acetylsalicylic acid (aspirin)
ASCUS	atypical squamous cells of undetermined significance (abnormal Pap smear finding that does not fully meet the criteria for a cancerous lesion)
ASD	atrial septal defect
ASD	autistic spectrum disorder
ASHD	arteriosclerotic heart disease
AST	aspartate aminotransferase (elevated in liver and heart disease); formerly called serum glutamic-oxaloacetic transaminase (SGOT)
AU	both ears (*auris uterque*); better to specify "in each ear/for both ears," rather than abbreviating
Au	gold (*aurum*)
AUB	abnormal uterine bleeding
AV	arteriovenous; atrioventricular
AVM	arteriovenous malformation
AVR	aortic valve replacement
AZT	azidothymidine
A&W	alive and well
B cells	lymphocytes produced in the bone marrow
Ba	barium
BAL	bronchoalveolar lavage
bands	immature white blood cells (granulocytes)
baso	basophils
BBB	bundle branch block
BC	bone conduction
bcr	breakpoint cluster region
BE	barium enema
bid, b.i.d.	twice a day (*bis in die*)
BKA	below-knee amputation
BM	bowel movement
BMD	bone mineral density
BMR	basal metabolic rate
BMT	bone marrow transplantation
BP, B/P	blood pressure
BPH	benign prostatic hyperplasia/hypertrophy
BPPV	benign paroxysmal positional vertigo
BRBPR	bright red blood per rectum (hematochezia)
BRCA1, BRCA2	breast cancer 1, breast cancer 2 (genetic markers for disease risk)
bs	blood sugar; breath sound(s)
BSE	breast self-examination
BSO	bilateral salpingo-oophorectomy
BSP	Bromsulphalein (bromosulfophthalein)—dye used in liver function testing; its retention is indicative of liver damage or disease
BT	bleeding time
BUN	blood urea nitrogen
bw, BW	birth weight
Bx, bx	biopsy
C	carbon; calorie
°C	degrees Celsius (on "metric" temperature scale); degrees centigrade
c̄	with (*cum*)
C1, C2	first cervical vertebra, second cervical vertebra (and so on)
CA	cancer; carcinoma; cardiac arrest; chronologic age
Ca	calcium
CABG	coronary artery bypass graft/grafting (cardiovascular surgery)
CAD	coronary artery disease
CAO	chronic airway obstruction
cap	capsule
CAPD	continuous ambulatory peritoneal dialysis
Cath	catheter; catheterization
CBC	complete blood (cell) count
CBT	cognitive behavioral therapy
CC	chief complaint
cc	cubic centimeter (same as mL: 1/1000 of a liter)
CCr, CrCl	creatinine clearance
CCU	coronary care unit; critical care unit
CDC	Centers for Disease Control and Prevention
CDH	congenital dislocated hip

CEA	carcinoembryonic antigen
cf.	compare (*confer*)
CF	cystic fibrosis; complement fixation (test)
c.gl	with (*cum*) glasses
CGMS	continuous glucose monitoring system
cGy	centigray (1/100 of a gray; a rad)
CHD	coronary heart disease; chronic heart disease
chemo	chemotherapy
CHF	congestive heart failure
chol	cholesterol
chr	chronic
μCi	microcurie
CIN	cervical intraepithelial neoplasia
CIS	carcinoma in situ
CK	creatine kinase
CKD	chronic kidney disease
Cl	chlorine
CLD	chronic liver disease
CLL	chronic lymphocytic leukemia
cm	centimeter (1/100 of a meter)
CMA	certified medical assistant
CMC	carpometacarpal (joint)
CMG	cystometrogram
CML	chronic myelogenous leukemia
CMV	cytomegalovirus
CNS	central nervous system
CO	carbon monoxide; cardiac output
CO$_2$	carbon dioxide
Co	cobalt
c/o	complains of
COD	condition on discharge
COPD	chronic obstructive pulmonary disease
CP	cerebral palsy; chest pain
CPA	costophrenic angle
CPAP	continuous positive airway pressure
CPD	cephalopelvic disproportion
CPR	cardiopulmonary resuscitation
CR	complete response; cardiorespiratory
CRBSI	catheter-related bloodstream infection
CRF	chronic renal failure
C&S	culture and sensitivity (of sputum)
C-section	cesarean section
CSF	cerebrospinal fluid; colony-stimulating factor
C-spine	cervical spine (x-ray film)
CT	computed tomography (x-ray imaging in axial and other planes)
ct.	count
CTPA	CT pulmonary angiography
CTS	carpal tunnel syndrome
Cu	copper (*cuprum*)
CVA	cerebrovascular accident; costovertebral angle
CVP	central venous pressure
CVS	cardiovascular system; chorionic villus sampling
c/w	compare with; consistent with

CX, CXR	chest x-ray (film)
Cx	cervix
cysto	cystoscopy
D&C	dilatation/dilation and curettage
DCIS	ductal carcinoma in situ
DD	discharge diagnosis; differential diagnosis
Decub.	decubitus (lying down)
Derm.	dermatology
DES	diethylstilbestrol; diffuse esophageal spasm
DEXA *or* DXA	dual-energy x-ray absorptiometry (a test of bone mineral density)
DI	diabetes insipidus; diagnostic imaging
DIC	disseminated intravascular coagulation
DICOM	digital image communication in medicine
diff.	differential count (of kinds of white blood cells)
DIG	digoxin; digitalis
DKA	diabetic ketoacidosis
dL, dl	deciliter (1/10 of a liter)
DLco	diffusion capacity of the lung for carbon monoxide
DLE	discoid lupus erythematosus
DM	diabetes mellitus
DNA	deoxyribonucleic acid
DNR	do not resuscitate
D.O.	doctor of osteopathy
DOA	dead on arrival
DOB	date of birth
DOE	dyspnea on exertion
DPT	diphtheria-pertussis-tetanus (vaccine)
DRE	digital rectal examination
DRG	diagnosis-related group
DSA	digital subtraction angiography
DSM	*Diagnostic and Statistical Manual of Mental Disorders*
DT	delirium tremens (caused by alcohol withdrawal)
DTR	deep tendon reflex(es)
DUB	dysfunctional uterine bleeding
DVT	deep vein thrombosis
D/W	dextrose in water
Dx	diagnosis
EBV	Epstein-Barr virus (cause of mononucleosis)
ECC	endocervical curettage; extracorporeal circulation; emergency cardiac care
ECF	extended care facility
ECG	electrocardiogram
ECHO	echocardiography
ECMO	extracorporeal membrane oxygenation
ECT	electroconvulsive therapy
ED	erectile dysfunction; emergency department
EDC	estimated date of confinement
EEG	electroencephalogram
EENT	eyes, ears, nose, throat
EGD	esophagogastroduodenoscopy

EGFR	epidermal growth factor receptor
EKG	electrocardiogram
ELISA	enzyme-linked immunosorbent assay
EM	electron microscope
EMB	endometrial biopsy
EMG	electromyogram
EMLA	eutectic mixture of local anesthetics
EMT	emergency medical technician
ENT	ear, nose, throat
EOM	extraocular movement; extraocular muscles
eos	eosinophils (type of white blood cell)
EPO	erythropoietin
ER	emergency room; estrogen receptor
ERCP	endoscopic retrograde cholangiopancreatography
ERT	estrogen replacement therapy
ESR (sed rate)	erythrocyte sedimentation rate (increase indicates inflammation)
ESRD	end-stage renal disease
ESWL	extracorporeal shock wave lithotripsy
ETOH	ethyl alcohol
ETT	exercise tolerance test
EUS	endoscopic ultrasonography
F, ° F	Fahrenheit, degrees Fahrenheit
FB	fingerbreadth; foreign body
FBS	fasting blood sugar
FDA	U.S. Food and Drug Administration
FDG-PET	2-deoxy-2[F-18]fluoro-D-glucose positron emission tomography
Fe	iron (Latin, *ferrum*)
FEF	forced expiratory flow
FEV$_1$	forced expiratory volume in first second
FFR	fractional flow reserve
FH	family history
FHR	fetal heart rate
FNA	fine needle aspiration
FPG	fasting plasma glucose
FROM	full range of movement/motion
FSH	follicle-stimulating hormone
F/U	follow-up
5-FU	5-fluorouracil (a chemotherapy drug)
FUO	fever of undetermined origin
Fx	fracture
G	gravida (pregnant)
g, gm	gram
μg	microgram (one millionth of a gram)
g/dL	grams per deciliter
Ga	gallium
GABA	gamma-aminobutyric acid; also spelled γ-aminobutyric acid—a neurotransmitter
GB	gallbladder
GBS	gallbladder series (an x-ray study)
GC	gonococcus
G-CSF	granulocyte colony-stimulating factor (promotes neutrophil production)
Gd	gadolinium
GERD	gastroesophageal reflux disease
GFR	glomerular filtration rate
GH	growth hormone
GI	gastrointestinal
GIST	gastrointestinal stromal tumor
G6PD	glucose-6-phosphate dehydrogenase (enzyme missing in an inherited red blood cell disorder)
GP	general practitioner
GM-CSF	granulocyte-macrophage colony-stimulating factor (promotes myeloid progenitor cells with differentiation to granulocytes)
grav. 1, 2, 3	*gravida* 1, 2, 3—first, second, third pregnancy
gt, gtt	drop (*gutta*), drops (*guttae*)
GTT	glucose tolerance test
GU	genitourinary
Gy	gray—unit of radiation absorption (exposure); equal to 100 rad
GYN, gyn	gynecology
H	hydrogen
h., hr	hour
H$_2$ blocker	histamine type 2 receptor antagonist (inhibitor of gastric acid secretion)
HAART	highly active antiretroviral therapy (for AIDS)
HAI	hemagglutination inhibition
Hb, hgb	hemoglobin
HbA$_{1c}$	glycosylated hemoglobin test (for diabetes)
HBV	hepatitis B virus
HCC	hepatocellular carcinoma
hCG, HCG	human chorionic gonadotropin
HCl	hydrochloric acid
HCO$_3$	bicarbonate
Hct, HCT	hematocrit
HCV	hepatitis C virus
HCVD	hypertensive cardiovascular disease
HD	hemodialysis (performed by artificial kidney machine)
HDL	high-density lipoprotein
He	helium
HEENT	head, eyes, ears, nose, throat
H&E	hematoxylin and eosin
Hg	mercury (Latin *hydragyrum,* "liquid silver")
H&H	hematocrit and hemoglobin (measurement)—red blood cell tests
HIPAA	Health Insurance Portability and Accountability Act (of 1996)
HIV	human immunodeficiency virus
HLA	histocompatibility locus antigen (identifies cells as "self")
HNP	herniated nucleus pulposus
h/o	history of
H$_2$O	water
H&P	history and physical (examination)
HPF; hpf	high-power field (in microscopy)

HPI	history of present illness	**K**	potassium
HPV	human papillomavirus	**kg**	kilogram (equal to 1000 g)
HRT	hormone replacement therapy	**KJ**	knee jerk
h.s.	at bedtime (*hora somni*)—write out so as not to confuse with hs (half-strength)	**KS**	Kaposi sarcoma
		KUB	kidneys, ureters, bladder (x-ray study)
hsCRP	high-sensitivity C-reactive protein	**L, l**	liter; left; lower
HSG	hysterosalpingography	**μL**	microliter (one millionth of a liter)
HSV	herpes simplex virus	**L1, L2**	first lumbar vertebra, second lumbar vertebra (and so on)
ht	height		
HTN	hypertension (high blood pressure)	**LA**	left atrium
Hx	history	**LAD**	left anterior descending (coronary artery); lymphadenopathy
I	iodine		
^{131}I	a radioactive isotope of iodine	**LADA**	latent autoimmune diabetes in adults
I-123	isotope of radioactive iodine—used in thyroid scans	**laser**	light amplification by stimulated emission of radiation
IBD	inflammatory bowel disease (Crohn's and ulcerative colitis)	**lat**	lateral
		LB	large bowel
ICD	implantable cardioverter-defibrillator	**LBBB**	left bundle branch block (a form of heart block)
ICP	intracranial pressure		
ICSH	interstitial cell–stimulating hormone	**LBW**	low birth weight
ICU	intensive care unit	**LD**	lethal dose
ID	infectious disease	**LDH**	lactate dehydrogenase
ID	intellectual disability	**LDL**	low-density lipoprotein (high levels are associated with heart disease)
I&D	incision and drainage		
IgA, IgD, IgE, IgG, IgM	immunoglobulins (type of antibodies)	**L-dopa**	levodopa (a drug used to treat Parkinson disease)
		LE	lupus erythematosus
IGF	insulin-like growth factor	**LEEP**	loop electrocautery excision procedure
IGRT	intensity-modulated gated radiation therapy	**LES**	lower esophageal sphincter
		LFTs	liver function tests
IHC	immunohistochemistry	**LH**	luteinizing hormone
IHD	ischemic heart disease	**LLL**	left lower lobe (of lung)
IHSS	idiopathic hypertrophic subaortic stenosis	**LLQ**	left lower quadrant (of abdomen)
IL-1 to IL-15	interleukins	**LMP**	last menstrual period
		LMWH	low-molecular-weight heparin
IM	intramuscular; infectious mononucleosis	**LOC**	loss of consciousness
IMRT	intensity-modulated radiation therapy	**LOS**	length of (hospital) stay
inf.	infusion; inferior	**LP**	lumbar puncture
INH	isoniazid (a drug used to treat tuberculosis)	**lpf**	low-power field (in microscopy)
		LPN	licensed practical nurse
inj.	injection	**LS**	lumbosacral (spine)
INR	international normalized ratio (measures the time it takes for blood to clot and compares it to an average)	**LSD**	lysergic acid diethylamide (a hallucinogen)
		LSH	laparoscopic supracervical hysterectomy
		LSK	liver, spleen, kidneys
I&O	intake and output (measurement of patient's fluids)	**LTB**	laryngotracheal bronchitis (croup)
		LTC	long-term care
IOL	intraocular lens (implant)	**LTH**	luteotropic hormone (same as prolactin)
IOP	intraocular pressure	**LUL**	left upper lobe (of lung)
IORT	intraoperative radiation therapy	**LUQ**	left upper quadrant (of abdomen)
IPPB	intermittent positive-pressure breathing	**LV**	left ventricle
IQ	intelligence quotient	**LVAD**	left ventricular assist device
ITP	idiopathic thrombocytic purpura	**L&W**	living and well
IUD	intrauterine device	**lymphs**	lymphocytes
IUP	intrauterine pregnancy	**lytes**	electrolytes
IV	intravenous	**MA**	mental age
IVP	aptravenous pyelogram	**MAC**	monitored anesthesia care; *Mycobacterium avium* complex (a common cause of opportunistic pneumonia)
IVUS	intravascular ultrasound		
J-tube	jejunostomy tube		

MAI	*Mycobacterium avium-intracellulare*
MAOI	monoamine oxidase inhibitor (a type of antidepressant)
MBD	minimal brain dysfunction
mcg	microgram—also abbreviated µg; equal to one millionth of a gram
MCH	mean corpuscular hemoglobin (average amount in each red blood cell)
MCHC	mean corpuscular hemoglobin concentration (average concentration in a single red cell)
mCi	millicurie
µCi	microcurie
MCP	metacarpophalangeal (joint)
MCV	mean corpuscular volume (average size of a single red blood cell)
M.D., MD	doctor of medicine
MDD	major depressive disorder
MDI	multiple daily injections; metered-dose inhaler (used to deliver aerosolized medication to a patient)
MDR	minimum daily requirement
MDS	myelodysplastic syndrome (bone marrow disorder)
MED	minimum effective dose
mEq	milliequivalent
mEq/L	milliequivalent per liter (unit of measure for the concentration of a solution)
mets	metastases
MG	myasthenia gravis
Mg	magnesium
mg	milligram (1/1000 of a gram)
mg/cc³	milligram per cubic centimeter
mg/dL	milligram per deciliter
MH	marital history; mental health
MI	myocardial infarction; mitral insufficiency
mL, ml	milliliter (1/1000 of a liter)
mm	millimeter (1/1000 of a meter); 0.039 inch
mm Hg, mmHg	millimeters of mercury
MMPI	Minnesota Multiphasic Personality Inventory
MMR	measles-mumps-rubella (vaccine)
MMT	manual muscle testing
µm	micrometer (one millionth of a meter, or 1/1000 of a millimeter); sometimes seen in older sources as µ (for "micron," an outdated term)
MoAb	monoclonal antibody
MODS	multiple organ dysfunction syndrome
monos	monocytes (type of white blood cells)
MR	mitral regurgitation; magnetic resonance
MRA	magnetic resonance angiography
MRI	magnetic resonance imaging
mRNA	messenger RNA
MRSA	methicillin-resistant *Staphylococcus aureus*
MS	multiple sclerosis; mitral stenosis; morphine sulfate
MSL	midsternal line
MTD	maximum tolerated dose
MTX	methotrexate
MUGA	multiple-gated acquisition scan (of heart)
multip	multipara; multiparous
MVP	mitral valve prolapse
myop	myopia (nearsightedness)
N	nitrogen
NA, N/A	not applicable; not available
Na	sodium (*natrium*)
NASH	nonalcoholic steatohepatitis
NB	newborn
NBS	normal bowel sounds; normal breath sounds
NCD	neurocognitive disorder
ND	normal delivery; normal development
NED	no evidence of disease
neg.	negative
NF	neurofibromatosis
NG tube	nasogastric tube
NHL	non-Hodgkin lymphoma
NICU	neonatal intensive care unit
NK cells	natural killer cells
NKA	no known allergies
NKDA	no known drug allergies
NOAC	novel anticoagulant drug
NOTES	natural orifice transluminal endoscopic surgery
NPO	nothing by mouth (*nil per os*)
NSAID	nonsteroidal anti-inflammatory drug (often prescribed to treat musculoskeletal disorders)
NSCLC	non–small cell lung cancer
NSR	normal sinus rhythm (of heart)
NTP	normal temperature and pressure
NT-proBNP	N-terminal pro-peptide of BNP
O, O₂	oxygen
OA	osteoarthritis
OB/GYN	obstetrics and gynecology
OCPs	oral contraceptive pills
O.D.	doctor of optometry
OD	right eye (*oculus dexter*); better to specify "right eye," rather than abbreviating
OD	overdose
OMT	osteopathic manipulative treatment
OR	operating room
ORIF	open reduction plus internal fixation
ORTH; Ortho.	orthopedics
OS	left eye (*oculus sinister*); better to specify "left eye," rather than abbreviating
os	opening; bone
OT	occupational therapy (helps patients perform activities of daily living and function in work-related situations)
OU	both eyes (*oculus uterque*); better to specify "both eyes," rather than abbreviating

oz	ounce
P	phosphorus; posterior; pressure; pulse; pupil
p̄	after (post)
P2, P₂	pulmonary valve closure (a heart sound)
PA	pulmonary artery; posteroanterior
P-A	posteroanterior
P&A	percussion and auscultation
PAC	premature atrial contraction
PaCO₂	partial pressure of carbon dioxide in arterial blood
PACS	picture archival communications system
PAD	peripheral arterial disease
palp.	palpable; palpation
PALS	pediatric advanced life support
PaO₂	partial pressure of oxygen in blood
Pap smear	Papanicolaou smear (from cervix and vagina)
para 1, 2, 3	unipara, bipara, tripara (number of viable births)
pc, p.c.	after meals (*post cibum*)
PCA	patient-controlled anesthesia
PCI	percutaneous coronary intervention
PCO₂, pCO₂	partial pressure of carbon dioxide
PCP	*Pneumocystis* pneumonia; phencyclidine (a hallucinogen)
PCR	polymerase chain reaction (process that allows making copies of genes)
PD	peritoneal dialysis
PD	progressive disease
PDA	patent ductus arteriosus
PDR	*Physicians' Desk Reference*
PE	physical examination; pulmonary embolus
PEEP	positive end-expiratory pressure
PEG	percutaneous endoscopic gastrostomy (feeding tube placed in stomach)
PEJ	percutaneous endoscopic jejunostomy (feeding tube placed in small intestine)
per os	by mouth
PERRLA	pupils equal, round, reactive to light and accommodation
PET	positron emission tomography
PE tube	ventilating tube for eardrum
PFT	pulmonary function test
PG	prostaglandin
PH	past history
pH	potential hydrogen (scale to indicate degree of acidity or alkalinity)
PI	present illness
PICC	peripherally inserted central catheter
PID	pelvic inflammatory disease
PIN	prostatic intraepithelial neoplasia
PIP	proximal interphalangeal (joint)
PKU	phenylketonuria
PM, p.m.	in the afternoon (*post meridiem*)
PMH	past medical history
PMN	polymorphonuclear leukocyte
PMS	premenstrual syndrome

PND	paroxysmal nocturnal dyspnea
PNS	peripheral nervous system
PO, p.o.	by mouth (*per os*)
p/o	postoperative
PO₂, pO₂	partial pressure of oxygen
poly	polymorphonuclear leukocyte
postop	postoperative (after surgery)
PPBS	postprandial blood sugar
PPD	purified protein derivative (used in test for tuberculosis)
preop	preoperative
prep	prepare for
PR	partial response
primip	primipara
PRL	prolactin
p.r.n.	as needed; as necessary (*pro re nata*)
procto	proctoscopy
prot.	protocol
Pro. time	prothrombin time (test of blood clotting)
PSA	prostate-specific antigen
PSCT	peripheral stem cell transplantation
PSRS	proton stereotactic radiosurgery
PT	prothrombin time; physical therapy (helps patients regain use of muscles and joints after injury or surgery)
pt.	patient
PTA	prior to admission (to hospital)
PTC	percutaneous transhepatic cholangiography
PTCA	percutaneous transluminal coronary angioplasty
PTH	parathyroid hormone
PTHC	percutaneous transhepatic cholangiography
PTSD	post-traumatic stress disorder
PTT	partial thromboplastin time (a test of blood clotting)
PU	pregnancy urine
PUVA	psoralen ultraviolet A (a treatment for psoriasis)
PVC	premature ventricular contraction
PVD	peripheral vascular disease
PVT	paroxysmal ventricular tachycardia
PWB	partial weight-bearing
Px	prognosis
Q	blood volume; rate of blood flow (daily)
q	every (*quaque*, "each")
qAM	every morning; better to specify than to abbreviate
qd, q.d.	every day (*quaque die*); better to specify "each/every day," rather than confusing with qid or qod
qh	every hour (*quaque hora*); better to specify than to abbreviate
q2h	every 2 hours; better to specify than to abbreviate
qid, q.i.d.	four times daily (*quater in die*); better to specify than to abbreviate

q.n.s.	quantity not sufficient (*quantum non sufficit*)
qPM	every evening; better to specify than to abbreviate
QRS	a wave complex in an electrocardiographic study
q.s.	sufficient quantity (*quantum sufficit*)
qt	quart
R	respiration; right
RA	rheumatoid arthritis; right atrium
Ra	radium
rad	radiation absorbed dose
RAIU	radioactive iodine uptake test
RBBB	right bundle branch block
RBC, rbc	red blood count; red blood cell
RDDA	recommended daily dietary allowance
RDS	respiratory distress syndrome
REM	rapid eye movement
RF	rheumatoid factor
Rh (factor)	rhesus (monkey) factor in blood
RhoGAM	drug to prevent Rh factor reaction in Rh-negative women
RIA	radioimmunoassay (test for measuring minute quantities of a substance)
RLL	right lower lobe/lung
RLQ	right lower quadrant (abdomen)
RML	right middle lobe
RNA	ribonucleic acid
R/O	rule out
ROM	range of motion
ROS	review of systems
RRR	regular rate and rhythm (of heart)
RT	right; radiation therapy
RUL	right upper lobe (of lung)
RUQ	right upper quadrant (of abdomen)
RV	right ventricle
Rx	treatment; therapy; prescription
$\bar{s}$	without (*sine*)
S1, S2	first sacral vertebra, second sacral vertebra (and so on)
S-A node	sinoatrial node (pacemaker of heart)
SAD	seasonal affective disorder
SARS	severe acute respiratory syndrome
SBE	subacute bacterial endocarditis
SBFT	small bowel follow-through (x-ray study of small intestine function)
SD	stable disease—tumor does not shrink but does not grow
segs	segmented, mature white blood cells (neutrophils)
SERM	selective estrogen receptor modulator
s.gl	without (*sine*) glasses
SGOT	see AST
SGPT	see ALT
SIADH	syndrome of inappropriate antidiuretic hormone
SIDS	sudden infant death syndrome

Sig.	directions—medication instructions (*signa*, "mark")
SIRS	systemic inflammatory response syndrome (severe bacteremia)
SL	sublingual
SLE	systemic lupus erythematosus
SLT	selective laser trabeculoplasty
SMA-12	blood chemistry profile including 12 different studies/assays
SMAC	sequential multiple analyzer computer (automated analytical device for testing blood)
SMBG	self-monitoring of blood glucose
SOAP	subjective, objective, assessment, plan (format used for patient notes)
SOB	shortness of breath
s.o.s.	if necessary (*si opus sit,* "if there should be [such a] necessity")
S/P	status post (previous disease, condition, or procedure)
sp. gr.	specific gravity
SPECT	single photon emission computed tomography
SQ	subcutaneous
S/S, Sx	signs and symptoms
SSCP	substernal chest pain
SSRI	selective serotonin reuptake inhibitor (a type of antidepressant)
Staph.	staphylococci (berry-shaped bacteria occurring in clusters)
stat., stat	immediately (*statim*)
STD	sexually transmitted disease
STH	somatotropic hormone (somatotropin) (a growth hormone)
STI	sexually transmitted infection
Strep.	streptococci (berry-shaped bacteria occurring in twisted chains)
subcu, subcut	subcutaneous
SQ	subcutaneous
subQ, sub-Q	subcutaneous
SVC	superior vena cava
SVD	spontaneous vaginal delivery
Sx	symptoms; signs and symptoms
Sz	seizure
T	temperature; time
T cells	lymphocytes produced in the thymus gland
T tube	tube placed in biliary tract for drainage
T1, T2	first thoracic vertebra, second thoracic vertebra (and so on)
T_3	triiodothyronine (test)
T_4	thyroxine (test)
TA	therapeutic abortion
T&A	tonsillectomy and adenoidectomy
TAB	therapeutic abortion
TAH	total abdominal hysterectomy

TAT	Thematic Apperception Test	**UAO**	upper airway obstruction
TB	tuberculosis	**UC**	uterine contraction(s)
Tc	technetium	**UE**	upper extremity
TEE	transesophageal echocardiogram	**UGI**	upper gastrointestinal
TENS	transcutaneous electrical nerve stimulation	**umb.**	navel (umbilicus)
TFT	thyroid function test	**U/O**	urinary output
THR	total hip replacement (an arthroplasty procedure)	**URI**	upper respiratory infection
		U/S	ultrasound; ultrasonography
TIA	transient ischemic attack	**UTI**	urinary tract infection
tid, t.i.d.	three times daily (*ter in die*)	**UV**	ultraviolet
TKR	total knee replacement (an arthroplasty procedure)	**VA**	visual acuity
		VATS	video-assisted thoracic surgery (a thorascopy procedure)
TLC	total lung capacity	**VC**	vital capacity (of lungs)
TLE	temporal lobe epilepsy	**VCUG**	voiding cystourethrogram
TM	tympanic membrane	**VDRL**	Venereal Disease Research Laboratory (test for syphilis)
TMJ	temporomandibular joint		
TNF	tumor necrosis factor	**VEGF**	vascular endothelial growth factor
TNM	tumor-node-metastasis (cancer staging system)	**VF**	visual field; ventricular fibrillation
		V/Q scan	ventilation-perfusion scan (of lung)
tPA	tissue plasminogen activator	**V/S**	vital signs; versus
TPN	total parenteral nutrition	**VSD**	ventricular septal defect
TPR	temperature, pulse, respirations	**VT**	ventricular tachycardia (an abnormal heart rhythm)
TRUS	transrectal ultrasound (examination) (test to access the prostate and guide precise placement of a biopsy needle)		
		VTE	venous thromboembolism
		WAIS	Wechsler Adult Intelligence Scale
TSH	thyroid-stimulating hormone	**WBC, wbc**	white blood cell; white blood count
TSS	toxic shock syndrome	**WDWN**	well developed and well nourished
TUR, TURP	transurethral resection of the prostate	**WISC**	Wechsler Intelligence Scale for Children
TVH	total vaginal hysterectomy	**WNL**	within normal limits
Tx	treatment	**wt**	weight
UA	unstable angina (chest pain at rest or of increasing frequency)	**XRT**	radiation therapy
		y/o, yr	year(s) old

ACRONYMS

An *acronym* is the name for an abbreviation that forms a pronounceable word.

ACE ("ace") **a**ngiotensin-**c**onverting **e**nzyme

AIDS (ādz) **a**cquired **i**mmuno**d**eficiency **s**yndrome

APGAR (ĂP-gahr) **a**ppearance, **p**ulse, **g**rimace, **a**ctivity, **r**espiration

BUN ("bun" *or* bē-yū-ĔN) **b**lood **u**rea **n**itrogen

CABG ("cabbage") **c**oronary **a**rtery **b**ypass **g**raft/**g**rafting

CAT ("cat") **c**omputerized **a**xial **t**omography (*outdated term; use* CT)

CPAP ("SEE"-păp) **c**ontinuous **p**ositive **a**irway **p**ressure

DEXA (DECKS-ă) **d**ual **e**nergy **x**-ray **a**bsorptometry

ELISA ("eliza") **e**nzyme-**l**inked **i**mmuno**s**orbent **a**ssay

GERD (gĕrd) **g**astro**e**sophageal **r**eflux **d**isease

GIST (jĭst) **g**astro**i**ntestinal **s**tromal **t**umor

HAART ("heart") **h**ighly **a**ctive **a**ntiretroviral **t**herapy

HIPAA (HĬP-ă) **H**ealth **I**nsurance **P**ortability and **A**ccountability **A**ct of 1996

LASER (LĀ-zĕr) **l**ight **a**mplification by **s**timulated **e**mission of **r**adiation

LASIK (LĀ-sĭk) **l**aser **in** **s**itu **k**eratomileusis

LEEP ("leap") **l**oop **e**lectrocautery **e**xcision **p**rocedure

MAC (măk) **m**onitored **a**nesthesia **c**are; **M**ycobacterium **a**vium **c**omplex

MERS **M**iddle **E**ast **r**espiratory **s**yndrome

MICU (MĬK-yū) **m**edical **i**ntensive **c**are **u**nit

MIS ("miss") **m**inimally **i**nvasive **s**urgery

MODS (mōdz) **m**ultiple **o**rgan **d**ysfunction **s**yndrome

MUGA (MŪ-gă) **mu**ltiple-**g**ated **a**cquisition (scan)

NSAID (ĔN-sĕd) **n**onsteroidal **a**nti-**i**nflammatory **d**rug

NICU (NĬK-yū) **n**eonatal **i**ntensive **c**are **u**nit

PACS (păks) **p**icture **a**rchival **c**ommunications **s**ystem

PALS (pălz) **p**ediatric **a**dvanced **l**ife **s**upport

PANDAS (PĂN-dăz) **P**ediatric **A**utoimmune **N**europsychiatric **D**isorder(s) **A**ssociated with **S**treptococcal Infection(s)

PEEP ("peep") **p**ositive **e**nd-**e**xpiratory **p**ressure

PEG ("peg") **p**ercutaneous **e**ndoscopic **g**astrostomy

PERRLA (PĔR-lă) **p**upils **e**qual, **r**ound, **r**eactive to **l**ight and **a**ccommodation

PET ("pet") **p**ositron **e**mission **t**omography

PICU (PĬK-yŭ) **p**ediatric **i**ntensive **c**are **u**nit

PIP ("pip") **p**roximal **i**nter**p**halangeal (joint)
PUVA (poo-vă) **p**soralen **u**ltra**v**iolet **A**
REM (rĕm) **r**apid **e**ye **m**ovement
SAD ("sad") **s**easonal **a**ffective **d**isorder
SARS (sahrz) **s**evere **a**cute **r**espiratory **s**yndrome
SERM (sĕrm) **s**elective **e**strogen **r**eceptor **m**odulator
SIDS (sīdz) **s**udden **i**nfant **d**eath **s**yndrome
SIRS (sĕrz) **s**ystemic **i**nflammatory **r**esponse **s**yndrome

SMAC ("smack") **s**equential **m**ultiple **a**nalyzer **c**omputer (blood testing)
SOAP ("soap") **s**ubjective, **o**bjective, **a**ssessment, **p**lan
SPECT (spĕkt) **s**ingle **p**hoton **e**mission **c**omputed **t**omography
TENS (tĕnz) **t**rans**c**utaneous **e**lectrical **n**erve **s**timulation
TRUS ("truss") **t**rans**r**ectal **u**ltra**s**ound
TURP (tŭrp) **t**rans**u**rethral **r**esection of the **p**rostate
VATS (vătz) **v**ideo-**a**ssisted **t**horacic **s**urgery

EPONYMS

An *eponym* is a designation for a disorder, structure, or other medical entity derived from a person or place.

Achilles tendon (Achilles, Greek mythological hero)	This tendon connects the calf muscles to the heel. It lies at the only part of Achilles' body that was still vulnerable after his mother dipped him as an infant into the river Styx, when she held him by the heel.
Alzheimer disease (Alois Alzheimer, MD, German neurologist, 1864-1915)	Progressive mental deterioration marked by confusion, memory failure, and disorientation.
Apgar score (Virginia Apgar, MD, American anesthesiologist, 1909-1974)	Evaluation of an infant's physical condition, usually performed at 1 minute and then 5 minutes after birth. Highest score is 10. An Apgar rating of 9/10 is a score of 9 at 1 minute and 10 at 5 minutes.
Asperger syndrome (Hans Asperger, Austrian psychiatrist, 1906-1980)	A developmental disorder characterized by impairment of social interactions (resembling autism) but lacking in delays in language development and mental functioning.
Barrett esophagus (Norman Barrett, English physician, 1903-1979)	The lining of the esophagus is damaged by acid reflux. and may be a precancerous condition.
Bell palsy (Charles Bell, Scottish surgeon, 1774-1842)	Unilateral (one-sided) paralysis of the facial nerve.
Burkitt lymphoma (Denis Burkitt, English surgeon in Africa, 1911-1993)	Malignant tumor of lymph nodes; chiefly seen in central Africa. The Epstein-Barr virus is associated with this lymphoma.
Cheyne-Stokes respiration (John Cheyne, Scottish physician, 1777-1836; William Stokes, Irish physician 1804-1878)	Abnormal pattern of respirations with alternating periods of stoppage of breathing and deep, rapid breathing.
Colles fracture (Abraham Colles, Irish surgeon, 1773-1843)	A break (fracture) of the radius (outer forearm bone) near the wrist.
Crohn disease (Burrill B. Crohn, American physician, 1884-1983)	Chronic inflammatory bowel disease of unknown origin; usually affecting the ileum (last part of the small intestine), colon, or any part of the gastrointestinal tract.
Cushing syndrome (Harvey W. Cushing, American surgeon, 1869-1939)	A disorder resulting from chronic, excessive production of cortisol from the adrenal cortex. It also can result from administration of glucocorticoids (cortisone) in large doses for long periods.
Duchenne muscular dystrophy (Guillaume Benjamin Amand Duchenne, French neurologist, 1806-1875)	Abnormal, inherited condition marked by progressive hardening of muscles in the legs and hips (pelvis) beginning in infancy.
Epstein-Barr virus (Michael A. Epstein, English pathologist, born 1921; Yvonne M. Barr, English virologist, born 1932)	The herpesvirus that causes infectious mononucleosis and is associated with malignant conditions such as nose and throat cancer, Burkitt lymphoma, and Hodgkin disease.

eustachian tube (Bartolomeo Eustachio, Italian anatomist, 1524-1574)	Anatomic passageway that joins the throat and the middle ear cavity.
Ewing sarcoma (James Ewing, American pathologist, 1866-1943)	Malignant tumor that develops from bone marrow, usually in long bones or the hip (pelvis).
fallopian tube (Gabriele Falloppio, Italian anatomist, 1523-1562)	One of a pair of tubes or ducts leading from the ovary to the upper portion of the uterus.
Foley catheter (Frederic Foley, American physician, 1891-1966)	Rubber tube that is placed in the urethra to provide drainage of urine.
Giardia (Alfred Giardia, French biologist, 1846-1908)	One-celled organism (protozoan) that causes gastrointestinal infection with diarrhea, abdominal cramping, and weight loss. Cause of infection usually is fecally contaminated water.
Hodgkin lymphoma (Thomas Hodgkin lymphoma, English physician, 1798-1866)	Malignant tumor of the lymph nodes.
Huntington disease (George S. Huntington, American physician, 1851-1916)	Rare hereditary condition marked by chronic, progressively worsening dance-like movements (chorea) and mental deterioration, resulting in dementia.
Kaposi sarcoma (Moricz Kaposi, Austrian dermatologist, 1837-1902)	Malignant neoplasm of cells that line blood and lymph vessels. Soft brownish or purple papules appear on the skin. The tumor can metastasize to lymph nodes and internal organs. It is often associated with AIDS.
Marfan syndrome (Bernard-Jean A. Marfan, French pediatrician, 1858-1942)	Hereditary condition that affects bones, muscles, the cardiovascular system (leading to aneurysms), and eyes (lens dislocation). Affected people have overlong extremities with "spider-like" fingers (arachnodactyly), underdeveloped muscles, and easily movable joints.
Meniere disease (Prosper Ménière, French physician, 1799-1862)	Chronic disease of the inner ear with recurrent episodes of dizziness (vertigo), hearing loss, and ringing in the ears (tinnitus).
Neisseria gonorrhoeae (Albert L. S. Neisser, Polish dermatologist, 1855-1916)	A type of bacterium that causes gonorrhea (a sexually transmitted disease).
Paget disease (James Paget, English surgeon, 1814-1899)	Disease of bone, often affecting middle-aged or elderly people; marked by bone destruction and poor bone repair.
Pap test (George Papanicolaou, Greek physician in the United States, 1883-1962)	Method of examining stained cells obtained from the cervix and vagina. It is a common way to detect cervical cancer.
Parkinson disease (James Parkinson, English physician, 1755-1824)	Slowly progressive degenerative neurologic disorder marked by tremors, mask-like facial appearance, shuffling gait (manner of walking), and muscle rigidity and weakness.
Raynaud phenomenon (Maurice Raynaud, French physician, 1834-1881)	Intermittent attacks of loss of blood flow (ischemia) of the extremities of the body (fingers, toes, ears, and nose). Episodes most often are caused by exposure to cold.
Reye syndrome (R. Douglas Reye, Austrian pathologist, 1912-1978)	Acute brain disease (encephalopathy) and disease of internal organs following an acute viral infection.
Rinne test (Heinrich A. Rinne, German otologist, 1819-1868)	Hearing test using a vibrating tuning fork placed against a bone behind the patient's ear (mastoid bone).
Rorschach test (Herman Rorschach, Swiss psychiatrist, 1884-1922)	Personality test based on a patient's interpretation of 10 standard ink blots.

Salmonella (Daniel E. Salmon, American pathologist, 1850-1914)	Type of bacteria (rod-shaped) that causes typhoid fever and types of gastroenteritis (inflammation of the stomach and intestines).
Shigella (Kiyoshi Shiga, Japanese bacteriologist, 1870-1957)	Type of bacteria that causes severe infectious gastroenteritis (inflammation of stomach and intestines) and dysentery (diarrhea, abdominal pain, and fever).
Sjögren syndrome (Heinrik S.C. Sjögren, Swedish ophthalmologist, 1899-1986)	Abnormal dryness of the mouth, eyes, and mucous membranes, caused by deficient fluid production. It is a disorder of the immune system.
Snellen test (Herman Snellen, Dutch ophthalmologist, 1834-1908)	Test of visual clarity (acuity) using a special chart. Letters, numbers, or symbols are arranged on the chart in decreasing size from top to bottom.
Tay-Sachs disease (Warren Tay, English ophthalmologist, 1843-1927; Bernard Sachs, American neurologist, 1858-1944)	Inherited disorder of nerve degeneration caused by deficiency of an enzyme. Most affected children die between the ages of 2 and 4 years.
Tourette syndrome (Georges Gilles de la Tourette, French neurologist, 1857-1927)	Condition marked by abnormal facial grimaces, inappropriate speech, and involuntary movements of eyes, arms, and shoulders (tics).
von Willebrand disease (Erick A. von Willebrand, Finnish physician, 1870-1949)	Inherited blood disorder marked by abnormally slow blood clotting; caused by deficiency in a blood clotting factor (factor VIII).
Weber tuning fork test (Hermann D. Weber, English physician, 1823-1918)	Test of hearing using a vibrating tuning fork with the stem placed in the center of the patient's forehead.
Whipple procedure (Allen O. Whipple, American surgeon, 1881-1963)	A surgical procedure to remove a portion of the pancreas and the stomach and the entire first part of the small intestine (duodenum). Used in the treatment of pancreatic cancer and other conditions.
Wilms tumor (Max Wilms, German surgeon, 1867-1918)	Malignant tumor of the kidney occurring in young children.

SYMBOLS

=	equals		%	percent
≠	does not equal		°	degree; hour
+	positive		:	ratio; "is to"
−	negative		±	plus or minus (either positive or negative)
↑	above, increase		′	foot
↓	below, decrease		″	inch
♀	female		∴	therefore
♂	male		@	at, each
→	to (in direction of)		c̄	with
>	is greater than		s̄	without
<	is less than		#	pound; number
1°	primary to		≅	approximately equals, "is about"
2°	secondary to		Δ	change
ʒ	dram		p	short arm of a chromosome
℥	ounce		q	long arm of a chromosome

APPENDIX III

Normal Hematologic Reference Values and Implications of Abnormal Results

The implications of abnormal results included in this Appendix are major ones in each category. SI units are those used in the International System of Units, which generally are accepted for all scientific and technical uses. All laboratory values should be interpreted with caution because normal values differ widely among clinical laboratories. The following units are commonly seen in hematologic test reports.

dL = deciliter (1/10 of a liter *or* 100 mL)
g = gram
L = liter
mg = milligram (1/1000 of a gram)
mL = milliliter
mEq = milliequivalent

mm = millimeter (1/1000 of a meter)
mm^3 = cubic millimeter (cu mm)
mmol = millimole
U = unit
µL = microliter
µmol = micromole (one millionth of a mole)

BLOOD CELL COUNTS

Cell Category	Conventional Units	Si Units	Implications	
Erythrocytes (RBCs)				
Females	4.0-5.5 million/mm³ *or* μL	$4.0\text{-}5.5 \times 10^{12}/L$	*High*	♦ Polycythemia
				♦ Dehydration
Males	4.5-6.0 million/mm³ *or* μL	$4.5\text{-}6.0 \times 10^{12}/L$		
			Low	♦ Iron deficiency anemia
				♦ Blood loss
Leukocytes (WBCs)				
Total	5000-10,000/mm³ *or* μL	$5.0\text{-}10.0 \times 10^{9}/L$	*High*	♦ Bacterial infection
				♦ Leukemia
				♦ Eosinophils high in allergy
Differential (%)				
Neutrophils	54-62			
Lymphocytes	20-40		*Low*	♦ Viral infection
Monocytes	3--7			♦ Aplastic anemia
Eosinophils	1-3			♦ Chemotherapy
Basophils	0-1			
Platelets	150,000-350,000/mm³ *or* μL	$200\text{-}400 \times 10^{9}/L$	*High*	♦ Hemorrhage
				♦ Infections
				♦ Malignancy
				♦ Splenectomy
			Low	♦ Aplastic anemia
				♦ Chemotherapy
				♦ Hypersplenism

COAGULATION TESTS

Test	Conventional Units	Si Units	Implications	
Bleeding time (template method)	2.75-8.0 min	2.7-8.0 min	*Prolonged*	♦ Aspirin ingestion
				♦ Low platelet count
Coagulation time	5-15 min	5-15 min	*Prolonged*	♦ Heparin therapy
Prothrombin time (PT)*	11-12.5 sec	11-12.5 sec	*Prolonged*	♦ Vitamin K deficiency
				♦ Hepatic disease
				♦ Oral anticoagulant therapy (warfarin)
Partial thromboplastin time (PTT)	25-34 sec	25-37 sec	*Prolonged*	♦ Intravenous heparin therapy

*The INR (international normalized ratio) is a standard tool for monitoring the effects of an anticoagulant, warfarin; the normal INR value is <1.5.

RED BLOOD CELL TESTS

Test	Conventional Units	Si Units	Implications	
Hematocrit (Hct)				
Females	37%-47%	0.37-0.47	High	♦ Polycythemia
				♦ Dehydration
Males	40%-54%	0.40-0.54		
			Low	♦ Loss of blood
				♦ Anemia
Hemoglobin (Hb, Hgb)				
Females	12.0-14.0 g/dL *or* 120-140 g/L	1.86-2.48 mmol/L	High	♦ Polycythemia
				♦ Dehydration
Males	14.0-16.0 g/dL	2.17-2.79 mmol/L	Low	♦ Anemia
				♦ Blood loss

SERUM TESTS

Test	Conventional Units	Si Units	Implications	
Alanine aminotransferase (ALT; SGPT)	5-30 U/L	5-30 U/L	High	♦ Hepatitis
Albumin	3.5-5.5 g/dL	35-55 g/L	Low	♦ Hepatic disease
				♦ Malnutrition
				♦ Nephritis and nephrosis
Alkaline phosphatase (ALP)	20-90 U/L	20-90 U/L	High	♦ Bone disease
				♦ Hepatitis or tumor infiltration of liver
				♦ Biliary obstruction
Aspartate aminotransferase (AST; SGOT)	10-30 U/L	10-30 U/L	High	♦ Hepatitis
				♦ Cardiac and muscle injury
Bilirubin			High	♦ Hemolysis
Total	0.3-1.0 mg/dL	5.1-17 μmol/L		♦ Neonatal hepatic immaturity
Neonates	1-12 mg/dL	17-205 μmol/L		♦ Cirrhosis
				♦ Biliary tract obstruction
Blood urea nitrogen (BUN)	10-20 mg/dL	3.6-7.1 mmol/L	High	♦ Renal disease
				♦ Reduced renal blood flow
				♦ Urinary tract obstruction
			Low	♦ Hepatic damage
				♦ Malnutrition
Calcium	9.0-10.5 mg/dL	2.2-2.6 mmol/L	High	♦ Hyperparathyroidism
				♦ Multiple myeloma
				♦ Metastatic cancer
			Low	♦ Hypoparathyroidism
				♦ Total parathyroidectomy
Cholesterol (desirable range)				
Total	<200 mg/dL	<5.2 mmol/L	High	♦ High-fat diet
LDL cholesterol	<130 mg/dL	<3.36 mmol/L		♦ Inherited hypercholesterolemia
HDL cholesterol	>60 mg/dL	>1.55 mmol/L	Low	♦ Starvation

Test	Conventional Units	Si Units	Implications	
Creatine kinase (CK)				
Females	30-135 U/L	30-135 U/L	*High*	◆ Myocardial infarction
Males	55-170 U/L	55-170 U/L		◆ Muscle disease
Creatinine	<1.5 mg/dL	<133 µmol/L	*High*	◆ Renal disease
Glucose (fasting)	75-115 mg/dL	4.2-6.4 mmol/L	*High*	◆ Diabetes mellitus
			Low	◆ Hyperinsulinism
				◆ Fasting
				◆ Hypothyroidism
				◆ Addison disease
				◆ Pituitary insufficiency
Iron (Fe)				
Females	30-160 µg/dL	5.4-31.3 µmol/L	*High*	◆ Hemochromatosis
Males	45-160 µg/dL	8.1-31.3 µmol/L		◆ Transfusions
			Low	◆ Anemia
				◆ Bleeding
Lactate dehydrogenase (LDH)	100-190 U/L	100-190 U/L	*High*	◆ Tissue necrosis
				◆ Lymphomas
				◆ Muscle disease
Phosphate (PO_4^-)	3.0-4.5 mg/dL	1.0-1.5 mmol/L	*High*	◆ Renal failure
				◆ Bone metastases
				◆ Hypoparathyroidism
			Low	◆ Malnutrition
				◆ Malabsorption
				◆ Hyperparathyroidism
Potassium (K^+)	3.5-5.0 mEq/L	3.5-5.0 mmol/L	*High*	◆ Burn injury
				◆ Renal failure
				◆ Diabetic ketoacidosis
			Low	◆ Cushing syndrome
				◆ Loss of body fluids
Sodium (Na^+)	136-145 mEq/L	136-145 mmol/L	*High*	◆ Inadequate water intake
				◆ Water loss in excess of sodium
			Low	◆ Adrenal insufficiency
				◆ Inadequate sodium intake
				◆ Excessive sodium loss
Thyroxine (T4)	5-12 µg/dL	64-154 nmol/L	*High*	◆ Graves disease (hyperthyroidism)
			Low	◆ Hypothyroidism
Uric acid				
Females	2.5-8.0 mg/dL	150-480 µmol/L	*High*	◆ Gout
Males	1.5-6.0 mg/dL	90-360 µmol/L		◆ Leukemia

Drugs

Following is an alphabetized list of the drugs referred to in Chapter 21 (tables), with brand name(s) in parentheses and explanation of their use, including drug category and/or class. This Appendix, along with drugs listed alphabetically by brand name, also appears on the Evolve website.

Generic Name (Brand Name)	Explanation of Use
abiraterone (Zytiga)	Endocrine/antiandrogen
acarbose (Precose)	Antidiabetic (type 2 diabetes)/alpha-glucosidase inhibitor
acetaminophen (Tylenol)	Analgesic/mild
acyclovir (Zovirax)	Antiviral
adalimumab (Humira)	Gastrointestinal/anti-TNF
albuterol (Proventil, Ventolin, HFA)	Bronchodilator
alendronate (Fosamax)	Antiosteoporosis/bisphosphonate
alprazolam (Xanax)	Tranquilizer/minor/benzodiazepine
aluminum antacid (Rolaids)	GI/antacid
aluminum + magnesium antacid (Gaviscon)	GI/antacid
amiodarone (Cordarone)	Cardiovascular/antiarrhythmic
amlodipine (Norvasc)	Cardiovascular/calcium blocker
amoxicillin trihydrate (Amoxil, Trimox)	Antibiotic/penicillin
amoxicillin + clavulanate (Augmentin)	Antibiotic/penicillin
anastrozole (Arimidex)	Endocrine/aromatase inhibitor
apixaban (Eliquis)	Anticoagulant
aripiprazole (Abilify)	Tranquilizer/major
aspirin (Anacin, Ascription, Excedrin)	Analgesic/NSAID
atenolol (Tenormin)	Cardiovascular/beta blocker
atorvastatin (Lipitor)	Cardiovascular/cholesterol-lowering statin
azithromycin (Zithromax)	Antibiotic/macrolide
budesonide (Pulmicort)	Respiratory/steroid inhaler
bumetanide (Bumex)	Cardiovascular/diuretic
buspirone (BuSpar)	Tranquilizer/minor
caffeine	Stimulant
calcitonin (Cibacalcin)	Endocrine/thyroid
carbamazepine (Tegretol)	Anticonvulsant
cefprozil (Cefzil)	Antibiotic/cephalosporin
ceftazidime (Fortaz)	Antibiotic/cephalosporin
cefuroxime axetil (Ceftin)	Antibiotic/cephalosporin

Generic Name (Brand Name)	Explanation of Use
celecoxib (Celebrex)	Analgesic/NSAID
cephalexin (Keflex)	Antibiotic/cephalosporin
certolizumab pegol (Cimzia)	Gastrointestinal/anti-TNF
cetirizine (Zyrtec)	Antihistamine
chlorpheniramine maleate (Chlor-Trimeton)	Antihistamine
chlorpromazine (Thorazine)	Tranquilizer/major/phenothiazine
cholestyramine (Questran)	Cardiovascular/cholesterol-binding agent
cimetidine (Tagamet)	GI/antiulcer/anti-GERD
ciprofloxacin (Cipro)	Antibiotic/quinolone
clarithromycin (Biaxin)	Antibiotic/macrolide
clopidogrel (Plavix)	Antiplatelet
clotrimazole (Lotrimin, Mycelex)	Antifungal
codeine	Analgesic/narcotic
colestipol (Colestid)	Cardiovascular/cholesterol-binding agent
dabigatran (Pradaxa)	Anticoagulant
dalteparin (Fragmin)	Anticoagulant
denosumab (Prolia)	Antiosteoporosis
dexamethasone (Decadron)	Respiratory/steroid, intravenous or oral
dextroamphetamine + amphetamine (Adderall)	Stimulant
dextroamphetamine sulfate (Dexedrine)	Stimulant
diazepam (Valium)	Tranquilizer/minor/benzodiazepine
diclofenac sodium (Voltaren)	Analgesic/NSAID
digoxin (Lanoxin)	Cardiovascular/anti-CHF
diltiazem (Cardizem CD)	Cardiovascular/calcium antagonist
diphenhydramine (Benadryl)	Antihistamine
diphenoxylate + atropine (Lomotil)	GI/antidiarrheal
donepezil (Aricept)	Anti-Alzheimer disease
doxycycline	Antibiotic/tetracycline
duloxetine (Cymbalta)	Antidepressant
econazole, topical (Spectazole)	Antifungal
efavirenz + tenoforvir + emtricitabine (Atripla)	Antiviral/anti-HIV—all-in-one combination
efavirenz (Sustiva)	Anti-HIV
enalapril maleate (Vasotec)	Cardiovascular/ACE inhibitor
enoxaparin sodium (Lovenox)	Anticoagulant
enzalutamide (XTANDI)	Endocrine/antiandrogen
epinephrine	Bronchodilator
erythromycin (Ery-Tab)	Antibiotic/macrolide
escitalopram (Lexapro)	Antidepressant
estrogen (Premarin, Prempro, Estradiol)	Endocrine/estrogen
etanercept (Enbrel)	Gastrointestinal/anti-TNF
ethambutol (Myambutol)	Antitubercular
ether	Anesthetic/general
famotidine (Pepcid)	GI/antiulcer/anti-GERD
felbamate (Felbatol)	Anticonvulsant
fentanyl patch (Duragesic)	Analgesic/narcotic
fexofenadine (Allegra)	Antihistamine
fluconazole (Diflucan)	Antifungal
flunisolide (AeroBid)	Respiratory/steroid inhaler
fluoxymesterone (Halotestin)	Endocrine/androgen
flutamide (Eulexin)	Endocrine/antiandrogen
fluticasone propionate (Flovent)	Respiratory/steroid inhaler

Generic Name (Brand Name)	Explanation of Use
formoterol (Foradil)	Bronchodilator
formoterol + budesonide (Symbicort)	Bronchodilator
fulvestrant (Faslodex)	Endocrine/aromatase inhibitor
furosemide (Lasix)	Cardiovascular/diuretic
gabapentin (Neurontin)	Anticonvulsant
glipizide (Glucotrol XL)	Antidiabetic (type 2 diabetes)/sulfonylurea
glyburide (Diabeta, Micronase)	Antidiabetic (type 2 diabetes)/sulfonylurea
golimumab (Simponi)	Anti-TNF
goserelin (Zoladex)	Endocrine/antiandrogen
haloperidol (Haldol)	Tranquilizer/major
halothane (Fluothane)	Anesthetic/general
hydrochlorothiazide (HydroDIURIL)	Cardiovascular/diuretic
hydrocodone w/APAP (Lortab, Vicodin)	Analgesic/narcotic
hydrocortisone	Glucocorticoid
hydromorphone (Dilaudid)	Analgesic/narcotic
ibuprofen (Motrin, Advil)	Analgesic/NSAID
ibutilide (Corvert)	Antiarrhythmic
indinavir (Crixivan)	Antiviral/protease inhibitor/anti-HIV
infliximab (Remicade)	Gastrointestinal/anti-TNF
insulin aspart (NovoLog)	Antidiabetic (type 1 diabetes)
insulin detemir (Levemir)	Antidiabetic (type 1 diabetes)
insulin glargine (Lantus)	Antidiabetic (type 1 diabetes)
insulin glulisine (Apidra)	Antidiabetic (type 1 diabetes)
insulin lispro (Humalog)	Antidiabetic (type 1 diabetes)
insulin NPH (Humulin N)	Antidiabetic (type 1 diabetes)
insulin regular (Humulin R)	Antidiabetic (type 1 diabetes)
insulin zinc suspension (Ultralente)	Antidiabetic (type 1 diabetes)
interferon alfa-n1 (Wellferon)	Antiviral/anticancer drug
ipratropium bromide + albuterol (Combivent)	Bronchodilator
irbesartan (Avapro)	Cardiovascular/angiotensin II receptor blocker
isoniazid *or* INH (Nydrazid)	Antitubercular
itraconazole (Sporanox)	Antifungal
ketorolac (Toradol)	Analgesic/NSAID
lamivudine (Epivir)	Antiviral/reverse transcriptase inhibitor/anti-HIV
lansoprazole (Prevacid)	GI/antiulcer/anti-GERD
lepirudin (Refludan)	Anticoagulant
letrozole (Femara)	Endocrine/aromatase inhibitor
leuprolide (Lupron)	Endocrine/antiandrogen
levalbuterol (Xopenex)	Bronchodilator
levetiracetam (Keppra)	Anticonvulsant
levofloxacin (Levaquin)	Antibiotic
levothyroxine (Levothroid, Synthroid)	Endocrine/thyroid hormone
lidocaine (Xylocaine)	Anesthetic/local
lidocaine + prilocaine (EMLA)	Anesthetic/local
liothyronine (Cytomel)	Endocrine/thyroid hormone
lisdexamfetamine (Vyvanse)	Stimulant
lisinopril (Prinivil, Zestril)	Cardiovascular/ACE inhibitor
lithium carbonate (Eskalith)	Tranquilizer/major
loperamide (Imodium)	GI/antidiarrheal
loratadine (Claritin)	Antihistamine
lorazepam (Ativan)	Tranquilizer/minor/benzodiazepine

Generic Name (Brand Name)	Explanation of Use
losartan (Cozaar)	Cardiovascular/angiotensin II receptor blocker
lovastatin (Mevacor)	Cardiovascular/cholesterol-lowering statin
magnesium antacid (milk of magnesia)	GI/antacid
meclizine (Antivert)	Antihistamine
medroxyprogesterone acetate (Cycrin, Provera)	Endocrine/progestin
megestrol (Megace)	Endocrine/progestin
memantine (Namenda)	Anti-Alzheimer disease
meperidine (Demerol)	Analgesic/narcotic
metaproterenol (Alupent)	Bronchodilator
metformin (Glucophage)	Antidiabetic (type 2 diabetes)/biguanide
methaqualone (Quaalude)	Sedative-hypnotic
methylphenidate (Ritalin)	Stimulant
methylprednisolone (Medrol)	Respiratory/steroid, intravenous or oral
methyltestosterone (Virilon)	Endocrine/androgen
metoclopramide (Reglan)	GI/antinauseant
metoprolol (Lopressor, Toprol-XL)	Cardiovascular/beta blocker
miconazole (Monistat)	Antifungal
midazolam (Versed)	Sedative-hypnotic
modafinil (Provigil)	Stimulant/sleep antagonist
mometasone (Asmanex)	Respiratory/inhaler
montelukast sodium (Singulair)	Respiratory/leukotriene modifier
nafcillin (Unipen)	Antibiotic/penicillin
naproxen (Aleve)	Analgesic/NSAID
nifedipine (Adalat CC, Procardia)	Cardiovascular/calcium antagonist
nilutamide (Casodex)	Endocrine/antiandrogen
nitroglycerin	Cardiovascular/antianginal
nitrous oxide	Anesthetic/general
nystatin (Nilstat)	Antifungal
octreotide (Sandostatin)	Endocrine/growth
ofloxacin (Floxin)	Antibiotic/quinolone
olanzapine (Zyprexa)	Tranquilizer/major/antipsychotic
omeprazole (Prilosec)	GI/antiulcer/anti-GERD
ondansetron (Zofran)	GI/antinauseant
oxacillin (Bactocill)	Antibiotic/penicillin
oxycodone (OxyContin, Roxicodone)	Analgesic/narcotic
oxycodone with APAP (Roxicet, Endocet, Percocet)	Analgesic/narcotic
pamidronate disodium (Aredia)	Antiosteoporosis/bisphosphonate
p-aminosalicylic acid granules (PASER)	Antiubercular
paregoric	GI/antidiarrheal
phenytoin sodium (Dilantin)	Anticonvulsant
pioglitazone (Actos)	Antidiabetic (type 2 diabetes)
pirbuterol (Maxair)	Bronchodilator
prasugrel (Effient)	Antiplatelet
pravastatin (Pravachol)	Cardiovascular/cholesterol-lowering statin
prednisone	Respiratory/steroid, intravenous or oral
pregabalin (Lyrica)	Anticonvulsant
promethazine (Phenergan)	Antihistamine
procaine (Novocain)	Anesthetic, local
prochlorperazine maleate (Compazine)	GI/antinauseant
propofol (Diprivan)	Anesthetic/general
propranolol (Inderal)	Cardiovascular/beta blocker

Generic Name (Brand Name)	Explanation of Use
quinapril (Accupril)	Cardiovascular/ACE inhibitor
raloxifene (Evista)	Endocrine/SERM/antiosteoporosis
ramipril (Altace)	Cardiovascular/ACE inhibitor
ranitidine (Zantac)	GI/antiulcer/anti-GERD
repaglinide (Prandin)	Antidiabetic (type 2 diabetes)/meglitinide
ribavirin (Copegus, Rebetol)	Antiviral
rifampin (Rifadin)	Antitubercular
risperidone (Risperdal)	Tranquilizer/major
rivaroxaban (Xarelto)	Anticoagulant
rosiglitazone (Avandia)	Antidiabetic (type 2 diabetes)
rosuvastatin (Crestor)	Cardiovascular/cholesterol-lowering statin
salmeterol (Serevent)	Bronchodilator
salmeterol + fluticasone (Advair Diskus)	Corticosteroid anti-inflammatory–bronchodilator combination
Simeprevir (Olysio)	Antiviral
simvastatin (Zocor)	Cardiovascular/cholesterol-lowering statin
sofosbuvir (Sovaldi)	Antiviral
sotalol (Betapace)	Cardiovascular/beta blocker
spironolactone (Aldactone)	Cardiovascular/diuretic
sulfamethoxazole + trimethoprim (Bactrim)	Antibiotic/sulfonamide—antibacterial combination
sulfisoxazole (Gantrisin)	Antibiotic/sulfonamide
tamoxifen (Nolvadex)	Endocrine/SERM
temazepam (Restoril)	Sedative-hypnotic/benzodiazepine
terbinafine (Lamisil)	Antifungal
teriparatide (Forteo)	Antiosteoporosis
teriparatide (Forteo)	Endocrine/parathyroid
tetracycline (Sumycin, Terramycin)	Antibiotic/tetracycline
theophylline (Theo-Dur)	Bronchodilator
thiopental (Pentothal)	Anesthetic/general
thioridazine (Mellaril)	Tranquilizer/major/phenothiazine
ticagrelor (Brilinta)	Antiplatelet
tiotropium (Spiriva)	Bronchodilator
tissue plasminogen activator *or* tPA	Anticoagulant
tramadol (Ultram)	Analgesic/narcotic
triamcinolone (Aristocort)	Glucocorticoid
triamcinolone (Azmacort)	Respiratory/steroid inhaler
triamterene (Dyazide)	Cardiovascular/diuretic
triazolam (Halcion)	Sedative-hypnotic/benzodiazepine
trifluoperazine (Stelazine)	Tranquilizer/major/phenothiazine
valdecoxib (Bextra)	Analgesic/NSAID
valproic acid (Depakote)	Anticonvulsant
valsartan (Diovan)	Cardiovascular/angiotensin II receptor blocker
valsartan + sacubitril (Entresto; formerly LCZ696)	Cardiovascular/angiotensin II receptor blocker
warfarin (Coumadin)	Anticoagulant
zafirlukast (Accolate)	Respiratory/leukotriene modifier
zidovudine *or* AZT (Retrovir)	Antiviral/reverse transcriptase inhibitor/anti-HIV
zidovudine + lamivudine (Combivir)	Anti-HIV
zileuton (Zyflo)	Respiratory/leukotriene modifier
zoledronic acid (Zometa)	Antiosteoporosis/bisphosphonate
zolpidem tartrate (Ambien)	Sedative-hypnotic

ILLUSTRATIONS CREDITS

Figure 10-19B, from Albert D: *Albert & Jakobiec's Principles & Practice of Ophthalmology*, ed 3, Philadelphia, 2008, Saunders.

Figure 11-10, from Applegate E: *The Anatomy and Physiology Learning System*, ed 2, Philadelphia, 2000, Saunders.

Figure 16-9A, from Barkauskas VH et al: *Health and Physical Assessment*, ed 2, St. Louis, 1998, Mosby.

Figure 20-15, from Beare PG, Myers JL: *Adult Health Nursing*, ed 3, St. Louis, 1998, Mosby.

Figure 5-20F, from Bird D, Robinson D: *Modern Dental Assisting*, ed 10, Philadelphia, 2012, Saunders.

Unnumbered Figure 2-3, Figures 6-8B, 12-13A, 12-18B, 13-15, 16-11, 17-13, 20-9C, from Black J, Hawks J: Medical-Surgical Nursing, 8th ed., Philadelphia, 2009, Elsevier/Saunders.

Figures 20-4, 20-8B, from Braunwald E: *Heart Disease: A Textbook of Cardiovascular Medicine*, ed 4, Philadelphia, 1992, Saunders.

Figures 5-20E, 9-6A, 10-19A, 16-5B, 16-6B, 16-8D, 16-10B, 16-12B, 16-13A, from Callen JP et al: *Color Atlas of Dermatology*, ed 2, Philadelphia, 2002, Saunders.

Figure 15-38B & E, from Canale ST, Beaty JH: *Campbell's Operative Orthopaedics*, ed 11, St. Louis, 2008, Mosby.

Figures 13-4, 13-6, from Carr JH, Rodak BF: *Clinical Hematology Atlas*, ed 2, St. Louis, 2004, Mosby.

Figures 12-13B, 21-2A, from Chabner DE: *Medical Terminology: A Short Course*, ed 5, Philadelphia, 2009, Saunders.

Figure 16-16A, reprinted from Clinical Slide Collection on the Rheumatic Diseases.

Figure 16-8C, from Cohen BA: *Atlas of Pediatric Dermatology*, London, 1993, Wolfe.

Figure 5-19, from Christensen B, Kockrow E: *Foundations and Adult Health Nursing*, ed 5, St. Louis, 2006, Elsevier/Mosby.

Figure 5-20A, from Christensen GJ: *A Consumer's Guide to Dentistry*, St. Louis, 2002, Mosby.

Figure 18-20, from Clinical Pathological Conference, *Am J Med* 20:133, 1956.

Figure 15-33, from Coughlin M et al: *Surgery of the Foot and Ankle*, ed 8, St. Louis, 2007, Mosby.

Figure 11-23B, from Crawford MH, DiMarco JP, Paulus WJ: *Cardiology*, ed 2, St. Louis, 2004, Mosby.

Figures 5-14, 5-21A, 5-23, 5-24, 5-26, 5-29B, 7-7, 7-12A, 8-15, 8-16A, 11-1, from Damjanov I: *Pathology for the Health-Related Professions*, ed 4, Philadelphia, 2012, Elsevier/Saunders.

Figure 15-17, from Dempster DW, Shane E, Horbert W, et al: A Simple Method for Correlative Light and Scanning Electron Microscopy Of Human Iliac Crest Bone Biopsies: Qualitative Observations in Normal and Osteoporotic Subjects, *J Bone Miner Res* 1:15, 1986.

Figure 10-21, from Drake RL et al: Gray's Anatomy for Students, Philadelphia, Churchill Livingstone, 2005.

Figure 16-8L, from Farrar WE: *Atlas of Infections of the Nervous System*, London, 1993, Mosby-Wolfe.

Figure 5-20B, from Feldman M et al: *Sleisenger and Fordtran's Gastrointestinal and Liver Disease*, ed 8, Philadelphia, 2006, Saunders.

Figure 17-24D, from Fireman P, Slavin RG: *Atlas of Allergies*, ed 2, London, 1996, Glower Medical Publishing.

Figure 11-22B, from Forbes CD, Jackson WF: *Color Atlas and Text of Clinical Medicine*, ed 3, London, 2003, Mosby.

Figures 8-24, 20-13, from Frank ED et al: *Merrill's Atlas of Radiographic Positioning & Procedures*, ed 11, St. Louis, 2007, Mosby.

Figures 10-14B, 17-6A, from Frazier MS, Drzymkowski JW: *Essentials of Human Diseases and Conditions*, ed 3, Philadelphia, 2004, Saunders.

Figure 9-1B, from Gartner L: *Color Textbook of Histology*, ed 3, Philadelphia, 2007, Saunders.

Figure 20-8A, from Gill KA: *Abdominal Ultrasound: A Practitioner's Guide*, Philadelphia, 2001, Saunders.

Figure 22-2, from Gleitman H: *Psychology*, New York, 1991, WW Norton.

Figure 3-2, from Goering R et al: *Mims' Medical Microbiology*, ed 4, Edinburgh, 2008, Elsevier/Mosby Ltd.

Figures 2-3, 6-2A, 11-24A, from Goldman L, Schafer A: *Goldman's Cecil Medicine*, ed 24, Philadelphia, 2012, Elsevier/Saunders.

Figures 5-21B, 13-13, 16-8J, from Gould BE, Dyer R: *Pathophysiology for Health Professions*, ed 4, Philadelphia, 2011, Elsevier/Saunders.

Figure 15-36, from Greer I et al: *Mosby's Color Atlas and Text of Obstetrics and Gynecology*, London, 2001, Mosby.

Figures 2-14B, 10-16B, from Haaga J: *CT and MR Imaging of the Whole Body*, ed 4, St. Louis, 2003, Elsevier/Mosby.

Figures 16-8F, 16-15A, 16-18A, from Habif TP: *Clinical Dermatology*, ed 4, St. Louis, 2004, Mosby.

Figure 11-26, from Hicks GH: *Cardiopulmonary Anatomy and Physiology*, Philadelphia, 2000, Saunders.

Figure 13-5, from Hirsch JG: Cinemicrophotographic Observations of Granule Lysis in Polymorphonuclear Leucocytes during Phagocytosis, *J Exp Med*;116:827, 1962, by copyright permission of Rockefeller University Press.

Figure 1-5, from His E: *Hematopathology*, ed 1, Philadelphia, 2007, Elsevier/Churchill Livingstone.

Figures 6-3, 6-4A, 6-5, from Heuman DM, Mills AS, McGuire HH: *Gastroenterology*, Philadelphia, 1997, Elsevier/Saunders.

Figures 2-4B, 16-14A, from Huether S, McCance K: *Understanding Pathophysiology*, ed 5, St. Louis, 2012, Elsevier/Mosby.

Figures 10-20, 16-19B, 16-20A, 17-20, from Ignatavicius DD, Workman ML: *Medical-Surgical Nursing: Critical Thinking for Collaborative Care*, ed 4, Philadelphia, 2002, Saunders.

Figure 16-15B, from James W et al: *Andrews' Diseases of the Skin*, ed 11, Philadelphia, 2012, Saunders.

Figures 16-18B, 17-14, 17-16, 18-15A, from Jarvis C: *Physical Examination and Health Assessment*, ed 3, Philadelphia, 2000, Saunders.

Figure 15-34A, from Jebson LR, Coons DD: Total Hip Arthroplasty, *Surg Technol* October: 30(10):12-21, 1998.

Figure 7-5, from Joffe SA et al. *Radiographics* 23(6):1441-1455, 2003.

Figure 17-12A, from Kanski J, Bowling B: *Clinical Ophthalmology*, ed 7, Philadelphia, 2012, Saunders.

Figure 16-5A, from Kanski JJ: *Systemic Diseases and the Eye*, St. Louis, 2001, Mosby.

Figures 4-9, 6-8A, from Kliegman R et al: *Nelson Textbook of Pediatrics*, ed 19, Philadelphia, 2012, Elsevier/Saunders.

Figures 9-7, 10-15A, 11-17, 11-19A, 12-10, 12-11B, 12-12B, 19-2, 19-7B, from Kumar V, Cotran RS, Robbins SL: *Basic Pathology*, ed 8, Philadelphia, 2007, Saunders.

Figures 5-25C, 5-28B, 6-1, 7-12B, 8-18, 12-11A, 16-20C, 16-21B, 19-6B, 19-7A, 19-8, from Kumar V, Abbas A, Aster J: *Robbins & Cotran Pathologic Basis of Disease*, ed 8, Philadelphia, 2010, Elsevier/Saunders.

Figure 14-11B, from Lemmi FO, Lemmi CAE: *Physical Assessment Findings* CD-ROM, Philadelphia, 2000, Saunders.

Figures 5-18, 7-15A, 11-13, 11-19B & C, 12-8, 15-28, 16-17A, 16-22, 17-15, 17-19, 17-27B, from Lewis SM et al: *Medical-Surgical Nursing*, ed 8, St. Louis, 2011, Elsevier/Mosby.

Figure 10-22, from Lundy-Ekman L: *Neuroscience*, ed 3, St. Louis, 2008, Mosby.

Figure 16-16B, from Marcdante K et al: *Nelson Essentials of Pediatrics*, ed 5, Philadelphia, 2006, Saunders.

Figure 16-20B, from Marks J and Miller J: *Lookingbill and Marks' Principles of Dermatology*, ed 4, Philadelphia, 2007, Saunders.

Figure 15-34B, from Mercier LR: *Practical Orthopedics*, ed 5, St. Louis, 2000, Mosby.

Figure 20-3, from Mettler FA: *Essentials of Radiography*, ed 2, Philadelphia, 2004, Saunders.

Figure 15-35, from Miller MD, Howard RF, Plancher KD: *Surgical Atlas of Sports Medicine*, Philadelphia, 2003, Saunders.

Figures 15-38F, 18-17, from Moll JMH: *Rheumatology*, ed 2, London, 1997, Churchill Livingstone.

Figure 9-12A, from Morse SA et al: *Atlas of Sexually Transmitted Diseases and AIDS*, ed 2, 2003, London, Gower.

Figures 16-9C, 16-19A, 16-21A, from *Mosby's Medical, Nursing and Allied Health Dictionary*, ed 5, St. Louis, 1998, Mosby.

Figure 17-6B, from Newell FW: *Ophthalmology: Principles and Concepts*, ed 8, St. Louis, 1996, Mosby.

Figure 5-29A, from Odze R, Goldblum J: *Surgical Pathology of the GI Tract, Liver, Biliary Tract and Pancreas*, ed 2, Philadelphia, Saunders, 2009.

Figure 8-22, from O'Toole M [ed]: *Miller-Keane Encyclopedia & Dictionary of Medicine, Nursing & Allied Health*, ed 7, Philadelphia, 2003, Saunders.

Figure 17-12B, from Palay D and Krachmer J: *Primary Care Ophthalmology*, ed 2, St. Louis, 2006, Mosby.

Figure 16-14B, from Phipps WJ et al: *Medical-Surgical Nursing*, ed 7, St. Louis, 2003, Mosby.

Figure 6-2B, 7-10B, from Roberts J, Hedges J: *Clinical Procedures in Emergency Medicine*, ed 5, Philadelphia, 2010, Elsevier/Saunders.

Figure 8-16B, from Salvo S: *Mosby's Pathology for Massage Therapists*, ed 2, St. Louis, 2009, Mosby.

Figures 3-4, 16-3B, 16-7B, 16-8A, 18-15B, 18-16, from Seidel HM, et al: *Mosby's Guide to Physical Examination*, ed 5, St. Louis, 2003, Elsevier/Mosby.

Figure 1-3, from Soyer HP et al: *Dermoscopy*, ed 2, Philadelphia, 2012, Elsevier/Saunders.

Figures 5-20D, 9-12B, 14-10, 14-11A, 15-38A, from Swartz MH: *Textbook of Physical Diagnosis, History and Examination*, ed 5, Philadelphia, 2006, Saunders.

Figures 13-2A, 13-9, 16-2B, 17-2, 17-3, 17-7A, 19-1A, from Thibodeau GA, Patton KT: *Anatomy &Physiology*, ed 6, St. Louis, 2007, Mosby.

Figure 8-4, 12-9, from Thibodeau G, Patton K: *The Human Body in Health & Disease*, ed 4, St. Louis, 2005, Mosby.

Figure 13-10, from Tkachuk DC, Hirschmann JV, McArthur JR: *Atlas of Clinical Hematology*, Philadelphia, 2002, Saunders.

Figure 15-27B, US Centers for Disease Control and Prevention.

Figure 15-37, from Walter JB: *An Introduction to the Principles of Disease*, ed 3, Philadelphia, 1992, Saunders.

Figure 7-10A, from Warekois R and Robinson R: *Phlebotomy*, ed 2, Philadelphia, 2008, Saunders.

Figure 7-14B, from Wein A et al: *Campbell-Walsh Urology*, ed 10, Philadelphia, 2012, Saunders.

Figure 6-10, from Weinstein WM, Hawkey CJ, Bosch J: *Clinical Gastroenterology and Hepatology*, St. Louis, 2005, Mosby.

Unnumbered Figure 2-1, from Weir J et al: *An Imaging Atlas of Human Anatomy*, ed 4, Philadelphia, 2011, Elsevier/Mosby.

Figure 16-8E & I, from Weston WL et al: *Color Textbook of Pediatric Dermatology*, ed 3, 2002, St. Louis, Mosby.

Figure 16-8K, from White GM: *Color Atlas of Regional Dermatology*, London, 1994, Times-Mirror.

Figure 21-2, B to E, from Young AP, Kennedy DB: *Kinn's The Medical Assistant*, ed 9, Philadelphia, 2003, Saunders.

Figures 3-8, 9-6B, 14-12, 15-13B & C, 15-40D, 16-6A, 16-8B, 16-12, from Zitelli BJ, Davis HW: *Atlas of Pediatric Physical Diagnosis*, ed 2, St. Louis, 1992, Mosby.

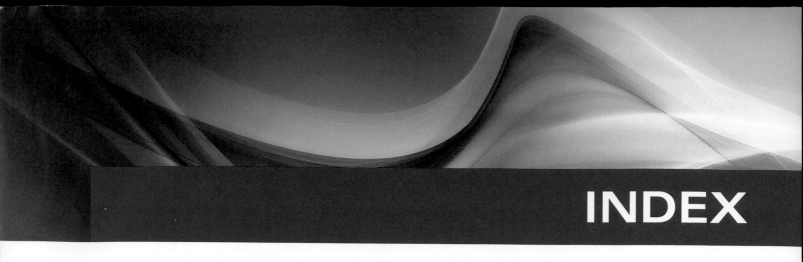

INDEX

A

A-, 14, 111, 941
AAAs (Abdominal aortic aneurysm), 423, 423f, 434
Ab-, 111, 618
AB (abortion), 121, 263, 285, 285f, 286, 288
Ab (antibody). *See* Antibodies (Ab).
Abbreviations
    for blood system, 526-527
    for cardiovascular system, 434-435
    for digestive system, 200
    "Do Not Use" list of, 904
    for ears, 727
    for endocrine system, 779
    for eyes, 718
    for female reproductive system, 288
    for lymphatic and immune systems, 565
    for male reproductive system, 326
    for musculoskeletal system, 623
    for nervous system, 374
    for oncology, 829
    for pharmacology, 903-904
    for psychiatry, 942
    for radiology and nuclear medicine, 867
    for respiratory system, 483-484
    for skin, 676
    for urinary system, 237
ABCDEs of melanoma (asymmetry, border, color, diameter, evolution), 675f, 676
Abdomen, 47, 48-49, 159
    combining forms for, 55, 76, 153, 156
    laparoscopy of, 199
Abdominal, 55
Abdominal aortic aneurysm (AAA), 423, 423f, 434
Abdominal cavity, 42f, 44f, 47, 259, 259f, 286, 286f
Abdominal ultrasonography, 196
Abdominal viscera, 40, 196
Abdomin/o, 55, 76
Abdominocentesis, 78, 199
Abdominopelvic cavity, 44, 45f, 46f, 72
Abdominopelvic quadrants, 49, 49f, 51, 72
Abdominopelvic regions, 48, 48f, 51, 72
Abdominoplasty, 82, 188
Abducens nerve (CN VI), 346f
Abduction, 615, 616, 616f, 618, 860
Abductor, 111
ABGs (arterial blood gases), 483
Abilify. *See* Aripiprazole.
Abl oncogene, 804, 821
Ablation
    catheter, 416, 432, 432f
    radiofrequency, 856, 867

ABMT (autologous bone marrow transplantation), 522, 526, 526f, 826
Abnormal, 111
    prefix for, 111, 114, 116, 929, 940, 942
    suffix for, 516
Abnormal involuntary movement scale (AIMS), 936, 942
Abnormal motor behavior, 929, 932t
ABO (blood types), 510, 526
Abortion (AB), 121, 263, 285, 285f, 286, 288
Abrasion, 660
    corneal, 705
Abruptio placentae, 280
Abscess, 87, 164
    pulmonary, 475
Absence seizures, 365, 371
Absolute neutrophil count (ANC), 526
Absorption, 140, 150
-ac, 13, 85
A.c., ac (*ante cibum;* before meals), 112, 903
AC (acromioclavicular) joint, 591, 620, 623
Acarbose, 890t
Accessory nerve (CN XI), 346f
Accessory organs of reproduction, 261, 261f
Accessory structures of skin, 656-659, 657f, 658f
Accommodation, 699, 702
Accupril. *See* Quinapril.
ACE (angiotensin-converting enzyme) inhibitors, 419, 421, 426, 434, 892, 893t, 899
Acetabular, 598
Acetabular components of total hip arthroplasty, 620f
Acetabul/o, 598
Acetabulum, 592, 593t, 594, 598
Acetaminophen (APAP), 377, 887t, 903
Acetone, 226, 229
Acetylcholine, 344, 349, 355
Achalasia, 162
Achilles tendon, 614f
Achlorhydria, 158
Achondroplasia, 82, 82f, 606
Acid phosphatase, 826
Acid-fast bacillus (AFB), 483
ACL (anterior cruciate ligament), 605f, 623, 626
ACLS (advanced cardiac life support), 434
Acne, 658, 666-667, 667f
Acne vulgaris, 666-667, 667f
Acous/o, 722
Acoustic, 722
Acoustic neuroma, 724
Acquired immunodeficiency syndrome (AIDS), 368, 559-561, 561f, 561t, 564, 565, 674
    opportunistic infections with, 560t
Acr/o, 76, 591, 925
Acromegaly, 81, 89, 90f, 775, 775f
Acromioclavicular (AC) joint, 591, 620, 623
Acromion, 591, 594
Acrophobia, 81, 925, 941t

ACSs (acute coronary syndromes), 420, 421f, 426, 434
ACTH (adrenocorticotropic hormone), 758, 759f, 760t, 761, 770-771, 779
Actinic keratoses, 672, 673f, 674
Activities of daily living (ADLs), 942
Actos. *See* Pioglitazone.
-acusis, 723
Acute, 85
Acute bacterial conjunctivitis, 704f
Acute coronary syndromes (ACSs), 420, 421f, 426, 434
Acute cystitis, 223, 223f
Acute lymphoid leukemia (ALL), 521, 521f, 524, 526, 818t, 819
Acute myeloid leukemia (AML), 520, 520f, 524, 526, 818t
Acute myocardial infarction (AMI), 420, 420f, 434
Acute otitis media (AOM), 724f, 725, 727
Acute paronychia, 663f
Acute renal failure (ARF), 231
Acute respiratory distress syndrome (ARDS), 483
Acute rheumatic mitral valvulitis, 422f
Acyclovir, 889t
Ad-, 112, 618, 754
AD (Alzheimer disease), 364, 364f, 372f, 374, 398, 927, 942
AD (right ear), 727
Ad lib (freely, as desired; *ad libitum*), 903
Ad libitum (freely, as desired; ad lib), 903
Adaptive immunity, 553-554, 553f, 554f, 555, 555f
Addiction, 886, 897
Addictive disorders, substance-related and, 930-931, 932f, 932t, 938
Addison disease, 771, 771f
Additive action of drugs, 886, 897
Adduction, 615, 616, 616f, 618, 860
Adductor, 112
Adenitis, 7, 764
Aden/o, 7, 76, 764, 806
Adenocarcinoma, 825
    of colon and/or rectum, 164, 165f, 196f
    cystic ovarian, 276, 808f
    gastric, 806
Adenohypophysis, 757, 757f, 761
Adenoid hypertrophy, 465
Adenoidectomy, 465
Adenoid/o, 465
Adenoids, 85, 91, 91f, 460, 461f, 464, 465, 550f, 551, 555
Adenoma, 7, 196f, 806
Adenomatous goiter, 768
Adenomatous polyposis coli syndrome, 804-805
Adenomatous polyposis of colon, 809f
Adenopathy, 14
Adenosine diphosphate (ADP), 434